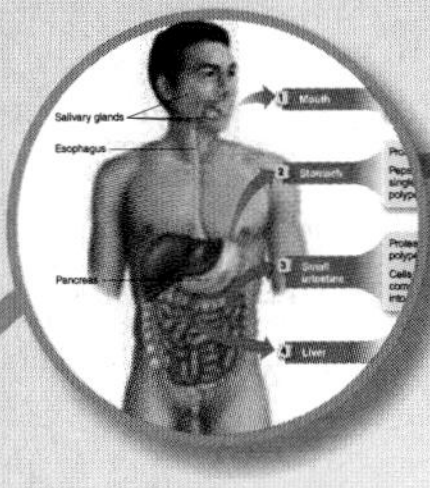

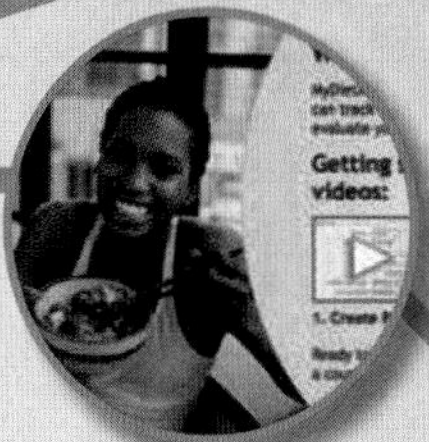

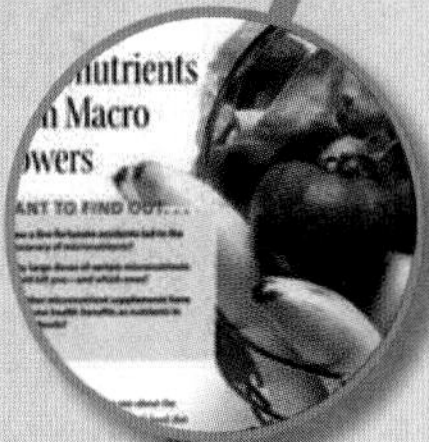

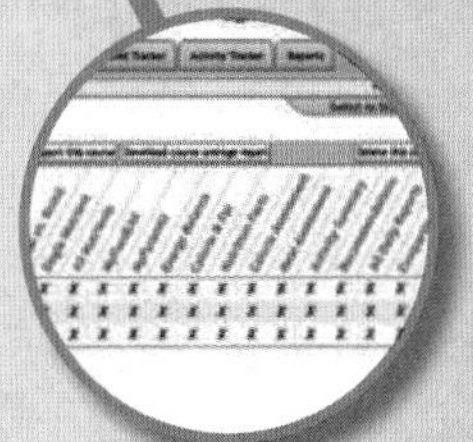

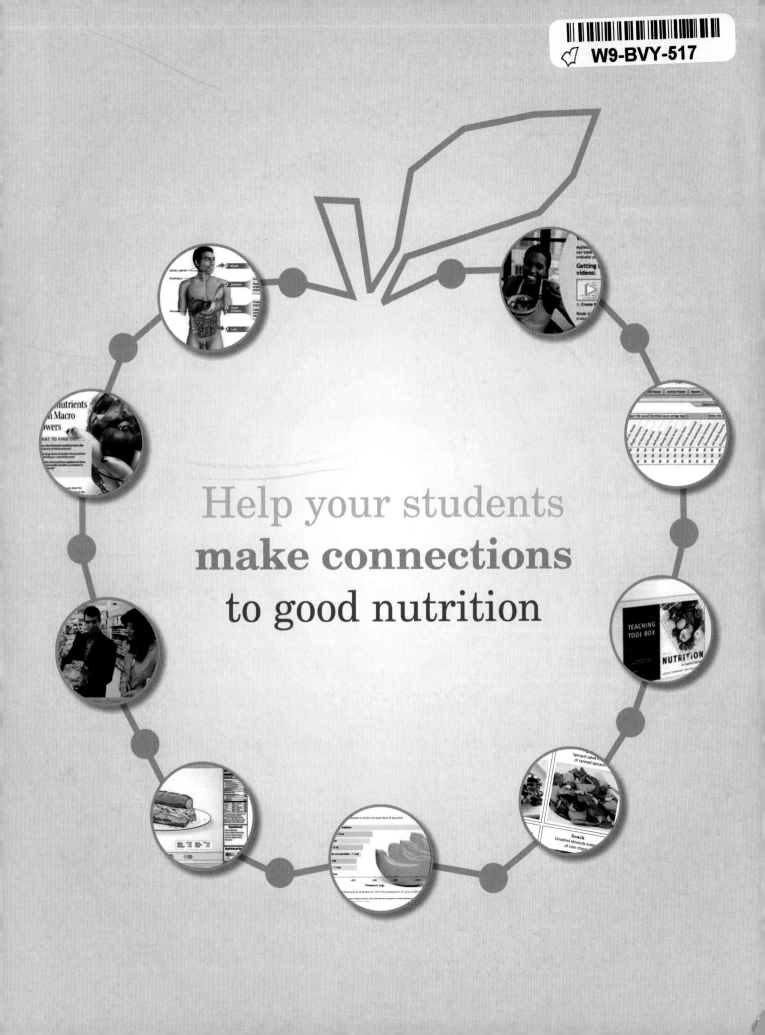

Help your students **make connections** to good nutrition

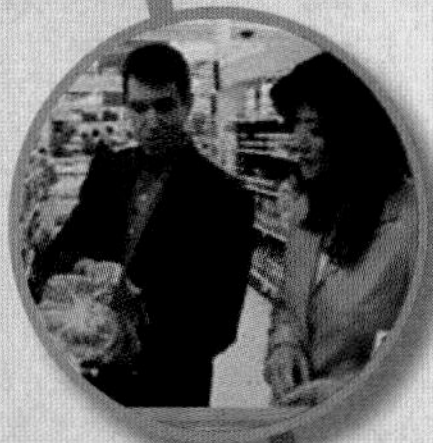

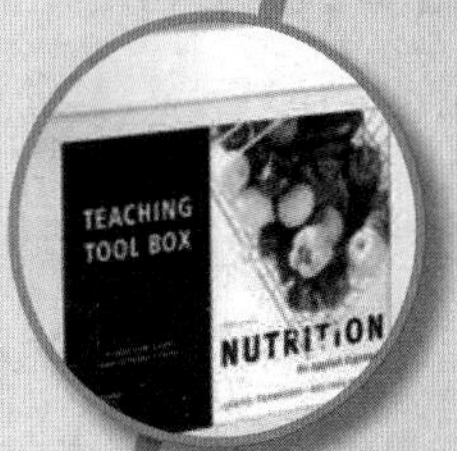

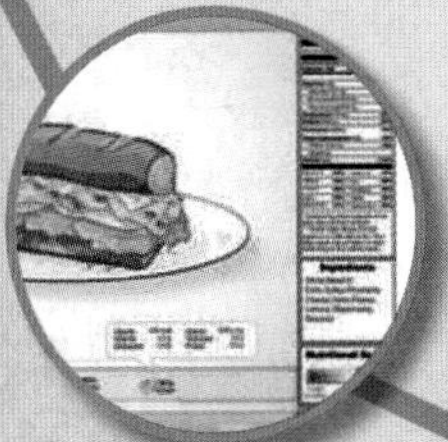

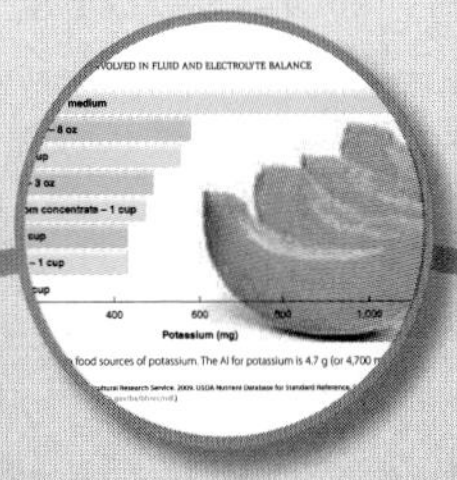

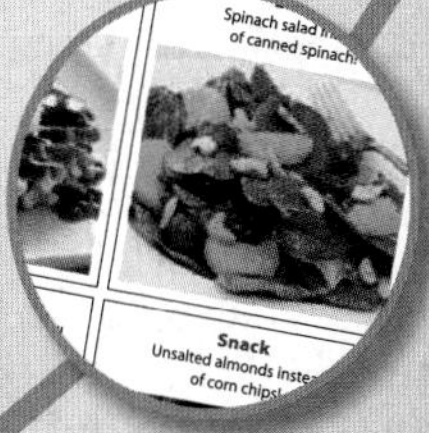

Help students make important nutrition connections

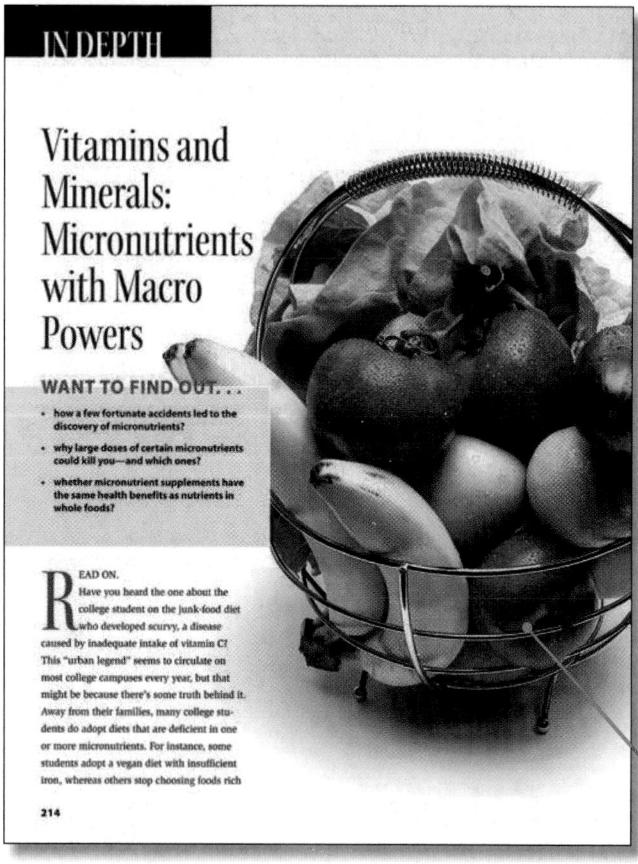
IN DEPTH

Vitamins and Minerals: Micronutrients with Macro Powers

WANT TO FIND OUT...

- how a few fortunate accidents led to the discovery of micronutrients?
- why large doses of certain micronutrients could kill you—and which ones?
- whether micronutrient supplements have the same health benefits as nutrients in whole foods?

READ ON.
Have you heard the one about the college student on the junk-food diet who developed scurvy, a disease caused by inadequate intake of vitamin C? This "urban legend" seems to circulate on most college campuses every year, but that might be because there's some truth behind it. Away from their families, many college students do adopt diets that are deficient in one or more micronutrients. For instance, some students adopt a vegan diet with insufficient iron, whereas others stop choosing foods rich

214

NEW! In Depth mini chapters

Eleven targeted In Depth mini chapters have been added to the Third Edition, with every main chapter now followed by a corresponding In Depth treatment of key concepts.

- **NEW! The New In Depth** structure creates a clearer presentation of compelling content that focuses on the important connections between nutrition, health, and disease.
- **The In Depth on Vitamins and Minerals** gives instructors flexibility with micronutrient material by presenting it in the traditional way, to serve as a quick overview prior to the first functional chapter.

Thompson and Manore build on students' natural interest in nutrition by demonstrating in a clear, conversational style how key nutritional information relates to their health, and how to debunk commonly held misconceptions.

CHAPTER 1: The Role of Nutrition in Our Health
In Depth: Alcohol

CHAPTER 2: Designing a Healthful Diet
In Depth: Phytochemicals

CHAPTER 3: The Human Body: Are We Really What We Eat?
In Depth: Disorders Related to Specific Foods

CHAPTER 4: Carbohydrates: Plant-Derived Energy Nutrients
In Depth: Diabetes

CHAPTER 5: Fats: Essential Energy-Supplying Nutrients
In Depth: Cardiovascular Disease

CHAPTER 6: Proteins: Crucial Components of All Body Tissues
In Depth: Vitamins and Minerals: Micronutrients with Macro Powers

CHAPTER 7: Nutrients Involved in Fluid and Electrolyte Balance
In Depth: Dehydration and Fluid Imbalance

CHAPTER 8: Nutrients Involved in Antioxidant Function
In Depth: Cancer

CHAPTER 9: Nutrients Involved in Bone Health
In Depth: Osteoporosis

CHAPTER 10: Nutrients Involved in Energy Metabolism and Blood Health
In Depth: Dietary Supplements: Necessity or Waste?

CHAPTER 11: Achieving and Maintaining a Healthful Body Weight
In Depth: Obesity

CHAPTER 12: Nutrition and Physical Activity: Keys to Good Health
In Depth: Disordered Eating

CHAPTER 13: Food Safety, Systems, and Technology
In Depth: Global Nutrition

CHAPTER 14: Nutrition Through the Life Cycle: Pregnancy and the First Year of Life
In Depth: The Fetal Environment: A Lasting Impression

CHAPTER 15: Nutrition Through the Life Cycle: Childhood to Late Adulthood
In Depth: Searching for the Fountain of Youth

NEW! Quick Tips

This feature provides helpful suggestions for incorporating better nutrition into daily life, in a succinct list format. Examples include shopping advice, cooking suggestions, food preparation tips, eating out ideas, exercise-related topics, food sources, and other creative ways to apply what readers have learned.

QUICK TIPS

Increasing Your Potassium Intake

✔ Avoid processed foods that are high in sodium and low in potassium. Check the Nutrition Facts Panel of the food before you buy it!

✔ For breakfast, look for cereals containing bran and/or wheat germ.

✔ Sprinkle wheat germ on yogurt and top with banana slices.

✔ Add wheat germ to baked goods, such as homemade pancakes and muffins.

✔ Drink milk! If you don't like milk, try one of the new drinkable yogurts. Many brands of soy milk are also good sources of potassium.

✔ Make a smoothie by blending ice cubes and low-fat vanilla ice cream or yogurt with a banana.

✔ Pack a can of low-sodium vegetable or tomato juice in your lunch in place of a soft drink.

✔ Serve avocado or bean dip with veggie slices.

✔ Replace the meat in your sandwich with thin slices of avocado or marinated tofu.

✔ Replace the meat in tacos and burritos with black or pinto beans.

✔ For a healthful alternative to french fries, toss slices of sweet potato in olive oil, place on a cookie sheet, and oven bake at 400° for 10–15 minutes.

✔ Toss a banana, some dried apricots, or a bag of sunflower seeds into your lunch bag.

✔ Make a fruit salad with apricots, bananas, cantaloupe, honeydew melon, mango, or papaya.

✔ Bake and enjoy a pumpkin pie!

What About You?

How Pure Is Your Favorite Bottled Water?

The next time you reach for a bottle of water, check the label. To find out how pure it is, consider the following factors:

1. Find out where it comes from. If no location is identified, even a bottle labeled "spring water" may actually contain tap water with minerals added to improve the taste. What you're looking for are the words "Bottled at the source." Water that comes from a protected groundwater source is less likely to have contaminants, such as disease-causing microbes. If the label doesn't identify the water's source, it should at least provide contact information, such as a phone number or website of the bottled water company, so that you can track down the source.

2. Find out how the water in the bottle has been treated. There are several ways of treating water, but what you're looking for is either of the following two methods, which have been proven to be effective against the most common waterborne disease-causing microorganisms:

💧 *Micron filtration* is a process whereby water is filtered through screens with various-sized microscopic holes. High-quality micron filtration can eliminate most chemical contaminants and microbes.

💧 *Reverse osmosis* is a process often referred to as *ultra-filtration* because it uses a membrane with microscopic openings that allow water to pass through but not larger compounds. Reverse osmosis membranes also utilize electrical charges to reject harmful chemicals.

If the label on your bottle of water says that the water was purified using any of the following methods, you might want to consider switching brands: filtered, carbon-filtered, particle-filtered, ozonated or ozone-treated, ultraviolet light, ion exchange, or deionized. These methods have not been proven to be effective against the most common waterborne disease-causing microorganisms.

3. Check the nutrient content on the label. Ideally, water should be high in magnesium (at least 20 mg per 8 fl. oz serving) and calcium but low in sodium (less than 5 mg per 8 fl. oz serving). Avoid bottled waters with sweeteners, as their "empty Calories" can contribute significantly to your energy intake. These products are often promoted as healthful beverage choices, with names including words such as *vitamins, herbs, nature,* and *life,* but they are essentially "liquid candy." Check the Nutrition Facts Panel and don't be fooled!

➡ Can you tell where the water in each bottle comes from?

NEW! What About You?

This self-assessment feature includes checklists, questionnaires and other engaging formats that present brief, targeted activities emphasizing active learning and applied thinking skills.

NEW! Eating Right All Day

Eating Right All Day visually highlights tasty suggestions students can use to improve their daily meals. The breakfast/lunch/dinner/snack format features appealing examples of satisfying everyday meals that are also good sources of nutrients.

Eating Right All Day

Breakfast
Whole-grain waffle with jam instead of a ham & cheese omlette!

Lunch
Spinach salad instead of canned spinach!

Dinner
Veggie pizza instead of pepperoni!

Snack
Unsalted almonds instead of corn chips!

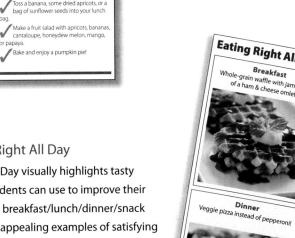

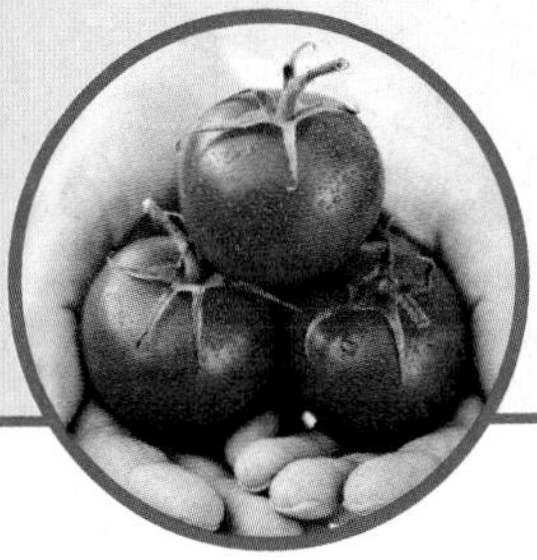

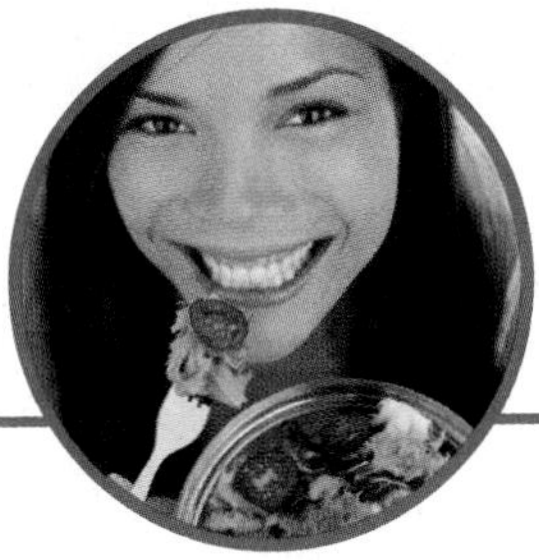

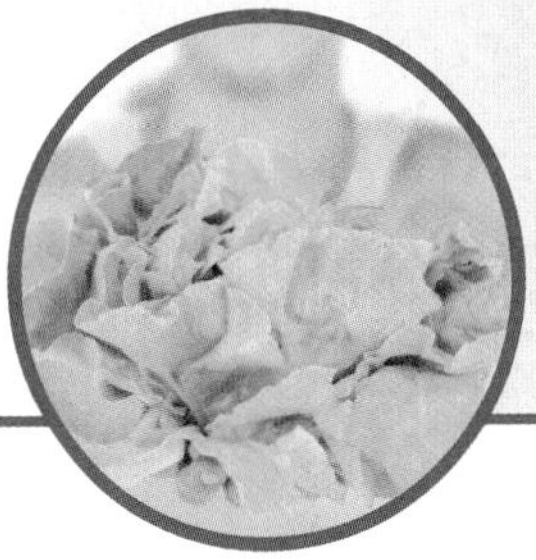

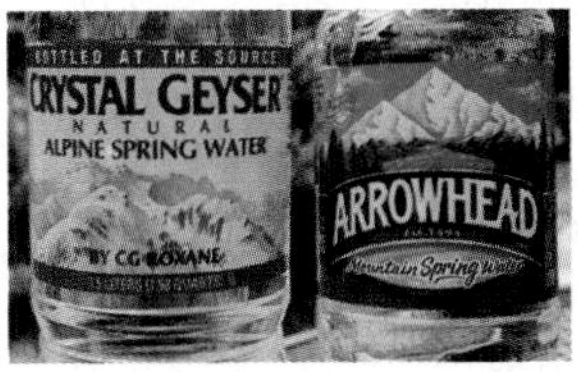

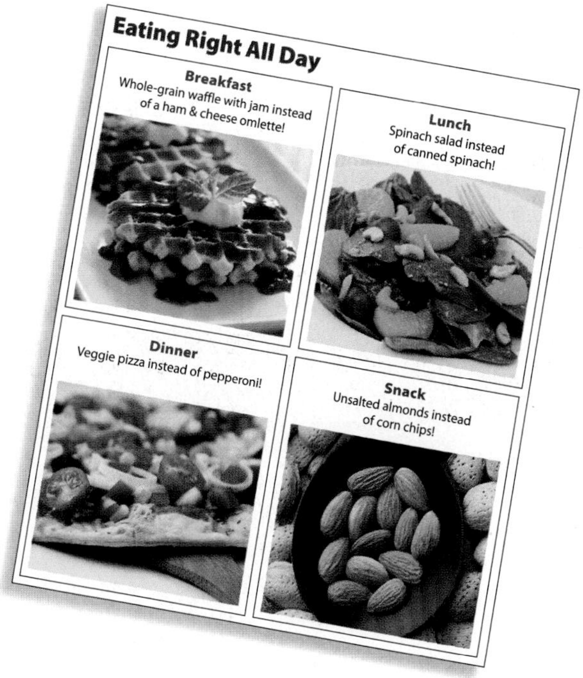

Make connections through media

PEARSON mynutritionlab

www.mynutritionlab.com

MyNutritionLab is the online course management system that makes it easy for you to organize your class, personalize your students' educational experience, and push their learning to the next level. MyDietAnalysis 5.0 will be available via single sign-on from MyNutritionLab. MyNutritionLab makes learning easy for students with its easy navigation on a chapter-by-chapter basis.

NutriTools

NutriTools

ABC News Videos

Author Videos

See It

NEW! NutriTools

21 new NutriTools interactive activities are available on MyNutritionLab. The Build-a-Sandwich, Build-a-Pizza, Build-a-Salad, and Build-a-Meal activities allow students to combine and experiment with different food options and learn first-hand how to build healthier meals. NutriTools activities include assignable and gradable questions.

NutriTools Include:

- Build-a-Meal
- Build-a-Salad
- Build-a-Sandwich
- Build-a-Pizza
- Know Your Calcium Sources
- Know Your Iron Sources
- Know Your Carbohydrate Sources
- Know Your Fat Sources
- Know Your Protein Sources
- Let's Go to Lunch—Fat Soluble Vitamins
- Let's Go to Lunch—Minerals
- Let's Go to Lunch—Water Soluble Vitamins
- Metabolism
- Vitamin Functionality
- Mineral Functionality
- Nutrients: Vitamin or Mineral?
- Food Label: What is Required?
- Digestion and Absorption
- Find the Carbohydrates

NEW! *ABC News* Videos

Nutrition topics come alive with 20 Lecture Launcher video clips, created in partnership with *ABC News*.

NEW! Author Videos

Instructional videos from author Janice Thompson cover key topics throughout the micronutrient chapters.

Animations

Created from the ground up, Nutrition animations spark student interest and bring to life complex physiological processes.

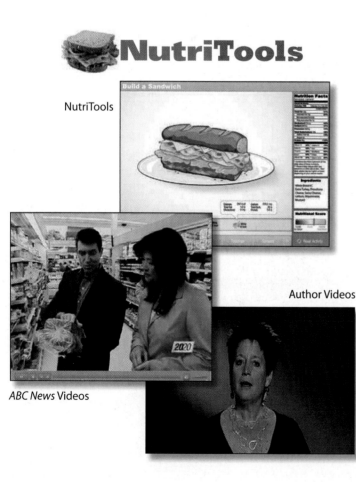

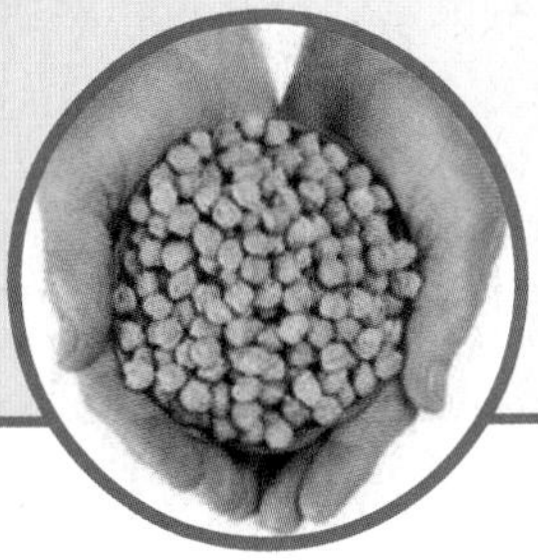
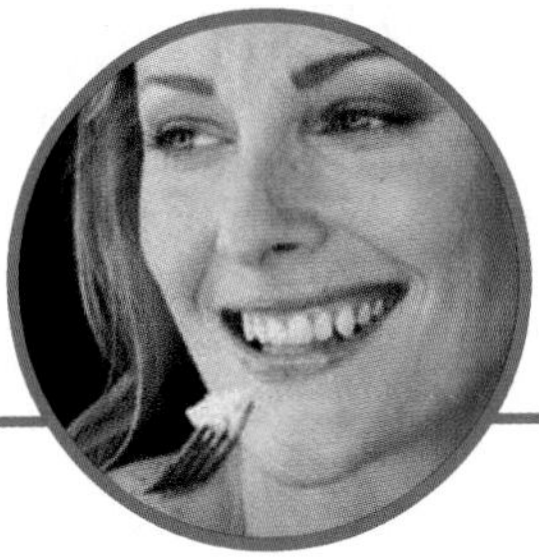
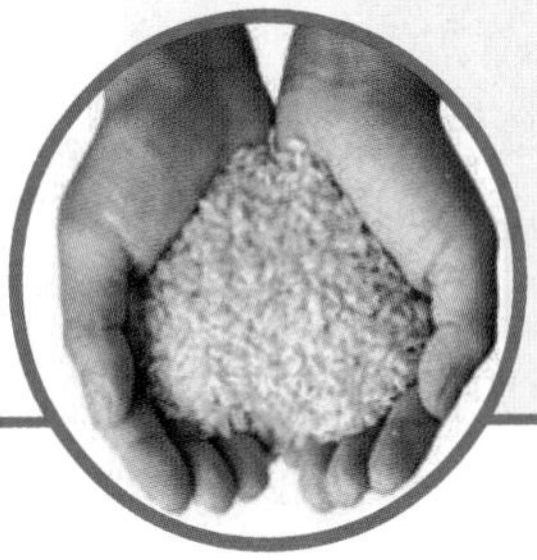

Read It

Pearson eText

Pearson eText is easy for students to read. Users can create notes, highlight text in different colors, create bookmarks, zoom, click hyperlinked words and phrases to review definitions, and view in single page or two-page mode. The eText also links students to associated media files, enabling them to view an animation as they read the text.

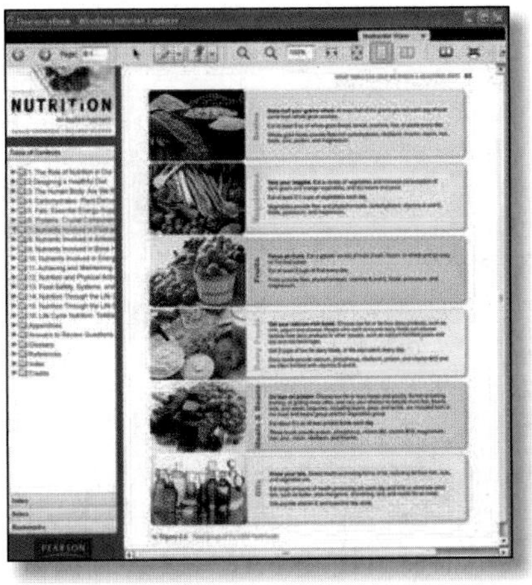

Pre- and Post-Quizzes

15 Pre-Reading Quiz questions and 30 Post-Reading Quiz questions are designed to help students measure their knowledge and progress.

Hear It

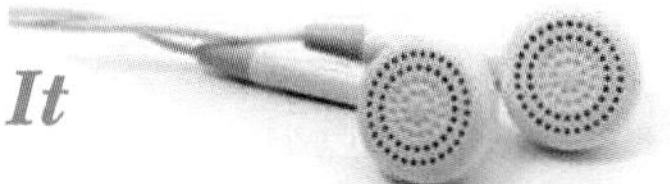

MP3 NutriCase Studies

These audio case studies walk listeners step-by-step through a true-to-life student nutrition challenge and pose compelling questions that apply the concepts from the chapter to the case study.

NutriCase Quiz Questions

90 brand new true-false and multiple choice, searchable questions related to the NutriCase study feature cover every angle on the real-life nutritional issues posed throughout the book.

Study It

This section contains access to extra math and chemistry nutrition-related content with ***Get Ready for Nutrition***. In addition, a PDF version of the Study Guide provides students with additional practice and help.

Review It

Do your students need extra study material that can be accessed from their computer or even their mobile device?

MyNutritionLab® makes studying for a quiz or exam easy:

- **The interactive flashcard** feature allows students to build a deck of flashcards from the key terms in every chapter, study them online, print them out to review, or even export them to their mobile phone.

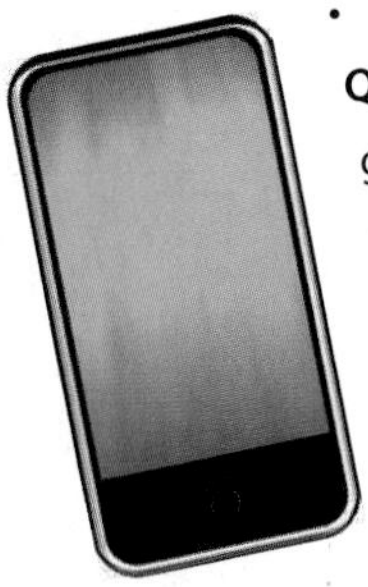

- **Multiple-Choice and True/False Practice Quizzes** for every chapter are automatically graded, so students can get feedback on their work and check their understanding of the material.
- **The online glossary** is a quick and easy resource for students to locate definitions for terms.

Do It

Promote active learning for your students by getting them to explore nutrition concepts through targeted activities. Learning tools focus on critical thinking scenarios that encourage students to become better consumers of nutrition information.

Make connections in the classroom

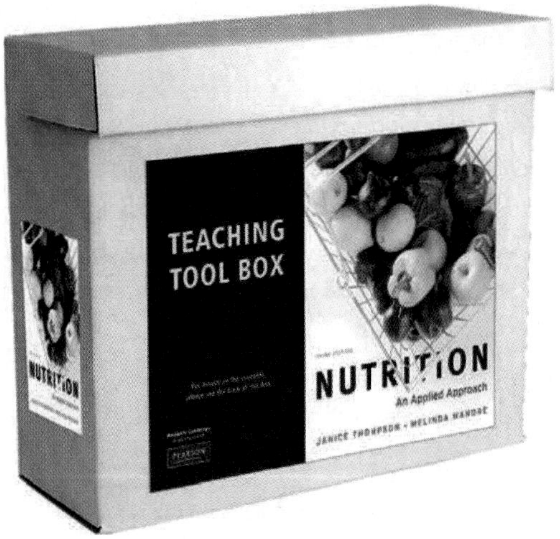

Everything You Need in One Convenient Place

Teaching Tool Box

Save hours of valuable planning time with one comprehensive course planning kit. In one handy box, adjunct, part-time, and full-time faculty will find a wealth of supplements and resources that reinforce key learning from the text and suit virtually any teaching style.

978-0-321-72123-5 • 0-321-72123-3

The Teaching Tool Box provides all the preparation and lecture tools instructors need, including:

- The **Course-at-a-Glance Quick Reference Guide** to easily locate resources
- ***Great Ideas: Active Ways to Teach Nutrition*** with suggestions for classroom activities
- **Instructor Resource and Support Manual**
- **Printed Test Bank**
- An **Instructor Resource DVD** including PowerPoint® Lecture Outlines, PRS Clicker Questions, Quiz Show questions, Video Clips, Transparency Masters, and the Computerized Test Bank
- A **MyNutritionLab with MyDietAnalysis access kit** so you can get online quickly
- The helpful ***Eat Right!*** student supplement
- **The Food Composition Table Supplement**

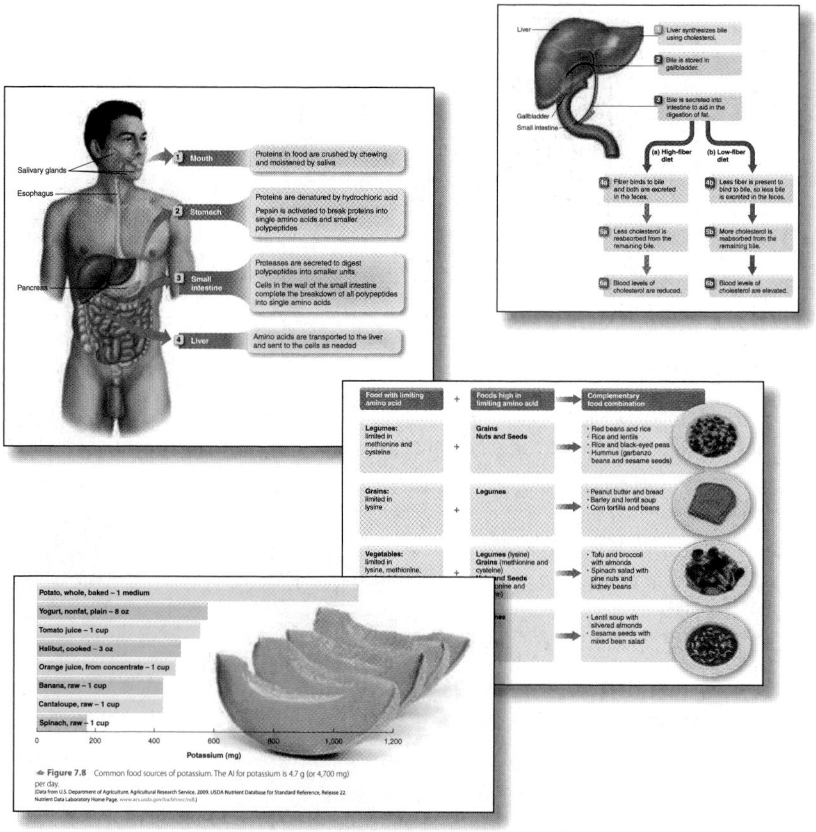

NEW! A **revitalized art and design program** enhances the text, making the Third Edition compelling and engaging for visually oriented non-major students. All 350 pieces of art have been refreshed, making them easier to read and communicating the right emphasis with the student in mind.

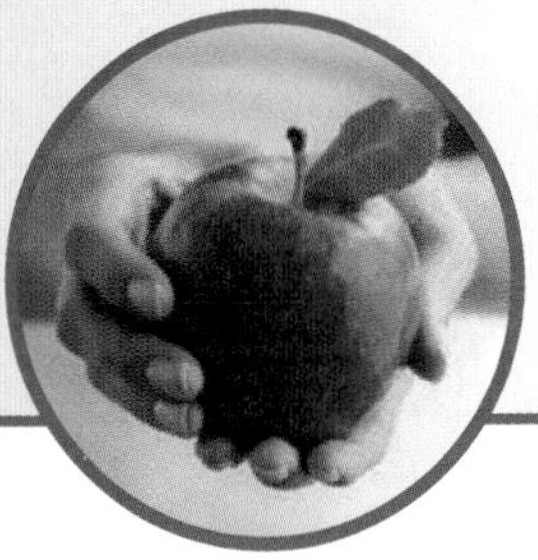
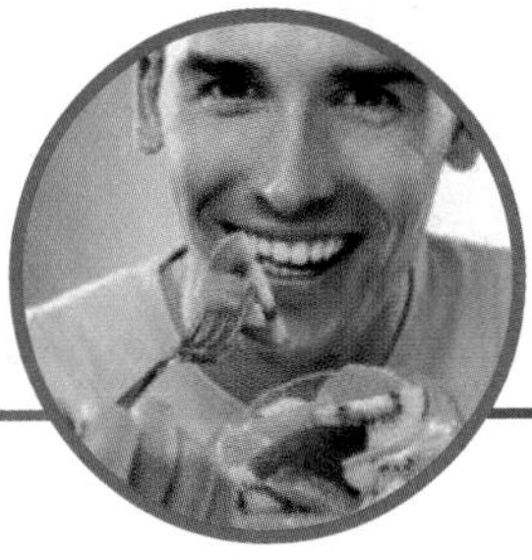
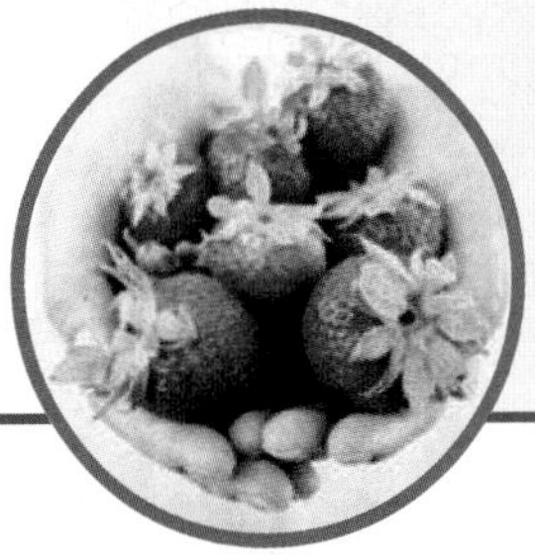

A Healthy Approach to Diet Analysis

MyDietAnalysis

www.mydietanalysis.com

MyDietAnalysis was developed by the nutrition database experts at ESHA Research, Inc. and is tailored for use in college nutrition courses. It offers an accurate, reliable, and easy-to-use program for your students' diet analysis needs. MyDietAnalysis features a database of nearly 20,000 foods and multiple reports. The program allows students to track their diet and activity, and generate and submit reports electronically. MyDietAnalysis is also available via single sign-on from MyNutritionLab®.

MyDietAnalysis 5.0 features **hundreds of NEW items**, including selections from popular brands and restaurants.

Restaurants include:

- Atlanta Bread
- Baja Fresh
- Mrs. Fields
- Caribou Coffee
- Jimmy John's
- White Castle Frozen Foods
- Golden Corral
- Red Robin Gourmet Burgers
- Chipotle
- Jersey Mike's
- Applebee's
- TGI Friday's
- Cracker Barrel

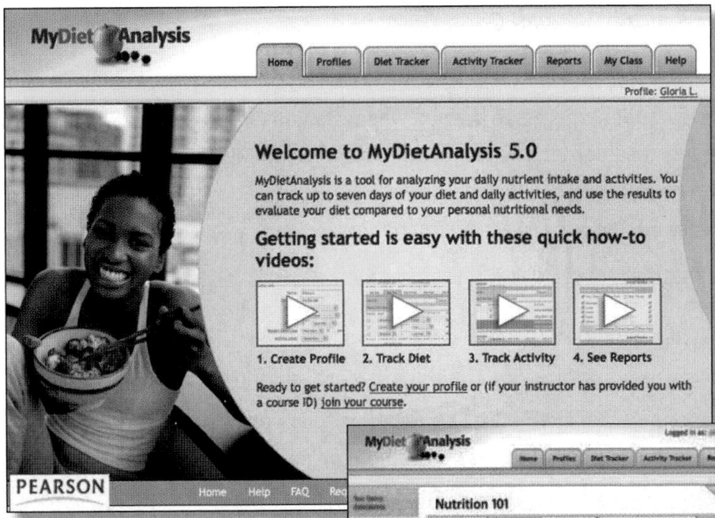

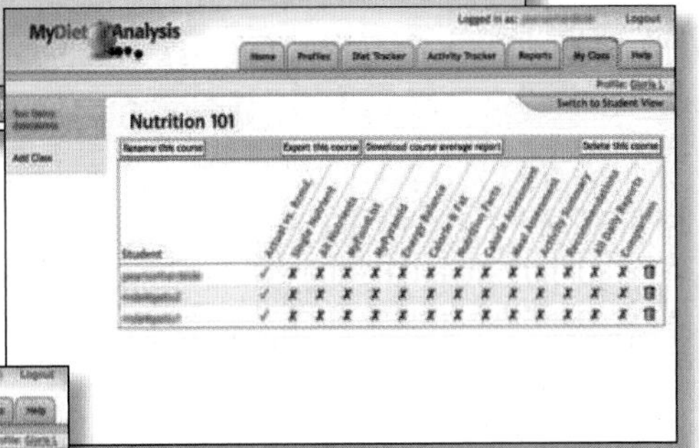

NEW! A Recipe Builder allows students to input all of the ingredients once and then call up the recipe for later entries.

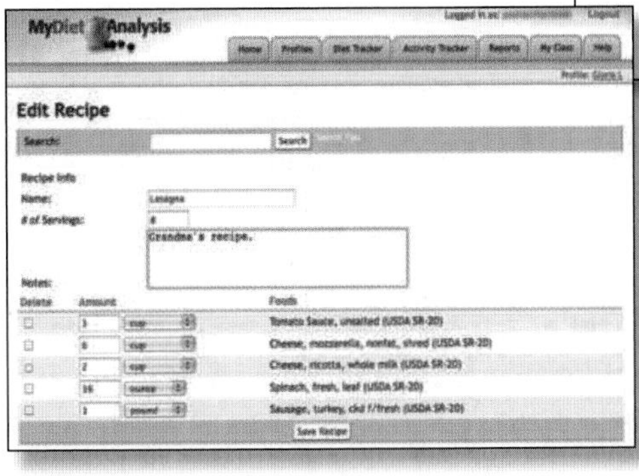

NEW! Improved My Class functionality for instructors includes the ability to assign certain reports, comment on student reports, and download all student reports.

Make connections with outstanding learning resources

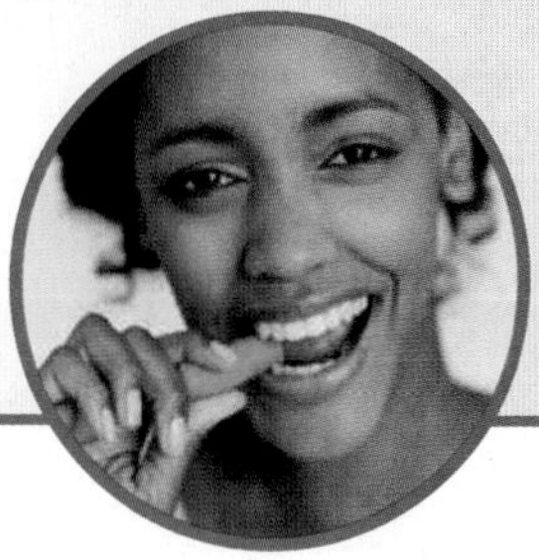

Flexible Options

Books a la Carte

978-0-321-72167-9 • 0-321-72167-5

This edition features the exact same content as ***Nutrition: An Applied Approach*, Third Edition** in a convenient, three-hole-punched, loose-leaf version. Books a la Carte also offer a great value for your students—this format costs 35% less than a new textbook.

Pearson eText Student Access Code Card

978-0-321-72130-3 • 0-321-72130-6

Pearson eText gives students access to the text whenever and wherever they can access the Internet. The eText pages look exactly like the printed text, and include powerful interactive and customization functions. This does not include the actual bound book.

CourseSmart eTextbook

978-0-321-72128-0 • 0-321-72128-4

CourseSmart eTextbooks are an exciting new choice for students looking to save money. As an alternative to purchasing the print textbook, students can subscribe to the same content online and save up to 40% off the suggested list price of the print text.

Student Supplements

Companion Website

www.pearsonhighered.com/thompsonmanore

The open access website features pre- and post-quizzes for each chapter, cumulative tests, Nutrition Debate assignments, Nutri-Cases, web links, flashcards, glossary, and a nutrition news feed. The multiple choice and essay questions help students prepare for exams, while other activities may be completed as homework or extra credit assignments. In addition, premium access to Study It, which provides students with ***Get Ready for Nutrition***, math and chemistry review, the student Study Guide, and access to the interactive NutriTools activities is provided with every new copy of the book.

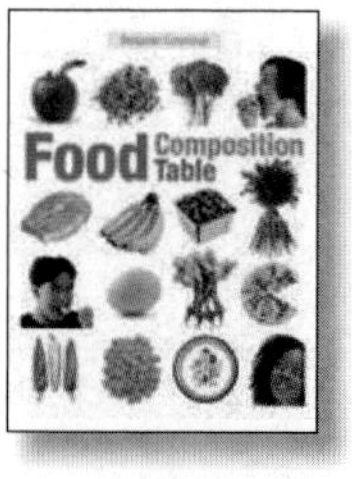

Food Composition Table

978-0-321-66793-9 • 0-321-66793-X

In the Second Edition, the USDA Nutrient Database for Standard Reference will be provided as a new practice supplement, offering the nutritional values of over 1,500 separate foods in an easy-to-follow format.

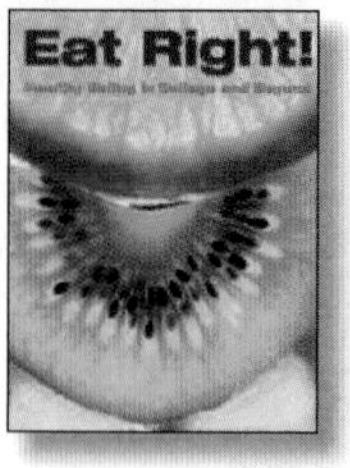

Eat Right! Healthy Eating in College and Beyond

978-0-8053-8288-4 • 0-8053-82887

This handy, full-color booklet provides students with practical guidelines, tips, shopper's guides, and recipes that turn healthy eating principles into blueprints for action. Topics include healthy eating in the cafeteria, dorm room, and fast food restaurants; planning meals on a budget; weight management; vegetarian alternatives; and how alcohol impacts health.

For a complete list of supplements available with this text, please visit our Web Catalog at www.pearsonhighered.com/nutrition

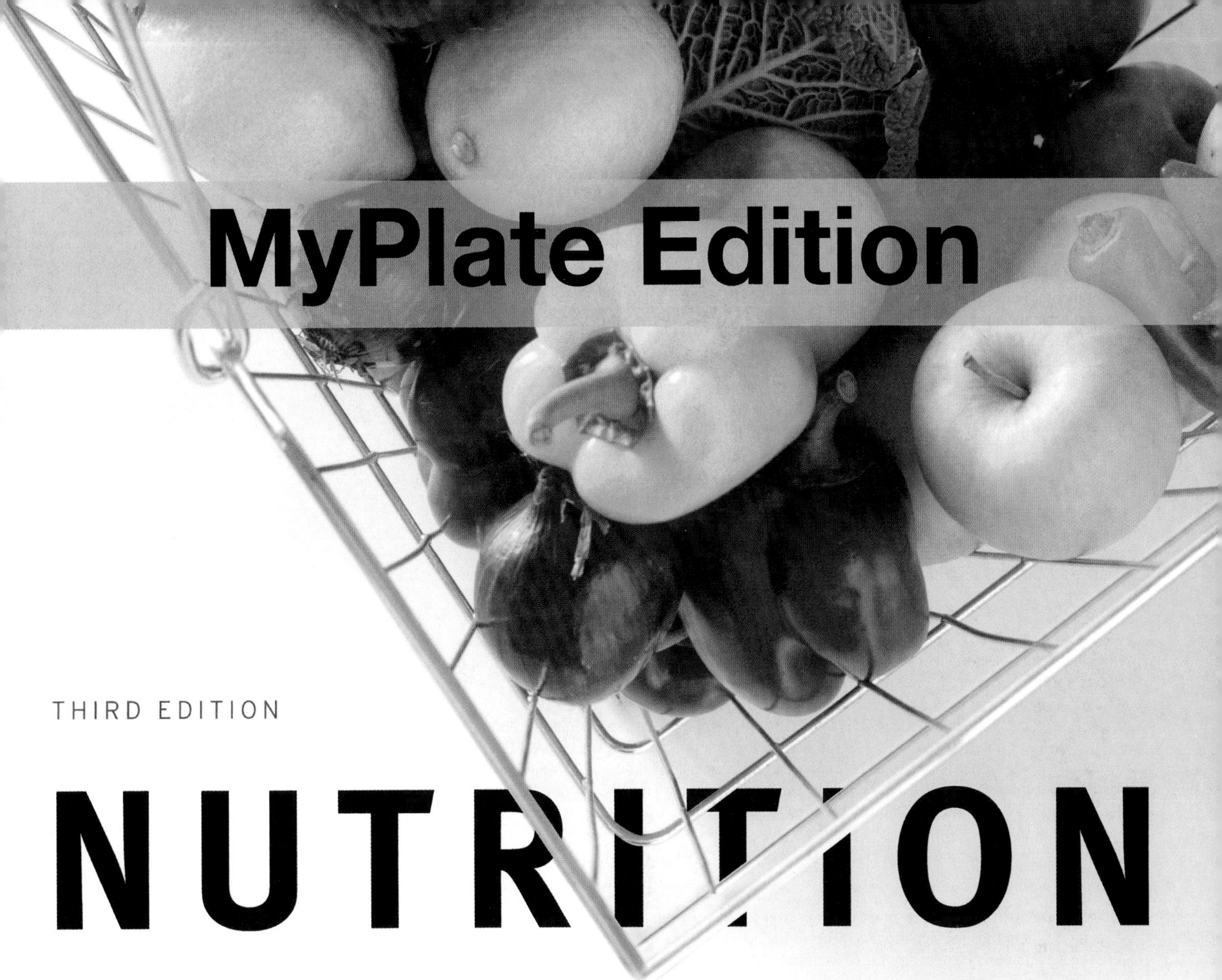

MyPlate Edition

THIRD EDITION

NUTRITION

An Applied Approach

Janice Thompson, Ph.D., FACSM

University of Bristol
University of New Mexico

Melinda Manore, Ph.D., RD, CSSD, FACSM

Oregon State University

PEARSON

Boston Columbus Indianapolis New York San Francisco Upper Saddle River Amsterdam
Cape Town Dubai London Madrid Milan Munich Paris Montreal Toronto Delhi
Mexico City São Paulo Sydney Hong Kong Seoul Singapore Taipei Tokyo

Executive Editor: Sandra Lindelof
Project Editor: Susan Scharf
Director of Development: Barbara Yien
Developmental Editor: Laura Bonazzoli
Art Development Editor: Kari Hopperstead
Editorial Assistant: Briana Verdugo
Senior Managing Editor: Deborah Cogan
Production Project Manager: Mary O'Connell
Media Producer: Susan Scharf
Production Management and Composition: S4Carlisle Publishing Services
Photo Manager: Donna Kalal
Interior Designer: Gary Hespenheide
Cover Designer: Yvo Riezebos Design
Illustrators: Precision Graphics
Photo Researcher: Regalle Jaramillo
Manufacturing Buyer: Stacey Weinberger
Executive Marketing Manager: Neena Bali

Cover Photo Credit: Peter Cade/Getty Images

Credits and acknowledgments borrowed from other sources and reproduced, with permission, in this textbook appear on the appropriate page within the text and on p. CR-1.

The Library of Congress has cataloged the earlier printing as follows:
Thompson, Janice,
Nutrition : an applied approach / Janice Thompson, Melinda Manore. – 3rd ed.
p. cm.
Includes bibliographical references and index.
ISBN 978-0-321-69664-9
1. Nutrition. I. Manore, Melinda, 1951- II. Title.
QP141.T467 2011
613.2–dc22

2010032841

ISBN 10: 0-321-81370-7; ISBN 13: 978-0-321-81370-1 (Student edition)
ISBN 10: 0-321-81438-X; ISBN 13: 978-0-321-81438-8 (Instructor Review copy)

1 2 3 4 5 6 7 8 9 10—**V303**—14 13 12 11

PEARSON

"To our Moms—your consistent love and support are the keys to our happiness and success. You have been incredible role models."

"To our Dads—you raised us to be independent, intelligent, and resourceful. We miss you and wish you were here to be proud of, and to brag about, our accomplishments."

About the Authors

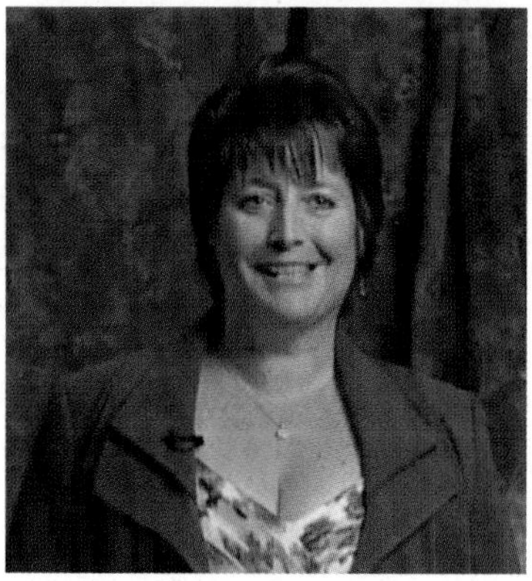

Janice Thompson, Ph.D., FACSM

University of Bristol
University of New Mexico

Janice Thompson earned a Ph.D. from Arizona State University in exercise physiology and nutrition. She is currently Bristol University's Head of the Centre of Exercise, Nutrition, and Health Sciences and Professor of Public Health Nutrition. Her research focuses on designing and assessing the impact of nutrition and physical activity interventions to reduce the risks for obesity, cardiovascular disease, and type 2 diabetes in high-risk populations. She also teaches nutrition and research methods courses, and mentors graduate research students.

Janice is a Fellow of the American College of Sports Medicine (ACSM) and a member of the American Society for Nutrition (ASN), the British Association of Sport and Exercise Science (BASES), The Nutrition Society in the United Kingdom, and the European College of Sports Science (ESS). Janice won an undergraduate teaching award while at the University of North Carolina, Charlotte. In addition to *Nutrition: An Applied Approach*, Janice co-authored the Pearson textbooks *Nutrition for Life* with Melinda Manore and *The Science of Nutrition* with Melinda Manore and Linda Vaughan. Janice loves traveling, yoga, hiking, and cooking and eating delicious food. She likes almost every vegetable except canned peas and believes chocolate should be listed as a food group.

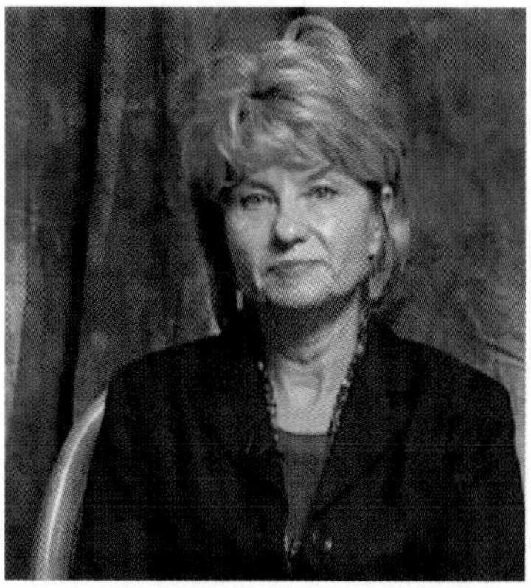

Melinda Manore, Ph.D., RD, CSSD, FACSM

Oregon State University

Melinda Manore earned a Ph.D. in human nutrition with a minor in exercise physiology at Oregon State University (OSU). She is the past chair of the Department of Nutrition and Food Management at OSU, and is currently a professor in the Department of Nutrition and Exercise Sciences. Prior to her tenure at OSU, she taught at Arizona State University for 17 years. Melinda's area of expertise is nutrition and exercise, especially the role of diet and exercise in health, exercise performance, weight control, and micronutrient needs. She focuses on the nutritional needs of active women and girls across the life cycle.

Melinda is an active member of the American Dietetic Association (ADA) and the American College of Sports Medicine (ACSM). She is the past chair of the ADA Research Committee and the Research Dietetic Practice Group, and served on the ADA Obesity Steering Committee. She is a Fellow, and currently Vice President, of ACSM, and is an active member of SCAN, a nutrition and exercise practice group of ADA. Melinda is also a member of the American Society of Nutrition (ASN) and the Obesity Society. She is the recent chair of UDSA's Nutrition and Health Planning and Guidance Committee. Melinda is the past nutrition column author and associate editor for ACSM's *Health and Fitness Journal* and *Medicine and Science in Sports and Exercise.* She serves on editorial boards of numerous research journals, and has won awards for excellence in research and teaching. She co-authored the Pearson textbooks *Nutrition for Life* with Janice Thompson and *The Science of Nutrition* with Janice Thompson and Linda Vaughan. Melinda is an avid walker, hiker, and former runner who loves to cook and eat great food. She is now trying her hand at gardening and birding.

Welcome to *Nutrition: An Applied Approach*, MyPlate Edition!

Why an Edition Update?

In late spring of 2010 the USDA released their new interactive food guidance system and visual reference, MyPlate, replacing the existing 2005 MyPyramid graphic and system. MyPlate (whose official online identity is www.ChooseMyPlate.gov) is based on the most recent (to date) 2010 Dietary Guidelines for Americans, designed to positively influence American's diets, eating habits, and understanding of and approach to the foods they consume.

MyPlate represents a significant shift from the prior MyPyramid template. It represents a major new direction in the way that basic nutrition guidelines are presented to the American public. For this reason, we felt an update to the Third Edition of *Nutrition: An Applied Approach* was necessary and useful. Nutrition is a constantly evolving science and practice, and our goal as authors is to provide students and instructors with the best, most current nutritional information and guidance available.

Why We Wrote the Book

Nutrition gets a lot of press. Pick up a magazine and you'll read the latest debate over which type of diet is best for weight loss; turn on the TV and you'll hear a Hollywood star describe how she lost 50 pounds without exercising; scan the headlines or read some blogs and you'll discover the politics surrounding the creation of new enhanced "designer" foods. How can you evaluate these sources of nutrition information and find out whether the advice they provide is reliable? How do you navigate through seemingly endless recommendations and come up with a way of eating that's right for *you*—one that supports your physical activity, allows you to maintain a healthful weight, and helps you avoid chronic diseases?

We Wrote This Book to Help You Answer These Questions

Our foundation text for this special edition, ***Nutrition: An Applied Approach,*** began with our conviction that both students and instructors would benefit from an accurate and clear textbook that links nutrients to their functional benefits. As authors and instructors, we know that students have a natural interest in their bodies, their health, their weight, and their success in sports and other activities. By demonstrating how nutrition relates to these interests, this text empowers students to reach their personal health and fitness goals. Throughout the text, material is presented in a lively narrative that continually links the facts to students' circumstances, lifestyles, and goals. Information on current events and research keeps the inquisitive spark alive, illustrating that nutrition is truly a "living" science, and a source of considerable debate. The content of ***Nutrition: An Applied Approach*** is appropriate for non-nutrition majors, but also includes information that will challenge students who have a more advanced understanding of chemistry and math. We present the "science side" in a contemporary narrative style that's easy-to-read and understand, with engaging features that reduce students' fears and encourage them to apply the material to their lives. Also, because this book is not a derivative of a majors text, the writing and the figures are cohesive and always level-appropriate.

As teachers, we are familiar with the myriad challenges of presenting nutrition information in the classroom, and we have included the most comprehensive ancillary package available to assist instructors in successfully meeting these challenges. We hope to contribute to the excitement of teaching and learning about nutrition: a subject that affects all of us, a subject so important and relevant that correct and timely information can make the difference between health and disease.

New in the Third Edition

Key goals for this edition included providing the most up-to-date and accurate nutrition information currently available, and optimizing students' ability to learn this information and apply it to their daily lives. To achieve this we have made some dramatic changes to our organization and material presentation, added several exciting new features, updated and integrated current information from recent scientific studies, and significantly enhanced the already excellent art program to ensure that ***Nutrition: An Applied Approach*** is the most up-to-date and easiest-to-use, comprehensive resource for nutrition students currently available.

In this special MyPlate edition, the entire text has been reviewed, and key chapters revised, to encompass the most current information available on the MyPlate food guidance system, and the 2010 Dietary Guidelines for Amercians. Eleven new **In Depth** "mini chapters" have been added to the four from the previous edition. These practical, topical, and graphically lively presentations now follow every chapter in the text, many with a dedicated focus on the links between nutrition and disease. In addition we have added several new features to this edition, aimed at making nutritional information more relevant and integrated into students' everyday lives. They include **Eating Right All Day**, a visual guide to suggested meal options tied to specific chapter content on micro- and macro-nutrients and key body systems; **Quick Tips**, brief lists appearing frequently throughout the text which, taken all together, provide an extensive array of simple suggestions and ideas for incorporating better eating habits into each student's day; **What About You?** a varied self-assessment feature that emphasizes active learning and content integration; and **Hot Topics**, informative snapshots of current issues students are undoubtedly encountering in sometimes less-reliable sources of popular information. Also note that detailed **Chapter Summaries** have been moved to the companion website for easier student access, and **References** are now located at the back of the text.

Additionally, this edition introduces four new full-page **NutriTools** activity overviews linked to the chapters on designing healthful diets (Build-a-Meal), carbohydrates (Build-a-Sandwich), fats (Build-a-Pizza), and antioxidants (Build-a-Salad), which tie-in with the extensive NutriTools content available on the Companion Website and MyNutritionLab™. Finally, in this new edition the **NutriCase** character of Hannah (daughter of the Judy character) has been updated and reimagined as a college-aged student, with new issues and struggles.

The Visual Walkthrough at the front of this text provides an overview of these and other important features in the Third Edition. For specific changes to each chapter, please see below.

Chapter 1 and accompanying In Depth:

- Revised and updated the Nutrition Debate on nutrigenomics, and moved the feature into the chapter.
- Moved and updated the In Depth mini chapter on Alcohol following Chapter 1
- Revised and updated chapter content on the evolution of nutrition as a science, and on the research into the role of nutrition in chronic diseases.
- Incorporated and updated content on pellagra into the Nutrition Myth or Fact? feature box.
- Created a new Figure 1.3 on the leading causes of death, from prior Table 1.1
- Added a new Hot Topic on nutrition-related email spam.

- Incorporated information on evaluating media hype into a new Quick Tips box.
- Revised and updated content on the scientific method, and on the CDC surveys (NHANES and BRFSS).
- Significantly revised and enhanced Figure 1.1, and added new photos.

Chapter 2 and accompanying In Depth:

- This entire chapter has been significantly revised and updated to reflect the new MyPlate logo and recommendations, as well as those of the 2010 Dietary Guidelines.
- Added a new Nutrition Debate on functional foods.
- Created a new In Depth mini chapter specifically on phytochemicals.
- Added new content on structure-function food label claims.
- Revised and updated content on MyPyramid.
- Revised and reorganized content on the Mediterranean Diet into a new Hot Topic.
- Expanded content on the nutritional costs of eating out, and added a related Quick Tip.
- Moved content on the DASH diet and related aspects to the In Depth following Chapter 5.
- Added a Nutrition Debate on functional foods.
- Significantly updated and enhanced Figures 2.2, 2.5 and 2.12, and added a new Figure 2.6 and new photos.
- Replaced Figure 2.5 with new MyPlate graphic.
- Replaced Figure 2.4 with a revised MyPlate version.

Chapter 3 and accompanying In Depth:

- Added a new Nutrition Debate on colon cleansing.
- Added a new Hot Topic on appetite suppressants.
- Revised and updated content on atoms, molecules, and cells.
- Created a new Nutrition Myth or Fact? box on the etiology of ulcers.
- Revised content on the neuromuscular regulation of digestion, and updated the terminology for GER and GERD.
- Reorganized content on traveler's diarrhea and created a new, related Quick Tips.
- Reorganized and revised content on food intolerances, allergies, and celiac disease into the new In Depth mini chapter.
- Revised Find the Quack content to cover extreme dieting.
- Significantly updated and enhanced Figures 3.1, 3.3, 3.5, 3.6, 3.7, 3.8, 3.9, 3.10, 3.11, 3.13, and 3.14, and added new photos.

Chapter 4 and accompanying In Depth:

- Revised and updated the Nutrition Debate on high fructose corn syrup, and moved the feature into the chapter.
- Added a new In Depth mini chapter on the links between nutrition and diabetes.
- Revised and updated content on artificial sweeteners.
- Removed content on lactose intolerance and incorporated it into the new In Depth mini chapter following Chapter 3.
- Revised and reorganized content on hypoglycemia into a new Hot Topic.
- Dropped the Shopper's Guide on complex carbohydrates and integrated the content into the text and other features.
- Expanded content on metabolic syndrome.

- Added clarifying content on the distinctions between the chemical structures related to "simple" and "complex" carbohydrates, and to definitions regarding "whole grain," "high fiber," and refined and unrefined carbohydrate sources.
- Added a new Eating Right All Day feature focusing on carbohydrates.
- Moved and expanded diabetes content into the new In Depth mini chapter.
- Significantly updated and enhanced Figures 4.5, 4.6, 4.8, and 4.13, and added new photos.

Chapter 5 and accompanying In Depth:

- Revised and updated the Nutrition Debate on fat blockers, and moved the feature into the chapter.
- Added a new In Depth mini chapter on the links between nutrition and cardiovascular disease.
- Incorporated and expanded prior Chapter 3 content on chitosan and fat blockers into the Nutrition Debate.
- Added a new Hot Topic on nuts.
- Added a new Nutrition Myth or Fact? box on the differences between margarine and butter.
- Added new NutriCase profiles for Hannah and Gustavo.
- Dropped the Shopper's Guide on dietary fats and integrated the content into the text and other features.
- Reorganized and revised content on cardiovascular disease and cancer into new In Depth mini chapters.
- Added a new Eating Right All Day feature focusing on dietary fats.
- Added new Quick Tips features on saturated and *trans* fats, food preparation, and eating out.
- Significantly updated and enhanced Figures 5.1, 5.3, and 5.10, and added new photos.

Chapter 6 and accompanying In Depth:

- Added a new Nutrition Debate on the connections between meat consumption and global warming.
- Revised and updated the In Depth mini chapter on vitamins and minerals.
- Revised content on vegetarian diets.
- Added a new Hot Topic on amino acid supplements.
- Revised and updated content on disorders related to inadequate protein intake.
- Dropped the Shopper's Guide on protein sources and integrated the content into the text and other features.
- Added a new Quick Tips on legumes.
- Added a new Eating Right All Day focusing on proteins.
- Revised the NutriCase profile for Liz.
- Moved content on high protein diets to Chapter 11.
- Significantly updated and enhanced Figures 6.8, 6.12, and 6.13, and added new photos.

Chapter 7 and accompanying In Depth:

- Revised and updated the Nutrition Debate on sports beverages, and moved the feature into the chapter.
- Added a new In Depth mini chapter on dehydration and fluid-balance disorders.
- Updated content in Figure 7.7 for calculations on water intake and output for the average adult female.
- Expanded content on fluid-related disorders to include heat-related illnesses.

- Added an overview of exercise-related hypoatremia to the Nutrition Myth or Fact? box.
- Dropped the Shopper's Guide on potassium sources and integrated the content into the text and other features.
- Expanded the food source graph figures to display 100% AI or RDA, to contextualize serving size vs. daily needs.
- Added a new Hot Topic on fluids and weight gain.
- Added a new Eating Right All Day focusing on sodium.
- Significantly updated and enhanced Figures 7.2, 7.6, and 7.7, and added new photos.

Chapter 8 and accompanying In Depth:
- Added a new Nutrition Debate on antioxidants.
- Added a new In Depth mini chapter on the links between nutrition and cancer.
- Revised and updated content on beta-carotene.
- Added a new Hot Topic on Vitamin A and acne.
- Revised and updated content on antioxidant minerals enzyme systems.
- Revised and refocused Table 8.1.
- Dropped the Shopper's Guide on vitamin E, vitamin A, and beta-carotene sources and integrated the content into the text and Quick Tips features.
- Moved and revised content on tobacco use damage and nutritional links cancer to the In Depth.
- Added a new Eating Right All Day focusing on antioxidants.
- Repositioned prior Nutrition Debate content on vitamin and mineral supplements into the Chapter 10 In Depth.
- Changed the NutriCase profile from Judy to Hannah.
- Significantly updated and enhanced Figures 8.3, 8.6, 8.7, 8.9, 8.12, and 8.14, and added new photos.

Chapter 9 and accompanying In Depth:
- Added a new Nutrition Debate on vitamin D deficiency.
- Added a new In Depth mini chapter on the links between nutrition and osetoporosis.
- Added a What About You? box on vitamin D.
- Revised Table 9.3 on the factors affecting vitamin D synthesis.
- Dropped the Shopper's Guide on calcium and vitamin D sources and integrated the content into the text and other features.
- Added a new Hot Topic on the connection between dairy foods and weight loss.
- Moved osteoporosis content to the new In Depth.
- Added a new Eating Right All Day focusing on calcium.
- Changed the NutriCase profile from Hannah to Theo.
- Significantly updated and enhanced Figures 9.4, 9.6, 9.7, 9.10, 9.12, and 9.13, and added new photos.

Chapter 10 and accompanying In Depth:
- Revised and updated the Nutrition Debate on the efficacy of zinc lozenges in fighting colds, and moved the feature into the chapter.
- Added a new In Depth mini chapter on dietary supplements.
- Revised Tables 10.1 and 10.2.
- Added a new Hot Topic on the role of vitamin B_6 and PMS.
- Dropped the Shopper's Guide on iron sources and integrated the content into the text and other features.

- Added a new Quick Tips on retaining vitamins in foods.
- Added a new Eating Right All Day focusing on iron.
- Significantly updated and enhanced Figures 10.3, 10.4, 10.5, 10.6, 10.7, 10.9, 10.11, 10.14, 10.16, and 10.17, and added new photos.

Chapter 11 and accompanying In Depth:

- Added a new Nutrition Debate on high protein diets.
- Added a new In Depth mini chapter on the links between nutriton and obesity.
- Added new content on brown fat and its potential association with energy expenditure.
- Revised content on healthful body weight.
- Added a new What About You? on readiness to lose weight.
- Added content on the relationship between cultural and economic factors and body weight.
- Added a new Nutrition Myth or Fact? on the costs of eating better.
- Expanded content on behavioral modification regarding weight loss.
- Revised and expanded content on low-carbohydrate diets.
- Added a new Hot Topic on dietary supplements for weight loss.
- Added new Quick Tips boxes on portion sizes, overcoming barriers to weight loss, and modifying behavior.
- Revised content on protein supplements and overweight/obesity, and moved it to several In Depths.
- Significantly updated and enhanced Figure 11.2, and added new photos.

Chapter 12 and accompanying In Depth:

- Revised and updated the Nutrition Debate on the amount of exercise needed to improve overall health, and moved the feature into the chapter.
- Revised and converted content from prior Chapter 13 on disordered eating into the new In Depth mini chapter.
- Added a new What About You? on increasing physical activity.
- Revised content on rates of physical activity in the U.S., and incorporated prior Table 12.1 content into the text.
- Revised and converted prior content on deceptive practices in marketing ergogenic aids into a new Hot Topic.
- Revised content on fluid/dehydration, and incorporated prior Table 12.7 content into the text.
- Added a new Hot Topic on muscle dysmorphia in men.
- Significantly updated and enhanced Figures 12.2, 12.3, 12.4, 12.5, and In Depth Figures 5 and 7, and added new photos.

Chapter 13 and accompanying In Depth:

- Revised and updated the Nutrition Debate on genetically modified organisms and moved the feature into the chapter.
- Adapted and updated content on global nutrition and created a new In Depth mini chapter.
- Content on food safety and global nutrition in the main chapter and In Depth was significantly revised and updated.
- Created a new Figure 13.1 on food safety issues "from farm to table."
- Dropped content from the prior Typhoid Mary feature.

- Added a new Nutrition Myth or Fact? on mad cow disease.
- Created a new Figure 2 on acute and long-term effects of malnutrition across the life cycle, in the In Depth.
- Added a new Hot Topic on the use of bisphenol A (BPA) in canned foods.
- Added a new Quick Tips on reducing exposure to pesticides.
- Added a new What About You? on ways to contribute to global food security.
- Significantly enhanced Figure 13.12, and added new photos.

Chapter 14 and accompanying In Depth:

- Introduced a new Nutrition Debate on breastfeeding throughout infancy and moved the feature into the chapter.
- Added a new In Depth mini chapter on the fetal environment.
- Introduced the MyPyramid for Moms logo and program.
- Added a new Hot Topic on breastfeeding adopted infants.
- Updated the recommendations for vitamin D supplementation for infants.
- Added new content on the lifelong effects of fetal and childhood exposure to famine, to the In Depth.
- Changed the NutriCase profile from Theo to Hannah.
- Added a new Figure 1, on the fetal origins of adult diseases, in the In Depth.
- Added web links related to parental preparedness.
- Significantly updated and enhanced Figures 14.6 and 14.9, and added new photos.

Chapter 15 and accompanying In Depth:

- Combined content on nutrition through the life cycle into a single, focused chapter spanning childhood through late adulthood.
- Added a new Nutrition Debate on the appropriate level of vigorous physical activity for older adults.
- Added a new In Depth mini chapter on longevity diets.
- Added a new Nutrition Myth or Fact? on the importance of breastfeeding.
- Added new content on childhood food insecurity.
- Revised and reorganized content on childhood and adolescent overweight and obesity.
- Added a new Quick Tips on stocking your first kitchen for independent teens and young adults.
- Added new content on bone density issues for adolescents.
- Introduced logos and content for the NICHHD's "Milk Matters" program.
- Added a new What About You? on longevity information resources.
- Changed the NutriCase profile from Hannah to Liz.
- Added new content on the marketing of supplements to seniors.
- Updated Figure 15.7 for the Tufts Modified MyPyramid for Older Adults, and added new photos.

Appendices and Back Matter:

- Dropped the previous Appendix A on the Nutrient Values of Foods as it is now a full, stand-alone supplement called the Food Composition Table.
- Added a new Appendix A—Dietary Guidelines, Upper Intake Levels, and Dietary Reference Intakes—which were previously located in the endpages at the front and back of the text.
- Data for Appendix C—Foods Containing Caffeine—has been revised and updated.
- Added a new Appendix G—The USDA Food Guide Evolution.

- References for all chapters and In Depth mini chapters are now located and centralized at the back of the text.
- Answers to Review Questions have been revised and updated to reflect the new edition's changes.
- Glossary terms have been revised, and expanded as needed.

Acknowledgments

It is always eye-opening to author a textbook and to realize that the work of so many people contributes to the final product. There are numerous people to thank, and we'd like to begin by extending our gratitude to our contributors. Our deep gratitude and appreciation goes to Dr. Linda Vaughan, of Arizona State University, who revised and condensed the fluid and electrolyte and the life cycle chapters; revised and updated the *In Depth* mini chapter on alcohol; and wrote all-new *In Depth* mini chapters on fluid imbalance disorders, the fetal environment and longevity diets. Our enduring thanks as well goes to the many contributors and colleagues who made important and lasting contributions to earlier editions of this text. We also extend our sincere thanks to the able reviewers who provided much important feedback and guidance for this revision.

We would like to thank the fabulous staff at Pearson Benjamin Cummings for their incredible support and dedication to this book. Our past and current Acquisitions Editors, Deirdre Espinoza and Sandra Lindelof, respectively, have provided unwavering support and guidance throughout the entire process of writing and publishing this book. We could never have written this text without the exceptional skills of Laura Bonazzoli, our Developmental Editor, whom we have been fortunate enough to have had on board for multiple editions. In addition to providing content guidance and writing the chapters on the role of nutrition and food safety, she also wrote original content for the In Depth on the role of supplements, and created numerous features and related content throughout this edition. Laura's energy, enthusiasm, and creativity significantly enhanced the quality of this textbook. Our Project Editor, Susan Scharf, kept us on course and sane with her sense of humor and excellent organizational skills, and made revising this book a pleasure instead of a chore, in addition to serving double-duty as the Media Producer for this edition. We are also deeply indebted to Art Development Editor Kari Hopperstead who significantly enhanced the art program in this edition and her cast skillful eye on every piece of art to review and improve it. Briana Verdugo, Editorial Assistant, provided the project with invaluable editorial and administrative support that we would have been lost without. Multiple talented players helped build this book in the production and design processes as well. Nancy Tabor, Senior Production Project Manager, and Mary O'Connell, Production Supervisor for the MyPlate edition, kept manuscripts and proofs moving, tracked every minute detail, and brought their considerable skills to bear on making the interior layout and flow of the book a thing of beauty. Donna Kalal skillfully supervised the photo program, assisted by Regalle Jaramillo who performed excellent research for hundreds of photos. Gary Hespenheide created both the beautiful interior design and our glorious cover. We would also like to thank the professionals at S4Carlisle Publishing Services, especially Tiffany Timmerman and Diane Kohnen, for their important contributions to this text.

We also can't go without thanking the marketing and sales teams, especially Neena Bali, Executive Marketing Manager, and her talented marketing team, who ensured that we directed our writing efforts to meet the needs of students and instructors, and who worked so hard to get this book out to those who will benefit most from it.

Our goal of meeting instructor and student needs could not have been realized without the team of educators and editorial staff who worked on the substantial supplements package for *Nutrition: An Applied Approach.* Linda Fleming, of

Middlesex Community College, authored the wonderful Instructor's Resource and Support Manual; Ruth Reilly of University of New Hampshire, and Carol Friesen of Ball State University, created the careful and comprehensive Test Bank, all of whom were ably guided by Karen Nein. Alex Streczyn provided important assistance for the media program, in addition to Liz Winer, Leslie Sumrall, and Sarah Young-Dualan.

We would also like to thank the many colleagues, friends, and family members who helped us along the way. Janice would like to thank her co-author Melinda Manore, who has provided unwavering support and guidance throughout her career and is a wonderful life-long friend and colleague. She would also like to thank her family and friends, who have been so incredibly supportive throughout her career. They are always there to offer a sympathetic ear and endless encouragement. She would also like to thank her students, as they are the reason she loves her job so much.

Melinda would specifically like to thank her husband, Steve Carroll, for the patience and understanding he has shown through this process—once again. He has learned that there is always another chapter due! Melinda would also like to thank her family, friends, graduate students, and professional colleagues for their support and listening ear throughout this whole process. They all helped make life a little easier during this incredibly busy time. Finally, she would like to thank Janice, a great friend and colleague, who makes working on the book fun and rewarding.

Reviewers

H. Giovanni Antunez
Health & Physical Education, Recreation & Sport Sciences, St. Cloud State University

Linda Armstrong, RD, LD, MBA
Dietetics & Health, Normandale Community College

Ms. Lenore L. Boccia, MS
Dean of Academic Affairs, The Restaurant School at Walnut Hill College

Melissa Chabot, MS, RD, CDN
Exercise and Nutritional Sciences, University at Buffalo

Eileen Daniel
Health Science, College at Brockport - SUNY

Ann Diker
Health Professions, Metropolitan State College of Denver

Urbi Ghosh
Biology, Oakton Community College

Janice Grover, MS, RD
Nutrition, Truckee Meadows Community College

Laura Hutchinson
Health, Fitness & Nutrition, Holyoke Community College

Jessica Hodge
Nutrition, Folsom Lake College

Beau Kjerulf Greer, Ph.D., CSCS
Physical Therapy & Human Movement Sciences, Sacred Heart University

Pauline A. Lizotte, Ph.D.
Math, Science & Health Careers, Manchester Community College

Alexandria Miller, PhD, RD/LD
Human and Family Sciences, Department of Health Professions, Northeastern State University

Rebecca Roach
Food Science & Human Nutrition, University of Illinois at Urbana Champaign

Vicki S. Schwartz, MS, RD, LDN
Nutrition Sciences, Drexel University

Andrea Villarreal
Applied Technology, Family & Consumer Sciences, Phoenix College

Diana Watson-Maile, Ed.D.
Family & Consumer Sciences, East Central University

Brief Contents

Chapter 1
The Role of Nutrition in Our Health 2
IN DEPTH Alcohol 28

Chapter 2
Designing a Healthful Diet 38
IN DEPTH Phytochemicals 67

Chapter 3
The Human Body: Are We Really What We Eat? 72
IN DEPTH Disorders Related to Specific Foods 100

Chapter 4
Carbohydrates: Plant-Derived Energy Nutrients 106
IN DEPTH Diabetes 137

Chapter 5
Fats: Essential Energy-Supplying Nutrients 142
IN DEPTH Cardiovascular Disease 173

Chapter 6
Proteins: Crucial Components of All Body Tissues 184
IN DEPTH Vitamins and Minerals: Micronutrients with Macro Powers 216

Chapter 7
Nutrients Involved in Fluid and Electrolyte Balance 226
IN DEPTH Fluid Imbalance 250

Chapter 8
Nutrients Involved in Antioxidant Function 254
IN DEPTH Cancer 281

Chapter 9
Nutrients Involved in Bone Health 290
IN DEPTH Osteoporosis 318

Chapter 10
Nutrients Involved in Energy Metabolism and Blood Health 326
IN DEPTH Dietary Supplements: Necessity or Waste? 360

Chapter 11
Achieving and Maintaining a Healthful Body Weight 368
IN DEPTH Obesity 402

Chapter 12
Nutrition and Physical Activity: Keys to Good Health 410
IN DEPTH Disordered Eating 442

Chapter 13
Food Safety and Technology: Impact on Consumers 454
IN DEPTH Global Nutrition 490

Chapter 14
Nutrition Through the Life Cycle: Pregnancy and the First Year of Life 500
IN DEPTH The Fetal Environment: A Lasting Impression 536

Chapter 15
Nutrition Through the Life Cycle: Childhood to Late Adulthood 540
IN DEPTH Searching for the Fountain of Youth 574

Appendices A-1
References R-1
Answers to Review Questions AN-1
Glossary G-1
Index IN-1
Credits CR-1

Contents

Chapter 1

The Role of Nutrition in Our Health 2

What Is Nutrition? 4

How Does Nutrition Contribute to Health? 4

NUTRITION MYTH OR FACT?:
Is Pellagra an Infectious Disease? 5

Nutrition Is One of Several Factors Supporting Wellness 5

A Healthful Diet Can Prevent Some Diseases and Reduce Your Risk for Others 6

What Are Nutrients? 8

Macronutrients Provide Energy 9

YOU DO THE MATH:
Calculating the Energy Contribution of Carbohydrates, Fats, and Proteins 10

Micronutrients Assist in the Regulation of Body Functions 11

Water Supports All Body Functions 13

How Much of Each Nutrient Do Most People Need? 13

Use the Dietary Reference Intakes to Check Your Nutrient Intake 13

Diets Based on the DRIs Promote Wellness 15

Research Study Results: Who Can We Believe? 16

Research Involves Applying the Scientific Method 16

Various Types of Research Studies Tell Us Different Stories 19

Use Your Knowledge of Research to Help You Evaluate Media Reports 20

Nutrition Advice: Whom Can You Trust? 21

Trustworthy Experts Are Educated and Credentialed 22

Government Sources of Information Are Usually Trustworthy 23

Professional Organizations Provide Reliable Nutrition Information 24

NUTRI-CASE:
Liz 24

NUTRITION DEBATE:
Nutrigenomics: Personalized Nutrition or Pie in the Sky? 25

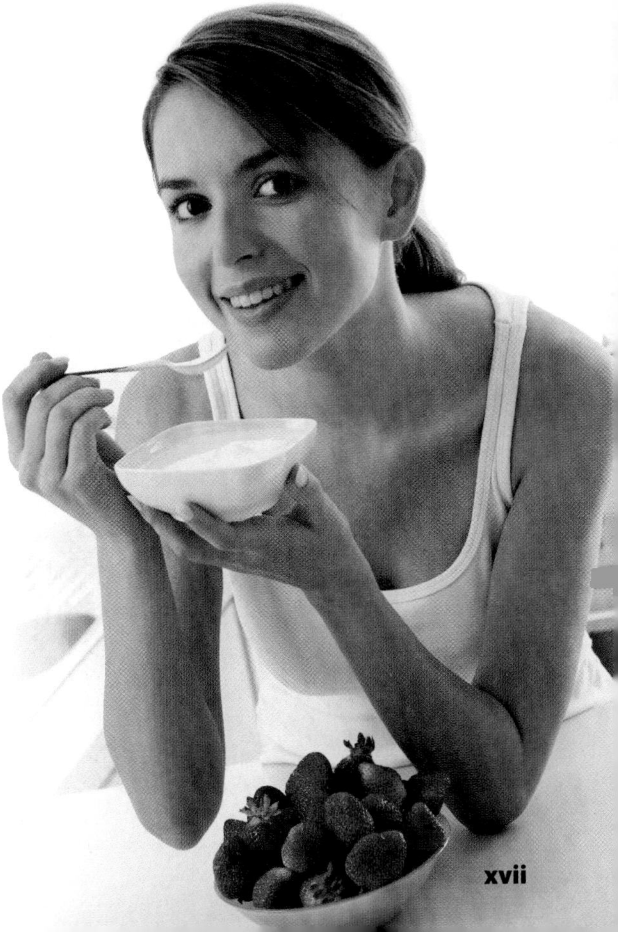

IN DEPTH: Alcohol 28

What Do We Know About Moderate Alcohol Intake? 29

Benefits of Moderate Alcohol Intake 29

Concerns About Moderate Alcohol Intake 30

What Happens to Alcohol in the Body? 30

Effects of Alcohol Abuse on Personal Health 31

Alcohol Hangovers 32

NUTRI-CASE: **Theo** 33

Reduced Brain Function 33

Alcohol Poisoning 33

Reduced Liver Function 33

Increased Risk for Chronic Disease 34

Malnutrition 34

Increased Risk for Traumatic Injury 34

Fetal and Infant Health Problems 35

WHAT ABOUT YOU?: **Do You Have a Problem with Alcohol Abuse?** 35

Should You Be Concerned About Your Alcohol Intake? 36

Talking to Someone About Alcohol Addiction 36

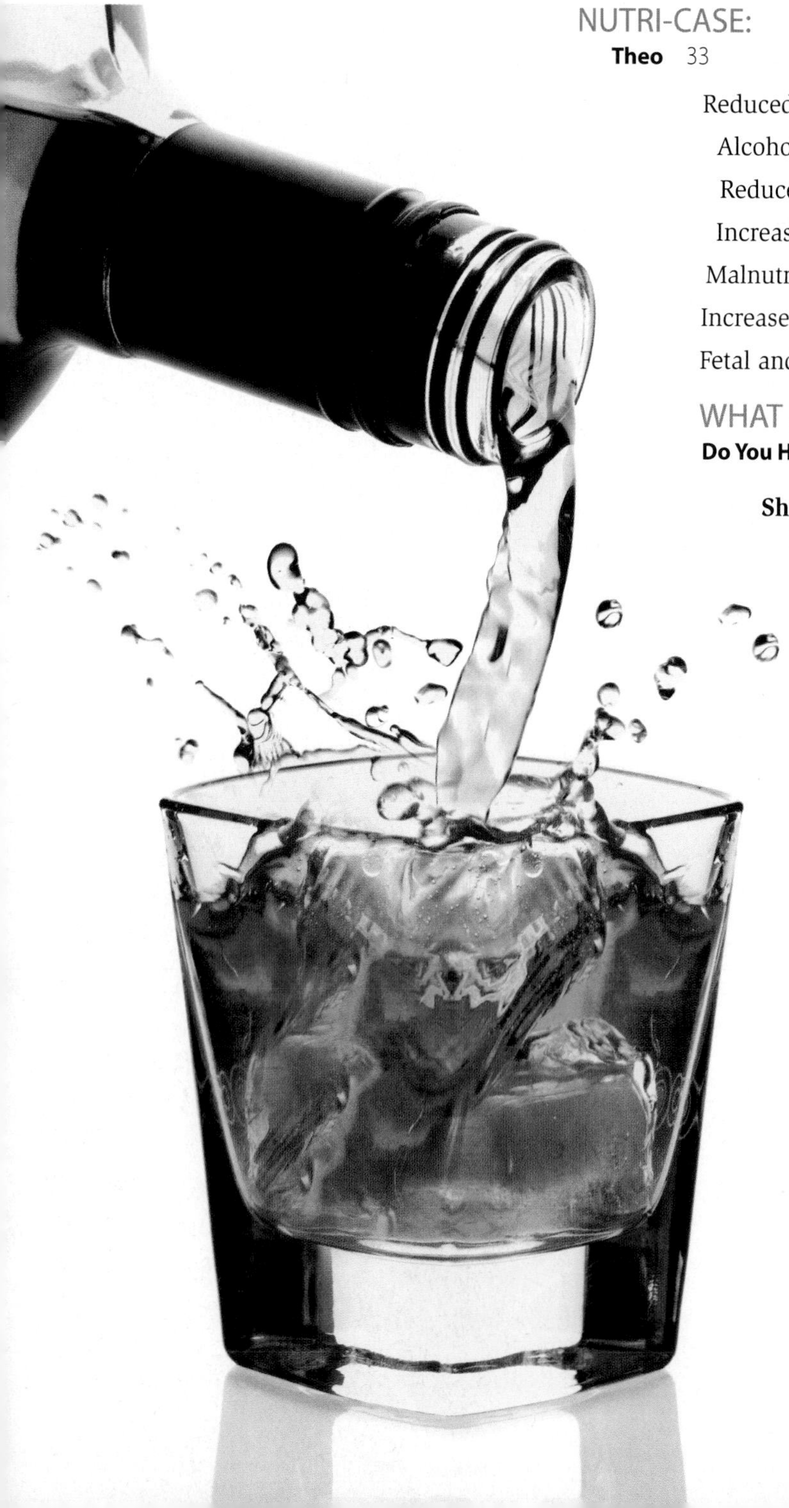

Chapter 2

Designing a Healthful Diet 38

What Is a Healthful Diet? 40

A Healthful Diet Is Adequate 40

A Healthful Diet Is Moderate 40

A Healthful Diet Is Balanced 41

A Healthful Diet Is Varied 41

What Tools Can Help Me Design a Healthful Diet? 41

Food Labels 41

NUTRITION LABEL ACTIVITY:
How Do Health Claims on Food Labels Measure Up? 47

NUTRI-CASE:
Gustavo 47

Dietary Guidelines for Americans 48

The USDA Food Patterns 51

NUTRITION LABEL ACTIVITY:
How Realistic Are the Serving Sizes Listed on Food Labels? 55

Can Eating Out Be Part of a Healthful Diet? 58

YOU DO THE MATH:
How Much Exercise Is Needed to Combat Increasing Food Portion Sizes? 59

The Hidden Costs of Eating Out 60

The Healthful Way to Eat Out 61

NUTRITION DEBATE:
Can Functional Foods Improve Our Health? 63

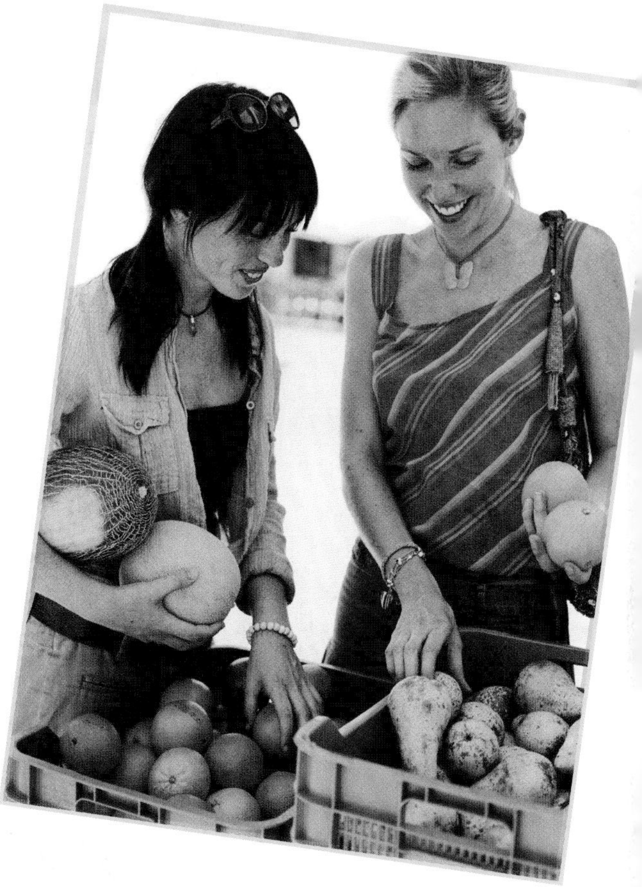

IN DEPTH: Phytochemicals 67

What Are Phytochemicals? 68

How Do Phytochemicals Reduce Our Risk for Disease? 68

NUTRI-CASE:
Hannah 70

Is There an RDA for Phytochemicals? 70

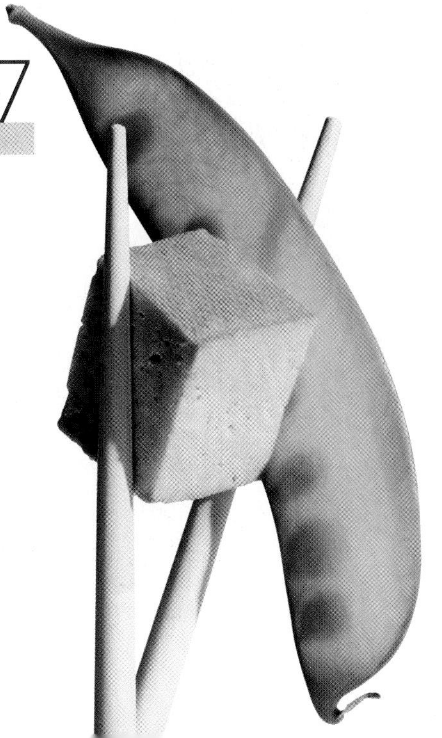

What Role Do Fats Play in Chronic Disease? 167

EATING RIGHT ALL DAY 167

NUTRITION DEBATE:
Fat Blockers—Help or Hype? 169

IN DEPTH: Cardiovascular Disease 173

What Is Cardiovascular Disease? 174

Atherosclerosis Is Narrowing of Arteries 174

Hypertension Signals an Increased Risk for Heart Attack and Stroke 175

NUTRI-CASE:
Gustavo 175

Who Is at Risk for Cardiovascular Disease? 176

Many Risk Factors Are Within Your Control 176

The Role of Dietary Fats in Cardiovascular Disease 177

WHAT ABOUT YOU?:
Blood Lipid Levels: How Do Yours Measure Up? 179

Calculating Your Risk for Cardiovascular Disease 179

Lifestyle Choices Can Help Prevent or Control Cardiovascular Disease 179

Recommendations to Improve Blood Lipid Levels 179

Recommendations to Reduce Blood Pressure 182

Prescription Medications Can Improve Blood Lipids and Blood Pressure 182

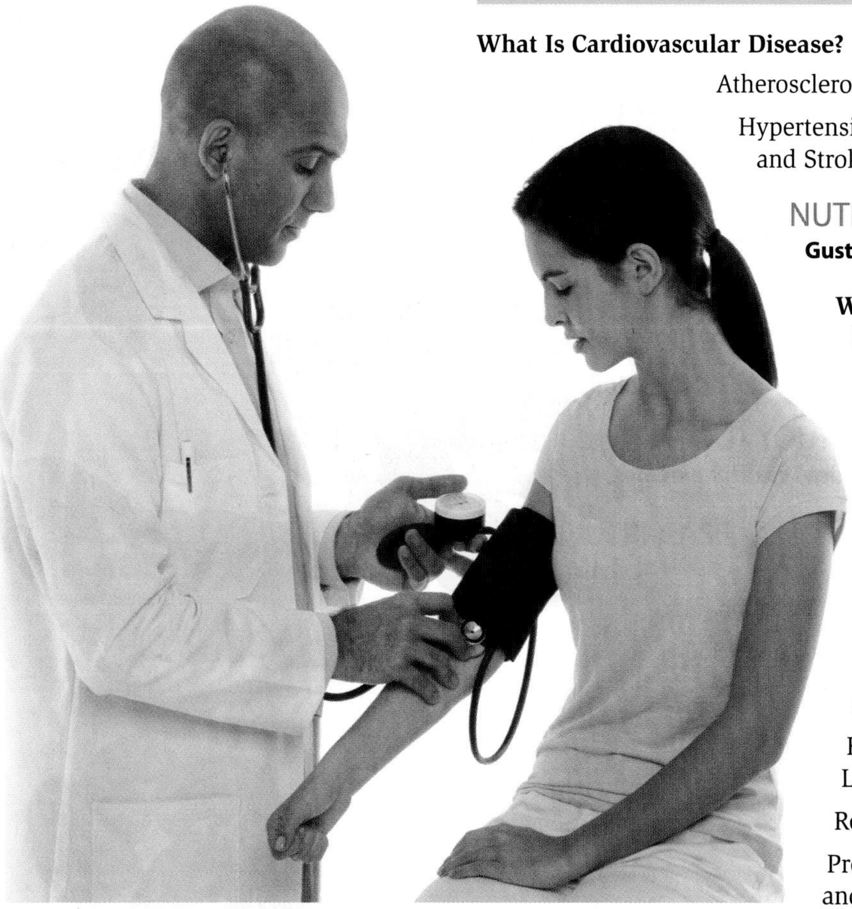

Chapter 6

Proteins: Crucial Components of All Body Tissues 184

What Are Proteins? 186

How Do Proteins Differ from Carbohydrates and Lipids? 186

The Building Blocks of Proteins Are Amino Acids 186

How Are Proteins Made? 188
Amino Acids Bond to Form a Variety of Peptides 188
Genes Regulate Amino Acid Binding 188
Protein Turnover Involves Synthesis and Degradation 189
Protein Organization Determines Function 190
Protein Synthesis Can Be Limited by Missing Amino Acids 192
Protein Synthesis Can Be Enhanced by Mutual Supplementation 192

Why Do We Need Proteins? 193
Proteins Contribute to Cell Growth, Repair, and Maintenance 193
Proteins Act as Enzymes and Hormones 194
Proteins Help Maintain Fluid and Electrolyte Balance 194
Proteins Help Maintain Acid–Base Balance 194
Proteins Help Maintain a Strong Immune System 195
Proteins Serve as an Energy Source 196

How Do Our Bodies Break Down Proteins? 197
Stomach Acids and Enzymes Break Proteins into Short Polypeptides 197
Enzymes in the Small Intestine Break Polypeptides into Single Amino Acids 197
Protein Digestibility Affects Protein Quality 198

How Much Protein Should We Eat? 199
Nitrogen Balance Is a Method Used to Determine Protein Needs 199

NUTRITION MYTH OR FACT?:
Do Athletes Need More Protein than Inactive People? 199

Recommended Dietary Allowance for Protein 201

YOU DO THE MATH:
Calculating Your Protein Needs 201

Most Americans Meet or Exceed the RDA for Protein 202
Protein: Much More than Meat! 202

WHAT ABOUT YOU?:
How Much Protein Do You Eat? 204

Can a Vegetarian Diet Provide Adequate Protein? 205

EATING RIGHT ALL DAY 206

Types of Vegetarian Diets 206
Why Do People Become Vegetarians? 206
What Are the Challenges of a Vegetarian Diet? 208

NUTRI-CASE:
Theo 209

Using the Vegetarian Food Guide Pyramid 209

What Health Problems Are Related to Protein Intake? 210

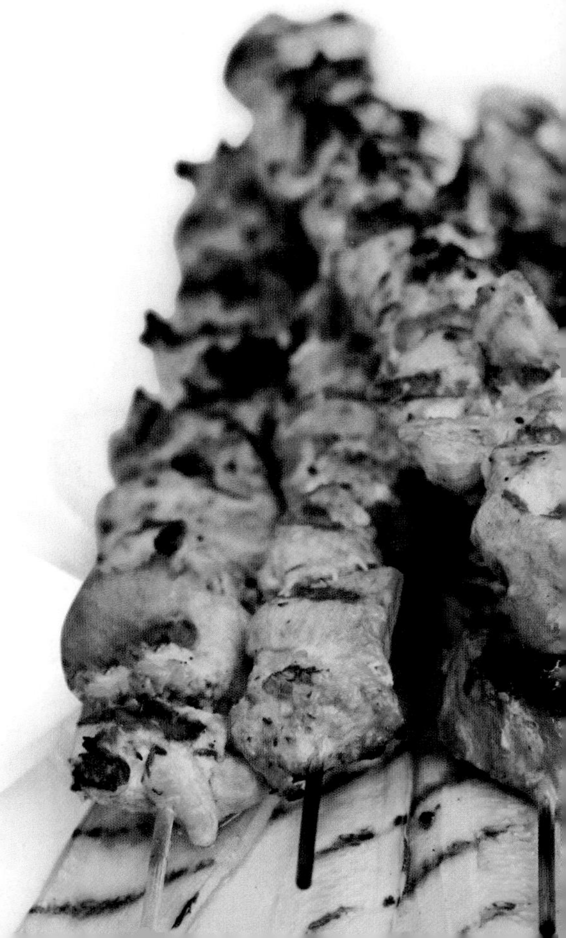

Too Much Dietary Protein Can Be Harmful 210
Protein-Energy Malnutrition Can Lead to Debility and Death 211
NUTRITION DEBATE:
Meat Consumption and Global Warming: Tofu to the Rescue? 213

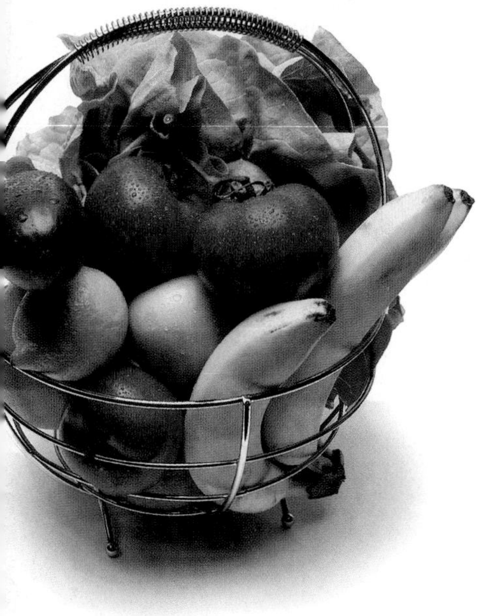

IN DEPTH: Vitamins and Minerals: Micronutrients with Macro Powers 216

Discovering the "Hidden" Nutrients 217
How Are Vitamins Classified? 217
Fat-Soluble Vitamins 217
Water-Soluble Vitamins 218
Same Vitamin, Different Names and Forms 220
How Are Minerals Classified? 220
Major Minerals 220
Trace Minerals 220
Same Mineral, Different Forms 221
How Do Our Bodies Use Micronutrients? 221
What We Eat Differs from What We Absorb 223
What We Eat Differs from What Our Cells Use 223
Controversies in Micronutrient Metabolism 223
NUTRI-CASE:
Liz 224
Are Supplements Healthful Sources of Micronutrients? 224
Can Micronutrients Really Prevent or Treat Disease? 225
Do More Essential Micronutrients Exist? 225

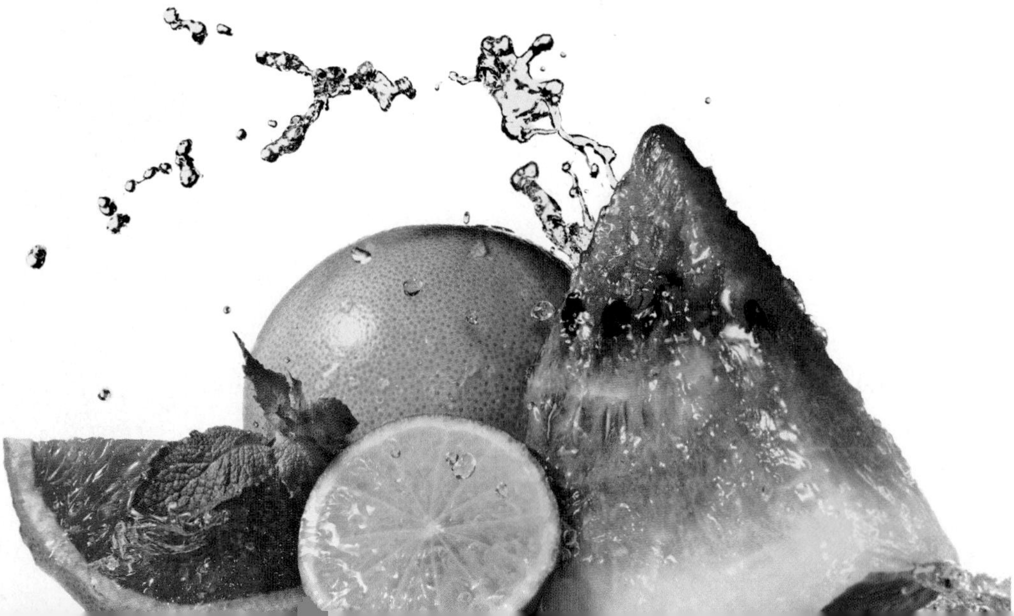

Chapter 7

Nutrients Involved in Fluid and Electrolyte Balance 226

What Are Fluids and Electrolytes, and What Are Their Functions? 228

- Body Fluid Is the Liquid Portion of Our Cells and Tissues 228
- Body Fluid Is Composed of Water and Salts Called Electrolytes 228
- Fluids Serve Many Critical Functions 230
- Electrolytes Support Many Body Functions 231

How Does Our Body Maintain Fluid Balance? 233

- Our Thirst Mechanism Prompts Us to Drink Fluids 233
- We Gain Fluids by Consuming Beverages and Foods and Through Metabolism 234
- We Lose Fluids Through Urine, Sweat, Evaporation, Exhalation, and Feces 234

A Profile of Nutrients Involved in Hydration and Neuromuscular Function 236

- Water 236
  - WHAT ABOUT YOU?: **How Pure Is Your Favorite Bottled Water?** 239
  - NUTRI-CASE: **Judy** 239
- Sodium 240
  - EATING RIGHT ALL DAY 241
- Potassium 242
  - NUTRITION MYTH OR FACT?: **Can Fluids Provide Too Much of a Good Thing?** 243
- Chloride 245
- Phosphorus 245
  - NUTRITION DEBATE: **Sports Beverages: Help or Hype?** 247

IN DEPTH: Fluid Imbalance 250

Dehydration 251

- Classifying Dehydration 251
- Preventing Dehydration During and After Physical Activity 251

Heat Illnesses 252

- Heat Cramps 252

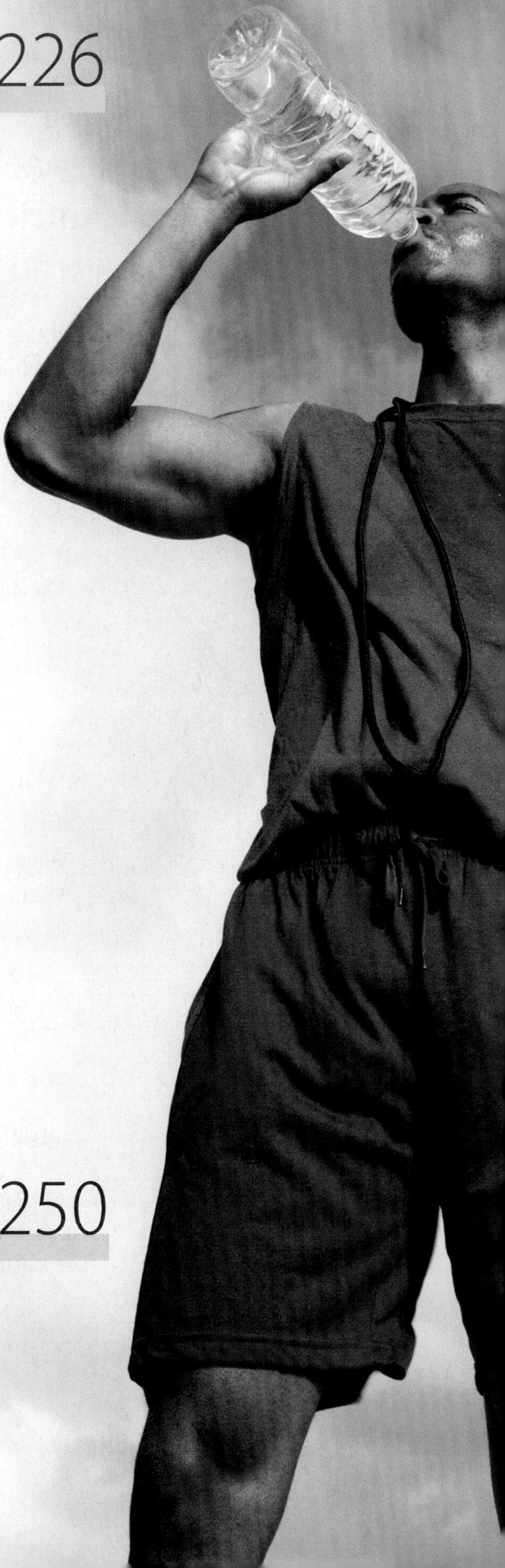

Heat Exhaustion 252

NUTRI-CASE:
Gustavo 253

Heat Stroke 253

Chapter 8

Nutrients Involved in Antioxidant Function 254

What Are Antioxidants, and How Does Our Body Use Them? 256
Oxidation Is a Chemical Reaction in Which Atoms Lose Electrons 256
Oxidation Sometimes Results in the Formation of Free Radicals 257
Free Radicals Can Destabilize Other Molecules and Damage Our Cells 258
Antioxidants Work by Stabilizing Free Radicals or Opposing Oxidation 258

A Profile of Nutrients That Function as Antioxidants 259
Vitamin E 260
Vitamin C 262

EATING RIGHT ALL DAY 263

NUTRITION MYTH OR FACT?:
Can Vitamin C Prevent the Common Cold? 264

NUTRI-CASE:
Hannah 266

Beta-Carotene 267
Vitamin A: Much More than an Antioxidant Nutrient 269
Selenium 274
Copper, Iron, Zinc, and Manganese Assist in Antioxidant Function 276

NUTRITION DEBATE:
Antioxidants: Food or Supplements? 277

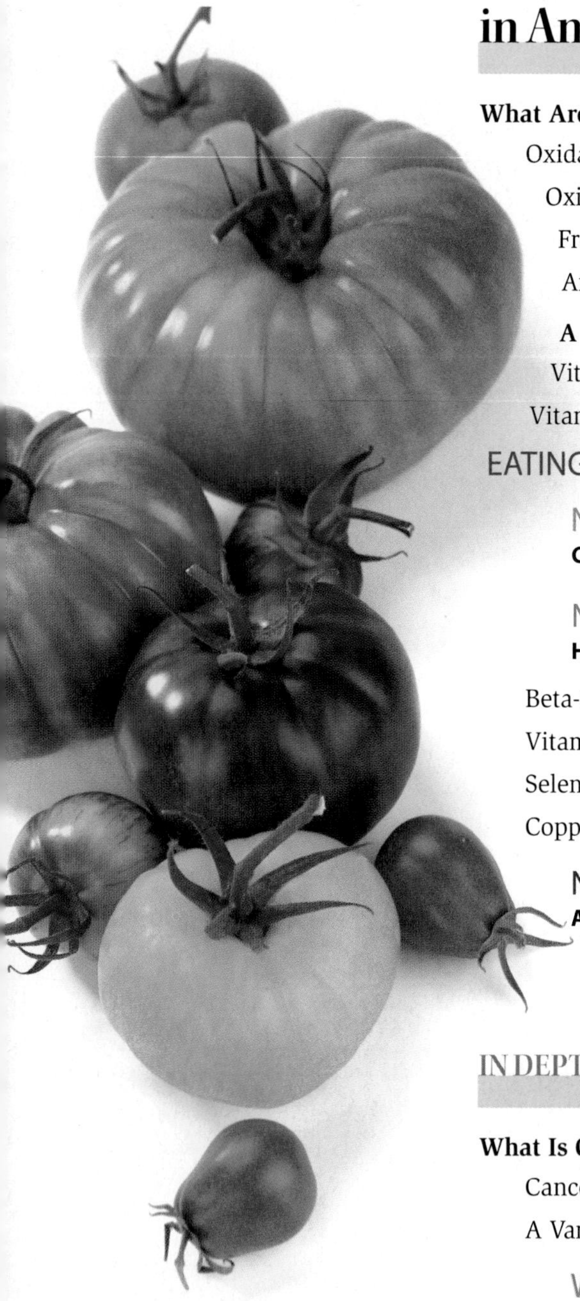

IN DEPTH: Cancer 281

What Is Cancer? 282
Cancer Progresses in Three Stages 282
A Variety of Factors Influence Cancer Risk 283

WHAT ABOUT YOU?:
Are You Living Smart? 285

Cancer Prompts a Variety of Signs and Symptoms 286

How Is Cancer Treated? 287

Can Cancer Be Prevented? 287

Check 287

Quit 287

Move 288

Nourish 288

Antioxidants Play a Role in Preventing Cancer 288

NUTRI-CASE:
Gustavo 289

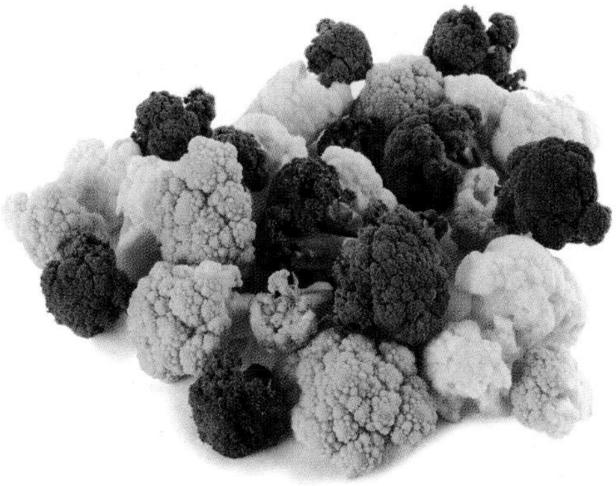

Chapter 9

Nutrients Involved in Bone Health 290

How Does Our Body Maintain Bone Health? 292

The Composition of Bone Provides Strength and Flexibility 292

The Constant Activity of Bone Tissue Promotes Bone Health 293

How Do We Assess Bone Health? 295

A Profile of Nutrients That Maintain Bone Health 296

Calcium 296

EATING RIGHT ALL DAY 301

Vitamin D 301

WHAT ABOUT YOU?:
Are You Getting Enough Vitamin D? 305

NUTRITION LABEL ACTIVITY:
How Much Calcium Am I Really Consuming? 306

NUTRI-CASE:
Theo 307

Vitamin K 308

Phosphorus 309

Magnesium 310

Fluoride 312

NUTRITION DEBATE:
Vitamin D Deficiency: Why the Surge, and What Can Be Done? 315

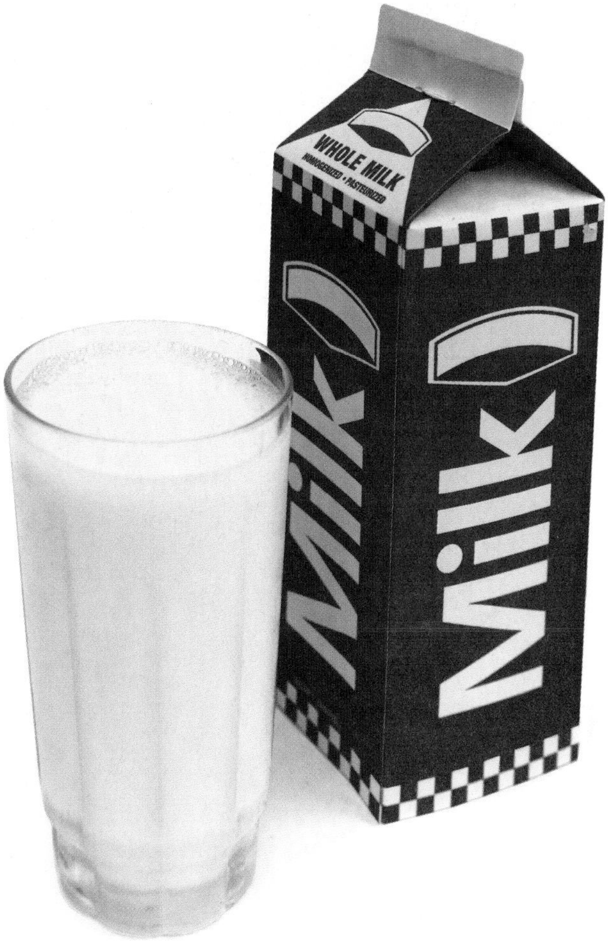

IN DEPTH: **Osteoporosis** 318

What Is Osteoporosis? 319

What Influences Osteoporosis Risk? 320

Aging Increases Osteoporosis Risk 320

Gender and Genetics Affect Osteoporosis Risk 320

Tobacco, Alcohol, and Caffeine Influence Osteoporosis Risk 320

Nutritional Factors Influence Osteoporosis Risk 321

Regular Physical Activity Reduces Osteoporosis Risk 322

How Is Osteoporosis Treated? 322

WHAT ABOUT YOU?:
Are You at Risk for Osteoporosis? 323

Can Osteoporosis Be Prevented? 324

Consider Supplements 324

NUTRI-CASE:
Gustavo 325

Other Preventive Measures 325

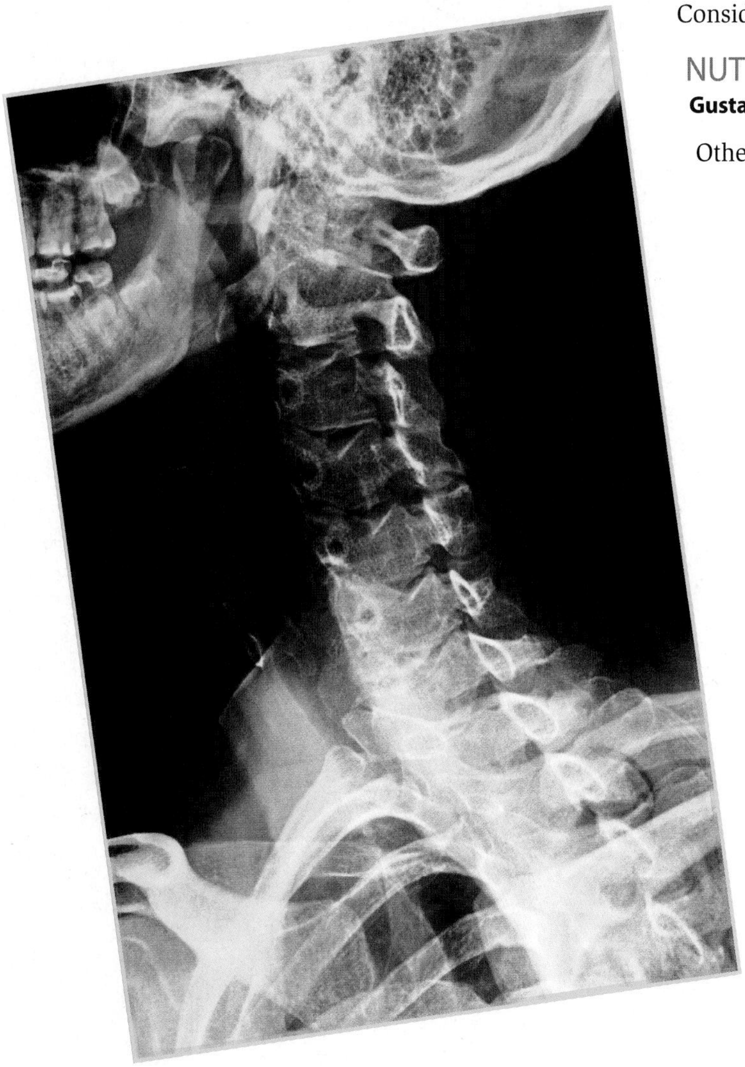

Chapter 10

Nutrients Involved in Energy Metabolism and Blood Health 326

How Does Our Body Regulate Energy Metabolism? 328

Our Body Requires Vitamins and Minerals to Produce Energy 328

Some Micronutrients Assist with Nutrient Transport and Hormone Production 329

A Profile of Nutrients Involved in Energy Metabolism 330

Thiamin (Vitamin B_1) 331

Riboflavin (Vitamin B_2) 332

Niacin 333

Vitamin B_6 (Pyridoxine) 334

Folate 336

Vitamin B_{12} (Cobalamin) 339

Pantothenic Acid 341

Biotin 341

Choline 343

Iodine 343

Chromium 344

Manganese 344

NUTRITION MYTH OR FACT?:
Can Chromium Supplements Enhance Body Composition? 345

Sulfur 345

What Is the Role of Blood in Maintaining Health? 346

A Profile of Nutrients That Maintain Healthy Blood 347

Vitamin K 347

Iron 348

EATING RIGHT ALL DAY 353

NUTRI-CASE:
Liz 353

Zinc 354

Copper 355

NUTRITION DEBATE:
Do Zinc Lozenges Help Fight the Common Cold? 357

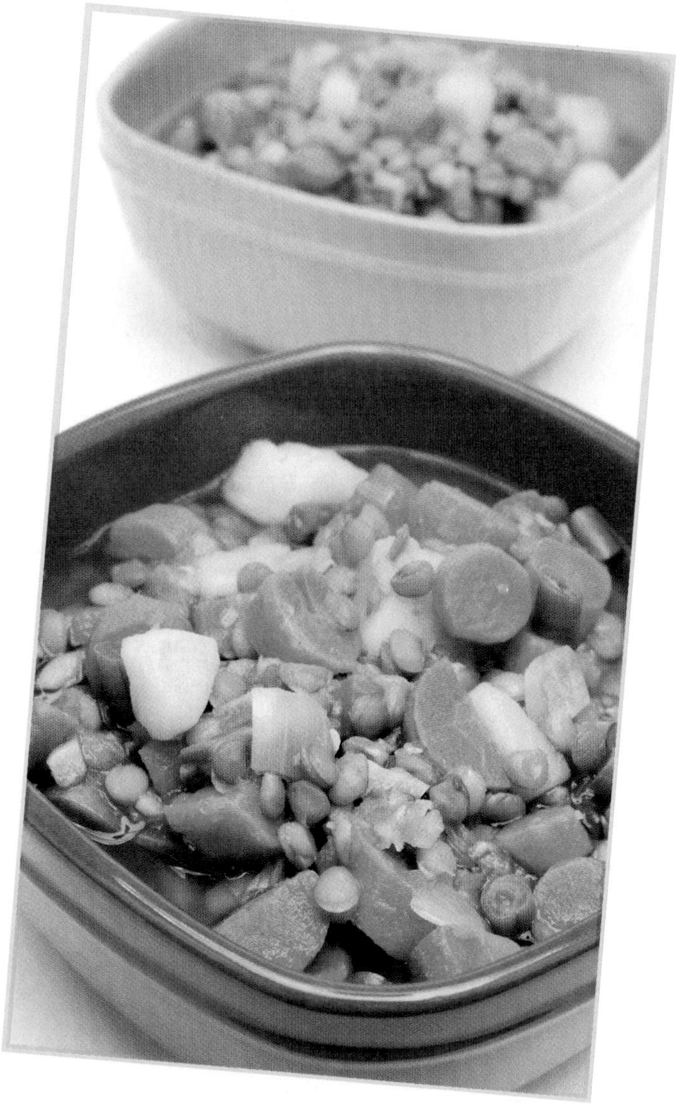

IN DEPTH: **Dietary Supplements: Necessity or Waste?** 360

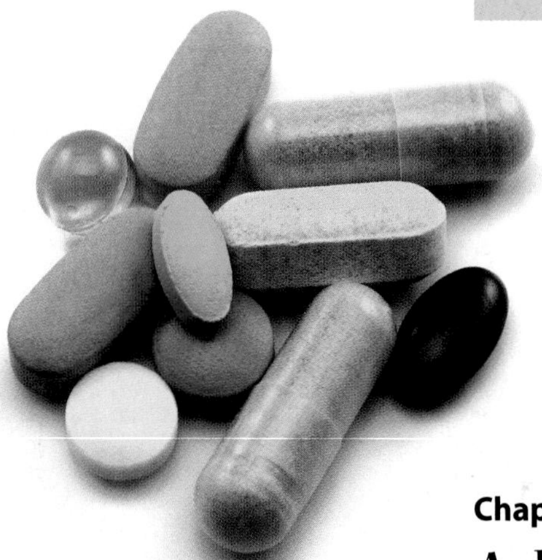

What Are Dietary Supplements? 361

How Are Dietary Supplements Regulated? 361

How Can You Avoid Fraudulent or Dangerous Supplements? 362

Are There Special Precautions for Herbal Supplements? 363

Should You Take a Dietary Supplement? 364

NUTRI-CASE:
Theo 366

Chapter 11

Achieving and Maintaining a Healthful Body Weight 368

How Can You Evaluate Your Body Weight? 370

Understand What a Healthful Body Weight Really Is 370

Determine Your Body Mass Index (BMI) 370

Measure Your Body Composition 372

YOU DO THE MATH:
Calculating Your Body Mass Index 374

Assess Your Fat Distribution Patterns 374

What Makes Us Gain and Lose Weight? 375

We Gain or Lose Weight When Our Energy Intake and Expenditure Are Out of Balance 375

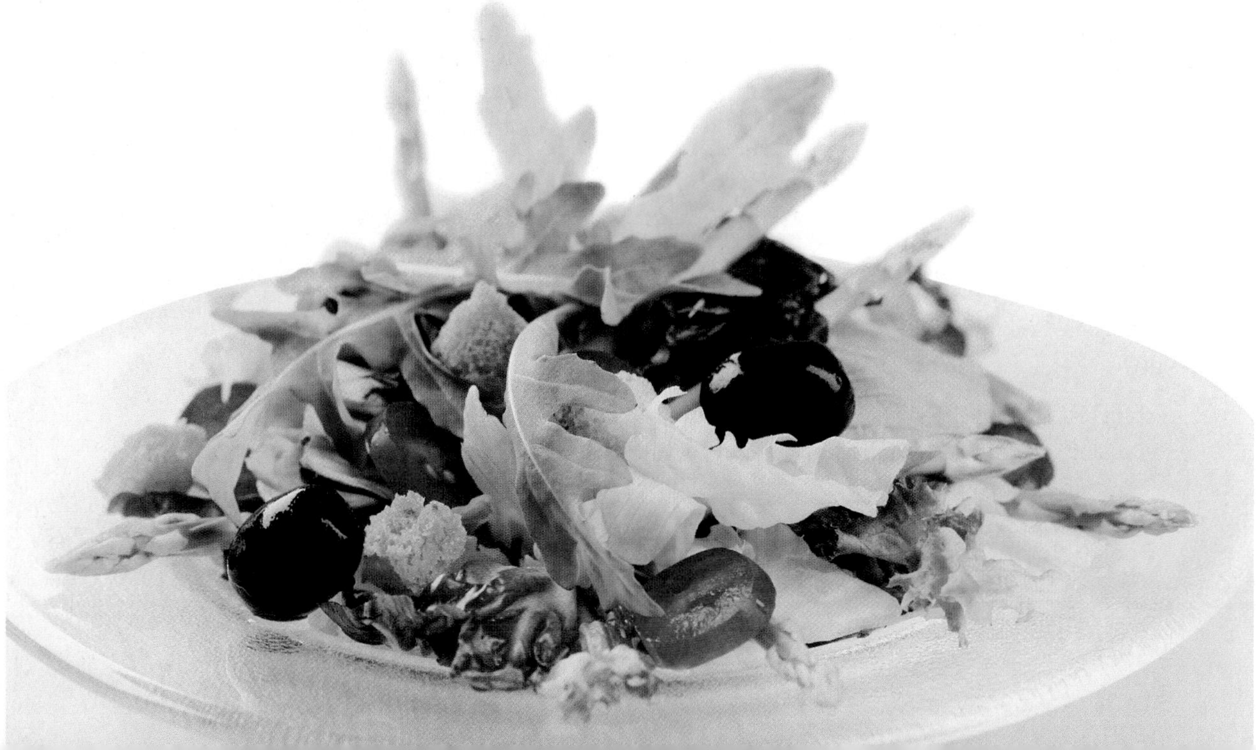

When Traveling to Other Countries 471

NUTRI-CASE:
Theo 472

How Is Food Spoilage Prevented? 472
Natural Methods Are Effective in Preserving Foods 473
Modern Techniques Improve Food Safety 473

What Are Food Additives, and Are They Safe? 476
Additives Can Enhance a Food's Taste, Appearance, Safety, or Nutrition 476
Are Food Additives Considered Safe? 478

How Is Genetic Modification Used in Food Production? 479

Do Residues Harm Our Food Supply? 480
Persistent Organic Pollutants Can Cause Illness 481
Pesticides Protect Against Crop Losses 482
Growth Hormones and Antibiotics Are Used in Animals 484
Are Organic Foods More Healthful? 485

NUTRITION DEBATE:
Genetically Modified Organisms: A Blessing or a Curse? 487

IN DEPTH: **Global Nutrition** 490

Malnutrition in the Developing World 491
What Causes Undernutrition in the Developing World? 491
What Health Problems Result from Undernutrition? 493
Why Is Obesity a Growing Problem in Developing Nations? 495

Malnutrition in the United States 495

What Can Be Done to Relieve Malnutrition? 496
Global Solutions 496
Local Solutions 496
Get Involved! 497

NUTRI-CASE:
Judy 497

WHAT ABOUT YOU?:
Do Your Actions Contribute to Global Food Security? 498

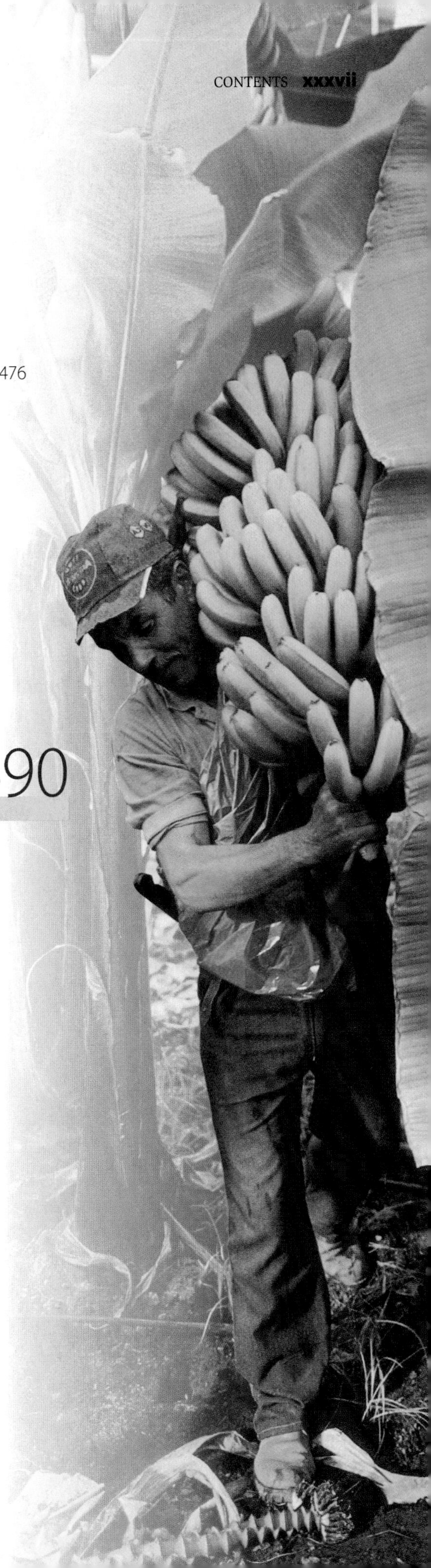

Chapter 14

Nutrition Through the Life Cycle: Pregnancy and the First Year of Life 500

Starting Out Right: Healthful Nutrition in Pregnancy 502

Is Nutrition Important Before Conception? 502

Why Is Nutrition Important during Pregnancy? 502

How Much Weight Should a Pregnant Woman Gain? 505

What Are a Pregnant Woman's Nutrient Needs? 508

Nutrition-Related Concerns for Pregnant Women 512

NUTRI-CASE:
Judy 517

Lactation: Nutrition for Breastfeeding Mothers 517

How Does Lactation Occur? 518

What Are a Breastfeeding Woman's Nutrient Needs? 519

Getting Real About Breastfeeding: Advantages and Challenges 521

Infant Nutrition: From Birth to 1 Year 525

Typical Infant Growth and Activity Patterns 525

Nutrient Needs for Infants 525

What Types of Formula Are Available? 528

When Do Infants Begin to Need Solid Foods? 528

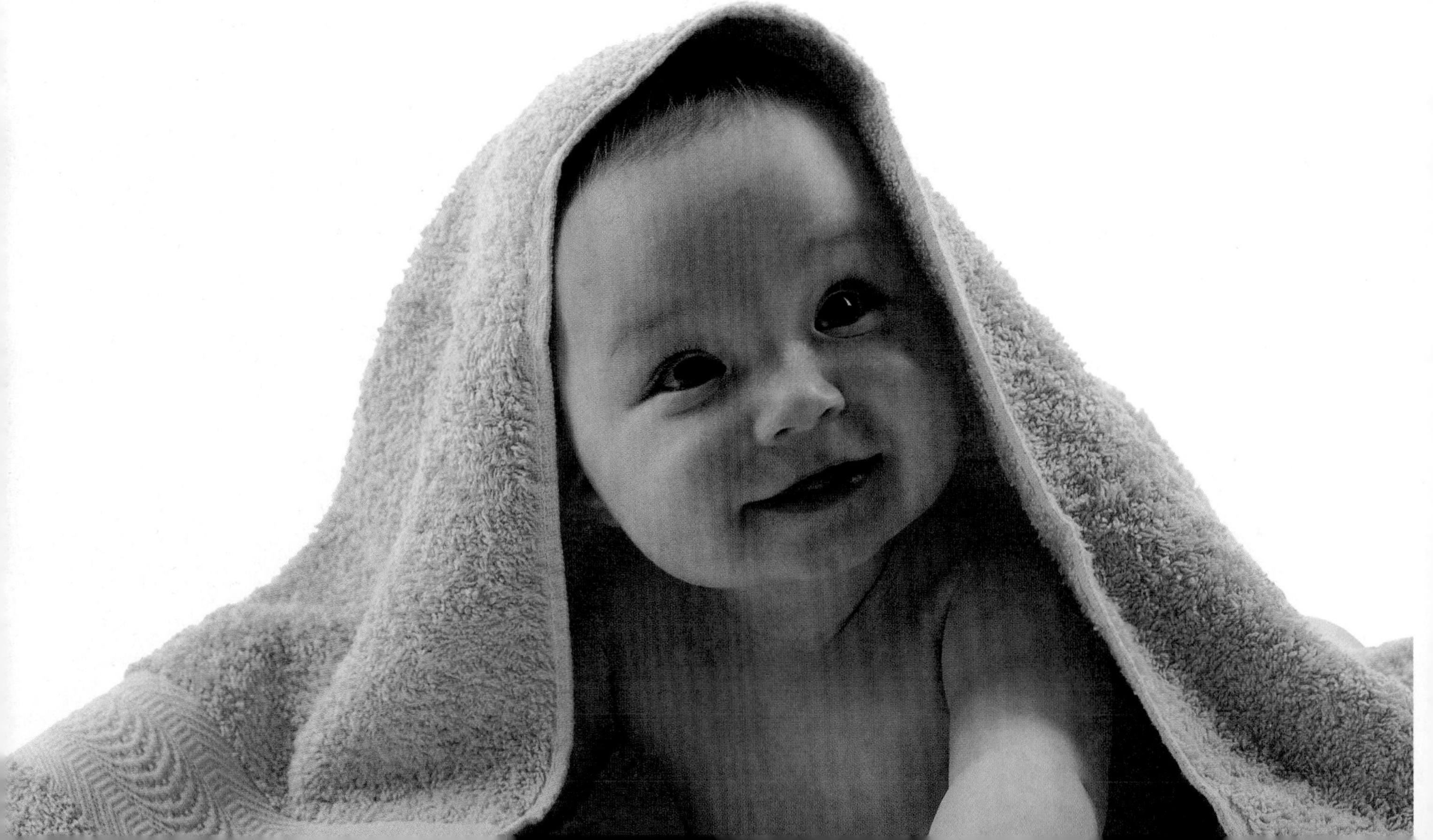

NUTRITION LABEL ACTIVITY:
Reading Infant Food Labels 529

What *Not* to Feed an Infant 530

Nutrition-Related Concerns for Infants 531

NUTRITION DEBATE:
Should Breastfeeding Throughout Infancy Be Mandatory? 533

IN DEPTH: **The Fetal Environment: A Lasting Impression** 536

Exposure to Famine 537

Exposure to Specific Nutrient Deficiencies 538

Exposure to Dietary Excesses 538

Exposure to Alcohol, Tobacco, and Other Toxic Agents 538

NUTRI-CASE:
Hannah 539

Implications for Your Health 539

Chapter 15

Nutrition Through the Life Cycle: Childhood to Late Adulthood 540

Nutrition for Toddlers 542

What Are a Toddler's Nutrient Needs? 542

YOU DO THE MATH:
Is This Menu Good for a Toddler? 544

Encouraging Nutritious Food Choices with Toddlers 545

Nutrition-Related Concerns for Toddlers 546

Nutrition for Preschool and School-Age Children 547

What Are a Child's Nutrient Needs? 547

NUTRITION MYTH OR FACT?:
Are Vegan Diets Appropriate for Young Children? 548

Encouraging Nutritious Food Choices with Children 551

NUTRITION MYTH OR FACT?:
Is Breakfast the Most Important Meal of the Day? 552

Nutrition-Related Concerns for Children 553

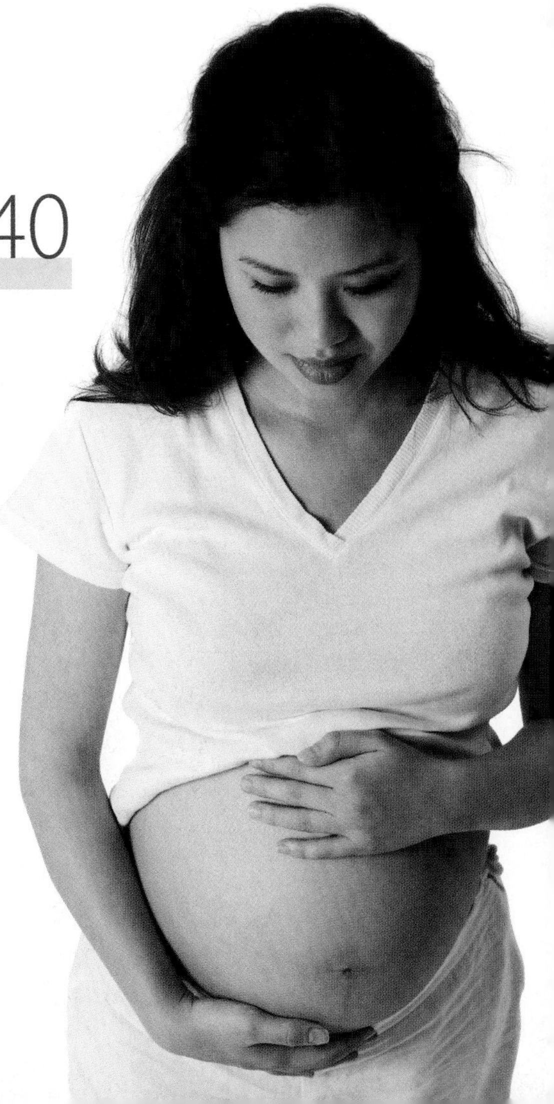

Nutrition for Adolescents 554
Adolescent Growth and Activity Patterns 554
What Are an Adolescent's Nutrient Needs? 555
Encouraging Nutritious Food Choices with Adolescents 556
Nutrition-Related Concerns for Adolescents 558
NUTRI-CASE:
Liz 559
Pediatric Obesity Watch: A Concern for Children and Adolescents 560
The Seeds of Pediatric Obesity 560
Prevention Through a Healthful Diet 560
Prevention Through an Active Lifestyle 561
Nutrition for Older Adults 561
What Physiologic Changes Accompany Aging? 562
What Are an Older Adult's Nutrient Needs? 564
Nutrition-Related Concerns for Older Adults 567
NUTRITION DEBATE:
Physical Activity in Older Adulthood: Should Seniors "Go for the Gold"? 571

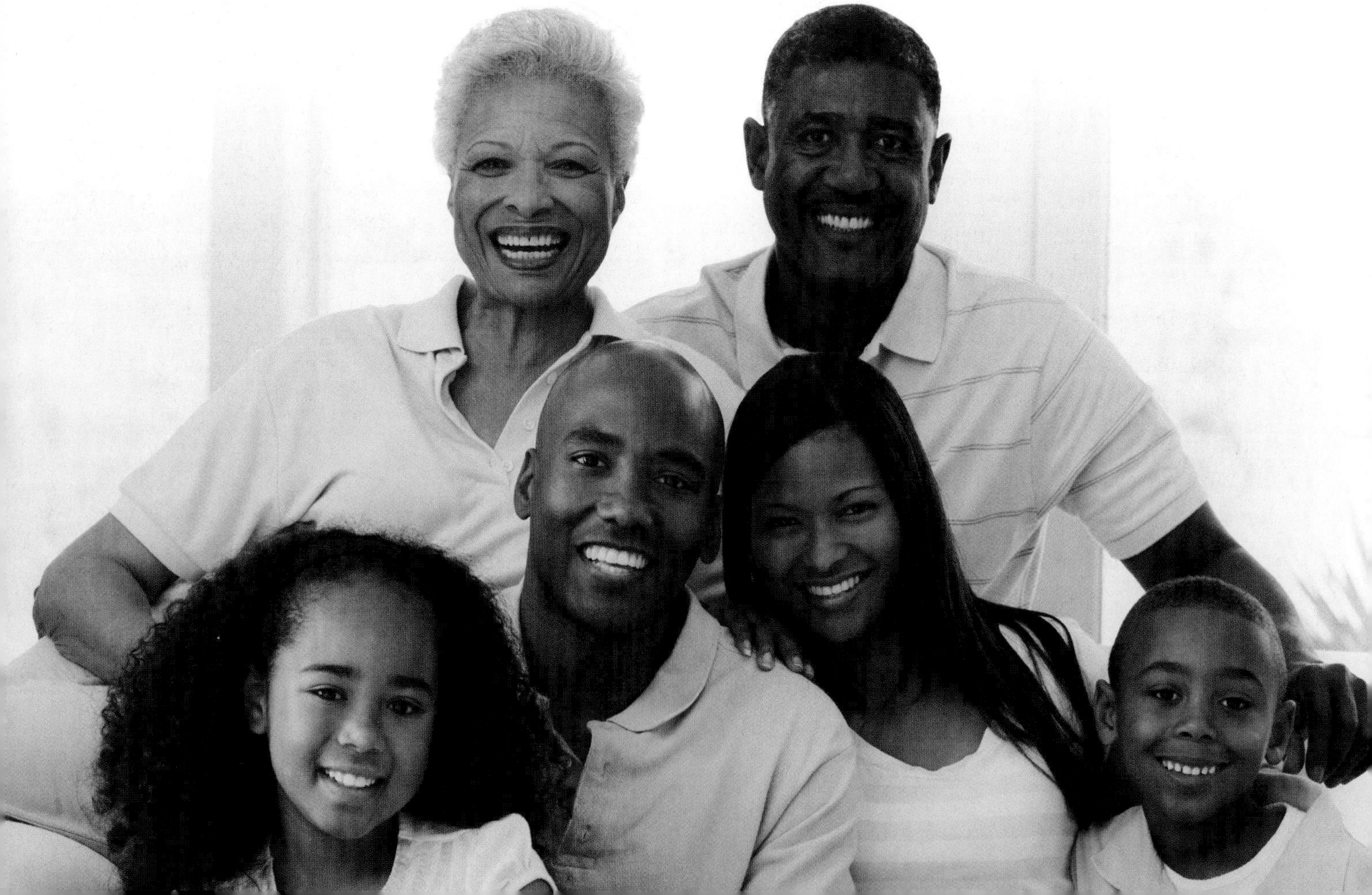

IN DEPTH: Searching for the Fountain of Youth 574

Does Calorie Restriction Increase Life Span? 575

Effects of Calorie Restriction 575

Challenges of Calorie Restriction 576

Alternatives to Calorie Restriction 577

Can Supplements Slow Aging? 577

NUTRI-CASE:
Gustavo 578

Are Your Actions Today Promoting a Longer, Healthier Life? 578

WHAT ABOUT YOU?:
How Long Are You Likely to Live? 579

Appendices

Appendix A
Dietary Guidelines, Upper Intake Levels, and Dietary Reference Intakes A-1

Appendix B
Calculations and Conversions B-1

Appendix C
Foods Containing Caffeine C-1

Appendix D
U.S. Exchange Lists for Meal Planning D-1

Appendix E
Stature-for-Age Charts E-1

Appendix F
Organizations and Resources F-1

Appendix G
The USDA Food Guide Evolution G-1

References R-1

Answers to Review Questions AN-1

Glossary G-1

Index IN-1

Credits CR-1

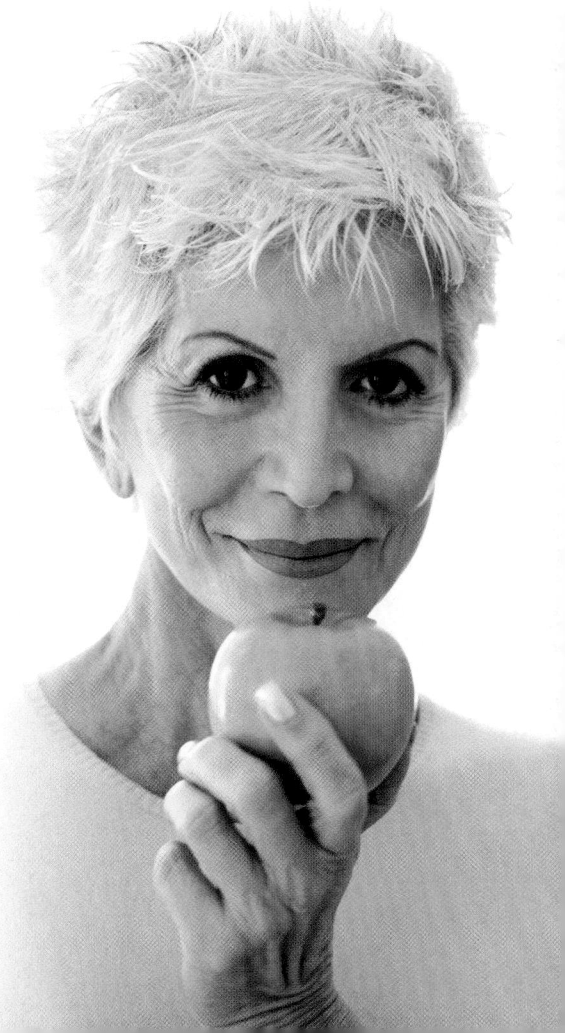

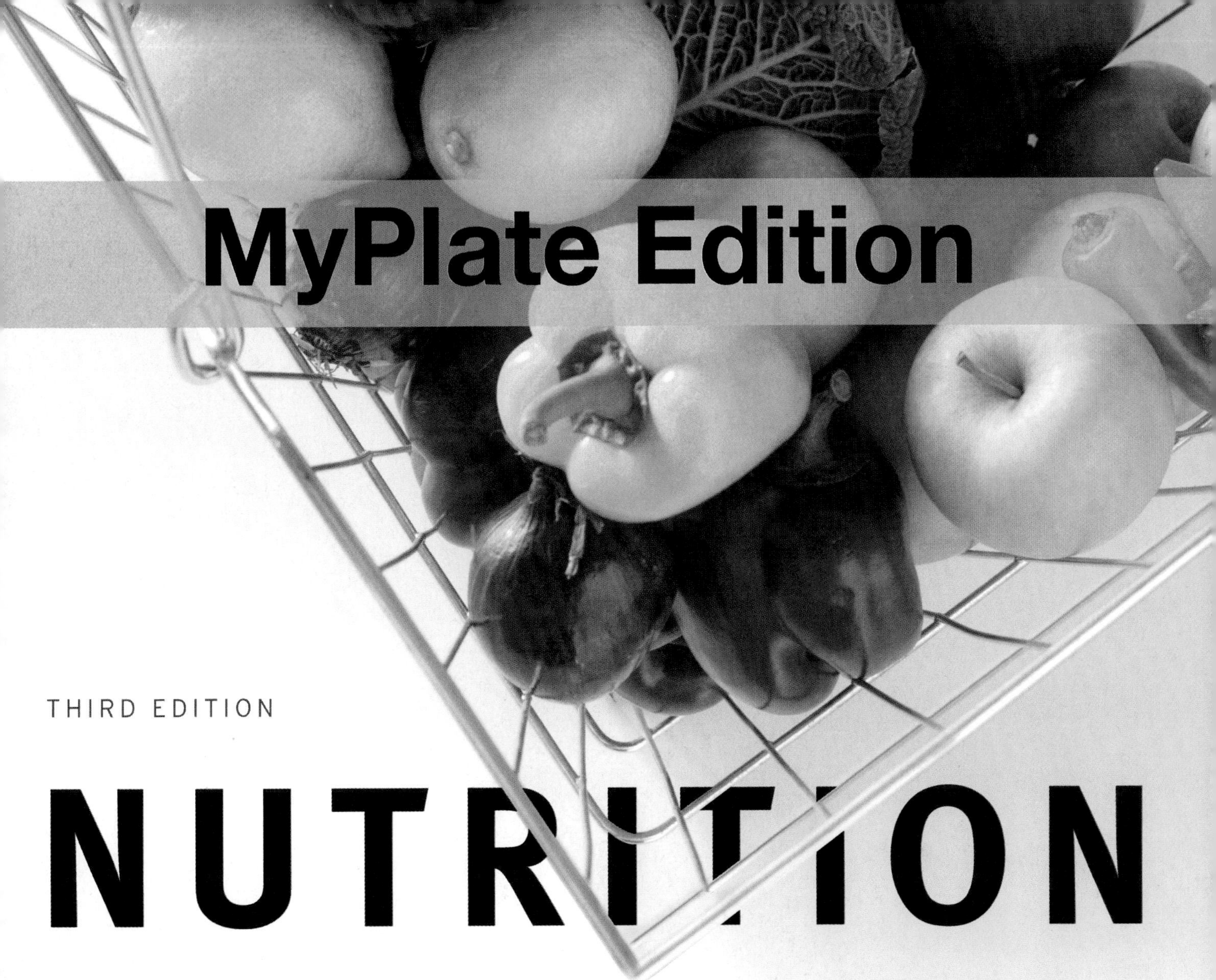

MyPlate Edition

THIRD EDITION

NUTRITION

An Applied Approach

1 The Role of Nutrition in Our Health

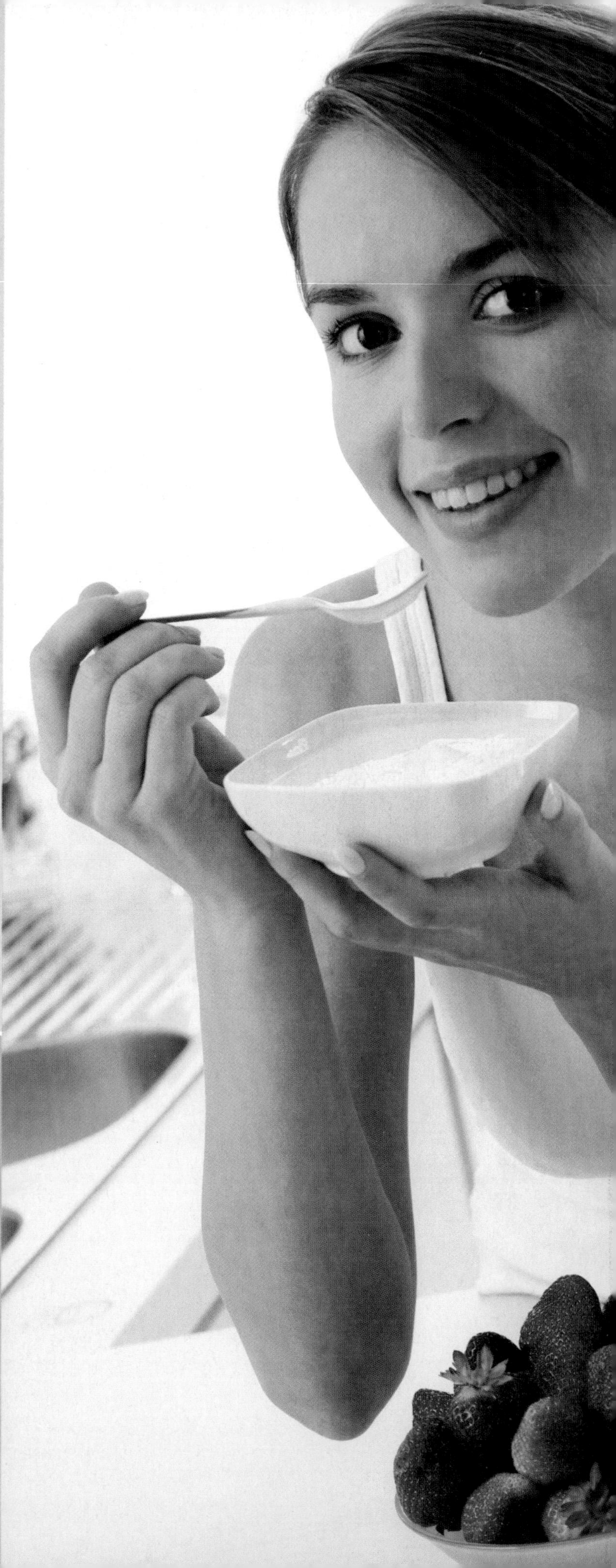

CHAPTER OBJECTIVES

After reading this chapter you will be able to:

1. **Define the term *nutrition,* p. 4.**
2. **Discuss why nutrition is important to health, pp. 4–7.**
3. **Identify the six classes of nutrients essential for health, p. 8.**
4. **Identify the Dietary Reference Intakes for nutrients, pp. 13–15.**
5. **Describe the four steps of the scientific method, pp. 16–17.**
6. **List at least four sources of reliable and accurate nutrition information, pp. 21–23.**

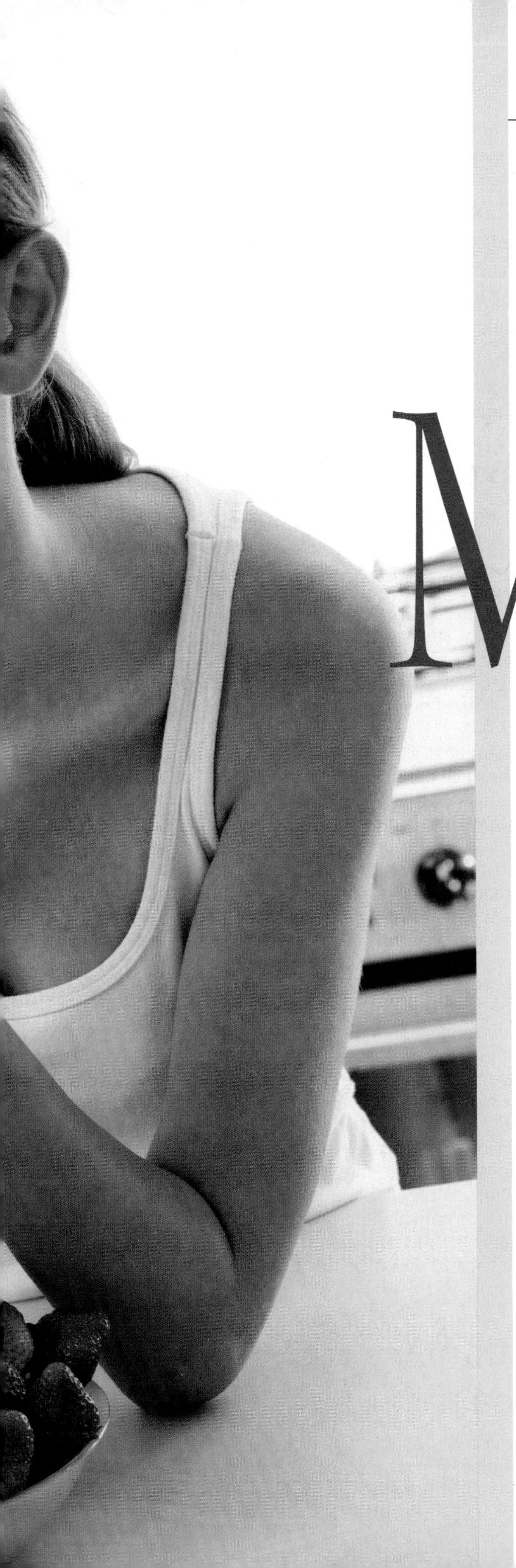

Test Yourself

1. **T F Calories are a measure of the amount of fat in foods.**
2. **T F Proteins are not a primary source of energy for our body.**
3. **T F The Recommended Dietary Allowance is the amount of a nutrient that meets the needs of almost all healthy people of a particular age and gender.**

Test Yourself answers can be found at the end of the chapter.

Miguel hadn't expected that college life would make him feel so tired. After classes, he just wanted to go back to his dorm and sleep. Plus, he had been having difficulty concentrating and was worried that his first-semester grades would be far below those he'd achieved in high school. Scott, his roommate, had little sympathy. "It's all that junk food you eat!" he insisted. "Let's go down to the organic market for some real food." Miguel dragged himself to the market with Scott but rested at the juice counter while his roommate went shopping. A middle-aged woman wearing a white lab coat approached him and introduced herself as the market's staff nutritionist. "You're looking a little pale," she said. "Anything wrong?" Miguel explained that he had been feeling tired lately. "I don't doubt it," the woman answered. "I can see from your skin tone that you're anemic. You need to start taking an iron supplement." She took a bottle of pills from a shelf and handed it to him. "This one is the easiest for you to absorb, and it's on special this week. Take it twice a day, and you should start feeling better in a day or two." Miguel purchased the supplement and began taking it that night with the meal his roommate had prepared. He took it twice the next day as well, just as the nutritionist had recommended, but didn't feel any better. After 2 more days, he visited the university health clinic, where a nurse drew some blood for testing. When the results of the blood tests came in, the physician told him that his thyroid gland wasn't making enough of the hormone that he needed to keep his body functioning properly. She prescribed a medication and congratulated Miguel for catching the problem early. "If you had waited," she said, "it would only have gotten worse, and you could have become seriously ill." Miguel asked if he should continue taking his iron supplements. The physician looked puzzled. "Where did you get the idea that you needed iron supplements?"

Like Miguel, you've probably been offered nutrition-related advice from well-meaning friends and self-professed "experts." Perhaps you found the advice helpful, or maybe, as in Miguel's case, it turned out to be all wrong. Where can you go for reliable advice about nutrition? What exactly *is* nutrition, anyway, and why does what we eat have such an influence on our health? In this chapter, we'll begin to answer these questions, and you'll gain a deeper understanding as you work through the rest of this book. Our goal is that, by the time you finish this course, you'll be the expert on your own nutritional needs!

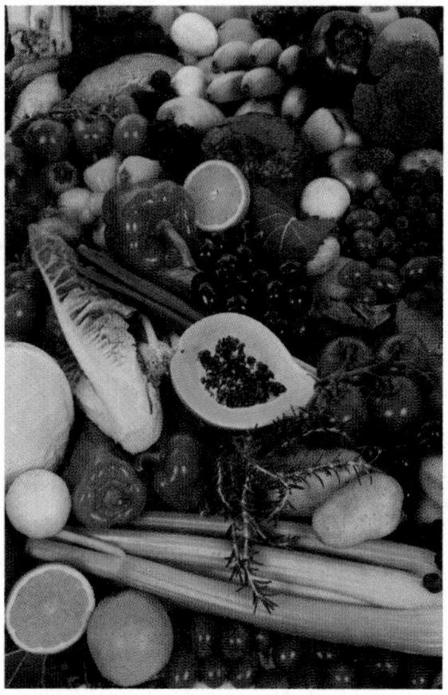

Nutrition is the science that studies all aspects of food.

What Is Nutrition?

If you think that the word *nutrition* means pretty much the same thing as *food*, you're right—partially. But the word has a broader meaning, which will gradually become clear as you make your way in this course. Specifically, **nutrition** is the science that studies food and how food nourishes our body and influences our health. It encompasses how we consume, digest, metabolize, and store nutrients and how these nutrients affect our body. Nutrition also involves studying the factors that influence our eating patterns, making recommendations about the amount we should eat of each type of food, attempting to maintain food safety, and addressing issues related to the global food supply. You can think of nutrition, then, as the discipline that encompasses everything about food.

Nutrition is a relatively new scientific discipline. Although food has played a defining role in the lives of humans since the evolution of our species, the importance of nutrition to our health has been formally recognized and studied over only the past 100 years or so. Early research in nutrition focused on making the link between nutrient deficiencies and illness. For instance, the cause of scurvy, which is a vitamin C deficiency, was discovered in the mid-1700s. At that time, however, vitamin C had not been identified—what was known was that some ingredient found in citrus fruits could prevent scurvy. Another example of early discoveries in nutrition is presented in the accompanying Nutrition Myth or Fact? box about a disease called pellagra.

Nutrition research continued to focus on identifying and preventing deficiency diseases through the first half of the 20th century. Then, as the higher standard of living after World War II led to an improvement in the American diet, nutrition research began pursuing a new objective: supporting wellness and preventing and treating **chronic diseases**—that is, diseases that come on slowly and can persist for years, often despite treatment. Chronic diseases of particular interest to nutrition researchers include obesity, heart disease, type 2 diabetes, and various cancers. This new research has raised as many questions as it has answered, and we still have a great deal to learn about the relationship between nutrition and chronic disease.

In the closing decades of the 20th century, an exciting new area of nutrition research began to emerge. Reflecting our growing understanding of genetics, *nutrigenomics* seeks to uncover links between our genes, our environment, and our diet. The Nutrition Debate on page 25 describes this new field of research in detail.

nutrition The science that studies food and how food nourishes our body and influences our health.

chronic diseases Diseases that come on slowly and can persist for years, often despite treatment.

How Does Nutrition Contribute to Health?

Think about it: if you eat three meals a day, by this time next year, you'll have had more than a thousand chances to influence your body's makeup! As you'll learn in this text, you are what you eat: the substances you take into your body are broken

NUTRITION MYTH OR FACT?

Is Pellagra an Infectious Disease?

In the first few years of the 20th century, Dr. Joseph Goldberger successfully controlled outbreaks of several fatal infectious diseases, from yellow fever in Louisiana to typhus in Mexico. So it wasn't surprising that, in 1914, the Surgeon General of the United States chose him to tackle another disease, thought to be infectious, that was raging throughout the South. Called *pellagra,* the disease was characterized by a skin rash, diarrhea, and mental impairment. At the time, it afflicted more than 50,000 people each year, and in about 10% of cases it resulted in death.[1]

Goldberger began studying the disease by carefully observing its occurrence in groups of people. He asked, if it is infectious, then why would it strike children in orphanages and prison inmates yet leave their nurses and guards unaffected? Why did it overwhelmingly affect impoverished millworkers and sharecroppers while leaving their affluent (and well-fed) neighbors healthy? Could a dietary deficiency cause pellagra?

To confirm his hunch, he conducted a series of trials in which he fed afflicted orphans and prisoners, who had been consuming a limited, corn-based diet, a variety of nutrient-rich foods, including meats. They recovered. Moreover, orphans and inmates who did not have pellagra and ate the new diet did not develop the disease. Finally, Goldberger recruited eleven healthy prison inmates, who, in return for a pardon of their sentence, agreed to consume a corn-based diet. After 5 months, six of the eleven developed pellagra.

Still, many skeptics were unable to give up the idea that pellagra was an infectious disease. To prove that pellagra was not spread by germs, Goldberger and his colleagues deliberately injected themselves with and ingested patients' scabs, nasal secretions, and other bodily fluids. He and his team remained healthy.

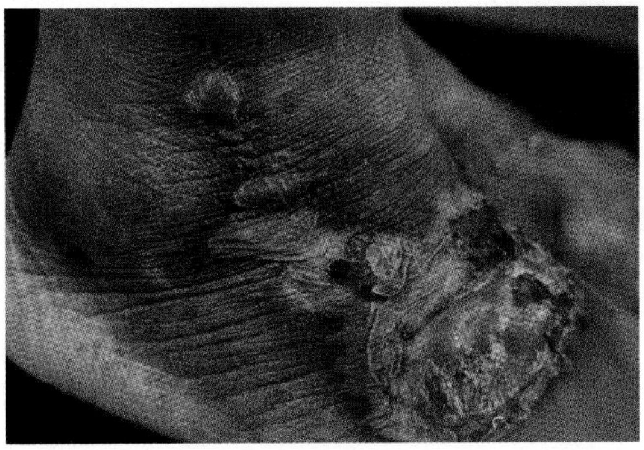

Pellagra is often characterized by a scaly skin rash.

Although Goldberger could not identify the precise component in the new diet that cured pellagra, he eventually found an inexpensive and widely available substance, brewer's yeast, that when added to the diet prevented or reversed the disease. Shortly after Goldberger's death in 1937, scientists identified the nutrient that is deficient in the diet of pellagra patients: niacin, one of the B-vitamins, which is plentiful in brewer's yeast.[1]

down and reassembled into your brain cells, bones, muscles—all of your tissues and organs. The foods you eat also provide your body with the energy it needs to function properly. In addition, we know that proper nutrition can help us improve our health, prevent certain diseases, achieve and maintain a desirable weight, and maintain our energy and vitality. Let's take a closer look at how nutrition supports health and wellness.

Nutrition Is One of Several Factors Supporting Wellness

Wellness can be defined in many ways. Traditionally considered simply the absence of disease, wellness has been redefined as we have learned more about our body and what it means to live a healthful lifestyle. Wellness is now considered to be a multidimensional process, one that includes physical, emotional, social, occupational, and spiritual health **(Figure 1.1)**. Wellness is not an endpoint in our lives, but is an active process we work on every day.

In this book, we focus on two critical aspects of physical health: nutrition and physical activity. The two are so closely related that you can think of them as two sides of the same coin: our overall state of nutrition is influenced by how much energy we expend doing daily activities, and our level of physical activity has a major impact on how we use the nutrients in our food. We can perform more strenuous activities for longer periods of time when we eat a nutritious diet, whereas an inadequate or excessive food intake can make us lethargic. A poor diet, inadequate or

wellness A multidimensional, lifelong process that includes physical, emotional, social, occupational, and spiritual health.

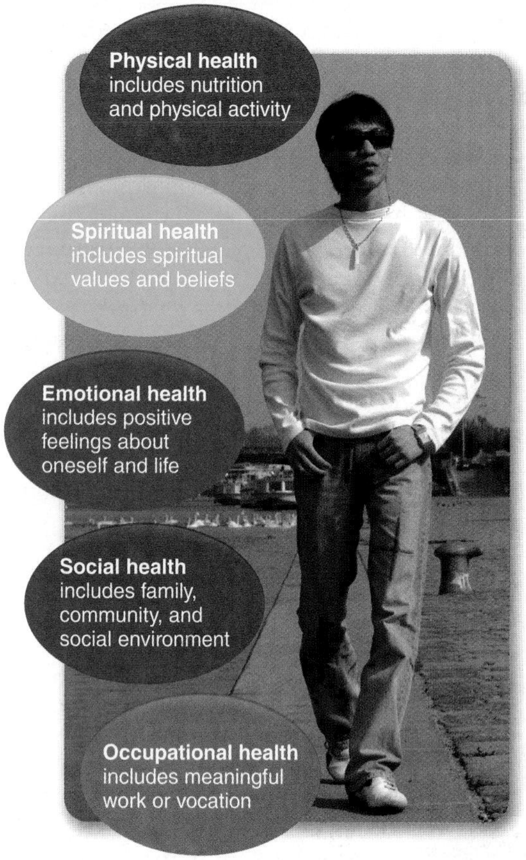
Physical health
includes nutrition and physical activity
Spiritual health
includes spiritual values and beliefs
Emotional health
includes positive feelings about oneself and life
Social health
includes family, community, and social environment
Occupational health
includes meaningful work or vocation

Figure 1.1 Many factors contribute to wellness. Primary among these are a nutritious diet and regular physical activity.

excessive physical activity, or a combination of these also can lead to serious health problems. Finally, several studies have suggested that healthful nutrition and regular physical activity can increase feelings of well-being and reduce feelings of anxiety and depression. In other words, wholesome food and physical activity just plain feel good!

A Healthful Diet Can Prevent Some Diseases and Reduce Your Risk for Others

Nutrition appears to play a role—from a direct cause to a mild influence—in the development of many diseases (**Figure 1.2**). As we noted earlier, poor nutrition is a direct cause of deficiency diseases, such as scurvy and pellagra. Early nutrition research focused on identifying the missing nutrient behind such diseases and on developing guidelines for nutrient intakes that are high enough to prevent them. Over the years, nutrition scientists successfully lobbied for the fortification of foods with the nutrients of greatest concern. These measures, along with a more abundant and reliable food supply, have almost completely wiped out the majority of nutrient-deficiency diseases in developed countries. However, they are still major problems in many developing nations.

In addition to causing disease directly, poor nutrition can have a more subtle influence on our health. For instance, it can contribute to the development of brittle bones (a disease called *osteoporosis*), as well as to the progression of some forms of cancer. These associations are considered mild; however, poor nutrition is also strongly associated with three chronic diseases—heart disease, stroke, and diabetes—which are among the top ten causes of death in the United States (**Figure 1.3**).

It probably won't surprise you to learn that the primary link between poor nutrition and mortality is obesity. That is, obesity is fundamentally a consequence of eating more Calories than are expended. At the same time, obesity is a well-

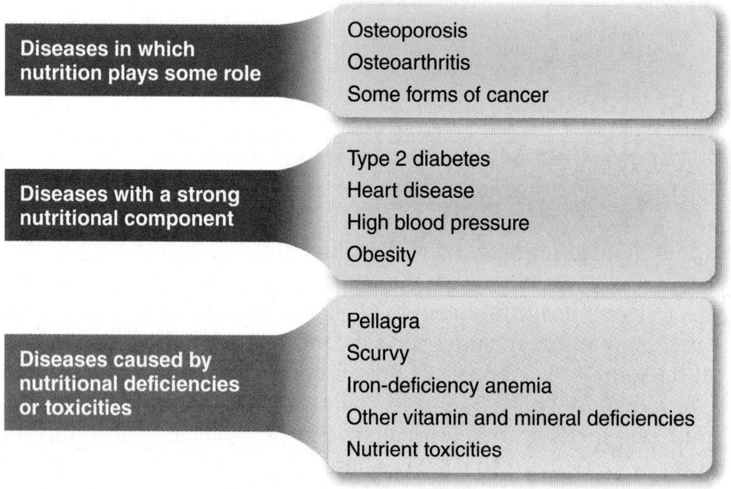
Diseases in which nutrition plays some role
Osteoporosis
Osteoarthritis
Some forms of cancer
Diseases with a strong nutritional component
Type 2 diabetes
Heart disease
High blood pressure
Obesity
Diseases caused by nutritional deficiencies or toxicities
Pellagra
Scurvy
Iron-deficiency anemia
Other vitamin and mineral deficiencies
Nutrient toxicities

Figure 1.2 The relationship between nutrition and human disease. Notice that whereas nutritional factors are only marginally implicated in the diseases of the top row, they are strongly linked to the development of the diseases in the middle row and truly causative of those in the bottom row.

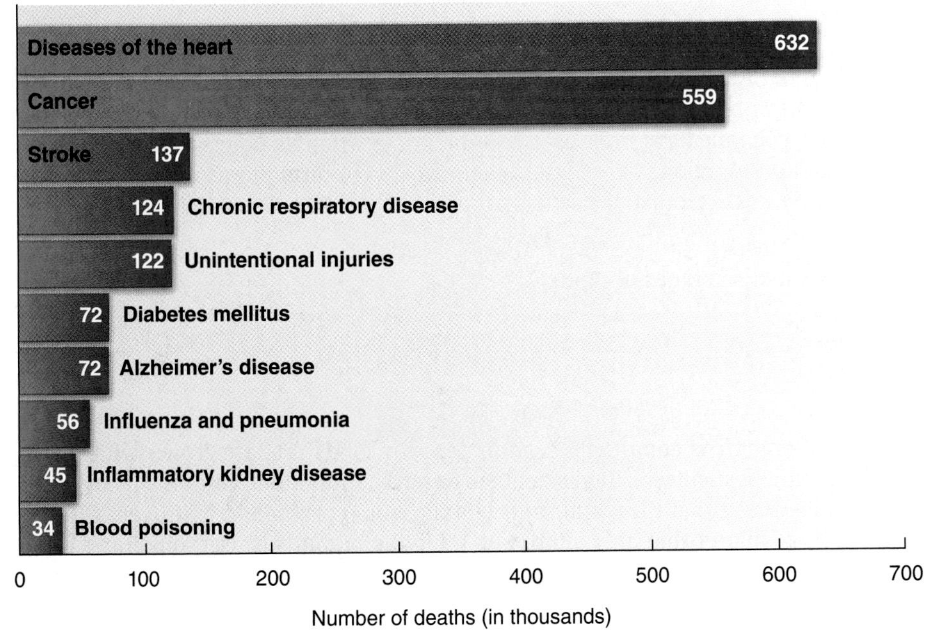

Figure 1.3 Of the ten leading causes of death in the United States in 2005, three—heart disease, stroke, and diabetes—are strongly associated with poor nutrition. In addition, nutrition plays a more limited role in the development of some forms of cancer.
Data from U.S. Dept. of Health and Human Services, CDC, NCHS, *National Vital Statistics Reports,* Vol. 57. No. 14, April 17, 2009.

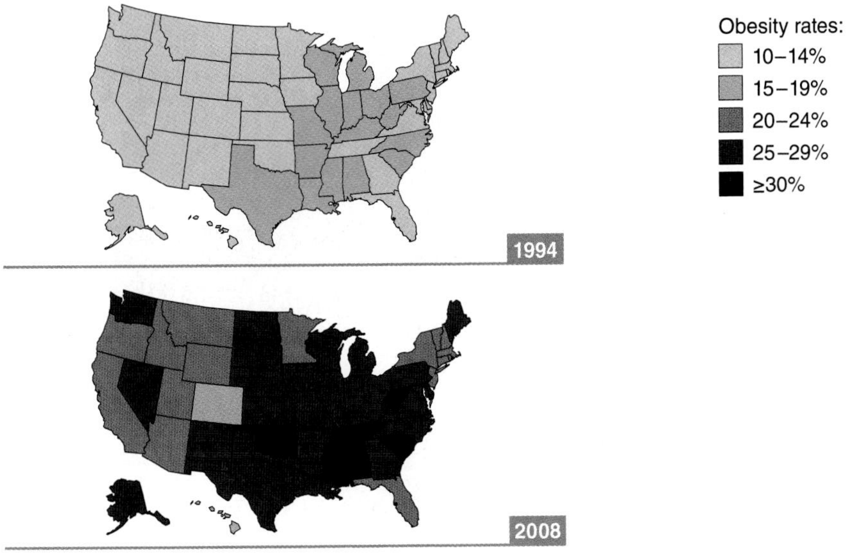

Figure 1.4 These diagrams illustrate the increase in obesity rates across the United States from 1994 to 2008 as documented in the Behavioral Risk Factor Surveillance System. Obesity is defined as a body mass index greater than or equal to 30, or approximately 30 lb overweight for a 5′4″ woman.
Graphics from Centers for Disease Control and Prevention, U.S. Obesity Trends 1985 to 2008. Available at www.cdc.gov/obesity/data/trends.html#State.

established risk factor for heart disease, stroke, type 2 diabetes, and some forms of cancer. Unfortunately, the prevalence of obesity has dramatically increased throughout the United States during the past 20 years (**Figure 1.4**). Throughout this text, we will discuss in detail how nutrition and physical activity affect the development of obesity.

RECAP Nutrition is the science that studies food and how food affects our body and our health. Nutrition is an important component of wellness and is strongly associated with physical activity. One goal of a healthful diet is to prevent nutrient-deficiency diseases, such as scurvy and pellagra; a second goal is to lower the risk for chronic diseases, such as type 2 diabetes and heart disease.

What Are Nutrients?

A glass of milk or a spoonful of peanut butter may seem to be made up of only one substance, but in reality most foods are a combination of many different chemicals. Some of these chemicals are not useful to the body, whereas others are critical to human growth and function. These latter chemicals are referred to as **nutrients.** The following are the six groups of nutrients found in the foods we eat **(Figure 1.5)**:

- carbohydrates
- fats and oils (two types of lipids)
- proteins
- vitamins
- minerals
- water

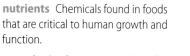

nutrients Chemicals found in foods that are critical to human growth and function.

organic A substance or nutrient that contains the elements carbon and hydrogen.

The term *organic* is commonly used to describe foods that are grown without the use of synthetic pesticides. When scientists describe individual nutrients as **organic,** however, they mean that these nutrients contain both carbon and hydrogen, fundamental units of matter that are common to all living organisms. Carbohydrates, lipids, proteins, and vitamins are organic. Minerals and water are not. Organic and inorganic

Figure 1.5 The six groups of essential nutrients found in the foods we consume.

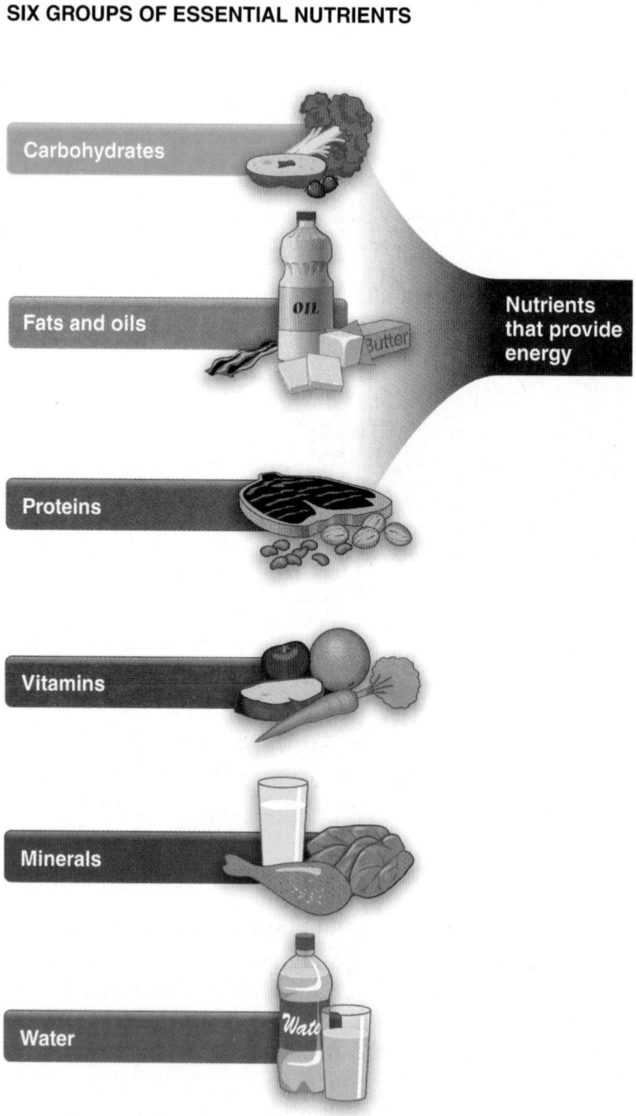

nutrients are equally important for sustaining life but differ in their structures, functions, and basic chemistry.

Alcohol is a chemical commonly consumed in beverages and that may also be added to some foods as a flavoring or preservative. But it is not considered a nutrient because it is not critical for body functioning or the building or repairing of tissues. In fact, alcohol is considered to be both a drug and a toxin. We discuss alcohol ***In Depth*** on pages 28–37.

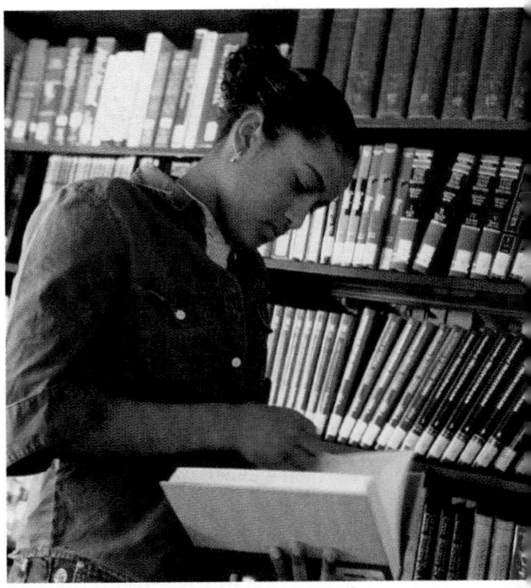

Carbohydrates are the primary source of fuel for our body, particularly for our brain.

Macronutrients Provide Energy

Carbohydrates, fats, and proteins are the only nutrients that provide energy. By this we mean that our body breaks down these nutrients and reassemble their components into a fuel that supports physical activity and basic functioning. Although taking a multivitamin might be beneficial in other ways, it will not provide you with the energy for a 20-minute session on the stair-climber! The energy nutrients are also referred to as **macronutrients.** *Macro* means "large," and our body needs relatively large amounts of these nutrients to support normal function and health.

Energy Is Measured in Kilocalories

The energy in foods is measured in units called *kilocalories (kcal)*. A kilocalorie is the amount of heat required to raise the temperature of 1 kilogram (about 2.2 pounds) of water by 1 degree Celsius. We can say that the energy found in 1 gram of carbohydrate is equal to 4 kcal.

You've certainly also seen the term *Calorie*. What's the difference? Well, technically, 1 kilocalorie is equal to 1,000 Calories. *Kilo-* is a prefix used in the metric system to indicate 1,000 (think of *kilometer*). For the sake of simplicity, nutrition labels use the term *Calories* to indicate kilocalories. Thus, if the wrapper on an ice cream bar states that it contains 150 Calories, it actually contains 150 kilocalories.

In this textbook, we use the term *energy* when referring to the general concept of energy intake or energy expenditure. We use the term *kilocalories (kcal)* when discussing units of energy. We use the term *Calories* only when presenting information about foods.

Both carbohydrates and proteins provide 4 kcal per gram, alcohol provides 7 kcal per gram, and fats provide 9 kcal per gram. Thus, for every gram of fat we consume, we obtain more than twice the energy derived from a gram of carbohydrate or protein. Refer to the You Do the Math box on page 10 to learn how to calculate the energy contribution of carbohydrates, fats, and proteins in a given food.

macronutrients Nutrients that our body needs in relatively large amounts to support normal function and health. Carbohydrates, fats, and proteins are macronutrients.

Carbohydrates Are a Primary Fuel Source

Carbohydrates are the primary source of fuel for our body, particularly for our brain and during physical exercise **(Figure 1.6)**. *Carbo-* refers to carbon, and *-hydrate* refers to water. You may remember that water is made up of hydrogen and oxygen. Thus, carbohydrates are composed of chains of carbon, hydrogen, and oxygen.

Carbohydrates encompass a wide variety of foods; rice, wheat, and other grains as well as vegetables are carbohydrates, and fruits contain natural sugars that are

carbohydrates The primary fuel source for our body, particularly for our brain and for physical exercise.

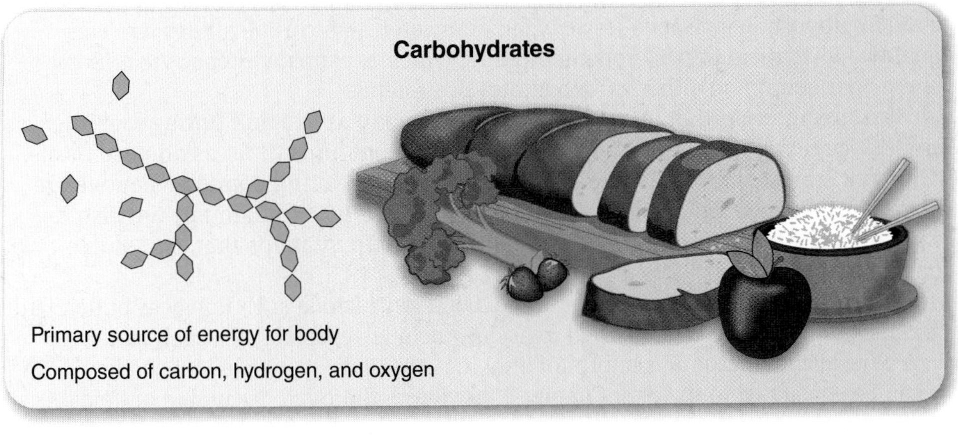
Carbohydrates
Primary source of energy for body
Composed of carbon, hydrogen, and oxygen

Figure 1.6 Carbohydrates are a primary source of energy for our body and are found in a wide variety of foods.

YOU DO THE MATH

Calculating the Energy Contribution of Carbohydrates, Fats, and Proteins

The energy in food is used for everything from maintaining normal body functions—such as breathing, digesting food, and repairing damaged tissues and organs—to enabling you to perform physical activity and even to read this text. So how much energy is produced from the foods you eat?

Carbohydrates are the main energy source for your body and should make up the largest percentage of your nutrient intake, about 45–65%; they provide 4 kcal of energy per gram of carbohydrate consumed. Proteins also provide 4 kcal of energy per gram, but they should be limited to no more than 10–35% of your daily energy intake. Fats provide the most energy, 9 kcal per gram. Fats should make up approximately 20–35% of your total energy intake per day. In order to figure out whether you're taking in the appropriate percentages of carbohydrates, fats, and proteins, you will need to use a little math.

1. Let's say you have completed a personal diet analysis, and you consume 2,500 kcal per day. From your diet analysis, you also find that you consume 300 g of carbohydrates, 90 g of fat, and 123 g of protein.
2. To calculate your percentage of total energy that comes from carbohydrate, you must do two things:
   a. Take your total grams of carbohydrate and multiply by the energy value for carbohydrate to give you how many kcal of carbohydrate you have consumed.

      300 g of carbohydrate × 4 kcal/g
      = 1,200 kcal of carbohydrate

   b. Take the number of kcal of carbohydrate you have consumed, divide this number by the total number of kcal you consumed, and multiply by 100. This will give you the percentage of the total energy you consume that comes from carbohydrate.

      (1,200 kcal/2,500 kcal) × 100 × = 48%
      of total energy comes from carbohydrate

3. To calculate your percentage of total energy that comes from fat, you follow the same steps but incorporate the energy value for fat:
   a. Take your total grams of fat and multiply by the energy value for fat to find the kcal of fat you consumed.

      90 g of fat × 9 kcal/g = 810 kcal of fat

   b. Take the number of kcal of fat you have consumed, divide this number by the total number of kcal you consumed, and multiply by 100 to get the percentage of total energy you consume that comes from fat.

      (810 kcal/2,500 kcal) × 100 = 32.4%
      of total energy comes from fat

Now try these steps to calculate the percentage of the total energy you consume that comes from protein.

Also, have you ever heard that alcohol provides "empty Calories"? Alcohol contributes 7 kcal per gram. You can calculate the percentage of kcal from alcohol in your daily diet, but remember that it is not considered an energy nutrient.

These calculations will be very useful throughout this course as you learn more about how to design a healthful diet and how to read labels to assist you in meeting your nutritional goals. Later in this book you will learn how to estimate your unique energy needs.

carbohydrates. Carbohydrates are also found in legumes (including lentils, dry beans, and peas), milk and other dairy products, seeds, and nuts. Carbohydrates and their role in health are the subject of Chapter 4.

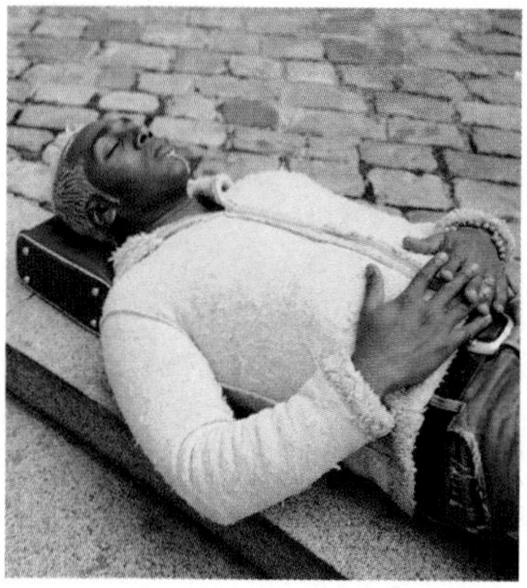

▲ Fats are an important source of energy for our body, especially when we are at rest.

fats An important energy source for our body at rest and during low-intensity exercise.

Fats Provide Energy and Other Essential Nutrients

Fats are another important source of energy for our body **(Figure 1.7)**. They are a type of *lipids,* a diverse group of organic substances that are insoluble in water. Like carbohydrates, fats are composed of carbon, hydrogen, and oxygen; however, they contain proportionally much less oxygen and water than carbohydrates do. This quality allows them to pack together tightly, which explains why they yield more energy per gram than either carbohydrates or proteins.

Fats are an important energy source for our body at rest and during low-intensity exercise. Our body is capable of storing large amounts of fat as adipose tissue. These fat stores can then be broken down for energy during periods when we are not eating—for example, while we are asleep. Foods that contain fats are also essential for the transportation into our body of certain vitamins that are soluble only in fat.

Dietary fats come in a variety of forms. Solid fats include such things as butter, lard, and margarine. Liquid fats, referred to as *oils,* include vegetable oils, such as canola and olive oils. Cholesterol is a form of lipid that our body can make independently, and it can be consumed in the diet. Chapter 5 provides a thorough discussion of lipids.

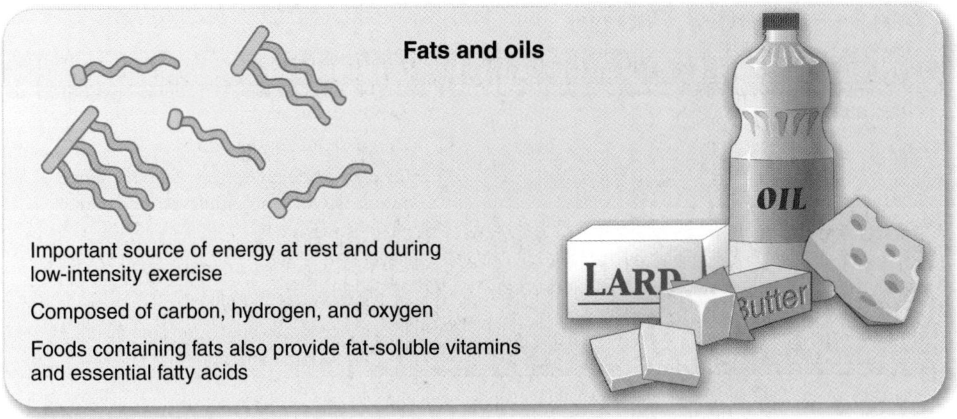
Fats and oils
Important source of energy at rest and during low-intensity exercise
Composed of carbon, hydrogen, and oxygen
Foods containing fats also provide fat-soluble vitamins and essential fatty acids
OIL
LARD
Butter

Figure 1.7 Fats are an important energy source during rest and low-intensity exercise. Foods containing fats also provide other important nutrients.

Proteins Support Tissue Growth, Repair, and Maintenance

Proteins also contain carbon, hydrogen, and oxygen, but they are different from carbohydrates and fats in that they contain the element *nitrogen* (**Figure 1.8**). Within proteins, these four elements assemble into small building blocks known as amino acids. We break down dietary proteins into amino acids and reassemble them to build our own body proteins—for instance, the proteins in our muscles and blood.

Although proteins can provide energy, they are not a primary source of energy for our body. Instead, the main role of proteins is in building new cells and tissues. Proteins are also important in regulating the breakdown of foods and our fluid balance.

Proteins are found primarily in meats and dairy products, but seeds, nuts, and legumes are also good sources, and we obtain small amounts from vegetables and whole grains. Proteins are the subject of Chapter 6.

proteins The only macronutrient that contains nitrogen; the basic building blocks of proteins are amino acids.

micronutrients Nutrients needed in relatively small amounts to support normal health and body functions. Vitamins and minerals are micronutrients.

vitamins Organic compounds that assist us in regulating our body's processes.

metabolism The process by which large molecules, such as carbohydrates, fats, and proteins, are broken down via chemical reactions into smaller molecules that can be used as fuel, stored, or assembled into new compounds the body needs.

Micronutrients Assist in the Regulation of Body Functions

Vitamins and minerals are referred to as **micronutrients.** That's because we need relatively small amounts of these nutrients to support normal health and body functions.

Vitamins are organic compounds that help regulate our body's functions. Contrary to popular belief, vitamins do not contain energy (kilocalories); however, they are essential to energy **metabolism,** the process by which the macronutrients are

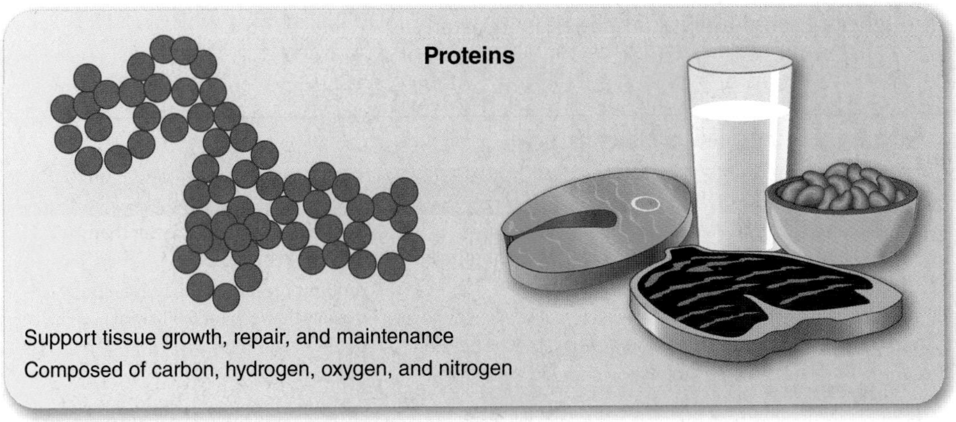
Proteins
Support tissue growth, repair, and maintenance
Composed of carbon, hydrogen, oxygen, and nitrogen

Figure 1.8 Proteins contain nitrogen in addition to carbon, hydrogen, and oxygen. Proteins support the growth, repair, and maintenance of body tissues.

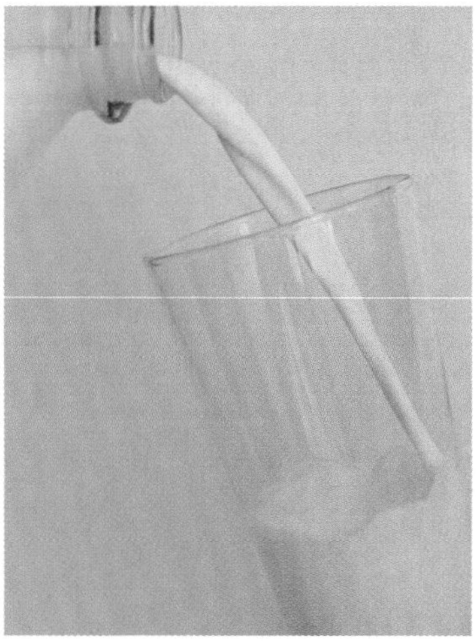

Fat-soluble vitamins are found in a variety of fat-containing foods, including dairy products.

fat-soluble vitamins Vitamins that are not soluble in water but are soluble in fat. These include vitamins A, D, E, and K.

water-soluble vitamins Vitamins that are soluble in water. These include vitamin C and the B-vitamins.

minerals Inorganic substances that are not broken down during digestion and absorption and are not destroyed by heat or light. Minerals assist in the regulation of many body processes and are classified as major minerals or trace minerals.

major minerals Minerals we need to consume in amounts of at least 100 mg per day and of which the total amount in our body is at least 5 g.

trace minerals Minerals we need to consume in amounts less than 100 mg per day and of which the total amount in our body is less than 5 g.

TABLE 1.1 Overview of Vitamins

Type	Names	Distinguishing Features
Fat-soluble	A, D, E, and K	Soluble in fat Stored in the human body Toxicity can occur from consuming excess amounts, which accumulate in the body
Water-soluble	C, B-vitamins (thiamin, riboflavin, niacin, vitamin B_6, vitamin B_{12}, pantothenic acid, biotin, and folate)	Soluble in water Not stored to any extent in the human body Excess excreted in urine Toxicity generally only occurs as a result of vitamin supplementation

broken down into the smaller molecules that our body can absorb and use. So vitamins assist with releasing and using the energy in carbohydrates, fats, and proteins. They are also critical in building and maintaining healthy bone, muscle, and blood; supporting our immune system, so that we can fight infection and disease; and ensuring healthy vision.

Vitamins are classified as two types: **fat-soluble vitamins** and **water-soluble vitamins** (Table 1.1). This classification affects how vitamins are absorbed, transported, and stored in our body. Both types of vitamins are essential for our health and are found in a variety of foods. Learn more about vitamins in the ***In Depth*** examination following Chapter 6. Chapters 7 through 10 discuss individual vitamins in detail.

Minerals are inorganic substances because they do not contain carbon and hydrogen. In fact, minerals are not compounds made up of smaller components; instead, they are fundamental units of matter themselves. Some important dietary minerals are sodium, potassium, calcium, magnesium, and iron. Because minerals are already in the most fundamental form possible, they cannot be broken down during digestion or when our body uses them to promote normal function; they are also not destroyed by heat or light. Thus, all minerals maintain their structure, no matter what environment they are in. This means that the calcium in our bones is the same as the calcium in the milk we drink, and the sodium in our cells is the same as the sodium in our table salt.

Minerals have many important functions in our body. They assist in fluid regulation and energy production, are essential to the health of our bones and blood, and help rid our body of the harmful by-products of metabolism.

Minerals are classified according to the amounts we need in our diet and according to how much of the mineral is found in our body. The two categories of minerals in our diet and body are the **major minerals** and the **trace minerals** (Table 1.2). Learn more about minerals in the ***In Depth*** following Chapter 6. Chapters 7 through 10 discuss individual minerals in detail.

TABLE 1.2 Overview of Minerals

Type	Names	Distinguishing Features
Major minerals	Calcium, phosphorus, sodium, potassium, chloride, magnesium, sulfur	Needed in amounts greater than 100 mg/day in our diets Amount present in the human body is greater than 5 g (or 5,000 mg)
Trace minerals	Iron, zinc, copper, manganese, fluoride, chromium, molybdenum, selenium, iodine	Needed in amounts less than 100 mg/day in our diets Amount present in the human body is less than 5 g (or 5,000 mg)

Water Supports All Body Functions

Water is an inorganic nutrient (it contains oxygen and hydrogen, but not carbon) that is vital for our survival. We consume water in its pure form; in juices, soups, and other liquids; and in solid foods, such as fruits and vegetables. Adequate water intake ensures the proper balance of fluid both inside and outside our cells, and it assists in the regulation of nerve impulses, muscle contractions, nutrient transport, and the excretion of waste products. Because of the key role that water plays in our health, Chapter 7 focuses on water and its function in our body.

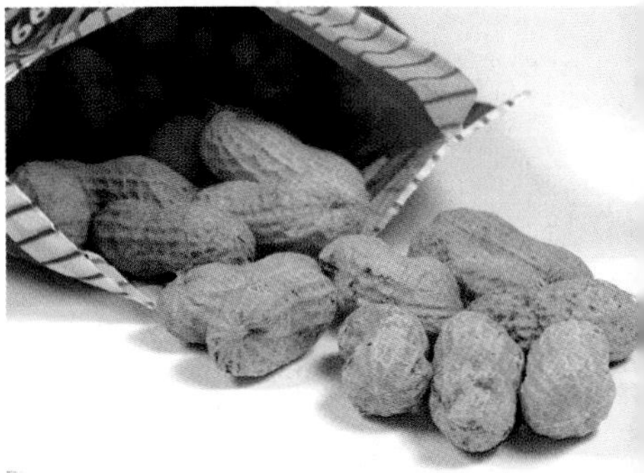

Peanuts are a good source of magnesium and phosphorus, which play important roles in the formation and maintenance of our skeleton.

RECAP **The six essential nutrient groups found in foods are carbohydrates, fats, proteins, vitamins, minerals, and water. Carbohydrates, fats, and proteins are macronutrients. Often referred to as energy nutrients, they provide our body with energy. Carbohydrates and fats are our main energy sources; proteins primarily support tissue growth, repair, and maintenance. Vitamins and minerals are micronutrients. Vitamins are organic compounds that assist in breaking down the macronutrients for energy and in maintaining many other functions. Minerals are inorganic units of matter that play critical roles in virtually all aspects of human health and function. Water is critical for our survival and is important for regulating nervous impulses, muscle contractions, nutrient transport, and the excretion of waste products.**

How Much of Each Nutrient Do Most People Need?

Now that you know what the six classes of nutrients are, you're probably wondering how much of each you need each day. That depends on your gender, your age, your activity level, and many other factors. In Chapter 2, you'll learn how to plan a healthful diet that's just right for you. To get ready, you need to become familiar with the current standard intake recommendations that apply to most healthy people.

Use the Dietary Reference Intakes to Check Your Nutrient Intake

The United States and Canada share a set of standards defining the recommended intake values for various nutrients. These are called the **Dietary Reference Intakes (DRIs)** (**Figure 1.9**). The DRIs are dietary standards for healthy people only; they do not apply to people with diseases or to those who are suffering from nutrient deficiencies. For each nutrient (such as vitamin C or iron), the DRIs identify the amount

Dietary Reference Intakes (DRIs) A set of nutritional reference values for the United States and Canada that applies to healthy people.

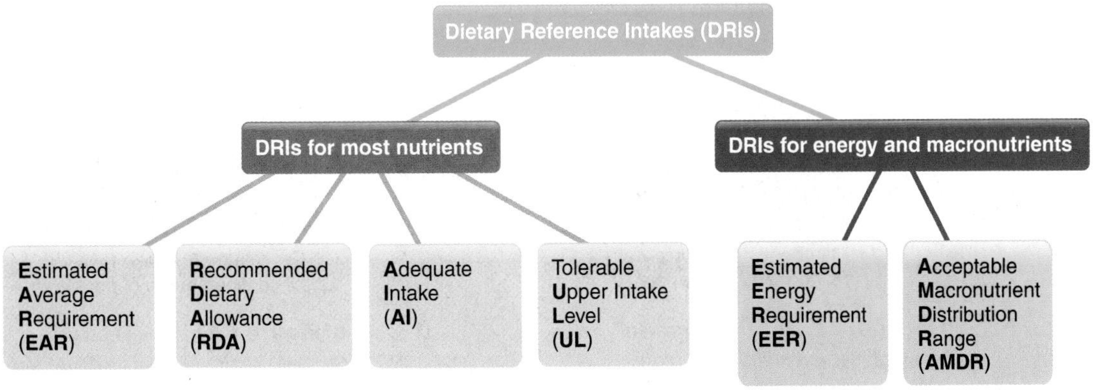

Figure 1.9 The Dietary Reference Intakes (DRIs) for all nutrients. Note that the Estimated Energy Requirement (EER) applies only to energy, and the Acceptable Macronutrient Distribution Range (AMDR) applies only to the macronutrients and alcohol.

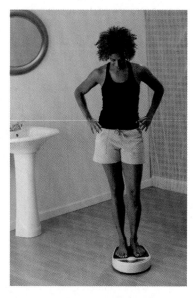

Knowing your daily Estimated Energy Requirement (EER) is a helpful way to maintain a healthy body weight.

needed to prevent deficiency diseases in healthy individuals, as well as the amount that may reduce the risk for chronic diseases in healthy people. The DRIs also establish an upper level of safety for nutrient intake.

The DRIs for most nutrients consist of four values:

- Estimated Average Requirement (EAR)
- Recommended Dietary Allowance (RDA)
- Adequate Intake (AI)
- Tolerable Upper Intake Level (UL)

For total energy and the macronutrients, different standards are used. We'll identify those shortly.

The Estimated Average Requirement Guides the Recommended Dietary Allowance

The **Estimated Average Requirement (EAR)** represents the average daily intake level estimated to meet the requirement of half the healthy individuals in a particular life stage and gender group.[2] **Figure 1.10** is a graph representing this value. As an example, the EAR for phosphorus for women between the ages of 19 and 30 years represents the average daily intake of phosphorus that meets the requirement of half the women in this age group. Scientists use the EAR to define the Recommended Dietary Allowance (RDA) for a given nutrient. Obviously, if the EAR meets the needs of only half the people in a group, then the recommended intake will be higher.

The Recommended Dietary Allowance Meets the Needs of Nearly All Healthy People

The **Recommended Dietary Allowance (RDA)** represents the average daily nutrient intake level that meets the requirements of 97–98% of healthy individuals in a particular life stage and gender group (**Figure 1.11**).[2] For example, the RDA for phosphorus is 700 mg per day for women between the ages of 19 and 30 years. This amount of phosphorus will meet the nutrient requirements of almost all women in this age category.

Again, scientists use the EAR to establish the RDA. In fact, if an EAR cannot be determined for a nutrient, then this nutrient cannot have an RDA. When this occurs, an Adequate Intake value is determined for the nutrient.

The Adequate Intake Is Based on Estimates of Nutrient Intakes

The **Adequate Intake (AI)** value is a recommended average daily nutrient intake level assumed to be adequate. It is based on observations or experiments involving healthy

Estimated Average Requirement (EAR) The average daily nutrient intake level estimated to meet the requirement of half the healthy individuals in a particular life stage or gender group.

Recommended Dietary Allowance (RDA) The average daily nutrient intake level that meets the nutrient requirements of 97–98% of healthy individuals in a particular life stage and gender group.

Adequate Intake (AI) A recommended average daily nutrient intake level based on observed or experimentally determined estimates of nutrient intake by a group of healthy people.

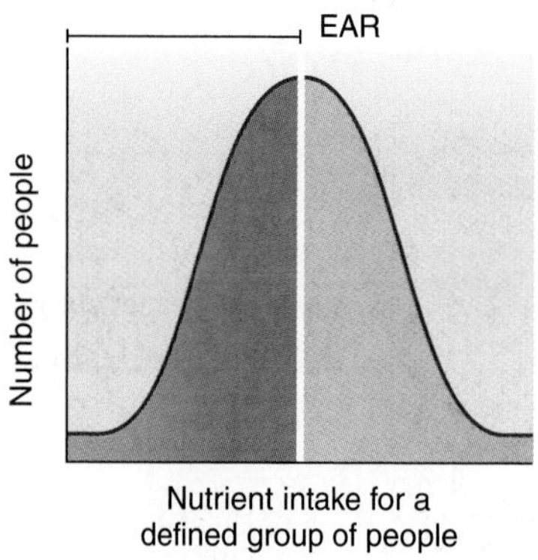

Figure 1.10 The Estimated Average Requirement (EAR) represents the average daily nutrient intake level that meets the requirements of half the healthy individuals in a given group.

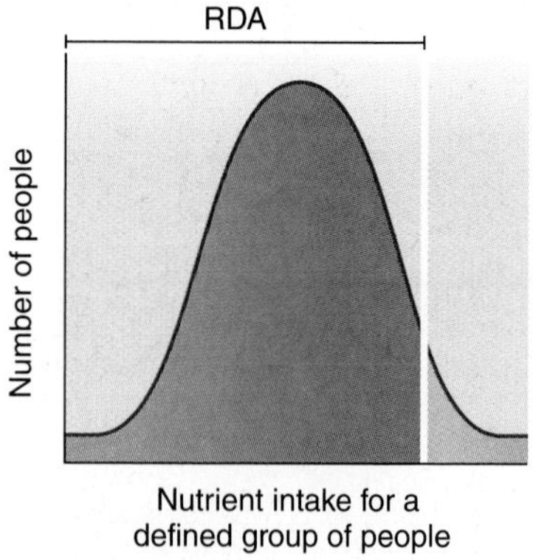

Figure 1.11 The Recommended Dietary Allowance (RDA) represents the average daily nutrient intake level that meets the requirements of almost all (97–98%) healthy individuals in a given life stage or gender group.

TABLE 1 Myths About Alcohol Metabolism

The Claim	The Reality
Physical activity, such as walking around, will speed up the breakdown of alcohol.	Muscles don't metabolize alcohol; the liver does.
Drinking a lot of coffee will keep you from getting drunk.	Coffee does not cause alcohol to be excreted in the urine.
Using a sauna or steam room will force the alcohol out of your body.	Very little alcohol is lost in the sweat; the alcohol will remain in your bloodstream.
Herbal and nutritional products are available that speed up the breakdown of alcohol.	There is no scientific evidence that commercial supplements will increase the rate of alcohol metabolism; they will not lower blood alcohol levels.

Despite what you may have heard, there is no effective intervention to speed up the breakdown of alcohol **(Table 1)**. The key to keeping your BAC below the legal limit is to drink alcoholic beverages while eating a meal or large snack; to drink very slowly, no more than one drink per hour; and to limit your total consumption of alcohol on any one occasion.

It also helps to fully quench your thirst with a nonalcoholic beverage *before* having your first alcoholic drink, and to make every other beverage nonalcoholic. More tips for controlling your alcohol intake are in the Quick Tips feature below.

A person who steadily increases his or her alcohol consumption over time becomes more tolerant of a given intake of alcohol. Chronic drinkers experience *metabolic tolerance,* a condition in which the liver becomes more efficient in its breakdown of alcohol. This means that the person's BAC rises more slowly after consuming a certain number of drinks. In addition, chronic drinkers develop what is called *functional tolerance,* meaning that they show few, if any, signs of impairment or intoxication even at high BACs. As a result, these individuals may need to consume twice as much alcohol as when they first started drinking in order to reach the same state of euphoria.

QUICK TIPS

Taking Control of Your Alcohol Intake

✓ Think about WHY you are planning to drink. Is it to relax and socialize, or are you using alcohol to release stress? If the latter, try some stress-reduction techniques that don't involve alcohol, such as exercise, yoga, meditation, or simply talking with a friend.

✓ Make sure you have a protein-containing meal or snack before your first alcoholic drink; having food in the stomach delays its emptying. This gives more of the alcohol a chance to be broken down and means that less is available to be absorbed into the bloodstream.

✓ Before you drink alcohol, have a large glass of water, iced tea, or soda. Once your thirst has been satisfied, your rate of fluid intake will drop. After that, rotate between alcoholic and nonalcoholic drinks.

✓ Dilute hard liquor with large amounts of diet soda, water, or juice. Remember, a glass of pure orange juice doesn't look any different from one laced with vodka, so no one will even know what it is you are or are not drinking! These diluted beverages are cheaper and lower in Calories, too!

✓ Whether or not your drink is diluted, sip slowly to allow your liver time to keep up with your alcohol intake.

✓ If your friends pressure you to drink, volunteer to be the designated driver. You'll have a "free pass" for the night in terms of saying no to alcoholic drinks.

✓ Decide in advance what your alcohol intake will be, and plan some strategies for sticking to your limit. If you are going to a bar, for example, take only enough money to buy two beers and two sodas. If you are at a party, stay occupied dancing, sampling the food, or talking with friends, and stay as far away from the keg as you can.

Effects of Alcohol Abuse on Personal Health

Alcohol is a drug. It exerts a narcotic effect on virtually every part of the brain, acting as a sedative and depressant. Excessive intake of this drug, whether occasional or chronic, is generally referred to as **alcohol abuse** and can lead to alcoholism.

Binge drinking, the consumption of five or more alcoholic drinks on one occasion (within a 3- to 5-hour span, for example) for men, or four or more for women, occurs in about 15% of U.S. adults and in youth as young as 12 years of age.[6] Young males between the ages of 18 and 25 have the highest rate of binge drinking.[6,7] Binge drinking by college students and other young adults (or even underage adolescents) increases the risk for potentially fatal falls, drownings, and automobile accidents. Acts of physical violence, including vandalism and physical and sexual assault, are also associated with binge drinking. The physiologic consequences also carry over beyond the actual binge: hangovers, which are

alcohol abuse The excessive consumption of alcohol, whether chronically or occasionally.

binge drinking The consumption of five or more alcoholic drinks on one occasion for men, or four or more for women.

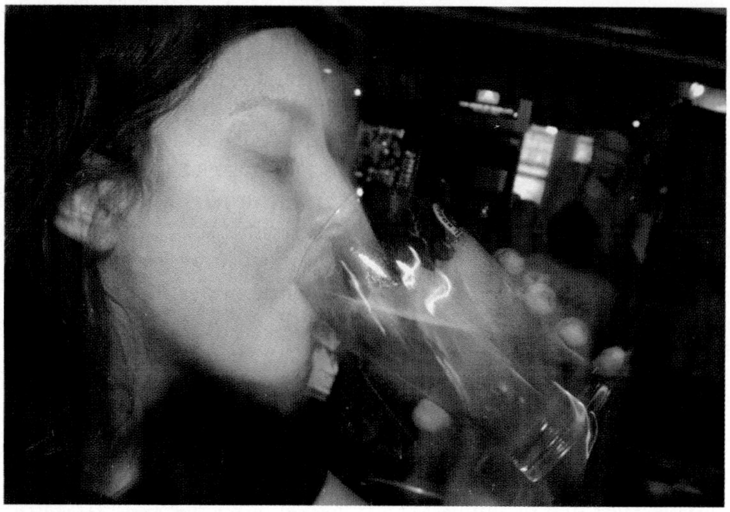

Binge drinking or excessive drinking can lead to a number of negative consequences.

discussed shortly, are practically inevitable, given the amount of alcohol consumed.

Alcoholism (also called *chronic alcohol dependence*) is a disease characterized by chronic dependence on alcohol, with the following symptoms:

- *craving:* a strong need or urge to drink alcoholic beverages
- *loss of control:* the inability to stop once drinking has begun
- *physical dependence:* the presence of nausea, sweating, shakiness, and other signs of withdrawal after stopping alcohol intake
- *tolerance:* the need to drink larger and larger amounts of alcohol to get the same "high," or pleasurable sensations, associated with alcohol intake

Alcohol Hangovers

Alcohol hangover is a frequent and extremely unpleasant consequence of drinking too much alcohol. It lasts up to 24 hours, and its symptoms include headache, fatigue, dizziness, muscle aches, nausea and vomiting, sensitivity to light and sound, and extreme thirst. Some people also experience depression, anxiety, irritability, and other mood disturbances.

Some of the symptoms occur because of alcohol's effect as a *diuretic,* a compound that increases urine output. Alcohol inhibits the release of the hormones that normally regulate urine production, so the body loses excessive fluid and minerals, such as sodium. This results in headache, thirst, dizziness, and light-headedness. The strategies suggested earlier—quenching your thirst with a nonalcoholic beverage before drinking alcohol and switching between alcoholic and nonalcoholic drinks—can help you avoid dehydration.

Alcohol irritates the lining of the stomach and increases the production of stomach acid. This may account for the abdominal pain, nausea, and vomiting seen in most hangovers.

Alcohol also disrupts normal body metabolism, leading to low levels of blood glucose and elevated levels of blood acidity. These disturbances contribute to the characteristic fatigue, weakness, and mood changes seen after excessive alcohol intake. Finally, alcohol disrupts various biological rhythms, such as sleep patterns and cycles of hormone secretion, leading to a jet lag type of effect.

While many folk remedies, including various herbal products, are claimed to prevent or reduce hangover effects, few have been proven effective. Drinking water or other nonalcoholic beverages will minimize the risk for dehydration, while the consumption of toast or dry cereal will bring blood glucose levels back to normal. Getting adequate sleep can counteract the fatigue, and the use of antacids may reduce nausea and abdominal pain. Although acetaminophen, aspirin, and ibuprofen might be useful for headaches, they may worsen stomach pain, increase the risk for gastrointestinal bleeding, and over time increase the risk for liver damage.

alcoholism A disease state characterized by chronic dependence on alcohol.

alcohol hangover A consequence of drinking too much alcohol; symptoms include headache, fatigue, dizziness, muscle aches, nausea and vomiting, sensitivity to light and sound, extreme thirst, and mood disturbances.

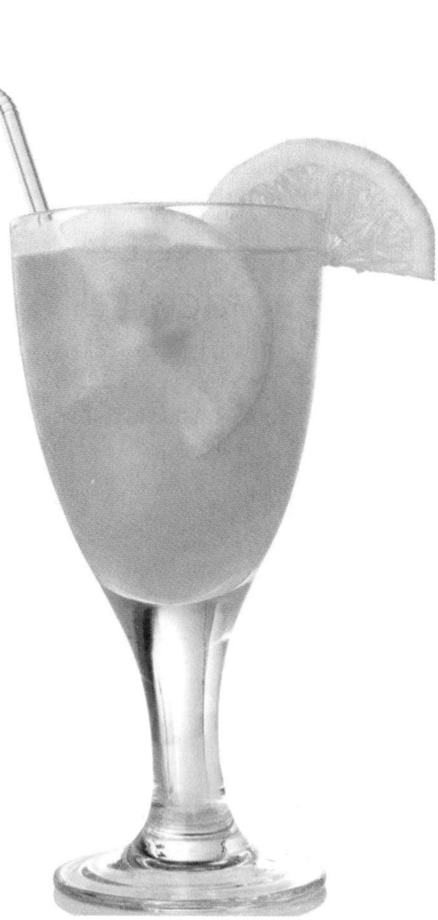

Is it wine or juice? The only way to tell if this glass holds an alcoholic or a nonalcoholic drink is to take a sip! At a party, fruit juices and sodas can be socially acceptable substitutes for alcoholic drinks.

NUTRI-CASE THEO

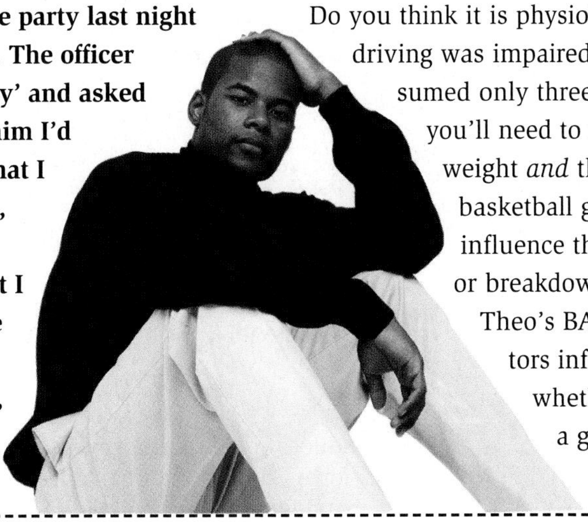

"I was driving home from a post-game party last night when I was pulled over by the police. The officer said I seemed to be driving 'erratically' and asked me how many drinks I'd had. I told him I'd only had three beers and explained that I was pretty tired from the game. Then, just to prove I was fine, I offered to count backwards from a hundred, but I must have sounded sober, because he didn't make me do it. I can't believe he thought I was driving drunk! Still, maybe three beers after a game really is too much."

Do you think it is physiologically possible that Theo's driving was impaired even though he had consumed only three beers? Before you answer, you'll need to factor in both Theo's body weight *and* the effect of playing a long basketball game. What other factors that influence the rate of alcohol absorption or breakdown could have affected Theo's BAC? How can all of these factors influence a decision about whether or not "three beers after a game really is too much"?

Reduced Brain Function

Alcohol is well known for its ability to alter behavior, mainly through its effects on the brain. Even at low intakes, alcohol impairs reasoning and judgment (**Table 2**). For college students, the academic consequences of drinking include falling behind in classes, doing poorly on exams and papers, missing classes, and getting lower grades overall.[8] Alcohol also interferes with normal sleep patterns, alters sight and speech, and leads to loss of fine and gross motor skills, such as handwriting, hand–eye coordination, and balance. Many people who drink experience unexpected mood swings, intense anger, or unreasonable irritation. Others react in the opposite direction, becoming sad, withdrawn, and lethargic. When teens or young adults chronically consume excessive amounts of alcohol, they may permanently damage brain structure and function.[9] Intellectual functioning and memory can be lost. In addition, early exposure to alcohol increases the risk for future alcohol addiction and may contribute to lifelong deficits in memory, motor skills, and muscle coordination.[10,11]

Alcohol Poisoning

At very high intakes of alcohol, a person is at risk for **alcohol poisoning**, a metabolic state that occurs in response to binge drinking. At high BACs, the respiratory center of the brain is depressed and cardiac function shuts down, leading to loss of consciousness, heart failure, and death. Like Todd in our opening story, many binge drinkers lose consciousness before alcohol poisoning becomes fatal, but emergency care is often essential.

If someone passes out after a night of hard drinking, he or she should never be left alone to "sleep it off." Instead, the person should be placed on his or her side to prevent aspiration if vomiting occurs. The person should also be watched carefully for cold and clammy skin, a bluish tint to the skin, or slow, irregular breathing. If any of these signs become evident, or there is any reason to believe he or she has alcohol poisoning, seek emergency healthcare immediately.

TABLE 2 Effects of Blood Alcohol Concentration (BAC) on Brain Activity

Blood Alcohol Concentration	Typical Response
0.02–0.05%	Feeling of relaxation, euphoria, relief
0.06–0.10%	Impaired judgment, fine motor control, and coordination; loss of normal emotional control; legally drunk in many states (at the upper end of the range)
0.11–0.15%	Impaired reflexes and gross motor control; staggered gait; legally drunk in all states; slurred speech
0.16–0.20%	Impaired vision; unpredictable behavior; further loss of muscle control
0.21–0.35%	Total loss of coordination; stupor
0.40% and above	Loss of consciousness; coma; suppression of respiratory response; death

Reduced Liver Function

In addition to its effects on the brain, alcohol can damage the liver, which is the main site of alcohol metabolism.

alcohol poisoning A potentially fatal condition in which an overdose of alcohol results in cardiac and/or respiratory failure.

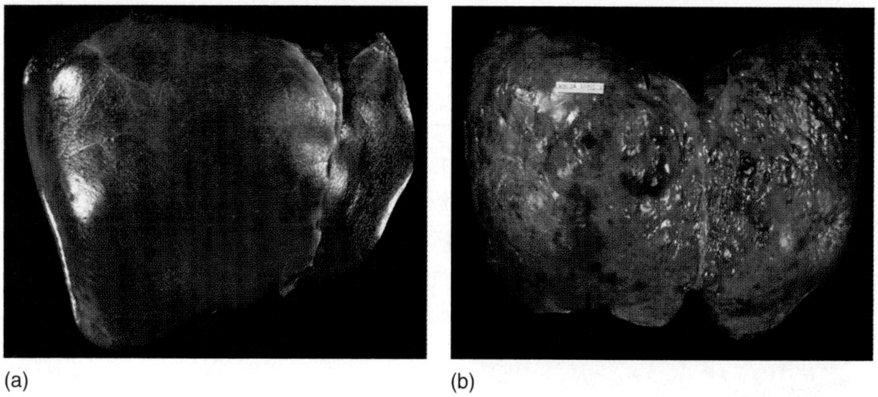

Figure 2 Cirrhosis of the liver, caused by chronic alcohol abuse. **(a)** A healthy liver. **(b)** A liver damaged by cirrhosis.

Liver cells are damaged or destroyed during periods of excessive alcohol intake; the longer the alcohol abuse, the greater the damage to the liver. **Fatty liver,** a condition in which abnormal amounts of fat build up in the liver, is an early yet reversible sign of alcohol-related liver damage. **Alcoholic hepatitis** causes loss of appetite, nausea and vomiting, abdominal pain, and jaundice (a yellowing of the skin and eyes, reflecting loss of liver function). **Cirrhosis of the liver** is often the result of long-term alcohol abuse; liver cells are scarred, blood flow through the liver is impaired, and liver function declines **(Figure 2)**.

Increased Risk for Chronic Disease

Heavy drinking has been associated with a number of diseases. For example, it damages the pancreas, which produces insulin, a hormone essential for blood glucose regulation. It also decreases the body's ability to respond properly to insulin. The result is chronically elevated blood glucose levels and an increased risk for diabetes. Research has strongly linked heavy alcohol intake to increased risk for cancer of the mouth and throat, esophagus, stomach, liver, colon, and female breast.[12] A recent study estimated that as many as 13% of cancers in a group of Japanese men were due to heavy drinking, complicated by smoking.[13] So, although moderate drinking may provide some health benefits, it is clear that chronically high intakes of alcohol damage a number of body organs and systems, increasing a person's risk for chronic disease and death.

Malnutrition

As alcohol intake increases to 30% or more of total energy intake, appetite is lost and the intake of healthful foods declines. Over time, the diet becomes deficient in protein, fats, carbohydrates, vitamins A and C, and minerals such as iron, zinc, and calcium. Even if food intake is maintained, the toxic effects of alcohol damage many digestive organs, including the stomach, small intestine, pancreas, and liver. The digestion of foods and absorption of nutrients become inadequate, leading to malnutrition and inappropriate weight loss.

Increased Risk for Traumatic Injury

Excessive alcohol intake is the leading cause of death for Americans under the age of 21. It is also the third leading cause of all U.S. deaths.[14] It has been estimated that as many as 6,000 young Americans die each year from alcohol-related motor vehicle accidents, suicides, and homicides. As previously noted, rates of physical and sexual assaults, vandalism, accidental falls, and drownings also increase when people are under the influence of alcohol.

fatty liver An early and reversible stage of liver disease often found in people who abuse alcohol and characterized by the abnormal accumulation of fat within liver cells; also called alcoholic steatosis.

alcoholic hepatitis Inflammation of the liver caused by alcohol; other forms of hepatitis can be caused by a virus or toxin.

cirrhosis of the liver Endstage liver disease characterized by significant abnormalities in liver structure and function; may lead to complete liver failure.

teratogen A compound known to cause fetal harm or danger.

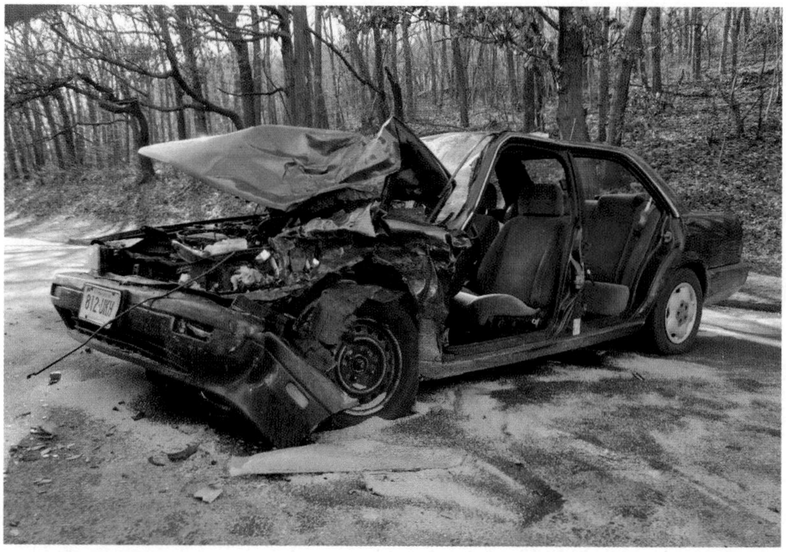

Excessive alcohol intake greatly increases the risks for car accidents and other traumatic injuries.

Fetal and Infant Health Problems

The March of Dimes estimates that more than 40,000 babies are born each year with some type of alcohol-related defect.[15] Alcohol is a known **teratogen** (a substance that causes fetal harm) that readily crosses the placenta into the fetal bloodstream. Since the immature fetal liver cannot effectively break down the alcohol, it accumulates in the fetal blood and tissues, increasing the risk for various birth defects. The effects of maternal alcohol intake are dose-related: the more the mother drinks, the greater the potential harm to the fetus. Drinking early in the pregnancy—even before the woman realizes she is pregnant—can cause particularly severe harm.

Fetal Alcohol Spectrum Disorder is an umbrella term used to describe the range of complications that develop when a woman consumes alcohol while pregnant. The diagnosis of *Alcohol Related Birth Defects* (ARBD) is made when an infant is born with one or more congenital defects, including malformations of the heart, bone, kidney, eyes, or ears as the result of prenatal exposure to alcohol. Alcohol consumption during pregnancy can also result in *Alcohol Related Neurodevelopmental Disorders* (ARND), which lead to central nervous system damage, learning impairments, and behavioral problems throughout life, including hyperactivity, attention deficit disorder, or other related disorders.

Fetal alcohol syndrome (FAS) is the most severe of these conditions and is characterized by malformations of the face, limbs, heart, and nervous system. The characteristic facial features persist throughout the child's life (**Figure 3**). Newborn and infant death rates are abnormally high, and those who do survive may suffer from emotional, behavioral, social, learning, and developmental problems throughout life. FAS is one of the most common causes of mental retardation in the United States and the only one that is completely preventable.

Fetal alcohol effects (FAE) are a more subtle set of consequences related to maternal alcohol intake. Although usually not identified at birth, this condition often becomes evident when the child enters preschool or kindergarten. The child may exhibit hyperactivity, attention deficit disorder, or impaired learning abilities. It is estimated that the incidence of FAE may be ten times greater than that of FAS.

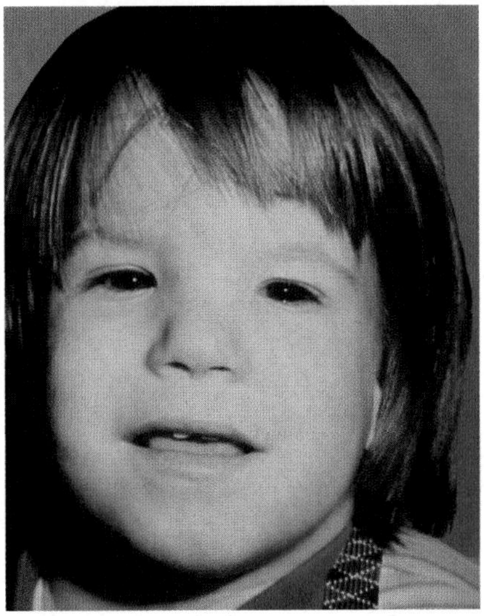

Figure 3 A child with fetal alcohol syndrome (FAS). The facial features typical of children with FAS include a short nose with a low, wide bridge; drooping eyes with an extra skinfold; and a flat, thin upper lip. These external traits are typically accompanied by behavioral problems and learning disorders. The effects of FAS are irreversible.

fetal alcohol syndrome (FAS) A set of serious, irreversible alcohol-related birth defects characterized by certain physical and mental abnormalities.

fetal alcohol effects (FAE) A set of subtle consequences of maternal intake of alcohol, such as impaired learning and behavioral problems.

What About You?

Do You Have a Problem with Alcohol Abuse?

Have you ever felt you should cut down on your drinking?	Yes/No
Have people annoyed you by criticizing your drinking?	Yes/No
Have you ever felt bad or guilty about your drinking?	Yes/No
Do you drink alone when you feel angry or sad?	Yes/No
Has your drinking ever made you late for school or work?	Yes/No
Have you ever had a drink first thing in the morning to steady your nerves or get rid of a hangover?	Yes/No
Do you ever drink after promising yourself you won't?	Yes/No

If you answered "yes" to one or more of these questions, provided by the National Institute on Alcohol Abuse and Alcoholism, you may have a problem with alcohol abuse and should consult your primary healthcare provider or a specialized counselor to explore it in more detail.

There is no known safe level of alcohol consumption for pregnant women. Women who are pregnant, think they may be pregnant, or are trying to become pregnant should abstain from all alcoholic beverages.

Women who are breastfeeding should also abstain from alcohol, since it easily passes into the breast milk at levels equal to blood alcohol concentrations. If consumed by the infant, the alcohol in breast milk can slow motor development, depress the central nervous system, and increase sleepiness in the child. Alcohol also reduces the mother's ability to produce milk, putting the infant at risk for malnutrition.

Should You Be Concerned About Your Alcohol Intake?

Even if you are not dependent on alcohol, you should be concerned about your alcohol intake if you engage in binge drinking or drink at inappropriate times (such as while pregnant, before or while driving a car, to deal with negative emotions, or while at work/school). If you do, complete the self-assessment quiz to become more aware of recognizing a potential problem; recognizing a problem is the first step toward overcoming it.

If you think you have an alcohol problem, it is important for you to speak with a trusted friend, counselor, or healthcare provider. There are many effective support groups that can help you plan a course of action to cut down or eliminate your alcohol intake. Taking control of your alcohol intake will allow you to take control of your life.

Talking to Someone About Alcohol Addiction

You may suspect that a close friend or relative is one of the nearly 14 million Americans who abuse alcohol or are dependent on alcohol.[16] If you notice that your friend or relative uses alcohol as the primary way to calm down, cheer up, or relax, that may be a sign of alcohol dependency or addiction. The appearance of tremors or other signs of withdrawal and the initiation of secretive behaviors when consuming alcohol are other indications that alcohol has become a serious problem.

Many people become defensive or hostile when asked about their use of alcohol; denial is very common. The single hardest step toward sobriety is often the first: accepting the fact that help is needed. Some people respond well when confronted by one person, whereas others benefit more from a group intervention. There should be no blaming or shaming; alcohol addiction and dependency are medical conditions with a strong genetic component. The National Institute on Alcoholism and Alcohol Abuse suggests the following approaches when trying to get a friend or relative into treatment.

Stop covering up and making excuses Many times, family and friends will make excuses to others to protect the person from the results of his or her drinking. It is important, however, to stop covering for that person, so that he or she can experience the full consequences of inappropriate alcohol consumption.

Intervene at a vulnerable time The best time to talk to someone about problem drinking is shortly after an alcohol-related incident, such as a DUI arrest, an alcohol-related traffic accident, or a public scene. Wait until the person is sober and everyone is relatively calm.

Be specific Tell the person exactly why you are concerned; use examples of specific problems associated with his or her drinking habits (such as poor school or work performance, legal problems, or inappropriate behaviors). Explain what will happen if the person chooses not to get help—for example, no longer going out with the person if alcohol will be available, no longer riding with him or her in motor vehicles, or moving out of a shared home.

Get help Professional help is available from community agencies, healthcare providers, online sites, school or worksite wellness centers, and some religious organizations. Several contacts and websites are listed at the end of this ***In Depth*** essay. If the person indicates a willingness to get help, call immediately for an appointment and/or immediately take him or her to a treatment center. The longer the delay, the more likely it is that the person will experience a change of heart.

Enlist the support of others Whether or not the person agrees to get help, calling on other friends and relatives can often be effective, especially if you have had alcohol-related problems of your own. Formal support groups, such as Al-Anon and Alateen, can provide additional information and guidance.

Treatment for alcohol-related problems works for many, but not all, individuals. "Success" is measured in small steps, and relapses are common. Most scientists agree that people who abuse alcohol cannot just "cut down." Complete avoidance of all alcoholic beverages is the only way for most people who abuse alcohol to achieve full and ongoing recovery.

Web Resources

www.aa.org
Alcoholics Anonymous, Inc.

This site provides links to local AA groups and provides information on the AA program.

www.al-anon.alateen.org
Al-Anon Family Group Headquarters, Inc.

This site provides links to local Al-Anon and Alateen groups, which provide support for spouses, children, and other loved ones of people addicted to alcohol.

www.ncadd.org
National Council on Alcoholism and Drug Dependence, Inc.

Educational materials and information on alcoholism can be obtained from this site.

www.niaaa.nih.gov
National Institute on Alcohol Abuse and Alcoholism

Visit this website for information on the prevalence, consequences, and treatments of alcohol-related disorders. Information for healthcare providers, people struggling with alcohol abuse, and family members is available free of charge.

www.collegedrinkingprevention.gov
College Drinking: Changing the Culture

The NIAAA developed this website specifically for college students seeking information and advice on the subject of college drinking. Services include self-assessment questionnaires, answers to frequently asked questions, news articles, research, and links to support groups.

www.madd.org
Mothers Against Drunk Driving

Links to local chapters, statistics related to drunk driving, and prevention strategies are easily accessed from this site.

www.marchofdimes.com
March of Dimes

Find information on fetal alcohol syndrome and fetal alcohol effects at this website.

2 Designing a Healthful Diet

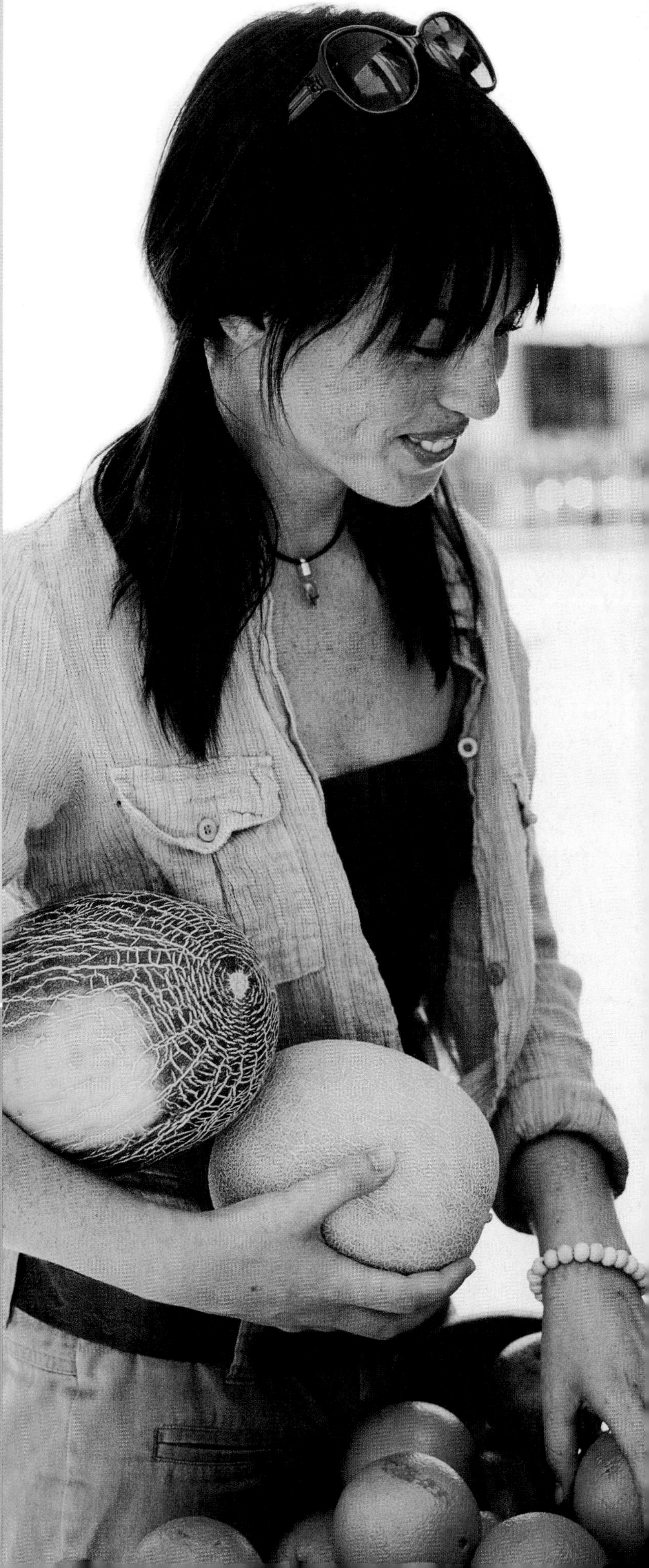

CHAPTER OBJECTIVES

After reading this chapter you will be able to:

1. **Identify the characteristics of a healthful diet, pp. 40–41.**
2. **Name five components that must be included on food labels and use the Nutrition Facts Panel to determine the nutritional adequacy of a given food, p. 42.**
3. **Describe the Dietary Guidelines for Americans and discuss how these Guidelines can be used to design a healthful diet, pp. 48–51.**
4. **Identify the food groups and recommended equivalent amounts included in MyPlate, pp. 51–56.**
5. **Explain how MyPlate can be used to design a healthful ethnic diet, pp. 57–60.**
6. **List at least four ways to practice moderation and apply healthful dietary guidelines when eating out, pp. 61–62.**

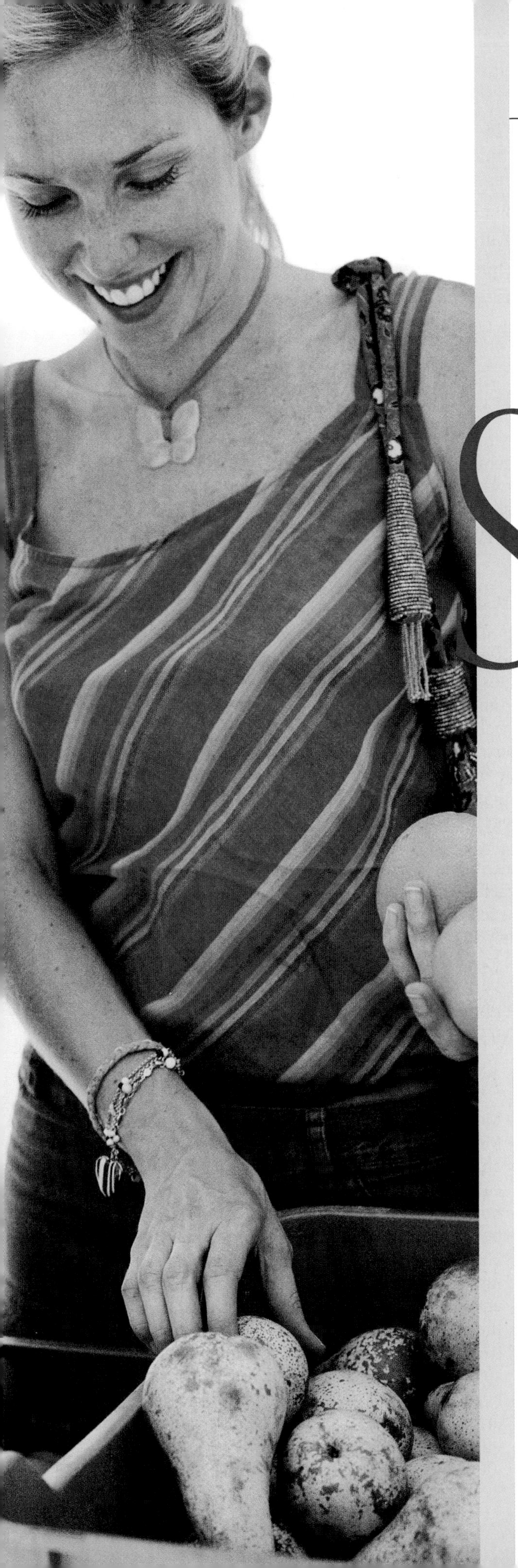

Test Yourself

1. T F A healthful diet should always include vitamin supplements.
2. T F If it says so on the label, it has to be true.
3. T F A plain cup of coffee and a café mocha have about the same number of Calories.

Test Yourself answers can be found at the end of the chapter.

Shivani and her parents moved to the United States from India when she was 6 years old. Although she was delicate in comparison to her American peers, Shivani was healthy and energetic, excelling in school and riding her new bike in her suburban neighborhood. By the time Shivani entered high school, her weight had caught up to that of her American classmates. Now a college freshman, she has joined the more than 16% of U.S. teens who are overweight.[1] Shivani explains, "In India, the diet is mostly rice, lentils, and vegetables. Many people are vegetarians, and many others eat meat only once or twice a week, and very small portions. Desserts are only for special occasions. When we moved to America, I wanted to eat like all the other kids: hamburgers, french fries, sodas, and sweets. I gained a lot of weight on that diet, and now my doctor says my cholesterol level, my blood pressure, and my blood sugar level are all too high. I wish I could start eating like my relatives back in India again, but they don't serve rice and lentils at the dorm cafeteria."

What influence does diet have on health? What exactly qualifies as a "poor diet," and what makes a diet healthful? Is it more important to watch how much we eat or what kinds of foods we choose? Is low-carb better, or low-fat? What do the national Dietary Guidelines advise, and do they apply to real people (like you)?

The truth is, there's no one way to eat that's right for everyone. We're individuals with unique preferences, needs, and cultural influences. You may love broccoli, whereas your roommate can't stand it. A person with diabetes may need to eat less added sugar and more protein than a person without diabetes.

People following certain religious practices may avoid specific meats and dairy products. Thus, there are literally millions of ways to design a healthful diet to fit individual needs.

Given all this potential confusion, it's a good thing there are nutritional tools to guide us in designing our own healthful diet. In this chapter, we'll discover these tools, including the Dietary Guidelines for Americans, the USDA's MyPlate, and others. Before we explore the question of how to design a healthful diet, however, we should first make sure we understand what a healthful diet *is*.

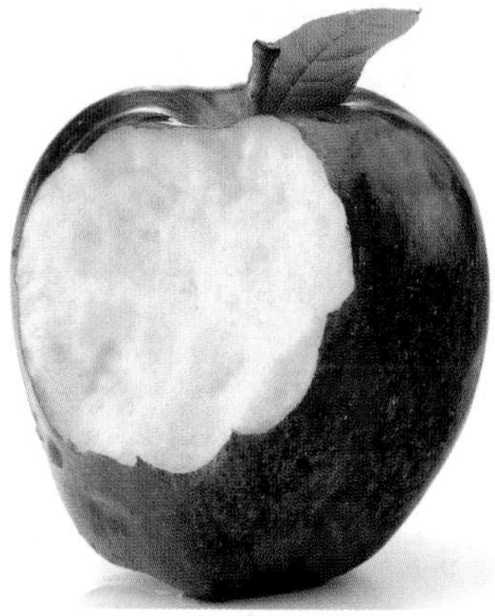

A healthful diet can help prevent disease.

What Is a Healthful Diet?

A **healthful diet** provides the proper combination of energy and nutrients. It has four characteristics: it is adequate, moderate, balanced, and varied. No matter if you are young or old, overweight or underweight, healthy or ill, if you keep these characteristics in mind, you will be able to select foods that provide you with the optimal combination of nutrients and energy each day.

A Healthful Diet Is Adequate

An **adequate diet** provides enough of the energy, nutrients, and fiber to maintain a person's health. A diet may be inadequate in only one area, or many areas. For example, many people in the United States do not eat enough vegetables and therefore are not consuming enough of the fiber and micronutrients vegetables provide. However, their intake of protein, fat, and carbohydrate may be adequate. In fact, some people who eat too few vegetables are overweight or obese, which means that they are eating a diet that, although inadequate in one area, exceeds their energy needs. On the other hand, a generalized state of undernutrition can occur if an individual's diet contains an inadequate level of several nutrients for a long period of time.

healthful diet A diet that provides the proper combination of energy and nutrients and is adequate, moderate, balanced, and varied.

adequate diet A diet that provides enough of the energy, nutrients, and fiber needed to maintain a person's health.

moderation Eating any foods in moderate amounts—not too much and not too little.

A diet that is adequate for one person may not be adequate for another. For example, the energy needs of a small woman who is lightly active are approximately 1,700 to 2,000 kilocalories (kcal) each day, whereas a highly active male athlete may require more than 4,000 kcal each day to support his body's demands. These two individuals differ greatly in their activity level and in their quantity of body fat and muscle mass, which means they require very different levels of fat, carbohydrate, protein, and other nutrients to support their daily needs.

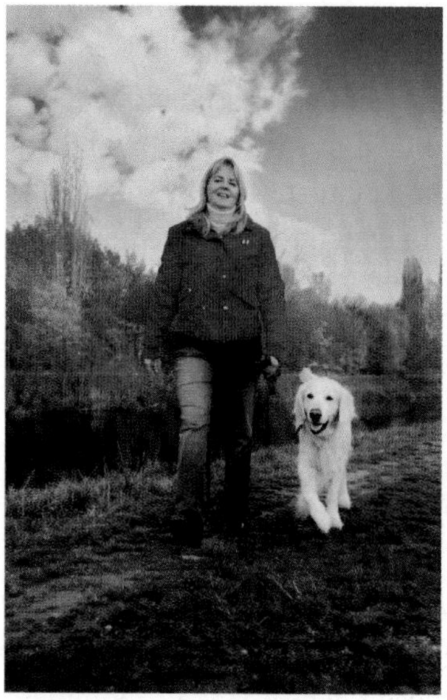

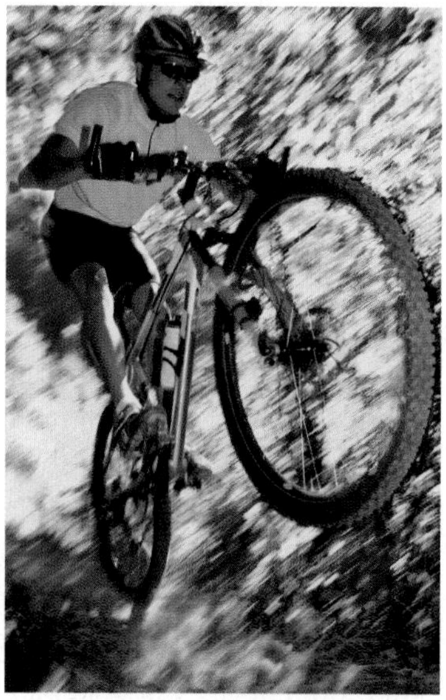

A diet that is adequate for one person may not be adequate for another. A woman who is lightly active may require fewer kilocalories of energy per day than a highly active male.

A Healthful Diet Is Moderate

Moderation is one of the keys to a healthful diet. **Moderation** refers to eating any foods in moderate amounts—not too much and not too little. If we eat too much or too little of certain foods, we cannot reach our health goals. For example, some people drink as much as 60 fluid ounces (three 20-oz bottles) of soft drinks on some days. Drinking this much contributes an extra 765 kcal of energy to a person's diet. In order to allow for these extra kcal and avoid weight gain, most people would need to reduce their food intake significantly. This could mean eliminating many healthful food choices. In contrast, people who drink mostly water or other beverages that contain little or no energy can consume more nourishing foods that will support their wellness.

A Healthful Diet Is Balanced

A **balanced diet** contains the combinations of foods that provide the proper proportions of nutrients. As you will learn in this course, the body needs many types of foods in varying amounts to maintain health. For example, fruits and vegetables are excellent sources of fiber, vitamin C, potassium, and magnesium. In contrast, meats are not good sources of fiber and these nutrients. However, meats are excellent sources of protein, iron, zinc, and copper. By eating the proper balance of all healthful foods, including fruits, vegetables, and meats or meat substitutes, we can be confident that we're consuming the balanced nutrition we need to maintain health.

A Healthful Diet Is Varied

Variety refers to eating many different foods from the different food groups on a regular basis. With thousands of healthful foods to choose from, trying new foods is a fun and easy way to vary your diet. Eat a new vegetable each week or substitute one food for another, such as raw spinach on your turkey sandwich in place of iceberg lettuce. Selecting a variety of foods increases the likelihood that you will consume the multitude of nutrients your body needs. As an added benefit, eating a varied diet prevents boredom and helps you avoid the potential of getting into a "food rut." Later in this chapter, we'll provide suggestions for eating a varied diet.

RECAP **A healthful diet provides adequate nutrients and energy, and it includes sweets, fats, and salty foods in moderate amounts only. A healthful diet includes an appropriate balance of nutrients and a wide variety of foods.**

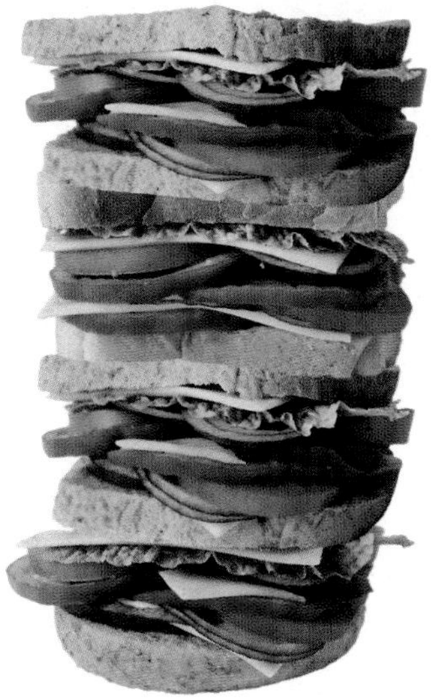

The serving size on a nutrition label may not be the same as the amount you eat.

What Tools Can Help Me Design a Healthful Diet?

Many people feel it is impossible to eat a healthful diet. They may mistakenly believe that the foods they would need to eat are too expensive or not available to them, or they may feel too busy to do the necessary planning, shopping, and cooking. Some people rely on dietary supplements to get enough nutrients instead of focusing on eating a variety of foods. But is it really that difficult to eat healthfully?

Although designing and maintaining a healthful diet is not as simple as eating whatever you want, most of us can improve our diets with a little practice and a little help. Let's look at some tools for designing a healthful diet.

Food Labels

To design and maintain a healthful diet, it's important to read and understand food labels. It may surprise you to learn that prior to the 1970s, there were no federal regulations for including nutrition information on food labels. The U.S. Food and Drug Administration (FDA) first established such regulations in 1973. Throughout the 1970s and 1980s, consumer interest in food quality grew substantially, leading the U.S. Congress to pass the Nutrition Labeling and Education Act in 1990. This act specifies which foods require a food label, provides detailed descriptions of the information that must be included on the label, and describes the companies and food products that are exempt from publishing complete nutrition information on food labels. For example, detailed food labels are not required for meat or poultry, as these products are regulated by the U.S. Department of Agriculture, not the FDA. In addition, foods such as coffee and most spices are not required to follow the FDA labeling guidelines, as they contain insignificant amounts of all nutrients that must be listed in nutrition labeling.

balanced diet A diet that contains the combinations of foods that provide the proper proportions of nutrients.

variety Eating a lot of different foods each day.

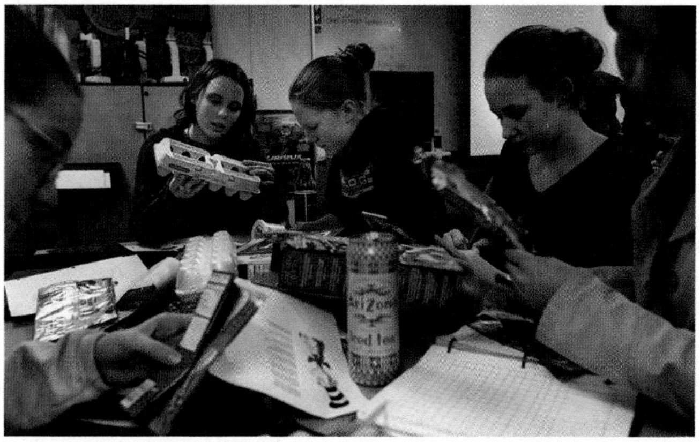

In this text, you will learn how to read food labels, a skill that can help you meet your nutritional goals.

Five Components Must Be Included on Food Labels

Five primary components of information must be included on food labels **(Figure 2.1)**:

1. *A statement of identity:* The common name of the product or an appropriate identification of the food product must be prominently displayed on the label. This information tells us very clearly what the product is.
2. *The net contents of the package:* The quantity of the food product in the entire package must be accurately described. Information may be listed as weight (such as "grams"), volume (such as "fluid ounces"), or numerical count (such as "4 each").
3. *Ingredient list:* The ingredients must be listed by their common names, in descending order by weight. This means that the first product listed is the predominant ingredient in that food. This information can be very useful in many situations, such as when you are looking for foods that are lower in fat or sugar or when you are attempting to identify foods that contain whole-grain flour instead of processed wheat flour.
4. *The name and address of the food manufacturer, packer, or distributor:* You can use this information to find out more details about a food product and to contact the company if there is something wrong with the product or you suspect that it has caused an illness.
5. *Nutrition information:* The Nutrition Facts Panel contains the nutrition information required by the FDA. This panel is the primary tool to assist you in choosing more healthful foods. An explanation of the components of the Nutrition Facts Panel follows.

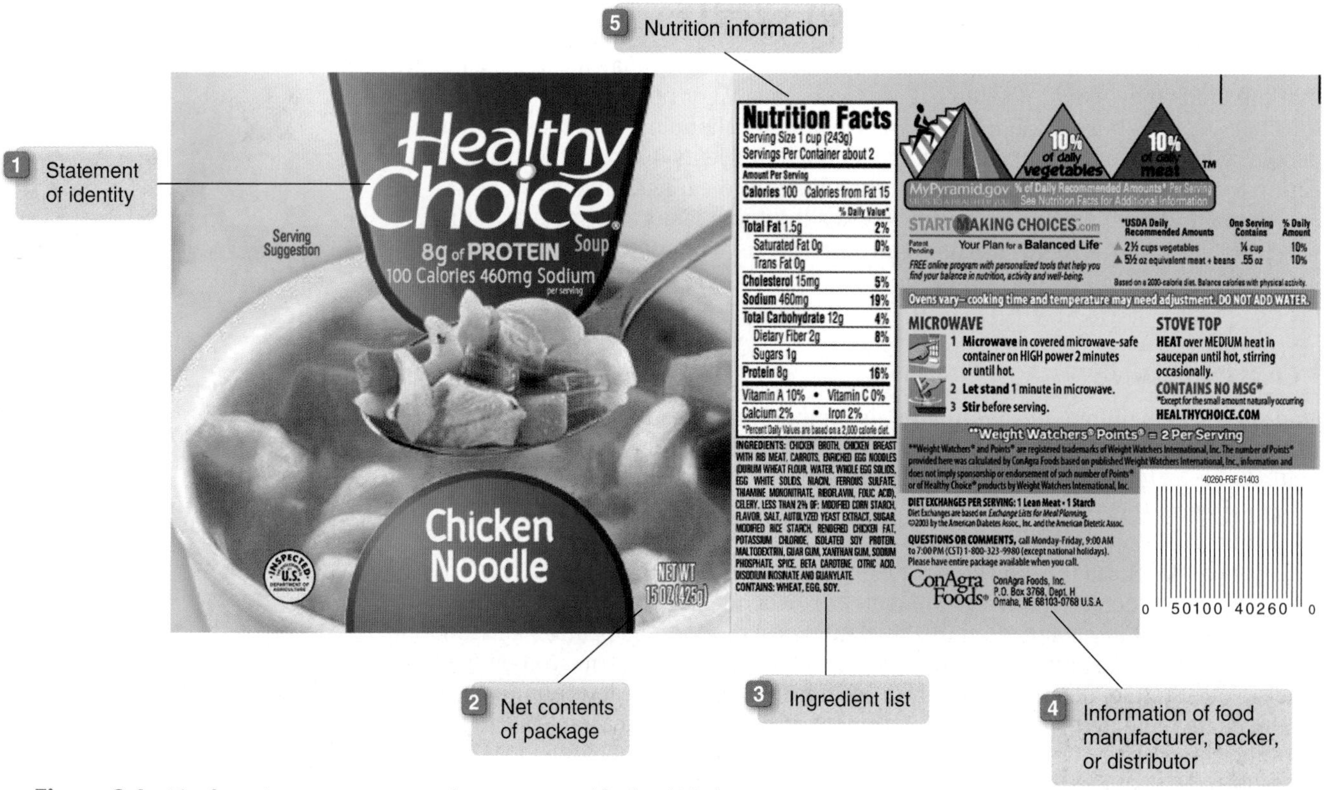

Figure 2.1 The five primary components that are required for food labels.

How to Read and Use the Nutrition Facts Panel on Foods

Figure 2.2 shows an example of a **Nutrition Facts Panel.** You can use the information on this panel to learn more about an individual food, and you can use the panel to compare one food to another. Let's start at the top of the panel and work our way down to better understand how to use this information.

1. *Serving size and servings per container:* This section describes the serving size in a common household measure (such as a cup) and a metric measure (such as grams), as well as how many servings are contained in the package. The FDA has defined serving sizes based on the amounts of each food people typically eat. However, keep in mind that the serving size listed on the package may not be the same as the amount *you* eat. You must factor in how much of the food you eat when determining the amount of nutrients that this food contributes to your diet.

2. *Calories and Calories from fat per serving:* This section describes the total number of Calories and the total number of Calories that come from fat in 1 serving of that food. By looking at this section of the label, you can determine whether a food is relatively high in fat. For example, 1 serving of the food on this label (as prepared) contains 320 total Calories, with 90 of those Calories coming from fat. This means that this food contains 28% of its total Calories as fat (90 fat Calories ÷ 320 total Calories).

3. *List of nutrients:* This section states the nutrients this food contains. In this food, the nutrients listed toward the top, including total fat, saturated fat, *trans* fat, cholesterol, and sodium, are generally the nutrients you should strive to limit in a healthful diet. Some of the nutrients listed toward the bottom, including fiber, vitamins A and C, calcium, and iron, are those you should try to consume more of.

Nutrition Facts Panel The label on a food package that contains the nutrition information required by the FDA.

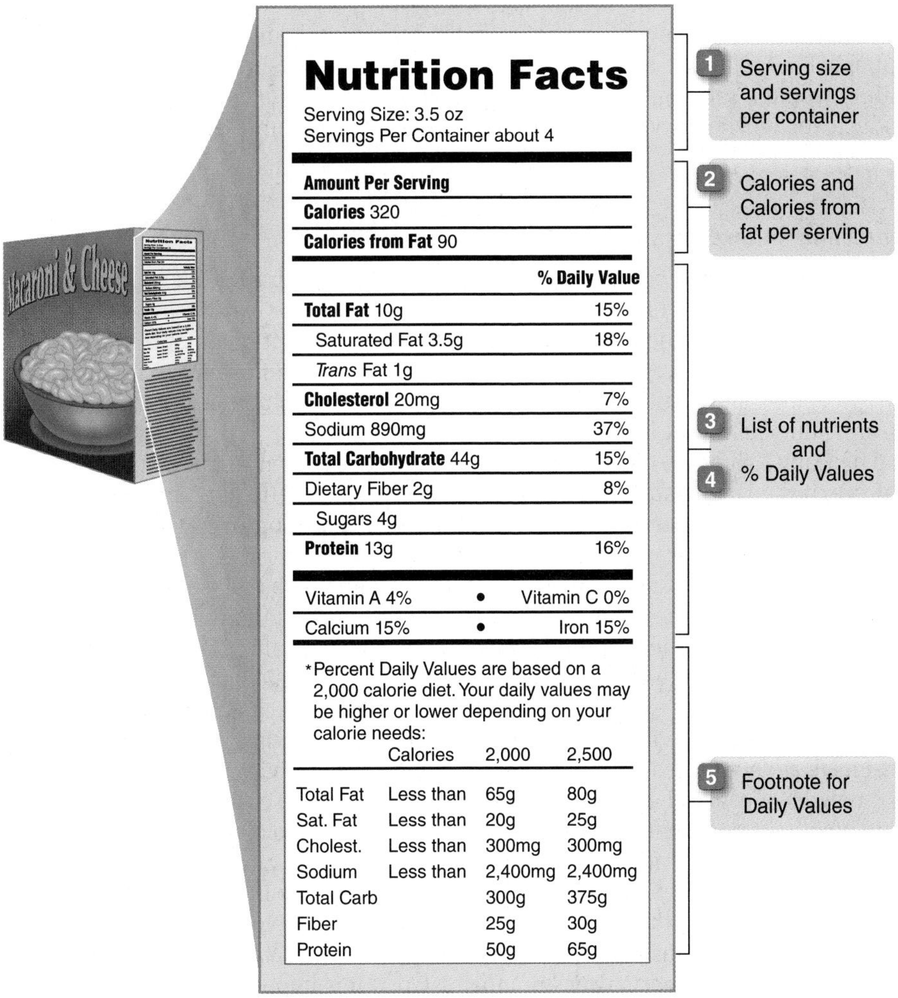

Figure 2.2 The Nutrition Facts Panel contains a variety of information to help you make more healthful food choices.

Nutrition Facts

Serving Size: 3.5 oz
Servings Per Container about 4

Amount Per Serving

Calories 320

Calories from Fat 90

	% Daily Value
Total Fat 10g	15%
Saturated Fat 3.5g	18%
Trans Fat 1g	
Cholesterol 20mg	7%
Sodium 890mg	37%
Total Carbohydrate 44g	15%
Dietary Fiber 2g	8%
Sugars 4g	
Protein 13g	16%

Vitamin A 4%	•	Vitamin C 0%
Calcium 15%	•	Iron 15%

*Percent Daily Values are based on a 2,000 calorie diet. Your daily values may be higher or lower depending on your calorie needs:

	Calories	2,000	2,500
Total Fat	Less than	65g	80g
Sat. Fat	Less than	20g	25g
Cholest.	Less than	300mg	300mg
Sodium	Less than	2,400mg	2,400mg
Total Carb		300g	375g
Fiber		25g	30g
Protein		50g	65g

1. Serving size and servings per container

2. Calories and Calories from fat per serving

3. List of nutrients and
4. % Daily Values

5. Footnote for Daily Values

4. ***Percent Daily Values (%DV):*** This section tells you how much a serving of food contributes to your overall intake of the nutrients listed on the label. For example, 10 grams of fat constitutes 15% of your total daily recommended fat intake. Because we are all individuals, with unique nutritional needs, it is impractical to include nutrition information that applies to each person consuming a food. That would require thousands of labels! Thus, when defining the %DV, the FDA based its calculations on a 2,000-Calorie diet. Even if you do not consume 2,000 Calories each day, you can still use the %DV to figure out whether a food is high or low in a given nutrient. For example, foods that contain less than 5% DV of a nutrient are considered low in that nutrient, whereas foods that contain more than 20% DV are considered high in that nutrient. If you are trying to consume more calcium in your diet, select foods that contain more than 20% DV for calcium. In contrast, if you are trying to consume lower-fat foods, select foods that contain less than 5% or 10% fat. By comparing the %DV of foods for any nutrient, you can quickly decide which food is higher or lower in that nutrient without having to know how many Calories you need.
5. *Footnote (lower part of the panel):* This section tells you that the %DV are based on a 2,000-Calorie diet and that your needs may be higher or lower based on your caloric needs. The remainder of the footnote includes a table with values that illustrate the differences in recommendations between 2,000-Calorie and 2,500-Calorie diets; for instance, someone eating 2,000 Calories should strive to eat less than 65 grams of fat per day, whereas a person eating 2,500 Calories should eat less than 80 grams of fat per day. The table may not be present if the food label is too small. When present, the footnote and table are always the same, because the information refers to general dietary advice for all Americans, rather than to a specific food.

By comparing labels from various foods, you can start designing a more healthful diet today. Let's assume you are trying to limit your intake of sodium. Look at the soup label in Figure 2.1 and the macaroni and cheese label in Figure 2.2. How much sodium would a serving of these foods provide? If you had a choice of either of these products for lunch or a veggie burrito with 280 mg of sodium, which would you choose?

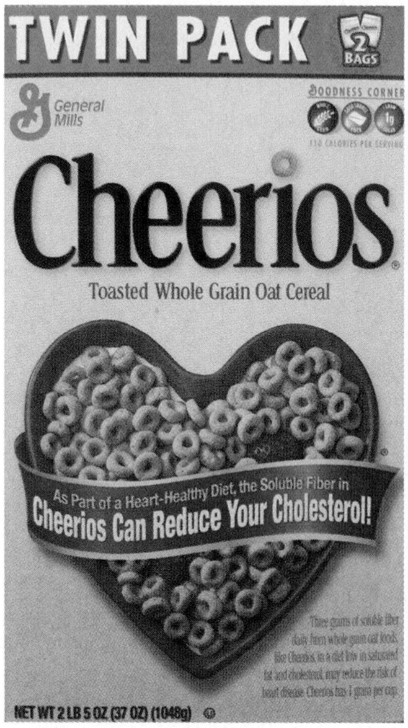

▲ This Cheerios box is an example of an approved health claim.

Food Labels Can Contain a Variety of Nutrient Claims

Have you ever noticed a food label displaying a claim such as "This food is low in sodium" or "This food is part of a heart-healthy diet"? The claim may have influenced you to buy the food, even if you weren't sure what it meant. Let's take a look.

The FDA regulates two types of claims that food companies put on food labels: nutrient claims and health claims. Food companies are prohibited from using a nutrient or health claim that is not approved by the FDA.

The Daily Values on the food labels serve as a basis for nutrient claims. For instance, if the label states that a food is "low in sodium," the food contains 140 mg or less of sodium per serving. **Table 2.1** defines the terms approved for use in nutrient claims.

The FDA also allows food labels to display certain claims related to health and disease **(Table 2.2)**. To help consumers gain a better understanding of nutritional information related to health, the FDA has developed a Health Claims Report Card **(Figure 2.3)**, which grades the level of confidence in a health claim based on current scientific evidence. For example, if current scientific evidence about a particular health claim is not convincing, the label may have to include a disclaimer, so that consumers are not misled. Complete the Nutrition Label Activity (page 47) to determine the strengths of certain health claims made for foods that are commonly consumed.

In addition to nutrient and health claims, labels may also contain structure–function claims. These are claims that can be made without approval from the FDA. While these claims can be generic statements about a food's impact on the body's structure and function, they cannot refer to a specific disease or symptom. Examples of structure–function claims include "Builds stronger bones," "Improves memory," "Slows signs of aging," and "Boosts your immune system." It is important to remember that

percent Daily Values (%DV) Information on a Nutrition Facts Panel that identifies how much a serving of food contributes to your overall intake of the nutrients listed on the label; based on an energy intake of 2,000 Calories per day.

TABLE 2.1 United States Food and Drug Administration (FDA)–Approved Nutrient-Related Terms and Definitions

Nutrient	Claim	Meaning
Energy	Calorie free	Less than 5 kcal per serving
	Low Calorie	40 kcal or less per serving
	Reduced Calorie	At least 25% fewer kcal than reference (or regular) food
Fat and Cholesterol	Fat free	Less than 0.5 g of fat per serving
	Low fat	3 g or less fat per serving
	Reduced fat	At least 25% less fat per serving than reference food
	Saturated fat free	Less than 0.5 g of saturated fat **AND** less than 0.5 g of *trans* fat per serving
	Low saturated fat	1 g or less saturated fat and less than 0.5 g *trans* fat per serving **AND** 15% or less of total kcal from saturated fat
	Reduced saturated fat	At least 25% less saturated fat **AND** reduced by more than 1 g saturated fat per serving as compared to reference food
	Cholesterol free	Less than 2 mg of cholesterol per serving **AND** 2 g or less saturated fat and *trans* fat combined per serving
	Low cholesterol	20 mg or less cholesterol **AND** 2 g or less saturated fat per serving
	Reduced cholesterol	At least 25% less cholesterol than reference food **AND** 2 g or less saturated fat per serving
Fiber and Sugar	High fiber	5 g or more fiber per serving*
	Good source of fiber	2.5 g to 4.9 g fiber per serving
	More or added fiber	At least 2.5 g more fiber per serving than reference food
	Sugar free	Less than 0.5 g sugars per serving
	Low sugar	Not defined; no basis for recommended intake
	Reduced/less sugar	At least 25% less sugars per serving than reference food
	No added sugars or without added sugars	No sugar or sugar-containing ingredient added during processing
Sodium	Sodium free	Less than 5 mg sodium per serving
	Very low sodium	35 mg or less sodium per serving
	Low sodium	140 mg or less sodium per serving
	Reduced sodium	At least 25% less sodium per serving than reference food
Relative Claims	Free, without, no, zero	No or a trivial amount of given nutrient
	Light (or lite)	This term can have three different meanings: (1) a serving provides 1/3 fewer kcal than or half the fat of the reference food; (2) a serving of a low-fat, low-Calorie food provides half the sodium normally present; or (3) lighter in color and texture, with the label making this clear (for example, light molasses)
	Reduced, less, fewer	Contains at least 25% less of a nutrient or kcal than reference food
	More, added, extra, or plus	At least 10% of the Daily Value of nutrient as compared to reference food (may occur naturally or be added); may be used only for vitamins, minerals, protein, dietary fiber, and potassium
	Good source of, contains, or provides	10% to 19% of Daily Value per serving (may not be used for carbohydrate)
	High in, rich in, or excellent source of	20% or more of Daily Value per serving for protein, vitamins, minerals, dietary fiber, or potassium (may not be used for carbohydrate)

Data from U.S. Food and Drug Administration. 2008. Food Labeling Guide. Available at www.fda.gov/Food/GuidanceComplianceRegulatoryInformation/GuidanceDocuments/FoodLabelingNutrition/FoodLabelingGuide/default.htm.

*High fiber claims must also meet the definition of low fat; if not, then the level of total fat must appear next to the high fiber claim.

these claims can be made with no proof, and thus there are no guarantees that any benefits identified in structure–function claims are true about that food. Thus, just because something is stated on the label doesn't guarantee it is always true!

In recent years, a variety of foods referred to as functional foods have become available to consumers. The Institute of Food Technologists defines a **functional food** as a food or food component that provides a health benefit beyond basic nutrition. You may be wondering what some examples of functional foods are, if they are safe, and if they are effective. Find the answers in the Nutrition Debate (page 63).

functional food A food or food component that provides a health benefit beyond basic nutrition.

TABLE 2.2 U.S. Food and Drug Administration–Approved Health Claims on Labels

Disease/Health Concern	Nutrient	Example of Approved Claim Statement
Osteoporosis	Calcium	Regular exercise and a healthy diet with enough calcium help teens and young white and Asian women maintain good bone health and may reduce their high risk for osteoporosis later in life.
Coronary heart disease	Saturated fat and cholesterol Fruits, vegetables, and grain products that contain fiber, particularly soluble fiber Soluble fiber from whole oats, psyllium seed husk, and beta glucan soluble fiber from oat bran, rolled oats (or oatmeal), and whole-oat flour Soy protein Plant sterol/stanol esters Whole-grain foods	Diets low in saturated fat and cholesterol and rich in fruits, vegetables, and grain products that contain some types of dietary fiber, particularly soluble fiber, may reduce the risk for heart disease, a disease associated with many factors.
Cancer	Dietary fat Fiber-containing grain products, fruits, and vegetables Fruits and vegetables Whole-grain foods	Low-fat diets rich in fiber-containing grain products, fruits, and vegetables may reduce the risk for some types of cancer, a disease associated with many factors.
Hypertension and stroke	Sodium Potassium	Diets containing foods that are a good source of potassium and that are low in sodium may reduce the risk of high blood pressure and stroke.*
Neural tube defects	Folate	Healthful diets with adequate folate may reduce a woman's risk of having a child with a brain or spinal cord defect.
Dental caries	Sugar alcohols	Frequent between-meal consumption of foods high in sugars and starches promotes tooth decay. The sugar alcohols in [name of food] do not promote tooth decay.

Data from U.S. Food and Drug Administration. 2008. Food Labeling Guide. Available at www.fda.gov/Food/GuidanceComplianceRegulatoryInformation/GuidanceDocuments/FoodLabelingNutrition/FoodLabelingGuide/default.htm.

*Required wording for this claim. Wordings for other claims are recommended model statements but not required verbatim.

Figure 2.3 The U.S. Food and Drug Administration's Health Claims Report Card.

Health Claims Report Card

FDA category		Required disclaimer
A	**High** Significant scientific agreement	Applies to claims listed in Table 2.2 No disclaimer needed
B	**Moderate** Evidence is not conclusive	"... although there is scientific evidence supporting the claim, the evidence is not conclusive."
C	**Low** Evidence is limited and not conclusive	"Some scientific evidence suggests ... however, FDA has determined that this evidence is limited and not conclusive."
D	**Extremely Low** Little scientific evidence supporting this claim	"Very limited and preliminary scientific research suggests ... FDA concludes that there is little scientific evidence supporting this claim."

RECAP The ability to read and interpret food labels is important for planning and maintaining a healthful diet. Food labels must list the identity of the food, the net contents of the package, the contact information for the food manufacturer or distributor, the ingredients in the food, and a Nutrition Facts Panel. The Nutrition Facts Panel provides specific information about Calories, macronutrients, and selected vitamins and minerals. Food labels may also contain claims related to nutrients, health, and body structure and function.

NUTRITION LABEL ACTIVITY

How Do Health Claims on Food Labels Measure Up?

The U.S. Food and Drug Administration has published a Health Claims Report Card to assist consumers in deciphering health claims on food labels (Figure 2.3). It is important to note that the claims that are based on high scientific agreement do not require a label disclaimer. The claims reported in Table 2.2 are those that are based on high scientific agreement. Included here is a food label listing health claims: based on the Health Claims Report Card criteria listed in Figure 2.3, what level of confidence do scientists currently have about these health claims? Taking this level of confidence into consideration, would you recommend this product to relatives or friends if they were concerned about heart disease? Why or why not?

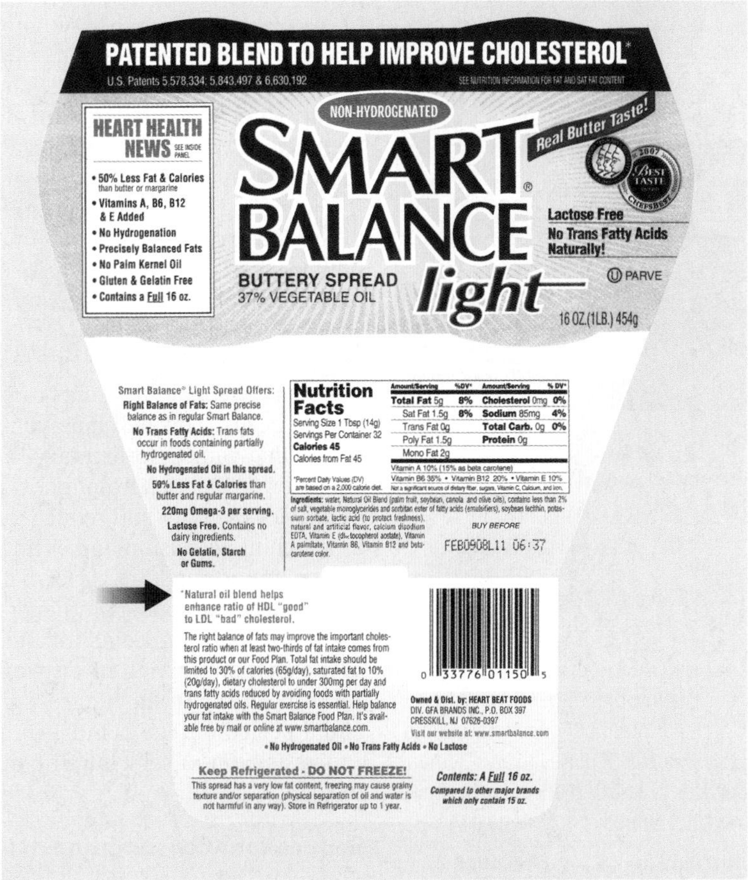

NUTRI-CASE GUSTAVO

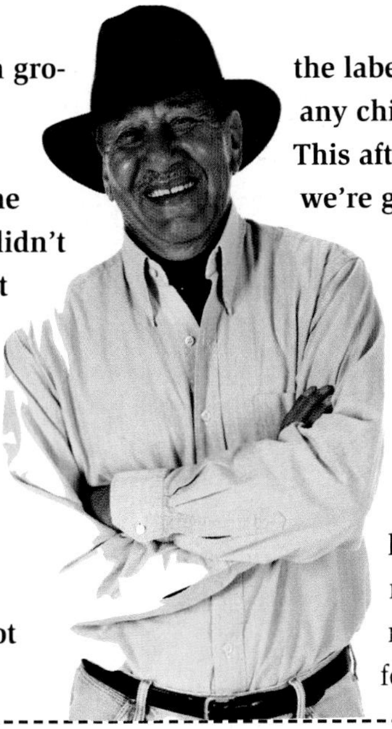

"Until last night, I hadn't stepped inside a grocery store for 10 years, maybe more. But then my wife fell and broke her hip and had to go to the hospital. On my way home from visiting her, I remembered that we didn't have much food in the house, so I thought I'd do a little shopping. Was I ever in for a shock. I don't know how my wife does it, choosing between all the different brands, reading those long labels. She never went to school past sixth grade, and she doesn't speak English very well, either! I bought a frozen chicken pie for my dinner, but it didn't taste right, so I got the package out of the trash and read all the labels, and that's when I realized there wasn't any chicken in it at all! It was made out of tofu! This afternoon, my daughter is picking me up, and we're going to do our grocery shopping together!"

Given what you've learned about FDA food labels, what parts of a food package would you advise Gustavo to be sure to read before he makes a choice? What other advice might you give him to make his grocery shopping easier? Imagine that, like Gustavo's wife, you have only limited skills in mathematics and reading. In that case, what other strategies might you use when shopping for nutritious foods?

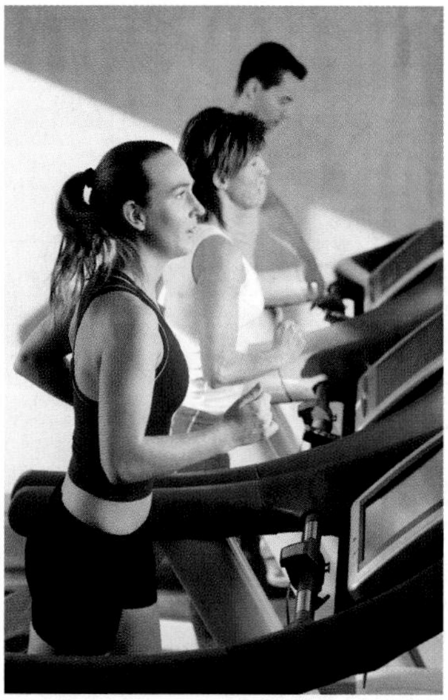

Being physically active for at least 30 minutes each day can reduce your risk for chronic diseases.

Dietary Guidelines for Americans

The **Dietary Guidelines for Americans** are a set of principles developed by the U.S. Department of Agriculture and the U.S. Department of Health and Human Services to promote health, reduce the risk for chronic diseases, and reduce the prevalence of overweight and obesity among Americans through improved nutrition and physical activity.[2] They are updated approximately every 5 years, and the current Guidelines were published in 2010. The 2010 Dietary Guidelines for Americans include twenty-three recommendations for the general population, but you don't have to remember all twenty-three! Instead, they encourage you to focus on the following four main ideas.

Following is a brief description of each of the chapters and key recommendations of the Dietary Guidelines for Americans. Refer to **Table 2.3** for specific examples of how you can alter your current diet and physical activity habits to meet some of the recommendations in the Dietary Guidelines.

Dietary Guidelines for Americans A set of principles developed by the U.S. Department of Agriculture and the U.S. Department of Health and Human Services to assist Americans in designing a healthful diet and lifestyle.

nutrient-dense foods Foods that provide the most nutrients for the least amount of energy (Calories).

nutrient density The relative amount of nutrients per amount of energy (or number of Calories).

Balance Calories to Maintain Weight

Consume adequate nutrients to promote your health while staying within your energy needs. This will help you maintain a healthful weight. You can achieve this by controlling your Calorie intake; if you are overweight or obese, you will need to consume fewer Calories from foods and beverages. At the same time, increase your level of physical activity and reduce the time that you spend in sedentary behaviors, such as watching television and sitting at the computer.

An important strategy for balancing your Calories is to consistently choose **nutrient-dense** foods and beverages—that is, foods and beverages that supply the highest level of nutrients for the lowest level of Calories. **Figure 2.4** compares 1 day of meals that are high in **nutrient density** to meals that are low in nutrient density. As you can see in this figure, skim milk is more nutrient dense than whole milk, and a peeled orange is more nutrient dense than an orange soft drink. This example can assist you in selecting the most nutrient-dense foods when planning your meals.

Reduce Your Consumption of Foods and Food Components of Concern

The Dietary Guidelines suggest that we reduce our consumption of the following foods and food components. Doing so will help us maintain a healthy weight and lower our risks for chronic diseases.

Sodium Excessive consumption of sodium, a major mineral found in salt, is linked to high blood pressure in some people. Eating a lot of sodium also can cause some

TABLE 2.3 Ways to Incorporate the Dietary Guidelines for Americans into Your Daily Life

If You Normally Do This	Try Doing This Instead
Watch television when you get home at night	Do 30 minutes of stretching or lifting of hand weights in front of the television
Drive to the store down the block	Walk to and from the store
Go out to lunch with friends	Take a 15- or 30-minute walk with your friends at lunchtime 3 days each week
Eat white bread with your sandwich	Eat whole-wheat bread or some other bread made from whole grains
Eat white rice or fried rice with your meal	Eat brown rice or try wild rice
Choose cookies or a candy bar for a snack	Choose a fresh nectarine, peach, apple, orange, or banana for a snack
Order french fries with your hamburger	Order a green salad with low-fat salad dressing on the side
Spread butter or margarine on your white toast each morning	Spread fresh fruit compote on whole-grain toast
Order a bacon double cheeseburger at your favorite restaurant	Order a turkey burger or grilled chicken sandwich without the cheese and bacon, and add lettuce and tomato
Drink nondiet soft drinks to quench your thirst	Drink iced tea, ice water with a slice of lemon, seltzer water, or diet soft drinks
Eat regular potato chips and pickles with your favorite sandwich	Eat carrot slices and crowns of fresh broccoli and cauliflower dipped in low-fat or nonfat ranch dressing

Meals with Foods High in Nutrient Density	Meals with Foods Low in Nutrient Density

Breakfast
1 cup cooked oatmeal with
 1/2 cup skim milk
1 slice whole-wheat toast with
 1 tsp. butter
6 fl. oz grapefruit juice

Breakfast
1 cup puffed rice cereal with
 1/2 cup whole milk
1 slice white toast with
 1 tsp. butter
6 fl. oz grape drink

Snack
1 peeled orange
1 cup nonfat yogurt

Snack
1 12-oz can orange soft drink
1.5 oz cheddar cheese

Lunch
Turkey sandwich
 3 oz turkey breast
 2 slices whole-grain bread
 2 tsp. Dijon mustard
 3 slices fresh tomato
 2 leaves red leaf lettuce
1 cup baby carrots with
 broccoli crowns
20 fl. oz (2.5 cups) water

Lunch
Hamburger
 3 oz regular ground beef
 1 white hamburger bun
 2 tsp. Dijon mustard
 1 tbsp. tomato ketchup
 2 leaves iceberg lettuce
1 snack-sized bag potato chips
20 fl. oz cola soft drink

Snack
1/2 whole-wheat bagel
1 tbsp. peanut butter
1 medium apple

Snack
3 chocolate sandwich cookies
1 12-oz can diet soft drink
10 Gummi Bears candy

Dinner
Spinach salad
 1 cup fresh spinach leaves
 1/4 cup sliced tomatoes
 1/4 cup diced green pepper
 1/2 cup kidney beans
 1 tbsp. fat-free Italian
 salad dressing
3 oz broiled chicken breast
1/2 cup cooked brown rice
1/2 cup steamed broccoli
8 fl. oz (1 cup) skim milk

Dinner
Green salad
 1 cup iceberg lettuce
 1/4 cup diced tomatoes
 1 tsp. green onions
 1/4 cup bacon bits
 1 tbsp. regular Ranch
 salad dressing
3 oz beef round steak,
 breaded and fried
1/2 cup cooked white rice
1/2 cup sweet corn
8 fl. oz (1 cup) iced tea

Figure 2.4 A comparison of 1 day's meals containing foods high in nutrient density to meals with foods low in nutrient density.

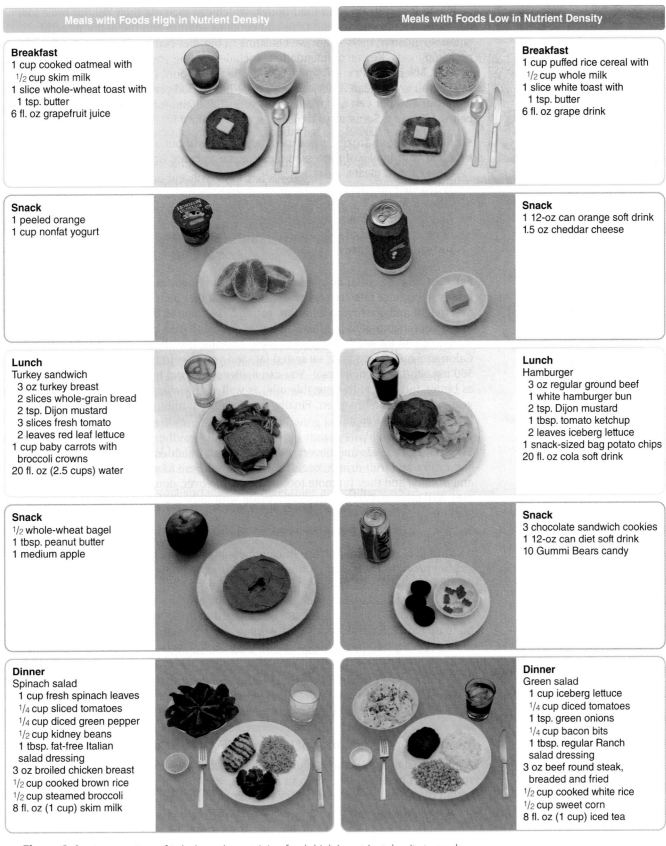

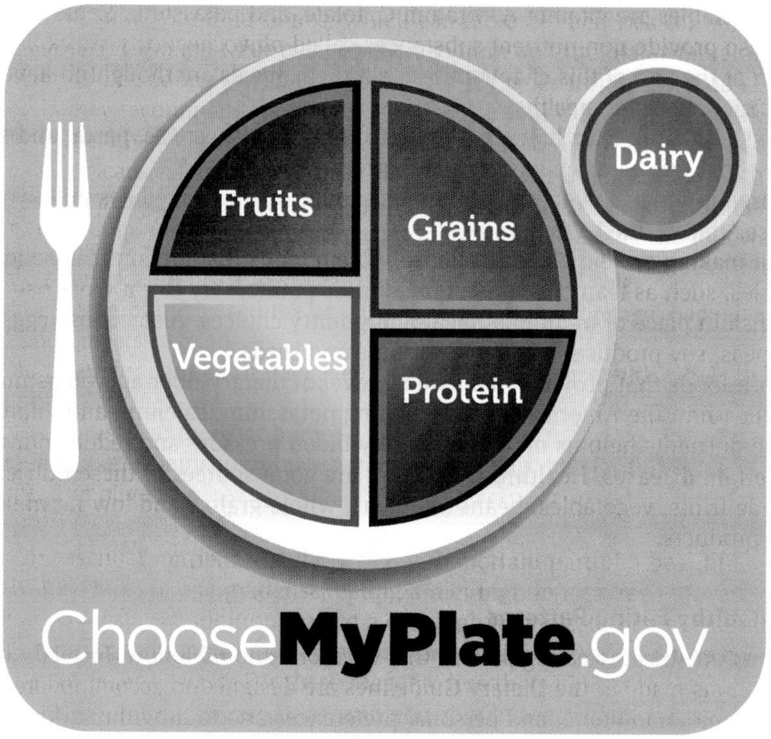

Figure 2.5 The USDA MyPlate graphic. MyPlate is an interactive food guidance system based on the 2010 Dietary Guidelines for Americans and the Dietary Reference Intakes from the National Academy of Sciences. Eating more fruits, vegetables, and whole grains and choosing foods low in fat, sugar, and sodium from the five food groups in MyPlate will help you balance your Calories and consume a healthier food pattern overall.

Data adapted from: HYPERLINK "http://www.nal.usda.gov/fnic/history/hist" www.nal.usda.gov/fnic/history/hist.htm and http://www.choosemyplate.gov/downloads/MyPlate/ABriefHistoryOfUSDAFoodGuides.pdf.

continue to be promoted until new MyPlate versions can be developed. MyPlate is intended to help Americans:

- eat in moderation to balance Calories
- eat a variety of foods
- consume the right proportion of each recommended food group
- personalize their eating plan
- increase their physical activity
- set goals for gradually improving their food choices and lifestyle.

Food Groups in the USDA Food Patterns

The food groups emphasized in the USDA Food Patterns, MyPlate graphic, and its online tools are grains, vegetables, fruits, dairy, and protein foods. These food groups are represented in the plate graphic with segments of five different colors. **Figure 2.6** illustrates each of these food groups and provides more detailed information on the nutrients they provide and recommended amounts to be consumed each day.

The Concept of Empty Calories

One concept introduced in the USDA Food Patterns is that of **empty Calories.** These are Calories from solid fats and/or added sugars that provide few or no nutrients. The USDA recommends that you limit the empty Calories you eat to a small number that fits your Calorie and nutrient needs depending on your age, gender, and level of physical activity. Foods that contain the most empty Calories include cakes, cookies, pastries, doughnuts, soft drinks, fruit drinks, cheese, pizza, ice cream, sausages, hot dogs, bacon, and ribs. High-sugar foods, such as candies, desserts, gelatin, soft drinks, and alcoholic beverages, are called *empty Calorie foods*, as all of the Calories in these foods are empty! However, some foods that contain empty Calories from solid fats and added sugars also provide important nutrients. Examples are sweetened applesauce, sweetened breakfast cereals, regular ground beef, and whole milk. To reduce your intake of empty Calories but ensure you get adequate nutrients, choose the unsweetened or lean or nonfat versions of these foods.

empty Calories A term used by the USDA to indicate Calories from solid fats and/or added sugars.

NUTRITION LABEL ACTIVITY

How Realistic Are the Serving Sizes Listed on Food Labels?

Many people read food labels to determine the energy (caloric) value of foods, but it is less common to pay close attention to the actual serving size that corresponds to the listed caloric value. To test how closely your "naturally selected" serving size matches the actual serving size of certain foods, try these label activities:

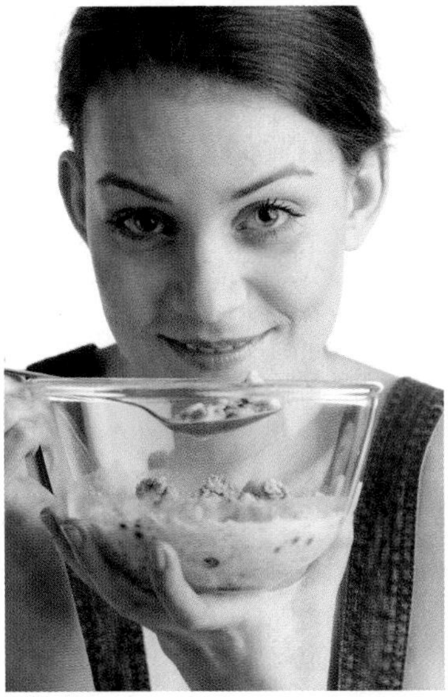

- Choose a breakfast cereal that you commonly eat. Pour the amount of cereal you would normally eat into a bowl. Before adding milk, use a measuring cup to measure the amount of cereal you poured. Now read the label of the cereal to determine the serving size (for example, 1/2 cup or 1 cup) and the caloric value listed on the label. How do your "naturally selected" serving size and the label-defined serving size compare?
- At your local grocery store, locate various boxes of snack crackers. Look at the number of crackers and total Calories per serving listed on the labels of crackers such as regular Triscuits, reduced-fat Triscuits, Vegetable Thins, and Ritz crackers. How do the number of crackers and total Calories per serving differ for the serving size listed on each box? How do the serving sizes listed in the Nutrition Facts Panel compare to how many crackers you would usually eat?

These activities are just two examples of ways to understand how nutrition labels can help you make balanced and healthful food choices. As many people do not know what constitutes a serving size, they are inclined to consume too much of some foods (such as snack foods and meat) and too little of other foods (such as fruits and vegetables).

Figure 2.7 identifies the number of cups or oz-equivalent servings recommended for a 2,000-kcal diet and gives examples of amounts equal to 1 cup or 1 oz-equivalent for foods in each group. As you study this figure, notice the variety of examples for each group. For instance, an oz-equivalent serving from the grains group can mean one slice of bread or two pancakes. Because of their low density, 2 cups of raw, leafy vegetables, such as spinach, actually constitutes a 1-cup serving from the vegetables group. Although an oz-equivalent serving of meat is actually 1 oz, 1/2 oz of nuts also qualifies. One egg, 1 tablespoon of peanut butter, and 1/4 cup cooked legumes are also considered 1 oz-equivalents from the protein foods group. Although it may seem unnatural and inconvenient to measure foods, understanding equivalent amounts is important. **Figure 2.8** shows you a practical way to estimate food amounts.

It is important to understand that no nationally standardized definition for a serving size exists for any food. Thus, an amount that the USDA describes as an ounce may not be equal to a serving size identified on a food label. For instance, the serving size for crackers in MyPlate is 2 rye crispbreads, 5 whole-wheat crackers, or 7 small square or round crackers. In contrast, a serving size for crackers on a food label can range from 5 to 18 crackers, depending on the size and weight of the cracker. When comparing amounts in MyPlate to serving sizes on packaged foods, check the measurement used for a serving size at the top of the Nutrition Facts Panel. Try the Nutrition Label Activity to determine whether the serving sizes listed on assorted food labels match the serving sizes you normally eat.

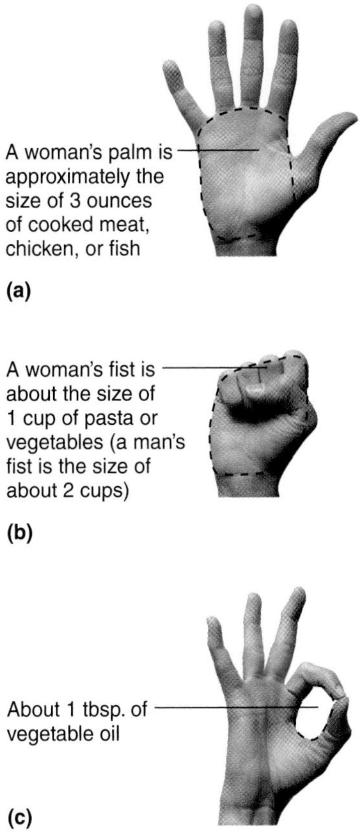
A woman's palm is approximately the size of 3 ounces of cooked meat, chicken, or fish
(a)
A woman's fist is about the size of 1 cup of pasta or vegetables (a man's fist is the size of about 2 cups)
(b)
About 1 tbsp. of vegetable oil
(c)

Figure 2.8 Use your hands to help you estimate the amounts of common foods.

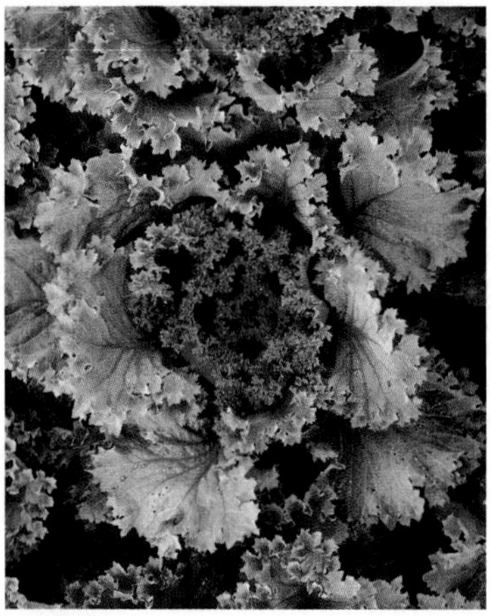

Nutrient-packed foods—such as kale, which is an excellent source of calcium—should be part of a well-rounded diet.

For items sold individually, such as muffins, burgers, bottled juices, and so on, the equivalent amounts in MyPlate vary—sometimes dramatically. For example, a "mini" bagel is 1 oz, whereas a typical large bagel served in delis is 4 oz! In addition, serving sizes in restaurants, cafes, and movie theatres have grown substantially over the past 30 years.[3] This "supersizing" phenomenon, now seen even at home, indicates a major shift in accessibility to foods and in accepted eating behaviors. It has also become an important contributor to the rise in obesity rates around the world. If you don't want to gain weight, it's important to become educated about portion size. In a study conducted by Young and Nestle,[9] introductory nutrition students were asked to take to class a "medium-sized" bagel, baked potato, muffin, apple, or cookie. The foods the students took to class were then weighed, and most well exceeded the amount that would be assumed to be consistent with the USDA's MyPlate recommendations. Thus, when using diet-planning tools, such as food labels and the USDA's ChooseMyPlate website, it is essential to learn the definition of an equivalent amount for the tool you are using and *then* measure your food intake to determine whether you are meeting the guidelines. Refer to the You Do the Math box (page 59) to estimate how much physical activity you would need to do to expend the excess energy you consume because of increasing food portion sizes.

Ethnic Variations of MyPyramid

As you know, the population of the United States is culturally and ethnically diverse, and this diversity influences our food choices. Foods that we may typically consider a part of an Asian, a Latin American, or a Mediterranean diet can also fit into a healthful diet. You can easily incorporate foods that match your specific ethnic, religious, or other preferences into your own personalized MyPlate daily food plan. You can also use one of the many ethnic and cultural variations of the previous USDA Food Guide Pyramid. These include the Latin American Diet Pyramid and the Asian Diet Pyramid, shown in **Figure 2.9**. There are also variations for Native Americans, African Americans, and many others.[4] These variations illustrate that anyone can design a healthful diet to accommodate his or her food preferences.

Of these variations, the Mediterranean diet has enjoyed considerable popularity. Does it deserve its reputation as a healthful diet? Check out the Hot Topic to learn more.

HOT TOPIC

The Mediterranean Diet

A Mediterranean-style diet has received significant attention in recent years, as the rates of cardiovascular disease in many Mediterranean countries are substantially lower than the rates in the United States. These countries include Portugal, Spain, Italy, France, Greece, Turkey, and Israel. Each country has unique dietary patterns; however, they share the following characteristics:

- Meat is eaten monthly, and eggs, poultry, fish, and sweets are eaten weekly, making the diet low in saturated fats and refined sugars.
- The fat used predominantly for cooking and flavor is olive oil, making the diet high in monounsaturated fats.
- Foods eaten daily include grains, such as bread, pasta, couscous, and bulgur; fruits; beans and other legumes; nuts; vegetables; and cheese and yogurt. These choices make this diet high in fiber and rich in vitamins and minerals.

Figure 2.10 illustrates the Mediterranean Diet Pyramid. It suggests daily physical activity and daily intake of breads, cereals, and other grains; fruits, legumes, and other vegetables; and nuts. It also includes frequent consumption of meat, fish, poultry, and eggs. Cheese and yogurt, rather than milk, are the primary dairy sources. A unique feature of the Mediterranean diet is the consumption of wine and olive oil daily.

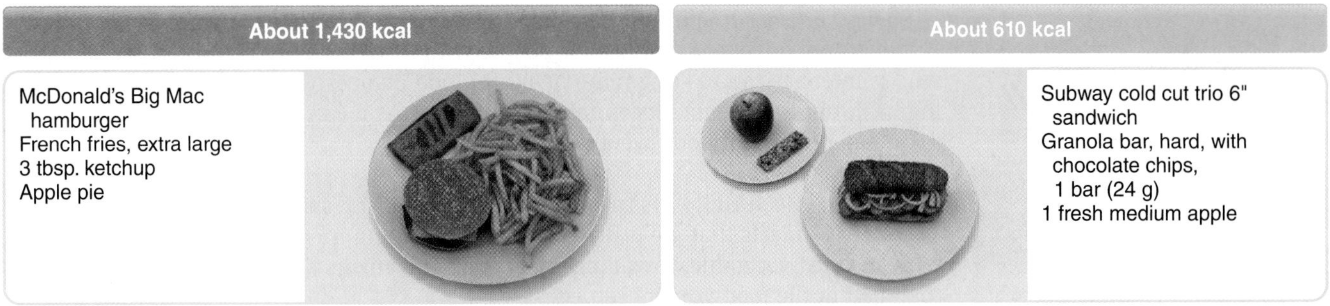
About 1,430 kcal
McDonald's Big Mac hamburger
French fries, extra large
3 tbsp. ketchup
Apple pie
About 610 kcal
Subway cold cut trio 6" sandwich
Granola bar, hard, with chocolate chips, 1 bar (24 g)
1 fresh medium apple

Figure 2.12 The energy density of two fast-food meals. The meal on the left is higher in total kilocalories and fat, while the meal on the right is lower in kilocalories and fat and is the preferred choice for someone trying to lose weight.

The Healthful Way to Eat Out

Most restaurants, even fast-food restaurants, offer lower-fat menu items. For instance, eating a regular McDonald's hamburger, a small order of french fries, and a diet beverage or water provides 480 kcal and 19 g of fat (35% of kcal from fat). To provide some vegetables for the day, you can add a side salad with low-fat or nonfat salad dressing. Other fast-food restaurants also offer smaller portions, sandwiches made with whole-grain bread, grilled chicken or other lean meats, and side salads. Many sit-down restaurants offer "lite" menu items, such as grilled chicken and a variety of vegetables, which are usually a much better choice than foods from the regular menu.

Here are some other suggestions on how to eat out in moderation. Practice some of these Quick Tips every time you eat out.

QUICK TIPS

Eating Right When You're Eating Out

- Avoid all-you-can-eat buffet-style restaurants.
- Avoid appetizers that are breaded, fried, or filled with cheese or meat, or skip the appetizer completely.
- Order a healthful appetizer as an entrée instead of a larger meal.
- Order your meal from the children's menu.
- Share an entrée with a friend.
- Order broth-based soups instead of cream-based soups.
- Order any meat dish grilled or broiled, and avoid fried or breaded meat dishes.
- If you order a meat dish, select lean cuts of meat.
- Order a meatless dish filled with vegetables and whole grains. Avoid dishes with cream sauces and a lot of cheese.
- Instead of a beef burger, order a chicken burger, fish burger, or veggie burger.
- Order a salad with low-fat or nonfat dressing served on the side.
- Order steamed vegetables on the side instead of potatoes or rice. If you order potatoes, make sure to get a baked potato (with very little butter or sour cream, on the side).
- Order beverages with few or no Calories, such as water, tea, or diet drinks. Avoid coffee drinks made with syrups, as well as those made with cream, whipping cream, or whole milk.
- Don't feel you have to eat everything you're served. If you feel full, take the rest home for another meal.
- Skip dessert or share one dessert with a lot of friends, or order fresh fruit for dessert.
- Watch out for those "yogurt parfaits" offered at some fast-food restaurants. Many are loaded with sugar, fat, and Calories.

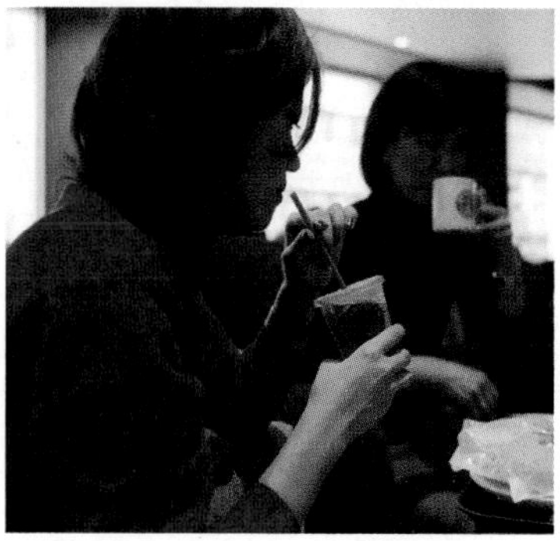

When ordering your favorite coffee drink, avoid flavored syrups, cream, and whipping cream and request reduced-fat or skim milk instead.

Table 2.5 lists some examples of low-fat foods you can choose when you eat out.[7] Although provided as examples for people with diabetes, they are useful for anyone who is interested in making more healthful food choices while eating out. By choosing healthful foods and appropriate portion sizes, you can eat out regularly and still maintain a healthful body weight.

RECAP **Healthful ways to eat out include choosing smaller menu items, ordering meats that are grilled or broiled, avoiding fried foods, choosing items with steamed vegetables, avoiding energy-rich appetizers and desserts, and eating less than half of the food you are served.**

TABLE 2.5 Low-Fat Food Choices Available in Restaurants

Appetizers	Salads	Breads	Entrées	Fats	Desserts
Minestrone soup	Tossed with mixed greens, lettuce, tomato, and cucumber	Whole-grain rolls	Baked halibut with thyme and fresh-squeezed lemon	Diet margarine	Fresh fruit
Chicken soup with vegetables		Corn tortillas		Low-fat/ low-Calorie salad dressing	Fruit sorbet
Raw celery and carrots with low-fat or nonfat ranch dressing	Spinach salad with crab meat, raw vegetables, and nonfat salad dressing	Whole-wheat or pumpernickel bread	Grilled skinless chicken breast with tomato salsa	Low-fat sour cream or yogurt	Fat-free or low-fat yogurt

Data from American Diabetes Association. 2007. Your Guide to Eating Out. www.diabetes.org/nutrition-and-recipes/nutrition/eatingoutguide.jsp. Printed with permission.

Nutrition DEBATE

Can Functional Foods Improve Our Health?

Many conventional foods "provide a health benefit beyond basic nutrition" and therefore qualify as functional foods. For example, oatmeal provides carbohydrates, but its soluble fiber also improves bowel function. Other types of functional foods (also called *nutraceuticals*) are processed to create fortified, enriched, or enhanced foods, which provide a higher level of micronutrients than the same foods would supply in an unprocessed form. For example, iodine is added to salt, orange juice is fortified with calcium, and milk is enriched with extra calcium. Sometimes, the health-promoting substances are developed in a functional food by altering the way in which the food is produced. For example, eggs with higher levels of omega-3 fatty acids result from feeding hens a special diet. And produce can be genetically engineered to contain higher levels of nutrients. Dietary supplements also qualify as functional foods.[7]

Are Functional Foods Safe?

The FDA regulates functional foods in the same way it regulates conventional foods. This means that in order for a food to be allowed on the market, any "functional" ingredient added to that food must be generally recognized as safe.

Recently, other federal agencies and consumer advocacy groups have petitioned the FDA to reevaluate the way it regulates functional foods.[8] They contend that many food companies are making unsubstantiated health claims for their products. They also warn that dozens of products currently sold as foods contain ingredients, such as herbs, that are not FDA approved for use in foods. They caution that such products could have adverse health effects on vulnerable consumers.

In response to these and other concerns, the FDA is considering a new regulatory system by which any product bearing health claims would be subject to FDA oversight. Thus, not only herbs, but even conventional food ingredients promoted for use in the treatment or prevention of disease in humans, would be subject to FDA control.[9] But until such a system is in effect, consumers should remain skeptical about the safety and effectiveness of functional foods.

Are Functional Foods Effective?

Is there any research to support the claims of health benefits made by manufacturers of functional foods? That depends on the product. So if you're considering regular consumption of a functional food, do your homework. To give you some practice, let's consider one currently on the market—designer yogurt.

People have been consuming yogurt for thousands of years. Yogurt contains live bacteria, called *probiotics* ("pro-life"), which are known to benefit human health. These helpful bacteria reproduce in the food naturally during the production process. Probiotics are also available in supplement form.

How do probiotics work? When a person consumes a product containing probiotics, the bacteria adhere to the intestinal wall for a few days, exerting their beneficial effects. Although their exact actions are currently being researched, it is believed that some crowd out harmful bacterial, viral, and fungal species; some produce nutrients and other helpful substances; and others influence the immune system.[10] They may be beneficial for conditions such as some forms of diarrhea, irritable bowel syndrome, inflammatory bowel disease, lactose intolerance, and certain types of infections.[10–12]

It is important to remember that, in order to be effective, foods containing probiotics must provide an adequate number of bacteria, thought to be 1 to 10 billion.[13] In the United States, the National Yogurt Association has created a "Live Active Culture" seal to be placed on yogurt containers to indicate that the yogurt has an adequate amount of active bacteria per gram. Also, because they can survive in the body for only a limited period of time, probiotics should be consumed daily, and they must be stored properly (usually refrigerated) and consumed within a relatively brief period of time.

Some food manufacturers are employing researchers to find and cultivate strains of probiotic bacteria that have specific health benefits. For example, Activia, a yogurt made by Dannon, contains a probiotic species said to promote regular bowel movements by reducing the time stool stays in the colon. The longer fecal matter remains in the colon, the more water is removed from it, and the harder it gets, so reduced transit time means softer bowel movements. Is this claim valid?

Four studies published in peer-reviewed journals found that consuming three 4-oz servings of Activia a day for 10 to 14 days sped up stool transit time by 10% to 40%. This effect was seen in both men and women. Convinced? If constipation were a problem for you, would you eat Activia three times a day?

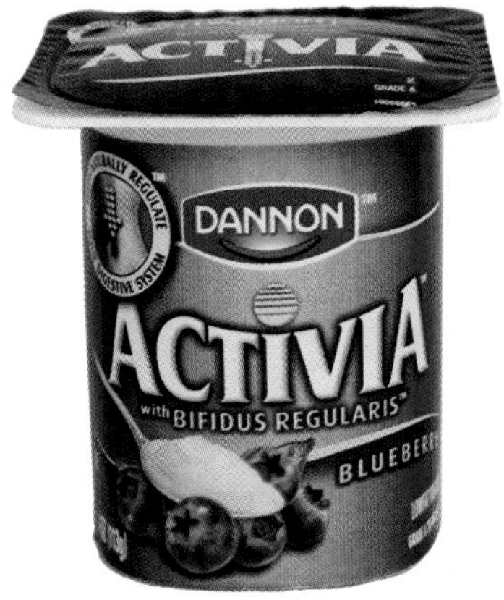

Consuming Activia yogurt may improve bowel function.

Chapter Review

Test Yourself ANSWERS

1. False. A healthful diet can be achieved by food alone; particular attention must be paid to adequacy, variety, moderation, and balance. However, some individuals may need to take vitamin supplements under certain circumstances.

2. False. The fact that something is stated on a food label doesn't guarantee it is true! Structure–function claims—such as "Supports healthy bones!" and "Promotes regularity!"—are not regulated by the FDA and may or may not be backed with solid research evidence.

3. False. A cup of black coffee has about 2 kcal. Adding a teaspoon of sugar and a tablespoon of whole milk would increase that amount to about 27 kcal. In contrast, a coffee mocha might contain from 350 to 500 kcal, depending on its size and precise contents.

Find the Quack

Jimena is a 19-year-old sophomore in a small liberal arts college. Everyone in Jimena's family is either overweight or obese, but now that she is away from home and living at an out-of-state school, Jimena has become determined to break out of her "family pattern" and lose weight. In a fashion magazine, she reads about a grapefruit diet called the Mayo Clinic Diet. Jimena figures that any diet with a medical clinic behind it must be reputable, so she decides to try it. The diet requires that Jimena eat two eggs and two slices of bacon every morning with an 8-oz glass of grapefruit juice or half a grapefruit; eat a salad, red meat or poultry, and another serving of grapefruit at lunch; and eat a salad, red meat or poultry, and another serving of grapefruit at dinner. No snacks between meals are allowed. The diet is to be followed for 8 weeks: 12 days on the diet followed by 2 days off, then resumption of the diet again.

The magazine article makes the following claims:

- The consumption of grapefruit or grapefruit juice is absolutely essential because the grapefruit "is a catalyst that starts the fat-burning process."
- The consumption of bacon and eggs at breakfast and salad at lunch and dinner is also absolutely essential because these foods combine to promote fat burning.
- Anyone following the diet will lose 52 lb in 8 weeks. No weight loss will occur during the first 4 days, but the average weight loss for the remainder of the 8-week period will be 1 lb a day.
- The diet is safe and healthful if followed as described for 8 weeks.

1. Although you have not yet studied digestion and the absorption of food, do you believe the article's claim that there is something unique about grapefruit that catalyzes (initiates and speeds up) fat burning? Why or why not?
2. If the loss of 1 lb of body weight requires the body to expend 3,500 kcal more than it takes in, do you think it is possible for anyone trying the grapefruit diet to lose 52 lb in 56 days, without any prescribed physical activity and the daily consumption of two eggs, two strips of bacon, three servings of grapefruit, two salads, and two servings of meat or poultry? Why or why not?
3. What two food groups are entirely missing from this diet? Do you think this is problematic for some dieters? Why or why not?
4. Do you believe that this grapefruit diet, which the article refers to as the Mayo Clinic Diet, is truly endorsed by the Mayo Clinic—the medical institution based in Rochester, Minnesota, and known internationally for its high-quality healthcare? Go online and, using your favorite search engine, type in the search terms "grapefruit diet" and "Mayo Clinic." What do you discover?

Answers can be found on the companion website, at www.pearsonhighered.com/thompsonmanore.

NutriTools

Check out the companion website at www.pearsonhighered.com/thompsonmanore, or use MyNutritionLab.com, to access interactive animations, including:

- What's Missing on This Label?

Review Questions

1. The Nutrition Facts Panel identifies which of the following?
   a. all of the nutrients and Calories in the package of food
   b. the Recommended Dietary Allowance for each nutrient in the package of food
   c. a footnote identifying the Tolerable Upper Intake Level for each nutrient in the package of food
   d. the % Daily Values of select nutrients in a serving of the packaged food
2. An adequate diet
   a. provides enough energy to meet minimum daily requirements.
   b. provides enough energy, nutrients, and fiber to maintain a person's health.
   c. provides a sufficient variety of nutrients to maintain a healthful weight and to optimize the body's metabolic processes.
   d. contains combinations of foods that provide healthful proportions of nutrients.
3. The Dietary Guidelines for Americans recommend which of the following?
   a. choosing and preparing foods without salt
   b. consuming two alcoholic beverages per day
   c. replacing solid fats with vegetable oils
   d. following the Mediterranean diet
4. Of the five food groups in MyPlate, which should make up half of your plate?
   a. grains
   b. vegetables
   c. fruits and dairy
   d. fruits and vegetables
5. What does it mean to choose foods for their nutrient density?
   a. Dense foods, such as peanut butter and chicken, are more nutritious choices than transparent foods, such as mineral water and gelatin.
   b. Foods with a lot of nutrients per Calorie, such as fish, are more nutritious than foods with fewer nutrients per Calorie, such as candy.
   c. Calorie-dense foods, such as cheesecake, should be avoided.
   d. Fat makes foods dense; thus, foods high in fat should be avoided.
6. True or false? For most foods, the USDA has established a standardized definition of a serving size.
7. True or false? Structure–function claims on food labels must be approved by the FDA.
8. True or false? Empty Calories are the extra amount of energy a person can consume after meeting all essential needs through eating nutrient-dense foods.
9. True or false? The USDA classifies beans, peas, and lentils in both the vegetables group and the protein foods group.
10. True or false? More than half of all Americans eat out at least once a week.

Answers to Review Questions can be found at the back of this text, and additional essay questions and answers are located on the companion website, at www.pearsonhighered.com/thompsonmanore.

Web Resources

www.fda.gov
U.S. Food and Drug Administration (FDA)

Learn more about the government agency that regulates our food and first established regulations for nutrition information on food labels.

www.nccam.nih.gov/health/probiotics
National Center for Complementary and Alternative Medicine

The brochure "An Introduction to Probiotics" provides additional information on probiotics.

www.healthierus.gov/dietaryguidelines
Dietary Guidelines for Americans

Use these guidelines to make healthful changes in your food choices and physical activity habits to help reduce your risk for chronic disease.

www.chooseMyPlate.gov
The USDA's MyPlate home page.

www.oldwayspt.org
Oldways Preservation and Exchange Trust

Find variations of ethnic and cultural food pyramids.

www.hp2010.nhlbihin.net/portion
The National Institutes of Health (NIH) Portion Distortion Quiz

Take this fun quiz to see if you know how today's food portions compare to those of 20 years ago.

www.eatright.org
The American Dietetic Association

Visit the food and nutrition information section of this website for additional resources to help you achieve a healthful lifestyle.

NutriTools

Build a Meal

See live updates of Nutritional Facts based on your selections!

Nutrition Facts

Serving Size 1 Meal

Amount Per Serving

Calories 481	Calories from Fat 45

	% Daily Value**
Total Fat 5g	8%
Saturated Fat 1g	20%
Monosaturated *Fat* 1g	
Polyunsaturated Fat 7g	
Cholesterol 72mg	24%
Sodium 696mg	29%
Potassium 517mg	15%
Total Carbohydrate 47g	16%
Dietary Fiber 6g	24%
Sugars 10g	
Protein 31g	62%

Vitamin A	3%	•	Vitamin C	15%
Calcium	30%	•	Iron	16%
Thiamin	17%	•	Riboflavin	17%
Niacin	33%	•	Folate	11%
Vitamin B6	21%	•	Vitamin B12	20%

* Contains less than 2 percent of the daily value of these nutrients.
** Percent Daily Values (DV) are based on a 2,000 calorie diet. Your daily values may be higher or lower depending on your calorie needs.

Ingredients

Roasted chicken, Cooked broccoli, Mixed vegetables, Brown rice, Strawberries, Apple, Iced tea

Nutritional Score

Could be better — Good — Highly Nutritous

Calories	7 kcal	Sodium	24 mg
Total Fat	.1 g	Total Carb.	0 g
Cholesterol	0 mg	Protein	.9 g

Soda | Ice tea | 2% Milk | Sports drink | Apple Juice

Main Course | Side Dish | Starter | Fast Food | Beverages | ○ Reset Activity

Build a virtual meal by choosing food icons in many combinations!

Learn the nutritional values of your food choices as you build them!

Score your meal's nutritional value!

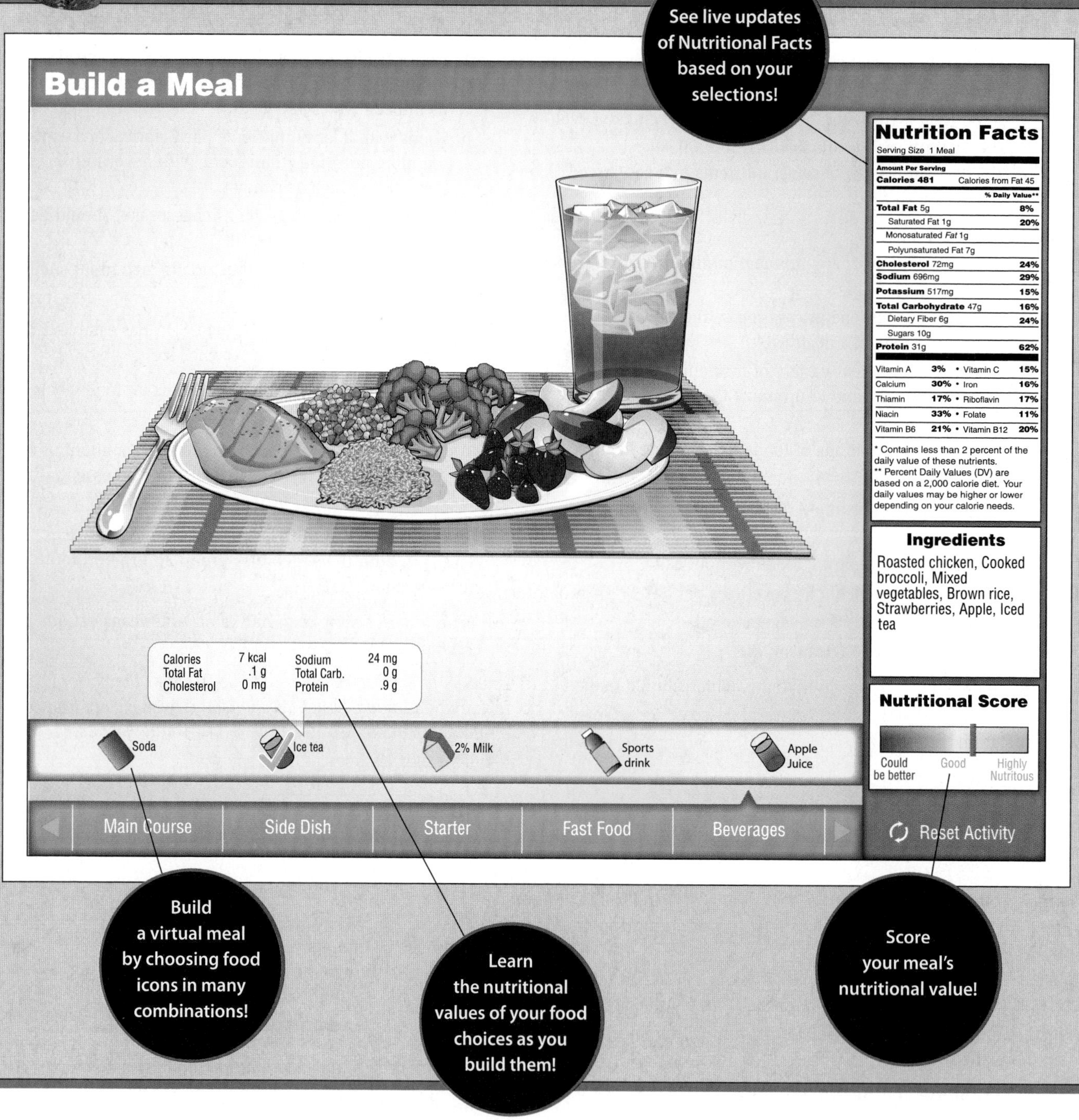

To build your meal, just visit www.pearsonhighered.com/thompsonmanore **or** www.mynutritionlab.com

After building your meal, you should be able to answer these questions:

1. Is your meal meeting your kcal needs as well as your nutrient needs?
2. How can you build a highly nutritious meal when you do not eat meat?
3. How do you know you're selecting the best options for fruits and vegetables?
4. In what ways can your meal meet your calcium needs if you do not drink milk?
5. Is your beverage choice adding to or subtracting from your overall nutritional score?

Phytochemicals

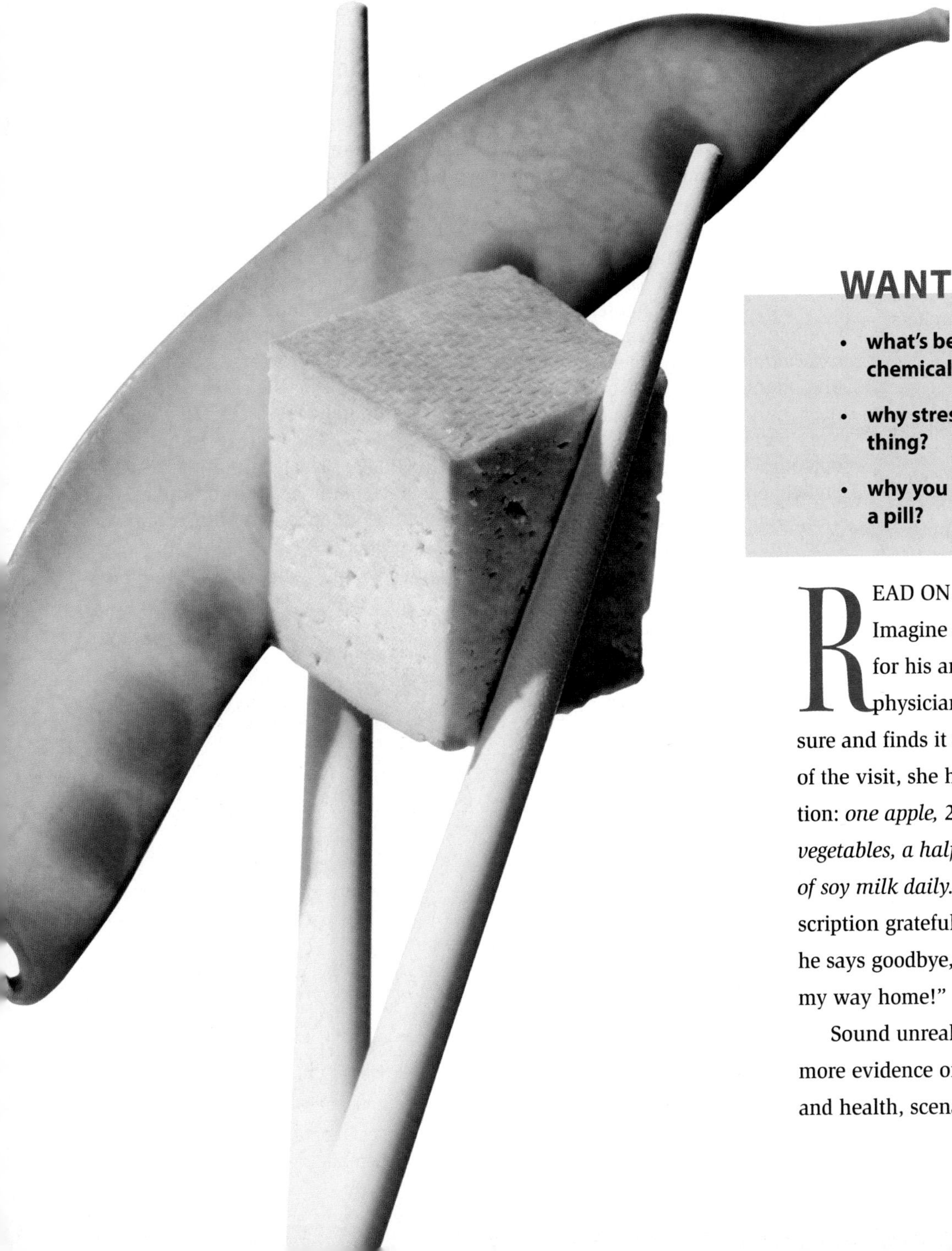

WANT TO FIND OUT . . .

- **what's behind all the fuss about phytochemicals?**
- **why stressing your cells can be a *good* thing?**
- **why you can't put fruits and veggies into a pill?**

READ ON.

Imagine a patient seeing his physician for his annual physical exam. The physician measures his blood pressure and finds it slightly elevated. At the close of the visit, she hands the patient a prescription: *one apple, 2 servings of dark-green leafy vegetables, a half cup of oatmeal, and 2 cups of soy milk daily.* The patient accepts the prescription gratefully, assuring his physician as he says goodbye, "I'll stop at the market on my way home!"

Sound unreal? As researchers provide more evidence on the link between nutrition and health, scenarios like this might become familiar. Here, we explore *In Depth* some of the reasons that certain chemicals that occur naturally in plant foods are thought to promote health. Who knows? When you finish reading, you might find yourself writing up your own health-promoting grocery list!

What Are Phytochemicals?

Phyto- means "plant," so **phytochemicals** are plant chemicals. These naturally occurring compounds are believed to protect plants from a variety of injurious agents, including insects, microbes, the oxygen they produce, and the UV light they capture and transform into the nutrients we need. Although more than 5,000 different phytochemicals have already been identified, researchers believe there are thousands more.[1] Any one food can contain hundreds. **Figure 1** on page 69 shows some groups of only a few of the most common.

Phytochemicals are not considered nutrients—that is, substances necessary for sustaining life. Even for carotenoids, a well-studied class of phytochemicals, the Food and Nutrition Board of the Institute of Medicine concluded in 2000 that there is not enough evidence to establish a daily recommended intake.[2] So, whereas a total lack of vitamin C or iron is incompatible with life, a total lack of lutein or allylic sulfur compounds is not known to be fatal. On the other hand, eating an abundance of phytochemical-rich foods has been shown to reduce the risk for cardiovascular disease, cancer, diabetes, Alzheimer's disease, cataracts, and age-related functional decline.[1,3]

The evidence supporting this observation of a reduced disease risk stems mainly from large epidemiological studies in which people report their usual food intake to researchers, who then look for relationships between specific dietary patterns and common diseases. These large studies often find that the reduced disease risk from high intakes of plant foods cannot be attributed solely to differences in intake of macronutrients and micronutrients. This suggests that other compounds in plant foods may be reducing the risk for disease.

As we noted in Chapter 1, epidemiological studies can only reveal *associations* between general patterns of food intake and health conditions; they cannot prove that a food or dietary pattern directly *causes* a health outcome. To better understand how phytochemicals influence health and disease, researchers have turned to biochemical, cellular, and animal studies.

How Do Phytochemicals Reduce Our Risk for Disease?

For decades, laboratory experiments have shown that, at least in the test tube, many phytochemicals have antioxidant properties. As you will learn in Chapter 8, antioxidants can neutralize certain unstable, highly reactive compounds, called *free radicals*, that damage our cells. Free radicals are an unavoidable by-product of normal metabolism, but they are also produced in response to radiation, air pollution, industrial chemicals, tobacco smoke, infections, and even intense exercise.

The health effects of this damage, also known as oxidative damage, typically don't arise until later in life. Many **diseases of aging**, such as cardiovascular disease, cancer, cataracts, arthritis, and certain neurologic disorders, have been linked to oxidative damage that accumulates over years. It's no surprise, therefore, that antioxidant-rich foods reduce the risk for these conditions.

Unfortunately, biology is not fully explained by a few simple chemical reactions. In fact, the latest research evidence on phytochemicals suggests that their health-promoting properties are largely unrelated to the antioxidant activity measured in the test tube.[4,5] This is in part because phytochemicals can be modified during digestion and after absorption, so that cells are exposed to **metabolites** that are structurally different from the phytochemicals found in foods.[5] Clearly, the test tube cannot explain what is happening inside the body.

Fortunately, researchers have also done cellular and animal studies, which have revealed that phytochemicals have many health-promoting functions independent of their antioxidant properties. For example, phytochemicals are thought to

phytochemicals Compounds found in plants that are believed to have health-promoting effects in humans.

diseases of aging Conditions that typically occur later in life as a result of lifelong accumulated risk, such as exposure to high-fat diets, a lack of physical activity, and excess sun exposure.

metabolites The form that nutrients take when they have been used by the body. For example, lactate is a metabolite of carbohydrate that is produced when we use carbohydrate for energy.

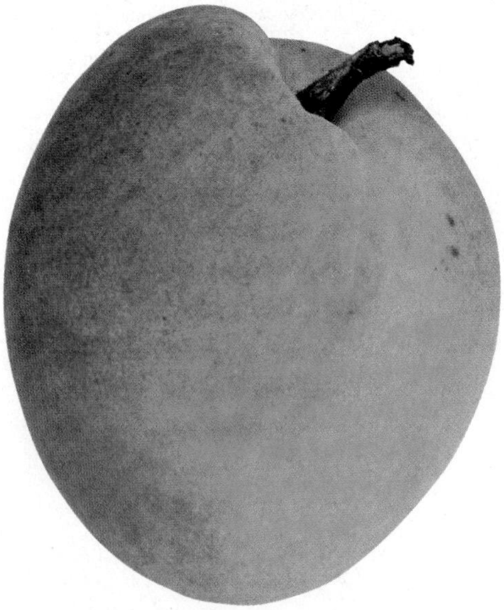

Apricots contain carotenoids, a type of phytochemical.

Phytochemical	Health Claims	Food Source	
Carotenoids: alpha-carotene, beta-carotene, lutein, lycopene, zeaxanthin, etc.	Diets with foods rich in these phytochemicals may reduce the risk for cardiovascular disease, certain cancers (e.g., prostate), and age-related eye diseases (cataracts, macular degeneration).	Red, orange, and deep-green vegetables and fruits, such as carrots, cantaloupe, sweet potatoes, apricots, kale, spinach, pumpkin, and tomatoes	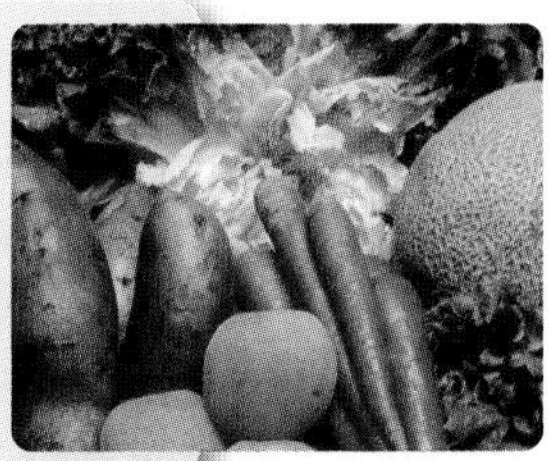
Flavonoids:[1] flavones, flavonols (e.g., quercetin), catechins (e.g., epigallocatechin gallate or EGCG), anthocyanidins, isoflavonoids, etc.	Diets with foods rich in these phytochemicals are associated with lower risk for cardiovascular disease and cancer, possibly because of reduced inflammation, blood clotting, and blood pressure and increased detoxification of carcinogens or reduction in replication of cancerous cells.	Berries, black and green tea, chocolate, purple grapes and juice, citrus fruits, olives, soybeans and soy products (soy milk, tofu, soy flour, textured vegetable protein), flaxseed, whole wheat	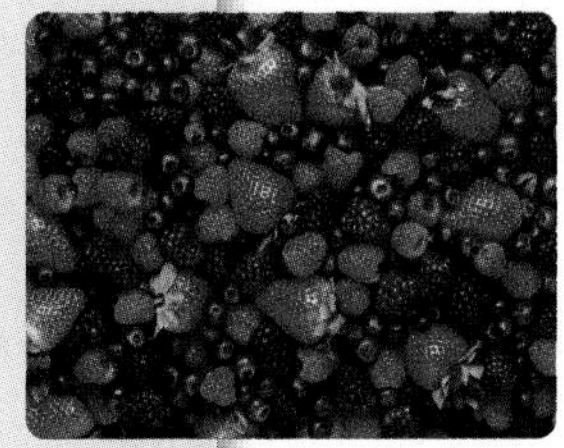
Phenolic acids:[1] ellagic acid, ferulic acid, caffeic acid, curcumin, etc.	Similar benefits as flavonoids.	Coffee beans, fruits (apples, pears, berries, grapes, oranges, prunes, strawberries), potatoes, mustard, oats, soy	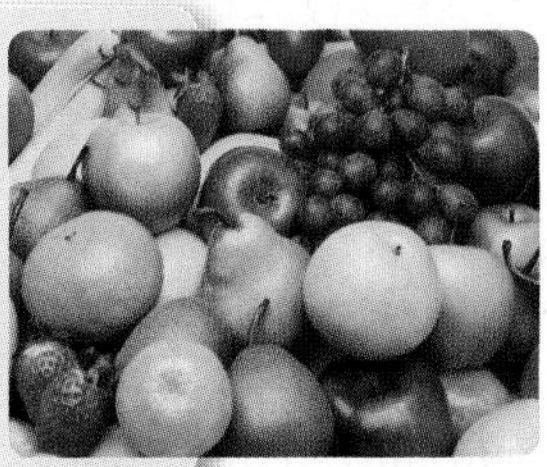
Phytoestrogens:[2] genistein, diadzein, lignans	Foods rich in these phytochemicals may provide benefits to bones and reduce the risk for cardiovascular disease and cancers of reproductive tissues (e.g., breast, prostate).	Soybeans and soy products (soy milk, tofu, soy flour, textured vegetable protein), flaxseed, whole grains	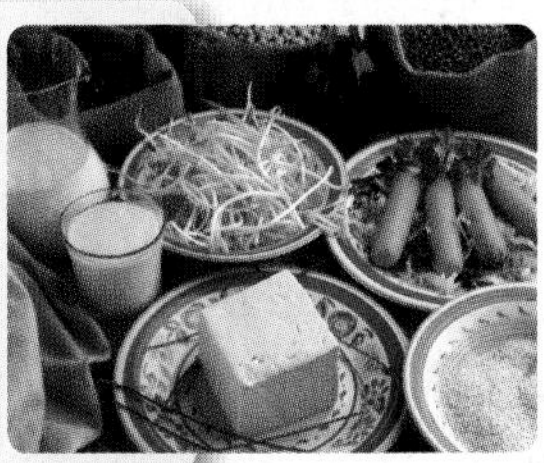
Organosulfur compounds: allylic sulfur compounds, indoles, isothiocyanates, etc.	Foods rich in these phytochemicals may protect against a wide variety of cancers.	Garlic, leeks, onions, chives, cruciferous vegetables (broccoli, cabbage, cauliflower), horseradish, mustard greens	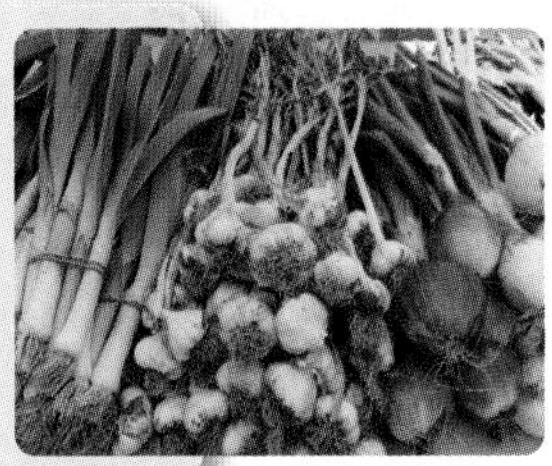

[1] Flavonoids, phenolic acids, and stilbenes are three groups of phytochemicals called phenolics. The phytocemical resveratrol is a stilbene. Flavonoids and phenolic acids are the most abundant phenolics in our diet.

[2] Phytoestrogens include phytochemicals that have mild or anti-estrogenic action in our body. They are grouped together based on this similarity in biological function, but they also can be classified into other phytochemical groups, such as isoflavonoids.

Figure 1 Health claims and food sources of phytochemicals.

NUTRI-CASE HANNAH

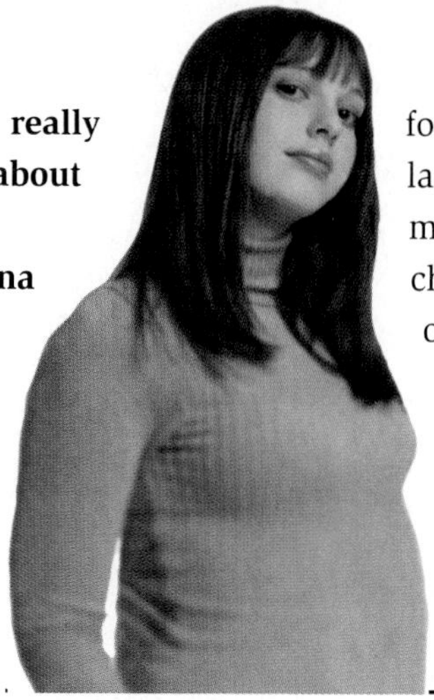

"On my way home from campus today, I was really hungry, and when I passed by a Quick Stop about halfway home, I just had to go in. I looked around for something nutritious, like a banana or an apple or something, but they didn't have anything fresh. So I bought some pretzels. I know pretzels aren't exactly health food, but at least they're low fat."

Hannah and her mother live in an urban neighborhood that has eleven different fast-food outlets and four convenience stores, but lacks a grocery store. There is no local farmer's market or community garden. In order to purchase fresh produce, they have to travel to one of the more affluent neighborhoods several miles away. Given the importance of phytochemicals to a healthful diet, can you think of at least two strategies Hannah and her mother could use to increase their access to affordable produce?

- reduce inflammation,[6] which is linked to the development of Alzheimer's disease and cardiovascular disease and is symptomatic of arthritis.
- protect against cancer by slowing tumor cell growth, instructing cancer cells to die, and enhancing the activity of enzymes that detoxify cancer-promoting agents, called carcinogens.[7]
- protect against infections indirectly by enhancing immune function and directly by acting as antibacterial and antiviral agents.[7]
- reduce the risk for cardiovascular disease by lowering blood lipids, blood pressure, and blood clotting.[1]

It is not yet known which of these roles is most important in reducing disease risk. Many other issues are also not well understood yet, such as which phytochemicals are needed and how much.

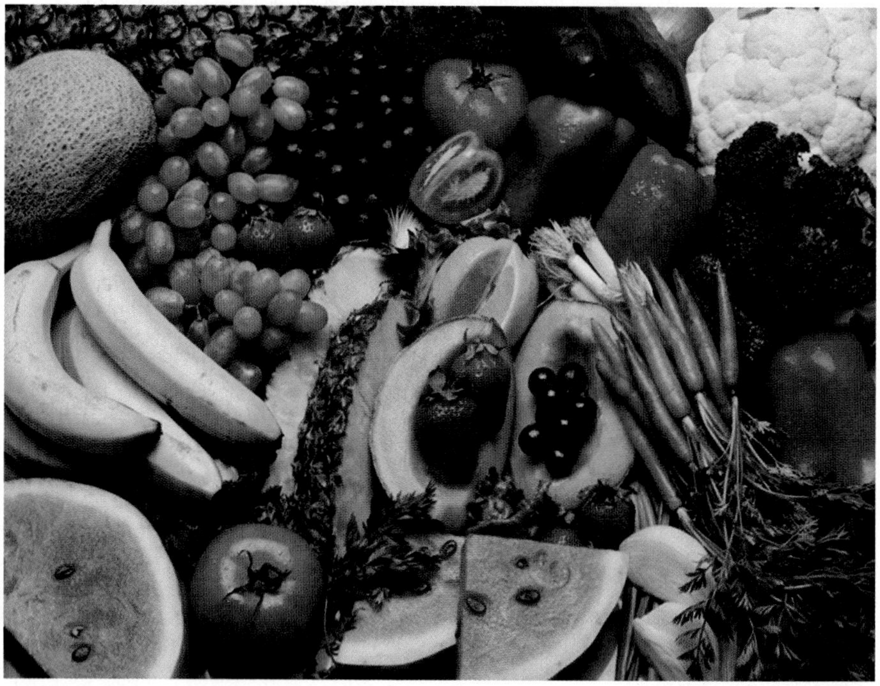

Choose whole foods as sources of phytochemicals, rather than supplements, whenever possible.

Is There an RDA for Phytochemicals?

Most well-controlled studies research only one phytochemical or food at a time. When the results are published, we read about them in the popular press: one day we're advised to eat tomatoes, another day blueberries, then pomegranates. But these individual findings can be misleading. As scientists begin to "map" more and more phytochemicals, they're making the following discoveries:

- Phytochemicals interact with each other in the body to produce a synergistic effect, which is greater than the sum of the effects of individual phytochemicals.[1] This may explain why whole tomatoes were found to reduce prostate cancer in rats, whereas a phytochemical called lycopene that is present in tomatoes, when given alone, did not.[8]
- Phytochemicals interact with macronutrients and vitamins and minerals. For example, the anticancer effect of garlic is enhanced by vitamin A, selenium, and certain fats.[9]
- Phytochemicals can act in different ways under different circumstances in the body. For example,

HOT TOPIC

Will a PB&J Keep the Doctor Away?

Whole-grain bread, natural peanut butter, and grape jelly: how could a food that tastes so good be good for the body, too? We've known for decades about the fiber, micronutrients, and healthful fats a PB&J provides. But recently, research has revealed that the comforting PB&J is a good source of *resveratrol*, a phytochemical being studied in labs worldwide. Research has linked resveratrol to protective effects against cancer, heart disease, obesity, viral infections, and neurologic diseases, such as Alzheimer's disease; however, so far, the effects have been demonstrated only in mice.[15,16]

A flavonoid, resveratrol is found in the skins of dark grapes, in dark grape juice, in most red wines, and in dark berries, such as blueberries and cranberries. But fruits are not the only source: resveratrol also happens to be plentiful in peanuts, including peanut butter. Still, no one knows what an effective "dose" of resveratrol looks like, or whether the amounts in a PB&J qualify. We also don't yet know whether high doses, such as those found in supplements, can be harmful.

If you decide to add resveratrol to your diet, we hope you'll bypass supplements in favor of the humble PB&J. Although the jury is still out on the benefits of its resveratrol content, it makes a highly nutritious meal or snack, doesn't need refrigeration, is inexpensive, and tastes great.

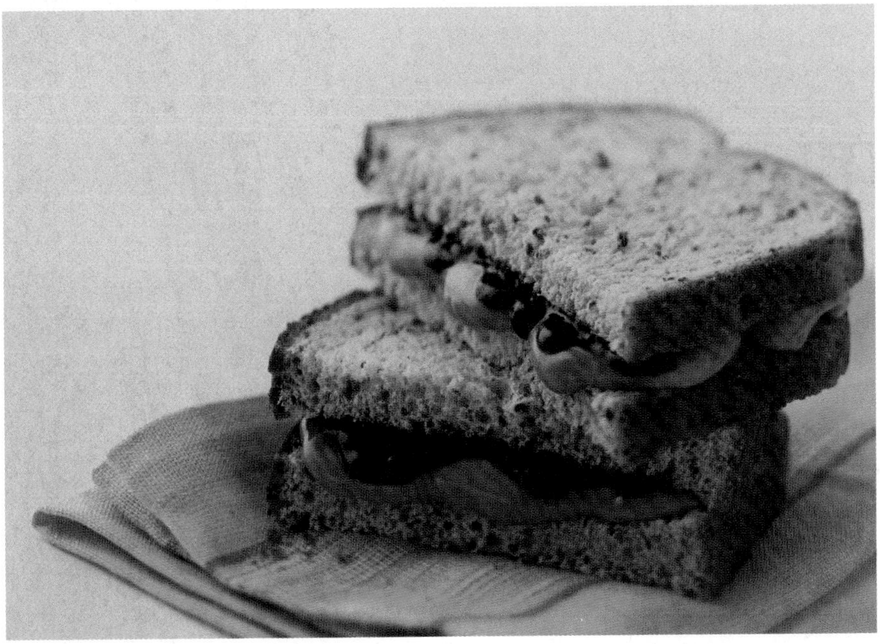

- phytoestrogens in soy appear to reduce the incidence of breast cancer in healthy women, but they may enhance cancer development when the disease is already present.[10]

For these reasons, no RDA for phytochemicals can safely be established for any life-stage group.

In addition, although epidemiological studies suggest that the more phytochemicals we consume, the better our health, this benefit appears to be limited to the phytochemicals consumed in foods. That is, phytochemicals appear to be protective in the low doses commonly provided by foods, but they may have very different effects as supplements. This may be due to their mode of action: scientists now believe that, instead of *protecting* our cells, phytochemicals might benefit our health by *stressing* our cells, causing them to rev up their internal defense systems.[4] Cells are very well equipped to deal with minor stresses, but not with excessive stress, which may explain why clinical trials with phytochemical supplements rarely show the same benefits as high intakes of plant foods.[4,11]

So, are phytochemical supplements harmful? Generally speaking, taking high doses of anything is risky. A basic principle of toxicology is that any compound can be toxic if the dose is high enough. Dietary supplements are no exception to this rule. For example, clinical trials found that supplementing with 20 to 30 mg/day of beta-carotene for 4 to 6 years increased lung cancer risk by 16% to 28% in smokers.[12,13] Based on these and other results, experts recommend against beta-carotene supplementation.[14]

In short, whereas there is ample evidence to support the health benefits of diets rich in fruits, vegetables, legumes, whole grains, and nuts, no recommendation for precise phytochemical amounts can be given, and phytochemical supplements should be avoided. The best advice for optimal health is to consume a plant-based diet consisting of as many whole foods as possible.

Web Resources

www.aicr.org
American Institute for Cancer Research

Search for "phytochemicals" to learn about the AICR's stance on and recommendations about phytochemicals and their roles in cancer prevention.

www.lpi.oregonstate.edu
Linus Pauling Institute

This extensive website covers not only phytochemicals but also nutrients and other cutting-edge health and nutrition topics.

3 The Human Body: Are We Really What We Eat?

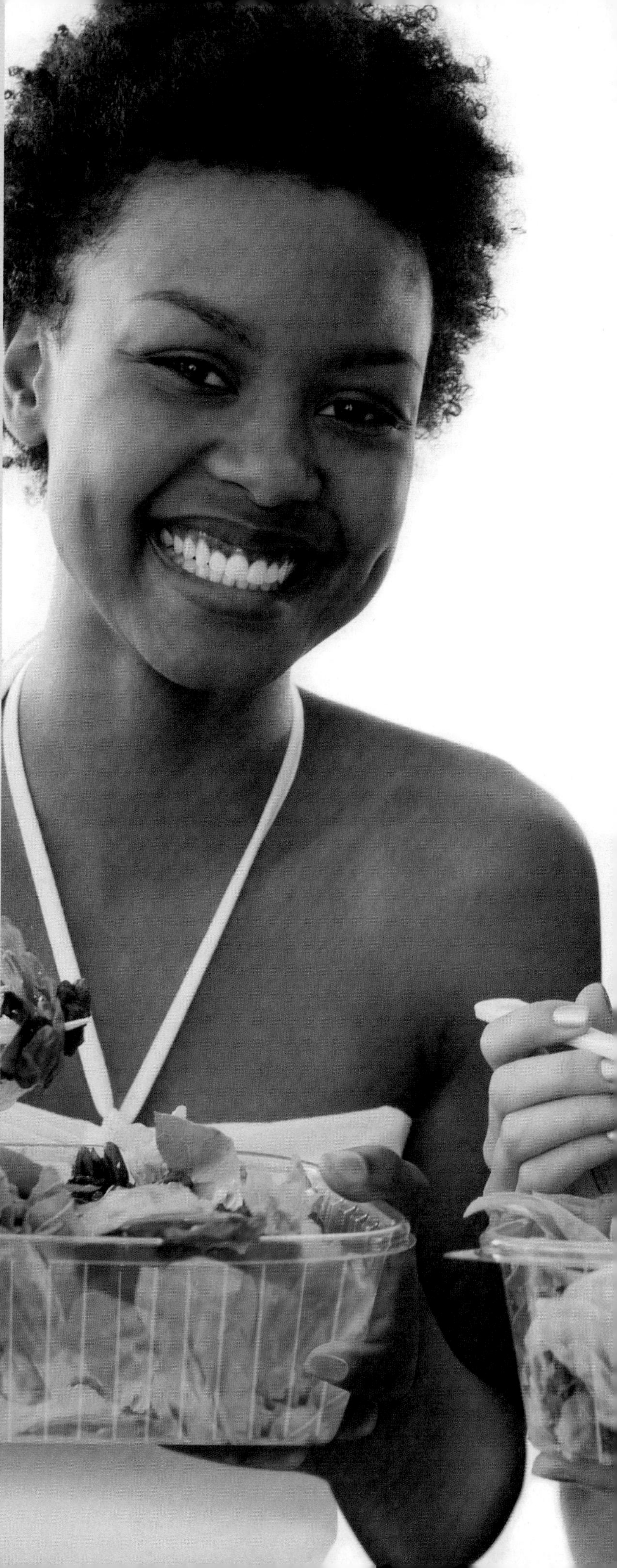

CHAPTER OBJECTIVES

After reading this chapter you will be able to:

1. **Distinguish between appetite and hunger, describing the mechanisms that stimulate each, pp. 74–75.**
2. **Describe what is meant by the expression "You are what you eat," pp. 79–81.**
3. **Identify two functions of the cell membrane, p. 80.**
4. **Draw a picture of the gastrointestinal tract, labeling all major and accessory organs, p. 82.**
5. **Describe the contribution of each organ of the gastrointestinal system to the digestion, absorption, and elimination of food, pp. 83–92.**
6. **Discuss the causes, symptoms, and treatments of gastroesophageal reflux disease, ulcers, diarrhea, constipation, and irritable bowel syndrome, pp. 92–96.**

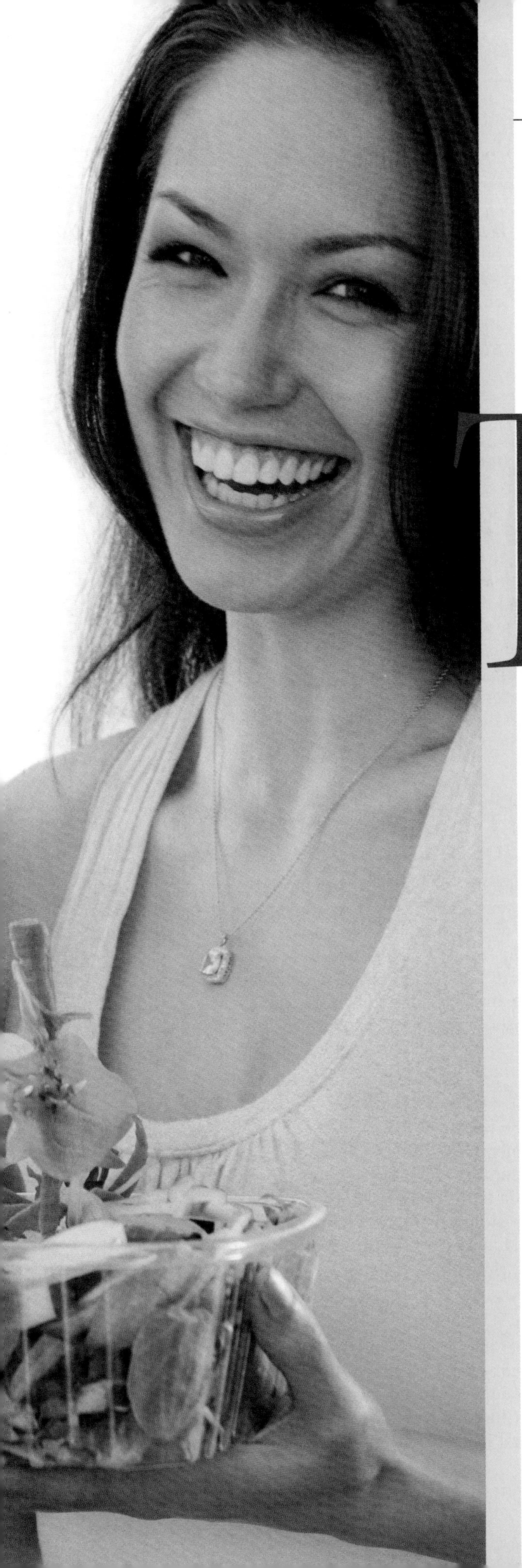

Test Yourself

1. T F Sometimes we have an appetite even though we are not hungry.
2. T F The entire process of the digestion and absorption of one meal takes about 24 hours.
3. T F Most ulcers result from a type of infection.

Test Yourself answers can be found at the end of the chapter.

Two months ago, Andrea's lifelong dream of becoming a lawyer came one step closer to reality: she moved out of her parents' home in the Midwest to attend law school in Boston. Unfortunately, adjusting to a new city and new friends, and her intensive course work, has been more stressful than she'd imagined, and Andrea has been experiencing insomnia and exhaustion. What's more, her always "sensitive stomach" has been getting worse: after almost every meal, she gets cramps so bad she can't stand up, and twice she has missed classes because of sudden attacks of pain and diarrhea. She suspects that the problem is related to stress and wonders if she is going to experience it throughout her life. She is even thinking of dropping out of school if that would make her feel well again.

Almost everyone experiences brief episodes of abdominal pain, diarrhea, or other symptoms from time to time. Such episodes are usually caused by food poisoning or an infection, such as influenza. But do you know anyone who experiences these symptoms periodically for days, weeks, or even years? If so, has it made you wonder why? What are the steps in normal digestion and absorption of food, and at what points can the process break down?

We begin this chapter with a look at some of the factors that make us feel as if we want to eat. We'll then discuss the physiologic processes by which the body digests and absorbs food and eliminates waste products. Finally, we'll look at some disorders that affect these processes.

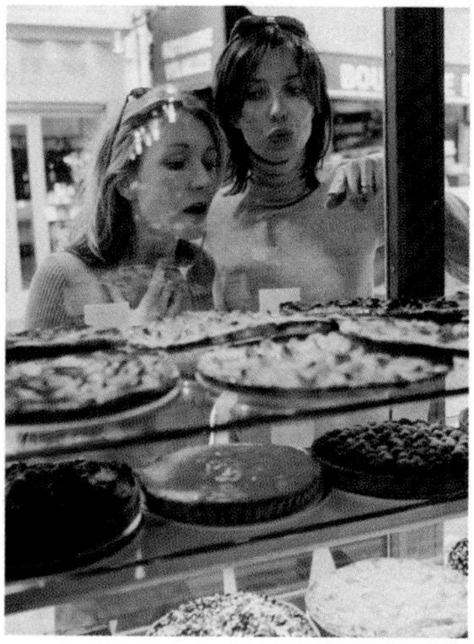

Food stimulates our senses.

Why Do We Want to Eat What We Want to Eat?

You've just finished eating at your favorite Thai restaurant. As you walk back to the block where you parked your car, you pass a bakery window displaying several cakes and pies, each of which looks more enticing than the last, and through the door wafts a complex aroma of coffee, cinnamon, and chocolate. You stop. You know you're not hungry, but you go inside and buy a slice of chocolate torte and an espresso, anyway. Later that night, when the caffeine from the chocolate and espresso keeps you awake, you wonder why you succumbed.

Two mechanisms prompt us to seek food: hunger and appetite. **Hunger** is a physiologic drive for food that occurs when our body senses that we need to eat. The drive is *nonspecific;* when you're hungry, a variety of foods could satisfy you. If you've recently finished a nourishing meal, then hunger probably won't compel you toward a slice of chocolate torte. Instead, the culprit is likely to be **appetite,** a psychological desire to consume *specific* foods. It is aroused when environmental cues—such as the sight of chocolate cake or the smell of coffee—stimulate your senses, triggering pleasant emotions and memories.

People commonly experience appetite in the absence of hunger. That's why you can crave cake and coffee even after eating a full meal. On the other hand, it is possible to have a physiologic need for food yet have no appetite. This state, called **anorexia,** can accompany a variety of illnesses, from infectious diseases to mood disorders. It can also occur as a side effect of certain medications, such as the chemotherapy used in treating cancer patients. Although the following sections describe hunger and appetite as separate entities, ideally the two states coexist: we seek specific, appealing foods to satisfy a physiologic need for nutrients.

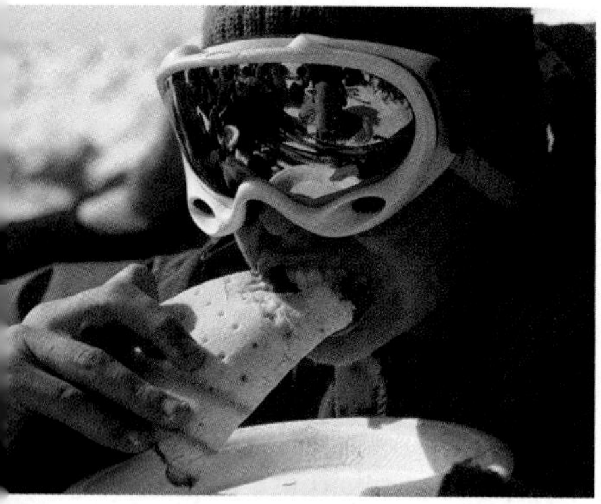

Hunger is a physiologic stimulus that prompts us to find food and eat.

The Hypothalamus Prompts Hunger in Response to Various Signals

Because hunger is a physiologic stimulus that drives us to find food and eat, we often feel it as a negative or unpleasant sensation. The primary organ producing that sensation is the brain. That's right—it's not our stomach but our brain that tells us when we're hungry. The region of brain tissue responsible for prompting us to seek food is called the **hypothalamus** (**Figure 3.1**). It's located above the pituitary gland in the forebrain, a region that regulates many types of involuntary activity. The hypothalamus triggers feelings of either hunger or satiation (fullness) by integrating signals from three sources: nerve cells, chemicals called *hormones,* and the amount and type of food we eat. Let's review these three types of signals.

The Role of Nerve Cells

One important signal comes from nerve cells lining the stomach and small intestine that detect changes in pressure according to whether the organ is empty or distended with food. The cells relay these data to the hypothalamus. For instance, if you have not eaten for many hours and your stomach and small intestine do not contain food, these data are sent to the hypothalamus, which in turn prompts you to experience the sensation of hunger.

The Role of Hormones

Hormones are chemical messengers that are secreted into the bloodstream by one of the many *glands* of the body. The presence of different hormones in the blood helps regulate body functions. Insulin and glucagon are two hormones responsible for maintaining blood glucose levels. Glucose is our body's most readily available fuel supply. It's not surprising, then, that its level in the blood is an important signal af-

hunger A physiologic sensation that prompts us to eat.

appetite A psychological desire to consume specific foods.

anorexia An absence of appetite.

hypothalamus A region of the forebrain above the pituitary gland, where visceral sensations, such as hunger and thirst, are regulated.

hormone A chemical messenger secreted into the bloodstream by one of the many glands of the body, which acts as a regulator of physiologic processes at a site remote from the gland that secreted it.

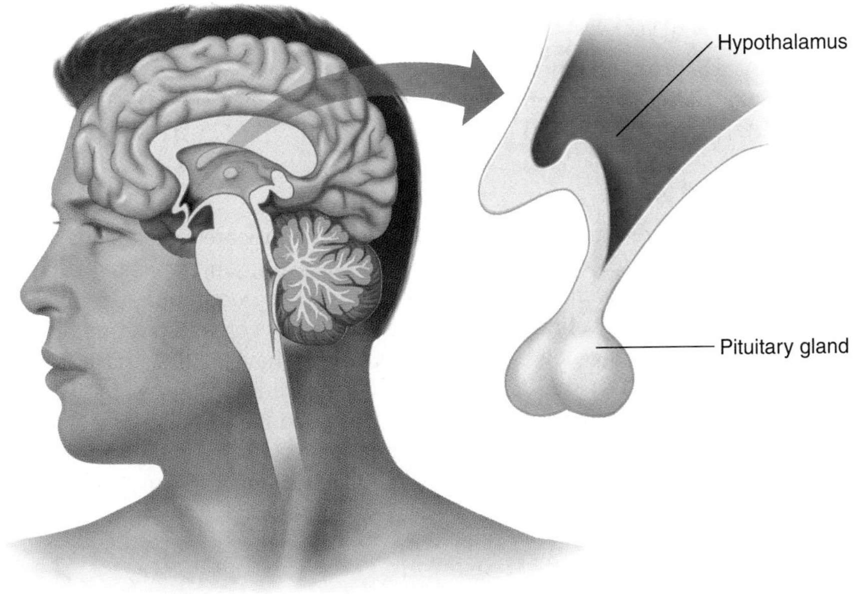

Figure 3.1 The hypothalamus triggers hunger by integrating signals from nerve cells throughout the body, as well as from messages carried by hormones.

fecting hunger. When we have not eaten for a while, our blood glucose levels fall, prompting a change in the level of insulin and glucagon. This chemical message is relayed to the hypothalamus, which then prompts us to eat in order to supply our body with more glucose.

After we eat, the hypothalamus picks up the sensation of a distended stomach, other signals from the gut, and a rise in blood glucose levels. When it integrates these signals, you have the experience of feeling full, or *satiated*. However, as we have noted, even though our brain sends us clear signals about hunger, most of us become adept at ignoring them and eat when we are not truly hungry.

In addition to insulin and glucagon, a variety of other hormones and hormone-like substances signal the hypothalamus to cause us to feel hungry or satiated. More details about the hormones involved in digestion are provided later in this chapter. For more information about the role of hormones in weight management, see Chapter 11.

The Role of the Amount and Type of Food

Although the reason behind this observation is not understood, researchers have long recognized that foods containing protein have the highest satiety value.[1] This means that a ham and egg breakfast will cause us to feel satiated for a longer period of time than will pancakes with maple syrup, even if both meals have exactly the same number of Calories.

Another factor affecting hunger is how bulky the meal is—that is, how much fiber and water is within the food. Bulky meals tend to stretch the stomach and small intestine, which sends signals back to the hypothalamus telling us that we are full, so we stop eating. Beverages tend to be less satisfying than semisolid foods, and semisolid foods have a lower satiety value than solid foods. For example, if you were to eat a bunch of grapes, you would feel a greater sense of fullness than if you drank a glass of grape juice.

RECAP **In contrast to appetite, hunger is a physiologic sensation triggered by the hypothalamus in response to cues about stomach and intestinal distention and the levels of certain hormones and hormone-like substances. High-protein foods make us feel satiated for longer periods of time, and bulky meals fill us up quickly, causing the distention that signals us to stop eating.**

Environmental Cues Trigger Appetite

Whereas hunger is prompted by internal signals, appetite is triggered by aspects of our environment. The most significant factors influencing our appetite are sensory data, social and cultural cues, and learning **(Figure 3.2)**.

The Role of Sensory Data

Foods stimulate our five senses. Foods that are artfully prepared, arranged, or ornamented, with several different shapes and colors, appeal to our sense of sight. The aromas of foods such as freshly brewed coffee and baked goods can also be powerful stimulants. Much of our ability to taste foods actually comes from our sense of smell. This is why foods are not as appealing when we have a stuffy nose due to a cold. Certain tastes, such as sweetness, are almost universally appealing, while others, such as the astringent taste of some foods (for instance, spinach and kale), are quite individual. Texture, or "mouth feel," is also important in food choices, as it stimulates nerve endings sensitive to touch in our mouth and on our tongue. Even our sense of hearing can be stimulated by foods, from the fizz of cola to the crunch of pretzels.

The Role of Social and Cultural Cues

In addition to sensory cues, our brain's association with certain social events, such as birthday parties and holiday gatherings, can stimulate our appetite. At these times, our culture gives us permission to eat more than usual or to eat "forbidden" foods. Even when we feel full, these cues can motivate us to accept a second helping.

For some people, being in a certain location, such as at a baseball game or a movie theatre, can trigger appetite. Others may be influenced by activities such as watching television or at certain times of the day associated with mealtimes. Many people feel an increase or a decrease in appetite according to whom they are with; for example, they may eat more when at home with family members and less when out on a date.

In some people, appetite masks an emotional response to an external event. For example, a person might experience a desire for food rather than a desire for emo-

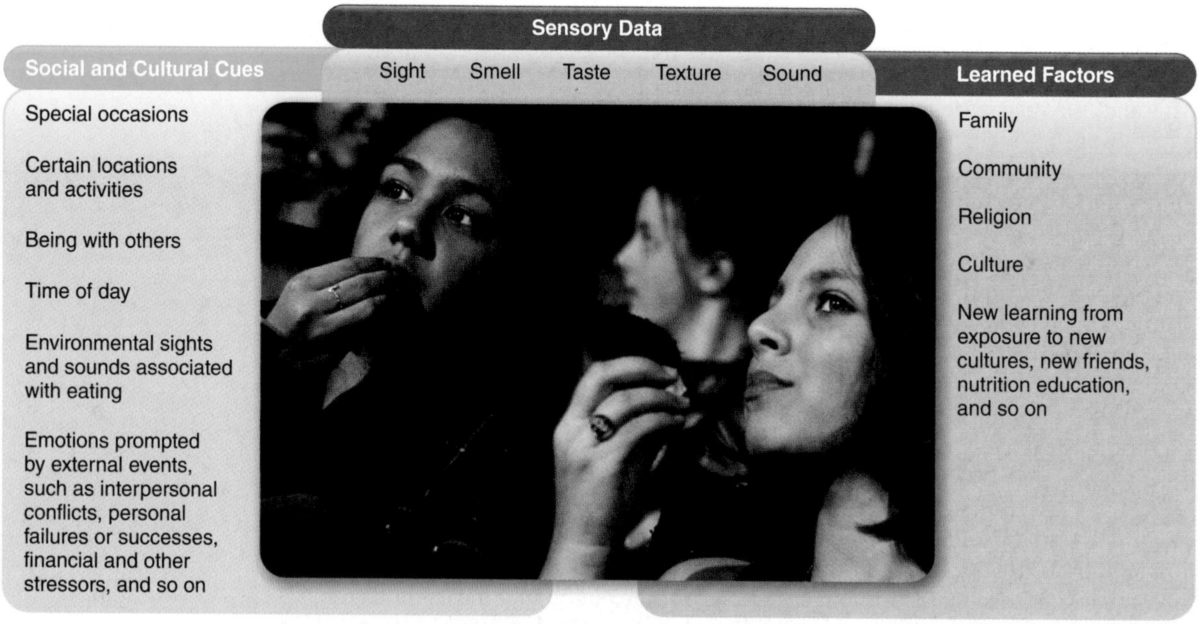
Sensory Data
Sight
Smell
Taste
Texture
Sound
Social and Cultural Cues
Special occasions
Certain locations and activities
Being with others
Time of day
Environmental sights and sounds associated with eating
Emotions prompted by external events, such as interpersonal conflicts, personal failures or successes, financial and other stressors, and so on
Learned Factors
Family
Community
Religion
Culture
New learning from exposure to new cultures, new friends, nutrition education, and so on

Figure 3.2 Appetite is a drive to consume specific foods, such as popcorn at the movies. It is aroused by social and cultural cues and sensory data and is influenced by learning.

tional comfort after receiving a failing grade or arguing with a close friend. Many people crave food when they're frustrated, worried, or bored or when they're at a gathering where they feel anxious or awkward. Others subconsciously seek food as a "reward." For example, have you ever found yourself heading out for a burger and fries after handing in a term paper?

The Role of Learning

Pigs' feet, anyone? What about blood sausage, stewed octopus, or snakes? These are delicacies in various cultures. Would you eat grasshoppers? If you'd grown up in certain parts of Africa or Central America, you might. That's because your preference for particular foods is largely a learned response. The culture in which you are raised teaches you what plant and animal products are appropriate to eat. If your parents fed you cubes of plain tofu throughout your toddlerhood, then you are probably still eating tofu.

That said, early introduction to foods is not essential: we can learn to enjoy new foods at any point in our lives. For instance, many immigrants adopt a diet typical of their new home, especially when their traditional foods are not readily available. This happens temporarily when we travel: the last time you were away from home, you probably sampled a variety of dishes that are not normally part of your diet.

Food preferences also change when people learn what foods are most healthful. Since reading Chapter 1, has your diet changed at all? Chances are, as you learn more about the health benefits of specific types of carbohydrates, fats, and proteins, you'll start incorporating more of these foods in your diet.

We can also "learn" to dislike foods we once enjoyed. For example, if we experience an episode of food poisoning after eating undercooked scrambled eggs, we might develop a strong distaste for all types of eggs. Many adults who become vegetarians do so after learning about the treatment of animals in slaughterhouses: they might have eaten meat daily when young but no longer have any appetite for it.

Now that you understand the differences between appetite and hunger, as well as the influence of learning on food choices, you might be curious to investigate your own reasons for eating what and when you do. If so, check out the self-assessment box What About You: Do You Eat in Response to External or Internal Cues?

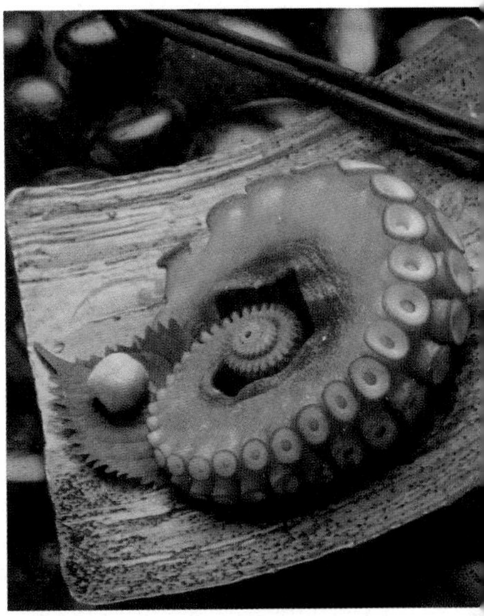

Food preferences are influenced by the family and culture you are raised in.

HOT TOPIC

Prescription Appetite Suppressants: Help or Harm?

The manufacturers of three new appetite suppressants are hoping for Food and Drug Administration (FDA) approval of their drugs, but smooth sailing isn't guaranteed. Such drugs typically work by influencing the central nervous system, and they can cause serious psychological side effects. In 2007, for example, a similar drug failed to win FDA approval because of its links to depression and suicidal thoughts. Another concern related to appetite suppressants is their effect on the heart and circulatory system. In the 1990s, two were removed from the market because of drug-related damage to heart valves, and one drug currently on the market, Meridia, can increase blood pressure and heart rate. Another problem is the drugs' limited effectiveness: many work for a short while, but, when weight goes down, appetite surges back again.[2]

RECAP **In contrast to hunger, appetite is a psychological desire to consume specific foods. It is triggered when external stimuli arouse our senses, and it often occurs in combination with social and cultural cues. Our preference for certain foods is largely learned from the culture in which we were raised, but our food choices can change with exposure to new foods or through new learning experiences.**

What About You?

Do You Eat in Response to External or Internal Cues?

Whether you're trying to lose weight, gain weight, or maintain your current weight, you might find it intriguing to keep a log of the reasons behind your decisions about what, when, where, and why you eat. Are you eating in response to internal sensations telling you that your body needs food, or in response to your emotions, your situation, or a prescribed diet? Keeping a "cues" log for 1 full week would give you the most accurate picture of your eating habits, but even logging 2 days of meals and snacks should increase your cue awareness.

Each day, every time you eat a meal, snack, or beverage other than water, make a quick note of the following:

- **When you eat:** Many people eat at certain times (for example, 6 PM), whether they are hungry or not.
- **What you eat, and how much:** Do you choose a cup of yogurt and a 6-oz glass of orange juice or a candy bar and a 20-oz cola?
- **Where you eat:** At home, watching television; on the subway; and so on.
- **With whom you eat:** Are you alone or with others? If with others, are they also eating? Have they offered you food?
- **Your emotions:** Some people overeat when they are happy, others when they are anxious, depressed, bored, or frustrated. Still others eat as a way of denying feelings they don't want to identify and deal with. For some, food becomes a substitute for emotional fulfillment.
- **Your sensations—what you see, hear, or smell:** Are you eating because you just saw a TV commercial for pizza, or smelled homemade cookies?
- **Any dietary restrictions:** Are you choosing a particular food because it is allowed on your current diet plan? Or are you hungry for a meal but drinking a diet soda to stay within a certain allowance of Calories? Are you restricting yourself because you feel guilty about having eaten too much at another time?
- **Your physiologic hunger:** Finally, rate your hunger on a scale from 1 to 5 as follows:
  - 1 = you feel uncomfortably full or even stuffed
  - 2 = you feel satisfied but not uncomfortably full
  - 3 = neutral; you feel no discernible satiation or hunger
  - 4 = you feel hungry and want to eat
  - 5 = you feel strong physiologic sensations of hunger and need to eat

After keeping a log for 2 or more days, you might become aware of patterns you'd like to change. For example, maybe you notice that you often eat when you are not actually hungry but are worried about homework or personal relationships. Or maybe you notice that you can't walk past the snack bar without going in. This self-awareness may prompt you to change those patterns. For instance, instead of stifling your worries with food, you could write down exactly what you are worried about, including steps you can take to address your concerns. And the next time you approach the snack bar, you could check with your gut: are you truly hungry? If so, then purchase a healthful snack, maybe a piece of fruit or a bag of peanuts. If you're not really hungry, then take a moment to acknowledge the strength of this visual cue—and then walk on by.

NUTRI-CASE JUDY

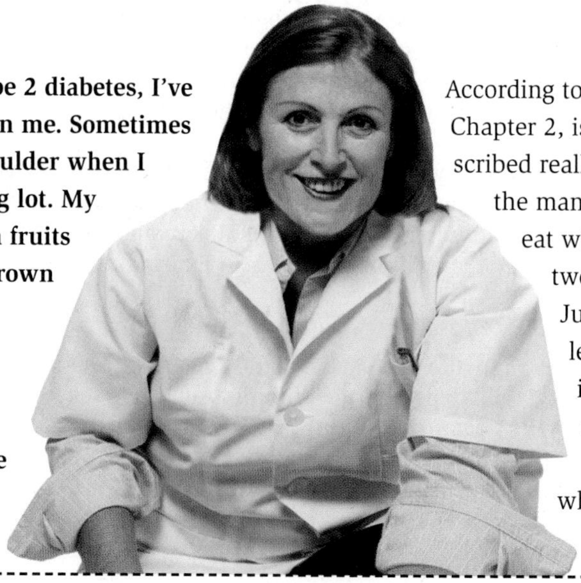

"Ever since I was diagnosed with type 2 diabetes, I've felt as if there's a 'food cop' spying on me. Sometimes I feel like I have to look over my shoulder when I pull into the Dunkin' Donuts parking lot. My doctor says I'm supposed to eat fresh fruits and vegetables, fish, brown bread, brown rice . . . I didn't bother telling him I don't like that stuff and I don't have the money to buy it or the time to cook it even if I did. Besides, that kind of diet is for movie stars. All the real people I know eat the same way I do."

According to what you learned in Chapter 2, is the diet Judy's doctor described really just for "movie stars"? Of the many factors influencing why we eat what we eat, identify at least two that might be affecting Judy's food choices. If you learned that Judy had not finished high school, would that fact have any bearing on your answer? If so, in what way?

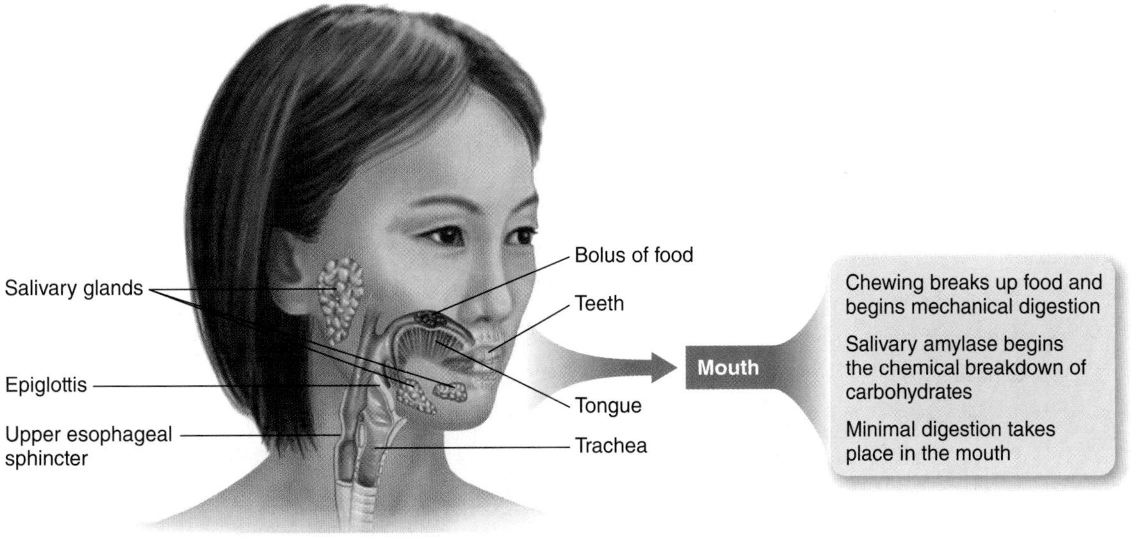
Salivary glands
Epiglottis
Upper esophageal sphincter
Bolus of food
Teeth
Tongue
Trachea
Mouth
Chewing breaks up food and begins mechanical digestion
Salivary amylase begins the chemical breakdown of carbohydrates
Minimal digestion takes place in the mouth

Figure 3.6 Where your food is now: the mouth. Chewing moistens food and mechanically breaks it down into pieces small enough to swallow, while salivary amylase begins the chemical digestion of carbohydrates.

digestion—as well as many other biochemical processes that go on in our body—could not happen without them. By the way, enzyme names typically end in *-ase* (as in *amylase*), so they are easy to recognize as we look at the digestive process.

In reality, very little digestion occurs in the mouth. This is because we do not hold food in the mouth for very long and because not all of the enzymes needed to break down food are present in saliva. Salivary amylase starts the digestion of carbohydrates in the mouth, and this digestion continues until food reaches the stomach. There, salivary amylase is destroyed by the acidic environment of the stomach.

RECAP **Digestion, absorption, and elimination take place in the gastrointestinal (GI) tract. In the cephalic phase of digestion, hunger and appetite work together to prepare the GI tract for digestion and absorption. Chewing initiates mechanical digestion by breaking the food mass apart and mixing it together. The release of saliva moistens food and starts the process of chemical digestion of carbohydrates through the action of the enzyme salivary amylase.**

The Esophagus Propels Food into the Stomach

The mass of food that has been chewed and moistened in the mouth is referred to as a **bolus.** This bolus is swallowed **(Figure 3.7)** and propelled to the stomach through the esophagus. Most of us take swallowing for granted. However, it is a very complex process involving voluntary and involuntary motion. A tiny flap of tissue called the *epiglottis* acts as a trapdoor covering the entrance to the trachea (windpipe). The epiglottis is normally open, allowing us to breathe freely even while chewing (Figure 3.7a). As a food bolus moves to the very back of the mouth, the brain is sent a signal to temporarily raise the soft palate and close the openings to the nasal passages, preventing the aspiration of food or liquid into the sinuses (Figure 3.7b). The brain also signals the epiglottis to close during swallowing, so that food and liquid cannot enter the trachea.

Sometimes this protective mechanism goes awry—for instance, when we try to eat and talk at the same time. When this happens, food or liquid enters the trachea. Typically, this causes us to cough involuntarily and repeatedly until the offending food or liquid is expelled.

As the trachea closes, the sphincter muscle at the top of the esophagus, called the *upper esophageal sphincter*, opens to allow the passage of food. The **esophagus** is a

bolus A mass of food that has been chewed and moistened in the mouth.

esophagus A muscular tube of the GI tract connecting the back of the mouth to the stomach.

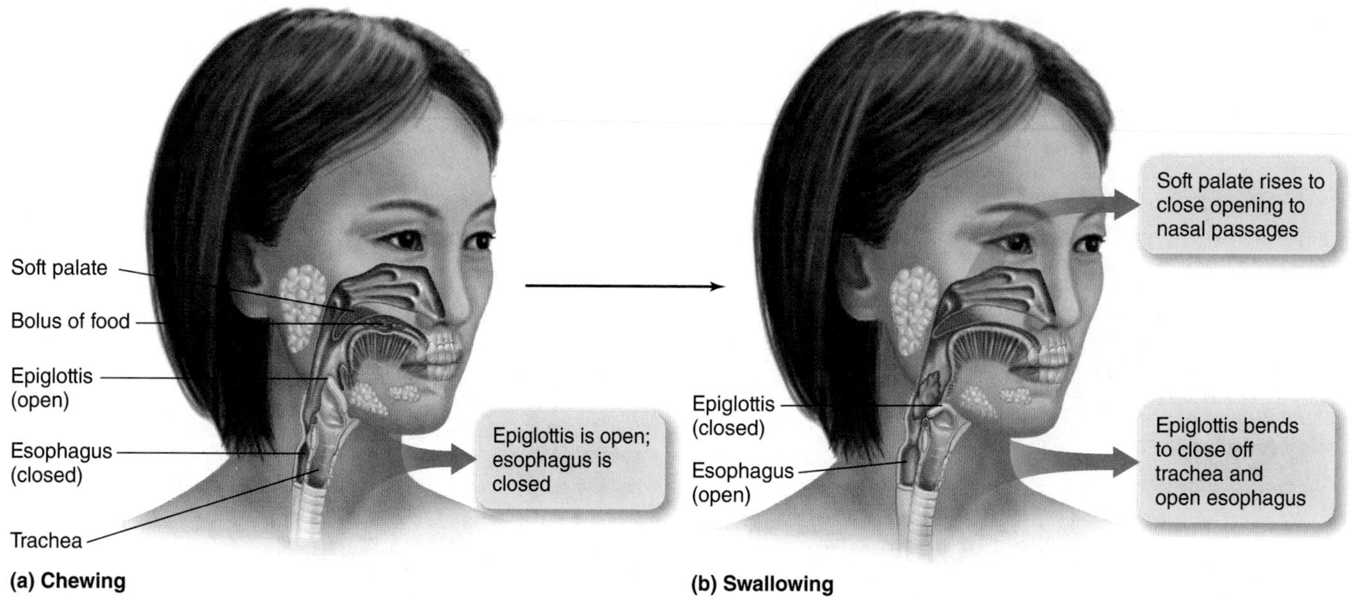

Figure 3.7 Chewing and swallowing are complex processes. **(a)** During the process of chewing, the epiglottis is open and the esophagus is closed, so that we can continue to breathe as we chew. **(b)** During swallowing, the epiglottis closes, so that food does not enter the trachea and obstruct our breathing. Also, the soft palate rises to seal off our nasal passages to prevent the aspiration of food or liquid into the sinuses.

muscular tube that connects and transports food from the mouth to the stomach (**Figure 3.8**). It does this by contracting two sets of muscles: inner sheets of circular muscle squeeze the food while outer sheets of longitudinal muscle push food along the length of the tube. Together, these rhythmic waves of squeezing and pushing are called **peristalsis.** We will see later in this chapter that peristalsis occurs throughout the GI tract.

Gravity also helps transport food down the esophagus, which explains why it is wise to sit or stand upright while eating. Together, peristalsis and gravity can transport a bite of food from our mouth to the opening of the stomach in 5 to 8 seconds. At the end of the esophagus is a sphincter muscle, the *gastroesophageal sphincter* (*gastro-* means "stomach"), which is normally tightly closed. When food reaches the end of the esophagus, this sphincter relaxes to allow the food to pass into the stomach. In some people, this sphincter is continually somewhat relaxed. Later in the chapter, we'll discuss this disorder and the unpleasant symptoms it causes.

peristalsis Waves of squeezing and pushing contractions that move food in one direction through the length of the GI tract.

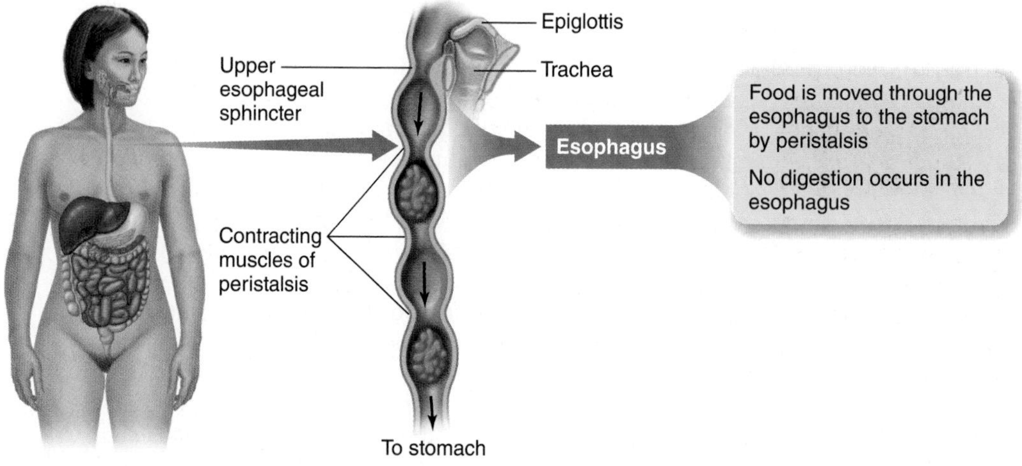

Figure 3.8 Where your food is now: the esophagus. Peristalsis, the rhythmic contraction and relaxation of both circular and longitudinal muscles in the esophagus, propels food toward the stomach. Peristalsis occurs throughout the GI tract.

The Stomach Mixes, Digests, and Stores Food

The **stomach** is a J-shaped organ. Its size is fairly individual; in general, its volume is about 6 fl. oz (3/4 cup) when it is empty. When the stomach is full, it can expand to hold about 32 fl. oz, or about 4 cups. Before any food reaches the stomach, the brain sends signals, telling it to be ready for the food to arrive. This causes an increased secretion of **gastric juice,** which contains several important compounds:

- *Hydrochloric acid (HCl)* keeps the stomach interior very acidic—more so than many citrus juices. This acidic environment kills many of the bacteria that may have entered your body with your sandwich. HCl also starts to **denature** proteins, which means it uncoils the bonds that maintain their structure. This is an important preliminary step in protein digestion.
- HCl also converts *pepsinogen,* an inactive substance, into the active enzyme *pepsin,* which begins to digest proteins into smaller components. In addition, pepsin activates many other GI enzymes needed to digest your meal.
- *Gastric lipase* is an enzyme responsible for fat (lipid) digestion. It begins to break apart the fat in the turkey and the mayonnaise in your sandwich; however, only minimal digestion of fat occurs in the stomach.
- Your stomach also secretes *mucus,* which protects its lining from being digested by the HCl and pepsin.

With these gastric juices already present, the chemical digestion of proteins and fats begins as soon as food enters your stomach (**Figure 3.9**). In this *gastric phase* of digestion, the hormone *gastrin* is secreted. Gastrin increases the secretions of the gastric cells, making the gastric juices even more acidic. It also stimulates stomach contractions, which begin to mix and churn the food until it becomes a liquid called **chyme.** This physical mixing and churning of food is another example of mechanical digestion. Enzymes can access the liquid chyme more readily than solid forms of food. This access facilitates chemical digestion.

Although most absorption occurs in the small intestine, the stomach lining does begin absorbing a few substances. These include water, some medium-chain fatty acids (components of certain types of fats), some minerals, and some drugs, including aspirin and alcohol.[3]

Another of your stomach's jobs is to store your sandwich (or what's left of it!) while the next part of the digestive tract, the small intestine, gets ready for the next wave of food. Remember that the stomach can hold about 4 cups of food. If this amount were to move suddenly into the small intestine all at once, it would overwhelm it. Instead, chyme stays in your stomach about 2 to 4 hours (a high-fat meal

stomach A J-shaped organ where food is partially digested, churned, and stored until it is released into the small intestine.

gastric juice Acidic liquid secreted within the stomach; it contains hydrochloric acid, pepsin, and other compounds.

denature The action of the unfolding of proteins in the stomach. Proteins must be denatured before they can be digested.

chyme A semifluid mass consisting of partially digested food, water, and gastric juices.

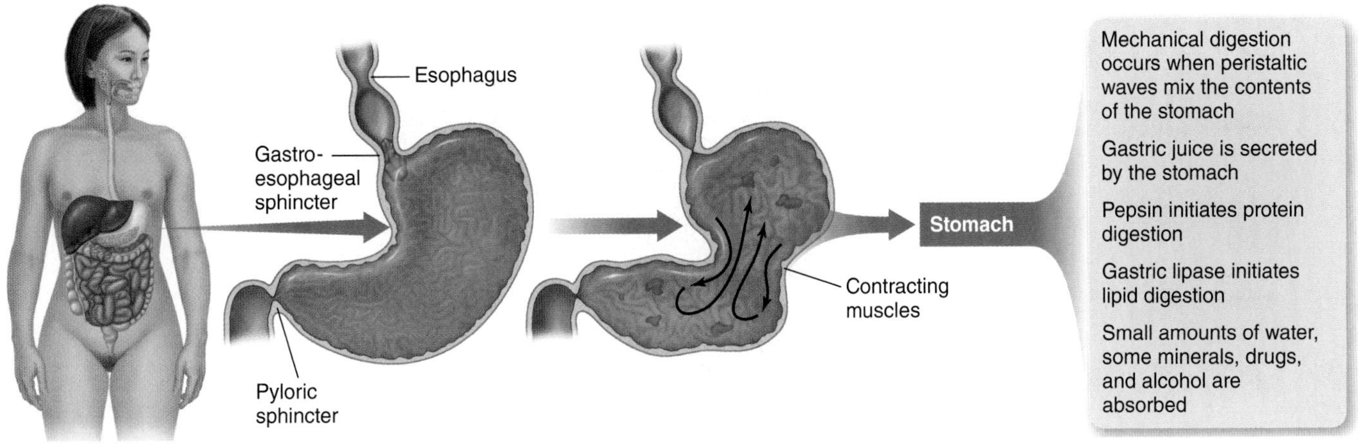

Figure 3.9 Where your food is now: the stomach. In the stomach, the protein and fat in your sandwich begin to be digested. Your meal is churned into chyme and stored until released into the small intestine.

may remain for up to 6 hours) before being released periodically in spurts into the duodenum, which is the first part of the small intestine. Regulating this release is the *pyloric sphincter* (Figure 3.9).

RECAP **The esophagus is a muscular tube that transports food from the mouth to the stomach via waves of peristalsis. The stomach prepares itself for digestion by secreting gastric juice. It also secretes mucus to protect its lining. As the hormone gastrin causes the stomach to churn food into a liquid called chyme, the digestion of proteins and fats begins. The stomach stores chyme and releases it periodically into the small intestine through the pyloric sphincter.**

Most Digestion and Absorption Occurs in the Small Intestine

The **small intestine** is the longest portion of the GI tract, accounting for about two-thirds of its length. However, it is called "small" because it is only an inch in diameter.

The small intestine is composed of three sections (**Figure 3.10**). The *duodenum* is the section that is connected via the pyloric sphincter to the stomach. The *jejunum* is the middle portion, and the last portion is the *ileum*. It connects to the large intestine at another sphincter, called the *ileocecal valve*.

Most digestion and absorption takes place in the small intestine. Here, food is broken down into its smallest components, molecules that the body can then absorb into its internal environment. In the next section, we'll identify a variety of accessory organs, enzymes, and unique anatomical features of the small intestine that permit maximal absorption of most nutrients.

small intestine The longest portion of the GI tract, where most digestion and absorption take place.

gallbladder A tissue sac beneath the liver that stores bile and secretes it into the small intestine.

The Gallbladder and Pancreas Aid in Digestion

We left your sandwich as chyme, being released periodically into the small intestine. As the chyme enters the duodenum, a hormone-like substance called cholecystokinin (CCK) is released in response to the presence of protein and fat from the turkey and mayonnaise. The **gallbladder,** an accessory organ located beneath the

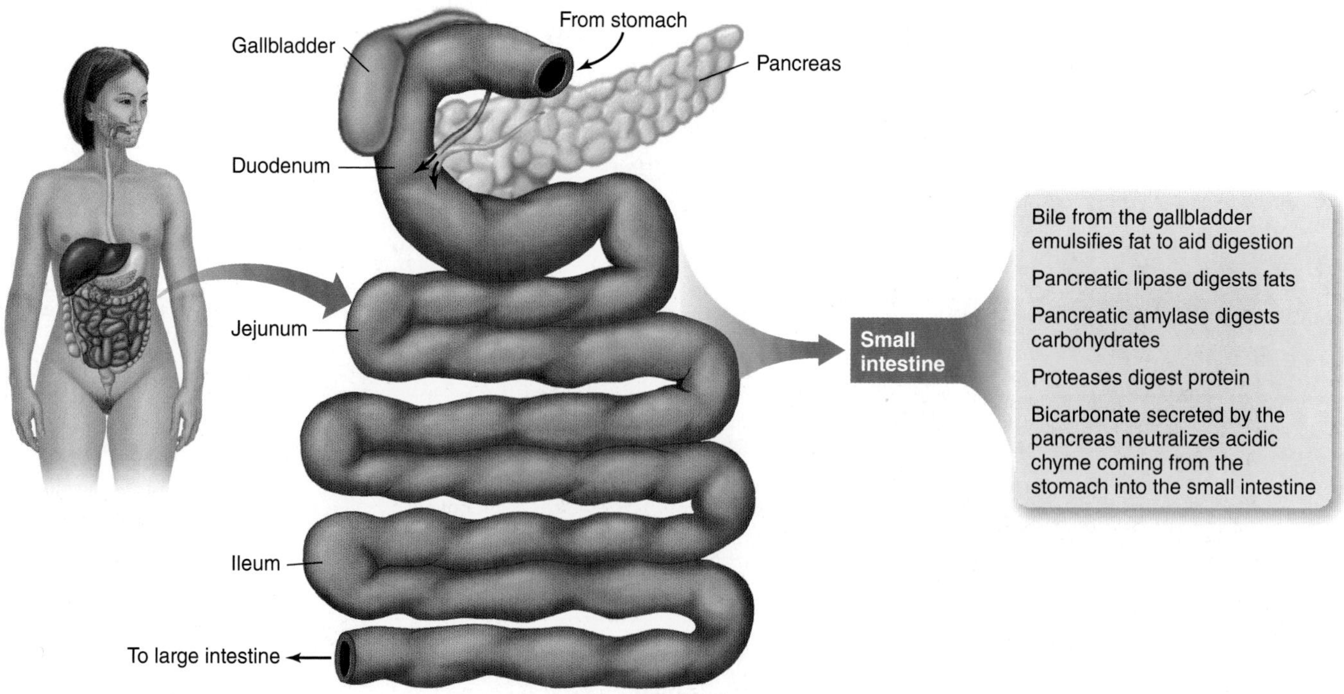
Gallbladder
From stomach
Pancreas
Duodenum
Jejunum
Ileum
To large intestine
Small intestine
Bile from the gallbladder emulsifies fat to aid digestion
Pancreatic lipase digests fats
Pancreatic amylase digests carbohydrates
Proteases digest protein
Bicarbonate secreted by the pancreas neutralizes acidic chyme coming from the stomach into the small intestine

Figure 3.10 Where your food is now: the small intestine. Here, most of the digestion and absorption of the nutrients in your sandwich take place.

liver (see Figures 3.5 and 3.10), stores a greenish fluid called **bile,**which the liver produces. The release of CCK signals the gallbladder to contract, sending bile through the *common bile duct* into the duodenum. Bile then *emulsifies* the fat; that is, it reduces the fat into smaller globules and disperses them, so that they are more accessible to digestive enzymes. If you've ever noticed how a drop of liquid detergent breaks up a film of fat floating at the top of a basin of greasy dishes, you understand the function of bile.

The **pancreas,** another accessory organ, manufactures, holds, and secretes different digestive enzymes. It is located behind the stomach (see Figures 3.5 and 3.10). Enzymes secreted by the pancreas include *pancreatic amylase,* which continues the digestion of carbohydrates, and *pancreatic lipase,* which continues the digestion of fats. *Proteases* secreted in pancreatic juice digest proteins. The pancreas is also responsible for manufacturing hormones that are important in metabolism. Earlier we mentioned insulin and glucagon, two pancreatic hormones that help regulate the amount of glucose in the blood.

Another essential role of the pancreas is to secrete bicarbonate into the duodenum. Bicarbonate is a base; like all bases, it is capable of neutralizing acids. Recall that chyme leaving the stomach is very acidic. The pancreatic bicarbonate neutralizes the acidic chyme. This action helps the pancreatic enzymes work more effectively. It also ensures that the lining of the duodenum is not eroded.

Now the protein, carbohydrate, and fat in your sandwich have been processed into a liquid that contains molecules of nutrients small enough for absorption. This molecular "soup" continues to move along the small intestine via peristalsis, encountering the absorptive cells of the intestinal lining all along the way.

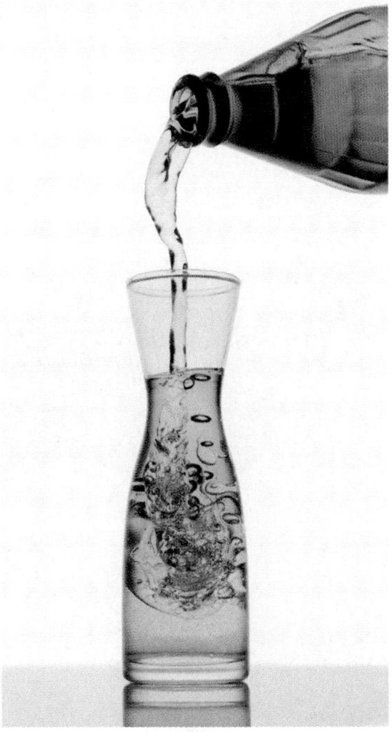

A small amount of vinegar emulsifies the oil in this container.

A Specialized Lining Enables the Small Intestine to Absorb Food

The lining of the GI tract is especially well suited for absorption. If you were to look at the inside of the lining, which is also referred to as the mucosal membrane, you would notice that it is heavily folded (**Figure 3.11**). This feature increases the surface area of the small intestine and allows it to absorb more nutrients than if it were smooth. Within these larger folds, you would notice even smaller, finger-like projections called *villi,* whose constant movement helps them encounter and trap nutrient molecules. Inside each villus are *capillaries,* or tiny blood vessels, and a **lacteal,** which is a small lymph vessel. (The role of the lymphatic system is presented on pages 88–89.) The capillaries absorb water-soluble nutrients directly into the bloodstream, whereas lacteals absorb fat-soluble nutrients into a watery fluid called *lymph.*

Covering the villi are specialized cells carpeted with hairlike structures called *microvilli.* Since this makes them look like tiny scrub brushes, these cells are sometimes referred to collectively as the **brush border.** The carpet of microvilli multiplies the surface area of the small intestine more than 500 times, tremendously increasing its absorptive capacity.

Intestinal Cells Readily Absorb Vitamins, Minerals, and Water

The turkey sandwich you ate contained several vitamins and minerals in addition to protein, carbohydrate, and fat. The vitamins and minerals are not really "digested" in the same way that macronutrients are. Vitamins do not have to be broken down because they are small enough to be readily absorbed by the small intestine. For example, fat-soluble vitamins, such as vitamins A, D, E, and K, are soluble in lipids and are absorbed into the intestinal cells along with the fats in our foods. Water-soluble vitamins, such as the B-vitamins and vitamin C, typically use some type of transport process to cross the intestinal lining. Minerals don't need to be digested because they are already the smallest possible units of matter. Thus, they are absorbed all along the small intestine, and in some cases in the large intestine as well, by a wide variety of mechanisms.

Finally, a large component of food is water, and, of course, you also drink lots of water throughout the day. Water is readily absorbed along the entire length of the GI tract because it is a small molecule that can easily pass through the cell membrane. However, as we will see shortly, a significant percentage of water is absorbed in the large intestine.

bile Fluid produced by the liver and stored in the gallbladder; it emulsifies fats in the small intestine.

pancreas A gland located behind the stomach that secretes digestive enzymes.

lacteal A small lymph vessel located inside the villi of the small intestine.

brush border The microvilli-covered lining cells of the small intestine's villi. These microvilli tremendously increase the small intestine's absorptive capacity.

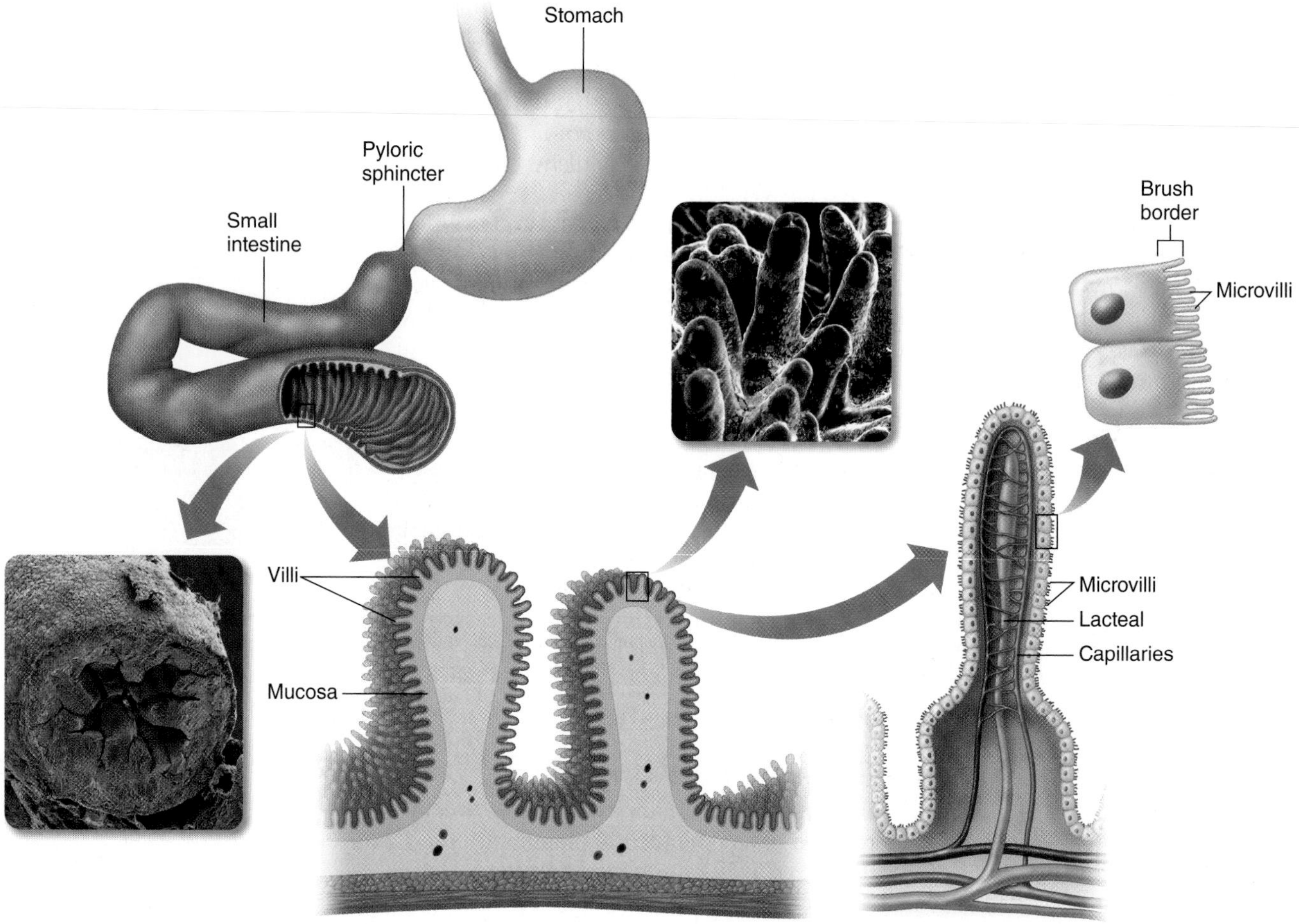

Figure 3.11 Absorption of nutrients occurs via the specialized lining of the small intestine. The lining of the small intestine is heavily folded and has thousands of finger-like projections called *villi*. The cells covering the villi end in hairlike projections called *microvilli*, which together form the brush border. These features significantly increase the absorptive capacity of the small intestine.

Blood and Lymph Transport Nutrients and Fluids

We noted earlier that, within the intestinal villi, capillaries and lacteals absorb water-soluble and fat-soluble nutrients, respectively, into blood and lymph. These two fluids then transport the nutrients throughout the body. Blood travels through the cardiovascular system, and lymph travels through the lymphatic system (**Figure 3.12**).

The oxygen we inhale into our lungs is absorbed by our red blood cells. This oxygen-rich blood then travels to the heart, where it is pumped out to the rest of the body. Blood travels to all of our tissues to deliver nutrients and other materials and pick up waste products. As blood travels through the GI tract, it picks up most of the nutrients, including water, that are absorbed through the mucosal membrane of the small intestine. This nutrient-rich blood is then transported to the liver. The role of the liver in packaging the arriving nutrients is described in the following section.

The lymphatic vessels pick up most fats, fat-soluble vitamins, and fluids that have escaped from the cardiovascular system and transport them in lymph. In its journey through the lymphatic vessels of the body, this lymph is filtered through *lymph nodes*, clusters of immune and other cells that trap particles and destroy harmful microbes. Eventually, lymph returns to the bloodstream in an area near the heart where the lymphatic and blood vessels join together.

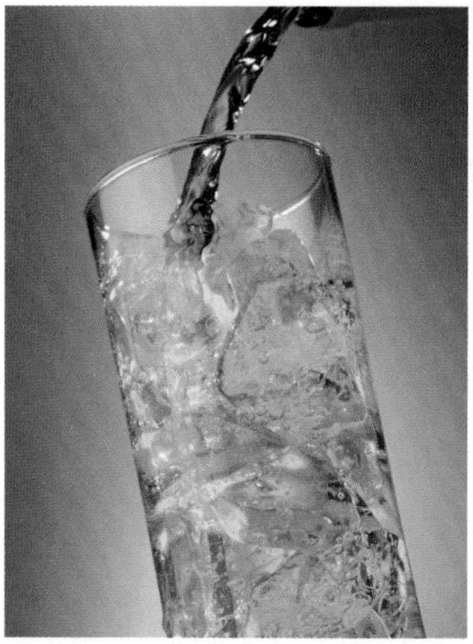

Water is readily absorbed along the entire length of the GI tract.

Bear in mind that circulation also allows for the elimination of metabolic wastes. The waste products picked up by the blood as it circulates around the body are filtered and excreted by the kidneys in urine. In addition, much of the carbon dioxide remain-

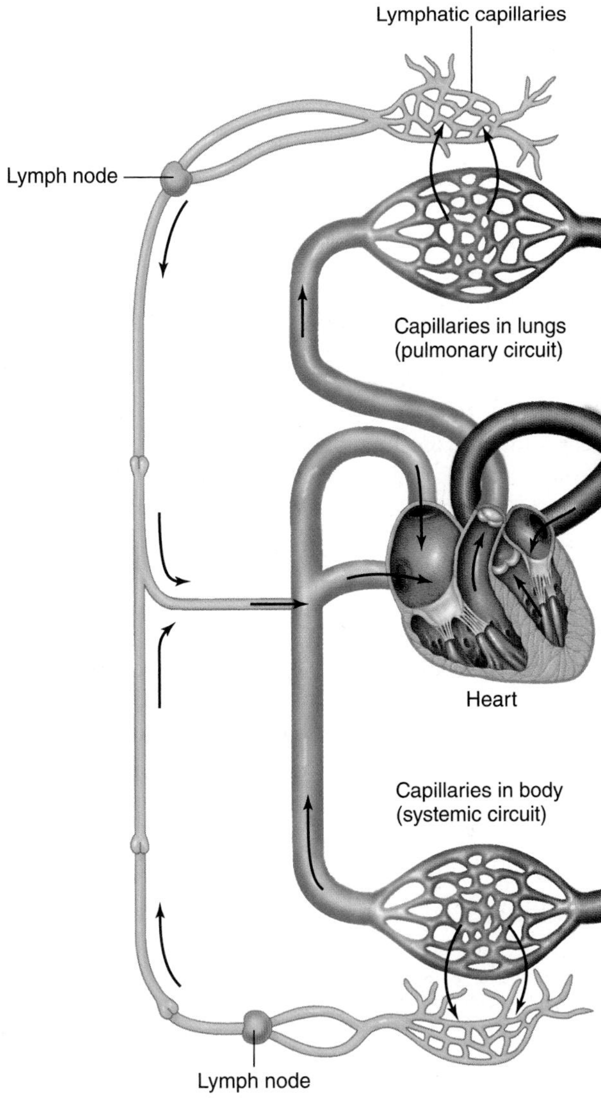

Figure 3.12 Blood travels through the cardiovascular system to transport nutrients and fluids and pick up waste products. Lymph travels through the lymphatic system and transports most fats and fat-soluble vitamins.

ing in the blood once it reaches the lungs is exhaled into the outside air, making room for oxygen to attach to the red blood cells and repeat this cycle of circulation.

The Liver Regulates Blood Nutrients

Once nutrients are absorbed from the small intestine, most enter the *portal vein,* which carries them to the **liver.** The liver is a triangular, wedge-shaped organ weighing about 3 pounds and resting almost entirely within the protection of the rib cage on the right side of the body (see Figure 3.5). It is not only the largest digestive organ but also one of the most important organs in the body, performing more than 500 discrete functions.

One function of the liver is to receive the products of digestion and then release into the bloodstream those nutrients needed throughout the body. The liver also processes and stores simple sugars, fats, and amino acids and plays a major role in regulating their levels in the bloodstream. For instance, after we eat a meal, the liver picks up excess glucose (a simple sugar) from the blood and stores it as glycogen, releasing it into the bloodstream when we need energy later in the day. It also stores certain vitamins. But the liver is more than a nutrient warehouse: it also manufactures blood proteins and can even make glucose when necessary to keep our blood glucose levels constant.

Have you ever wondered why people who abuse alcohol are at risk for liver damage? It's because another of the liver's functions is to filter the blood, removing wastes and toxins such as alcohol, medications, and other drugs. When you drink,

liver The largest auxiliary organ of the GI tract and one of the most important organs of the body. Its functions include the production of bile and processing of nutrient-rich blood from the small intestine.

your liver works hard to break down the alcohol; but with heavy drinking over time, liver cells become damaged and scar tissue forms. The scar tissue blocks the free flow of blood through the liver, so that any further toxins accumulate in the blood, causing confusion, coma, and ultimately death.

Another important job of the liver is to synthesize many of the chemicals the body uses to carry out metabolic processes. For example, the liver synthesizes bile, which, as we just discussed, is then stored in the gallbladder until the body needs it to emulsify fats.

RECAP **Most digestion and absorption occurs in the small intestine. Its three sections are the duodenum, the jejunum, and the ileum. The gallbladder stores bile, which emulsifies fats, and the pancreas synthesizes and secretes digestive enzymes that break down carbohydrates, fats, and proteins. The lining of the small intestine is heavily folded, with the surface area expanded by villi and microvilli. Nutrients are absorbed across the mucosal membrane. The liver processes all the nutrients absorbed from the small intestine and stores and regulates energy nutrients.**

The Large Intestine Stores Food Waste Until It Is Excreted

The **large intestine** (also called the *colon*) is a thick, tubelike structure that frames the small intestine on three-and-a-half sides (**Figure 3.13**). It begins with a tissue sac called the *cecum,* which explains the name of the sphincter—the *ileocecal valve*—that connects it to the ileum of the small intestine. From the cecum, the large intestine continues up along the left side of the small intestine as the *ascending colon*. The *transverse colon* runs across the top of the small intestine, and then the *descending colon* comes down on the right. The *sigmoid colon* is the last segment of the colon; it extends from the bottom right corner to the *rectum*. The last segment of the large intestine is the *anal canal,* which is about an inch and a half long.

What has happened to your turkey sandwich? The undigested food components in the chyme finally reach the large intestine. By this time, the digestive mass entering the large intestine does not resemble the chyme that left the stomach several hours before. This is because most of the nutrients have been absorbed, leaving mainly nondigestible food material, such as fiber, bacteria, and water. As in the stomach, cells lining the large intestine secrete mucus, which helps protect it from the abrasive materials passing through it.

large intestine The final organ of the GI tract, consisting of the cecum, colon, rectum, and anal canal and in which most water is absorbed and feces are formed.

Bacteria colonizing the large intestine are normal and helpful residents, since they finish digesting some of the nutrients from your sandwich. The by-products of this digestion, such as short-chain fatty acids, are reabsorbed into the body, where they re-

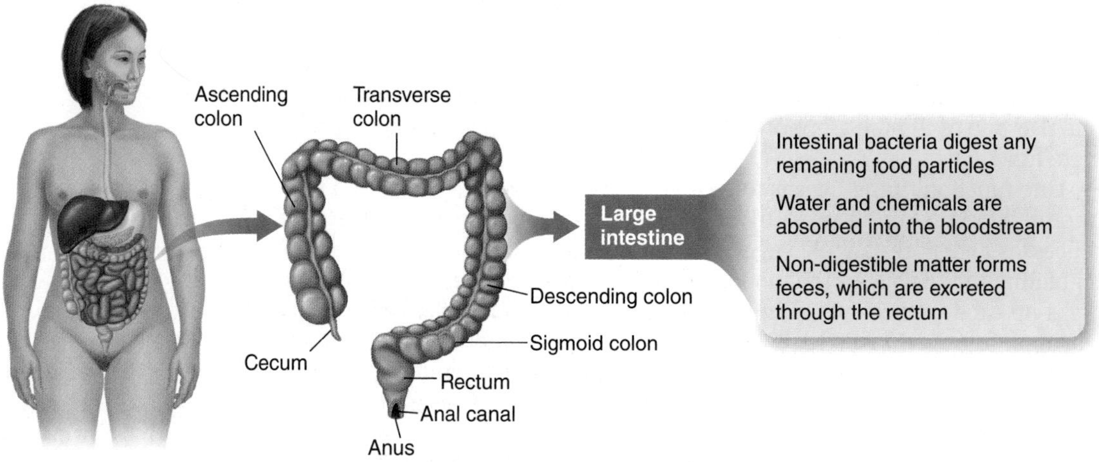

Figure 3.13 Where your food is now: the large intestine. Most water absorption occurs here, as does the formation of food wastes into semisolid feces. Peristalsis propels the feces to the body exterior.

turn to the liver and are either stored or used as needed. Intestinal bacteria, called *intestinal flora,* also help synthesize certain vitamins and are thought to promote intestinal motility. In fact, as we discussed in the Nutrition Debate in Chapter 2, the types of bacteria that thrive in our large intestine are so helpful that many people consume them deliberately in yogurt and probiotics supplements!

No other digestion occurs in the large intestine. Instead, its main functions are to store the digestive mass for 12 to 24 hours and, during that time, to absorb nutrients and water from it, leaving a semisolid mass called *feces*. Peristalsis occurs weakly to move the feces through the colon, except for one or more stronger waves of peristalsis each day, which force the feces more powerfully toward the rectum for elimination.

Some people believe that so-called toxins in the colon are responsible for a wide variety of health problems. They say that colon cleansing—in which the person consumes a liquid "detox" diet, takes laxatives, uses a series of enemas, or undergoes a procedure called colonic irrigation—flushes away these toxins and restores health. What do the experts say? Check out the Nutrition Debate near the end of this chapter to find out!

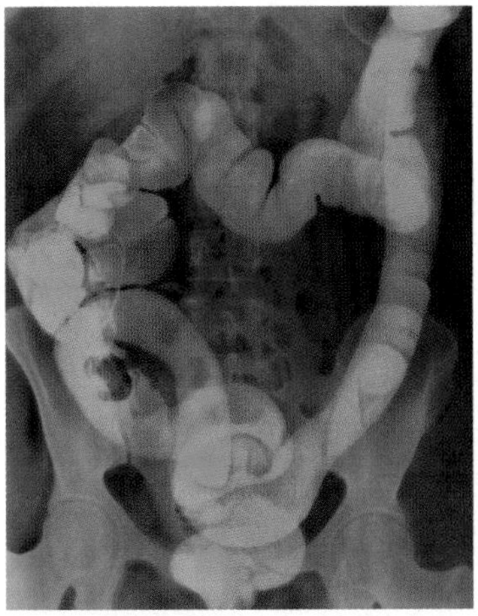

The large intestine is a thick, tubelike structure that stores the undigested mass exiting the small intestine, and also absorbs any remaining nutrients and water.

RECAP **The large intestine is composed of six sections: the cecum, ascending colon, descending colon, sigmoid colon, rectum, and anal canal. Small amounts of undigested and indigestible food material, bacteria, and water enter the large intestine. Intestinal bacteria accomplish the final digestion of any remaining digestible food products. The main functions of the large intestine are to store the digestive mass and to absorb any remaining nutrients and water. A semisolid mass, called feces, is then eliminated from the body.**

The Neuromuscular System Regulates the Activities of the GI Tract

Now that you can identify the organs involved in digestion, absorption, and elimination, and the job each performs, you might be wondering—who's the boss? In other words, what organ or system directs and coordinates all of these interrelated processes? The answer is the neuromuscular system. Both of its components, the nervous and muscular systems, are essential partners in regulating the activities of the GI tract.

The Muscles of the Gastrointestinal Tract Mix and Move Food

The purpose of the muscles of the GI tract is to mix food and move it in one direction—that is, from the mouth toward the anus. When food is present, nerves respond to the stretching of the tract walls and send signals to its muscles, stimulating peristalsis. As with an assembly line, the entire GI tract functions together so that materials are moved in one direction in a coordinated manner and wastes are removed as needed.

In order to process the large amount of food we consume daily, we use both voluntary and involuntary muscles. Muscles in the mouth are primarily voluntary; that is, they are under our conscious control. Once we swallow, involuntary muscles largely take over to propel food through the rest of the GI tract. This enables us to continue digesting and absorbing our food while we're working, exercising, and even sleeping. Let's now reveal the master controller behind these involuntary muscular actions.

The Enteric Nerves Coordinate and Regulate Digestive Activities

The nervous system in your body is like the communications system in a manufacturing plant. Within this communications system, the central nervous system (CNS), composed of the brain and spinal cord, is like the main control desk. For example, as discussed earlier in this chapter, the hypothalamus of the brain plays an important role in the control of hunger and satiation.

An intricate system of nerves branches out from the CNS; this system is called the peripheral nervous system. It includes the nerves of the GI tract, which are collectively known as the **enteric nervous system.**

enteric nervous system The nerves of the GI tract.

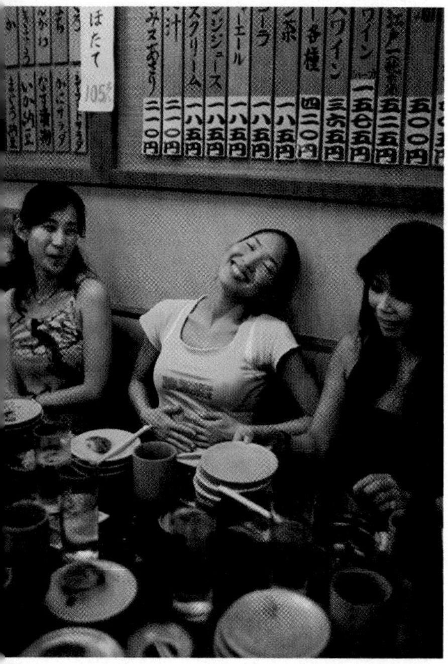

When we eat, both voluntary and involuntary muscles help us digest the food.

Enteric nerves work both independently of and in collaboration with the CNS. For example, they can respond independently to signals produced within the GI tract without first relaying them to the CNS for interpretation or assistance. On the other hand, many jobs require the involvement of the CNS. For instance, as we discussed earlier, special nerves in the GI tract pick up mechanical signals indicating how far the tract wall is stretched—that is, how full it is. These receptors signal the brain that your digestive tract is full, and then your brain sends out messages that prompt you to stop eating. Another type of enteric nerve picks up chemical signals about how acidic the digestive environment is or if there is protein or fat present. The CNS receives and responds to these signals; for example, it may send out a message to the pancreas to secrete enzymes for fat digestion.

All along the GI tract are a series of glands whose actions are also controlled by the nervous system. When food digestion products reach various locations within the GI tract, these glands are stimulated to release digestive enzymes, mucus, or water and electrolytes. For example, as chyme moves from the stomach into the small intestine, nerve signals are sent to stimulate the pancreas, gallbladder, and mucosal cells lining the intestinal tract. These signals cause these glands and cells to secrete digestive enzymes, bile, bicarbonate, and water, secretions necessary to continue digestion in the small intestine.

RECAP **The coordination and regulation of digestion are directed by the neuromuscular system. Voluntary muscles assist us with chewing and swallowing. Once food is swallowed, the involuntary muscles along the entire length of the GI tract function together, so that materials are moved in one direction in a coordinated manner and wastes are removed as needed. The enteric nerves of the GI tract work with the central nervous system to achieve the digestion, absorption, and elimination of food.**

What Disorders Are Related to Digestion, Absorption, and Elimination?

Considering the complexity of digestion, absorption, and elimination, it's no wonder that sometimes things go wrong. Clinical disorders can disturb gastrointestinal functioning, as can merely consuming the wrong types or amounts of food for our unique needs. Whenever there is a problem with the GI tract, the absorption of nutrients can be affected and, over time, malnutrition can result. Let's look more closely at some GI tract disorders and what you might be able to do if they affect you.

Heartburn and Gastroesophageal Reflux Disease (GERD) Are Caused by Reflux of Stomach Acid

When you eat food, your stomach secretes hydrochloric acid to start the digestive process. In many people, the amount of HCl secreted is occasionally excessive, or the gastroesophageal sphincter opens too soon. In either case, the result is that HCl seeps back up into the esophagus (**Figure 3.14**). Although the stomach is protected from HCl by a thick coat of mucus, the esophagus does not have this mucous coating. Thus, the HCl burns it. When this happens, a person experiences a painful sensation in the region of the chest behind the sternum (breastbone). This condition, clinically known as *gastroesophageal reflux* (*GER*), is commonly called **heartburn**. Many people take over-the-counter antacids to neutralize the HCl, thereby relieving the heartburn. A nondrug approach is to repeatedly swallow: this action causes any acid within the esophagus to be swept down into the stomach, eventually relieving the symptoms.

Gastroesophageal reflux disease (GERD) is a more painful type of GER that occurs more than twice per week. Although people who experience occasional GER

heartburn (gastroesophageal reflux [GER]) A painful sensation that occurs over the sternum when hydrochloric acid backs up into the lower esophagus.

gastroesophageal reflux disease (GERD) A more painful type of GER that occurs more than twice per week.

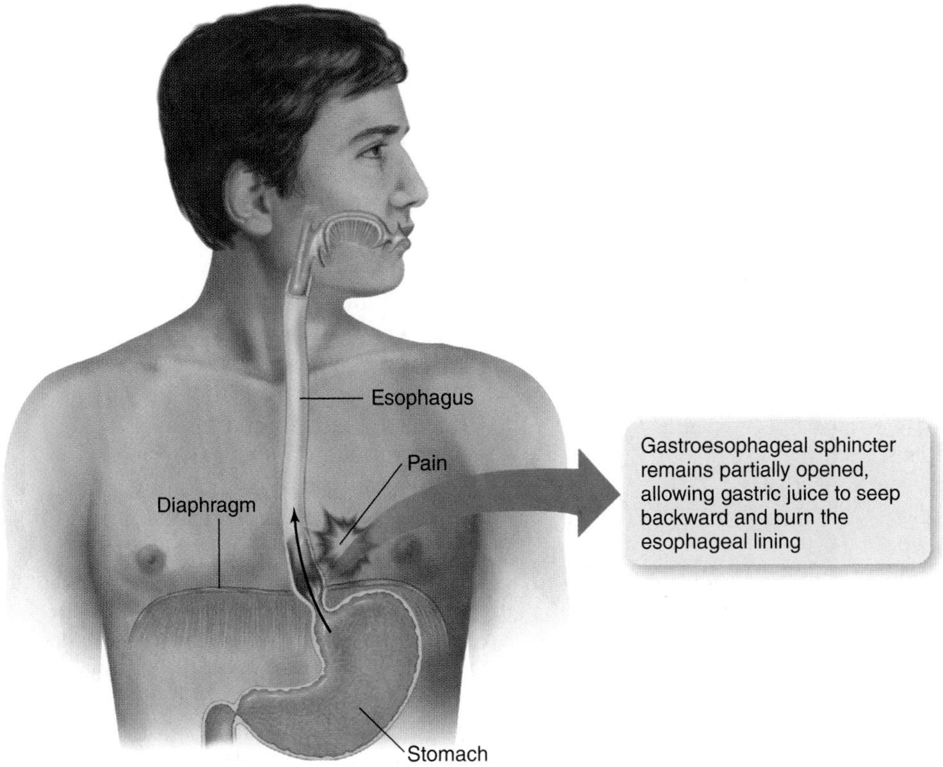
Esophagus
Pain
Diaphragm
Gastroesophageal sphincter remains partially opened, allowing gastric juice to seep backward and burn the esophageal lining
Stomach

Figure 3.14 The mechanism of gastroesophageal reflux: acidic gastric juices seep backward through an open or relaxed sphincter into the lower portion of the esophagus, burning its lining. The pain is felt behind the sternum (breastbone), over the heart.

usually have no structural abnormalities, many people with GERD have an overly relaxed or damaged esophageal sphincter or damage to the esophagus itself. Although the classic symptom of GERD is GER, some people instead experience chest pain, trouble swallowing, burning in the mouth, the feeling that food is stuck in the throat, or hoarseness in the morning.[4]

The exact causes of GERD are unknown. However, a number of factors may contribute, including the following:[4]

- A hiatal hernia, which occurs when the upper part of the stomach lies above the diaphragm muscle. Normally, the horizontal diaphragm muscle separates the stomach from the chest cavity and helps keep acid from seeping into the esophagus. Stomach acid can more easily enter the esophagus in people with a hiatal hernia.
- Cigarette smoking
- Alcohol use
- Overweight
- Pregnancy
- Foods such as citrus fruits, chocolate, caffeinated drinks, fried foods, garlic and onions, spicy foods, and tomato-based foods, such as chili, pizza, and spaghetti sauce.
- Large, high-fat meals. These meals stay in the stomach longer and increase stomach pressure, making it more likely that acid will be pushed up into the esophagus.
- Lying down soon after a meal. In susceptible people, this is almost certain to bring on symptoms, since it positions the body so it is easier for the stomach acid to back up into the esophagus.

One way to reduce the symptoms of GERD is to identify the types of foods or situations that trigger episodes, and then avoid them. Eating smaller meals also helps. After a meal, wait at least 3 hours before lying down. Some people relieve their nighttime symptoms by elevating the head of their bed 4 to 6 inches—for instance, by placing a wedge between the mattress and the box spring. This keeps the chest area elevated and minimizes the amount of acid that can back up into the esophagus. People with GERD who smoke should stop, and, if they are overweight, they should lose

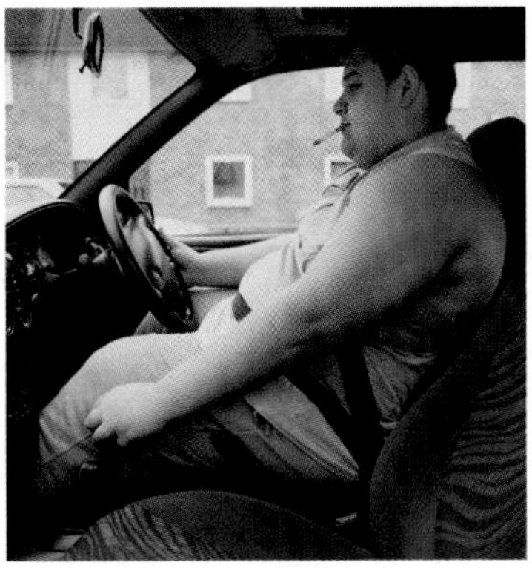

Although the exact causes of gastroesophageal reflux disease (GERD) are unknown, smoking and being overweight may be contributing factors.

NUTRITION MYTH OR FACT?

Are Ulcers Caused by Stress, Alcohol, or Spicy Foods?

For decades, physicians believed that experiencing high levels of stress, drinking alcohol, and eating spicy foods were the primary factors responsible for ulcers. But in 1982, Australian gastroenterologists Robin Warren and Barry Marshall detected the same species of bacteria in the majority of their ulcer patients' stomachs.[5] Treatment with an antibiotic effective against the bacterium *Helicobacter pylori* (*H. pylori*) cured the ulcers. It is now known that *H. pylori* plays a key role in the development of most peptic ulcers. The hydrochloric acid in gastric juice kills most bacteria, but *H. pylori* is unusual in that it thrives in acidic environments. Approximately 40% of people have this bacterium in their stomachs, but most people do not develop ulcers. The reason for this is not known.[6]

Prevention of infection with *H. pylori*, as with any infectious microorganism, includes regular hand washing and safe food-handling practices. Because of the role of *H. pylori* in ulcer development, treatment usually involves antibiotics and acid-suppressing medications. Special diets and stress-reduction techniques are no longer typically recommended because they do not reduce acid secretion. However, people with ulcers should avoid specific foods they identify as causing them discomfort.

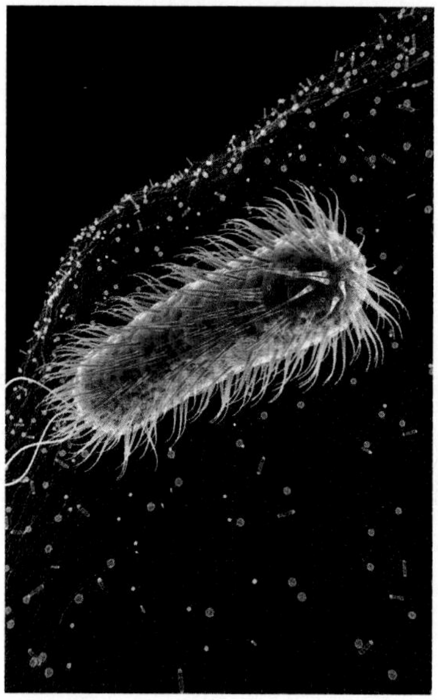

The *Helicobacter pylori* (*H. pylori*) bacterium plays a key role in the development of most peptic ulcers.

Although most peptic ulcers are caused by *H. pylori* infection, some are caused by prolonged use of nonsteroidal anti-inflammatory drugs (NSAIDs); these drugs include pain relievers, such as aspirin, ibuprofen, and naproxen sodium. They appear to cause ulcers by suppressing the secretion of mucus and bicarbonate, which normally protect the stomach from its acidic gastric juice. Ulcers caused by NSAID use generally heal once a person stops taking the medication.[7]

weight. Taking an antacid before a meal can help prevent symptoms, and many other medications are now available to treat GERD.

It is important to treat GERD, as it can cause serious health problems. GERD can lead to bleeding and ulcers in the esophagus. Scar tissue can develop in the esophagus, making swallowing very difficult. Some people can also develop a condition called Barrett's esophagus, which can lead to cancer. Asthma can also be aggravated or even caused by GERD.

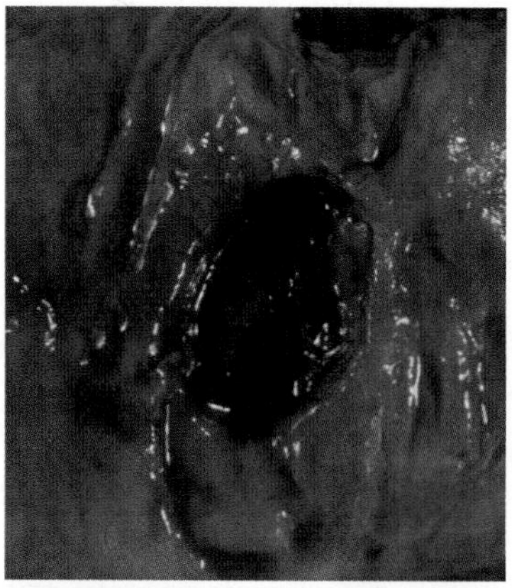

Figure 3.15 A peptic ulcer.

An Ulcer Is an Area of Erosion in the GI Tract

A **peptic ulcer** is an area of the GI tract that has been eroded away by a combination of hydrochloric acid and the enzyme pepsin (**Figure 3.15**). In almost all cases, it is located in the stomach area (*gastric ulcer*) or the part of the duodenum closest to the stomach (*duodenal ulcer*). It causes a burning pain in the abdominal area, typically 1 to 3 hours after eating a meal. In serious cases, eroded blood vessels bleed into the GI tract, causing vomiting of blood and/or blood in the stools, as well as anemia. If the ulcer entirely perforates the tract wall, stomach contents can leak into the abdominal cavity, causing a life-threatening infection.

You might have heard the advice that people with an ulcer should try to reduce their stress and avoid caffeine and spicy foods. But do these factors really cause or contribute to ulcers? Find the answer in the Nutrition Myth or Fact? box.

peptic ulcer An area of the GI tract that has been eroded away by the acidic gastric juice of the stomach.

RECAP **Heartburn is clinically known as gastroesophageal reflux (GER). It is caused by the seepage of gastric juices into the esophagus. Gastroesophageal reflux disease (GERD) is a more painful type of GER that occurs more than twice per week. Peptic ulcers are caused by erosion of the GI tract by hydrochloric acid and pepsin.**

Some Disorders Affect Intestinal Function

GERD and ulcers involve the upper GI tract. In this section, we'll discuss disorders affecting intestinal function.

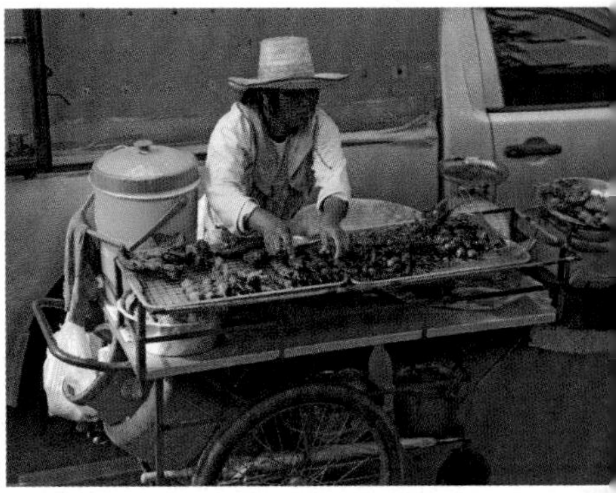

When traveling, it is wise to avoid food from street vendors.

Diarrhea

Diarrhea is the frequent passage (more than three times in 1 day) of loose, watery stools. Other symptoms may include cramping, abdominal pain, bloating, nausea, fever, and blood in the stools. Diarrhea is usually caused by an infection of the gastrointestinal tract, a chronic disease, stress, or reactions to medications.[8] It can also occur as a reaction to a particular food or food ingredient. Disorders related to specific foods include food intolerances, allergies, and celiac disease. These are discussed ***In Depth*** following this chapter.

Whatever the cause, diarrhea can be harmful if it persists for a long period of time because the person can lose large quantities of water and minerals and become severely dehydrated. **Table 3.1** reviews the signs and symptoms of dehydration, which is particularly dangerous in infants and young children. In fact, a child can die from dehydration in just a few days. Adults, particularly the elderly, can also become dangerously ill if severely dehydrated. A doctor should be seen immediately if diarrhea persists for more than 24 hours in children or more than 3 days in adults or if diarrhea is bloody, fever is present, or there are signs of dehydration.

A condition referred to as *traveler's diarrhea* has become a common health concern due to the expansion in global travel. *Traveler's diarrhea* is experienced by people traveling to countries outside of their own and is usually caused by viral or bacterial infections. Diarrhea represents the body's way of ridding itself of an invasive agent. The large intestine and even some of the small intestine become irritated by the microbes and the body's defense against them. This irritation leads to increased secretion of fluid and increased motility of the large intestine, causing watery and frequent bowel movements. In some cases, the person may also experience nausea, vomiting, and low-grade fever. Usually, people who are otherwise healthy recover completely within 4 to 6 days.[9]

People generally get traveler's diarrhea from consuming water or food that is contaminated with fecal matter. Very risky foods include any raw or undercooked fish, meats, and raw fruits and vegetables. Tap water, ice made from tap water, and unpasteurized milk and dairy products are also common sources of infection.

What can you do to prevent traveler's diarrhea? The following Quick Tips from the National Institutes of Health should help.[10]

If you do suffer from traveler's diarrhea, it is important to replace the fluid and nutrients lost as a result of the illness. Specially formulated oral rehydration solutions are available in most countries. Antibiotics may also be taken to kill bacteria. Once treatment is initiated, the diarrhea should cease within 2 to 3 days. If the diarrhea persists for more than 10 days after the initiation of treatment, or if there is blood in your stools, you should see a physician immediately.

diarrhea A condition characterized by the frequent passage of loose, watery stools.

constipation A condition characterized by the absence of bowel movements for a period of time that is significantly longer than normal for the individual. When a bowel movement does occur, stools are usually small, hard, and difficult to pass.

Constipation

At the opposite end of the spectrum from diarrhea is **constipation,** which is typically defined as a condition in which no stools are passed for 2 or more days; however, it is important to recognize that some people normally experience bowel movements only every second or third day. Thus, the definition of constipation varies from one person to another. In addition to being infrequent, the stools are usually hard, small, and somewhat difficult to pass.

Many people experience temporary constipation at some point in their lives, such as when they travel,

TABLE 3.1 Signs and Symptoms of Dehydration in Adults and Children

Symptoms in Adults	Symptoms in Children
Thirst	Dry mouth and tongue
Light-headedness	No tears when crying
Less frequent urination	No wet diapers for 3 hours or more
Dark-colored urine	High fever
Fatigue	Sunken abdomen, eyes, or cheeks
Dry skin	Irritable or listless
	Skin does not rebound when pinched and released

Data from National Digestive Diseases Information Clearinghouse (NDDIC). 2003. *Diarrhea.* NIH Publication No. 04–2749. http://digestive.niddk.nih.gov/ddiseases/pubs/diarrhea/index.htm.

QUICK TIPS

Avoiding Traveler's Diarrhea

✓ Do not drink tap water or use it to brush your teeth.

✓ Do not drink unpasteurized milk or dairy products.

✓ Do not use ice made from tap water. Freezing does not kill all microbes.

✓ Avoid raw or rare meats, and raw fruits and vegetables, including lettuce and fruit salads, unless they can be peeled and you peel them yourself.

✓ Do not eat meat or shellfish that is not hot when served.

✓ Do not eat food from street vendors.

✓ Do drink bottled water. Make sure you are the one to break the seal, and wipe the top of the bottle clean before doing so. You can also safely choose canned carbonated soft drinks and hot drinks made with boiling water, such as coffee or tea.

✓ Consult your doctor when planning your trip. Depending on where you are going and how long you will stay, your doctor may recommend that you take antibiotics before leaving to protect you from possible infection.

when their schedule is disrupted, if they change their diet, or if they are on certain medications. Many healthcare providers suggest increasing fiber and fluid in the diet. Five to nine servings of fruits and vegetables each day and six or more servings of whole grains is recommended. If you eat breakfast cereal, make sure you buy a cereal containing at least 2 to 3 g of fiber per serving. The dietary recommendation for fiber and the role it plays in maintaining healthy elimination are discussed in detail in Chapter 4. Staying well hydrated is important when increasing your fiber intake. Regular exercise may also help reduce your risk for constipation.

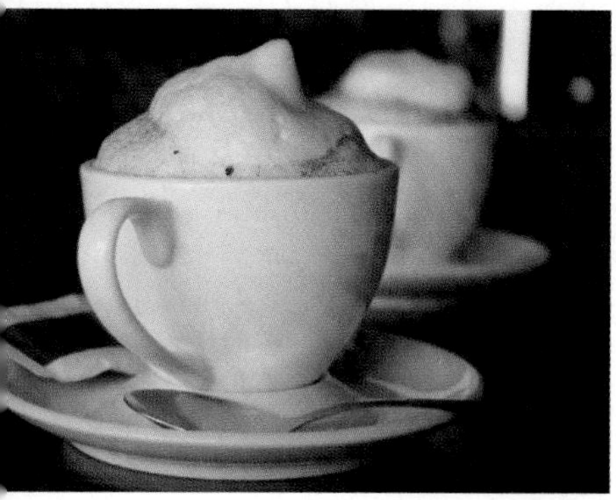

Consuming caffeinated drinks is one of several factors that have been linked with irritable bowel syndrome.

Irritable Bowel Syndrome

Irritable bowel syndrome (IBS) is a disorder that interferes with the normal functions of the colon (commonly referred to as the "large bowel"). It is one of the most common medical diagnoses, applied to approximately 20% of the U.S. population, and it affects more women than men.[11,12] Symptoms include abdominal cramps, bloating, and either constipation or diarrhea: in some people with IBS, food moves too quickly through the colon and fluid cannot be absorbed fast enough, which causes diarrhea. In others, the movement of the colon is too slow and too much fluid is absorbed, leading to constipation.

IBS shows no sign of underlying disease that can be observed or measured. However, it appears that the colon is more sensitive to physiologic or emotional stress in people with IBS than in healthy people. Some researchers believe that the problem stems from conflicting messages between the central nervous system and the enteric nervous system. The immune system may also trigger symptoms of IBS. Some of the foods thought to cause physiologic stress linked to IBS include caffeinated tea, coffee, and colas; chocolate; alcohol; dairy products; and wheat. Certain medications may also increase the risk.

If you think you have IBS, it is important to have a complete physical examination to rule out any other health problems, including celiac disease (see the ***In Depth*** essay following this chapter). Treatment options include taking certain medications to treat diarrhea or constipation, managing stress, engaging in regular physical activity, eating smaller meals, avoiding foods that exacerbate symptoms, eating a higher-fiber diet, and drinking at least six to eight glasses of water each day.[15] Although IBS is uncomfortable, it does not appear to endanger long-term health. However, severe IBS can be disabling and can prevent people from leading normal lives; thus, an accurate diagnosis and effective treatment are critical.

RECAP **Diarrhea is the frequent passage of loose or watery stools. It should be treated quickly to avoid dehydration or even death. Constipation is failure to have a bowel movement within a time period that is normal for the individual. Irritable bowel syndrome (IBS) causes abdominal cramps, bloating, and constipation or diarrhea. The causes of IBS are unknown; however, physiologic and emotional stress is implicated.**

irritable bowel syndrome (IBS) A bowel disorder that interferes with normal functions of the colon.

NUTRI-CASE LIZ

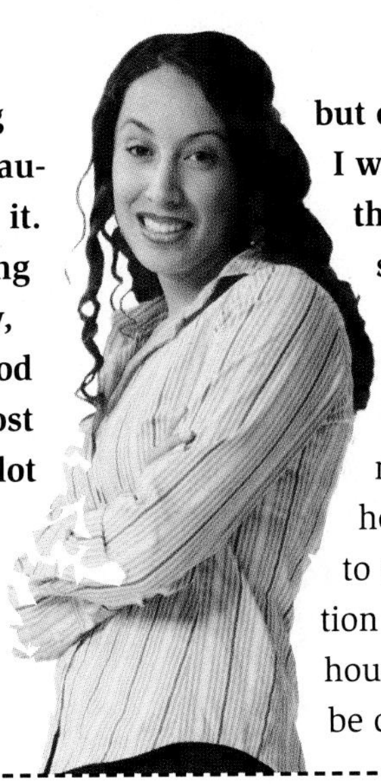

"I used to think of my peanut allergy as no big deal, but ever since my experience at that restaurant last year, I've been pretty obsessive about it. For months afterwards, I refused to eat anything that I hadn't prepared myself. I do eat out now, but I always insist that the chef prepare my food personally, with clean utensils, and I avoid most desserts. They're just too risky. Shopping is a lot harder, too, because I have to check every label. The worst, though, is eating at my friends' houses. I have to ask them, "Do you keep peanuts or peanut butter in your house? Some of them are really sympathetic, but others look at me as if I'm a hypochondriac! I wish I could think of something to say to them to make them understand that this isn't something I have any control over."

What could Liz say in response to friends who don't understand the cause and seriousness of her food allergy? Do you think it would help Liz to share her fears with her doctor and to discuss possible strategies? If so, why? In addition to shopping, dining out, and eating at friends' houses, what other situations might require Liz to be cautious about her food choices?

all of her body systems and sending her into a state called *anaphylactic shock*. Left untreated, anaphylactic shock is nearly always fatal, so many people with known food allergies carry with them a kit containing an injection of a powerful stimulant called epinephrine. This drug can reduce symptoms long enough to buy the victim time to get emergency medical care.

Physicians use a variety of tests to diagnose food allergies. Usually, the physician orders a skin test, commonly known as a "scratch test," in which a clinician swabs a small amount of fluid containing the suspected allergen onto the patient's skin, then lightly scratches or pricks the area so that the fluid seeps under the patient's skin. After 15–20 minutes, the clinician checks the area: redness and/or swelling indicates that the patient is allergic to the substance. However, people can have a positive response with allergy skin testing yet not have any problems with the specific substance in daily life.[4] Thus, some physicians will perform a blood test, in which a sample of the patient's blood is tested for the presence of unique proteins, called *antibodies*, that the immune system produces in a person with an allergy. In Liz's case, the blood test detected antibodies specific to peanut allergen.

Beware of e-mail spam, Internet websites, and ads in popular magazines attempting to link a vast assortment of health problems to food allergies. Typically, these ads offer allergy-testing services for exorbitant fees, then make even more money by selling "nutritional counseling" and sometimes supplements and other products they say will help you cope with your allergies. If you suspect you might have a food allergy, consult an MD.

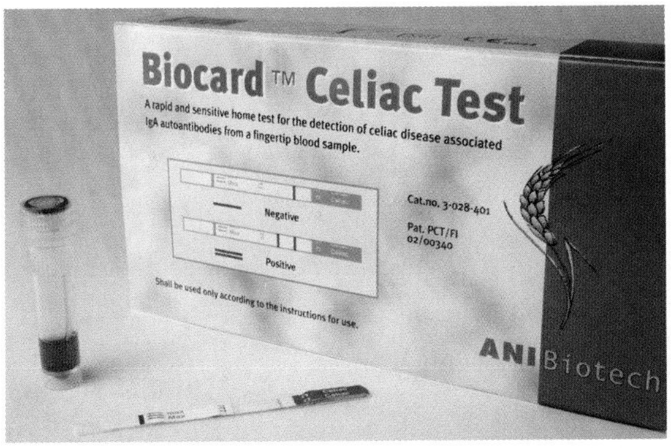

A simple blood test can identify celiac disease.

Celiac Disease

Celiac disease, also known as *celiac sprue,* is a disease that severely damages the lining of the small intestine and interferes with the absorption of nutrients. It is classified as an *autoimmune* disease; that is, the body's own immune system causes the destruction. Because there is a strong genetic predisposition to celiac disease, with the risk now linked to specific gene markers, it is also considered a genetic disorder. Specifically, celiac disease occurs in about 1 of 133 Americans, but in 1 of 22 Americans with a close relative diagnosed with the disorder.[5]

In celiac disease, the offending food component is *gliadin,* a fraction of a protein, called *gluten,* that is found in wheat, rye, barley, and triticale. When people with celiac disease eat one of these grains, their immune system triggers an inflammatory response that erodes the villi of the small intestine. If the person is unaware of the disorder and continues

celiac disease An autoimmune disorder characterized by an inability to absorb a component of gluten called gliadin. This causes an inflammatory immune response that damages the lining of the small intestine.

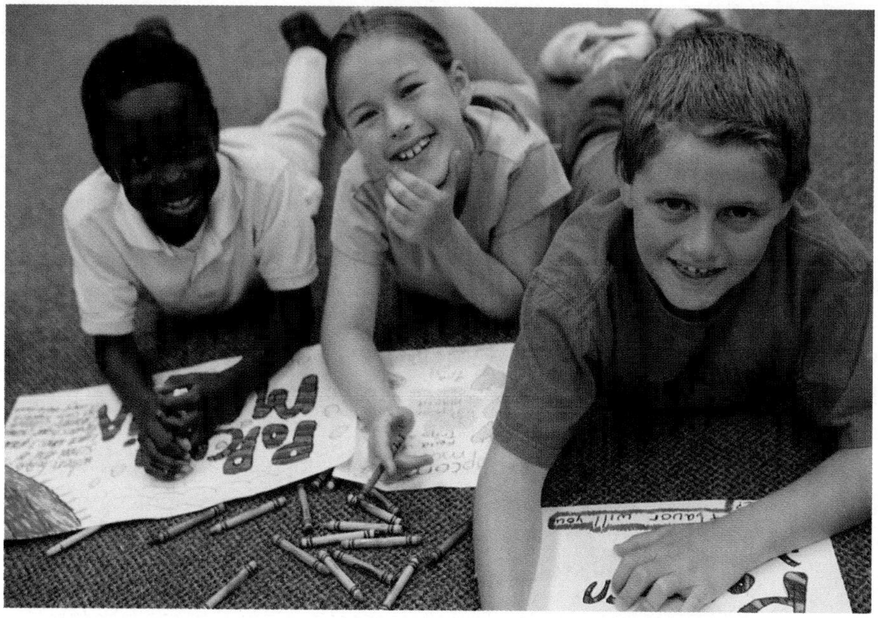

Schoolchildren may have celiac disease and not know it. Undiagnosed celiac disease can lead to physical and mental disorders as children grow.

to eat gluten, repeated immune reactions cause the villi to become greatly decreased, and there is less absorptive surface area. As a result, the person becomes unable to absorb certain nutrients properly—a condition known as *malabsorption*. Over time, malabsorption can lead to malnutrition (poor nutrient status). Deficiencies of iron, folic acid, calcium, and vitamins A, D, E, and K are common in those suffering from celiac disease, as are inadequate intakes of protein and total energy.[6]

Symptoms of celiac disease often mimic those of other intestinal disturbances, such as irritable bowel syndrome, so the condition is often misdiagnosed. Some of the symptoms of celiac disease are fatty stools (due to poor fat absorption); frequent stools, either watery or hard, with an odd odor; cramping; anemia; pallor; weight loss; fatigue; and irritability. However, other puzzling symptoms do not appear to involve the GI tract. These include an intensely itchy rash called *dermatitis herpetiformis,* osteoporosis (poor bone density), infertility, seizures, anxiety, irritability, depression, and migraine headaches, among others.[6]

Diagnostic tests for celiac disease include a variety of blood tests that screen for the presence of antibodies to gluten, or for the genetic markers of the disease. Although the antibody test is considered generally reliable for diagnosing celiac disease, false negatives are not uncommon. Thus, the "gold standard" for diagnosis is a biopsy of the small intestine showing atrophy of the intestinal villi. Because one of the long-term complications of undiagnosed celiac disease is an increased risk for intestinal cancer, early diagnosis can be life-saving. Unfortunately, celiac disease is widely underdiagnosed in the United States.[6] This is one reason that some researchers and healthcare professionals favor screening school-age children for celiac disease, as is common in several European countries.

Currently, there is no cure for celiac disease. Treatment is with a special diet that excludes all forms of wheat, rye, barley, and triticale. Oats are allowed, but they are often contaminated with wheat flour from processing, and even a microscopic amount of gluten can cause

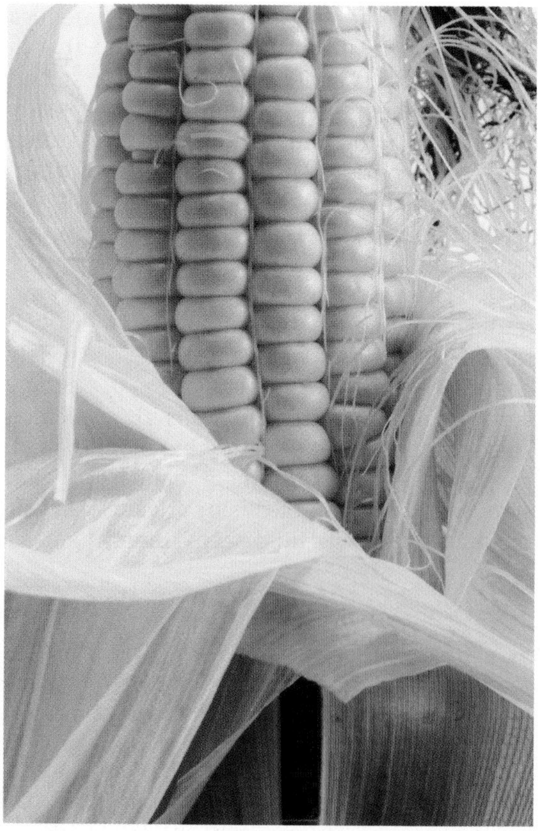

For people with celiac disease, corn is a gluten-free source of carbohydrates.

an immune response. The diet is made even more challenging by the fact that many binding agents and other unfamiliar ingredients in processed foods are derived from gluten. Thus, nutritional counseling is essential. Fortunately, more gluten-free foods are becoming available, including breads made from corn, rice, tapioca, potato, arrowroot, cassava, soy, and even garbanzo bean flours.

To meet the need for comprehensive and current information about celiac disease, in 2007 the National Digestive Diseases Information Clearinghouse, part of the National Institutes of Health (NIH), launched the Celiac Disease Awareness Campaign. One goal of the campaign is to raise awareness of celiac disease among physicians, registered dietitians, and other healthcare providers.[5]

If you suspect you have celiac disease, consult your physician. Do not simply attempt to eliminate gluten from your diet, since if you then decide to undergo antibody screening, being on a gluten-free diet will invalidate the results of the test. Moreover, a gluten-free diet is notoriously difficult to maintain without appropriate nutritional counseling and support.

Web Resources

www.nlm.nih.gov/medlineplus
MEDLINE Plus Health Information

Search for "food allergies" to obtain additional resources as well as the latest news about food allergies.

www.healthfinder.gov
Health Finder

Search this site to learn more about disorders related to digestion, absorption, and elimination.

www.ific.org
International Food Information Council Foundation (IFIC)

Scroll down to "Food Safety Information" and click on the link for "Food Allergies and Asthma" for additional information on food allergies.

www.foodallergy.org
The Food Allergy and Anaphylaxis Network (FAN)

Visit this site to learn more about common food allergens.

www.americanceliac.org/cd
American Celiac Disease Alliance

Learn more about the diagnosis and treatment of celiac disease, ongoing research, and living with celiac disease.

www.csaceliacs.org
Celiac Sprue Association—National Celiac Disease Support Group

Get information on the Celiac Sprue Association, a national educational organization that provides information and referral services for persons with celiac disease.

www.gfmall.com
Gluten-Free Mall

Find out where you can buy gluten-free products.

4 Carbohydrates: Plant-Derived Energy Nutrients

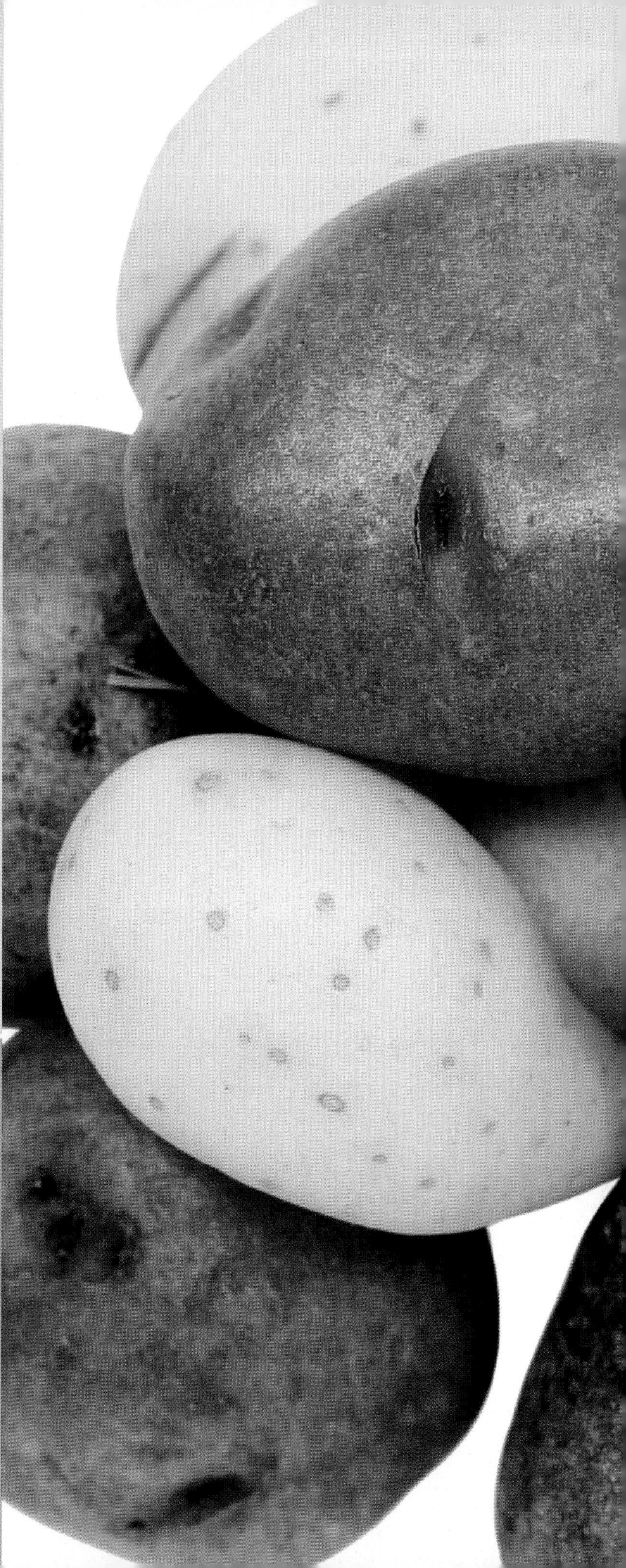

CHAPTER OBJECTIVES

After reading this chapter you will be able to:

1. **Describe the difference between simple and complex carbohydrates, pp. 108–110.**
2. **List four functions of carbohydrates in our body, pp. 113–115.**
3. **Discuss how carbohydrates are digested and absorbed by our body, pp. 116–118.**
4. **Define the Acceptable Macronutrient Distribution Range for carbohydrates, and the Adequate Intake for fiber, pp. 122, 125–126, 128.**
5. **Identify the potential health risks associated with diets high in refined sugars, pp. 123–125.**
6. **List five foods that are good sources of carbohydrates, pp. 125–128.**
7. **Identify three alternative sweeteners, pp. 130–132.**

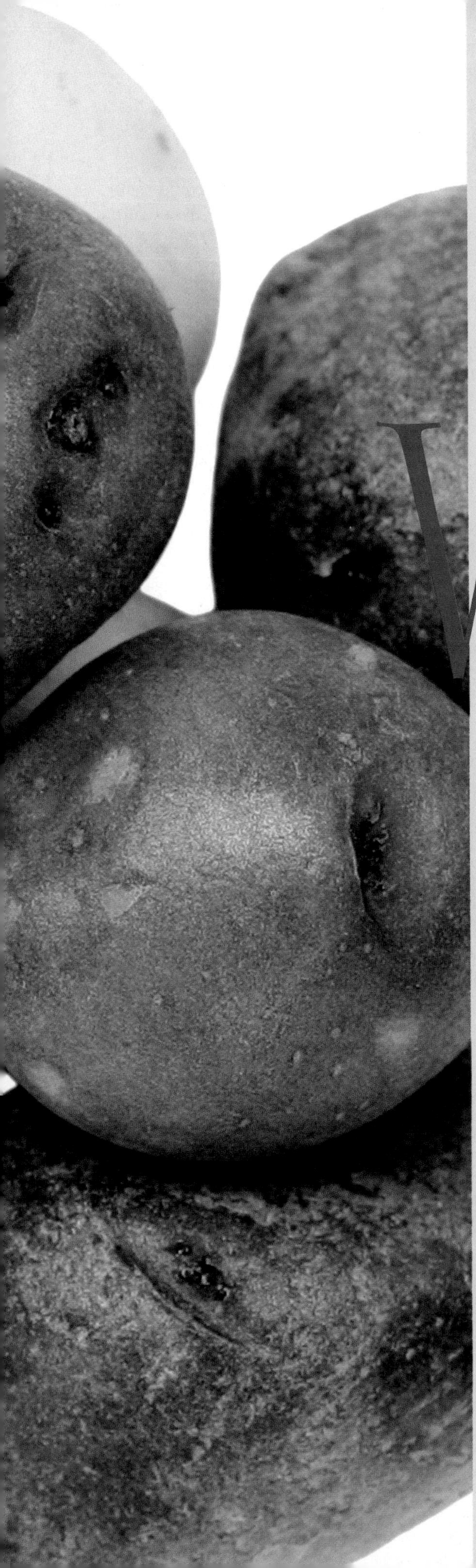

Test Yourself

1. **T F Diets high in sugar cause hyperactivity in children.**
2. **T F Carbohydrates are fattening.**
3. **T F Alternative sweeteners, such as aspartame, are safe for us to consume.**

Test Yourself answers can be found at the end of the chapter.

When Khalil lived at home, he snacked on whatever was around. That typically meant fresh fruit or his mom's homemade flatbread, and either plain water or skim milk. His parents never drank soda, and the only time he ate sweets was on special occasions. Now Khalil is living on campus. When he gets hungry between classes, he visits the snack shack in the Student Union for one of their awesome chocolate-chunk cookies, a cinnamon roll, or a brownie and washes it down with a large cola. Studying at night, he munches on cheese curls or corn chips and drinks more cola to help him stay awake. Not suprisingly, Khalil has noticed lately that his clothes feel tight. When he steps on the scale, he's shocked to discover that, since starting college 3 months ago, he's gained 7 pounds!

Several popular diets—including the Zone Diet, Sugar Busters, and Dr. Atkins' New Diet Revolution—claim that carbohydrates are bad for your health. They recommend reducing carbohydrate consumption and eating more protein and fat.[1–3] Is this good advice? If you had a friend like Khalil who regularly consumed several soft drinks a day, plus chips, cookies, candy, and other high-carbohydrate snacks, would you say anything? Are carbohydrates a health menace, and is one type of carbohydrate as bad as another?

In this chapter, we'll explore the differences between simple and complex carbohydrates and learn why some carbohydrates really are better than others. We'll also learn how the human body breaks down carbohydrates and uses them to maintain our health and to fuel our activity and exercise. In the ***In Depth*** essay following this chapter, we'll discuss the relationship between carbohydrate intake and diabetes.

What Are Carbohydrates?

As we mentioned in Chapter 1, carbohydrates are one of the three macronutrients. As such, they are an important energy source for the entire body and are the preferred energy source for nerve cells, including those of the brain. We will say more about their functions later in this chapter.

The term **carbohydrate** literally means "hydrated carbon." Water (H_2O) is made of hydrogen and oxygen, and, when something is said to be *hydrated*, it contains water. Thus, the chemical abbreviation for carbohydrate (CHO) indicates the atoms it contains: **c**arbon, **h**ydrogen, and **o**xygen.

We obtain carbohydrates predominantly from plant foods, such as fruits, vegetables, and grains. Plants make the most abundant form of carbohydrate, called **glucose**, through a process called **photosynthesis**. During photosynthesis, the green pigment of plants, called *chlorophyll*, absorbs sunlight, which provides the energy needed to fuel the manufacture of glucose. As shown in **Figure 4.1**, water absorbed from the earth by the roots of plants combines with the carbon dioxide present in the leaves to produce the carbohydrate glucose. Plants continually store glucose and use it to support their own growth. Then, when we eat plant foods, our body digests, absorbs, and uses the stored glucose.

Carbohydrates can be classified as *simple* or *complex*. These terms are used to describe carbohydrates based on the number of molecules of sugar present.[4] Simple carbohydrates contain either one or two molecules, whereas complex carbohydrates contain hundreds to thousands of molecules.

carbohydrate One of the three macronutrients, a compound made up of carbon, hydrogen, and oxygen that is derived from plants and provides energy.

glucose The most abundant sugar molecule, a monosaccharide generally found in combination with other sugars; it is the preferred source of energy for the brain and an important source of energy for all cells.

photosynthesis The process by which plants use sunlight to fuel a chemical reaction that combines carbon and water into glucose, which is then stored in their cells.

Energy from sun

Carbon dioxide from air

Glucose stored in plant

Water

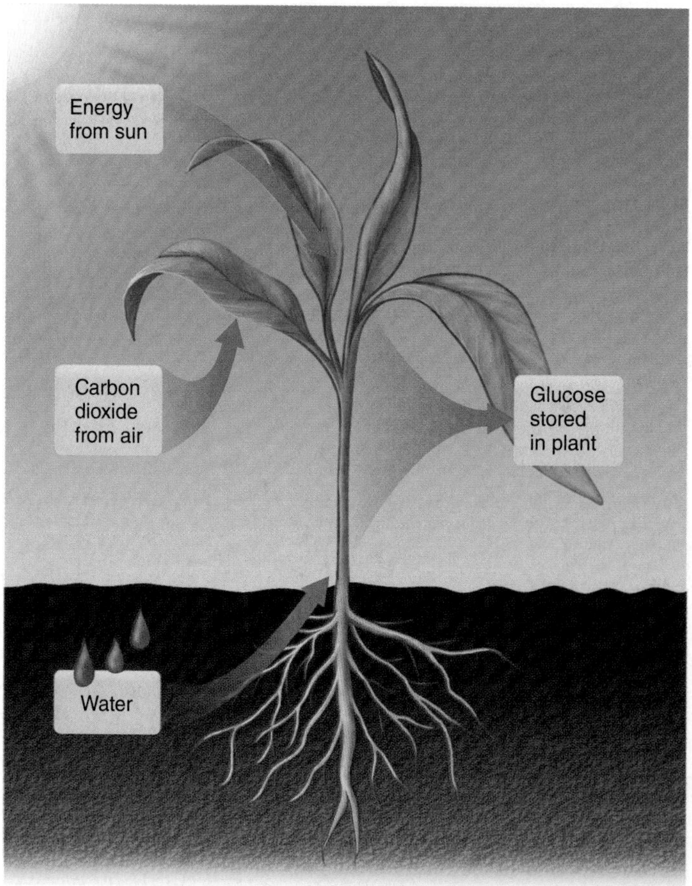

Figure 4.1 Plants make carbohydrates through the process of photosynthesis. Water, carbon dioxide, and energy from the sun are combined to produce glucose.

Simple Carbohydrates Include Monosaccharides and Disaccharides

Simple carbohydrates are commonly referred to as *sugars*. Four of these sugars are called **monosaccharides** because they consist of a single sugar molecule (*mono* means "one," and *saccharide* means "sugar"). The other three sugars are **disaccharides**, which consist of two molecules of sugar joined together (*di* means "two").

Glucose, Fructose, Galactose, and Ribose Are Monosaccharides

Glucose, fructose, and *galactose* are the three most common monosaccharides in our diet. Each of these monosaccharides contains six carbon atoms, twelve hydrogen atoms, and six oxygen atoms **(Figure 4.2)**. Very slight differences in the arrangement of the atoms in these three monosaccharides cause major differences in their levels of sweetness.

Given what you've just learned about how plants manufacture glucose, it probably won't surprise you to discover that glucose is the most abundant sugar molecule in our diets and in our body. Glucose does not generally occur by itself in foods, but attaches to other sugars to form disaccharides and complex carbohydrates. In our body, glucose is the preferred source of energy for the brain, and it is a very important source of energy for all cells.

Fructose, the sweetest natural sugar, is found in fruits and vegetables. Fructose is also called *levulose,*or *fruit sugar*. In many processed foods, it comes in the form of *high-fructose corn syrup*. This syrup is manufactured from corn and is used to sweeten soft drinks, desserts, candies, and jellies.

Galactose does not occur alone in foods. It joins with glucose to create lactose, one of the three most common disaccharides.

Ribose is a five-carbon monosaccharide. Very little ribose is found in our diets; our body produces ribose from the foods we eat, and ribose is contained in the genetic material of our cells: deoxyribonucleic acid (DNA) and ribonucleic acid (RNA).

Lactose, Maltose, and Sucrose Are Disaccharides

The three most common disaccharides found in foods are *lactose, maltose,* and *sucrose* **(Figure 4.3)**. **Lactose** (also called *milk sugar*) consists of one glucose molecule and one galactose molecule. Interestingly, human breast milk has more lactose than cow's milk does, making human breast milk taste sweeter.

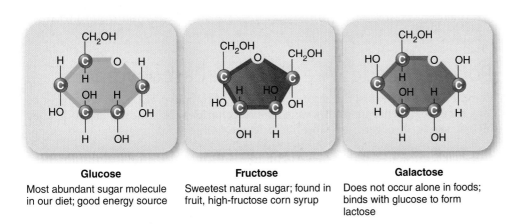

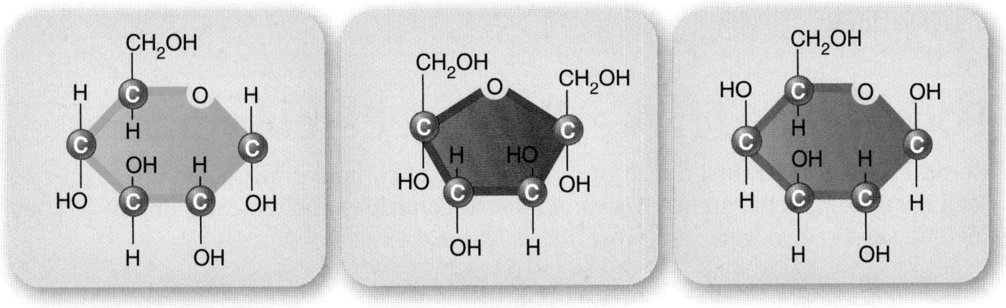

Glucose
Most abundant sugar molecule in our diet; good energy source

Fructose
Sweetest natural sugar; found in fruit, high-fructose corn syrup

Galactose
Does not occur alone in foods; binds with glucose to form lactose

Figure 4.2 The three most common monosaccharides. Notice that all three contain identical atoms: six carbon, twelve hydrogen, and six oxygen. It is only the arrangement of these atoms that differs among them.

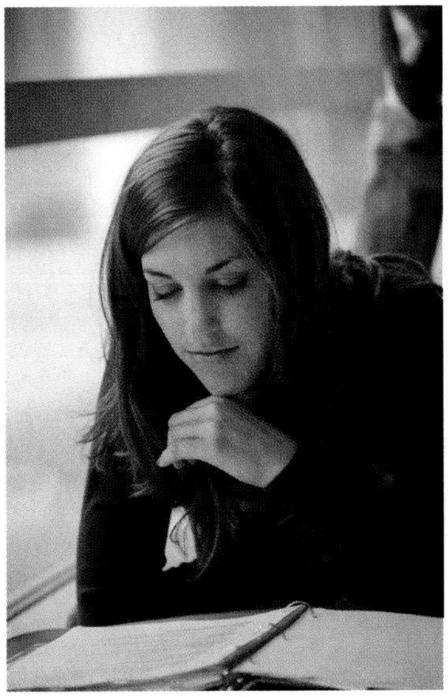

In our body, glucose is the preferred source of energy for the brain.

simple carbohydrate Commonly called *sugar;* can be either a monosaccharide (such as glucose) or a disaccharide.

monosaccharide The simplest of carbohydrates, consisting of one sugar molecule, the most common form of which is glucose.

disaccharide A carbohydrate compound consisting of two sugar molecules joined together.

fructose The sweetest natural sugar; a monosaccharide that occurs in fruits and vegetables; also called levulose, or fruit sugar.

galactose A monosaccharide that joins with glucose to create lactose, one of the three most common disaccharides.

ribose A five-carbon monosaccharide that is located in the genetic material of cells.

lactose A disaccharide consisting of one glucose molecule and one galactose molecule. It is found in milk, including human breast milk; also called *milk sugar*.

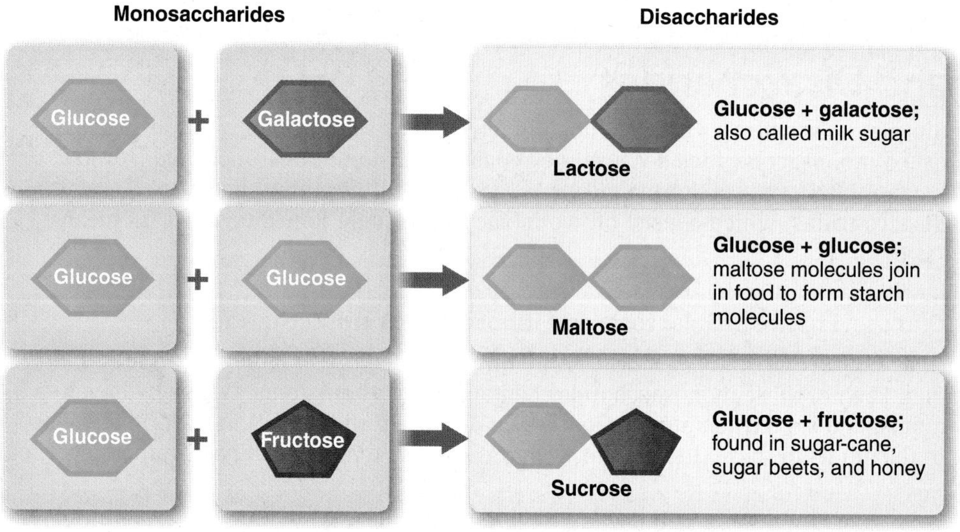

Figure 4.3 Galactose, glucose, and fructose join together to make the disaccharides lactose, maltose, and sucrose.

Maltose (also called *malt sugar*) consists of two molecules of glucose. It does not generally occur by itself in foods but, rather, is bound together with other molecules. As our body breaks these larger molecules down, maltose results as a by-product. Maltose is also the sugar that is fermented during the production of beer and liquor products. **Fermentation** is a process in which an agent, such as yeast, causes an organic substance to break down into simpler substances and results in the production of the energy molecule adenosine triphosphate (ATP). Maltose is formed during the breakdown of sugar in grains and other foods into alcohol. Contrary to popular belief, very little maltose remains in alcoholic beverages after the fermentation process is complete; thus, alcoholic beverages are not good sources of carbohydrate.

Sucrose is composed of one glucose molecule and one fructose molecule. Because sucrose contains fructose, it is sweeter than lactose or maltose. Sucrose provides much of the sweet taste found in honey, maple syrup, fruits, and vegetables. Table sugar, brown sugar, powdered sugar, and many other products are made by refining the sucrose found in sugarcane and sugar beets. Are honey and other naturally occurring forms of sucrose more healthful than manufactured forms? The Nutrition Myth or Fact? box investigates this question.

RECAP **Carbohydrates contain carbon, hydrogen, and oxygen. Plants make one type of carbohydrate, glucose, through the process of photosynthesis. Simple carbohydrates include monosaccharides and disaccharides. Glucose, fructose, and galactose are monosaccharides; lactose, maltose, and sucrose are disaccharides.**

Polysaccharides Are Complex Carbohydrates

Complex carbohydrates, the second major type of carbohydrate, generally consist of long chains of glucose molecules called **polysaccharides** (*poly* means "many"). They include starch, glycogen, and most fibers **(Figure 4.4)**.

Starch Is a Polysaccharide Stored in Plants

Plants store glucose not as single molecules but as polysaccharides in the form of **starch**. Excellent food sources of starch include grains (wheat, rice, corn, oats, and barley), legumes (peas, beans, and lentils), and tubers (potatoes and yams). Our cells cannot use the complex starch molecules exactly as they exist in plants. Instead, our body must break them down into the monosaccharide glucose, from which we can then meet our energy needs.

maltose A disaccharide consisting of two molecules of glucose. It does not generally occur independently in foods but results as a by-product of digestion; also called *malt sugar*.

fermentation A process in which an agent causes an organic substance to break down into simpler substances and results in the production of ATP.

sucrose A disaccharide composed of one glucose molecule and one fructose molecule; sucrose is sweeter than lactose or maltose.

complex carbohydrate A nutrient compound consisting of long chains of glucose molecules, such as starch, glycogen, and fiber.

polysaccharide A complex carbohydrate consisting of long chains of glucose.

starch A polysaccharide stored in plants; the storage form of glucose in plants.

NUTRITION MYTH OR FACT?

Is Honey More Nutritious Than Table Sugar?

Liz's friend Tiffany is dedicated to eating healthful foods. She advises Liz to avoid sucrose and to eat foods that contain honey, molasses, or raw sugar. Like many people, Tiffany believes these sweeteners are more natural and nutritious than refined table sugar. How can Liz sort sugar fact from fiction?

Remember that sucrose consists of one glucose molecule and one fructose molecule joined together. From a chemical perspective, honey is almost identical to sucrose, since honey also contains glucose and fructose molecules in almost equal amounts. However, enzymes in bees' "honey stomachs" separate some of the glucose and fructose molecules, resulting in honey looking and tasting slightly different than sucrose. As you know, bees store honey in combs and fan it with their wings to reduce its moisture content. This also alters the appearance and texture of honey.

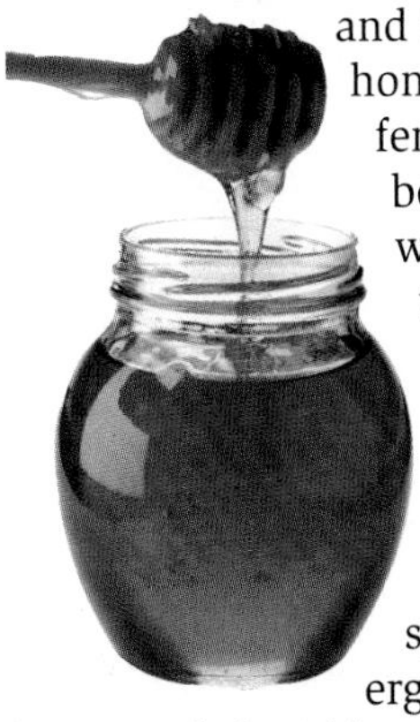

Honey does not contain any more nutrients than sucrose, so it is not a more healthful choice than sucrose. In fact, per tablespoon, honey has more Calories (energy) than table sugar. This is because the crystals in table sugar take up more space on a spoon than the liquid form of honey, so a tablespoon contains less sugar. However, some people argue that honey is sweeter, so you use less.

It is important to note that honey commonly contains bacteria that can cause fatal food poisoning in infants. The more mature digestive system of older children and adults is immune to the effects of these bacteria, but babies younger than 12 months should never be given honey.

Are raw sugar and molasses more healthful than table sugar? Actually, the "raw sugar" available in the United States is not really raw. Truly raw sugar is made up of the first crystals obtained when sugar is processed. Sugar in this form contains dirt, parts of insects, and other by-products that make it illegal to sell in the United States. The raw sugar products in American stores have actually gone through more than half of the same steps in the refining process used to make table sugar. Raw sugar has a coarser texture than white sugar and is unbleached; in most markets, it is also significantly more expensive.

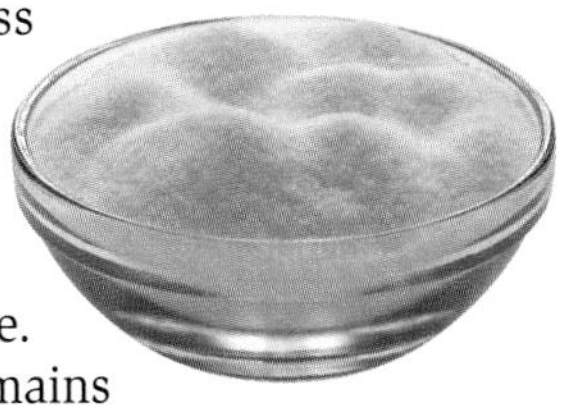

Molasses is the syrup that remains when sucrose is made from sugarcane. It is reddish brown in color with a distinctive taste that is less sweet than table sugar. It does contain some iron, but this iron does not occur naturally. It is a contaminant from the machines that process the sugarcane! Incidentally, blackstrap molasses is the residue of a third boiling of the syrup. It contains less sugar than light or dark molasses but more minerals.

Table 4.1 compares the nutrient content of white table sugar, raw sugar, honey, and blackstrap molasses. As you can see, none of them contains many nutrients that are important for health. This is why highly sweetened products are referred to as "empty Calories."

TABLE 4.1 Nutrient Comparison of Four Different Sugars

	Table Sugar	Raw Sugar	Honey	Molasses
Energy (kcal)	49	49	64	58
Carbohydrate (g)	12.6	12.6	17.3	14.95
Fat (g)	0	0	0	0
Protein (g)	0	0	0.06	0
Fiber (grams)	0	0	0	0
Vitamin C (mg)	0	0	0.1	0
Vitamin A (IU)	0	0	0	0
Thiamin (mg)	0	0	0	0.008
Riboflavin (mg)	0.002	0.003	0.008	0
Folate (µg)	0	0	0	0
Calcium (mg)	0	0.042	1	41
Iron (mg)	0	0	0.09	0.94
Sodium (mg)	0	0	1	7
Potassium (mg)	0	0.25	11	293

Data from U.S. Department of Agriculture, Agricultural Research Service. 2009. USDA National Nutrient Database for Standard Reference, Release 22. Nutrient Data Laboratory Home Page, www.ars.usda.gov/ba/bhnrc/ndl.

Note: Nutrient values are identified for 1 tablespoon of each product.

Our body easily digests most starches; however, some starches in plants are not digestible and are called *resistant*. Technically, resistant starch is classified as a type of fiber. When our intestinal bacteria ferment resistant starch, a fatty acid called *butyrate* is produced. Consuming resistant starch may be beneficial: some research suggests that butyrate consumption reduces the risk for cancer.[5] Legumes contain more resistant starch than do grains, fruits, or vegetables. This quality, plus their high protein and fiber content, makes legumes a healthful food.

Figure 4.4 Polysaccharides include starch, glycogen, and fiber.

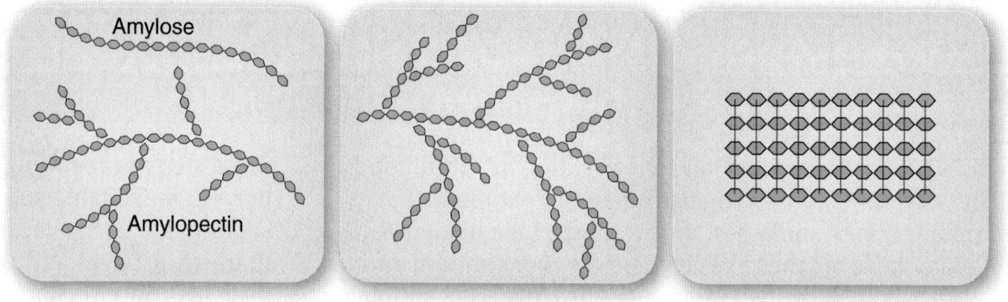

Starch
Storage form of glucose in plants; found in grains, legumes, and tubers

Glycogen
Storage form of glucose in animals; stored in liver and muscles

Fiber
Forms the support structures of leaves, stems, and plants

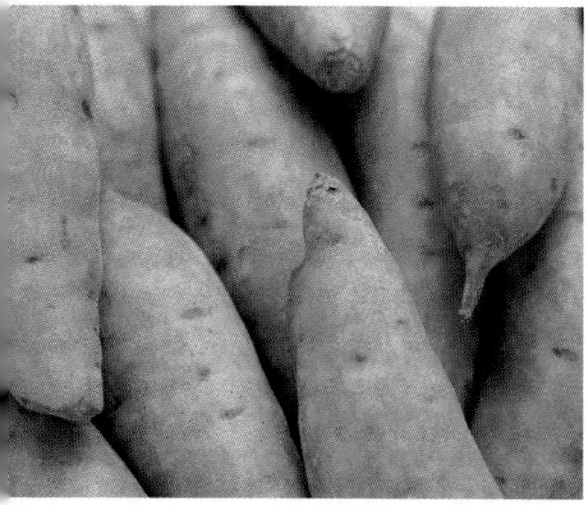

Tubers, such as these sweet potatoes, are excellent food sources of starch.

Glycogen Is a Polysaccharide Stored by Animals

Glycogen is the storage form of glucose for animals, including humans. After an animal is slaughtered, most of the glycogen is broken down by enzymes found in animal tissues. Thus, very little glycogen exists in meat. As plants contain no glycogen, it is not a dietary source of carbohydrate. As explained later in this chapter, we can break down glycogen into glucose when we need it for energy. We store glycogen in our liver and muscles; the storage and use of glycogen are discussed in more detail on pages 117–118.

Fiber Is a Polysaccharide That Gives Plants Their Structure

Like starch, fiber is composed of long polysaccharide chains; however, our body does not easily break down the bonds that connect fiber molecules. This means that most fibers pass through the digestive system without being digested and absorbed, so they contribute no energy to our diet. However, fiber offers many other health benefits, as we will see shortly (pages 114–115).

There are currently a number of definitions of fiber. Recently, the Food and Nutrition Board of the Institute of Medicine proposed three distinctions: *dietary fiber, functional fiber,* and *total fiber*.[6]

- **Dietary fiber** is the nondigestible parts of plants that form the support structures of leaves, stems, and seeds (see Figure 4.4). In a sense, you can think of dietary fiber as a plant's "skeleton."
- **Functional fiber** consists of the nondigestible forms of carbohydrates that are extracted from plants or manufactured in a laboratory and have known health benefits. Functional fiber is added to foods and is the form used in fiber supplements. Examples of functional fiber you might see on nutrition labels include cellulose, guar gum, pectin, and psyllium.
- **Total fiber** is the sum of dietary fiber and functional fiber.

Fiber can also be classified according to its chemical and physical properties as soluble or insoluble.

Soluble Fibers **Soluble fibers** dissolve in water. They are also **viscous**, forming a gel when wet, and fermentable; that is, they are easily digested by bacteria in the colon. Soluble fibers are typically found in citrus fruits, berries, oat products, and beans.

Research suggests that the regular consumption of soluble fibers reduces the risks for cardiovascular disease and type 2 diabetes by lowering blood cholesterol and blood glucose levels. The possible mechanisms by which fiber reduces the risk for various diseases are discussed in more detail on pages 115–116.

Soluble fibers include:

- *Pectins*, which contain chains of galacturonic acid and other monosaccharides. Pectins are found in the cell walls and intracellular tissues of many fruits and berries. They can be isolated and used to thicken foods, such as jams and yogurts.
- *Gums*, which contain galactose, glucuronic acid, and other monosaccharides. Gums are a diverse group of polysaccharides that are viscous. They are typically

glycogen A polysaccharide; the storage form of glucose in animals.

dietary fiber The nondigestible carbohydrate parts of plants that form the support structures of leaves, stems, and seeds.

functional fiber The nondigestible forms of carbohydrates that are extracted from plants or manufactured in a laboratory and have known health benefits.

total fiber The sum of dietary fiber and functional fiber.

soluble fibers Fibers that dissolve in water.

viscous Having a gel-like consistency; viscous fibers form a gel when dissolved in water.

isolated from seeds and are used as thickening, gelling, and stabilizing agents. Guar gum and gum arabic are common gums used as food additives.
- *Mucilages,* which are similar to gums and contain galactose, mannose, and other monosaccharides. Two examples are psyllium and carrageenan. Psyllium is the husk of psyllium seeds, which are also known as plantago or flea seeds. Carrageenan comes from seaweed. Mucilages are used as food stabilizers.

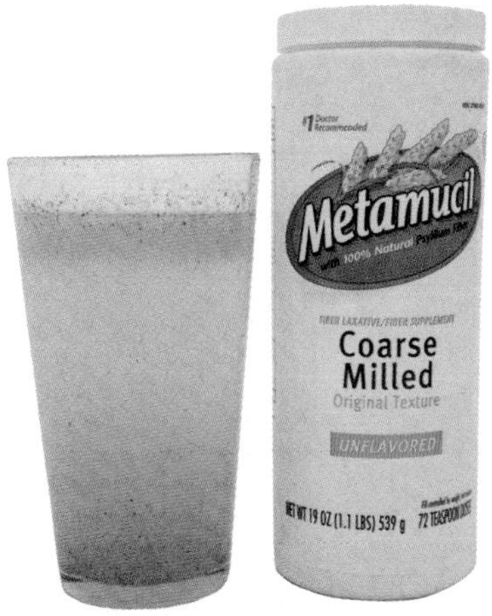

Dissolvable laxatives are an example of one type of soluble fiber.

Insoluble Fibers **Insoluble fibers** are those that do not typically dissolve in water. These fibers are usually nonviscous and typically cannot be fermented by bacteria in the colon. Insoluble fibers are generally found in whole grains, such as wheat, rye, and brown rice, and are found in many vegetables. These fibers are not associated with reducing cholesterol levels but are known for promoting regular bowel movements, alleviating constipation, and reducing the risk for diverticulosis (discussed later in this chapter). Examples of insoluble fibers include the following:

- *Lignins* are noncarbohydrate forms of fiber. Lignins are found in the woody parts of plant cell walls and in carrots and the seeds of fruits and berries. Lignins are also found in brans (the outer husk of grains such as wheat, oats, and rye) and other whole grains.
- *Cellulose* is the main structural component of plant cell walls. Cellulose is a chain of glucose units similar to amylose but, unlike amylose, cellulose contains bonds that are nondigestible by humans. Cellulose is found in whole grains, fruits, vegetables, and legumes. It can also be extracted from wood pulp or cotton, and it is added to foods as an agent for anticaking, thickening, and texturizing of foods.
- *Hemicelluloses* contain glucose, mannose, galacturonic acid, and other monosaccharides. Hemicelluloses are found in plant cell walls and they surround cellulose. They are the primary component of cereal fibers and are found in whole grains and vegetables. Although many hemicelluloses are insoluble, some are also classified as soluble.

RECAP **The three types of polysaccharides are starch, glycogen, and fiber. Starch is the storage form of glucose in plants, whereas glycogen is the storage form of glucose in animals. Fiber forms the support structures of plants. Soluble fibers dissolve in water, are viscous, and can be digested by bacteria in the colon, whereas insoluble fibers do not dissolve in water, are not viscous, and cannot be digested.**

Why Do We Need Carbohydrates?

We have seen that carbohydrates are an important energy source for our body. Let's learn more about this and discuss other functions of carbohydrates.

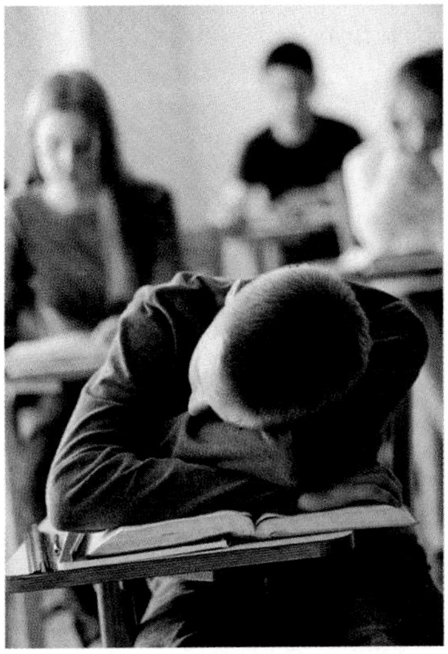

Our red blood cells can utilize only glucose and other monosaccharides, and our brain and other nervous tissues rely primarily on glucose. This is why we get tired, irritable, and shaky when we haven't eaten for a prolonged period of time.

Carbohydrates Provide Energy

Carbohydrates, an excellent source of energy for all our cells, provide 4 kilocalories (kcal) of energy per gram. Some of our cells can also use fat and even protein for energy if necessary. However, our red blood cells can utilize only glucose, and our brain and other nervous tissues primarily rely on glucose. This is why we get tired, irritable, and shaky when we haven't eaten any carbohydrate for a prolonged period of time.

Carbohydrates Fuel Daily Activity

Many popular diets—such as Dr. Atkins' New Revolution Diet and the Sugar Busters plan—are based on the idea that our body actually "prefers" to use fat and/or protein for energy. They claim that current carbohydrate recommendations are much higher than we really need.

In reality, the body relies mostly on both carbohydrates and fat for energy. In fact, as shown in **Figure 4.5**, our body always uses some combination of carbohydrates and fat to fuel daily activities. Fat is the predominant energy source used by our body at rest and during low-intensity activities, such as sitting, standing, and walking. Even during rest, however, our brain cells and red blood cells still rely on glucose.

insoluble fibers Fibers that do not dissolve in water.

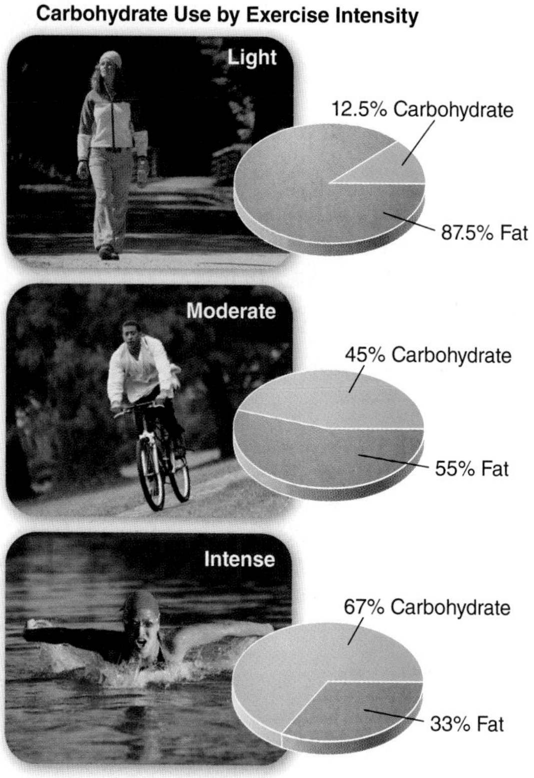

Figure 4.5 Amounts of carbohydrate and fat used during light, moderate, and intense exercise.[7]

Carbohydrates Fuel Exercise

When we exercise, whether running, briskly walking, bicycling, or performing any other activity that causes us to breathe harder and sweat, we begin to use more glucose than fat. Whereas fat breakdown is a slow process and requires oxygen, we can break down glucose very quickly either with or without oxygen. Even during very intense exercise, when less oxygen is available, we can still break down glucose very quickly for energy. That's why when you are exercising at maximal effort carbohydrates are providing most of the energy your body requires.

If you are physically active, it is important to eat enough carbohydrates to provide energy for your brain, red blood cells, and muscles. In Chapter 12, we discuss in more detail the carbohydrate recommendations for active people. In general, if you do not eat enough carbohydrate to support regular exercise, your body will have to rely on fat and protein as alternative energy sources. One advantage of becoming highly trained for endurance-type events, such as marathons and triathlons, is that our muscles are able to store more glycogen, which provides us with additional glucose we can use during exercise. (See Chapter 12 for more information on how exercise improves our use and storage of carbohydrates.)

Low Carbohydrate Intake Can Lead to Ketoacidosis

When we do not eat enough carbohydrate, our body seeks an alternative source of fuel for our brain and begins to break down stored fat. This process, called **ketosis**, produces an alternative fuel called **ketones**.

Ketosis is an important mechanism for providing energy to the brain during situations of fasting, low carbohydrate intake, or vigorous exercise.[5] However, ketones also suppress appetite and cause dehydration and acetone breath (the breath smells like nail polish remover). If inadequate carbohydrate intake continues for an extended period of time, the body will produce excessive amounts of ketones. Because many ketones are acids, high ketone levels cause the blood to become very acidic, leading to a condition called **ketoacidosis**. The high acidity of the blood interferes with basic body functions, causes the loss of lean body mass, and damages many body tissues. People with untreated diabetes are at high risk for ketoacidosis, which can lead to coma and even death. (See pages 137–141 for an ***In Depth*** look at diabetes.)

ketosis The process by which the breakdown of fat during fasting states results in the production of ketones.

ketones Substances produced during the breakdown of fat when carbohydrate intake is insufficient to meet energy needs. Ketones provide an alternative energy source for the brain when glucose levels are low.

ketoacidosis A condition in which excessive ketones are present in the blood, causing the blood to become very acidic, which alters basic body functions and damages tissues. Untreated ketoacidosis can be fatal. This condition is found in individuals with untreated diabetes mellitus.

gluconeogenesis The generation of glucose from the breakdown of proteins into amino acids.

Carbohydrates Spare Protein

If the diet does not provide enough carbohydrate, the body will make its own glucose from protein. This involves breaking down the proteins in blood and tissues into amino acids, then converting them to glucose. This process is called **gluconeogenesis** ("generating new glucose").

When our body uses amino acids for energy, they are not available to make new cells, repair tissue damage, support our immune system, or perform any of their other functions. During periods of starvation or when eating a diet that is very low in carbohydrate, our body will take amino acids from the blood first, and then from other tissues, such as muscles, heart, liver, and kidneys. Using amino acids in this manner over a prolonged period of time can cause serious, possibly irreversible, damage to these organs. (See Chapter 6 for more details on using protein for energy.)

Carbohydrates and Body Weight

Proponents of low-carbohydrate diets claim that eating carbohydrates makes you gain weight. However, anyone who consumes more Calories than he or she expends will gain weight, whether those Calories are in the form of simple or complex carbohydrates, protein, or fat. Moreover, fat is more energy dense than carbohydrate: it contains 9 kcal per gram, whereas carbohydrate contains only 4 kcal per gram. Thus, gram for gram, fat is twice as "fattening" as carbohydrate. In fact, eating carbohydrate sources that are high in fiber and other nutrients has been shown to reduce the overall risk for obesity, heart disease, and diabetes. Thus, all carbohydrates are not bad, and even a small amount of refined sugars can be included in a healthful diet.

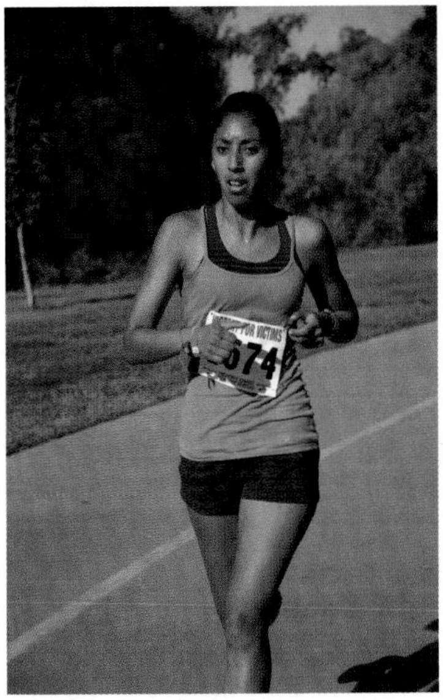

When we exercise or perform any activity that causes us to breathe harder and sweat, we begin to use more glucose than fat.

Fiber Helps Us Stay Healthy

The terms *simple* and *complex* can cause confusion when discussing the health effects of carbohydrates. As we explained earlier, these terms are used to designate the number of sugar molecules present in the carbohydrate. However, when distinguishing carbohydrates in terms of their effect on our health, it is more appropriate to talk about them in terms of their nutrient density and their fiber content. Although we cannot digest fiber, it is a very important substance in our diet. Research indicates that it helps us stay healthy and may prevent many digestive and chronic diseases. The following are potential benefits of fiber consumption:

- May reduce the risk of colon cancer. Although there is some controversy surrounding this issue, many researchers believe that fiber binds cancer-causing substances and speeds their elimination from the colon. However, recent studies of colon cancer and fiber have shown that the relationship between them is not as strong as previously thought.
- Helps prevent hemorrhoids, constipation, and other intestinal problems by keeping our stools moist and soft. Fiber gives gut muscles "something to push on" and makes it easier to eliminate stools.
- Reduces the risk for *diverticulosis,* a condition that is caused in part by trying to eliminate small, hard stools. A great deal of pressure must be generated in the large intestine to pass hard stools. This increased pressure weakens intestinal walls, causing them to bulge outward and form pockets **(Figure 4.6)**. Feces and fibrous materials can get trapped in these pockets, which become infected and inflamed. This is a painful condition that must be treated with antibiotics or surgery.
- May reduce the risk of heart disease by delaying or blocking the absorption of dietary cholesterol into the bloodstream **(Figure 4.7)**. In addition, when soluble fibers are digested, bacteria in the colon produce short-chain fatty acids that may lower the production of low-density lipoprotein (LDL) to healthful levels in our body.
- May enhance weight loss, as eating a high-fiber diet causes a person to feel more full. Fiber absorbs water, expands in the large intestine, and slows the movement of food through the upper part of the digestive tract. Also, people who eat a fiber-rich diet tend to eat fewer fatty and sugary foods.
- May lower the risk for type 2 diabetes. In slowing digestion and absorption, fiber also slows the release of glucose into the blood. It thereby improves the body's regulation of insulin production and blood glucose levels.

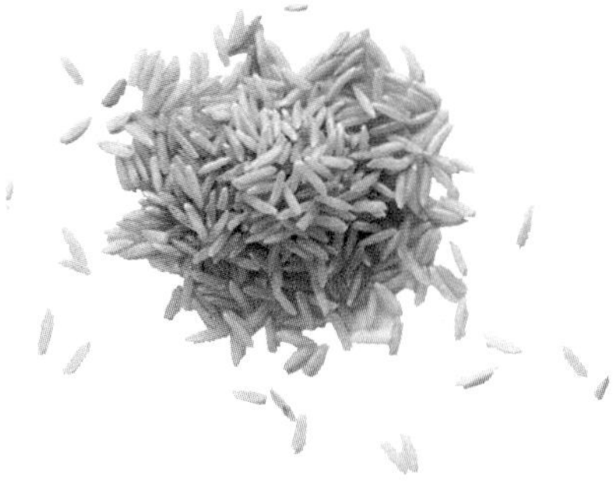

Brown rice is a good food source of dietary fiber.

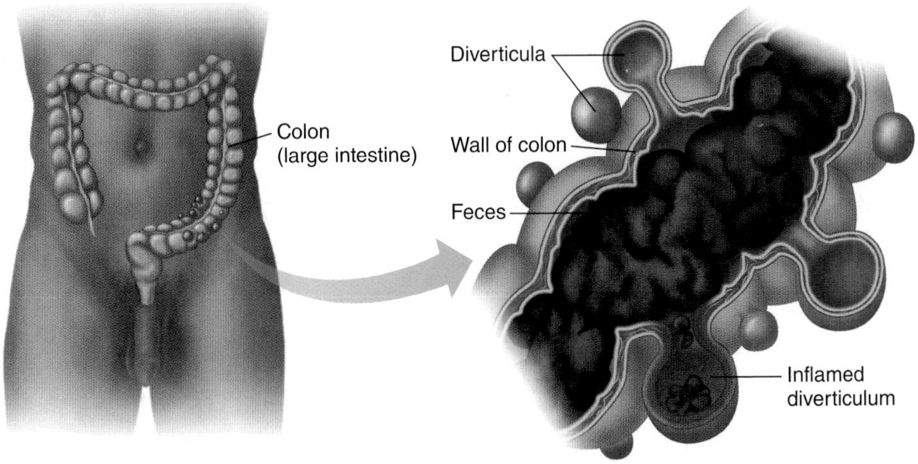

Figure 4.6 Diverticulosis occurs when bulging pockets form in the wall of the large intestine (colon). These pockets become infected and inflamed, requiring proper treatment.

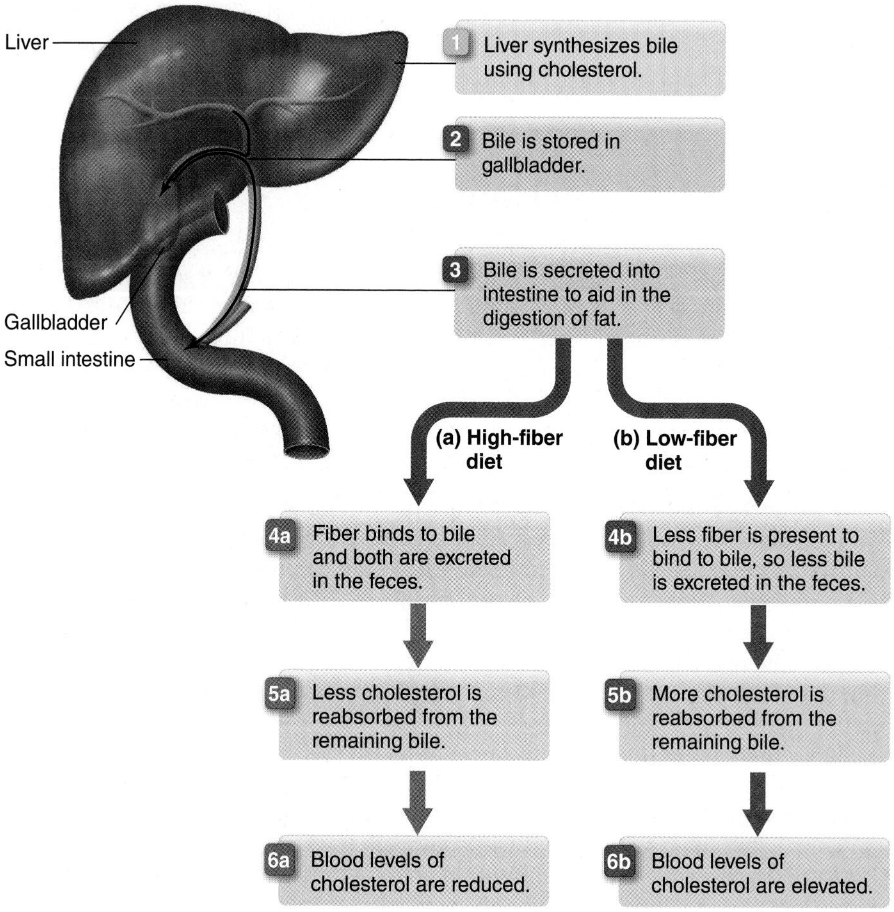
Liver
Gallbladder
Small intestine
1 Liver synthesizes bile using cholesterol.
2 Bile is stored in gallbladder.
3 Bile is secreted into intestine to aid in the digestion of fat.
(a) High-fiber diet
(b) Low-fiber diet
4a Fiber binds to bile and both are excreted in the feces.
4b Less fiber is present to bind to bile, so less bile is excreted in the feces.
5a Less cholesterol is reabsorbed from the remaining bile.
5b More cholesterol is reabsorbed from the remaining bile.
6a Blood levels of cholesterol are reduced.
6b Blood levels of cholesterol are elevated.

Figure 4.7 How fiber might help decrease blood cholesterol levels. **(a)** When eating a high-fiber diet, fiber binds to the bile that is produced from cholesterol, resulting in relatively more cholesterol being excreted in the feces. **(b)** When a lower-fiber diet is consumed, less fiber (and thus less cholesterol) is bound to bile and excreted in the feces.

RECAP **Carbohydrates are an important energy source at rest and during exercise, and they provide 4 kcal of energy per gram. Carbohydrates are necessary in the diet to spare body protein and prevent ketosis. Carbohydrate sources that contain fiber and other nutrients can reduce the risk for obesity, heart disease, and diabetes. Fiber helps prevent hemorrhoids, constipation, and diverticulosis; may reduce the risk for colon cancer and heart disease; and may assist with weight loss.**

How Does Our Body Break Down Carbohydrates?

Glucose is the form of sugar that our body uses for energy, and the primary goal of carbohydrate digestion is to break down polysaccharides and disaccharides into monosaccharides, which can then be converted to glucose. Chapter 3 provided an overview of digestion. Here, we focus specifically and in a bit more detail on the digestion and absorption of carbohydrates. **Figure 4.8** provides a visual tour of carbohydrate digestion.

Digestion Breaks Down Most Carbohydrates into Monosaccharides

Carbohydrate digestion begins in the mouth (Figure 4.8, step 1). As you saw in Chapter 3, the starch in the foods you eat mixes with your saliva during chewing. Saliva contains an enzyme called **salivary amylase,** which breaks starch into smaller particles and eventually into the disaccharide maltose. The next time you eat a piece of bread, notice that you can actually taste it becoming sweeter; this indicates the breakdown of starch into maltose. Disaccharides are not digested in the mouth.

salivary amylase An enzyme in saliva that breaks starch into smaller particles and eventually into the disaccharide maltose.

Salivary glands

Esophagus

1 Mouth
- Chewing stimulates secretion of saliva from salivary glands
- Salivary amylase breaks down starch into shorter polysaccharides and maltose

2 Stomach
- Salivary amylase is destroyed by acids
- No carbohydrate digestion takes place in the stomach

3 Pancreas
- Pancreatic amylase is secreted into small intestine

4 Small intestine
- Pancreatic amylase breaks down remaining starch into maltose
- Specific enzymes (maltase, sucrase, lactase) in small intestine break down disaccharides into monosaccharides
- All monosaccharides are absorbed by small intestine and enter bloodstream

5 Liver
- Monosaccharides travel in the bloodstream to the liver via the portal vein, are converted to glucose, and then transported to cells to provide energy
- Excess glucose is stored as glycogen in liver

6 Large intestine
- Some carbohydrates pass into large intestine undigested
- Bacteria ferment some undigested carbohydrate
- Remaining fiber is excreted in feces

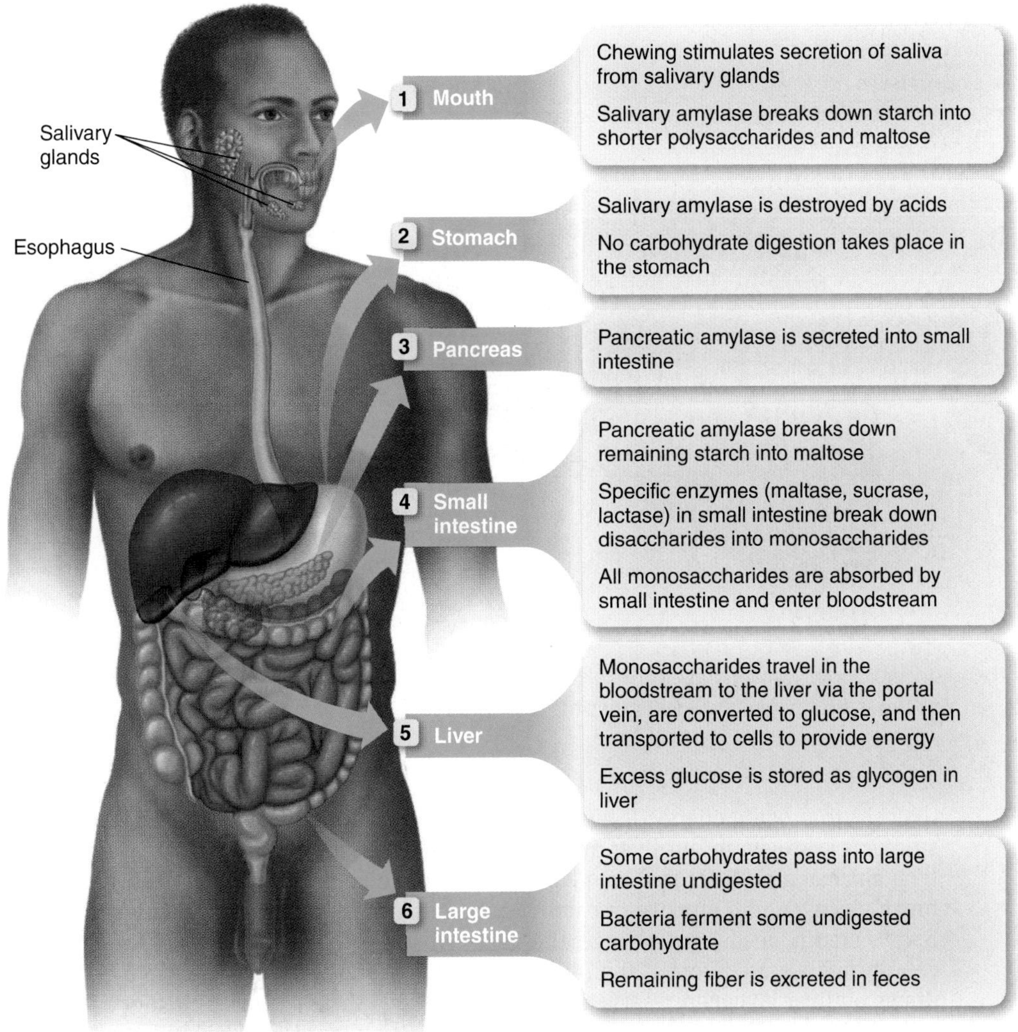

Figure 4.8 A review of carbohydrate digestion and absorption.

As the bolus of food leaves the mouth and enters the stomach, all digestion of carbohydrates ceases. This is because the acid in the stomach inactivates most of the salivary amylase enzyme (Figure 4.8, step 2).

The majority of carbohydrate digestion occurs in the small intestine. As the contents of the stomach enter the small intestine, the pancreas secretes an enzyme called **pancreatic amylase** into the small intestine (Figure 4.8, step 3). Pancreatic amylase continues to digest any remaining starch into maltose. Additional enzymes in the microvilli of the mucosal cells that line the intestinal tract work to break down disaccharides into monosaccharides. Maltose is broken down into glucose by the enzyme **maltase.** Sucrose is broken down into glucose and fructose by the enzyme **sucrase.** The enzyme **lactase** breaks down lactose into glucose and galactose (Figure 4.8, step 4). Notice that enzyme names are identifiable by the *–ase* suffix. All monosaccharides are then absorbed into the mucosal cells lining the small intestine, where they pass through and enter into the bloodstream.

The Liver Converts Most Non-Glucose Monosaccharides into Glucose

Once the monosaccharides enter the bloodstream, they travel to the liver, where fructose and galactose are converted to glucose (Figure 4.8, step 5). If needed immediately for energy, the glucose is released into the bloodstream, where it can travel to

pancreatic amylase An enzyme secreted by the pancreas into the small intestine that digests any remaining starch into maltose.

maltase A digestive enzyme that breaks maltose into glucose.

sucrase A digestive enzyme that breaks sucrose into glucose and fructose.

lactase A digestive enzyme that breaks lactose into glucose and galactose.

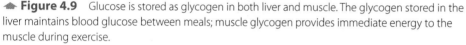

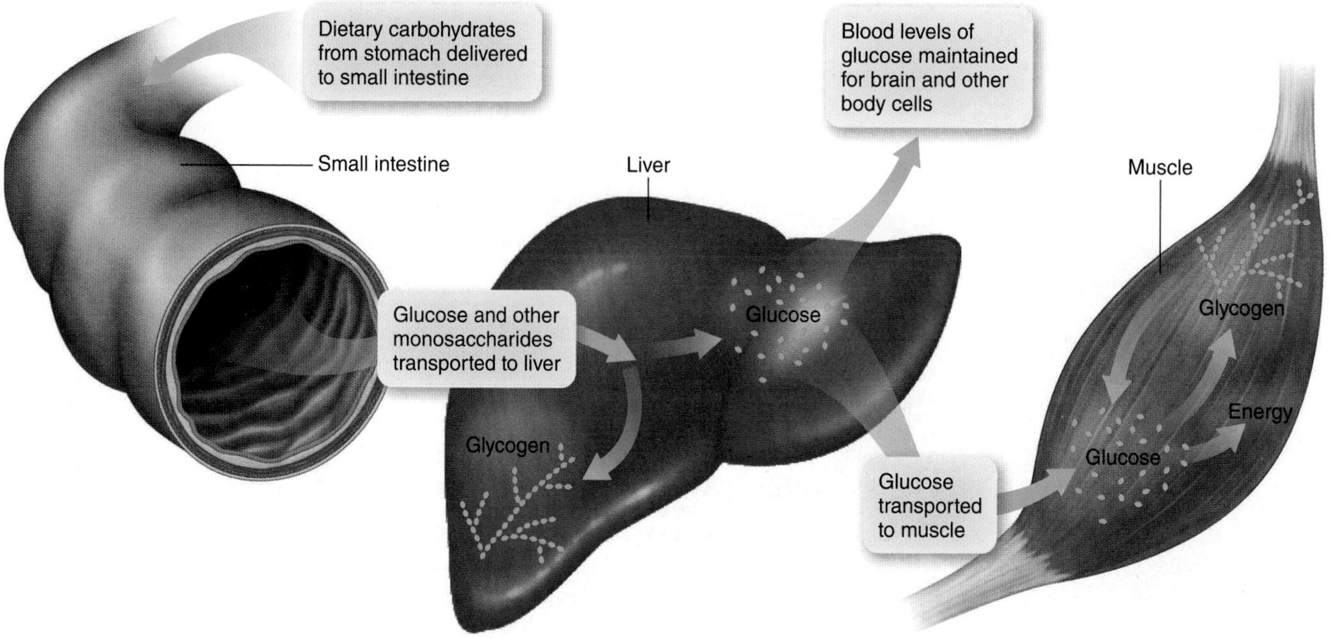
Dietary carbohydrates from stomach delivered to small intestine
Blood levels of glucose maintained for brain and other body cells
Small intestine
Liver
Muscle
Glucose and other monosaccharides transported to liver
Glucose
Glycogen
Glycogen
Energy
Glucose
Glucose transported to muscle

Figure 4.9 Glucose is stored as glycogen in both liver and muscle. The glycogen stored in the liver maintains blood glucose between meals; muscle glycogen provides immediate energy to the muscle during exercise.

the cells to provide energy. If glucose is not needed immediately for energy, it is stored as glycogen in our liver and muscles. Enzymes in liver and muscle cells combine glucose molecules to form glycogen (an anabolic, or building, process) and break glycogen into glucose (a catabolic, or destructive, process), depending on the body's energy needs. On average, the liver can store 70 g (280 kcal) and the muscles can normally store about 120 g (480 kcal) of glycogen. Between meals, our body draws on liver glycogen reserves to maintain blood glucose levels and support the needs of our cells, including those of our brain, spinal cord, and red blood cells **(Figure 4.9)**.

The glycogen stored in our muscles continually provides energy to our muscle cells, particularly during intense exercise. Endurance athletes can increase their storage of muscle glycogen from two to four times the normal amount through a process called *carbohydrate loading* (see Chapter 12). Any excess glucose is stored as glycogen in the liver and muscles and saved for such future energy needs as exercise. Once the storage capacity of the liver and muscles is reached, any excess glucose can be stored as fat in adipose tissue.

Fiber Is Excreted from the Large Intestine

As previously mentioned, humans do not possess enzymes in the small intestine that can break down fiber. Thus, fiber passes through the small intestine undigested and enters the large intestine, or colon. There, bacteria ferment some previously undigested carbohydrates, causing the production of gases and a few short-chain fatty acids. The cells of the large intestine use these short-chain fatty acids for energy. The fiber remaining in the colon adds bulk to our stools and is excreted (Figure 4.8, step 6) in feces. In this way, fiber assists in maintaining bowel regularity.

RECAP Carbohydrate digestion starts in the mouth and continues in the small intestine. Glucose and other monosaccharides are absorbed into the bloodstream and travel to the liver, where non-glucose sugars are converted to glucose. Glucose either is used by the cells for energy or is converted to glycogen and stored in the liver and muscle for later use.

HOT TOPIC

Is it Hunger—or Hypoglycemia?

After going for several hours without eating, have you ever felt spaced out, shaky, irritable, and weak? And did the symptoms subside once you'd eaten? If so, maybe you wondered if your symptoms were due to hypoglycemia.

In **hypoglycemia,** blood glucose falls to lower-than-normal levels. This commonly occurs in people with diabetes who aren't getting proper treatment, but it can also happen in people who don't have diabetes if their pancreas secretes too much insulin after a high-carbohydrate meal. The characteristic symptoms usually appear about 1 to 4 hours after the meal and occur because the body clears glucose from the blood too quickly. People with this form of hypoglycemia must eat smaller meals more frequently to level out their blood insulin and glucose levels.

The trouble is, ordinary hunger can make you experience symptoms just like those of true hypoglycemia. So which is it—hunger or hypoglycemia? You can only find out for sure by getting a blood test, but unless you have diabetes it's probably not necessary. For most healthy people, eating regular meals and healthy snacks is the only "treatment" needed.

A Variety of Hormones Regulate Blood Glucose Levels

Our body regulates blood glucose levels within a fairly narrow range to provide adequate glucose to the brain and other cells. A number of hormones, including insulin, glucagon, epinephrine, norepinephrine, cortisol, and growth hormone, assist the body with maintaining blood glucose.

When we eat a meal, our blood glucose level rises. But glucose in our blood cannot help our nerves, muscles, and other organs function unless it can cross into their cells. Glucose molecules are too large to cross cell membranes independently. To get in, glucose needs assistance from the hormone **insulin,** which is secreted by the pancreas **(Figure 4.10a)**. Insulin is transported in the blood throughout the body, where it stimulates special molecules located in cell membranes to transport glucose into the cell. Insulin can be thought of as a key that opens the gates of the cell membrane, enabling the transport of glucose into the cell interior, where it can be used for energy. Insulin also stimulates the liver and muscles to take up glucose and store it as glycogen.

When you have not eaten for a period of time, your blood glucose level declines. This decrease in blood glucose stimulates the pancreas to secrete another hormone, **glucagon** (Figure 4.10b). Glucagon acts in an opposite way to insulin: it causes the liver to convert its stored glycogen into glucose, which is then secreted into the bloodstream and transported to the cells for energy. Glucagon also assists in the breakdown of body proteins to amino acids, so that the liver can stimulate *gluconeogenesis,* the production of new glucose from amino acids.

Epinephrine, norepinephrine, cortisol, and growth hormone are additional hormones that work to increase blood glucose. Epinephrine and norepinephrine are secreted by the adrenal glands and nerve endings when blood glucose levels are low. They act to increase glycogen breakdown in the liver, resulting in a subsequent increase in the release of glucose into the bloodstream. They also increase gluconeogenesis. These two hormones are also responsible for our "fight-or-flight" reaction to danger; they are released when we need a burst of energy to respond quickly. Cortisol and growth hormone are secreted by the adrenal glands to act on liver, muscle, and adipose tissue. Cortisol increases gluconeogenesis and decreases the use of glucose by muscles and other body organs. Growth hormone decreases glucose uptake by our muscles, increases our mobilization and use of the fatty acids stored in our adipose tissue, and increases our liver's output of glucose.

Normally, the effects of these hormones balance each other to maintain blood glucose within a healthy range. An alteration in this balance can lead to health conditions such as diabetes (see the ***In Depth*** essay on pages 137–141) or hypoglycemia.

insulin The hormone secreted by the beta cells of the pancreas in response to increased blood levels of glucose; it facilitates the uptake of glucose by body cells.

glucagon The hormone secreted by the alpha cells of the pancreas in response to decreased blood levels of glucose; it causes the breakdown of liver stores of glycogen into glucose.

hypoglycemia A condition marked by blood glucose levels that are below normal fasting levels.

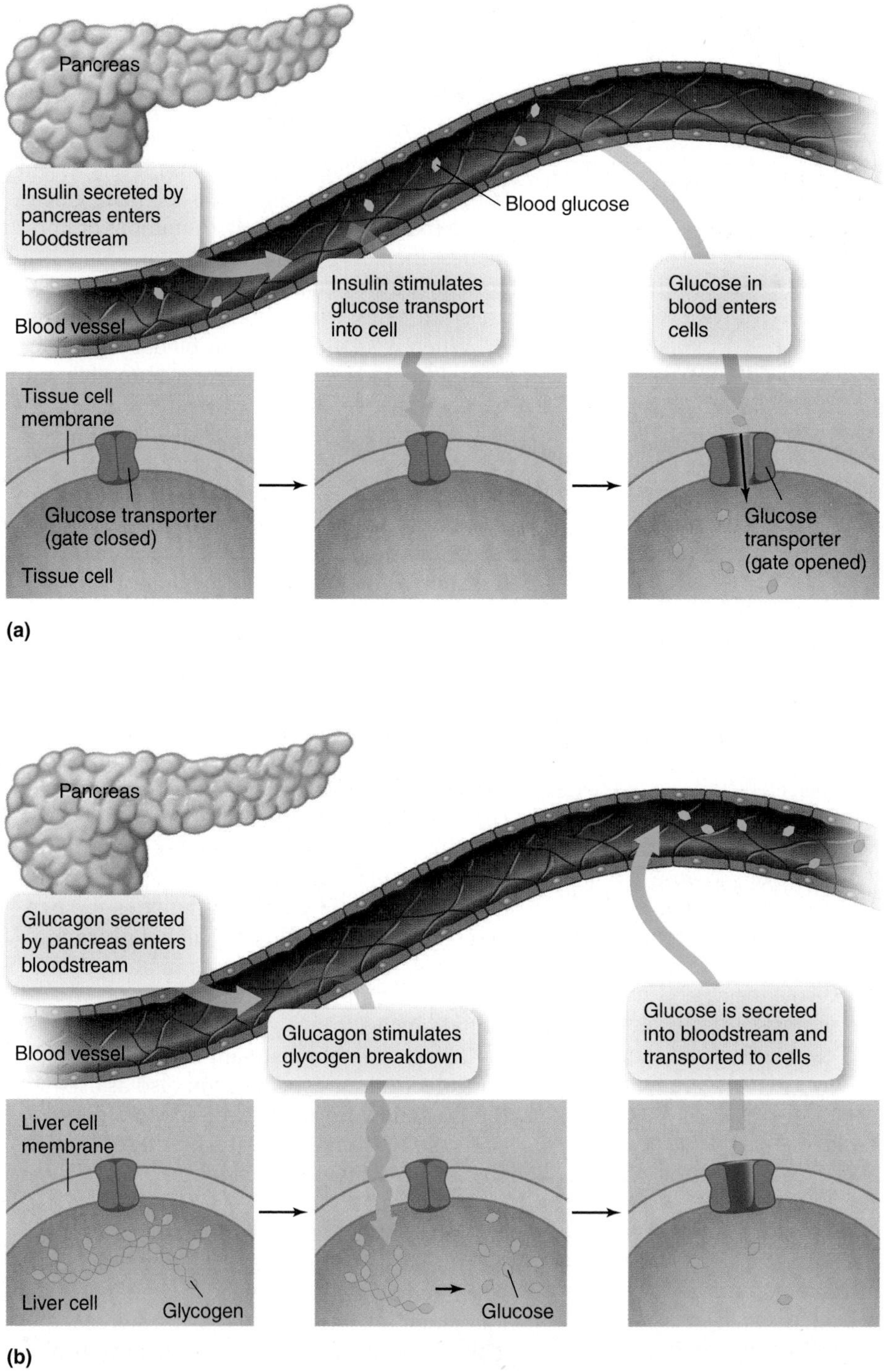

Figure 4.10 Regulation of blood glucose by the hormones insulin and glucagon. **(a)** When blood glucose levels increase after a meal, the pancreas secretes insulin. Insulin opens "gates" in the cell membrane to allow the passage of glucose into the cell. **(b)** When blood glucose levels are low, the pancreas secretes glucagon. Glucagon enters liver cells, where it stimulates the breakdown of stored glycogen into glucose. This glucose is then released into the bloodstream.

The Glycemic Index Shows How Foods Affect Our Blood Glucose Level

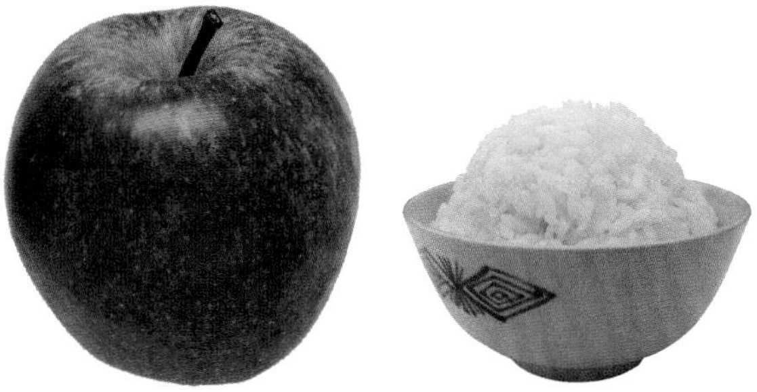

An apple has a lower glycemic index (38) than a serving of white rice (56).

The **glycemic index** is a measure of the potential of foods to raise blood glucose levels. Foods with a high glycemic index cause a sudden surge in blood glucose. This in turn triggers a surge in insulin, which may then be followed by a dramatic drop in blood glucose. Foods with a low glycemic index cause low to moderate fluctuations in blood glucose. When foods are assigned a glycemic index value, they are often compared to the glycemic effect of pure glucose.

The glycemic index of a food is not always easy to predict. **Figure 4.11** ranks certain foods according to their glycemic index. Do any of these rankings surprise you? Most people assume that foods containing simple sugars have a higher glycemic index than starches, but this is not always the case. For instance, compare the glycemic indexes for apples and instant potatoes. Although instant potatoes are a starchy food, they have a glycemic index value of 85, whereas the value for an apple is only 38!

The type of carbohydrate, the way the food is prepared, and its fat and fiber content can all affect how quickly the body absorbs it. It is important to note that we eat most of our foods combined into a meal. In this case, the glycemic index of the total meal becomes more important than the ranking of each food.

For determining the effect of a food on a person's glucose response, some nutrition experts believe that a food's **glycemic load** is more useful than the glycemic index. A food's glycemic load is the number of grams of carbohydrate it contains multiplied by the glycemic index of that carbohydrate. For instance, carrots are recognized as a vegetable having a relatively high glycemic index of about 68; however, the glycemic load of carrots is only 3.[8] This is because there is very little total carbohydrate in a serving of carrots. The low glycemic load of carrots means that carrot consumption is unlikely to cause a significant rise in glucose and insulin levels.

glycemic index The system that assigns ratings (or values) for the potential of foods to raise blood glucose and insulin levels.

glycemic load The amount of carbohydrate in a food multiplied by the glycemic index of the carbohydrate.

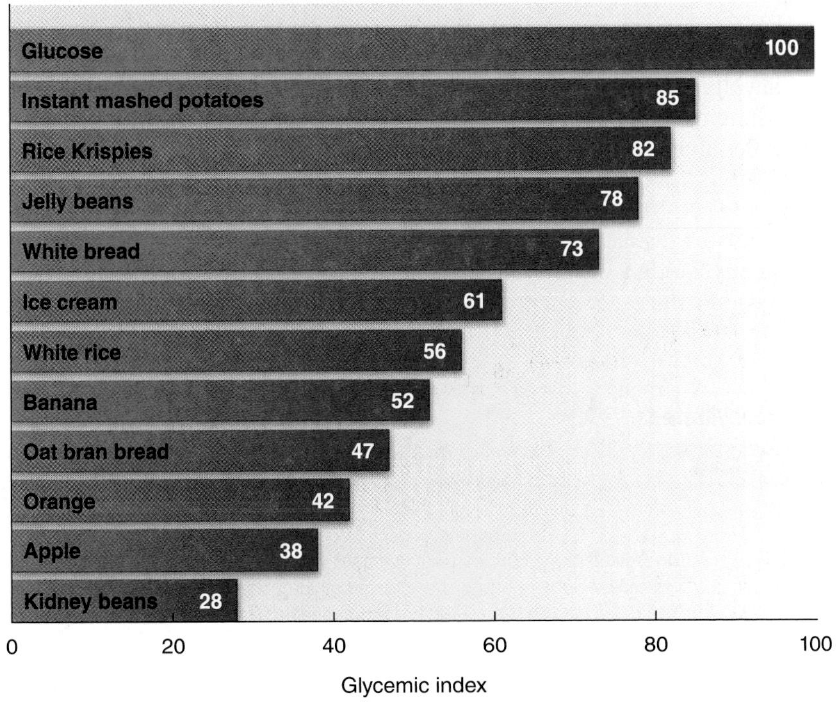

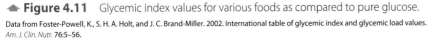

Figure 4.11 Glycemic index values for various foods as compared to pure glucose.

Data from Foster-Powell, K., S. H. A. Holt, and J. C. Brand-Miller. 2002. International table of glycemic index and glycemic load values. *Am. J. Clin. Nutr.* 76:5–56.

Why do we care about the glycemic index and glycemic load? Foods and meals with a lower glycemic load are better choices for someone with diabetes because they will not trigger dramatic fluctuations in blood glucose. They may also reduce the risk for heart disease and colon cancer because they generally contain more fiber, and fiber helps decrease fat levels in the blood. Recent studies have shown that people who eat lower glycemic index diets have more healthful blood lipid levels and their blood glucose values are more likely to be normal.[9–11] Diets with a low glycemic index and low glycemic load are also associated with a reduced risk for prostate cancer.[12] Despite some encouraging research findings, the glycemic index and glycemic load remain controversial. Many nutrition researchers feel that the evidence supporting their health benefits is weak. In addition, many believe the concepts of the glycemic index/load are too complex for people to apply to their daily lives. Other researchers insist that helping people choose foods with a lower glycemic index/load is critical in the prevention and treatment of many chronic diseases. Until this controversy is resolved, people are encouraged to eat a variety of fiber-rich and less-processed carbohydrates, such as beans and lentils, fresh vegetables, and whole-wheat bread, because these forms of carbohydrates have a lower glycemic load and they contain a multitude of important nutrients.

RECAP **Various hormones are involved in regulating blood glucose. Insulin lowers blood glucose levels by facilitating the entry of glucose into cells. Glucagon, epinephrine, norepinephrine, cortisol, and growth hormone raise blood glucose levels by a variety of mechanisms. The glycemic index is a value that indicates the potential of foods to raise blood glucose and insulin levels. The glycemic load is the amount of carbohydrate in a food multiplied by the glycemic index of the carbohydrate in that food. Foods with a high glycemic index/load cause surges in blood glucose and insulin, whereas foods with a low glycemic index/load cause more moderate fluctuations in blood glucose.**

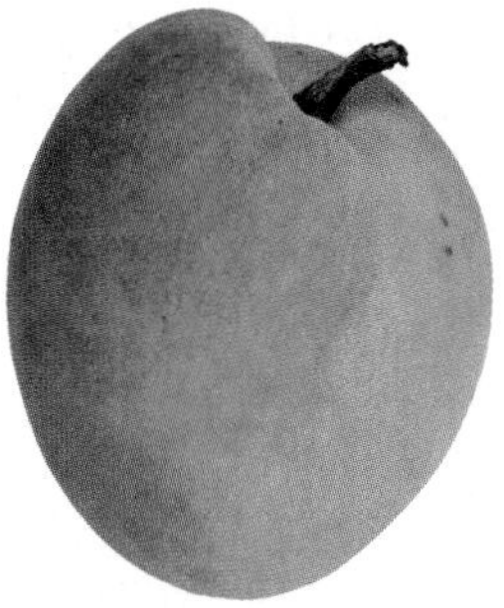

Eating the suggested daily amounts of vegetables and fruit, such as apricots, will ensure that you're getting enough fiber-rich carbohydrate in your diet.

How Much Carbohydrate Should We Eat?

Carbohydrates are an important part of a balanced, healthful diet. The Recommended Dietary Allowance (RDA) for carbohydrate is based on the amount of glucose the brain uses.[6] The current RDA for adults 19 years of age and older is 130 g of carbohydrate per day. It is important to emphasize that this RDA does not cover the amount of carbohydrate needed to support daily activities; it covers only the amount of carbohydrate needed to supply adequate glucose to the brain.

As we said in Chapter 1, carbohydrates have been assigned an Acceptable Macronutrient Distribution Range (AMDR) of 45% to 65% of total energy intake. **Table 4.2** compares the carbohydrate recommendations from the Institute of Medicine with the Dietary Guidelines for Americans related to carbohydrate-containing foods.[6,13] As you can see, the Institute of Medicine provides specific numeric recom-

TABLE 4.2 Dietary Recommendations for Carbohydrates

Institute of Medicine Recommendations*	Dietary Guidelines for Americans†
Recommended Dietary Allowance (RDA) for adults 19 years of age and older is 130 g of carbohydrate per day.	Choose fiber-rich fruits, vegetables, and whole grains often.
The Acceptable Macronutrient Distribution Range (AMDR) for carbohydrate is 45–65% of total daily energy intake.	Choose and prepare foods and beverages with little added sugars or caloric sweeteners, such as amounts suggested by the USDA Food Guide and the DASH eating plan (see Chapter 5 and its accompanying ***In Depth***).
Added sugar intake should be 25% or less of total energy intake each day.	Reduce the incidence of dental caries by practicing good oral hygiene and consuming sugar- and starch-containing foods and beverages less frequently.

* Data from "Dietary Reference Intakes for Energy, Carbohydrates, Fiber, Fat, Fatty Acids, Cholesterol, Protein, and Amino Acids (Macronutrients)," © 2002 by the National Academy of Sciences, courtesy of the National Academies Press, Washington, DC. Used by permission.

†U.S. Department of Health and Human Services (USDHHS) and U.S. Department of Agriculture (USDA). 2005. *Dietary Guidelines for Americans, 2005*. 6th ed. Washington, DC: U.S. Government Printing Office, www.healthierus.gov/dietaryguidelines.

mendations, whereas the Dietary Guidelines for Americans are general suggestions about foods high in fiber and low in added sugars. Most health agencies agree that most of the carbohydrates you eat each day should be high in fiber, whole grain, and unprocessed. As recommended in the USDA Food Guide, eating at least half your grains as whole grains and eating the suggested amounts of fruits and vegetables each day will ensure that you get enough fiber-rich carbohydrates in your diet. Keep in mind that fruits are predominantly composed of simple sugars and contain little or no starch. They are healthful food choices, however, as they are good sources of vitamins, some minerals, and fiber.

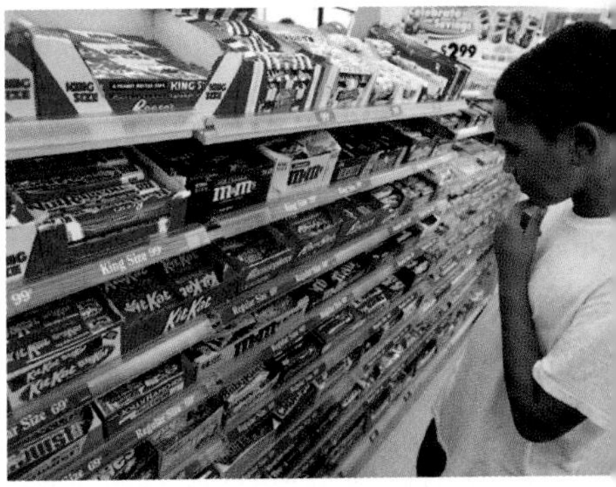

Foods with added sugars, such as candy, have lower levels of vitamins and minerals than foods that naturally contain simple sugars.

Most Americans Eat Too Much Sugar

The average carbohydrate intake per person in the United States is approximately 50% of total energy intake. For some people, almost half of this amount consists of sugars. Where does all this sugar come from? Some sugar comes from healthful food sources, such as fruit and milk. However, much of our sugar intake comes from *added sugars*. **Added sugars** are defined as sugars and syrups that are added to foods during processing or preparation.[6]

The most common source of added sugars in the U.S. diet is sweetened soft drinks; we drink an average of 40 gallons per person each year. Consider that one 12-oz cola contains 38.5 g of sugar, or almost 10 teaspoons. If you drink the average amount, you are consuming more than 16,420 g of sugar (about 267 cups) each year! Other common sources of added sugars include cookies, cakes, pies, fruit drinks, fruit punches, and candy. In addition, a surprising number of processed foods you may not think of as "sweet" actually contain a significant amount of added sugar, including many brands of peanut butter, flavored rice mixes, and even some canned soups!

Added sugars are not chemically different from naturally occurring sugars. However, foods and beverages with added sugars have lower levels of vitamins, minerals, and fiber than foods that naturally contain simple sugars. Given these nutrient limitations, it's best to choose and prepare foods and beverages with little added sugars. People who are very physically active are able to consume relatively more added sugars, whereas smaller or less active people should consume relatively less. The Nutrition Facts Panel includes a listing of total sugars, but a distinction is not generally made between added sugars and naturally occurring sugars. Thus, you may need to check the ingredients list. Refer to **Table 4.3** for a list of forms of sugar commonly used in foods. To maintain a diet low in added sugars, limit foods in which a form of added sugar is listed as one of the first few ingredients on the label.[14]

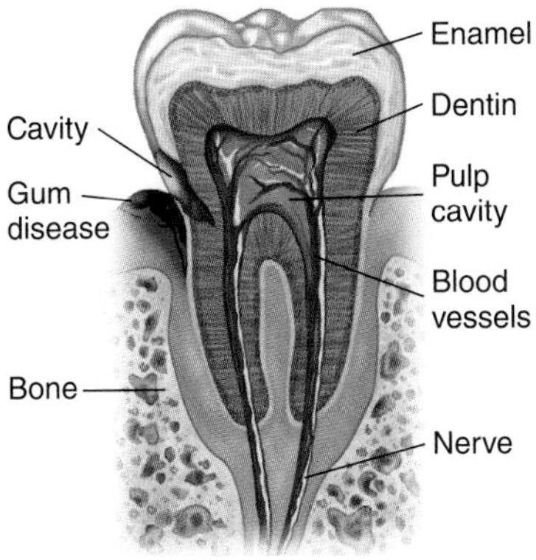

Figure 4.12 Eating simple carbohydrates can cause an increase in cavities and gum disease. This is because bacteria in the mouth consume simple carbohydrates present on the teeth and gums and produce acids, which eat away at these tissues.

Sugars Are Blamed for Many Health Problems

Why do sugars have such a bad reputation? First, they are known to cause tooth decay. Second, many people believe they cause hyperactivity in children. Third, eating a lot of sugar could increase the levels of unhealthful lipids, or fats, in our blood, increasing our risk for heart disease. High intakes of sugar have also been blamed for causing diabetes and obesity. Let's learn the truth about these accusations.

Sugar Causes Tooth Decay

Sugars do play a role in dental problems because the bacteria that cause tooth decay thrive on sugar. These bacteria produce acids, which eat away at tooth enamel and can eventually cause cavities and gum disease (**Figure 4.12**). Eating sticky foods that adhere to teeth—such as caramels, crackers, sugary cereals, and licorice—and sipping sweetened beverages over a period of time are two behaviors that increase the risk for tooth decay. This means that people shouldn't suck on hard candies or caramels, slowly sip soda or juice, or put babies to bed with a bottle unless it contains water. As we have seen, even breast milk contains sugar, which can slowly drip onto the baby's gums. As a result, infants should not routinely be allowed to fall asleep at the breast.

added sugars Sugars and syrups that are added to food during processing or preparation.

TABLE 4.3 Forms of Sugar Commonly Used in Foods

Name of Sugar	Definition
Brown sugar	A highly refined sweetener made up of approximately 99% sucrose and produced by adding to white table sugar either molasses or burnt table sugar for coloring and flavor.
Concentrated fruit juice sweetener	A form of sweetener made with concentrated fruit juice, commonly pear juice.
Confectioner's sugar	A highly refined, finely ground white sugar with added cornstarch to reduce clumping; also referred to as powdered sugar.
Corn sweetener	A general term for any sweetener made with cornstarch.
Corn syrup	A syrup produced by the partial hydrolysis of cornstarch.
Dextrose	An alternative term for glucose.
Fructose	A monosaccharide in fruits and vegetables, also called levulose or fruit sugar.
Glucose	The most abundant monosaccharide; it is the preferred source of energy for the brain and an important source of energy for all cells.
Granulated sugar	Another terms for white sugar, or table sugar.
High-fructose corn syrup	A type of corn syrup in which part of the sucrose is converted to fructose, making it sweeter than sucrose or regular corn syrup; most high-fructose corn syrup contains 42% to 55% fructose.
Honey	A sweet, sticky liquid sweetener made by bees from the nectar of flowers; contains glucose and fructose.
Invert sugar	A sugar created by heating a sucrose syrup with a small amount of acid; inverting sucrose results in its breakdown into glucose and fructose, which reduces the size of the sugar crystals; its smooth texture makes it ideal for use in making candies, such as fondant, and some syrups.
Lactose	A disaccharide formed by one molecule of glucose and one molecule of galactose; occurs naturally in milk and other dairy products.
Levulose	Another term for fructose, or fruit sugar.
Maltose	A disaccharide consisting of two molecules of glucose; it does not generally occur independently in foods but is a by-product of digestion; also called malt sugar.
Mannitol	A type of sugar alcohol.
Maple sugar	A sugar made by boiling maple syrup.
Molasses	A thick, brown syrup that is separated from raw sugar during manufacturing; it is considered the least refined form of sucrose.
Natural sweetener	A general term used for any naturally occurring sweetener, such as sucrose, honey, or raw sugar.
Raw sugar	The sugar that results from the processing of sugar beets or sugarcane; approximately 96% to 98% sucrose; true raw sugar contains impurities and is not stable in storage; the raw sugar available to consumers has been purified to yield an edible sugar.
Sorbitol	A type of sugar alcohol.
Turbinado sugar	The form of raw sugar that is purified and safe for human consumption; sold as "Sugar in the Raw" in the United States.
White sugar	Another name for sucrose, or table sugar.
Xylitol	A type of sugar alcohol.

To reduce your risk for tooth decay, brush your teeth after each meal, especially after drinking sugary drinks and eating candy. Drinking fluoridated water and using a fluoride toothpaste will also help protect your teeth.

There Is No Link Between Sugar and Hyperactivity in Children

Although many people believe that eating sugar causes hyperactivity and other behavioral problems in children, there is little scientific evidence to support this claim. Some children actually become less active shortly after a high-sugar meal! However, it is important to emphasize that most studies of sugar and children's behavior have only looked at the effects of sugar a few hours after ingestion. We know very little about the long-term effects of sugar intake on the behavior of children. Behavioral and learning problems are complex issues, most likely caused by a multitude of factors. Because of this complexity, the Institute of Medicine has stated that, overall, there does not appear to be enough evidence to state that eating too much sugar causes hyperactivity or other behavioral problems in children.[6] Thus, there is no Tolerable Upper Intake Level for sugar.

High Sugar Intake Can Lead to Unhealthful Levels of Blood Lipids

Research evidence suggests that consuming a diet high in sugars, particularly fructose, can lead to unhealthful changes in blood lipids. You will learn more about blood lipids (including cholesterol and lipoproteins) in Chapter 5. Briefly, higher intakes of sugars are associated with increases in our blood of both low-density lipoproteins (LDL, commonly referred to as "bad cholesterol") and triglycerides. At the same time, high sugar intake appears to *decrease* our high-density lipoproteins (HDL), which are protective and are often referred to as "good cholesterol."[6,15] These changes are of concern, as increased levels of triglycerides and LDL and decreased levels of HDL are risk factors for heart disease. However, there is not enough scientific evidence at the present time to state with confidence that eating a diet high in sugar causes heart disease. Still, based on current knowledge, it is prudent for a person at risk for heart disease to eat a diet low in sugars. Because fructose, especially in the form of high-fructose corn syrup, is a component of many processed foods and beverages, careful label reading is advised.

High Sugar Intake Does Not Cause Diabetes but May Contribute to Obesity

There is no scientific evidence that eating a diet high in sugar causes diabetes. In fact, studies examining the relationship between sugar intake and type 2 diabetes report no association between sugar intake and diabetes, or an increased risk for diabetes associated with increased sugar intake and weight gain, or a decreased risk for diabetes with increased sugar intake.[16–18] However, people who have diabetes need to moderate their intake of sugar and closely monitor their blood glucose levels.

There is somewhat more evidence linking sugar intake with obesity. For example, a recent study found that overweight children consumed more sugared soft drinks than did children of normal weight.[18] Another study found that for every extra sugared soft drink a child consumes per day, the risk for obesity increases by 60%.[19] We also know that if you consume more energy than you expend, you will gain weight. It makes intuitive sense that people who consume extra energy from high-sugar foods are at risk for obesity, just as people who consume extra energy from fat or protein gain weight. In addition to the increased potential for obesity, another major concern about high-sugar diets is that they tend to be low in nutrient density because the intake of high-sugar foods tends to replace that of more nutritious foods. The relationship between sugared soft drinks and obesity is highly controversial and is discussed in more detail in the Nutrition Debate on page 133.

RECAP **The RDA for carbohydrate is 130 g per day; this amount is only sufficient to supply adequate glucose to the brain. The AMDR for carbohydrate is 45% to 65% of total energy intake. Added sugars are sugars and syrups added to foods during processing or preparation. Sugar causes tooth decay but does not appear to cause hyperactivity in children. High intakes of sugars are associated with increases in unhealthful blood lipids. Diets high in sugar are not confirmed to cause diabetes but may contribute to obesity.**

Most Americans Eat Too Little Fiber-Rich Carbohydrates

Do you get enough fiber-rich carbohydrates each day? If you are like most people in the United States, you eat only about 2 servings of fruits or vegetables each day; this is far below the recommended amount.

Breads and cereals are another potential source of fiber-rich carbohydrates, and they're part of most Americans' diets. But are the breads and cereals you eat made with whole grains? If you're not sure, check out the ingredients lists on the labels of your favorite breads and breakfast cereals. Do they list *whole-wheat flour* or just

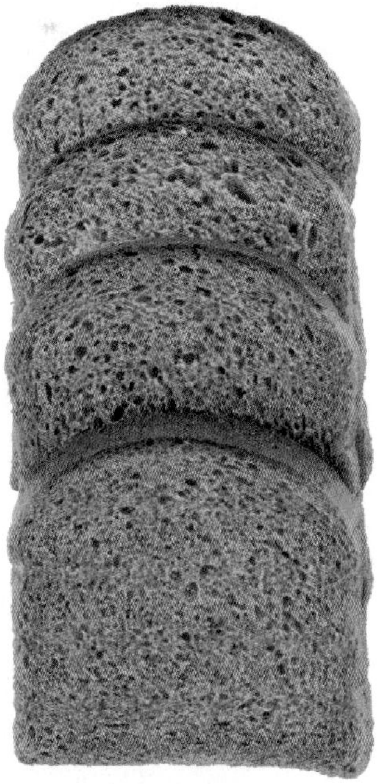

▲ Whole-grain foods provide more nutrients and fiber than foods made with enriched flour.

TABLE 4.4 Terms Used to Describe Grains and Cereals on Nutrition Labels

Term	Definition
Brown bread	Bread that may or may not be made using whole-grain flour. Many brown breads are made with white flour with brown (caramel) coloring added.
Enriched (or fortified) flour or grain	Enriching or fortifying grains involves adding nutrients back to refined foods. In order for a manufacturer to use this term in the United States, a minimum amount of iron, folate, niacin, thiamin, and riboflavin must be added. Other nutrients can also be added.
Refined flour or grain	Refining involves removing the coarse parts of food products; refined wheat flour is flour in which all but the internal part of the kernel has been removed. Refined sugar is made by removing the outer portions of sugar beets or sugarcane.
Stone ground	Refers to a milling process in which limestone is used to grind any grain. Stone ground does not mean that bread is made with whole grain, as refined flour can be stone ground.
Unbleached flour	Flour that has been refined but not bleached; it is very similar to refined white flour in texture and nutritional value.
Wheat flour	Any flour made from wheat, which includes white flour, unbleached flour, and whole-wheat flour.
White flour	Flour that has been bleached and refined. All-purpose flour, cake flour, and enriched baking flour are all types of white flour.
Whole-grain flour	A grain that is not refined; whole grains are milled in their complete form, with only the husk removed.
Whole-wheat flour	An unrefined, whole-grain flour made from whole-wheat kernels.

wheat flour? And what's the difference? To help you answer this question, in **Table 4.4** we've defined some terms commonly used on labels for breads and cereals. As you can see, whole-wheat flour is made from whole grains; only the husk of the wheat kernel has been removed. In contrast, the term *wheat flour* can be used to signify a flour that has been highly refined, with the bran and other fiber-rich portions removed.

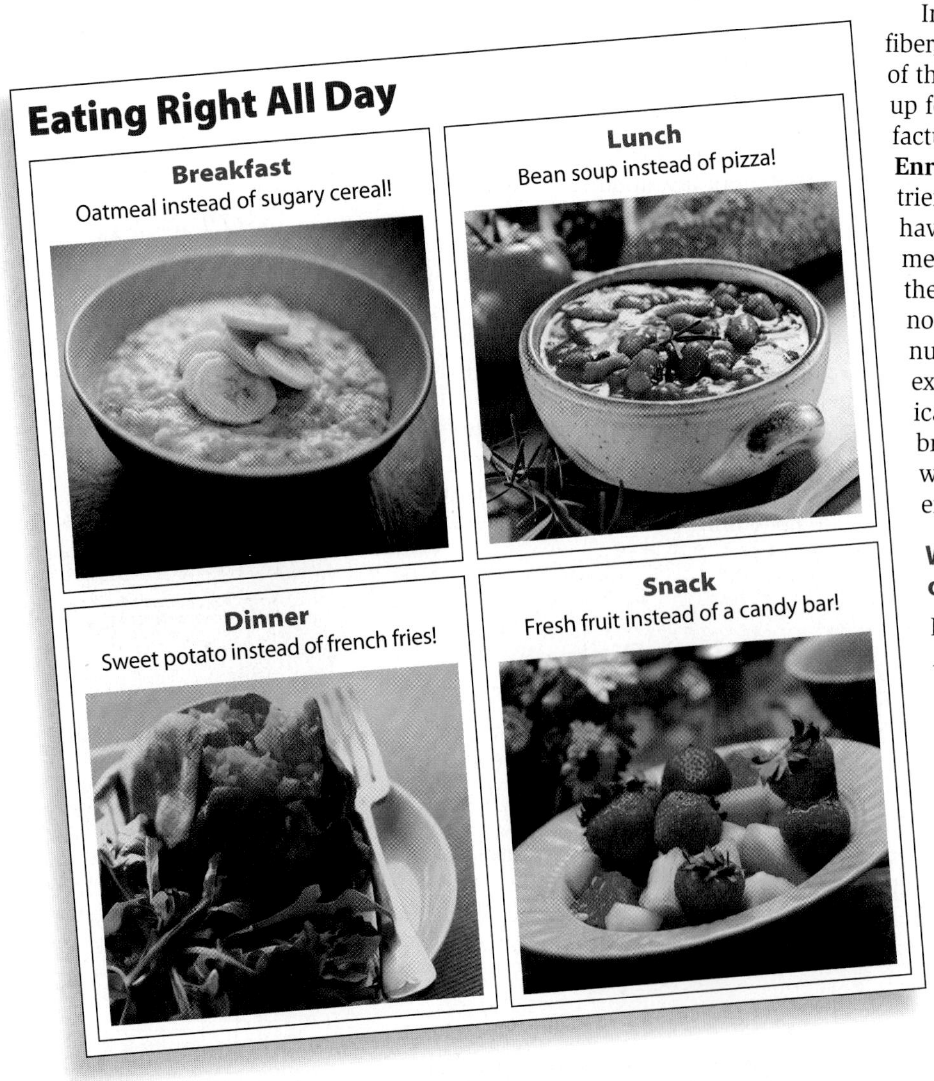
Eating Right All Day
Breakfast
Oatmeal instead of sugary cereal!
Lunch
Bean soup instead of pizza!
Dinner
Sweet potato instead of french fries!
Snack
Fresh fruit instead of a candy bar!

In addition to stripping a grain of its fiber, the refining process reduces many of the grain's original nutrients. To make up for some of the lost nutrients, manufacturers sometimes enrich the product. **Enriched foods** are foods in which nutrients that were lost during processing have been added back, so that the food meets a specified standard. Notice that the terms *enriched* and *fortified* are not synonymous: **fortified foods** have nutrients added that did not originally exist in the food (or existed in insignificant amounts). For example, some breakfast cereals have been fortified with iron, a mineral that is not present in cereals naturally.

We Need at Least 25 Grams of Fiber Daily

How much fiber do we need? The Adequate Intake for fiber is 25 g per day for women and 38 g per day for men, or 14 g of fiber for every 1,000 kcal per day that a person eats.[5] Most people in the United States eat only 12 to 18 g of fiber each day, getting only half of the fiber they need. Although fiber supplements are available, it is

QUICK TIPS

Hunting for Fiber

✓ Select breads made with *whole* grains, such as wheat, oats, barley, and rye. Two slices of whole-grain bread provide 4–6 grams of fiber.

✓ Switch from a low-fiber breakfast cereal to one that has at least 4 grams of fiber per serving.

✓ For a mid-morning snack, stir 1–2 tablespoons of whole ground flaxseed meal (4 grams of fiber) into a cup of low-fat or nonfat yogurt. Or choose an apple or a pear, with the skin left on (approximately 5 grams of fiber).

✓ Instead of potato chips with your lunchtime sandwich, have a side of carrot sticks or celery sticks (approximately 2 grams of fiber per serving).

✓ Eat legumes every day, if possible (approximately 6 grams of fiber per serving). Have them as your main dish, as a side, or in soups, chili, and other dishes.

✓ Don't forget the vegetables! A cup of cooked leafy greens provides about 4 grams of fiber, and a salad is rich in fiber.

✓ For dessert, try fresh, frozen, or dried fruit or a high-fiber granola with sweetened soy milk.

✓ When shopping, choose fresh fruits and vegetables whenever possible. Buy frozen vegetables and fruits when fresh produce is not available. Check frozen selections to make sure there is no sugar or salt added.

✓ Be careful when buying canned fruits, vegetables, and legumes, as they may be high in added sugar or sodium. Select versions without added sugar or salt, or rinse before serving.

best to get fiber from food because foods contain additional nutrients, such as vitamins and minerals.

It is also important to drink plenty of fluid as you increase your fiber intake, as fiber binds with water to soften stools. Inadequate fluid intake with a high-fiber diet can actually result in hard, dry stools that are difficult to pass through the colon. At least eight 8-oz glasses of fluid each day are commonly recommended.

Can you eat too much fiber? Excessive fiber consumption can lead to problems such as intestinal gas, bloating, and constipation. Because fiber binds with water, it causes the body to eliminate more water in the feces, so a very-high-fiber diet could result in dehydration. Fiber also binds many vitamins and minerals, so a high-fiber diet can reduce our absorption of important nutrients, such as iron, zinc, and calcium. In children, some elderly, the chronically ill, and other at-risk populations, extreme fiber intake can even lead to malnutrition—they feel full before they have eaten enough to provide adequate energy and nutrients. So, although some societies are accustomed to a very-high-fiber diet, most people in the United States find it difficult to tolerate more than 50 g of fiber per day.

Food Sources of Fiber

Eating the amounts of whole grains, vegetables, fruits, nuts, and legumes recommended in the USDA Food Guide will ensure that you eat enough fiber. **Figure 4.13** shows some common foods and their fiber content. You can use this information to design a diet that includes adequate fiber.

To help you eat right all day, see the menu choices high in fiber. Each of these choices is also packed with vitamins, minerals, and phytochemicals. For instance, a sweet potato is loaded with beta-carotene, a phytochemical the body converts to vitamin A.

See the Quick Tips box above for suggestions on selecting carbohydrate sources rich in fiber.

enriched foods Foods in which nutrients that were lost during processing have been added back, so that the food meets a specified standard.

fortified foods Foods in which nutrients are added that did not originally exist in the food, or which existed in insignificant amounts.

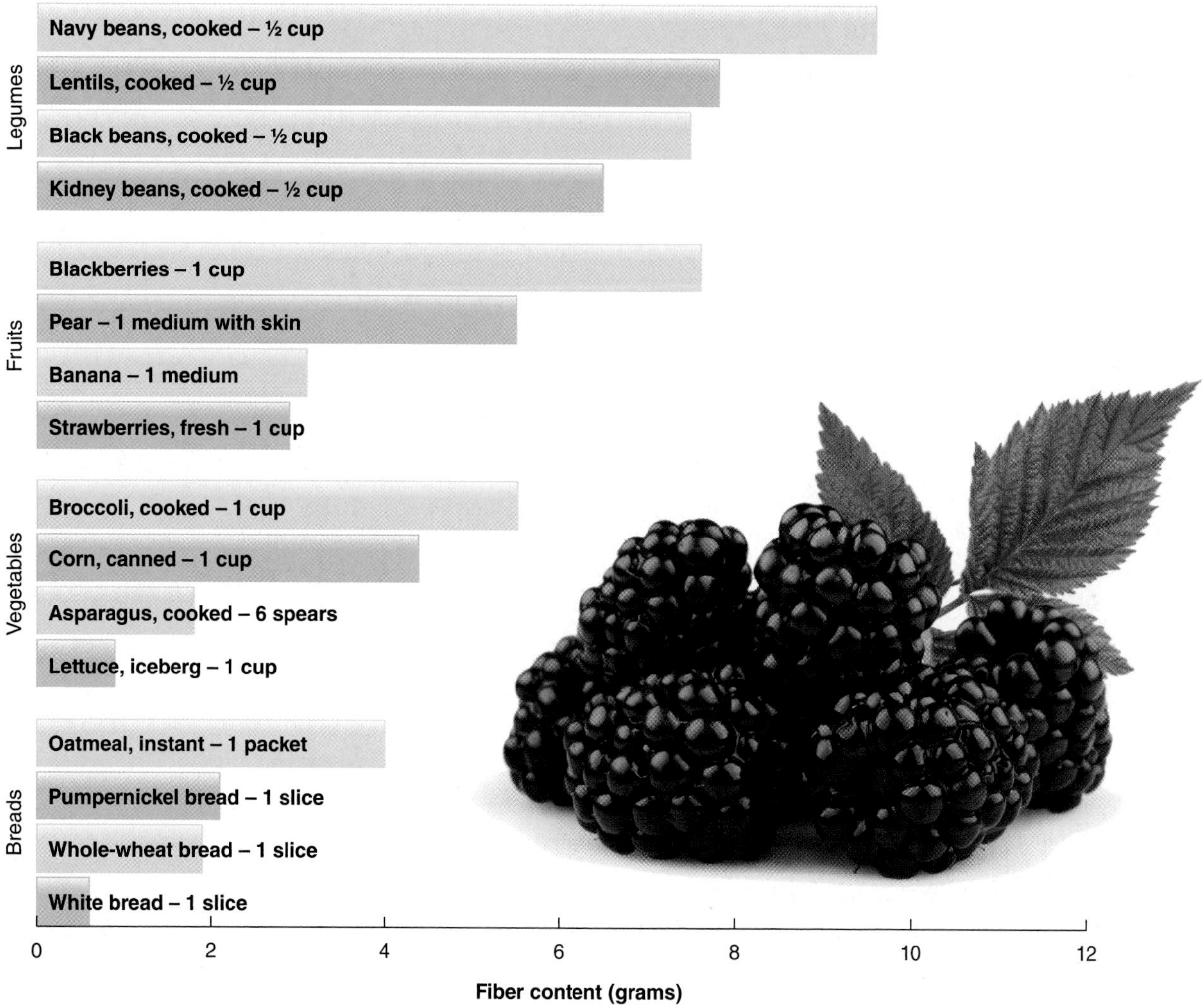

Figure 4.13 Fiber content of common foods. *Note:* The Adequate Intake for fiber is 25 g per day for women and 38 g per day for men.

Data from U.S. Department of Agriculture, Agricultural Research Service. 2009. USDA National Nutrient Database for Standard Reference, Release 22. Nutrient Data Laboratory Home Page, www.ars.usda.gov/ba/bhnrc/ndl.

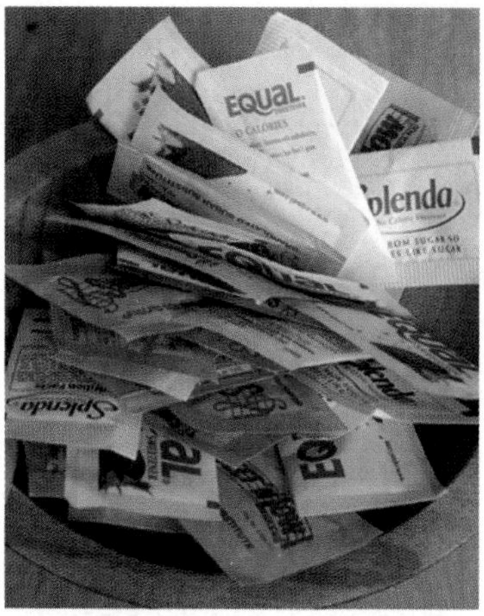

Contrary to reports claiming severe health consequences related to the consumption of alternative sweeteners, major health agencies have determined that they are safe to consume.

Try the Nutrition Label Activity coming up to learn how to recognize various carbohydrates on food labels. Armed with this knowledge, you are now ready to make more healthful food choices.

RECAP **The Adequate Intake for fiber is 25 g per day for women and 38 g per day for men. Most Americans eat only half of the fiber they need each day. Foods high in fiber and nutrient density include whole grains and cereals, fruits, and vegetables. The more processed the food, the fewer fiber-rich carbohydrates it contains.**

What's the Story on Alternative Sweeteners?

Most of us love sweets but want to avoid the extra Calories and tooth decay that go along with eating refined sugars. That's why we turn to alternative sweeteners.

NUTRITION LABEL ACTIVITY

Recognizing Carbohydrates on the Label

Figure 4.14 shows portions of labels for two breakfast cereals. The cereal on the left (a) is processed and sweetened, whereas the one on the right (b) is a whole-grain product with no added sugar.

- Check the center of each label to locate the amount of total carbohydrate. Notice that it is almost the same, although the sweetened cereal has a larger serving size.
- Now look at the information listed as subgroups under Total Carbohydrate. Notice that the sweetened cereal contains 13 g of sugar—half of its total carbohydrates—but only 1 g of dietary fiber. In contrast, the whole-grain cereal contains 4 g of fiber and only 1 g of sugar!
- Now look at the percent values listed to the right of the Total Carbohydrate section. For both cereals (without milk), their percent contribution to daily carbohydrate is 9%. This does not mean that 9% of the Calories in these cereals come from carbohydrates. Instead, it refers to the Daily Values listed at the bottom of each label. For a person who eats 2,000 kcal, the recommended amount of carbohydrate each day is 300 g. One serving of each cereal contains 26–27 g, which is about 9% of 300 g.

To compare the percent of total Calories that comes from carbohydrate in each cereal, do the following:

a. Calculate the *Calories* in 1 serving of the cereal that come from carbohydrate. Multiply the total grams of carbohydrate per serving by the energy value of carbohydrate. For the sweetened cereal:

$$26 \text{ g of carbohydrate} \times 4 \text{ kcal/g} = 104 \text{ kcal from carbohydrate}$$

b. Calculate the *percent of Calories* in the cereal that come from carbohydrate. Divide the Calories from carbohydrate by the total Calories for each serving and multiply by 100. For the sweetened cereal:

$$(104 \text{ kcal} \div 120 \text{ kcal}) \times 100 = 87\% \text{ Calories from carbohydrate}$$

c. Now do the same calculations for the whole-grain cereal and compare.

Which has a *lower* percentage of carbohydrate? What macronutrients does this cereal provide in *greater* amounts than the other product? Finally, check the ingredients for the sweetened cereal. Remember that they are listed in order from highest to lowest amount. The second and third ingredients listed are sugar and brown sugar, and the corn and oat flours are not whole-grain flours. Now look at the ingredients for the other cereal—whole-grain oats. Although the sweetened product is enriched with more B-vitamins, iron, and zinc, the whole-grain cereal packs 4 g of fiber per serving and contains no added sugars. Which cereal should you choose, and why?

Nutritive Sweeteners Include Sugars and Sugar Alcohols

Remember that all carbohydrates, including simple and complex, contain 4 kcal of energy per gram. Because sweeteners such as sucrose, fructose, honey, and brown sugar contribute Calories (or energy), they are called **nutritive sweeteners.**

Other nutritive sweeteners are the *sugar alcohols,* such as mannitol, sorbitol, isomalt, and xylitol. Popular in sugar-free gums and mints, sugar alcohols are less sweet than sucrose. Foods with sugar alcohols have health benefits that foods made with sugars do not have, such as a reduced glycemic response and a decreased risk for dental caries. Also, because sugar alcohols are absorbed slowly and incompletely from the small intestine, they provide less energy than sugar, usually 2 to 3 kcal of energy per gram. However, because they are not completely absorbed from the small intestine, they can attract water into the large intestine and cause diarrhea.

nutritive sweeteners Sweeteners, such as sucrose, fructose, honey, and brown sugar, that contribute Calories (energy).

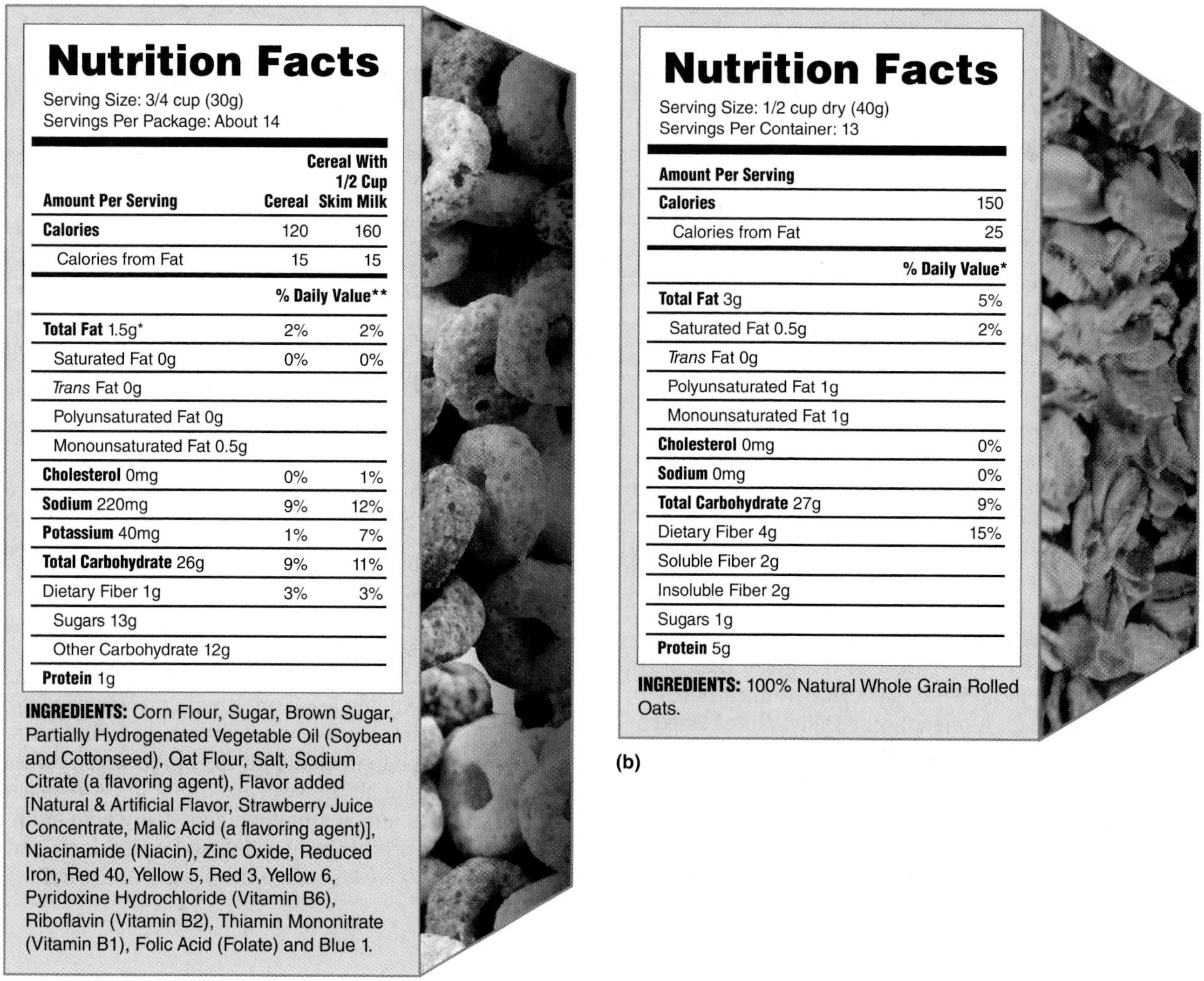

Nutrition Facts

Serving Size: 3/4 cup (30g)
Servings Per Package: About 14

Amount Per Serving	Cereal	Cereal With 1/2 Cup Skim Milk
Calories	120	160
Calories from Fat	15	15
	% Daily Value**	
Total Fat 1.5g*	2%	2%
Saturated Fat 0g	0%	0%
Trans Fat 0g		
Polyunsaturated Fat 0g		
Monounsaturated Fat 0.5g		
Cholesterol 0mg	0%	1%
Sodium 220mg	9%	12%
Potassium 40mg	1%	7%
Total Carbohydrate 26g	9%	11%
Dietary Fiber 1g	3%	3%
Sugars 13g		
Other Carbohydrate 12g		
Protein 1g		

INGREDIENTS: Corn Flour, Sugar, Brown Sugar, Partially Hydrogenated Vegetable Oil (Soybean and Cottonseed), Oat Flour, Salt, Sodium Citrate (a flavoring agent), Flavor added [Natural & Artificial Flavor, Strawberry Juice Concentrate, Malic Acid (a flavoring agent)], Niacinamide (Niacin), Zinc Oxide, Reduced Iron, Red 40, Yellow 5, Red 3, Yellow 6, Pyridoxine Hydrochloride (Vitamin B6), Riboflavin (Vitamin B2), Thiamin Mononitrate (Vitamin B1), Folic Acid (Folate) and Blue 1.

(a)

Nutrition Facts

Serving Size: 1/2 cup dry (40g)
Servings Per Container: 13

Amount Per Serving	
Calories	150
Calories from Fat	25
	% Daily Value*
Total Fat 3g	5%
Saturated Fat 0.5g	2%
Trans Fat 0g	
Polyunsaturated Fat 1g	
Monounsaturated Fat 1g	
Cholesterol 0mg	0%
Sodium 0mg	0%
Total Carbohydrate 27g	9%
Dietary Fiber 4g	15%
Soluble Fiber 2g	
Insoluble Fiber 2g	
Sugars 1g	
Protein 5g	

INGREDIENTS: 100% Natural Whole Grain Rolled Oats.

(b)

Figure 4.14 Labels for two breakfast cereals: **(a)** processed and sweetened cereal; **(b)** whole-grain cereal with no added sugar.

Alternative Sweeteners Are Non-Nutritive

A number of other products have been developed to sweeten foods without promoting tooth decay and weight gain. Because these products provide little or no energy, they are called **non-nutritive,** or *alternative,* **sweeteners.** Contrary to popular belief, alternative sweeteners have been determined to be safe for adults, children, and individuals with diabetes to consume. Although women who are pregnant should discuss the use of alternative sweeteners with their healthcare provider, in general, it appears safe for pregnant women to consume alternative sweeteners in amounts within the Food and Drug Administration (FDA) guidelines.[19] The **Acceptable Daily Intake (ADI)** is an FDA estimate of the amount of a sweetener that someone can consume each day over a lifetime without adverse effects. The estimates are based on studies conducted on laboratory animals, and they include a 100-fold safety factor. It is important to emphasize that actual intake by humans is typically well below the ADI.

The major alternative sweeteners currently available on the market are saccharin, acesulfame-K, aspartame, and sucralose.

non-nutritive sweeteners Manufactured sweeteners that provide little or no energy; also called *alternative sweeteners.*

Acceptable Daily Intake (ADI) An FDA estimate of the amount of a non-nutritive sweetener that someone can consume each day over a lifetime without adverse effects.

Saccharin

Discovered in the late 1800s, *saccharin* is about 300 times sweeter than sucrose. Evidence to suggest that saccharin may cause bladder tumors in rats surfaced in the 1970s; however, more than 20 years of scientific research has shown that saccharin is not related to bladder cancer in humans. Based on this evidence, in May of 2000 the National Toxicology Program of the U.S. government removed saccharin from its list of products that may cause cancer. No ADI has been set for saccharin, and it is used in foods and beverages and sold as a tabletop sweetener. Saccharin is sold as Sweet 'N Low (also known as "the pink packet") in the United States.

Acesulfame-K

Acesulfame-K (acesulfame potassium) is marketed under the names Sunette and Sweet One. It is a Calorie-free sweetener that is 200 times sweeter than sugar. It is used to sweeten gums, candies, beverages, instant tea, coffee, gelatins, and puddings. The taste of acesulfame-K does not change when it is heated, so it can be used in cooking. The body does not metabolize acesulfame-K, so it is excreted unchanged by the kidneys.

Aspartame

Aspartame, also called Equal ("the blue packet") and NutraSweet, is one of the most popular alternative sweeteners in foods and beverages. Aspartame is composed of two amino acids, phenylalanine and aspartic acid. When these amino acids are separate, one is bitter and the other has no flavor—but joined together they make a substance that is 180 times sweeter than sucrose. Although aspartame contains 4 kcal of energy per gram, it is so sweet that only small amounts are necessary; thus, it ends up contributing little or no energy. Because aspartame is made from amino acids, its taste is destroyed with heat (see Chapter 6), so it cannot be used in cooking.

A significant amount of research has been done to test the safety of aspartame. Although a number of false claims have been published, especially on the Internet, there is no scientific evidence to support the claim that aspartame causes brain tumors, Alzheimer's disease, or nerve disorders.

The ADI for aspartame is 50 mg per kg body weight per day. **Table 4.5** shows how many servings of aspartame-sweetened foods would have to be consumed to exceed the ADI. Although eating less than the ADI is considered safe, note that children who consume many powdered drinks, diet sodas, and other aspartame-flavored products could potentially exceed this amount. Drinks sweetened with aspartame are extremely popular among children and teenagers, but they are very low in nutritional value and should not replace healthful beverages, such as milk, water, and 100% fruit juice.

Some people should not consume any aspartame: those with the disease *phenylketonuria (PKU)*. This is a genetic disorder that prevents the breakdown of the

TABLE 4.5 The Amount of Food that a 50-Pound Child and a 150-Pound Adult Would Have to Consume Each Day to Exceed the ADI for Aspartame

Food	50-Pound Child	150-Pound Adult
12 fl. oz carbonated soft drink	7	20
8 fl. oz powdered soft drink	11	34
4 fl. oz gelatin dessert	14	42
Packets of tabletop sweetener	32	97

Data from International Food Information Council. 2003. *Everything You Need to Know About Aspartame.* Available at http://ific.org/publications/brochures/aspartamebroch.cfm.

amino acid phenylalanine. Because a person with PKU cannot metabolize phenylalanine, it builds up in the tissues of the body and causes irreversible brain damage. In the United States, all newborn babies are tested for PKU; those who have it are placed on a phenylalanine-limited diet. Some foods that are common sources of protein and other nutrients for growing children, such as meats and milk, contain phenylalanine. Thus, it is critical that children with PKU not waste what little phenylalanine they can consume on nutrient-poor products sweetened with aspartame.

Sucralose

The FDA has recently approved the use of *sucralose* as an alternative sweetener. It is marketed under the brand name Splenda and is known as "the yellow packet." It is made from sucrose, but chlorine atoms are substituted for the hydrogen and oxygen normally found in sucrose, and it passes through the digestive tract unchanged, without contributing any energy. It is 600 times sweeter than sucrose and is stable when heated, so it can be used in cooking. It has been approved for use in many foods, including chewing gum, salad dressings, beverages, gelatin and pudding products, canned fruits, frozen dairy desserts, and baked goods. Safety studies have not shown sucralose to cause cancer or to have other adverse health effects.

RECAP **Alternative sweeteners can be used in place of sugar to sweeten foods. Most of these products do not promote tooth decay and contribute little or no energy. The alternative sweeteners approved for use in the United States are considered safe when eaten in amounts less than the Acceptable Daily Intake.**

NUTRI-CASE HANNAH

"Last night, my mom called and said she'd be late getting home from work, so I made dinner. I made vegetarian quesadillas with flour tortillas, canned green chilies, cheese, and sour cream, plus a few baby carrots on the side. Later that night, I got really hungry, so I ate a package of sugar-free cookies. They're sweetened with sorbitol and taste just like real cookies! I ate maybe three or four, but I didn't think it was a big deal because they're sugar-free. When I checked the package label, I found out that each cookie has 90 Calories!

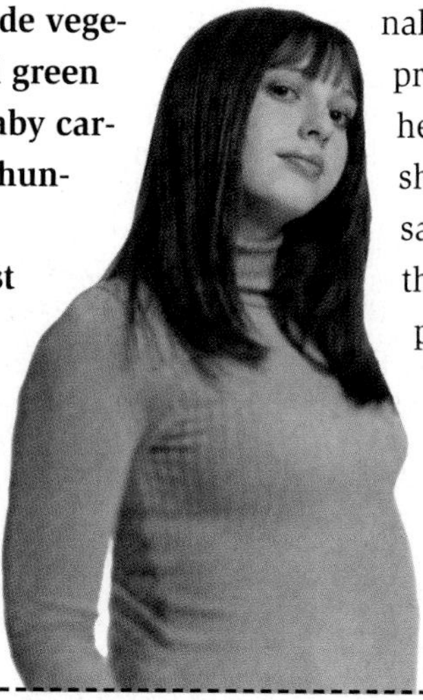

Without knowing the exact ingredients in Hannah's dinner and snack, would you agree that, prior to the cookies, she'd been making healthy choices? Why or why not? How might she have changed the ingredients in her quesadillas to increase their fiber content? And, if the cookies were sugar-free, how can you explain the fact that each cookie still contained 90 Calories?

Nutrition DEBATE

Is High-Fructose Corn Syrup the Cause of the Obesity Epidemic?

Over the past 30 years, obesity rates have increased dramatically for adults and children. Obesity has become public health enemy number one, as many chronic diseases, such as type 2 diabetes, heart disease, high blood pressure, and arthritis, go hand in hand with obesity.

Factors contributing to obesity include genetic influences, lack of adequate physical activity, and excessive consumption of energy. Genetics cannot be held solely responsible for the rapid rise in obesity that has occurred over the past 30 years. Our genetic makeup takes thousands of years to change; humans who lived 100 years ago had essentially the same genetic makeup as we do. We need to look at the effect of our lifestyle changes over the same period.

One lifestyle factor that has come to the forefront of nutrition research is the contribution of high-fructose corn syrup (HFCS) to overweight and obesity. HFCS is made by converting the starch in corn to glucose and then converting some of the glucose to fructose, which is sweeter. Unfortunately, fructose is metabolized differently than glucose, because it is absorbed farther down in the small intestine and, unlike glucose, it does not stimulate insulin release from the pancreas. Since insulin inhibits food intake in humans, this failure to stimulate insulin release could increase energy intake. In addition, fructose enters body cells via a transport protein not present in brain cells; thus, unlike glucose, fructose cannot enter brain cells and stimulate satiety signals. If we don't feel full, we are likely to continue eating or drinking.

However, the culprit in our increasing obesity rates may not be HFCS itself but, rather, the sweetened soft drinks and other products in which it is found. Bray et al.[20] emphasize that HFCS is the sole caloric sweetener in sugared soft drinks and represents more than 40% of caloric sweeteners added to other foods and beverages in the United States. These researchers have linked the increased use and consumption of HFCS with the rising rates of obesity since the 1970s, when HFCS first appeared.

The potential contribution of sweetened soft drink consumption to rising obesity rates in young people has received a great deal of attention. Studies show that girls and boys ages 6 to 11 years drank about twice as many soft drinks in 1998 as children did in 1977.[21] Equally alarming is the finding that one-fourth of a group of adolescents studied drank at least 26 oz of soft drinks each day. This intake is equivalent to almost 400 extra Calories daily![22] Another study found that replacing sweetened soft drinks with noncaloric beverages in 13- to 18-year-olds resulted in a significant decrease in body mass index in the those who were the most overweight when starting the study.[23]

This alarming information has led to dramatic changes in soft drink availability in schools and at school-sponsored events. In 2006, the soft drink industry agreed to a voluntary ban on sales of all sweetened soft drinks in elementary and high schools. Despite these positive changes, there is still ample availability of foods and beverages containing HFCS in the marketplace.

Although the evidence pinpointing HFCS as a major contributor to the obesity epidemic may appear strong, other nutrition professionals disagree. It has been proposed that soft drinks would have contributed to the obesity epidemic whether the sweetener was sucrose or fructose, and that their contribution to obesity is due to increased consumption as a result of advertising, increases in serving sizes, and virtually unlimited access to soft drinks.[24] Also, a recent study found that increased fructose consumption does not cause weight gain in humans.[25] It is possible that the obesity epidemic has resulted from increased consumption of energy (from sweetened soft drinks and other high-energy foods) *and* a reduction in physical activity levels, and HFCS itself is not to blame. Evidence to support this stems from the fact that obesity rates are rising around the world, and many countries experiencing this epidemic do not use HFCS as a sweetener.

This issue is extremely complex, and more research needs to be done in humans before we can fully understand how HFCS contributes to our diet and our health.[26]

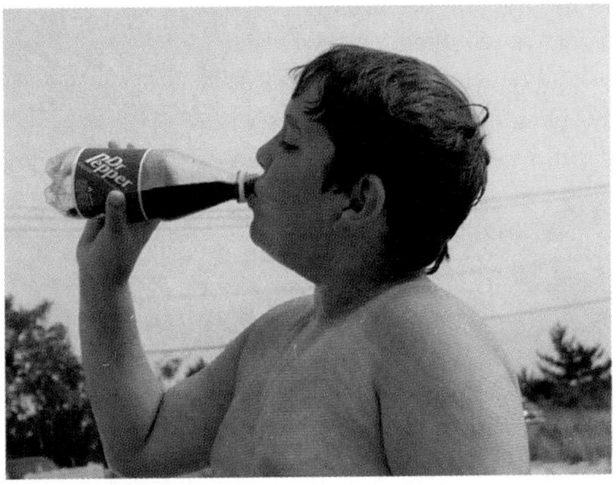

It is estimated that the rate of overweight in children has increased 100% since the mid-1970s.

Chapter Review

Test Yourself ANSWERS

1. **False.** There is no evidence that diets high in sugar cause hyperactivity or diabetes in children.
2. **False.** At 4 kcal/g, carbohydrates have less than half the energy of a gram of fat. Eating a high-carbohydrate diet will not cause people to gain body fat unless their total diet contains more energy (kcal) than they expend. In fact, eating a diet high in complex, fiber-rich carbohydrates is associated with a lower risk for obesity.
3. **True.** Contrary to recent reports claiming harmful consequences related to the consumption of alternative sweeteners, major health agencies have determined that these products are safe for most of us to consume in limited quantities.

Find the Quack

Christina is surfing the Internet looking for information for a report on carbohydrates for her nutrition class, when she spots something that intrigues her: Cure Diseases with Sugar! She wonders what it's all about and clicks to bring up the site. Glyconutrients! the homepage proclaims, stating that these special nutrients will reverse aging, increase sports performance, and help you achieve optimal health. Beside a photo of a slender, tanned couple walking along a beach are statements claiming that:

- "Processed foods are devoid of nourishment and have no nutritional value. They are also toxic. We both starve and poison ourselves by consuming these foods. This is why every degenerative disease condition is on the rise."
- "Pharmaceuticals (prescription and over-the-counter medications) do not work."
- "Glyconutrients are plant monosaccharides, essential plant sugars that have recently been shown to be essential to human life. We must consume glyconutrient supplements to protect our health. Without them, our cells will lose the ability to communicate with one another and perform the functions they were designed to do. We will then develop chronic diseases, such as cancer and diabetes."
- "A total of ninety-six patents have been filed on a range of glyconutrient products."
- "Just about every respected scientific journal has now published documents and articles on glycobiology and glyconutrients."
- "Your doctor will not know about glyconutrients because the topic is only just beginning to be taught in medical schools."

1. In Chapter 1, you learned how to spot false nutrition claims (pages 20–21). Discuss the validity of the website's statement about processed foods.
2. Comment on the website's definition of glyconutrients as plant monosaccharides that are essential for human life.
3. Are you impressed with the statement that "ninety-six patents have been filed on a range of glyconutrient products"? Why or why not?
4. What motive do you think might lurk behind the assertion that your doctor will not know about glyconutrients because the topic "is only just beginning to be taught in medical schools"?

Answers can be found on the companion website at www.pearsonhighered.com/thompsonmanore.

NutriTools Check out the companion website at www.pearsonhighered.com/thompsonmanore, or use MyNutritionLab.com, to access interactive animations, including:

- Food Label: Find the Carbohydrates
- Digestion and Absorption: Carbohydrates
- Know Your Carbohydrate Sources

Review Questions

1. The glycemic index rates
   a. the acceptable amount of alternative sweeteners to consume in 1 day.
   b. the potential of foods to raise blood glucose and insulin levels.
   c. the risk of a given food for causing diabetes.
   d. the ratio of soluble to insoluble fiber in a complex carbohydrate.
2. Carbohydrates contain
   a. carbon, nitrogen, and water.
   b. carbonic acid and a sugar alcohol.
   c. hydrated sugar.
   d. carbon, hydrogen, and oxygen.
3. The most common source of added sugar in the American diet is
   a. table sugar.
   b. white flour.
   c. alcohol.
   d. sweetened soft drinks.
4. Glucose, fructose, and galactose are
   a. monosaccharides.
   b. disaccharides.
   c. polysaccharides.
   d. complex carbohydrates.
5. Aspartame should not be consumed by people who have
   a. phenylketonuria.
   b. type 1 diabetes.
   c. lactose intolerance.
   d. diverticulosis.
6. True or false? Sugar alcohols are non-nutritive sweeteners.
7. True or false? Both insulin and glucagon are pancreatic hormones.
8. True or false? Adults need about 10 grams of fiber daily.
9. True or false? Plants store glucose as fiber.
10. True or false? Salivary amylase breaks down starches into galactose.

Answers to Review Questions can be found at the back of this text, and additional essay questions and answers are located on the companion website at www.pearsonhighered.com/thompsonmanore.

Web Resources

www.ific.org
International Food Information Council Foundation (IFIC)

Search this site to find out more about sugars and low-calorie sweeteners.

www.ada.org
American Dental Association

Go to this site to learn more about tooth decay as well as other oral health topics.

www.nidcr.nih.gov
National Institute of Dental and Craniofacial Research (NIDCR)

Find out more about recent oral and dental health discoveries and obtain statistics and data on the status of dental health in the United States.

NutriTools

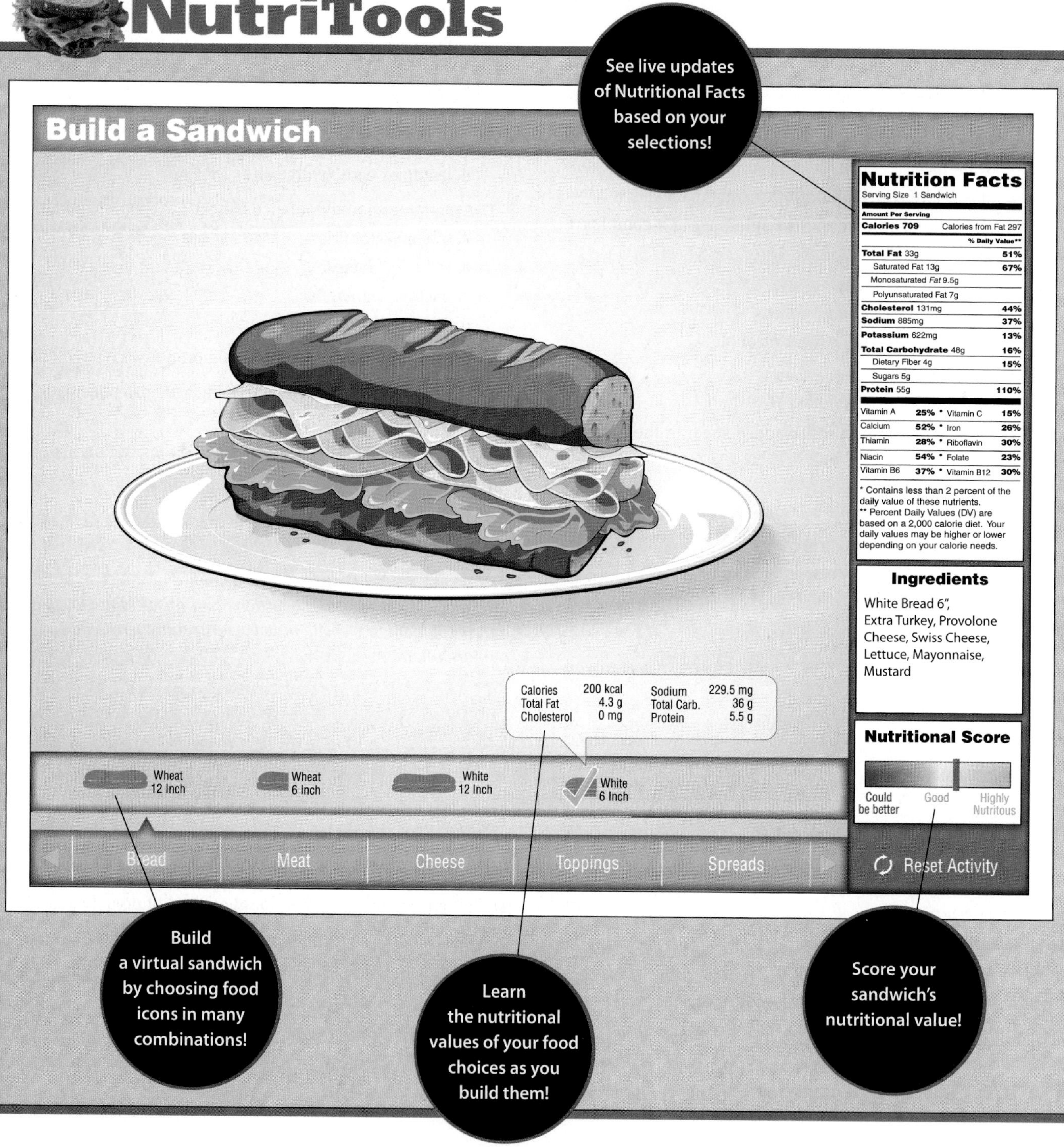

To build your sandwich, just visit www.pearsonhighered.com/thompsonmanore or www.mynutritionlab.com

After building your sandwich, you should be able to answer these questions:

1. How is your selection of combination toppings making your sandwich nutritious?
2. Is your sandwich higher or lower in kcalories than you need for one meal?
3. Which ingredients could you combine to build a sandwich with a nutritional score of 100?
4. How are the condiments added to your sandwich affecting its nutritional score?
5. Would a six-inch sandwich have half the nutritional score of a twelve-inch?

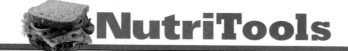

IN DEPTH

Diabetes

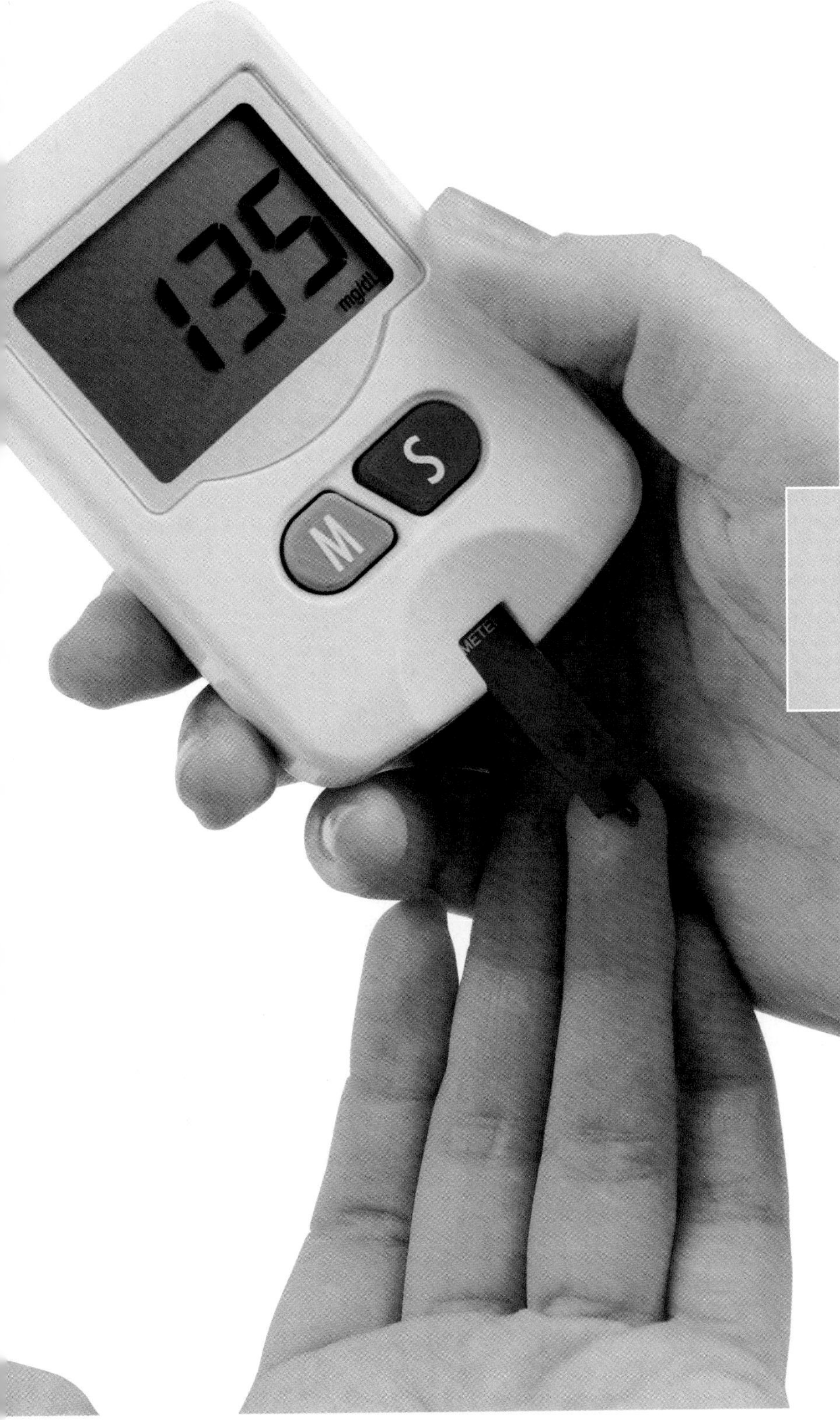

WANT TO FIND OUT. . .

- **if eating carbohydrates leads to diabetes?**
- **what the link is between diabetes and obesity?**
- **if you're at risk for diabetes?**

READ ON.

It was a typical day at a large medical center in the Bronx, New York: two patients were having toes amputated, another had nerve damage, one was being treated for kidney failure, another for infection, and another was blind. Despite their variety, these problems were due to just one disease: diabetes. On an average day, nearly half of the inpatients at the medical center have diabetes. And the problem isn't limited to the Bronx. Every day in the United States, 230 people with diabetes have surgery to remove toes, a foot, or an entire leg; 120 enter the final stage of kidney disease; and 55 go blind. A little over a decade ago, these complications, which typically develop about 10 to

15 years after the onset of the disease, were rarely seen in people younger than age 60. But now, as more and more children and adolescents are being diagnosed with diabetes, experts are predicting that the typical patient will be more like Iris, one of the patients with diabetes at the Bronx medical center this day. Iris is 26 years old.[1]

What is diabetes? Does eating carbohydrates lead to diabetes? Is obesity linked to diabetes? Here we'll explore ***In Depth*** the differences between type 1 and type 2 diabetes and the relationship between carbohydrates and a person's risk for diabetes. We'll also explore the link between diabetes, obesity, and other chronic diseases.

What Is Diabetes?

Diabetes is a chronic disease in which the body can no longer regulate glucose within normal limits, and blood glucose levels become dangerously high. It is imperative to detect and treat the disease as soon as possible because excessive fluctuations in glucose injure tissues throughout the body. As noted in the introduction, if not controlled, diabetes can lead to blindness, seizures, stroke, kidney failure, nerve disease, and cardiovascular disease. Damage to the body's nerves and blood vessels is especially problematic in the lower limbs. Along with an increased risk for infection, this increases the incidence of tissue death (necrosis), leading to a greatly increased number of toe, foot, and lower leg amputations in people with diabetes. Uncontrolled diabetes can also lead to ketoacidosis, which may result in coma and death.

As noted in Chapter 1, diabetes is the sixth leading cause of death in the United States.

Approximately 18 million people in the United States—7% of the total population, including adults and children—are diagnosed with diabetes. It is speculated that another 5.7 million people have diabetes but do not know it.[2]

Figure 1 shows the percentage of adults with diabetes from various ethnic groups in the United States.[2] As you can see, diabetes is more common in African Americans, Hispanic or Latino Americans, and American Indians and Alaska Natives than in Caucasians.

The two main forms of diabetes are type 1 and type 2. Some women develop a third form, *gestational diabetes*, during pregnancy; we will discuss this in more detail in Chapter 14.

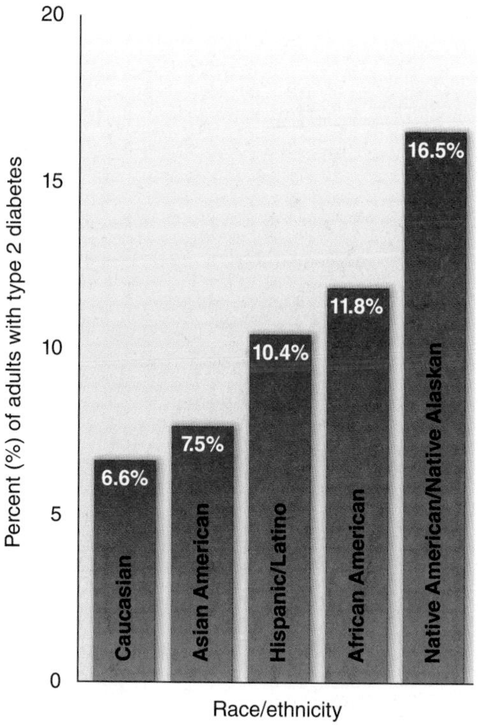

Figure 1 The percentage of adults from various ethnic and racial groups with type 2 diabetes.
Data from the National Diabetes Information Clearinghouse (NDIC). 2005. National Diabetes Statistics. National Institutes of Health [NIH] Publication No. 06-3892. http://diabetes.niddk.nih.gov/dm/pubs/statistics/index.htm.

In Type 1 Diabetes, the Body Does Not Produce Enough Insulin

Approximately 10% of people with diabetes have **type 1 diabetes**, in which the body cannot produce enough insulin. When people with type 1 diabetes eat a meal and their blood glucose rises, the pancreas is unable to secrete insulin in response. Glucose levels soar, and the body tries to expel the excess glucose by excreting it in the urine. In fact, the medical term for the disease is *diabetes mellitus* (from the Greek *diabainein*, "to pass through," and Latin *mellitus*, "sweetened with honey"), and frequent urination is one of its warning signs (see **Table 1** for other symptoms). If blood glucose levels are not controlled, a person with type 1 diabetes will become confused and lethargic and have trouble breathing. This is because the brain is not getting enough glucose to function properly. As discussed in Chapter 4, uncontrolled diabetes can lead to ketoacidosis; left untreated, the ultimate result is coma and death.

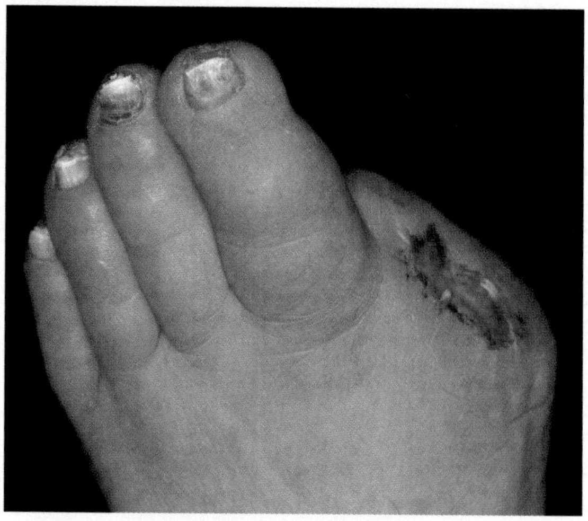

Amputations are a common complication of uncontrolled diabetes.

diabetes A chronic disease in which the body can no longer regulate glucose normally.

type 1 diabetes A disorder in which the body cannot produce enough insulin.

TABLE 1 Symptoms of Type 1 and Type 2 Diabetes

Type 1 Diabetes	Type 2 Diabetes*
Frequent urination	Any of the type 1 symptoms
Unusual thirst	Frequent infections
Extreme hunger	Blurred vision
Unusual weight loss	Cuts/bruises that are slow to heal
Extreme fatigue	Tingling/numbness in the hands or feet
Irritability	Recurring skin, gum, or bladder infections

Data from the American Diabetes Association, Diabetes Basics. Symptoms. www.diabetes.org/diabetes-basics/symptoms/.
*Some people with type 2 diabetes experience no symptoms.

HOT TOPIC

Diabetes Goes High-Tech

Vincent was diagnosed with type 1 diabetes when he was 10 years old. Now he's a college sophomore and has been living with the disease for 9 years. In that time, advances in diabetes monitoring and treatment have made Vincent's life just a little easier.

For instance, all people with diabetes have to test their blood glucose level many times each day. Until recently, Vincent had to prick his fingers to do this, and they would get tender and develop calluses. Now, the FDA has approved several devices that measure blood glucose without pricking the finger. Some of them can read glucose levels through the skin, and others take readings from a small needle implanted in the body. Also, during his first few years with diabetes, Vincent had to give himself two to four shots of insulin each day. Now he uses an insulin infusion pump, which looks like a small pager and delivers insulin into the body through a thin tube gradually throughout the day.

Sure, Vincent still has to watch his diet carefully, eating three nutritious meals a day and limiting snacks. But with his new high-tech devices, it's easier to control his blood glucose, and he can play sports, travel, and do most of the things he wants to do, just like his friends.

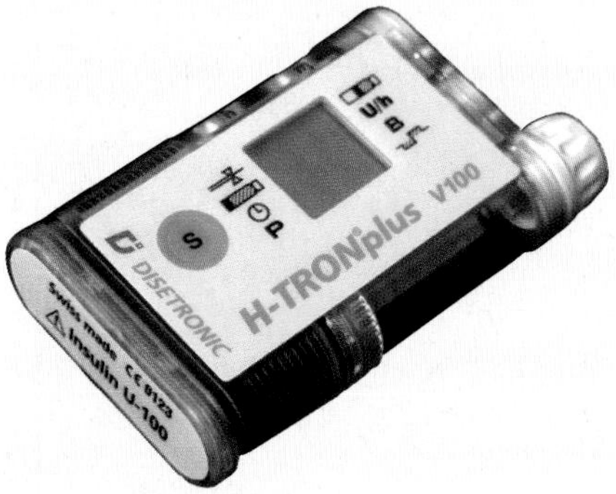

Insulin pumps can help those with diabetes eat a wider range of foods.

The cause of type 1 diabetes is unknown, but it may be an *autoimmune disease*. This means that the body's immune system attacks and destroys its own tissues—in this case, the insulin-producing cells of the pancreas.

Most cases of type 1 diabetes are diagnosed in adolescents around 10 to 14 years of age, although the disease can appear in infants, young children, and adults. It has a genetic link, so siblings and children of those with type 1 diabetes are at greater risk.[3]

The only treatment for type 1 diabetes is the administration of insulin by injection or pump several times daily. Insulin is a hormone composed of protein, so it would be digested in the small intestine if taken as a pill. Individuals with type 1 diabetes must monitor their blood glucose levels closely using a *glucometer* to ensure that they remain within a healthful range **(Figure 2)**.

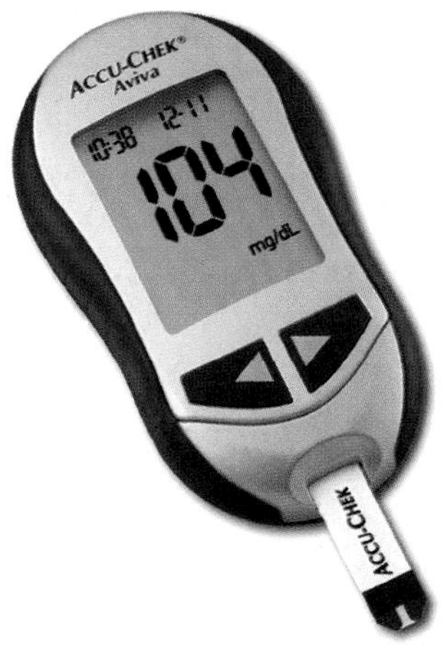

Figure 2 Monitoring blood glucose usually requires pricking the fingers and measuring the blood using a glucometer each day.

In Type 2 Diabetes, Cells Become Less Responsive to Insulin

In **type 2 diabetes**, body cells become resistant (less responsive) to insulin. This type of diabetes develops progressively, meaning that the biological changes resulting in the disease occur over a long period of time.

Obesity is the most common trigger for a cascade of changes that eventually results in this disorder. It is estimated that 80% to 90% of the people with type 2 diabetes are overweight or obese. Specifically, the cells of many obese people are less responsive to insulin, exhibiting a condition called *insulin insensitivity* (sometimes called insulin resistance). The pancreas attempts to compensate for this insensitivity by secreting more insulin. At first, the increased secretion of insulin is sufficient to maintain normal blood glucose levels. However, over time the blood of a person who is insulin insensitive will have to circulate very high levels of insulin to use glucose for energy. Eventually, this excessive production becomes insufficient for preventing a rise in fasting blood glucose. The resulting condition is referred to as **impaired fasting glucose**, meaning glucose levels are higher than normal but not high

type 2 diabetes A progressive disorder in which body cells become less responsive to insulin.

impaired fasting glucose Fasting blood glucose levels that are higher than normal but not high enough to lead to a diagnosis of type 2 diabetes; also called *pre-diabetes*.

enough to indicate a diagnosis of type 2 diabetes. Some health professionals refer to this condition as *pre-diabetes*, as people with impaired fasting glucose are more likely to get type 2 diabetes than people with normal fasting blood glucose levels. Ultimately, the pancreas becomes incapable of secreting these excessive amounts of insulin and stops producing the hormone altogether. Thus, blood glucose levels may be elevated because (1) of insulin insensitivity, (2) the pancreas can no longer secrete enough insulin, or (3) the pancreas has entirely stopped insulin production.

Who Is at Risk for Type 2 Diabetes?

As noted, obesity is the most common trigger for type 2 diabetes. But many other factors also play a role. For instance, relatives of people with type 2 diabetes are at increased risk, as are people with a sedentary lifestyle. A cluster of risk factors referred to as the *metabolic syndrome* is also known to increase the risk for type 2 diabetes. The criteria for metabolic syndrome are having a waist circumference ≥88 cm (35 in.)[4] for women and ≥102 cm (40 in.) for men, elevated blood pressure, and unhealthful levels of certain blood lipids and blood glucose.

Increased age is another risk factor for type 2 diabetes: most cases develop after age 45, and 23% of Americans 60 years and older have diabetes. Once commonly known as *adult-onset diabetes*, type 2 diabetes in children was virtually unheard of until recently. Unfortunately, the disease is increasing dramatically among children and adolescents, posing serious health consequences for them and their future children.[2]

In a 2004 study, more than 6% of college students were found to have pre-diabetes.[5] And each year, 3,700 people under age 20 are newly diagnosed with full-blown type 2 diabetes.[2] So what's your risk? Try the self-assessment What About You? and find out!

Lifestyle Choices Can Help Prevent or Control Diabetes

Type 2 diabetes is thought to have become an epidemic in the United States because of a combination of poor eating habits, sedentary lifestyles, increased obesity, and an aging population. We can't control our age, but we can and do control

What About You?

Calculate Your Risk for Type 2 Diabetes

To calculate your risk of developing type 2 diabetes, answer the following questions:

I am overweight.	Yes/No
I am sedentary (I exercise fewer than three times a week).	Yes/No
I have a close family member with type 2 diabetes.	Yes/No
I am a member of one of the following groups:	Yes/No
African American	
Hispanic American (Latino)	
Native American	
Pacific Islander	
(For women) I have been diagnosed with gestational diabetes, or I gave birth to at least one baby weighing more than 9 pounds.	Yes/No
My blood pressure is 140/90 or higher, or I have been told that I have high blood pressure.	Yes/No
My cholesterol levels are not normal.	Yes/No
(See the discussion of cholesterol in Chapter 5.)	

The more "yes" responses you give, the higher your risk of developing type 2 diabetes. You cannot change your ethnicity or your family members' health, but you can take steps to maintain a healthful weight and increase your physical activity. For tips, see Chapters 11 and 12.

Data from The National Diabetes Information Clearinghouse (NDIC). Available at **http://diabetes.niddk.nih.gov/dm/pubs/riskfortype2/**.

NUTRI-CASE JUDY

"My daughter, Hannah, has been pestering me about changing the way we eat and getting more exercise. She says she's just trying to lose weight, but ever since I learned I have type 2 diabetes I know she's been worried about me. What I didn't realize until last night is that she's worried about herself, too. All through dinner she was real quiet; then all of a sudden she says, 'Mom, I had my blood sugar tested at the health center, and guess what? They said I have pre-diabetes.' She said that's kind of like the first step toward diabetes and that, if she didn't make some serious changes, she'd end up just like me. So I guess we both need to change some things. Trouble is, I don't really know where to start."

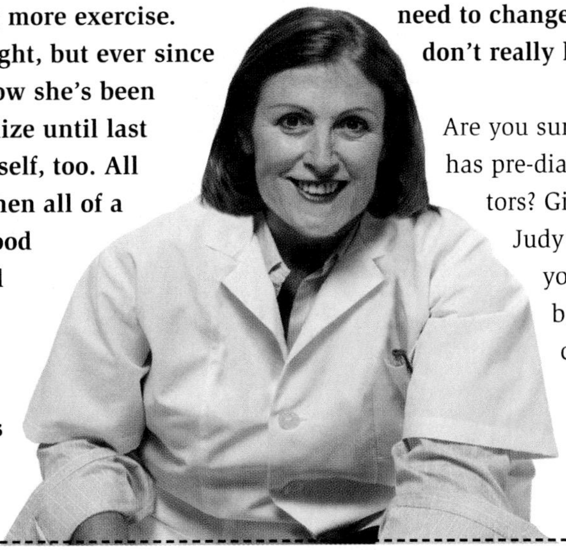

Are you surprised to learn that Hannah has pre-diabetes? What are her risk factors? Given what you know about Judy's and Hannah's lifestyle, can you think of any small changes both mother and daughter could make immediately to start addressing their high blood glucose levels?

how much and what types of foods we eat and how much physical activity we engage in—and that, in turn, influences our risk for obesity. Currently, over 30% of American college students are either overweight or obese.[6] Although adopting a healthful diet is important, moderate daily exercise may prevent the onset of type 2 diabetes more effectively than dietary changes alone.[7] (See Chapter 14 for examples of moderate exercise programs.) Exercise will also assist in weight loss, and studies show that losing only 10 to 30 pounds can reduce or eliminate the symptoms of type 2 diabetes.[8] In summary, by eating a healthy diet, staying active, and maintaining a healthful body weight, you should be able to keep your risk for type 2 diabetes low.

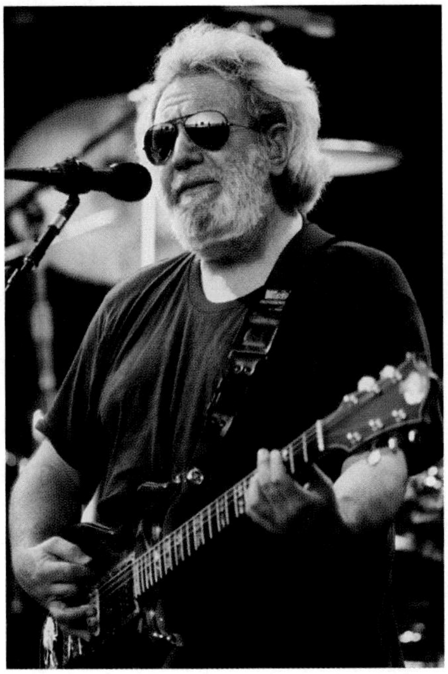

Jerry Garcia, a member of the Grateful Dead, had type 2 diabetes.

But what if you've already been diagnosed with type 2 diabetes? In general, you should follow many of the same dietary guidelines recommended for people without diabetes (see Chapter 2). One difference is that you may need to eat less carbohydrate and slightly more fat or protein to help regulate your blood glucose levels. Carbohydrates are still an important part of the diet, so, if you're eating less, make sure your choices are rich in nutrients and fiber. Precise nutritional recommendations vary according to each individual's responses to foods, so consulting with a registered dietician is essential.

In addition, people with diabetes should avoid alcoholic beverages, which can cause hypoglycemia. The symptoms of alcohol intoxication and hypoglycemia are very similar. People with diabetes, their companions, and even healthcare providers may confuse these conditions; this can result in a potentially life-threatening situation.

When blood glucose levels can't be adequately controlled with lifestyle changes, oral medications may be required. These drugs work in either of two ways: they improve body cells' sensitivity to insulin or reduce the amount of glucose the liver produces. Finally, if the pancreas can no longer secrete enough insulin, then people with type 2 diabetes must have daily insulin injections, just like people with type 1 diabetes.

Web Resources

www.diabetes.org
American Diabetes Organization

Find out more about the nutritional needs of people living with diabetes.

www.niddk.nih.gov
National Institute of Diabetes and Digestive and Kidney Diseases (NIDDK)

Learn more about diabetes, including treatment, complications, U.S. statistics, clinical trials, and recent research.

5

Fats: Essential Energy-Supplying Nutrients

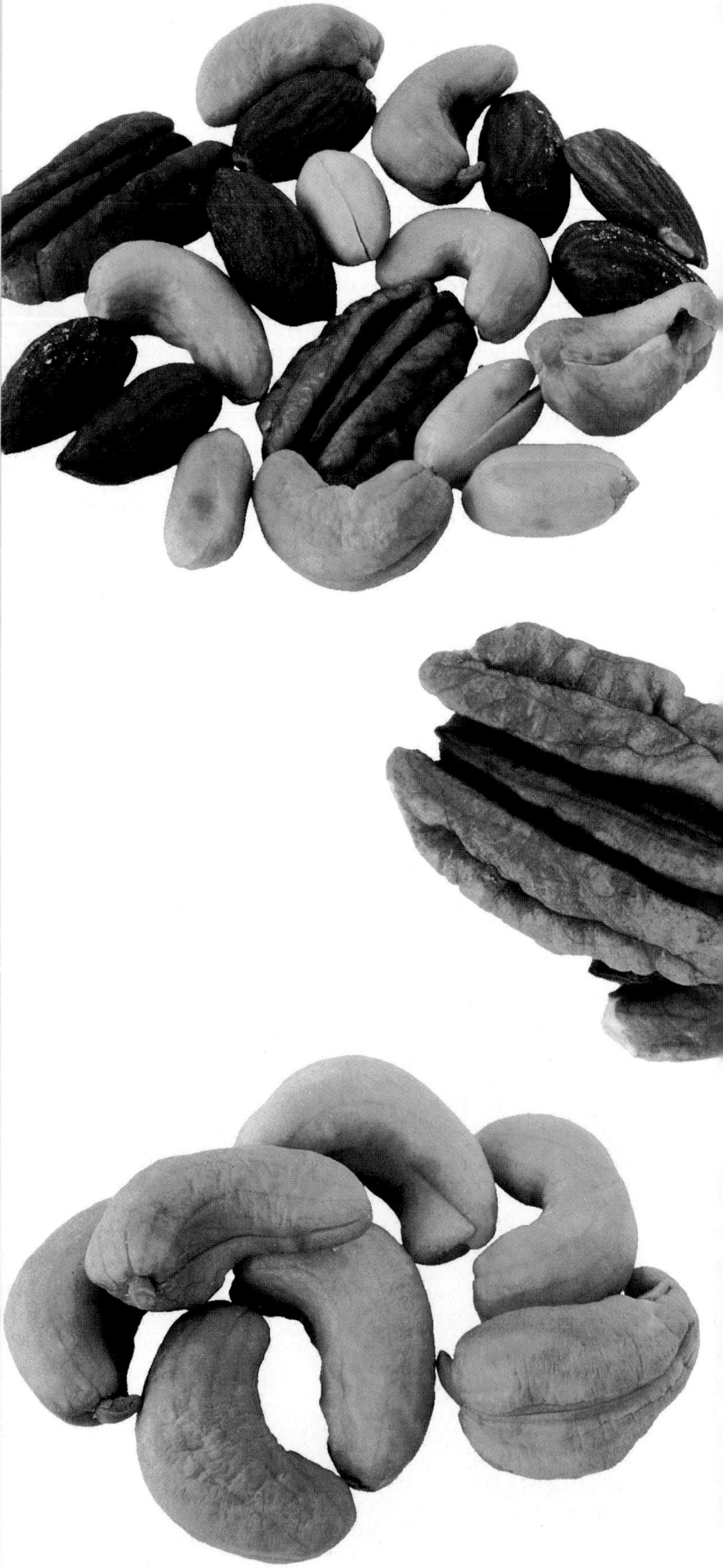

CHAPTER OBJECTIVES

After reading this chapter you will be able to:

1. **List and describe the three types of lipids found in foods, pp. 144–152.**
2. **Discuss how the level of saturation of a fatty acid affects its shape and the form it takes, pp. 145–150.**
3. **Explain the derivation of the term *trans* fatty acid and how *trans* fatty acids can negatively affect our health, pp. 147–152.**
4. **Identify the beneficial functions of the essential fatty acids, pp. 148–150.**
5. **List three functions of fat in our body, pp. 152–154.**
6. **Describe the steps involved in fat digestion, pp. 155–158.**
7. **Define the recommended dietary intakes for total fat, saturated fat, *trans* fats, and the two essential fatty acids, pp. 158–159.**
8. **Identify at least three common food sources of unhealthful fats and three common sources of beneficial fats, pp. 159–166.**

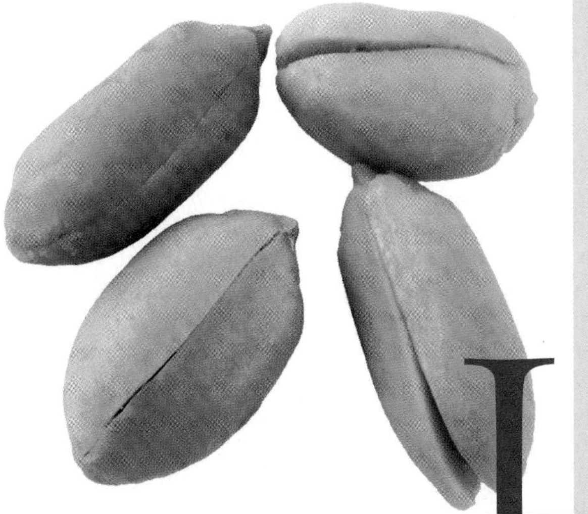

Test Yourself

1. **T F Some fats are essential for good health.**
2. **T F Fat is a primary source of energy during exercise.**
3. **T F Fried foods are relatively nutritious as long as vegetable shortening is used to fry the foods.**

Test Yourself answers can be found at the end of the chapter.

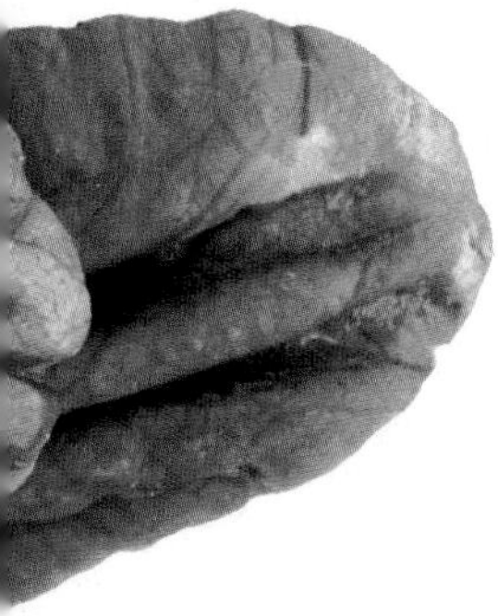

How would you feel if you purchased a bag of potato chips and were charged an extra 5% "fat tax"? What if you ordered fish and chips in your favorite restaurant, only to be told that, in an effort to avoid lawsuits, fried foods were no longer being served? Sound surreal? Believe it or not, these and dozens of similar scenarios are being proposed, threatened, and defended in the current "obesity wars" raging around the globe. From Maine to California, from Iceland to New Zealand, local and national governments and healthcare policy advisors are scrambling to find effective methods for combating their rising rates of obesity. For reasons we explore in this chapter, many of their proposals focus on limiting consumption of foods high in saturated fats—for instance, requiring food vendors and manufacturers to reduce the portion size of such foods; taxing or increasing their purchase price; levying fines on manufacturers who produce them; removing them from vending machines; banning advertisements of these foods to children; and using food labels and public service announcements to warn consumers away from these foods. At the same time, "food litigation" lawsuits have been increasing, including allegations against restaurant chains and food companies for failing to warn consumers of the health dangers of eating their energy-dense, high-saturated-fat foods.

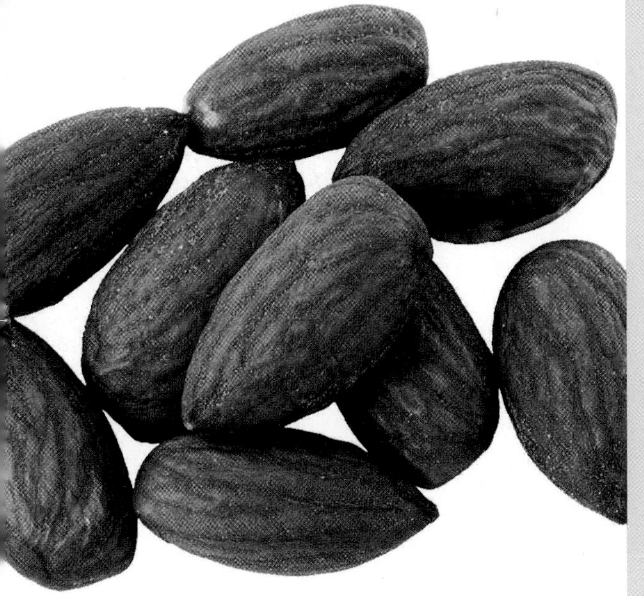

Is saturated fat really such a menace? If so, why? What is saturated fat, anyway? And are other fats just as bad? In this chapter, we'll answer these questions, plus identify some small changes you can make to shift your diet toward more healthful fats. The role of dietary fats in cardiovascular disease is discussed ***In Depth*** following this chapter.

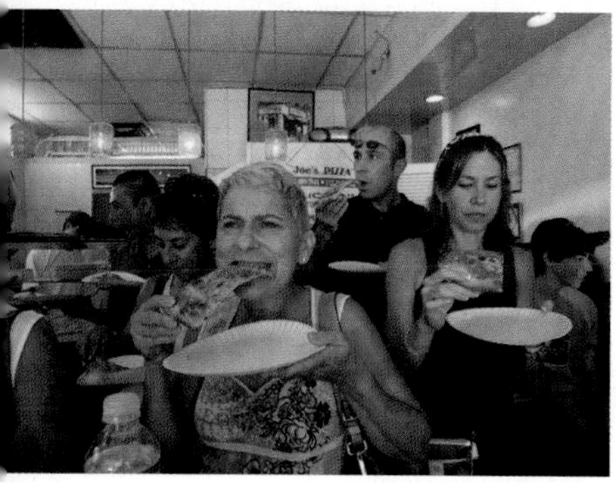

What Are Fats?

Fats are just one form of a much larger and more diverse group of organic substances called **lipids,** which are distinguished by the fact that they are insoluble in water. Think of a salad dressing made with vinegar, which is mostly water, and olive oil, which is a lipid. Shaking the bottle *disperses* the oil but doesn't *dissolve* it: that's why it separates back out again so quickly. Lipids are found in all sorts of living things, from bacteria to plants to human beings. In fact, their presence on your skin explains why you can't clean your face with water alone: you need some type of soap to break down the insoluble lipids before you can wash them away. In this chapter, we focus on the small group of lipids that are found in foods.

Fats and oils are two different types of lipids found in foods. Fats, such as butter, are solid at room temperature, whereas oils, such as olive oil, are liquid at room temperature. Because most people are more comfortable with the term *fats* instead of *lipids,* we will use that term generically throughout this book, including when we are referring to oils. Three types of fats are commonly found in foods: triglycerides, phospholipids, and sterols. Let's take a look at each.

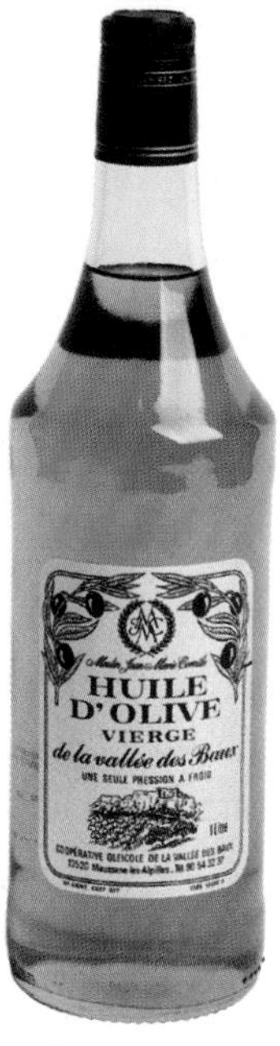

Some fats, such as olive oil, are liquid at room temperature.

Triglycerides Are the Most Common Food-Based Fat

Most of the fat we eat (95%) is in the form of triglycerides (also called *triacylglycerols*), which is the same form in which most body fat is stored. As reflected in the prefix *tri-,* a **triglyceride** is a molecule consisting of *three* fatty acids attached to a *three*-carbon glycerol backbone. **Fatty acids** are long chains of carbon atoms bound to each other as well as to hydrogen atoms. They are acids because they contain an acid group (carboxyl group) at one end of their chain. **Glycerol,** the backbone of a triglyceride molecule, is an alcohol composed of three carbon atoms. One fatty acid attaches to each of these three carbons to make the triglyceride **(Figure 5.1)**.

To understand why we want more of some fats than others, we need to know more about their properties and how they work in our body. In general, triglycerides can be classified by their chain length (number of carbons in each fatty acid), their level of saturation (how much hydrogen, H, is attached to each carbon atom in the fatty acid chain), and their shape, which is determined in some cases by how they

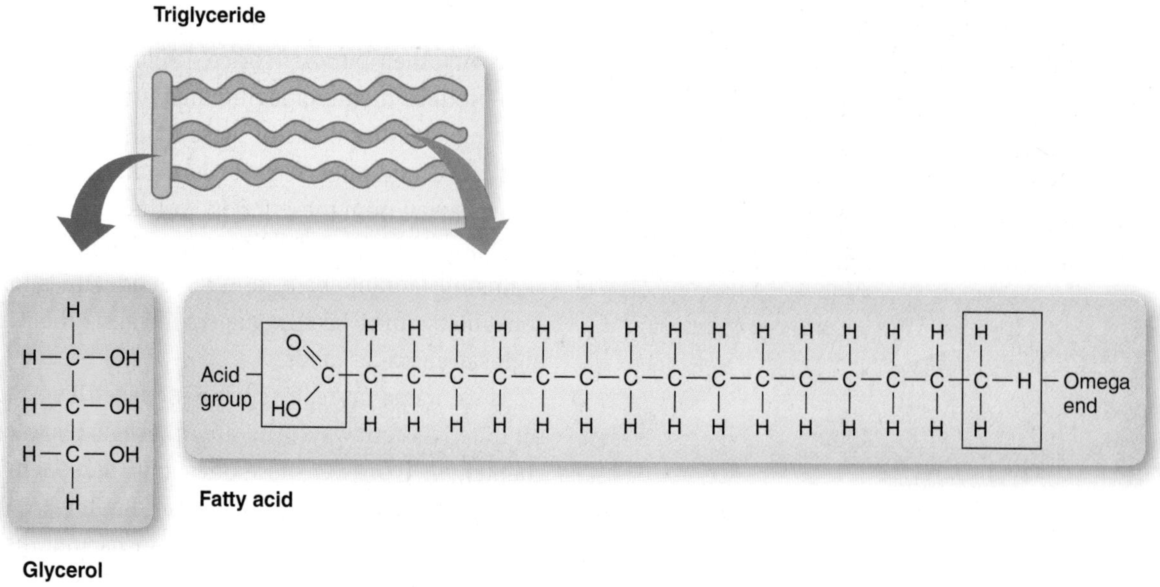

Figure 5.1 A triglyceride consists of three fatty acids attached to a three-carbon glycerol backbone.

are commercially processed. All of these factors influence how we use the triglycerides within our body.

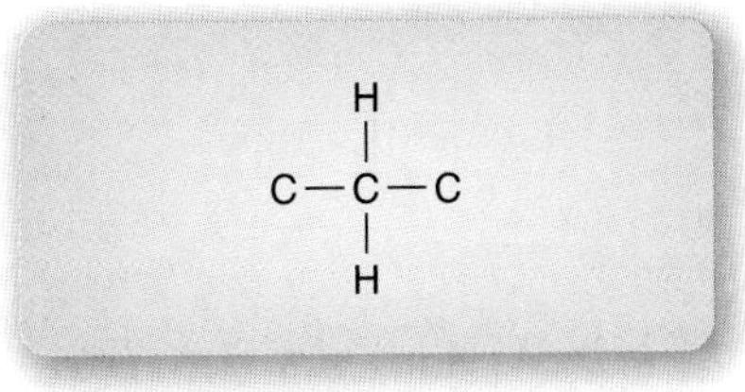

(a) Saturated fatty acid

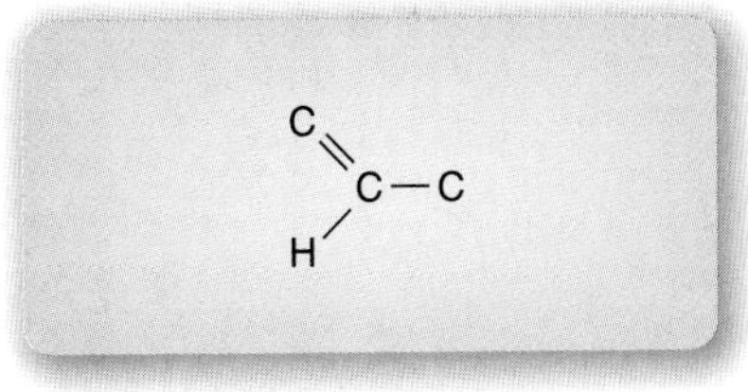

(b) Unsaturated fatty acid

Figure 5.2 An atom of carbon has four attachment sites. In fatty acid chains, two of these sites are filled by adjacent carbon atoms. **(a)** In saturated fatty acids, the other two sites are always filled by two hydrogen atoms. **(b)** In unsaturated fatty acids, at one or more points along the chain, a double bond to an adjacent carbon atom takes up one of the attachment sites that would otherwise be filled by hydrogen.

Chain Length Affects Triglyceride Function

The fatty acids attached to the glycerol backbone can vary in the number of carbons they contain, referred to as their *chain length*.

- Short-chain fatty acids are usually fewer than six carbon atoms in length.
- Medium-chain fatty acids are six to twelve carbons in length.
- Long-chain fatty acids are fourteen or more carbons in length.

Fatty acid chain length is important because it determines the method of fat digestion and absorption and affects how fats function within the body. For example, short- and medium-chain fatty acids are digested and transported more quickly than long-chain fatty acids. We will discuss the digestion and absorption of fats in more detail shortly. In addition, chain length can determine saturation, as discussed in the next section.

Saturated Fats Contain the Maximum Amount of Hydrogen

Triglycerides can also vary by the types of bonds found in the fatty acids. If a fatty acid has no carbons bonded together with a double bond, it is referred to as a **saturated fatty acid (SFA)** (**Figures 5.2a** and **5.3a**). This is because every carbon atom in the chain is *saturated* with hydrogen: each has the maximum amount of hydrogen bound to it. Some foods that are high in saturated fatty acids are coconut oil, palm kernel oil, butter, cream, whole milk, and beef.

Unsaturated Fats Contain Less Hydrogen

If, within the chain of carbon atoms, two carbons are bound to each other with a double bond, then this double carbon bond excludes hydrogen. This lack of hydrogen at *one* part of the molecule results in a fat that is referred to as *monounsaturated* (recall from Chapter 4 that the prefix *mono-* means "one"). A monounsaturated molecule is shown in Figures 5.2b and 5.3a. **Monounsaturated fatty acids (MUFAs)** are usually liquid at room temperature. Foods that are high in monounsaturated fatty acids are olive oil, canola oil, and cashew nuts.

If the fat molecules have *more than one* double bond, they contain even less hydrogen and are referred to as **polyunsaturated fatty acids (PUFAs).** (See Figure 5.3a.) Polyunsaturated fatty acids are also liquid at room temperature and include cottonseed, canola, corn, and safflower oils.

Although foods vary in the types of fatty acids they contain, in general we can say that animal-based foods tend to be high in saturated fats and plant foods tend to be high in unsaturated fats. Specifically, animal fats provide approximately 40–60% of their energy from saturated fats, whereas plant fats provide 80–90% of their energy from monounsaturated and polyunsaturated fats (**Figure 5.4**). Most oils are a good source of both MUFAs and PUFAs.

In general, saturated fats have a detrimental effect on our health, whereas unsaturated fats are protective. It makes sense, therefore, that diets high in plant foods—because they're low in saturated fats—are more healthful than diets high in animal products. We discuss the influence of various types of fatty acids on your risk for cardiovascular disease in the ***In Depth*** essay immediately following this chapter.

Carbon Bonding Affects Shape

Have you ever noticed how many toothpicks are packed into a small box? A hundred or more! But if you were to break a bunch of toothpicks into V shapes anywhere along their length, how many could you then fit into the same box? It would be very few because the bent toothpicks would jumble together, taking up much more space. Molecules of saturated fat are like straight toothpicks: they have no double carbon bonds and always form straight, rigid chains. As they have no kinks, these chains can pack together tightly (see Figure 5.3b). That is why saturated fats, such as the fat in meats, are solid at room temperature.

lipids A diverse group of organic substances that are insoluble in water; lipids include triglycerides, phospholipids, and sterols.

triglyceride A molecule consisting of three fatty acids attached to a three-carbon glycerol backbone.

fatty acids Long chains of carbon atoms bound to each other as well as to hydrogen atoms.

glycerol An alcohol composed of three carbon atoms; it is the backbone of a triglyceride molecule.

saturated fatty acids (SFAs) Fatty acids that have no carbons joined together with a double bond; these types of fatty acids are generally solid at room temperature.

monounsaturated fatty acids (MUFAs) Fatty acids that have two carbons in the chain bound to each other with one double bond; these types of fatty acids are generally liquid at room temperature.

polyunsaturated fatty acids (PUFAs) Fatty acids that have more than one double bond in the chain; these types of fatty acids are generally liquid at room temperature.

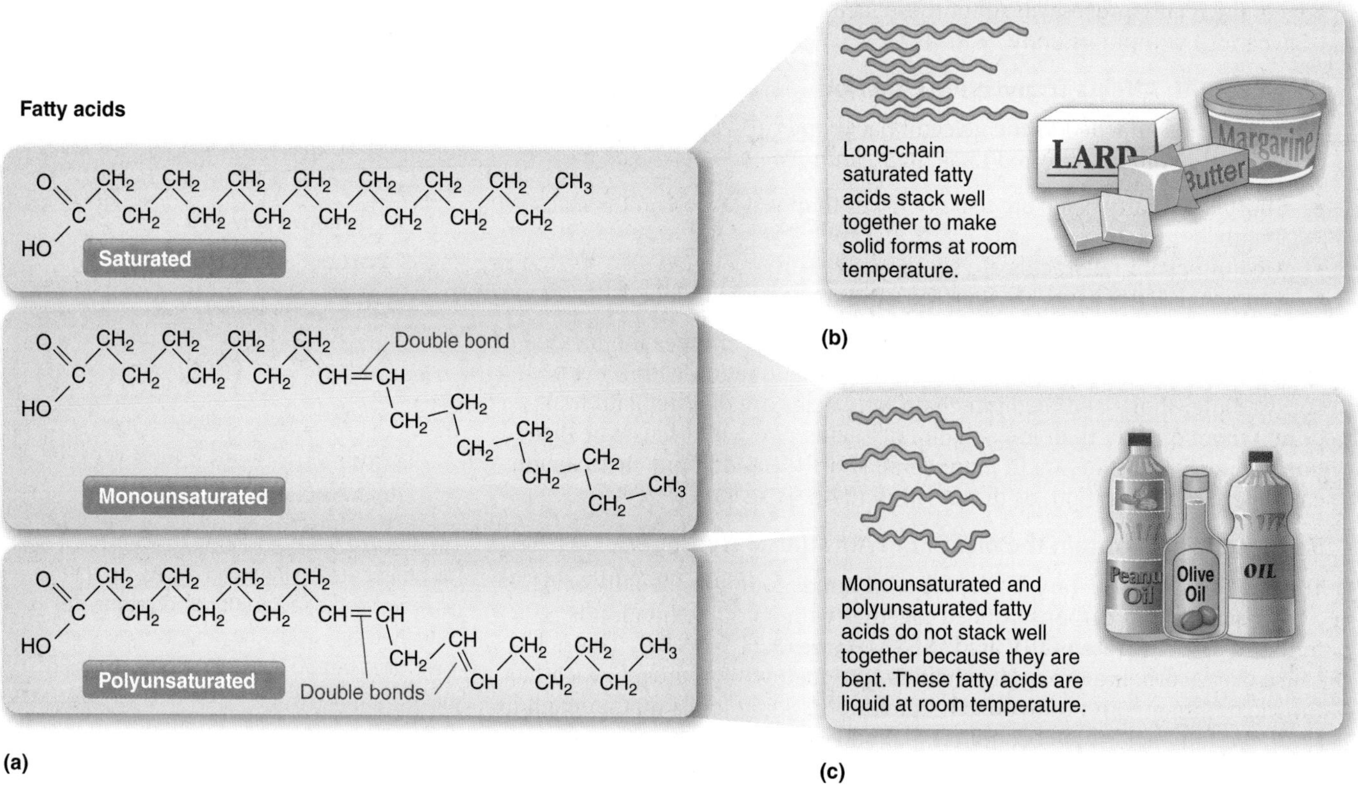

Figure 5.3 Examples of levels of saturation among fatty acids and how these levels of saturation affect the shape of fatty acids. **(a)** Saturated fatty acids are saturated with hydrogen, meaning they have no carbons bonded together with a double bond. Monounsaturated fatty acids contain two carbons bound by one double bond. Polyunsaturated fatty acids have more than one double bond linking carbon atoms. **(b)** Saturated fats have straight fatty acids packed tightly together and are solid at room temperature. **(c)** Unsaturated fats have "kinked" fatty acids at the area of the double bond, preventing them from packing tightly together; they are liquid at room temperature.

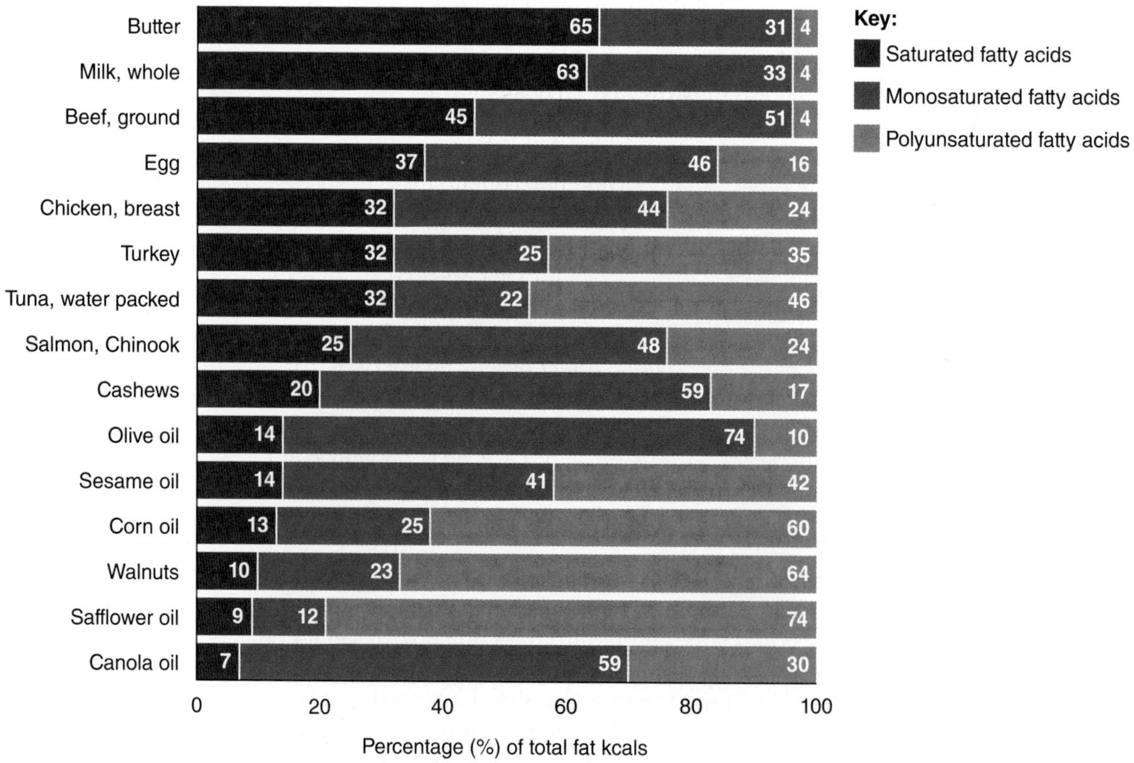

Figure 5.4 Major sources of dietary fat.

HOT TOPIC

The Nuts and Bolts on Nuts

Nuts are rich in healthful unsaturated fats, not to mention protein, some minerals, and fiber. But they're also high in energy: 160–180 kcal for a 1-ounce serving (about 4 tablespoons, depending on the nut). So why are nuts the new "in" food on popular diet plans?

Well, in several studies, when researchers fed people an ounce or two of nuts every day, the participants failed to gain the expected weight. And, in general, people who eat nuts are typically leaner than people who don't. No one has a definitive explanation for these findings. Some researchers speculate that people find nuts satiating and therefore eat less later on. Others propose that the energy in nuts may not be fully absorbed in the GI (gastrointestinal) tract.

Will nuts help you control your weight? Maybe—if you can limit yourself to an ounce or two a day. Trouble is, they taste so good, it's easy to overdo it.

In contrast, each double carbon bond of unsaturated fats gives them a kink along their length (see Figure 5.3c). This means that they are unable to pack together tightly—for example, to form a stick of butter—and instead are liquid at room temperature. In our body, unsaturated fatty acids are part of our cell membranes. They help keep the cell membranes flexible, allowing substances to move into and out of the cells.

We've just said that unsaturated fatty acids are kinked. That's true when they occur naturally in plant foods and plant oils. But unsaturated fatty acids can be manipulated by food manufacturers to create a type of straight, rigid fatty acid called a *trans* fat. Recall from Chapter 2 that the Dietary Guidelines for Americans suggest that you keep your *trans* fat intake as low as possible. In fact, *trans* fats are considered at least as harmful to your health as saturated fats. We'll explain why in a moment. For now, let's make sure we know what *trans* fats really are.

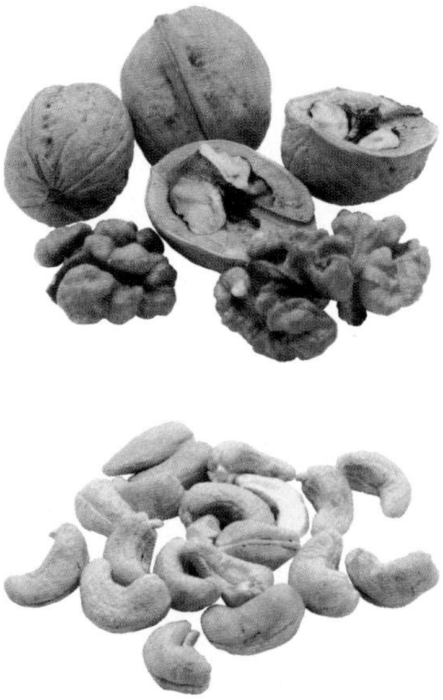

Walnuts and cashews are high in monounsaturated fatty acids.

Trans Fatty Acids Have Hydrogen Atoms on Opposite Sides

Unsaturated fatty acids can occur in either a *cis* or a *trans* shape. The prefix *cis* means things are located on the same side or near each other, whereas *trans* is a prefix that denotes across or opposite. These terms describe the positioning of the hydrogen atoms around the double carbon bond as follows:

- The prefix *cis* means "on the same side." A *cis fatty acid* has both hydrogen atoms located on the same side of the double bond **(Figure 5.5a)**. This positioning gives the *cis* molecule a pronounced kink at the double carbon bond. We typically find the *cis* fatty acids in nature, and thus in foods such as olive oil.
- In contrast, *trans* means "on the opposite side." In a *trans fatty acid,* the hydrogen atoms are attached on diagonally opposite sides of the double carbon bond (Figure 5.5b). This positioning makes *trans* fatty acid fats straighter and more rigid, just like saturated fats. Thus, "*trans* fats" is a collective term used to define fats with *trans* double bonds. Although a limited amount of natural *trans* fatty acids are found in cow's milk and meat, the majority of *trans* fatty acids in foods are produced by manipulating the fatty acids during food processing.

This process, called **hydrogenation,** was developed in the early 1900s in order to produce a type of cheap fat that could be stored in a solid form and would resist rancidity. During hydrogenation, pressurized hydrogen molecules are added directly to unsaturated fatty acids such as those found in corn and safflower oils. This causes the double bonds of the unsaturated fatty acids in the oil to be partially or totally removed. As a result, the fatty acid becomes more saturated and straighter.

The hydrogenation process can be controlled to make the oil more or less saturated: if only some of the double bonds are broken, the fat produced is called *partially hydrogenated,* a term you will see frequently on food labels. For example, corn oil margarine is a partially hydrogenated form of corn oil. Unless labeled as containing zero *trans* fatty acids, most margarines have more *trans* fatty acids than butter. So which is the more healthful choice—butter or margarine? Check out the Nutrition Myth or Fact? box on page 149 to find out!

hydrogenation The process of adding hydrogen to unsaturated fatty acids, making them more saturated and thereby more solid at room temperature.

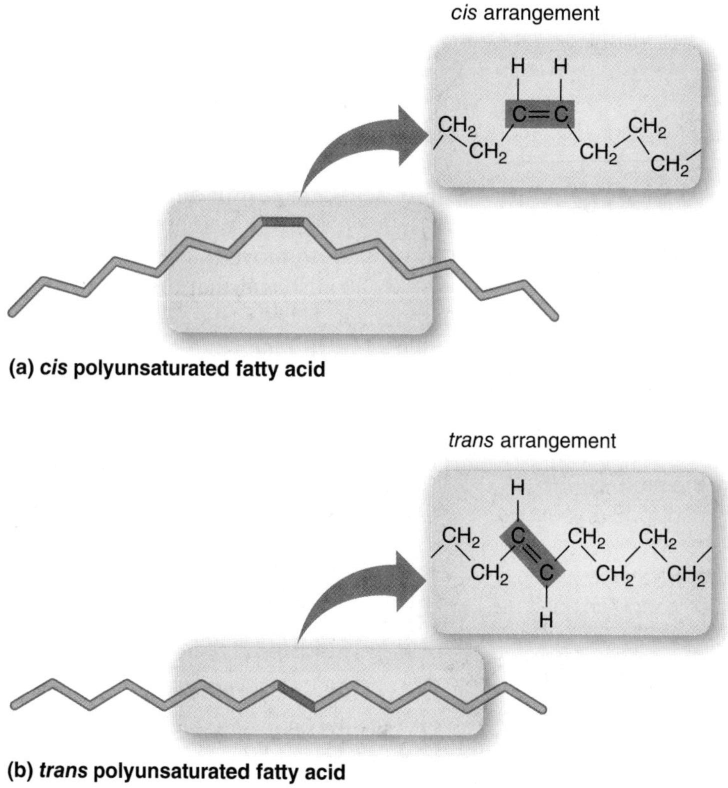

Figure 5.5 Structure of **(a)** a *cis* and **(b)** a *trans* polyunsaturated fatty acid. Notice that *cis* fatty acids have both hydrogen atoms located on the same side of the double bond. This positioning makes the molecule kinked. In the *trans* fatty acids, the hydrogen atoms are attached on diagonally opposite sides of the double carbon bond. This positioning makes them straighter and more rigid.

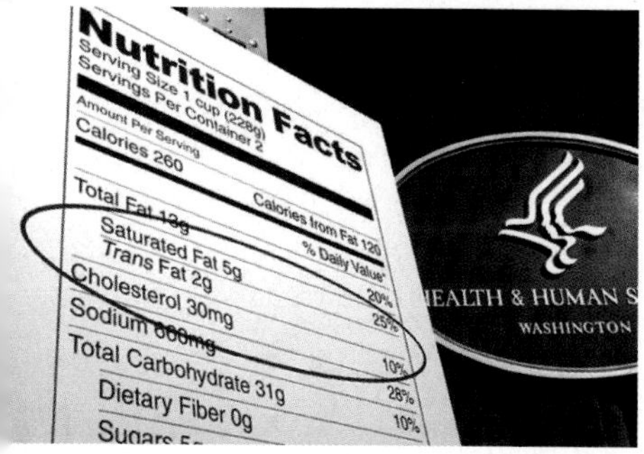

The U.S. FDA ruled that as of 2006, *trans* fatty acids, or *trans* fat, must be listed as a separate line item on the Nutrition Facts Panels for conventional foods and some dietary supplements.

Incidentally, even when a product *is* labeled as having "zero" *trans* fats, there can still be *trans* fatty acids in the product! That's because the U.S. Food and Drug Administration (FDA) allows products that have less than 1 g of *trans* fat per serving to claim that they are *trans* fat free. So, even if the Nutrition Facts Panel states 0 g *trans* fats, the product can still have 1/2 g of *trans* fat per serving. If the ingredients list states that the product contains partially hydrogenated oils, it contains *trans* fats.

For a period of several decades in the 20th century, partially hydrogenated oil products were in demand. Americans were being urged to reduce their intake of saturated fats and switched to partially hydrogenated oils, including spreadable margarines, assuming that these products were more healthful and could reduce the risk for heart disease. But as we discuss later in this chapter, this assumption did not turn out to be true.

Some Triglycerides Contain Essential Fatty Acids

There has been a lot of press lately about "omega" fatty acids, so you might be wondering what they are and why they're so important. First, let's explain the Greek name. As illustrated in **Figure 5.6**, one end of a fatty acid chain is designated the α (alpha) end (α is the first letter in the Greek alphabet). The other end of a fatty acid chain is called the ω (omega) end (ω is the last letter in the Greek alphabet). Two fatty acids with a unique structure are known to be essential to human growth and health: one of these has a double bond six carbons from the omega end (at ω-6), and the other has a double bond three carbons from the omega end (at ω-3). When synthesizing fatty acids, the body cannot insert double bonds before the ninth carbon from the omega end.[1] This means that we have to obtain ω-6 and ω-3 fatty acids from food. They are considered **essential fatty acids (EFAs)** because the body cannot make them, yet it requires them for healthy functioning.

essential fatty acids (EFAs) Fatty acids that must be consumed in the diet because they cannot be made by our body. The two essential fatty acids are linoleic acid and alpha-linolenic acid.

NUTRITION MYTH OR FACT?

Is Margarine More Healthful Than Butter?

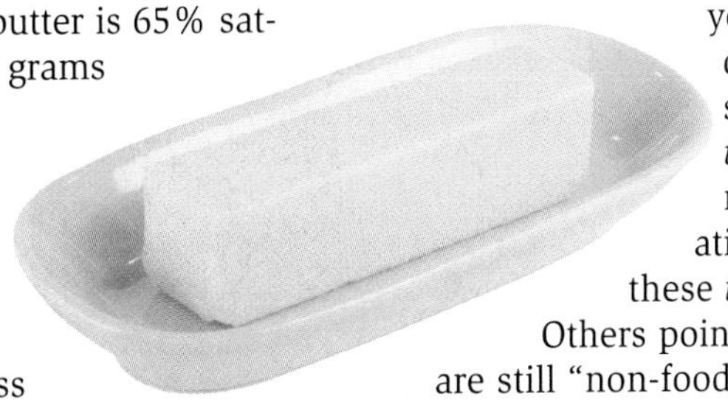

Your toast just popped up! Which will it be: butter or margarine? As you've just learned, butter is 65% saturated fat: 1 tablespoon provides 30 grams of cholesterol! In contrast, corn oil margarine is just 2% saturated fat, with no cholesterol. But how much *trans* fat does that margarine contain? And which is better—the more natural and more saturated butter or the more processed and less saturated margarine?

You're not the only one asking this question. Until recently, vegetable-based oils were hydrogenated to make margarines. These products were filled with *trans* fats that could increase the consumer's risk for heart disease, as well as harm cell membranes, weaken immune function, and inhibit the body's natural anti-inflammatory hormones. Some margarines also contained harmful amounts of toxic metals, such as nickel and aluminum, as by-products of the hydrogenation process. These are among some of the reasons researchers began warning consumers against using margarines several years ago.

So does that mean that the saturated-fat, cholesterol-rich butter is the better choice? A decade ago, that may have been the case, but, over the last ten years, food manufacturers have introduced "*trans* fat free margarines and spreads" that contain no cholesterol or *trans* fats and low amounts of saturated fats. The American Heart Association[2] advises that consumers choose these *trans* fat free margarines over butter.

Others point out that such manufactured products are still "non-foods" and recommend that those who prefer whole foods choose unprocessed nut butters (peanut, walnut, cashew, and almond butters). These natural alternatives are rich in essential fatty acids and other heart-healthy unsaturated fats but are still as energy-dense as butter.

Remember, a label claiming that a margarine has zero *trans* fatty acids doesn't guarantee that the product is *trans* fatty acid free (see the accompanying table). You have to look for margarines with no "partially hydrogenated" oil in them. That is the only way you will know your spread is entirely free of *trans* fatty acids. Check out the spreads listed in the table to help you decide which you're going to include in your diet.

Spreads for Your Bread*

Brand Name	Energy (kcal)	Sat fat (g)	*Trans* fat (g)	Sodium (mg)
Tubs and Squeezes Made Without Partially Hydrogenated Oil				
Promise Fat Free; I Can't Believe It's Not Butter (fat free)	5	0	0	90
Country Crock Omega Plus Light	50	1	0	80
Smart Balance Omega Light	50	1.5	0	80
Parkay Squeeze	70	1.5	0	110
Canola Harvest Original	100	1.5	0	100
Tubs Made with Partially Hydrogenated Oil				
Fleischmann's Light	50	0.5	NA	70
Blue Bonnet	60	1	0.4	130
I Can't Believe It's Not Butter! Original	80	2	0.3	90
Sticks				
Blue Bonnet Light	50	1	1	80
Fleischmann's Original	100	2	2.5	120
Butter				
Butter, any brand, stick	100	7.5	0.4	80
Land O'Lakes Light with Canola Oil	50	2	0	90
Shortening				
Crisco, stick or tub	100	3	0.5	0
Nut Butters				
Peanut butter	95	1.5	0	78
Almond butter	99	1	0	70

*All portion sizes are 1 tablespoon.
Data from Hurley, J., and B. Liebman. 2009. Covering the spreads: tracking down the butters and margarines. *Nutrition Action Healthletter*, Sept., pp. 13–15. Food Processor-SQL, Version 10.3, ESHA Research, Salem, OR.

Figure 5.6 The two essential fatty acids: linoleic acid (an omega-6 fatty acid) and alpha-linolenic acid (an omega-3 fatty acid).

Essential fatty acids

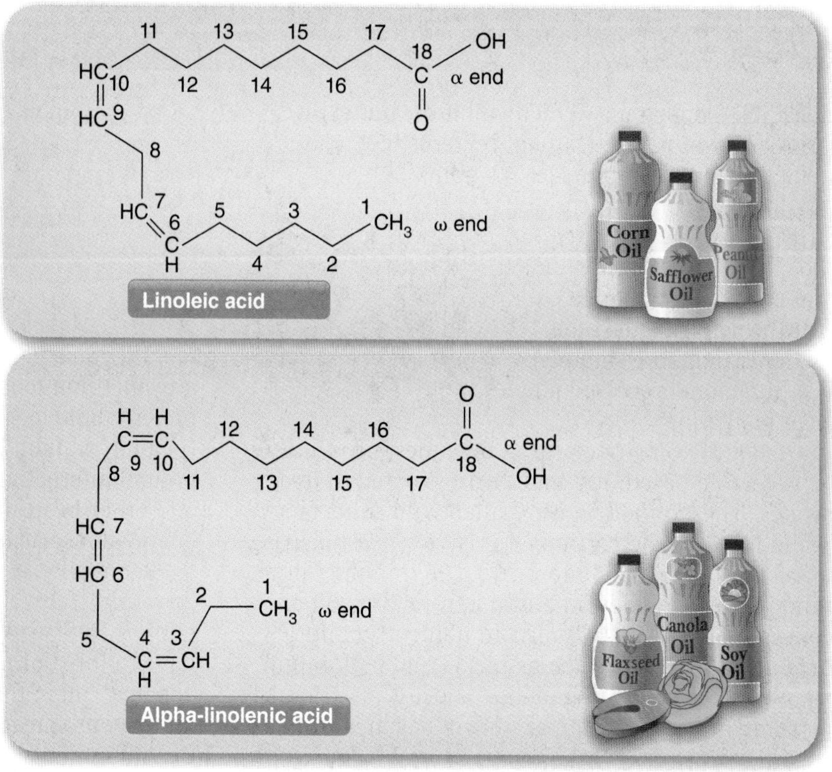

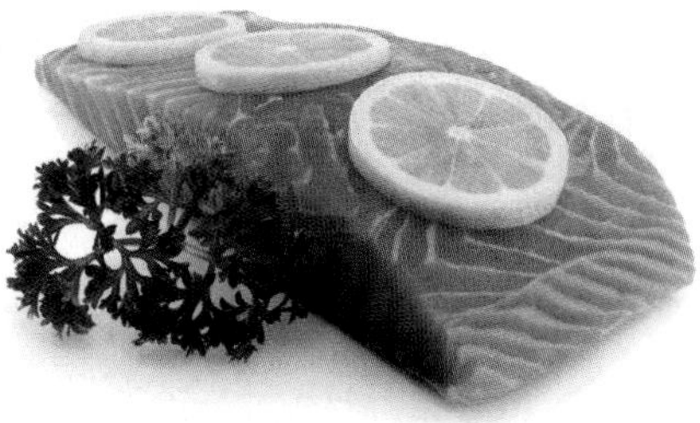

Salmon is high in omega-3 fatty acid content.

EFAs are essential to growth and health because they are precursors to important biological compounds called *eicosanoids,* which are produced in nearly every cell in the body.[3] Eicosanoids get their name from the Greek word *eicosa,* which means "twenty," as they are synthesized from fatty acids with twenty carbon atoms. In the body, eicosanoids are potent regulators of cellular function. For example, they help regulate gastrointestinal tract motility, blood clotting, blood pressure, the permeability of our blood vessels to fluid and large molecules, and the regulation of inflammation.

The body's synthesis of various eicosanoids depends in part on the abundance of the EFAs available as precursors. Since they play an important role in "regulating" biological processes, we need a balance of the various eicosanoids and thus a balance of EFAs. For example, we need just the right amount of blood clotting at the right time—too much and we get excessive blood clotting, and too little and we get excessive bleeding. As just noted, the two essential fatty acids in our diet are popularly known as omega-6 and omega-3 fatty acids. These are more technically referred to as linoleic acid and alpha-linolenic acid, respectively.

Linoleic Acid **Linoleic acid,** also known as an *omega-6 fatty acid,* is found in vegetable and nut oils, such as sunflower, safflower, corn, soy, and peanut oil. If you eat lots of vegetables or use vegetable-oil-based margarines or vegetable oils, you are probably getting adequate amounts of this essential fatty acid in your diet. Linoleic acid is metabolized in the body to arachidonic acid, which is a precursor to a number of eicosanoids. Linoleic acid is also needed for cell membrane structure and is required for the lipoproteins that transport fats in our blood.

linoleic acid An essential fatty acid found in vegetable and nut oils; also known as omega-6 fatty acid.

alpha-linolenic acid An essential fatty acid found in leafy green vegetables, flaxseed oil, soy oil, fish oil, and fish products; an omega-3 fatty acid.

Alpha-Linolenic Acid **Alpha-linolenic acid,** also known as an *omega-3 fatty acid,* was only recognized to be essential in the mid-1980s. It is found primarily in dark green, leafy vegetables, flaxseeds and flaxseed oil, soybeans and soybean oil, walnuts and walnut oil, and canola oil. You may also have read news reports of the health

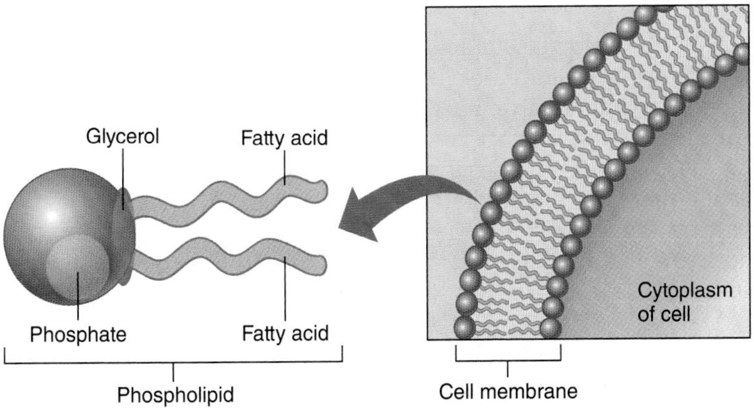

Figure 5.7 Structure of a phospholipid. Phospholipids consist of a glycerol backbone with two fatty acids and a compound that contains phosphate.

benefits of the omega-3 fatty acids found in many fish. The two omega-3 fatty acids found in fish, shellfish, and fish oils are **eicosapentaenoic acid (EPA)** and **docosahexaenoic acid (DHA)**. Fish that naturally contain more oil, such as salmon and tuna, are higher in EPA and DHA than lean fish, such as cod or flounder. Research indicates that diets high in EPA and DHA stimulate the production of regulatory compounds that reduce an individual's risk for heart disease.[4,5]

Phospholipids Combine Lipids with Phosphate

Along with the triglycerides just discussed, we also find phospholipids and sterols in the foods we eat. **Phospholipids** consist of two fatty acids and a glycerol backbone with another compound that contains phosphate (**Figure 5.7**). This addition of a phosphate compound makes phospholipids soluble in water, a property that enables phospholipids to assist in transporting fats in our bloodstream. We discuss this concept in more detail later in this chapter (page 153). Also, as you may recall from Chapter 3, phospholipids in our cell membranes regulate the transport of substances into and out of the cell. Phospholipids also help with the digestion of dietary fats: the liver uses phospholipids called *lecithins* to make bile. Note that our body manufactures phospholipids, so they are not essential for us to include in our diets. What *is* essential is phosphorus, a mineral that is combined with oxygen to make phosphate. See Chapter 9 to learn more about your requirements for phosphorus.

eicosapentaenoic acid (EPA) A metabolic derivative of alpha-linolenic acid.

docosahexaenoic acid (DHA) Another metabolic derivative of alpha-linolenic acid; together with EPA, it appears to reduce our risk for a heart attack.

phospholipids A type of lipid in which a fatty acid is combined with another compound that contains phosphate; unlike other lipids, phospholipids are soluble in water.

sterols A type of lipid found in foods and the body that has a ring structure; cholesterol is the most common sterol that occurs in our diets.

Sterols Have a Ring Structure

Sterols are also a type of lipid found in foods and in the body, but their multiple-ring structure is quite different from that of triglycerides (**Figure 5.8a**). Sterols are found in both plant and animal foods and are produced in the body. Plants contain some sterols, but these sterols are not very well absorbed and appear to block the absorption of dietary cholesterol, the most commonly occurring sterol in the diet (Figure 5.8b). Cholesterol is found only in the fatty part of animal products such as

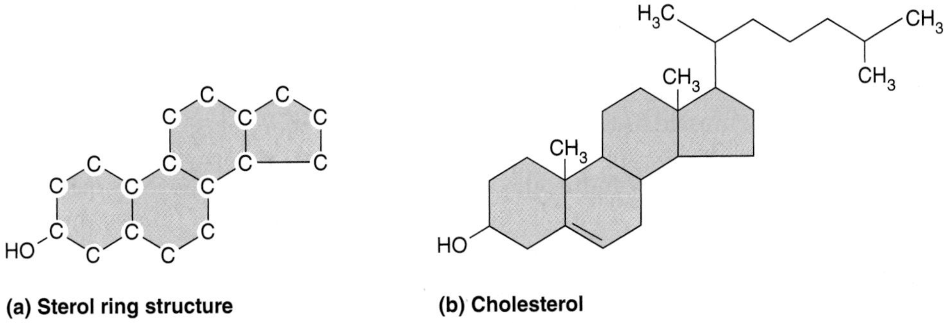

Figure 5.8 Sterol structure. **(a)** Sterols are lipids that contain multiple-ring structures. **(b)** Cholesterol is the most commonly occurring sterol in the diet.

butter, egg yolks, whole milk, meats, and poultry. Low- or reduced-fat animal products, such as lean meats and skim milk, have little cholesterol.

We don't need to consume cholesterol in our diet because our body continually synthesizes it, mostly in the liver and intestines. This continuous production is essential because cholesterol is part of every cell membrane, where it works in conjunction with fatty acids to help maintain cell membrane integrity. It is particularly plentiful in the neural cells that make up our brain, spinal cord, and nerves. The body also uses cholesterol to synthesize several important compounds, including sex hormones (estrogen, androgen, and progesterone), bile acids, adrenal hormones, and vitamin D. Thus, despite cholesterol's bad reputation, it is absolutely essential to human health.

RECAP **Fat is essential for health. Three types of fat are found in foods: triglycerides, phospholipids, and sterols. Triglycerides are the most common. A triglyceride is made up of glycerol and three fatty acids. These fatty acids can be classified based on chain length, level of saturation, and shape. Saturated and *trans* fatty acids increase our risk for cardiovascular disease, whereas unsaturated fatty acids, including the essential fatty acids, are protective. Phospholipids combine two fatty acids and a glycerol backbone with a phosphate-containing compound, making them soluble in water. Sterols have a multiple-ring structure; cholesterol is the most commonly occurring sterol in our diet.**

Why Do We Need Fats?

Dietary fat provides energy and helps our body perform some essential physiologic functions.

Fats Provide Energy

Dietary fat is a primary source of energy because fat has more than twice the energy per gram of carbohydrate or protein. Fat provides 9 kilocalories (kcal) per gram, whereas carbohydrate and protein provide only 4 kilocalories (kcal) per gram. This means that fat is much more energy dense. For example, 1 tbsp. of butter or oil contains approximately 100 kcal, whereas it takes 2.5 cups of steamed broccoli or 1 slice of whole-wheat bread to provide 100 kcal.

Fats Are a Major Fuel Source When We Are at Rest

At rest, we are able to deliver plenty of oxygen to our cells, so that metabolic functions can occur. Just as a candle needs oxygen for the flame to burn the tallow, our cells need oxygen to burn fat for energy. Thus, approximately 30–70% of the energy used at rest by the muscles and organs comes from fat.[6] The exact percentage varies, according to how much fat you are eating in your diet, how physically active you are, and whether you are gaining or losing weight. If you are dieting, more fat will be used for energy than if you are gaining weight. During times of weight gain, more of the fat consumed in the diet is stored in the adipose tissue, and the body uses more dietary protein and carbohydrate as fuel sources at rest.

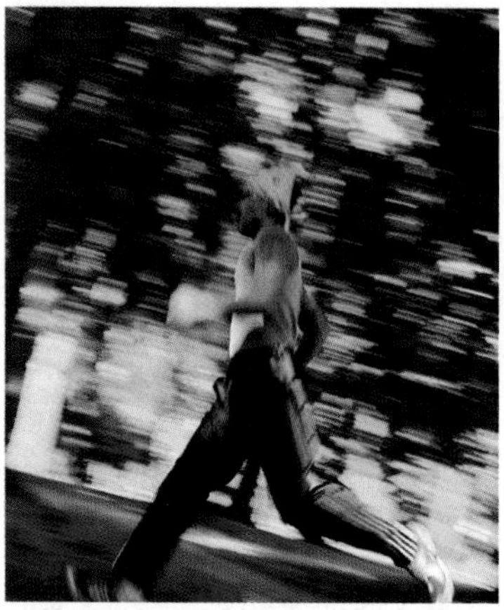

Dietary fat provides energy.

Fats Fuel Physical Activity

Fat is a major energy source during physical activity, and one of the best ways to lose body fat is to exercise. During exercise, fat can be mobilized from any of the following sources: muscle tissue, adipose tissue, blood lipoproteins, and/or any dietary fat consumed during exercise. A number of hormonal changes signal the body to break down stored energy to fuel the working muscles. The hormonal responses, and the amount and source of the fat used, depend on your level of fitness; the type, intensity, and duration of the exercise; and how well fed you are before you exercise.

For example, adrenaline strongly stimulates the breakdown of stored fat. Blood levels of adrenaline rise dramatically within seconds of beginning exercise, and this

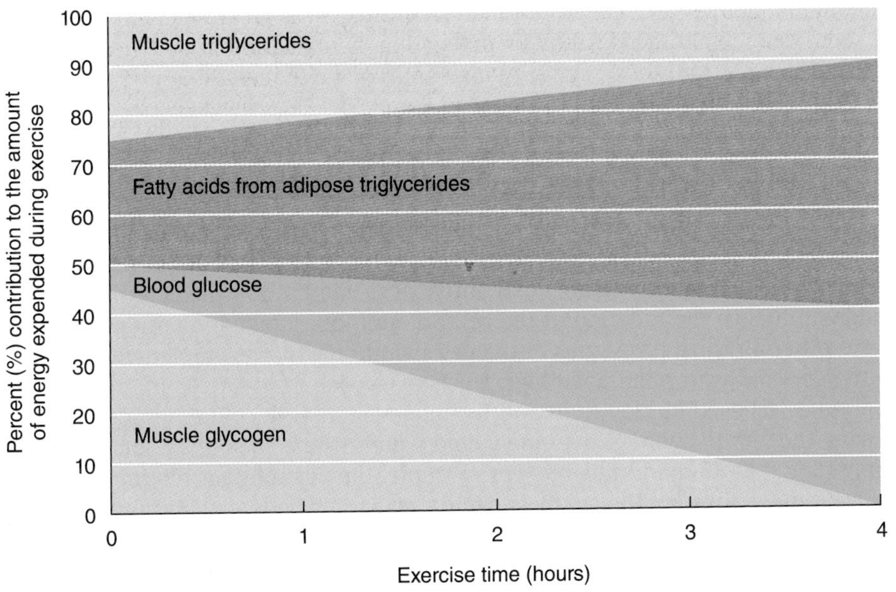

Figure 5.9 Various sources of energy used during exercise. As a person exercises for a prolonged period of time, fatty acids from adipose cells contribute relatively more energy than do carbohydrates stored in the muscle or circulating in our blood.

Data from Coyle, E. F. 1995. Substrate utilization during exercise in active people. *Am. J. Clin. Nutr.* 6[Suppl]: 958S–979S. Used with permission.

action activates additional hormones within the fat cell to begin breaking down fat. Adrenaline also signals the pancreas to *decrease* insulin production. This is important because insulin inhibits fat breakdown. Thus, when the need for fat as an energy source is high, blood insulin levels are typically low. As you might guess, blood insulin levels are high after eating, when our need for getting energy from stored fat is low and the need for fat storage is high.

Once fatty acids are released from the adipose cell, they travel in the blood attached to a protein, *albumin,* to the muscles, where they enter the mitochondria and use oxygen to produce ATP, which is the cell's energy source. Becoming more physically fit means you can deliver more oxygen to the muscle to use the fat that is delivered there. In addition, you can exercise longer when you are fit. Since the body has only a limited supply of stored carbohydrate as glycogen in muscle tissue, the longer you exercise, the more fat you use for energy. This point is illustrated in **Figure 5.9**. In this example, an individual is running for 4 hours at a moderate intensity. The longer the individual runs, the more depleted the muscle glycogen levels become and the more fat from adipose tissue is used as a fuel source for exercise.

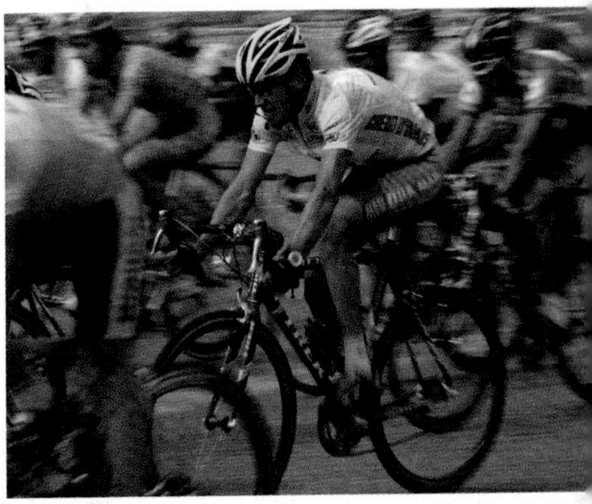

The longer you exercise, the more fat you use for energy. Cyclists in long-distance races use fat stores for energy.

Body Fat Stores Energy for Later Use

Our body stores extra energy in the form of body fat, which then can be used for energy at rest, during exercise, or during periods of low energy intake. Having a readily available energy source in the form of fat allows the body to always have access to energy, even when we choose not to eat (or are unable to eat), when we are exercising, and while we are sleeping. Our bodies have little stored carbohydrate—only enough to last about 1 to 2 days—and there is no place where our body can store extra protein. We cannot consider our muscles and organs as a place where "extra" protein is stored! For these reasons, the fat stored in our adipose and muscle tissues is necessary to keep the body going. Although we do not want too much stored adipose tissue, some fat storage is essential to good health.

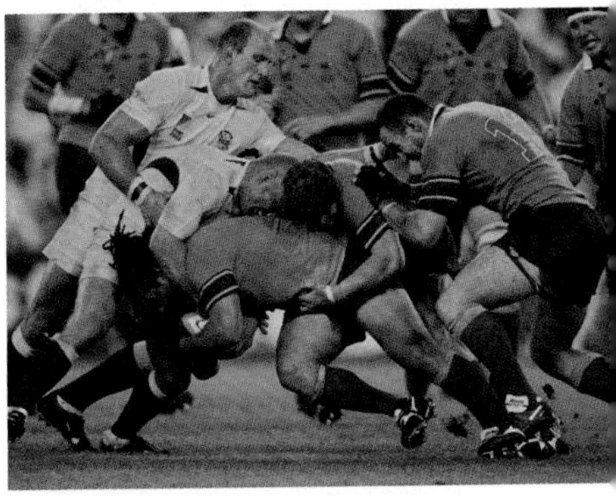

Adipose tissue pads our body and protects our organs when we fall or are bruised.

Fats Enable the Transport of Fat-Soluble Vitamins

Dietary fat enables the transport of the fat-soluble vitamins (A, D, E, and K) our body needs for many essential metabolic functions. For example, vitamin A is especially important for normal vision and gives us the ability to see at night. Vitamin D is important for regulating blood calcium and phosphorus concentrations within normal ranges, which indirectly helps maintain bone health. If vitamin D is low, blood calcium levels will drop below normal, and the body will draw calcium from the bones to maintain blood levels. Vitamin E functions primarily as an antioxidant in our body and keeps cell membranes healthy by preventing the oxidation of body fats. Finally, vitamin K is important for proteins involved in blood clotting and bone health. We discuss these vitamins in detail in Chapters 8 and 9.

Fats Help Maintain Cell Function

Fats are a critical part of every cell membrane. The types of fats in cell membranes help maintain membrane integrity, determine what substances are transported into and out of the cell, and regulate what substances can bind to the cell; thus, fats strongly influence the function of the cell. In addition, fats help maintain cell fluidity and other physical properties of the cell membrane. For example, wild salmon live in very cold water and have high levels of omega-3 fatty acids in their cell membranes. These fats stay fluid and flexible even in very cold environments, allowing the fish to swim in extremely cold water. In the same way, fats help our membranes stay fluid and flexible. For example, they enable our red blood cells to bend and move through the smallest capillaries in our body, delivering oxygen to all our cells.

Fats, especially PUFAs, are also primary components of the tissues of the brain and spinal cord, where they facilitate the transmission of information from one cell to another. We also need fats for the development, growth, and maintenance of these tissues.

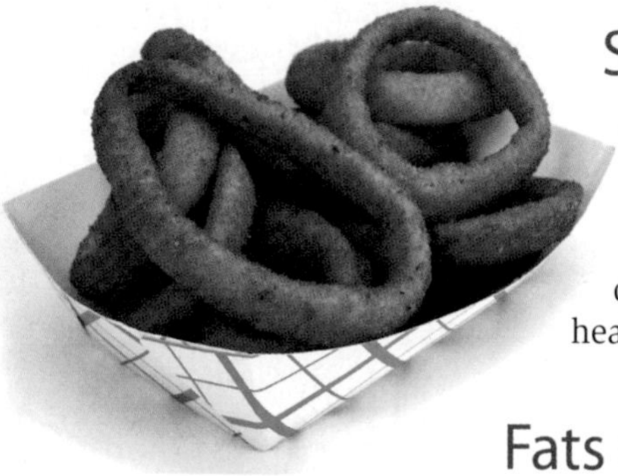

Fat adds texture and flavor to foods.

Stored Fat Provides Protection to the Body

Stored body fat also plays an important role in our body. Besides being the primary site of stored energy, adipose tissue pads our body and protects our organs, such as the kidneys and liver, when we fall or are bruised. The fat under our skin acts as insulation to help us retain body heat. Although we often think of body fat as "bad," it plays important roles in keeping our body healthy and functioning properly.

Fats Contribute to the Flavor and Texture of Foods

Dietary fat helps food taste good because it contributes to texture and flavor. Fat makes salad dressings smooth and ice cream "creamy," and it gives cakes and cookies their moist, tender texture. Frying foods in melted butter, lard, or oils gives them a crisp, flavorful coating; however, eating fried foods regularly is unhealthful because these foods are high in saturated and *trans* fatty acids.

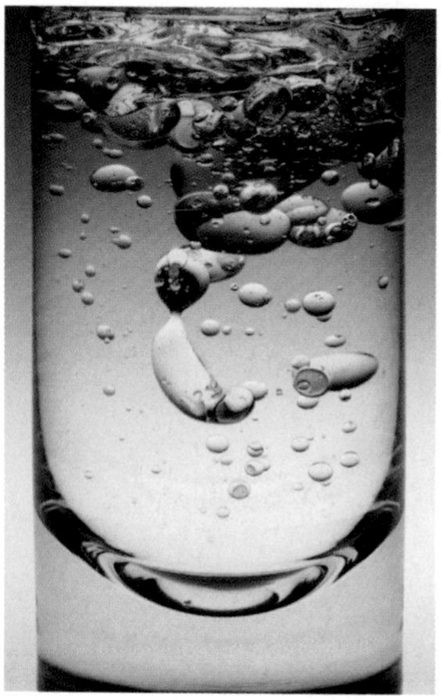

Fats and oils do not dissolve readily in water.

Fats Help Us Feel Satiated

Fats in foods help us feel satiated after a meal. Two factors probably contribute to this effect: first, fat has a much higher energy density than carbohydrate or protein. For example, a pat of butter weighing 5 g contains 35 kcal; 5 g of an apple contain only 3 kcal. For every gram of fat you consume, you get 2.25 times the amount of energy that you get with the same number of grams consumed in protein or carbohydrate.

Second, fat takes longer to digest than protein or carbohydrate because more steps are involved in the digestion process, which may make you feel fuller for a longer period of time because energy is slowly being released into your body.

On the other hand, you can eat more fat in a meal without feeling overfull because fat is generally compact in its size. Going back to our apple and butter example, one medium apple weighs 117 g (approximately 4 oz) and has 70 kcal, but the same number of Calories of butter—two pats—would hardly make you feel full! Looked at another way, an amount of butter weighing the same number of grams as a medium apple would contain 840 kcal!

TABLE 5.1 Omega-3 Fatty Acid Content of Selected Foods

Food Item	Total Omega-3	DHA	EPA*
		g/serving	
Flaxseed oil, 1 tbsp.	7.25	0.00	0.00
Salmon oil (fish oil), 1 tbsp.	4.39	2.48	1.77
Sardine oil, 1 tbsp.	3.01	1.45	1.38
Flaxseed, whole, 1 tbsp.	2.50	0.00	0.00
Herring, Atlantic, broiled, 3 oz	1.83	0.94	0.77
Anchovies w/oil, each	1.76	0.65	1.10
Herring oil, 1 tbsp.	1.53	0.57	0.85
Salmon, Coho, steamed, 3 oz	1.34	0.71	0.46
Canola oil, 1 tbsp.	1.28	0.00	0.00
Sardines, Atlantic, w/ bones and oil, 3 oz	1.26	0.43	0.40
Trout, rainbow fillet, baked, 3 oz	1.05	0.70	0.28
Walnuts, English, 1 tbsp.	0.66	0.00	0.00
Halibut, fillet, baked, 3 oz	0.53	0.31	0.21
Shrimp, canned, 3 oz	0.47	0.21	0.25
Tuna, white, in oil, 3 oz	0.38	0.19	0.04
Crab, Alaska King, steamed, 3 oz	0.36	0.10	0.25
Scallops, broiled, 3 oz	0.31	0.14	0.17
Tuna, light, in water, 3 oz	0.23	0.19	0.04
Avocado, Calif., fresh, whole	0.22	0.00	0.00
Spinach, cooked, 1 cup	0.17	0.00	0.00

Note: *EPA = eicosapentaenoic acid; DHA = docosahexaenoic acid
Data from Food Processor SQL, Version 10.3, ESHA Research, Salem, OR.

Dietary Reference Intakes for Essential Fatty Acids

Dietary Reference Intakes (DRIs) for the two essential fatty acids were set for the first time in 2002.[7]

- *Linoleic acid.* The Adequate Intake (AI) for linoleic acid (an omega-6 FA) is 14 to 17 g per day for adult men and 11 to 12 g per day for women 19 years and older. Using the typical energy intakes for adult men and women, this translates into an AMDR of 5–10% of total energy intake.
- *Alpha-linolenic acid.* The AI for alpha-linolenic acid (an omega-3 FA) is 1.6 g per day for adult men and 1.1 g per day for adult women. This translates into an AMDR of 0.6–1.2% of total energy. These recommendations are for omega-3 fatty acids as a group. No DRIs have been set for DHA or EPA specifically. So how do you know if you're getting enough in your diet? Look through **Table 5.1** to see if you are consuming any good food sources of these essential acids.

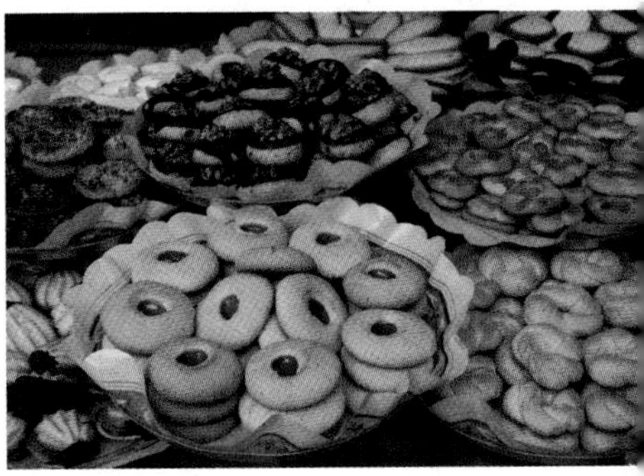

Baked goods are often high in hidden fats and may contain *trans* fats.

Following these recommendations, an individual consuming 2,000 kcal per day should consume about 11 to 22 g per day of linoleic acid and about 1.3 to 2.6 g per day of alpha-linolenic acid. Notice that the recommended intake of linoleic acid is close to ten times higher than the recommended intake of alpha-linolenic acid. This is in keeping with the 5:1 to 10:1 ratio of linoleic:alpha-linolenic acid recommended by the World Health Organization and supported by the Institute of Medicine.[7] Because these EFAs compete for the same enzymes to produce various eicosanoids, this ratio helps keep eicosanoid production in balance; that is, one isn't overproduced at the expense of the other.

RECAP The Acceptable Macronutrient Distribution Range (AMDR) for total fat is 20–35% of total energy. The Adequate Intake (AI) for linoleic acid is 14 to 17 g per day for adult men and 11 to 12 g per day for adult women. The AI for alpha-linolenic acid is 1.6 g per day for adult men and 1.1 g per day for adult women.

Don't Let the Fats Fool You!

Like many things, a little can be good, but too much can be harmful. We know that unsaturated fats are necessary for good health, but too much fat, regardless of type, can be unhealthful. That's one reason nutritionists have been recommending the reduction of dietary fat for over a decade. However, before you can make healthful reductions in your fat intake, you need to know where the fat in your diet is coming from.

Recognize the Fat in Foods

It is easy to eat a high-fat diet. First, we add fats, such as oils, butter, cream, shortening, margarine, mayonnaise, and salad dressings, to foods because they make food taste good. This type of fat is called **visible fat** because we can easily see that we are adding it to our food. When we add fat to foods ourselves, we generally know how much we are adding. Still, we may not be aware of the type of fat we're using and the number of Calories it adds to our meal. For instance, it's easy to make a salad into a high-fat meal by adding two or three tablespoons of full-fat salad dressing. Doing so also transforms the salad into a high-Calorie meal: concentrated fats, such as butter, oil, and salad dressings, have 100 kcal/tablespoon.

Limiting your intake of visible fats is important, but it's only the first step. You must also be on the lookout for **hidden fats**—that is, fats added to processed and prepared foods to improve taste and texture. Over the past decade, our intake of visible fats has decreased, while our intake of hidden fats has increased.[9] That's partly because, when fat exists naturally within a food, or is added during food preparation, we're less aware of how much or what type of fat is actually there. Do you read the information about fat on the Nutrition Facts Panel of the foods you buy? When eating out, do you look for or ask about the fat and Calorie content of the menu items you're considering?

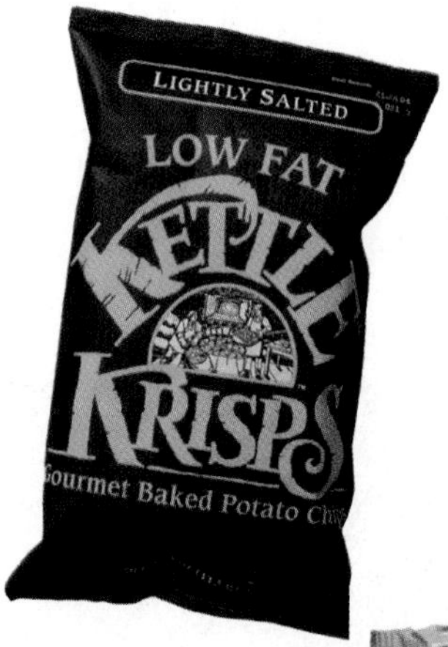

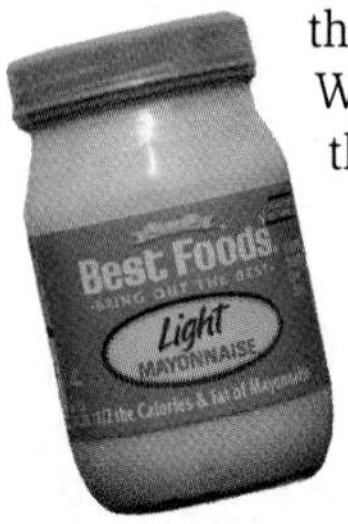

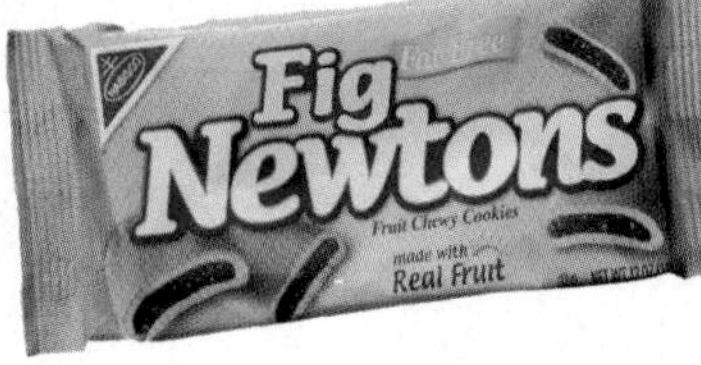

What's more, when fats are hidden, we're often tricked into choosing higher-fat foods over more healthful versions. For example, a slice of yellow cake is much higher in fat (40% of total energy) than a slice of angel food cake (1% of total energy), yet many consumers just assume the fat content of these foods is the same, since they are both cake. In addition to baked goods, foods that can be high in hidden fats include dairy products, frozen entrées, processed meats or meats that are not trimmed, and most convenience and fast foods, such as hamburgers, hot dogs, chips, ice cream, french fries, and other fried foods. When purchasing packaged foods, read the Nutrition Facts Panel and find out whether or not the product is high in hidden fats! The Nutrition Label Activity on page 161 shows you how to calculate the amount of fat hidden in packaged foods.

Decipher Label Claims

Since high-fat diets have been associated with obesity, many Americans are trying to reduce their total fat intake. Because of this concern, food manufacturers have been more than happy to provide consumers with low-fat alternatives to their favorite foods—so you can have your cake and eat it, too! The FDA and the USDA have set specific regulations on allowable product descriptions for reduced-fat products. The following claims are defined for 1 serving:

- Fat-free = less than 0.5 g of fat
- Low-fat = 3 g or less of fat
- Reduced or less fat: at least 25% less fat as compared to a standard serving
- Light: one-third fewer Calories or 50% less fat as compared with a standard serving amount

It is now estimated that there are more than 5,000 different fat-modified foods on the market.[14, 15] For example, you can purchase fat-modified dairy products, peanut butter, mayonnaise, cookies, crackers, and frozen meals. However, if you're choosing

visible fats Fat we can see in our foods or see added to foods, such as butter, margarine, cream, shortening, salad dressings, chicken skin, and untrimmed fat on meat.

hidden fats Fats that are hidden in foods, such as the fats found in baked goods, regular-fat dairy products, marbling in meat, and fried foods.

NUTRITION LABEL ACTIVITY

How Much Fat Is in This Food?

How can you figure out how much fat is in a food you buy? One way is to read the Nutrition Facts Panel on the label. By becoming a better label reader, you can make more healthful food selections. Two cracker labels are shown in **Figure 5.13**; one cracker is higher in fat than the other.

Let's review how you can use the label to find out what percentage of energy is coming from fat in each product. The calculations are relatively simple.

1. Divide the total Calories from fat by the total Calories per serving, and multiply the answer by 100.
   - For the regular wheat crackers: 50 kcal/150 kcal = 0.33 × 100 = 33%.

   Thus, for the regular crackers, the total energy coming from fat is 33%.
   - For the reduced-fat wheat crackers: 35 kcal/130 kcal = 0.269 × 100 = 27%.

   Thus, for the reduced-fat crackers, the total energy coming from fat is 27%.

   You can see that although the total amount of energy per serving is not very different between these two crackers, the percentage from fat is quite different.
2. If the total Calories per serving from fat are not given on the label, you can quickly calculate this value by multiplying the grams of total fat per serving by 9 (there are 9 kcal per gram of fat).
   - For the regular wheat crackers: 6 g fat × 9 kcal/gram = 54 kcal of fat.
   - To calculate the percentage of Calories from fat: 54 kcal/150 kcal = 0.36 × 100 = 36%.

   You can see that this value is not exactly the same as the 50 kcal reported on the label or the 33% of Calories from fat calculated in example 1. The values on food labels are rounded off, so your estimations may not be identical when you do this second calculation.

   In summary, you can quickly calculate the percentage of fat per serving for any packaged food in three steps: (1) multiply the grams of fat per serving by 9 kcal per gram; (2) divide this number by the total kcal per serving; (3) multiply by 100.

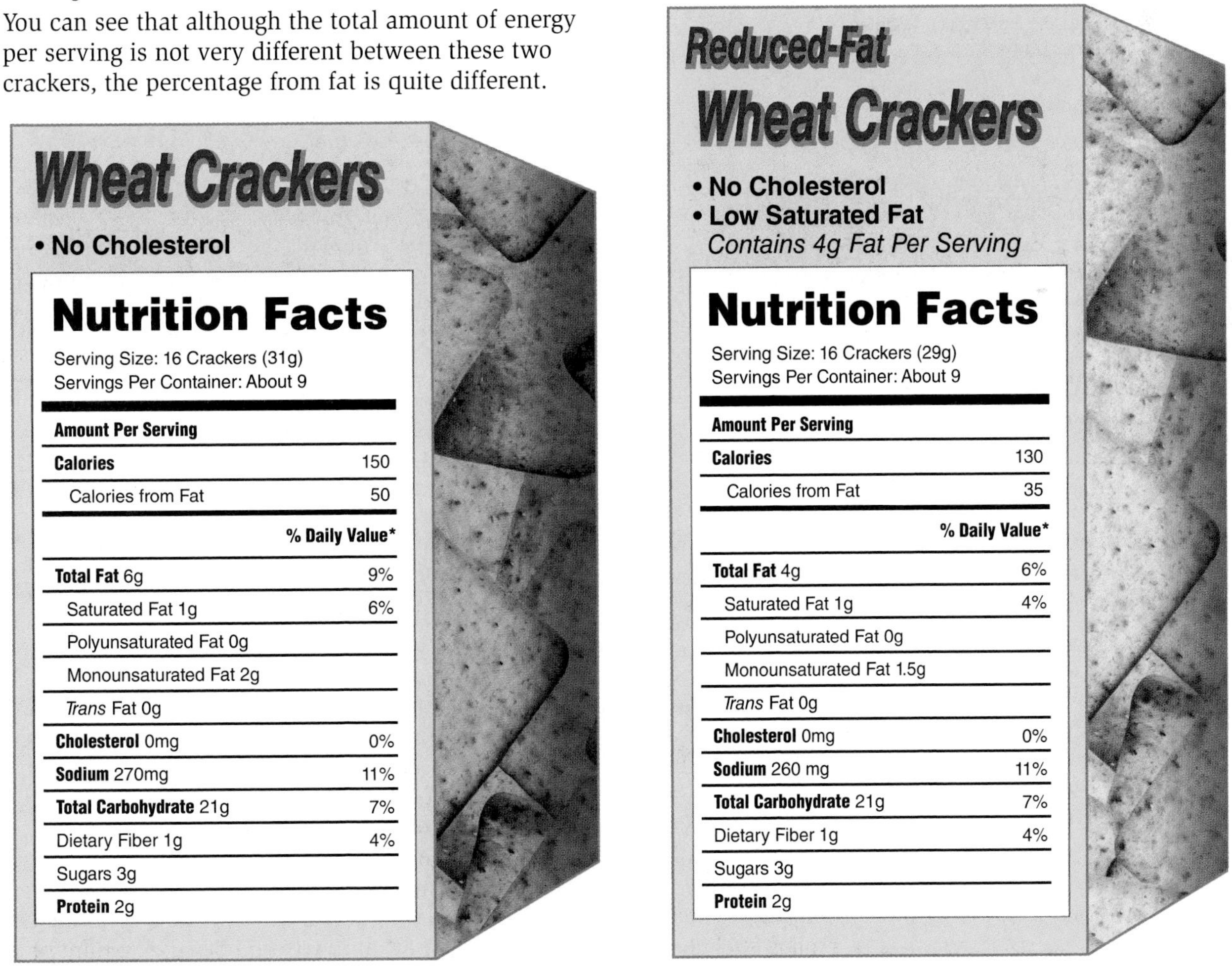

Wheat Crackers
• No Cholesterol
Nutrition Facts
Serving Size: 16 Crackers (31g)
Servings Per Container: About 9
Amount Per Serving
Calories 150
Calories from Fat 50
% Daily Value*
Total Fat 6g 9%
Saturated Fat 1g 6%
Polyunsaturated Fat 0g
Monounsaturated Fat 2g
Trans Fat 0g
Cholesterol 0mg 0%
Sodium 270mg 11%
Total Carbohydrate 21g 7%
Dietary Fiber 1g 4%
Sugars 3g
Protein 2g
Reduced-Fat
Wheat Crackers
• No Cholesterol
• Low Saturated Fat
Contains 4g Fat Per Serving
Nutrition Facts
Serving Size: 16 Crackers (29g)
Servings Per Container: About 9
Amount Per Serving
Calories 130
Calories from Fat 35
% Daily Value*
Total Fat 4g 6%
Saturated Fat 1g 4%
Polyunsaturated Fat 0g
Monounsaturated Fat 1.5g
Trans Fat 0g
Cholesterol 0mg 0%
Sodium 260 mg 11%
Total Carbohydrate 21g 7%
Dietary Fiber 1g 4%
Sugars 3g
Protein 2g

(a) (b)

Figure 5.13 Labels for two types of wheat crackers. **(a)** Regular wheat crackers. **(b)** Reduced-fat wheat crackers.

TABLE 5.2 Comparison of Full-Fat, Reduced-Fat, and Low-Fat Foods*

Product and Amount	Version	Energy (kcal)	Protein (g)	Carbohydrate (g)	Fat (g)	Saturated Fat (g)
Animal Products:						
Milk, 8 oz	Whole, 3.3% fat	150	8.0	11.4	8.2	4.6
	2% fat	121	8.1	11.7	4.7	3.0
	1% fat	102	8.0	11.7	2.6	1.5
	Skim (nonfat)	86	8.4	11.9	0.5	0.0
Cheese, cheddar, 1 oz	Regular	111	7.1	0.5	9.1	4.0
	Low-fat	81	9.1	0.0	5.1	2.7
	Nonfat	41	6.8	4.0	0.0	0.0
Cream cheese, 1 tbsp.	Soft regular	50	1.0	0.5	5.0	3.0
	Soft light	35	1.5	1.0	2.5	1.7
	Soft nonfat	15	2.5	1.0	0.0	0.0
Ground Beef, cooked (3 oz)	Regular (25% fat)	237	22	0	16	6.2
	Extra-lean (5% fat)	145	22	0	5.6	2.5
Chicken, frozen dinner (9–12 oz dinner cooked)	Fried breast with skin	470	20	30	30	10
	Grilled, skinless	360	20	38	14	4
Vegetable Spreads:						
Mayonnaise, 1 tbsp.	Regular	100	0.0	0.0	11.0	1.5
	Light	50	0.0	1.0	5.0	0.75
	Fat-free	10	0.0	2.0	0.0	0.08
Margarine, veg oil, 1 tbsp.	Regular	100	0.0	0.0	11.0	1.5
	Reduced-fat	60	0.0	0.0	7.0	1.3
Peanut butter, 1 tbsp.	Regular	95	4.1	3.1	8.0	1.5
	Reduced-fat	95	4.4	5.2	6.0	1.25
Grain Products:						
Cookies, Oreo, 3 cookies	Regular	160	2.0	24.0	7.0	1.5
	Reduced-fat	150	2.0	26.0	3.5	1.0
Cookies, Fig Newton, 3 cookies	Regular	174	3.0	29.0	4.4	1.45
	Fat-free	130	1.5	30.0	0.0	0.0
Muffin, 4 oz	Regular	429	6.0	54.0	21.0	3.0
	Low-fat	300	6.0	61.0	3.0	0.5

*The Food and Drug Administration and the U.S. Department of Agriculture have set specific regulations on allowable product descriptions for reduced-fat products. The following claims are defined for 1 serving amount: **fat-free**: less than 0.5 g of fat; **low-fat**: 3 g or less of fat; **reduced or less fat**: at least 25% less fat as compared to a standard serving; **light**: one-third fewer Calories or 50% less fat as compared with a standard serving amount.

Data from Food Processor-SQL, Version 10.3, ESHA Research, Salem, OR.

such foods because of a concern about your weight, let the buyer beware! Lower-fat versions of foods may not always be lower in Calories.

In **Table 5.2**, we list a number of full-fat foods with their lower-fat alternatives. If you were to incorporate such foods into your diet on a regular basis, you could significantly reduce the amount of fat you consume. Still, your choices may or may not reduce the amount of energy you consume. For example, as you can see in the table, drinking nonfat milk instead of whole milk would dramatically reduce both your fat and your energy intake. However, eating fat-free instead of regular Fig Newton cookies would not significantly reduce your energy intake.

Thus, if you think that eating fat-free foods means you're reducing your energy intake so significantly that you can eat all you want without gaining weight, you're mistaken. The reduced fat is often replaced with added carbohydrate, resulting in a very similar total energy intake. Thus, if you want to reduce both the amount of fat and energy you consume, you must read the labels of modified-fat foods carefully before you buy.[14]

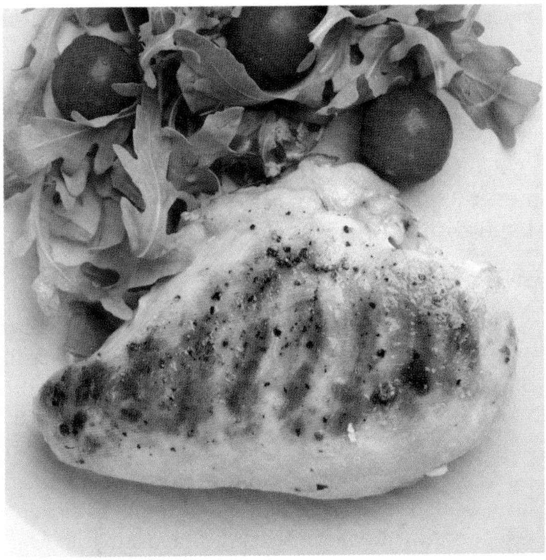

This skinless roasted chicken breast provides <1 g saturated fat and 131 kcal; with the skin, it would provide 3 g saturated fat and 235 kcal.

Limit Saturated and *Trans* Fats

Research over the last two decades has shown that diets high in saturated fatty acids negatively influence blood lipid levels, increasing our risk for heart disease. We now also know that *trans* fatty acids appear to function much like saturated fatty acids in our diet: both *trans* and saturated fatty acids lower "good" cholesterol and raise "bad" cholesterol, change cell membrane function, and alter the way cholesterol is removed from the blood. For these reasons, researchers believe that diets high in saturated and *trans* fatty acids can increase the risk for cardiovascular disease.

Reduce Your Intake of Saturated Fats

The recommended intake of saturated fats is less than 7–10% of our total energy; unfortunately, our average intake is between 11% and 12% of energy.[16] According to data from NHANES, about 64% of adults in the United States exceed the dietary recommendation for saturated fats.[17]

The last time you popped a frozen dinner into the microwave, did you stop and read the Nutrition Facts Panel on the box? If you had, you might have been shocked to learn how much saturated fat was in the meal. Where does it come from? Let's look at the primary sources of saturated fats in the American diet.

- *Animal products.* Meats contain saturated fats. The precise amount depends on the cut of the meat and how it is prepared. For example, red meats, such as beef, pork, and lamb, typically have more fat than skinless chicken or fish. Thus, lean meats are lower in saturated fat than regular cuts. In addition, broiled, grilled, or baked meats have less saturated fat than fried meats. Dairy products may also be high in saturated fat. Whole-fat milk has three times the saturated fat as low-fat milk, and nearly twice the energy. Whole eggs have just over a gram of saturated fat and are high in cholesterol.
- *Grain products.* Baked goods and snack foods are the main culprits in this food group. Pastries, cookies, and muffins may be filled with saturated fats, as well as *trans* fats, if they come from your local bakery. Tortilla chips, microwave and movie-theatre popcorn, snack crackers, and packaged rice and pasta mixes may also be high in saturated fat.

- *Vegetables and vegetable spreads/dressings.* We often don't think of plant foods as having high amounts of saturated fats, but if these foods are fried, breaded, or drenched in sauces they can become a source of saturated fat. For example, a small baked potato (138 g) has no fat and 134 kcal, whereas a medium serving (134 g) of french fries cooked in vegetable oil has 427 kcal, 23 g of fat, and 5.3 g of saturated fat. This is one-third of the saturated fat recommended for an entire day for a person on a 2,000-kcal/day diet. Some spreads, such as margarine, mayonnaise, and salad dressings, can also add saturated fats to your diet.

Avoid *Trans* Fatty Acids

The Institute of Medicine recommends that we keep our intake of *trans* fatty acids to an absolute minimum.[7] Currently, the average consumption of industrially produced *trans* fatty acids is only about 2–3% of total energy intake, with the majority coming from deep-fried fast or frozen foods, some tub margarines, and bakery products.[7, 18, 19] So, if our current consumption is already so low, why the advice to reduce it even further?

Although *trans* fatty acids make up only a small fraction of the average American diet, their negative effect on our health appears to be dramatic. Many health professionals feel that diets high in *trans* fatty acids increase the risk for heart disease even more than diets high in saturated fats.[20] A research review that involved over 140,000 individuals showed that for every 2% increase in energy intake from *trans* fatty acids, there was a 23% increase in incidence of heart disease.[20] Other researchers have concluded that the scientific evidence showing that *trans* fatty acids negatively affect health is so strong that it is unethical to do any additional long-term human research trials comparing the health effects of *trans* fatty acids to other types of fatty acids.

Because of the evidence linking *trans* fatty acid consumption to heart disease, the FDA requires manufacturers to list the amount of *trans* fatty acids per serving on the Nutrition Facts Panel. In addition, many cities are considering total bans on *trans* fatty acids in restaurants. For example, in New York City, an amendment to the health code has phased out all artificial *trans* fats in restaurants and other food establishments operating within the city limits.[21] Unfortunately, no such requirement exists for the majority of food establishments in the United States.

As we noted at the beginning of this chapter, legislators and food policy experts around the world are lobbying for the labeling of *trans* fatty acids on menus and/or the elimination of artificial *trans* fatty acids from restaurant foods and other ready-to-eat foods. Although this is a step in the right direction, if we are to achieve our goals for public health, we need to make sure that, in eliminating *trans* fatty acids from foods, we don't simply substitute saturated fats. Food establishments and food manufacturers need to switch to unsaturated fats if we are to reduce our risk for heart disease.

Shop Smart!

Next time you're at the grocery store, how can you limit the level of saturated and *trans* fats in the foods you buy? Try the Quick Tips on page 165 to help guide your choices.

Cook Smart!

You can also significantly reduce your intake of saturated fats by making smart choices when you cook. The Quick Tips on page 166 will help to guide you.

Select Beneficial Fats

As mentioned earlier, it's best to switch to healthful fats without increasing your total fat intake. Americans appear to get adequate amounts of omega-6 fatty acids, probably because of the large amount of salad dressings, vegetable oils, margarine, and mayonnaise we eat; however, our consumption of omega-3 fatty acids is more variable and can be low in the diets of people who do not eat leafy green vegetables, fish, or walnuts; drink soy milk; or use soybean, canola, or flaxseed oil.

How can you specifically increase your intake of omega-3 fatty acids? In Table 5.1 (page 159), we identified the omega-3 fatty acid content of various foods and supple-

QUICK TIPS

Shopping for Foods Low in Saturated and *Trans* Fats

✓ Read food labels. Look for foods with no hydrogenated oils and low amounts of saturated fats per serving.

✓ Select liquid or tub margarine/butters over hard stick forms. Fats that are solid at room temperature are usually high in *trans* or saturated fatty acids. Also, select margarines made from healthful fats, such as canola oil.

✓ Buy naturally occurring oils, such as olive and canola oil. These types of oils have not been hydrogenated and contain healthful unsaturated fatty acids and no *trans* fatty acids.

✓ Select reduced-fat baked products, such as crackers, chips, cookies, and muffins, over full-fat versions. If you are watching your weight, choose products with fewer Calories per serving as well.

✓ Cut back on packaged pastries, such as Danish, croissants, donuts, cakes, tarts, pies, and brownies. These baked goods are typically high in saturated and *trans* fatty acids.

✓ Select reduced-fat salad dressing and mayonnaise or select those made with healthful fats, such as olive oil and vinegar. If you select the full-fat versions, remember that a tablespoon of oil or full-fat mayonnaise contains 100 kcal.

✓ Add fish, especially those high in omega-3 fatty acids, to your shopping list. For example, select salmon, line-caught tuna, herring, and sardines. Many specialty markets now carry line-caught canned tuna, which is low in mercury. These tuna are smaller, usually less than 20 pounds, and have had less exposure to mercury in their lifetime.

✓ For other healthful sources of protein, select lean cuts of meat and skinless poultry, meat substitutes made with soy, or beans or lentils.

✓ Select low-fat or nonfat versions of milk, cheese, cottage cheese, yogurt, sour cream, cream cheese, and ice cream.

ments. Use this table to determine how you can increase your intake of omega-3 fatty acids. For example, consider including fish in your diet at least twice a week, use canola oil when baking, and add ground flaxseeds to your cereal or walnuts to your salad. You might also consider taking a daily fish oil supplement, using flaxseed oil, or buying products with omega-3 fatty acids added. As a consumer, you need to read the labels of these products carefully to determine if the omega-3 fatty acid content of the product is worth the extra cost.

It is important to recognize that there can be some risk associated with eating large amounts of certain fish on a regular basis. Some species of fish, including shark, swordfish, and king mackerel, contain high levels of mercury and other environmental contaminants. Women who are pregnant or breastfeeding, women who may become pregnant, and small children are at particularly high risk for toxicity from these contaminants. For more information on seafood contamination, see Chapter 13.

Of course, healthful fats include not only the essential fatty acids but also polyunsaturated and monounsaturated fats in general. Plant oils are excellent sources of unsaturated fats, as are avocados, olives, nuts and nut butters, and seeds. Substituting beneficial fats for saturated or *trans* fats isn't difficult. See the Eating Right All Day feature on page 167 for some simple menu choices to help you eat right all day.

Watch Out When You're Eating Out!

Many college students eat most of their meals in dining halls, fast-food restaurants, and other food establishments. If that describes you, watch out! The menu items you choose each day may be increasing the amount of fat in your diet, including your intake of saturated and *trans* fats. A high fat intake is especially difficult to avoid if you regularly eat fast food. Based on 2003–2004 NHANES data, fast-food consumers have

QUICK TIPS

Reducing Saturated Fats When Preparing and Cooking Foods

- ✓ Trim visible fat from meats before cooking.
- ✓ Remove the skin from poultry before cooking.
- ✓ Instead of frying meats, poultry, fish, or potatoes or other vegetables, bake or broil them.
- ✓ If you normally eat two eggs for breakfast, discard the yolk from one for half the cholesterol. Do the same in recipes calling for two eggs.
- ✓ Cook with olive oil or canola oil instead of butter.
- ✓ Use cooking spray instead of butter or oils for stir-frying and baking.
- ✓ Substitute hard cheeses (such as parmesan), which are naturally lower in fat, for softer cheeses that are higher in fat (such as cheddar).
- ✓ Substitute low-fat or nonfat yogurt for cream, cream cheese, mayonnaise, or sour cream in recipes; on baked potatoes, tacos, and salads; and in dips.

higher total energy, total fat, and saturated fat intake than those who eat fast food infrequently.[22] And although many fast food restaurants have eliminated *trans* fatty acids from their menus, McDonald's still has a few items, such as desserts and shakes, that contain *trans* fatty acids. In Chapter 2, we provided a list of general Quick Tips for Eating Right When You're Eating Out. The following are some specific strategies for improving the amount and type of fat in your menu choices.

Be Aware of Fat Replacers

One way to lower the fat content of foods such as chips, muffins, cakes, and cookies is by replacing the fat in a food with a *fat replacer*. Snack foods have been the primary target for fat replacers because it is more difficult to eliminate the fat from these types of products without dramatically changing the taste. In the mid-1990s, the food industry and nutritionists thought that fat replacers would be the answer to our growing obesity problem. They reasoned that if we substitute fat replacers for some of the traditional fats in snack and fast foods, we might be able to reduce both energy and fat intake and help Americans manage their weight better.

Products such as olestra (brand name Olean) hit the market in 1996 with a lot of fanfare, but the hype was short-lived. Initially, foods containing olestra had to bear a label warning of potential gastrointestinal side effects. In 2003, the FDA announced that this warning was no longer necessary, as research showed that olestra causes only mild, infrequent discomfort. However, even with the new labeling, only a limited number of foods in the marketplace contain olestra. It is also evident from our growing obesity problem that fat replacers, such as olestra, do not help Americans lose weight or even maintain their current weight.

RECAP **Visible fats are those foods that can be easily recognized as containing fat. Hidden fats are those fats added to our food during the manufacturing or cooking process, so we are not aware of how much fat has been added. By making simple substitutions when shopping and eating out, you can reduce the quantity of saturated and *trans* fatty acids in your diet and increase your intake of healthful fats. Fat replacers are substances used to replace the typical fats found in foods.**

What Role Do Fats Play in Chronic Disease?

There appears to be a generally held assumption that if you eat fat-free or low-fat foods you will lose weight and prevent chronic diseases. Certainly, we know that diets high in saturated and *trans* fatty acids can contribute to chronic diseases, including heart disease and cancer; however, as we have explored in this chapter, unsaturated fatty acids do not have this negative effect and some are essential to good health. Thus, a sensible health goal is to eat the appropriate amounts and types of fat.

The chronic disease most closely associated with diets high in saturated and *trans* fats is cardiovascular disease. This complex disorder is discussed ***In Depth*** following this chapter. In addition, high-fat diets have been linked to cancer. Is such a link supported by evidence?

Cancer develops as a result of a poorly understood interaction between the environment and genetic factors. In addition, most cancers take years to develop, so examining the impact of diet on cancer development can be a long and difficult process. Nevertheless, research does suggest that diet is one of several important environmental factors that influence the development of cancer.[23, 24]

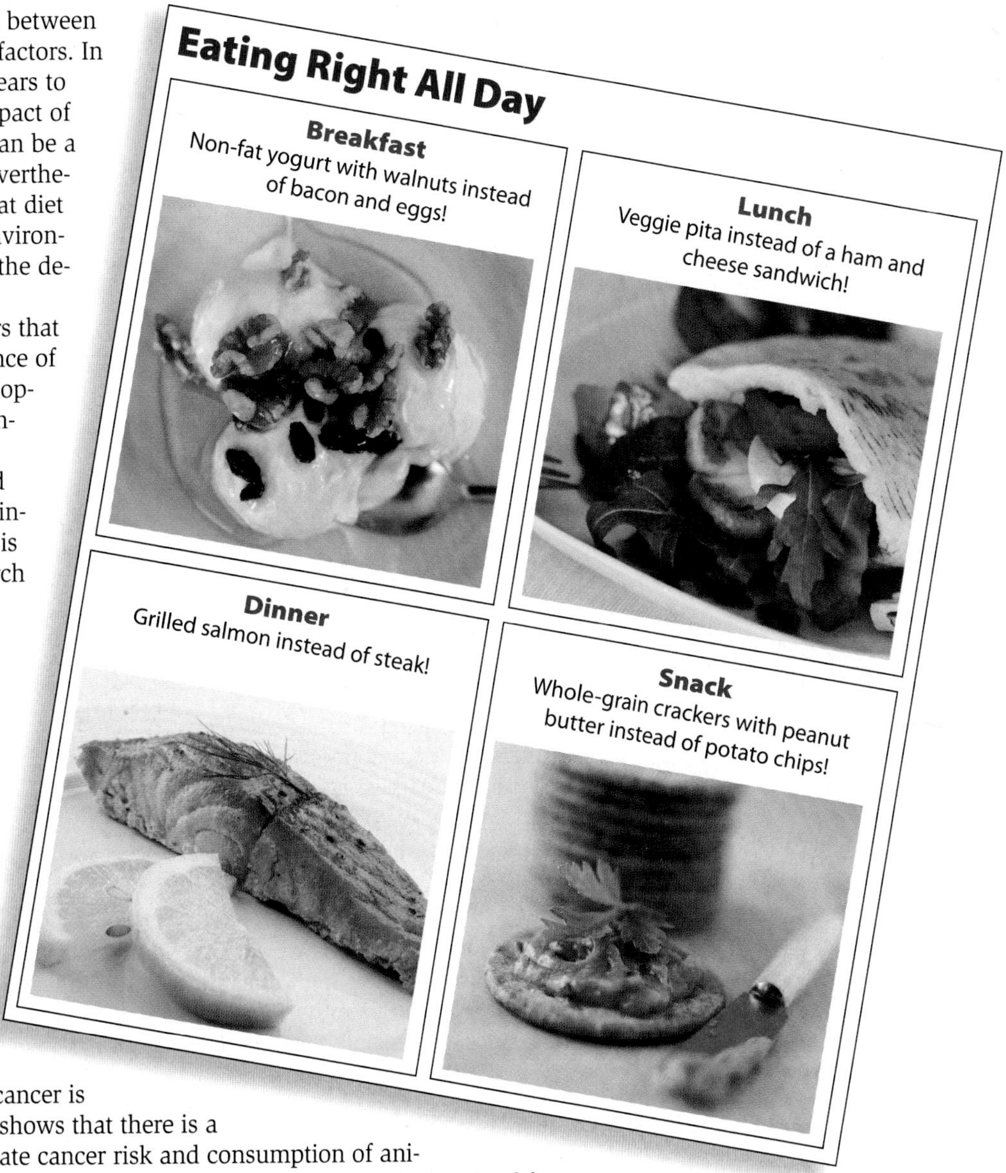
Eating Right All Day
Breakfast
Non-fat yogurt with walnuts instead of bacon and eggs!
Lunch
Veggie pita instead of a ham and cheese sandwich!
Dinner
Grilled salmon instead of steak!
Snack
Whole-grain crackers with peanut butter instead of potato chips!

Of the many dietary factors that have been studied, the influence of dietary fat intake on the development of cancer has been extensively researched. The relationship between type and amount of fat consumed and increased risk for breast cancer is controversial.[25, 26] Early research suggested an association between animal fat intake and increased risk for colon cancer, but more recent research indicates that the association involves factors other than fat that are found in red meat. Because we now know that physical activity can reduce the risk for colon cancer, earlier diet and colon cancer studies that did not control for this factor are now being questioned. The strongest association between dietary fat intake and cancer is for prostate cancer. Research shows that there is a consistent link between prostate cancer risk and consumption of animal fat, but not fat from plant sources. The exact mechanism by which animal fats may contribute to prostate cancer has not yet been identified.

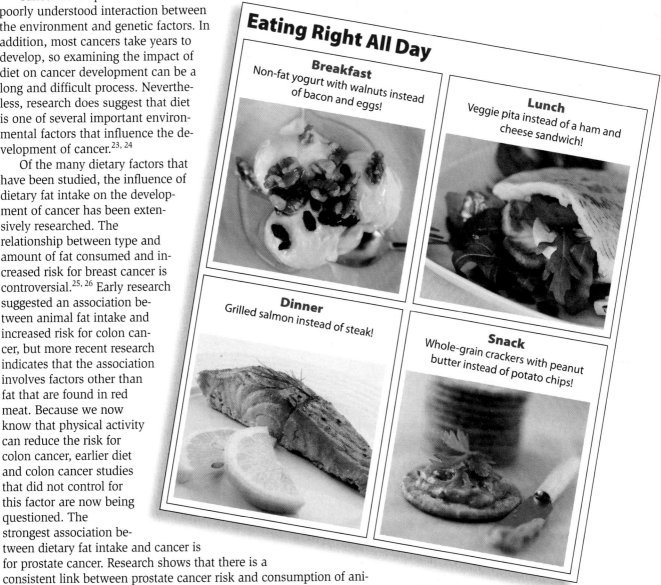

QUICK TIPS

Limiting Fat When You're Eating Out

✔ Find eating establishments that allow you to order alternatives to the usual menu items. For instance, if you like burgers, look for a restaurant that will grill your burger instead of frying it and will let you substitute a salad for french fries.

✔ Ask about the types of fats used in salad dressing, baked goods, and cooking processes. Many establishments are working to replace *trans* fatty acids with healthful fats in their menu items. If you have a favorite restaurant that you visit frequently, make sure you know the kinds of fats they use in their products.

✔ Select healthful appetizers, such as salads, broth-based soups, vegetables, or fruit, over white bread with butter, nachos, or fried foods such as chicken wings.

✔ Select broth-based soups, which are lower in fat and Calories than cream-based soups, which are typically made with cream, cheese, and/or butter.

✔ Ask that all visible fat be trimmed from meats and that poultry be served without the skin.

✔ Select menu items that use cooking methods that add little or no additional fat, such as broiling, grilling, steaming, and sautéing. Be alert to menu descriptions such as *fried, crispy, creamed, buttered, au gratin, escalloped*, and *parmesan*. Also avoid foods served in sauces such as butter sauce, alfredo, and hollandaise. All of these types of food preparation typically add more fat to a meal.

✔ Avoid meat and vegetable pot pies, quiches, and other items with a pastry crust, as these may be high in *trans* fats.

✔ Ask for spreads and condiments, such as butter, salad dressings, sauces, and sour cream, to be served on the side instead of added in the kitchen.

✔ Request low-fat spreads on your sandwiches, such as mustards or chutneys, over full-fat mayonnaise or butter.

✔ Substitute a salad, veggies, or fruit for the chips or french fries that come with the meal.

✔ Select lower-fat desserts, such as sorbet or a small cookie, over full-fat ice cream or a brownie. Alternatively, share a full-fat dessert with friends or family members, which will reduce both the Calories and fat you consume.

✔ Keep counting at your favorite cafe! Consider that a Starbucks tall cafe latte (12 oz) made with whole milk contains 200 kcal and 11 g of fat (7 g from saturated fat). Whipped cream can add 80–130 kcal and 8–12 g of fat. The same drink made with nonfat milk and no whipped cream contains 120 kcal and no fat. So ask for your coffee, hot chocolate, tea, or chai with nonfat milk and eliminate the whipped cream.

✔ Select lower-fat options to accompany your coffee drink. For example, choose a biscotti or a small piece of dark chocolate instead of a croissant, a scone, a muffin, coffee cake, or a large cookie.

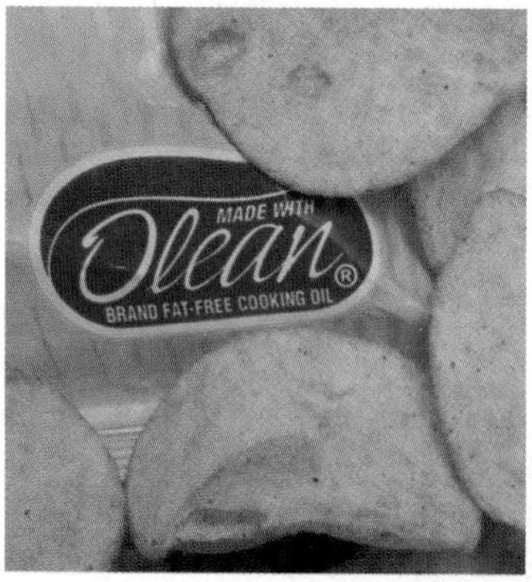

Snack foods have been the primary target for fat replacers, such as Olean, since it is more difficult to eliminate the fat from these types of foods without dramatically changing the taste.

RECAP **The types of fats we eat can significantly affect our health and risk for disease. Diets high in saturated and *trans* fatty acids increase our risk for heart disease. Selecting appropriate types of fat in the diet may also reduce your risk for some cancers, especially prostate cancer.**

Nutrition DEBATE
Fat Blockers—Help or Hype?

In the last thirty years, the rate of obesity has steadily increased among Americans. And growing right alongside our waistlines is the market for weight-loss supplements. It's a multibillion-dollar industry, with new products continually tempting us with promises of quick, effortless, and dramatic results. Currently, there's no regulation of weight-loss supplements, so consumers have no way of knowing if the product they're considering is effective, or safe.

One popular group of weight-loss supplements are the so-called fat blockers. Do these products really "block" fat? Can they really help you lose weight?

What Are the Claims?

One way to reduce energy intake and body weight would be to block the absorption of energy-containing macronutrients—such as fat, which contains 9 kcals/gram. If we could block fat absorption, then we could eat large portions of our favorite high-fat foods, including fast foods, snacks, and desserts, without worrying about gaining weight. Fat blockers are said to decrease the amount of fat absorbed in the small intestine, leaving more to be excreted from the body.

The main ingredient in many of these supplements is chitosan, a nondigestible substance extracted mainly from the exoskeletons of marine crustaceans.[27] Chitosan is said to bind up to four to six times its weight in fat. Thus, for every gram of chitosan consumed, 4–6 g of fat should be "blocked." If this were true, then consuming 3 g of chitosan a day would block 12–18 g of fat a day, or 108–162 kcal/day. Chitosan is also thought to block the absorption of bile acids. (Recall that bile is delivered to the small intestine to emulsify fats.) If bile absorption is blocked, then the liver must produce new supplies. Since

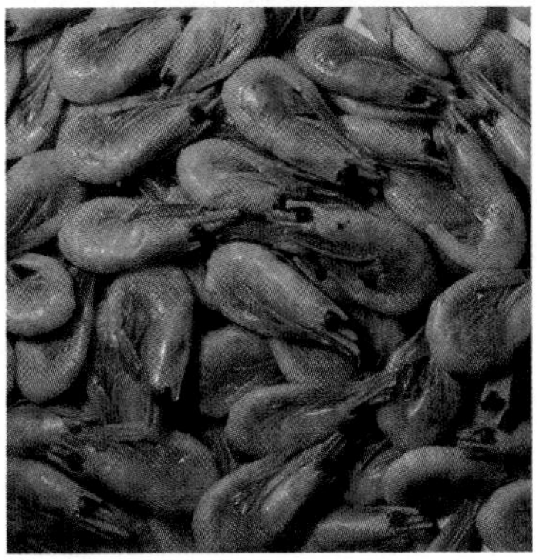

the liver takes cholesterol from the blood to make bile, fat blockers might reduce serum cholesterol as well.[27]

It all sounds good, but is there any evidence that fat blockers work? Let's review the research.

What Does the Research Say?

Chitosan has been studied extensively as a weight-loss aid. Two recent meta-analyses reviewing the efficacy of chitosan for weight loss from fourteen double-blind randomized controlled trials (RCT) involving over 1,000 participants concluded that there is some limited evidence that chitosan reduces body weight in humans.[28, 29, 30] The authors found that chitosan produced a small, but significant, greater average weight loss (1.7 kg, or 3.7 lb) over an average of 8.6 weeks compared to the placebo group (the group with no supplements). In considering these results, ask yourself, is such a small weight loss what you would expect from a weight-loss supplement?

In another study, researchers reported a slightly greater weight loss.[31] Overweight adults taking 3 grams of chitosan per day experienced a weight loss of 2.8 kg (6 pounds) in 8 weeks compared to the placebo group that gained weight (+0.8 kg, or +1.8 lb). However, participants were not consuming a controlled diet, but were only asked to record their food intake and physical activity. The average weight loss of less than a pound a week was still meager, but many people struggling with obesity might consider it significant—especially if, as indicated in this study, chitosan could help prevent further weight gain over time.

To learn more about the specific effects of chitosan, researchers at the University of California at Davis[32] studied its fat-trapping capacity in college students. They fed twelve men and twelve women a controlled diet for 4 days, followed by the same diet plus chitosan for 4 days. Fecal samples were collected to determine the amount of fat trapped by chitosan. They found that, with the control diet plus chitosan, fecal fat excretion increased by 1.8 g/day (16 kcal/day) for the men and 0.0 g/day for the women. They concluded that the amount of fat trapped by chitosan was clinically insignificant and that 7 weeks of supplementation (at 2.5 g/day) would be required for a 1-pound weight loss.

Are There Any Side Effects?

The most common side effects experienced by individuals using chitosan are gastrointestinal distress and flatulence. Also, some product formulations contain ingredients such as caffeine, herbs, and other substances that may cause problems in some people. Because chitosan is derived from shellfish, individuals who are allergic to shellfish should not use these products.

You Be the Judge

A quick Internet search reveals that chitosan-containing products range widely in price from five to forty dollars or more for a one-month supply. Would you want to try this product to prevent weight gain? How much is a potential weight loss of less than a pound a week worth to you?

Chapter Review

Test Yourself ANSWERS

1. True. Although eating too much fat, or too much of unhealthful fats (such as saturated and *trans* fatty acids), can increase our risk for diseases such as cardiovascular disease and obesity, some fats are essential to good health. We need to consume a certain minimum amount to provide adequate levels of essential fatty acids and fat-soluble vitamins.

2. True. Fat is our primary source of energy, both at rest and during low- and moderate-intensity exercise. Fat is also an important fuel source during prolonged exercise. During periods of high-intensity exercise, carbohydrate becomes the dominant fuel source.

3. False. Even foods fried in vegetable shortening can be unhealthful because they are higher in *trans* fatty acids. In addition, fried foods are high in fat and energy and can contribute to overweight and obesity.

Find the Quack

Like everyone else in his family, Luiz is overweight. In addition, both of Luiz's parents take prescription medications to manage their high blood pressure, and his paternal grandfather died at age 42 from a heart attack. Understandably, Luiz is concerned about his own risk for cardiovascular disease. On this morning's news broadcast, the health segment discusses the Dr. Dean Ornish Diet. It is supposed to be designed specifically for people at risk for cardiovascular disease. Luiz learns that the diet consists of the following:

- "Abundant consumption of legumes, fruits, vegetables, and whole grains"
- "Moderate consumption of nonfat dairy products and nonfat or very-low-fat processed foods (such as nonfat yogurt bars, very-low-fat frozen dinners, and so on)"
- "Avoidance of all of the following: meats, oils, oil-containing products (such as margarines and salad dressings), avocados, nuts, seeds, alcohol, and sugars (including honey, molasses, and high-fructose corn syrup)"
- "Adding 30 minutes a day of moderate physical activity or three 1-hour sessions per week"

The TV health segment states that the Dr. Dean Ornish Diet has been proven in clinical studies to reduce the risk factors for cardiovascular disease.

1. Compare the Dr. Dean Ornish Diet to the MyPlate graphic (fig. 2.5) in Chapter 2. What are the main similarities? What are the main differences you see?
2. Comment on the level of essential fatty acids the Dr. Dean Ornish Diet provides.
3. Based on the diet's recommendations, how much total fat do you think this diet provides?
4. Do you think the Dr. Dean Ornish Diet is a quack diet or a legitimate diet? If legitimate, do you think it is advisable for someone with a family history of cardiovascular disease, such as Luiz? Why or why not?

Answers can be found on the companion website at www.pearsonhighered.com/thompsonmanore.

NutriTools

Check out the companion website at www.pearsonhighered.com/thompsonmanore, or use MyNutritionLab.com, to access interactive animations, including:

- Know Your Fat Sources
- Digestion and Absorption

Review Questions

1. Omega-3 fatty acids are
   a. a form of *trans* fatty acid.
   b. metabolized in the body to arachidonic acid.
   c. synthesized in the liver and small intestine.
   d. found in leafy green vegetables, flaxseeds, soy milk, and fish.
2. One of the most sensible ways to reduce body fat is to
   a. limit intake of fat to less than 15% of total energy consumed.
   b. exercise regularly.
   c. avoid all consumption of *trans* fatty acids.
   d. restrict total Calories to 1,200 per day.
3. Fats in chylomicrons are taken up by cells with the help of
   a. lipoprotein lipase.
   b. micelles.
   c. sterols.
   d. pancreatic enzymes.
4. The risk for heart disease is increased in people who
   a. consume a diet high in saturated fats.
   b. consume a diet high in *trans* fats.
   c. consume a diet high in animal fats.
   d. all of the above.
5. Triglycerides with a double bond at one part of the molecule are referred to as
   a. monounsaturated fats.
   b. hydrogenated fats.
   c. saturated fats.
   d. sterols.
6. True or false? The Acceptable Macronutrient Distribution Range (AMDR) for fat is 20–35% of total energy.
7. True or false? During exercise, fat cannot be mobilized from adipose tissue for use as energy.
8. True or false? Triglycerides are the same as fatty acids.
9. True or false? *Trans* fatty acids are produced by food manufacturers; they do not occur in nature.
10. True or false? A serving of food labeled *reduced fat* has at least 25% less fat and 25% fewer Calories than a full-fat version of the same food.

Answers to Review Questions can be found at the back of this text, and additional essay questions and answers are located on the companion website at www.pearsonhighered.com/thompsonmanore.

Web Resources

www.americanheart.org
American Heart Association

Learn the best way to help lower your blood cholesterol level. Access the AHA's online cookbook for healthy-heart recipes and cooking methods.

www.caloriecontrol.org
Calorie Control Council

Go to this site to find out more about fat replacers.

www.nhlbi.nih.gov/chd
Live Healthier, Live Longer

Take a cholesterol quiz, and test your heart disease IQ. Create a diet using the Heart Healthy Diet or the TLC Diet online software.

www.nhlbi.nih.gov
National Heart, Lung, and Blood Institute

Learn how a healthful diet can lower your cholesterol levels. Use the online risk assessment tool to estimate your 10-year risk of having a heart attack.

www.nih.gov
The National Institutes of Health (NIH), U.S. Department of Health and Human Services

Search this site to learn more about dietary fats.

www.nlm.nih.gov/medlineplus
MEDLINE Plus Health Information

Search for "fats" or "lipids" to obtain additional resources and the latest news on dietary lipids, heart disease, and cholesterol.

www.hsph.harvard.edu/nutritionsource
The Nutrition Source: Knowledge for Healthy Eating Harvard School of Public Health

Go to this site and click on "Fats & Cholesterol" to find out how selective fat intake can be part of a healthful diet.

www.ific.org
International Food Information Council Foundation

Access this site to find out more about fats and dietary fat replacers.

NutriTools

See live updates of Nutrition Facts based on your selections!

Build a Pizza

Nutrition Facts

Serving Size 1 Slice

Amount Per Serving

Calories 250	Calories from Fat 116

	% Daily Value**
Total Fat 13g	**20%**
Saturated Fat 6g	**30%**
Monosaturated Fat 6g	**2**
Polyunsaturated Fat 4g	
Cholesterol 28mg	**1%**
Sodium 596mg	**25%**
Potassium 149mg	**<1%**
Total Carbohydrate 208g	**17%**
Dietary Fiber 1g	**1%**
Sugars 2g	
Protein 15g	**<1%**

Vitamin A	**14%**	•	Vitamin C	**0%**
Calcium	**38%**	•	Iron	**0%**
Thiamin	**13%**	•	Riboflavin	**15%**
Niacin	**1%**	•	Folate	**14%**
Vitamin B6	**0%**	•	Vitamin B12	**2%**

** Percent Daily Values (DV) are based on a 2,000 calorie diet. Your daily values may be higher or lower depending on your calorie needs.

Ingredients

Thin White Crust, Tomato Sauce, Extra Pepperoni, Olives

Calories	7 kcal	Sodium	24 mg
Total Fat	.1 g	Total Carb.	0 g
Cholesterol	0 mg	Protein	.9 g

Nutritional Score

Could be better — Good — Highly Nutritous

▶ Thick Wheat Crust	▶ Thin Wheat Crust	▶ Thick White Crust	✓ Thin White Crust

◀ | Crust | Meat | Cheese | Vegetables | Sauce | ▶ | ↻ Reset Activity

Build a virtual pizza by choosing food icons in many combinations!

Learn the nutritional values of your food choices as you build them!

Score your pizza's nutritional value!

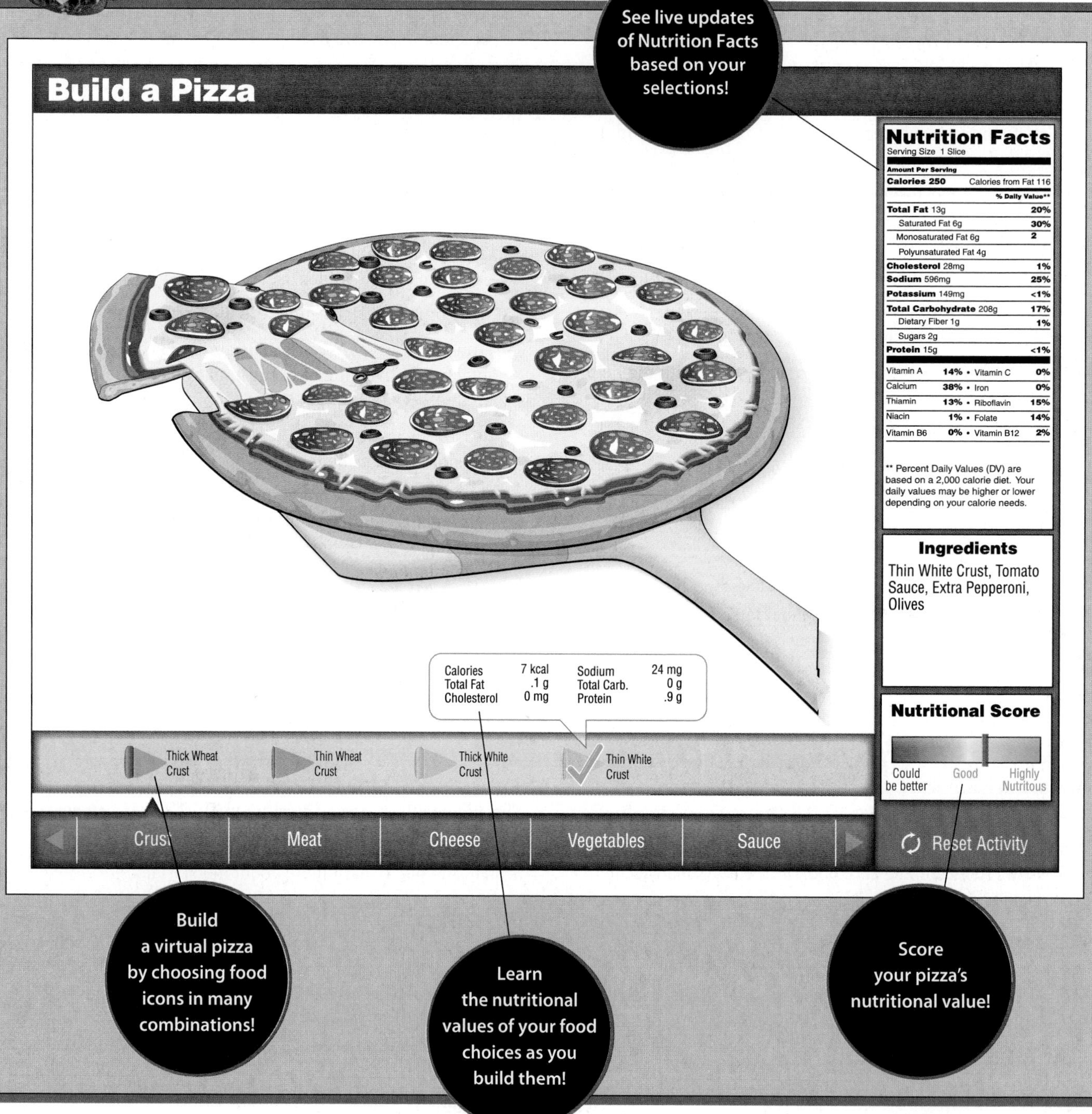

To build your pizza, just visit www.pearsonhighered.com/thompsonmanore **or** www.mynutritionlab.com

After building your pizza, you should be able to answer these questions:

1. How would you know if your pizza is "junk food" or a nutritious meal?
2. What toppings could you add to your pizza to make it highly nutritious?
3. In what ways is whole-wheat crust better than white crust?
4. How can you build a lowfat, nutritious pizza that also tastes good?
5. Which sauce and topping combinations can give you the best nutritional score?

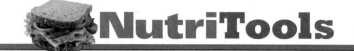

Cardiovascular Disease

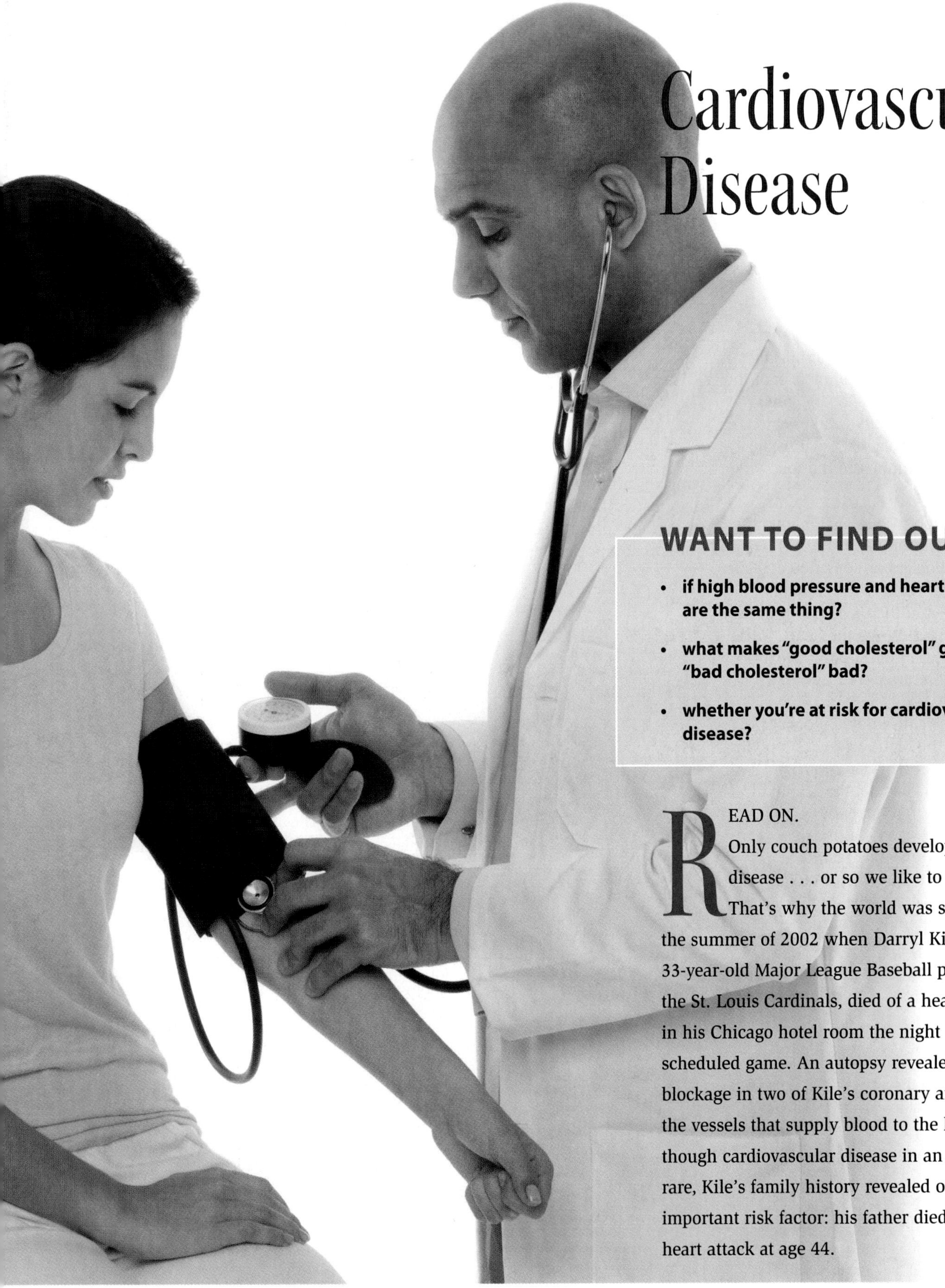

WANT TO FIND OUT. . .

- **if high blood pressure and heart disease are the same thing?**
- **what makes "good cholesterol" good and "bad cholesterol" bad?**
- **whether you're at risk for cardiovascular disease?**

READ ON.

Only couch potatoes develop heart disease . . . or so we like to think. That's why the world was stunned in the summer of 2002 when Darryl Kile, a 33-year-old Major League Baseball pitcher for the St. Louis Cardinals, died of a heart attack in his Chicago hotel room the night before a scheduled game. An autopsy revealed a 90% blockage in two of Kile's coronary arteries—the vessels that supply blood to the heart. Although cardiovascular disease in an athlete is rare, Kile's family history revealed one very important risk factor: his father died of a heart attack at age 44.

What causes a heart attack? Are genetics always to blame? If you have a family history of cardiovascular disease, is there anything you can do to reduce your risk? We explore these questions *In Depth* here.

What Is Cardiovascular Disease?

Cardiovascular disease is a general term used to refer to any abnormal condition involving dysfunction of the heart (*cardio-* means "heart") and blood vessels (*vasculature*). There are many forms of this disease, but the three most common are the following:

- *Coronary heart disease* occurs when blood vessels supplying the heart (the *coronary arteries*) become blocked or constricted; such blockage reduces the flow of blood—and the oxygen and nutrients it carries—to the heart. This can result in chest pain, called *angina pectoris*, and lead to a heart attack.
- *Stroke* is caused by a blockage of one of the blood vessels supplying the brain (the *cerebral arteries*). When this occurs, the region of the brain that depends on that artery for oxygen and nutrients cannot function. As a result, the movement, speech, or other body functions controlled by that part of the brain suddenly stop.
- *Hypertension*, also called *high blood pressure*, is a condition that may not cause any symptoms, but it increases your risk for a heart attack or stroke. If your blood pressure is high, it means that the force of the blood flowing through your arteries is above normal.

To understand cardiovascular disease, we need to look at a condition called *atherosclerosis*, which is responsible for the blockage of arteries that leads to heart attacks and strokes. What's more, hypertension is often a sign of underlying atherosclerosis. So let's take a closer look.

Atherosclerosis Is Narrowing of Arteries

Atherosclerosis is a disease in which arterial walls accumulate deposits of lipids and scar tissue that build up to such a degree that they impair blood flow. It's a complex process that begins with injury to the cells that line the insides of all arteries. Factors that commonly promote such injury are the forceful pounding of blood under high pressure and blood-vessel damage from irritants, such as the nicotine in tobacco or the excessive blood glucose in people with poorly controlled diabetes. Whatever the cause, the injury leads to vessel inflammation, which is increasingly being recognized as an important marker of cardiovascular disease.[1] Inflamed vessels become weakened, allowing lipids, mainly cholesterol, to seep through the layers of the vessel wall and eventually become trapped in thick, grainy deposits called *plaque*. The term *atherosclerosis* reflects the presence of these deposits: *athere* is a Greek word meaning "a thick porridge."

As plaques form, they narrow the interior of the blood vessel **(Figure 1)**. This slowly diminishes the blood supply to any tissues "downstream." As a result, these tissues—including heart muscle—wither, and gradually lose their ability to function. Alternatively, the blockage may occur suddenly, because a plaque ruptures and *platelets*,

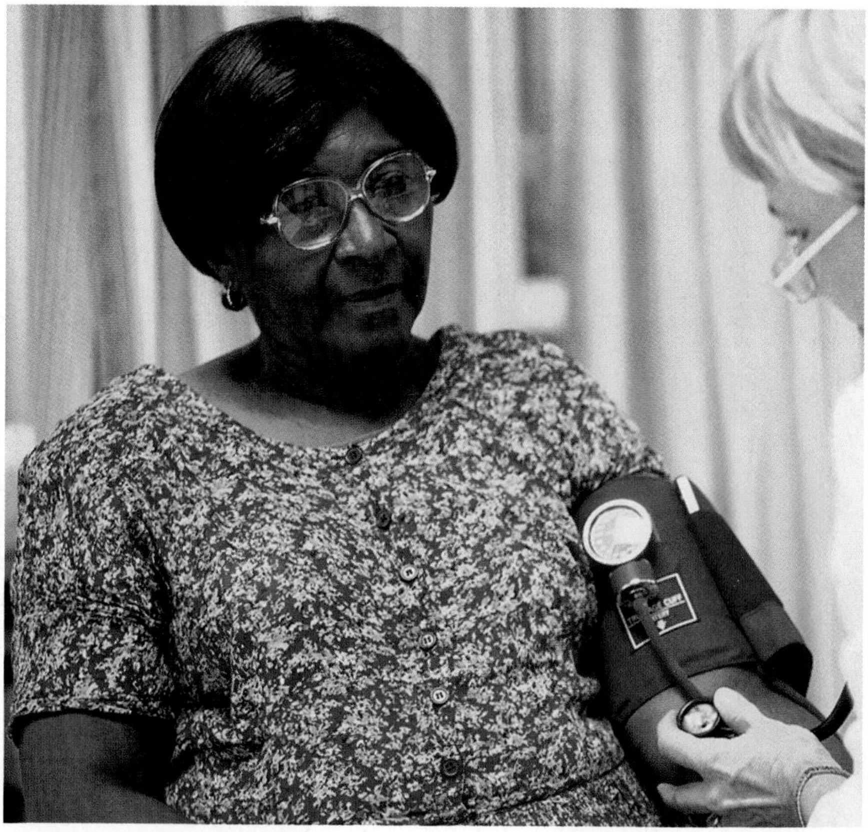

Hypertension is a major chronic disease in the United States, affecting more than 50% of adults over 65 years old.

cardiovascular disease A general term that refers to abnormal conditions involving dysfunction of the heart and blood vessels; cardiovascular disease can result in heart attack or stroke.

atherosclerosis A condition characterized by accumulation of deposits of lipids and scar tissue on artery walls. These deposits build up to such a degree that they impair blood flow.

TABLE 1 The DASH Eating Plan

Food Group	Daily Servings	Amount per Serving
Grains and grain products	7–8	1 slice bread 1 cup ready-to-eat cereal* 1/2 cup cooked rice, pasta, or cereal
Vegetables	4–5	1 cup raw leafy vegetables 1/2 cup cooked vegetable 6 fl. oz vegetable juice
Fruits	4–5	1 medium fruit 1/4 cup dried fruit 1/2 cup fresh, frozen, or canned fruit 6 fl. oz fruit juice
Low-fat or fat-free dairy foods	2–3	8 fl. oz milk 1 cup yogurt 1 1/2 oz cheese
Lean meats, poultry, and fish	2 or less	3 oz cooked lean meats, skinless poultry, or fish
Nuts, seeds, and dry beans	4–5 per week	1/3 cup or 1 1/2 oz nuts 1 tbsp. or 1/2 oz seeds 1/2 cup cooked dry beans
Fats and oils†	2–3	1 tsp. soft margarine 1 tbsp. low-fat mayonnaise 2 tbsp. light salad dressing 1 tsp. vegetable oil
Sweets	5 per week	1 tbsp. sugar 1 tbsp. jelly or jam 1/2 oz jelly beans 8 fl. oz lemonade

Note: The plan is based on 2,000-kcal/day. The number of servings in a food group may differ from the number listed, depending on your own energy needs.

*Serving amounts vary between 1/2 cup and 1 1/4 cups. Check the product's nutrition label.

†Fat content changes serving counts for fats and oils: for example, 1 tbsp. of regular salad dressing equals 1 serving; 1 tbsp. of a low-fat dressing equals 1/2 serving; 1 tablespoon of a fat-free dressing equals 0 servings.

Data from National Institutes of Health. Healthier Eating with DASH. www.nhlbi.nih.gov/health/public/heart/hbp/dash/new_dash.pdf.

pressure. When this is the case, a variety of medications can be prescribed. Some inhibit the body's production of cholesterol. Others prevent bile acids from being reabsorbed in the GI tract. Since bile is made from cholesterol, blocking its reabsorption means the liver must draw on cholesterol stores to make more. Diuretics may be prescribed to flush excess water and sodium from the body, reducing blood pressure. Other hypertension medications work to relax the blood vessel walls, giving more room for blood flow. Individuals taking such medications should also continue to practice the lifestyle changes listed earlier in this section, as these changes will continue to benefit their long-term health.

Web Resources

www.americanheart.org
American Heart Association

Learn the best way to help lower your blood cholesterol level. Access the AHA's online cookbook for healthy-heart recipes and cooking methods.

www.nhlbi.nih.gov
National Heart, Lung, and Blood Institute

Use this online risk assessment tool to estimate your 10-year risk of having a heart attack.

www.nlm.nih.gov/medlineplus
MEDLINE Plus Health Information

Find the latest news on dietary lipids and cardiovascular disease.

6 Proteins: Crucial Components of All Body Tissues

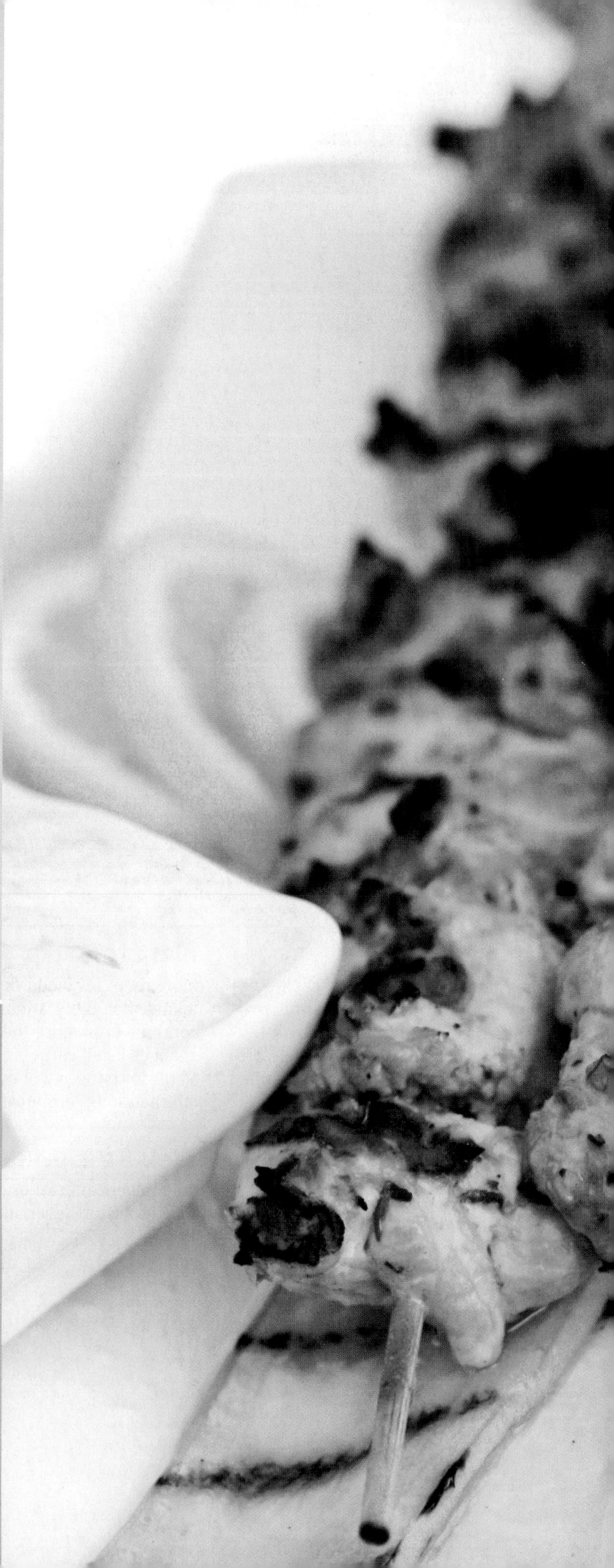

CHAPTER OBJECTIVES

After reading this chapter you will be able to:

1. Describe how proteins differ from carbohydrates and fats, p. 186.
2. Identify non-meat food combinations that are complete protein sources, pp. 192–193.
3. Describe four functions of proteins in our bodies, pp. 193–197.
4. Discuss how proteins are digested, absorbed, and synthesized by our bodies, pp. 197–199.
5. Calculate your recommended daily allowance for protein, p. 201.
6. List five foods that are good sources of protein, pp. 202–205.
7. Identify the potential health risks associated with high-protein diets, pp. 210–211.
8. Describe two disorders related to inadequate protein intake, pp. 211–212.

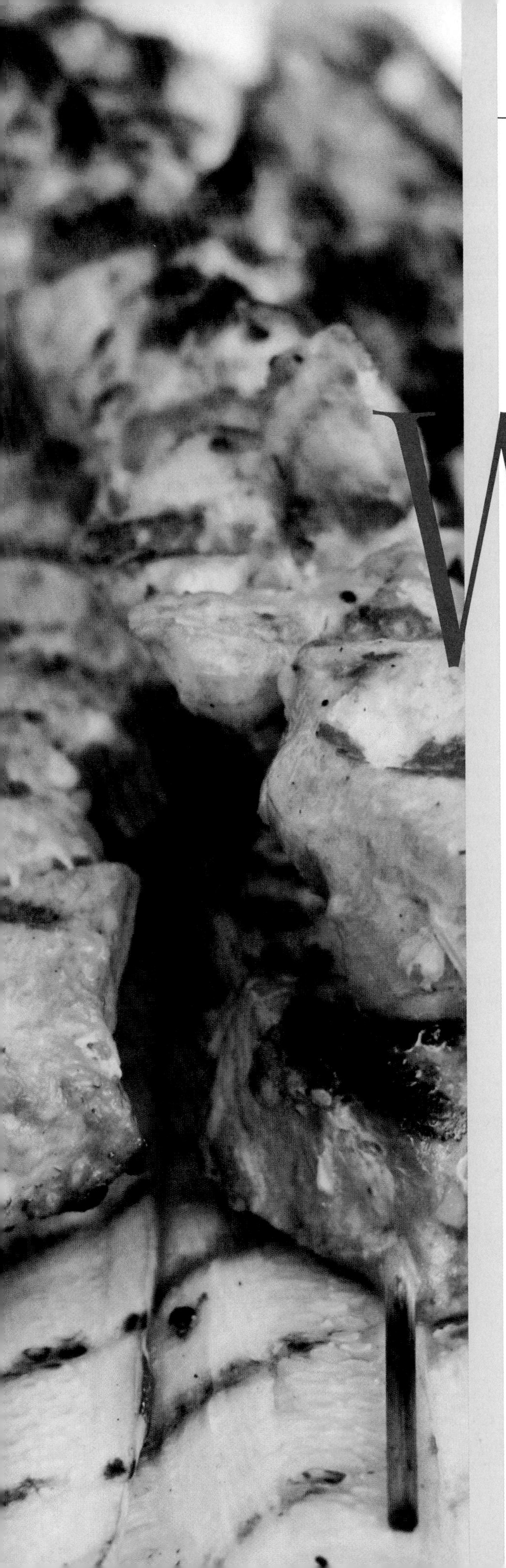

Test Yourself

1. T F Protein is a primary source of energy for our bodies.
2. T F Vegetarian diets are inadequate in protein.
3. T F Most people in the United States consume more protein than they need.

Test Yourself answers can be found at the end of the chapter.

What do professional skateboarder Forrest Kirby, Olympic figure skating champion Surya Bonaly, wrestler "Killer" Kowalski, and hundreds of other athletes have in common? They're all vegetarians! Olympic track icon Carl Lewis states: "I've found that a person does not need protein from meat to be a successful athlete. In fact, my best year of track competition was the first year I ate a vegan diet."[1] Although precise statistics on the number of vegetarian American athletes aren't available, a total of 3% of the U.S. population—approximately 6 to 8 million American adults—are estimated to be vegetarians.[2]

What is a protein, and what makes it so different from carbohydrates and fats? How much protein do you really need, and do you get enough in your daily diet? What exactly is a vegetarian, anyway? Do you qualify? If so, how do you plan your diet to include sufficient protein, especially if you play competitive sports? Are there real advantages to eating meat, or is plant protein just as good?

It seems as if everybody has an opinion about protein, both how much you should consume and from what sources. In this chapter, we'll address these and other questions to clarify the importance of protein in the diet and dispel common myths about this crucial nutrient.

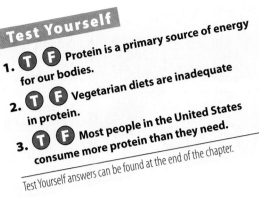

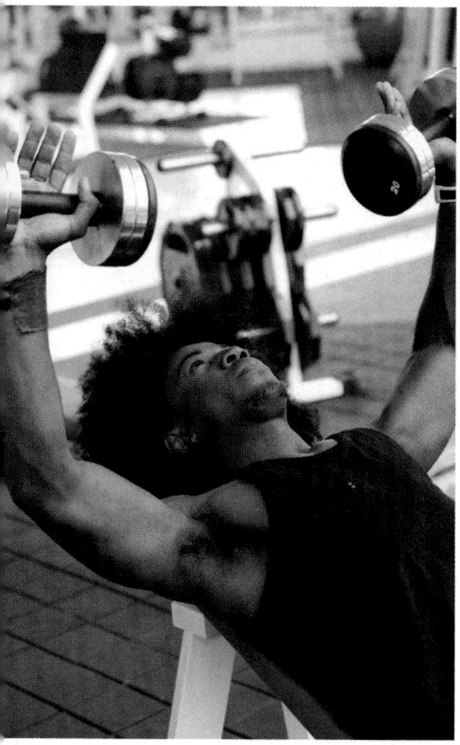

Proteins are an integral part of our body tissues, including our muscle tissue.

What Are Proteins?

Proteins are large, complex molecules found in the cells of all living things. Although proteins are best known as a part of our muscle mass, they are, in fact, critical components of all the tissues of the human body, including bones, blood, and skin. Proteins also function in metabolism, immunity, fluid balance, and nutrient transport, and they can provide energy in certain circumstances. The functions of proteins will be discussed in detail later in this chapter.

How Do Proteins Differ from Carbohydrates and Lipids?

As we saw in Chapter 1, proteins are one of the three macronutrients. Like carbohydrates and lipids, proteins are found in a wide variety of foods; plus, the human body is able to synthesize them. But unlike carbohydrates and lipids, proteins are made according to instructions provided by our genetic material, or DNA. We'll explore how DNA dictates the structure of proteins shortly.

Another key difference between proteins and the other macronutrients lies in their chemical makeup. In addition to the carbon, hydrogen, and oxygen also found in carbohydrates and lipids, proteins contain a special form of nitrogen that our bodies can readily use. Our bodies are able to break down the proteins in foods and utilize the nitrogen for many important processes. Carbohydrates and lipids do not provide nitrogen.

The Building Blocks of Proteins Are Amino Acids

The proteins in our bodies are made from a combination of building blocks called **amino acids,** molecules composed of a central carbon atom connected to four other groups: an amine group, an acid group, a hydrogen atom, and a side chain **(Figure 6.1a)**. The word *amine* means nitrogen-containing, and nitrogen is indeed the essential component of the amine portion of the molecule.

As shown in Figure 6.1b, the portion of the amino acid that makes each unique is its side chain. The amine group, acid group, and carbon and hydrogen atoms do not vary. Variations in the structure of the side chain give each amino acid its distinct properties.

The singular term *protein* is misleading, as there are potentially an infinite number of unique types of proteins in living organisms. Most of the proteins in our bodies are made from combinations of just twenty amino acids, identified in **Table 6.1**. By

proteins Large, complex molecules made up of amino acids and found as essential components of all living cells.

amino acids Nitrogen-containing molecules that combine to form proteins.

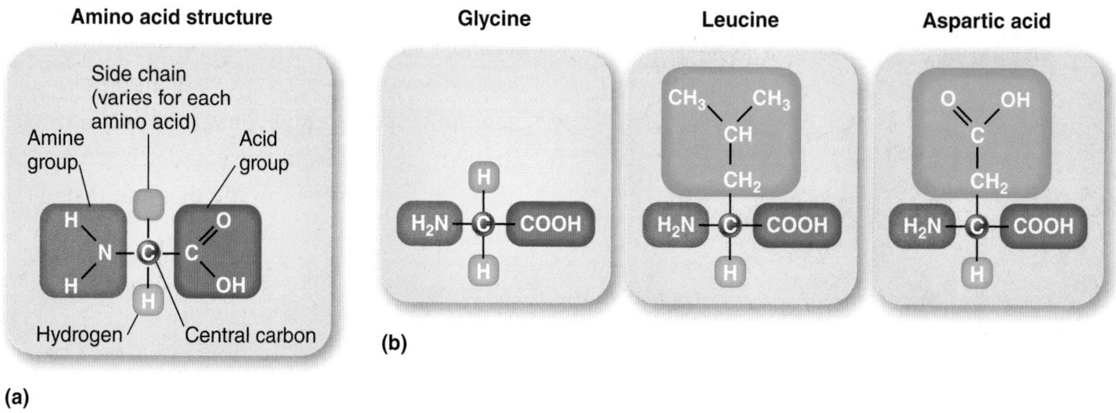

Figure 6.1 Structure of an amino acid. **(a)** All amino acids contain five parts: a central carbon atom, an amine group around the atom that contains nitrogen, an acid group, a hydrogen atom, and a side chain. **(b)** Only the side chain differs for each of the twenty amino acids, giving each its unique properties.

combining a few dozen to more than 300 copies of these twenty amino acids in various sequences, our bodies form an estimated 10,000 to 50,000 unique proteins. Two of the twenty amino acids listed in Table 6.1, cysteine and methionine, are unique in that, in addition to the components present in the other amino acids, they contain sulfur.

TABLE 6.1 Amino Acids of the Human Body

Essential Amino Acids	Nonessential Amino Acids
These amino acids must be consumed in the diet.	*These amino acids can be manufactured by the body.*
Histidine	Alanine
Isoleucine	Arginine
Leucine	Asparagine
Lysine	Aspartic acid
Methionine	Cysteine
Phenylalanine	Glutamic acid
Threonine	Glutamine
Tryptophan	Glycine
Valine	Proline
	Serine
	Tyrosine

We Must Obtain Essential Amino Acids from Food

Of the twenty amino acids in our bodies, nine are classified as essential. This does not mean that they are more important than the others. Instead, an **essential amino acid** is one that our bodies cannot produce at all or cannot produce in sufficient quantities to meet our physiologic needs. Thus, we must obtain essential amino acids from our food. Without the proper amount of essential amino acids in our bodies, we lose our ability to make the proteins and other nitrogen-containing compounds we need.

The Body Can Make Nonessential Amino Acids

Nonessential amino acids are just as important to our bodies as essential amino acids, but our bodies can make them in sufficient quantities, so we do not need to consume them in our diet. We make nonessential amino acids by transferring the amine group from an essential amino acid to a different acid group and side chain. This process is called **transamination,** and it is shown in **Figure 6.2**. The acid groups and side chains can be donated by amino acids, or they can be made from the breakdown products of carbohydrates and fats. Thus, by combining parts of different amino acids, the nonessential amino acids can be made.

Under some conditions, a nonessential amino acid can become an essential amino acid. In this case, the amino acid is called a *conditionally essential amino acid.* Consider what occurs in the disease known as phenylketonuria (PKU). As discussed in Chapter 4, someone with PKU cannot metabolize phenylalanine (an essential amino acid). Normally, the body uses phenylalanine to produce the nonessential amino acid tyrosine, so the inability to metabolize phenylalanine results in failure to make tyrosine. If PKU is not diagnosed immediately after birth, it results in irreversible brain damage. In this situation, tyrosine becomes a conditionally essential amino acid that must be provided by the diet. Other conditionally essential amino acids include arginine, cysteine, and glutamine.

RECAP Proteins are critical components of all the tissues of the human body. Like carbohydrates and lipids, they contain carbon, hydrogen, and oxygen. Unlike the other macronutrients, they also contain nitrogen and some contain sulfur, and their structure is dictated by DNA. The building blocks of proteins are amino acids. The amine group of the amino acid contains nitrogen. The portion of the amino acid that changes, giving each amino acid its distinct identity, is the side chain. The body cannot make essential amino acids, so we must obtain them from our diet. Our bodies can make nonessential amino acids from parts of other amino acids, carbohydrates, and fats.

essential amino acids Amino acids not produced by the body that must be obtained from food.

nonessential amino acids Amino acids that can be manufactured by the body in sufficient quantities and therefore do not need to be consumed regularly in our diet.

transamination The process of transferring the amine group from one amino acid to another in order to manufacture a new amino acid.

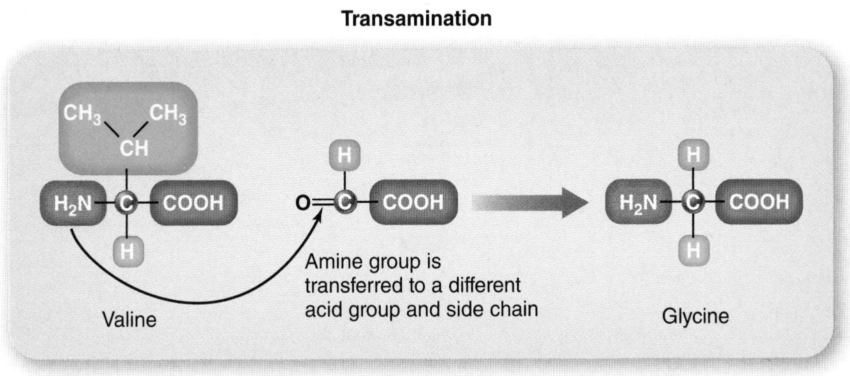

Figure 6.2 Transamination. Our bodies can make nonessential amino acids by transferring the amine group from an essential amino acid to a different acid group and side chain.

How Are Proteins Made?

As we have stated, our bodies can synthesize proteins by selecting the needed amino acids from the pool of all amino acids available at any given time. Let's look more closely at how this occurs.

Amino Acids Bond to Form a Variety of Peptides

Figure 6.3 shows that, when two amino acids join together, the amine group of one binds to the acid group of another in a unique type of chemical bond called a **peptide bond.** In the process, a molecule of water is released as a by-product.

Two amino acids joined together form a *dipeptide,* and three amino acids joined together are called a *tripeptide.* The term *oligopeptide* is used to identify a string of four to nine amino acids, while a *polypeptide* is ten or more amino acids bonded together. As a polypeptide chain grows longer, it begins to fold into any of a variety of complex shapes that give proteins their sophisticated structure.

Genes Regulate Amino Acid Binding

Each of us is unique because we inherited a specific genetic "code" that integrates the code from each of our parents. Each person's genetic code dictates minor differences in amino acid sequences, which in turn lead to differences in our bodies' individual proteins. These differences in proteins result in the unique physical and physiologic characteristics each one of us possesses.

As mentioned earlier, DNA dictates the structure of each protein our bodies synthesize. **Figure 6.4** shows how this process occurs. Cells use segments of DNA called *genes* as templates for assembling—or *expressing*—particular proteins. Thus, this process is referred to as **gene expression.** Since proteins are manufactured at the site of ribosomes in the cytoplasm, and DNA never leaves the nucleus, a special molecule is needed to copy, or transcribe, the information from DNA and carry it to the ribosome. This is the job of *messenger RNA* (*messenger ribonucleic acid,* or *mRNA*); during **transcription,** mRNA copies the genetic information from DNA in the nucleus and carries it to the ribosomes in the cytoplasm. Once this genetic information is at the ribosome, **translation** occurs: genetic information from the mRNA is translated into a growing chain of amino acids that are bonded together to make a specific protein.

Although the DNA for making every protein in our bodies is contained within each cell nucleus, not all genes are expressed and each cell does not make every type of protein. For example, each cell contains the DNA to manufacture the hormone insulin. However, only the cells of the pancreas express the insulin gene; that is, they are the only cells that produce insulin. Our physiologic needs alter gene expression, as do various nutrients. For instance, a cut in the skin that causes bleeding leads to the production of various proteins that clot the blood. If we consume more dietary iron than we need, the gene for ferritin (a protein that stores iron) is expressed, so

peptide bonds Unique types of chemical bonds in which the amine group of one amino acid binds to the acid group of another in order to manufacture dipeptides and all larger peptide molecules.

gene expression The process of using a gene to make a protein.

transcription The process through which messenger RNA copies genetic information from DNA in the nucleus.

translation The process that occurs when the genetic information carried by messenger RNA is translated into a chain of amino acids at the ribosome.

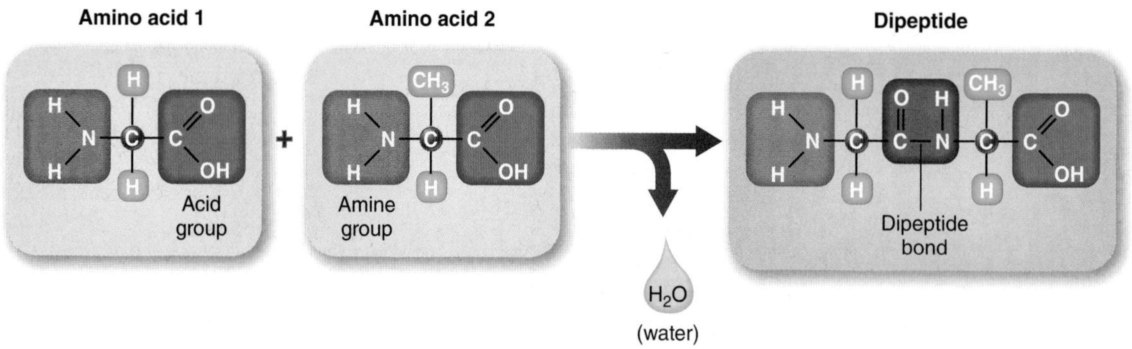

Figure 6.3 Amino acid bonding. Two amino acids join together to form a dipeptide. By combining multiple amino acids, proteins are made.

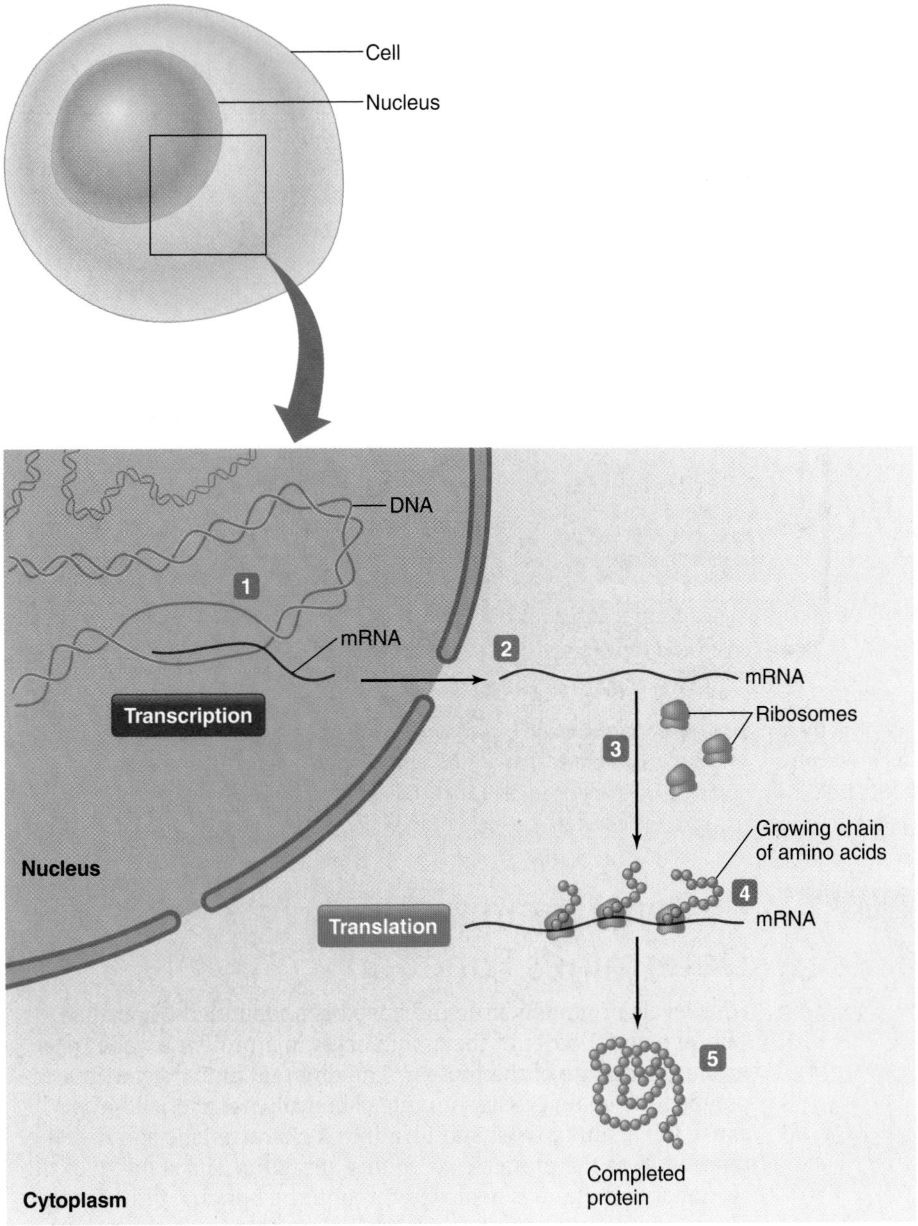
Cell
Nucleus
DNA
1
mRNA
2
mRNA
Transcription
Ribosomes
3
Growing chain
of amino acids
4
Nucleus
Translation
mRNA
5
Completed
protein
Cytoplasm
1 Part of the DNA unwinds, and a section of its genetic code is transcribed to the mRNA inside the nucleus.
2 The mRNA leaves the nucleus via a nuclear pore and travels to the cytoplasm.
3 Once the mRNA reaches the cytoplasm, it binds to a ribosome. The code on the mRNA is translated into the instructions for a specific order of amino acids.
4 Amino acids are added to the growing amino acid chain, and eventually a complete protein is produced.
5 Once the synthesis of the new protein is complete, the protein is released from the ribosome. The protein may go through further modifications in the cell, or can be functional in its current state.

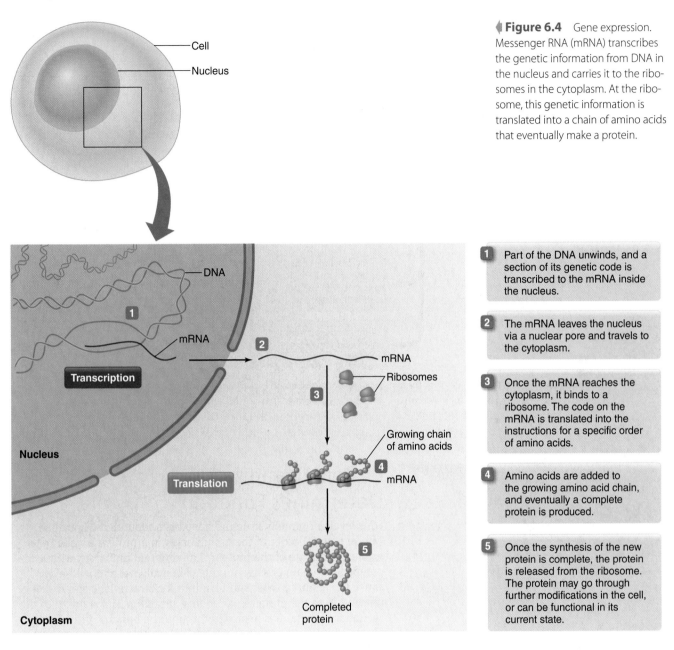

Figure 6.4 Gene expression. Messenger RNA (mRNA) transcribes the genetic information from DNA in the nucleus and carries it to the ribosomes in the cytoplasm. At the ribosome, this genetic information is translated into a chain of amino acids that eventually make a protein.

that we can store this excess iron. Our genetic makeup and how appropriately we express our genes are important factors in our health. The role of dietary factors in gene expression is discussed in more detail in the Chapter 1 Nutrition Debate on page 25.

Protein Turnover Involves Synthesis and Degradation

Our bodies constantly require new proteins to function properly. *Protein turnover* involves both the synthesis of new proteins and the degradation of existing proteins to provide the building blocks for those new proteins (**Figure 6.5**). This process allows the cells to respond to the constantly changing demands of physiologic functions. For instance, skin cells live for only about 30 days and must continually be replaced. The amino acids needed to produce these new skin cells can be obtained from the body's *amino acid pool,* which includes those amino acids we consume in our diet as well as those that are released from the breakdown of other cells in our bodies. The body's pool of amino acids is used to produce not only new amino acids but also other products, including glucose and fat.

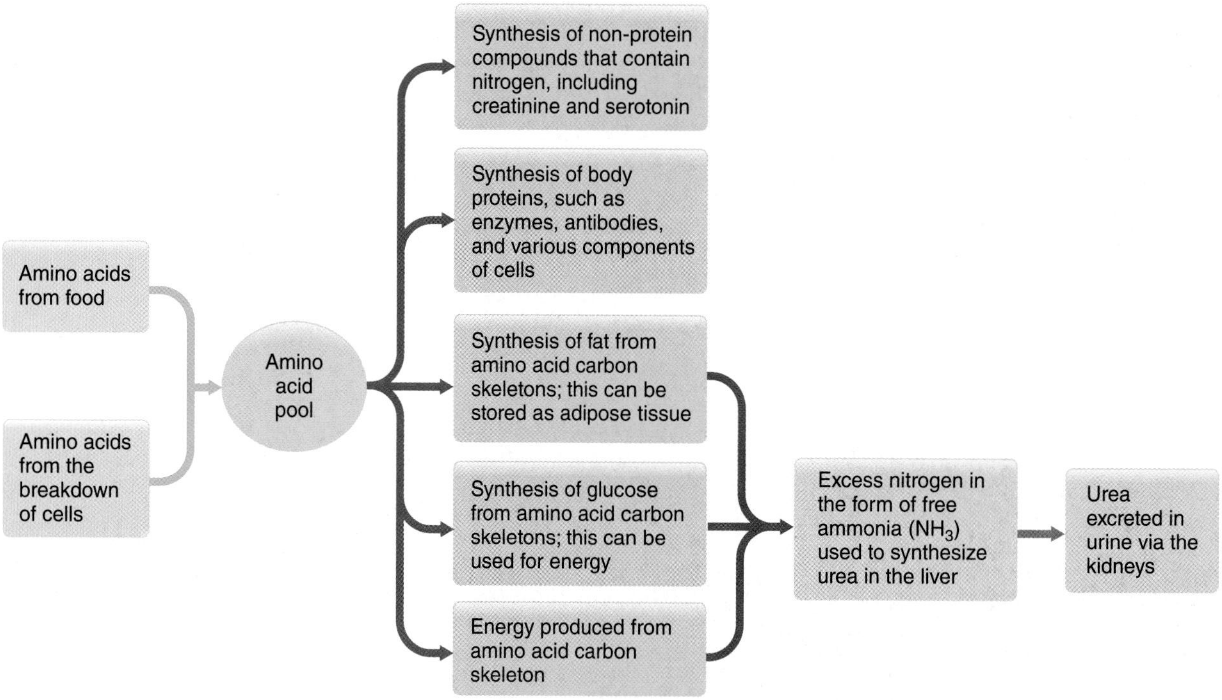

Figure 6.5 Protein turnover involves the synthesis of new proteins and breakdown of existing proteins to provide building blocks for new proteins. Amino acids are drawn from the body's amino acid pool and can be used to build proteins, fat, glucose, and non-protein nitrogen-containing compounds. Urea is produced as a waste product from any excess nitrogen, which is then excreted by the kidneys.

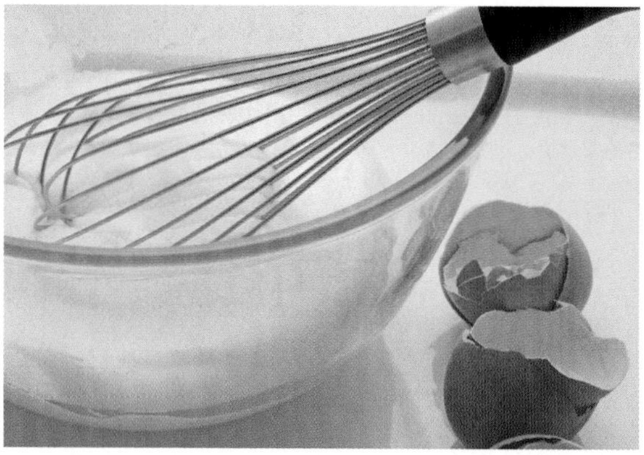

Stiffening egg whites denatures some of the proteins within them.

Protein Organization Determines Function

Four levels of protein structure have been identified **(Figure 6.6)**. The sequential order of the amino acids in a protein is called the *primary structure* of the protein. The different amino acids in a polypeptide chain possess unique chemical characteristics that cause the chain to twist and turn into a characteristic spiral shape, referred to as the protein's *secondary structure*. The stability of the secondary structure is achieved through the bonding of hydrogen atoms or sulfur atoms; these bonds create a bridge between two protein strands or two parts of the same strand of protein. The spiral of the secondary structure further folds into a unique three-dimensional shape, referred to as the protein's *tertiary structure;* this structure is critically important because it determines each protein's function in the body. Often, two or more separate polypeptides bond to form an even larger protein with a *quaternary structure*, which may be *globular* or *fibrous*.

The importance of the shape of a protein to its function cannot be overemphasized. For example, the protein strands in muscle fibers are much longer than they are wide (see Figure 6.6d). This structure plays an essential role in enabling muscle contraction and relaxation. In contrast, the proteins that form red blood cells are globular in shape, and they result in the red blood cells being shaped like flattened discs with depressed centers, similar to a miniature doughnut **(Figure 6.7)**. This structure and the flexibility of the proteins in the red blood cells permit them to change shape and flow freely through even the tiniest capillaries to deliver oxygen and still return to their original shape.

denaturation The process by which proteins uncoil and lose their shape and function when they are exposed to heat, acids, bases, heavy metals, alcohol, and other damaging substances.

Proteins can uncoil and lose their shape when they are exposed to heat, acids, bases, heavy metals, alcohol, and other damaging substances. The term used to describe this change in the shape of proteins is **denaturation.** Everyday examples of protein denaturation that we can see are the stiffening of egg whites when they are

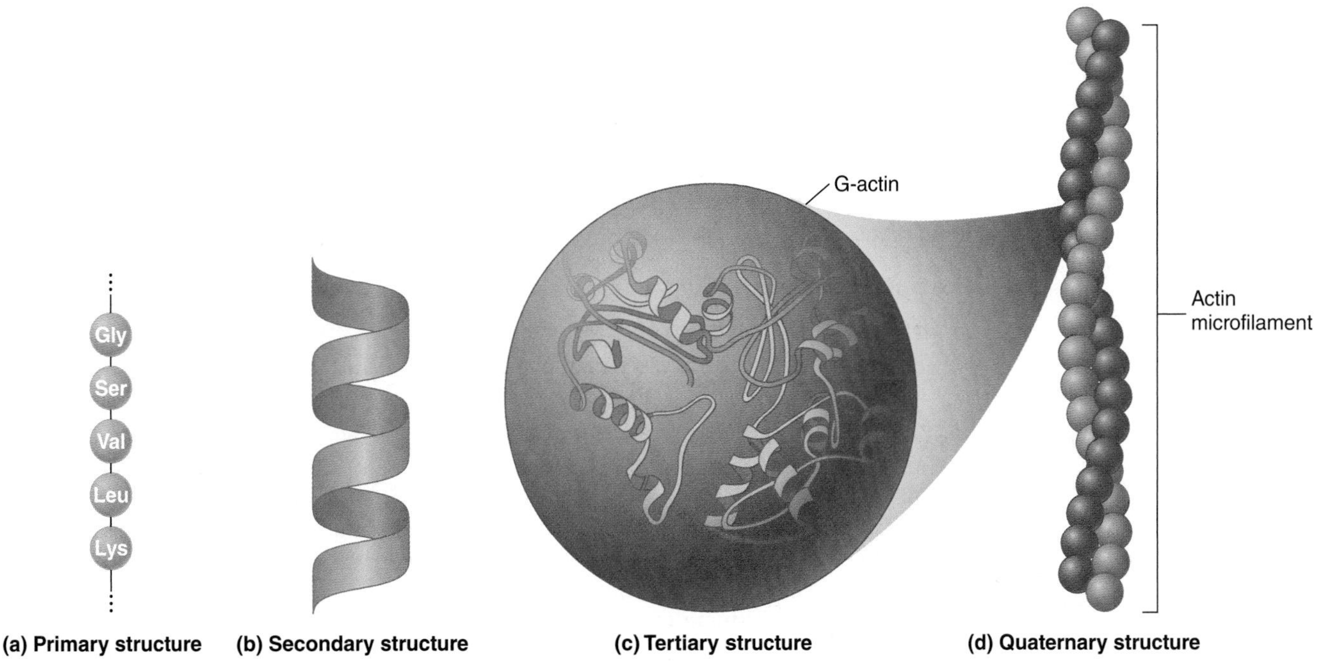

Figure 6.6 Levels of protein structure. **(a)** The primary structure of a protein is the sequential order of amino acids. **(b)** The secondary structure of a protein is the folding of the amino acid chain. **(c)** The tertiary structure is a further folding that results in the three-dimensional shape of the protein. **(d)** The quaternary structure of a protein refers to molecules containing two or more polypeptides that bond to form a larger protein, such as the actin molecule illustrated here. In this figure, strands of actin molecules intertwine to form contractile elements involved in generating muscle contractions.

whipped, the curdling of milk when lemon juice or another acid is added, and the solidifying of eggs as they cook.

Denaturation does not affect the primary structure of proteins. However, when a protein is denatured, its function is lost. For instance, denaturation of a critical enzyme on exposure to heat or acidity is harmful, because it prevents the enzyme from doing its job. This type of denaturation can occur during times of high fever or when the level of acid in the blood is out of the normal range. In some cases, denaturation

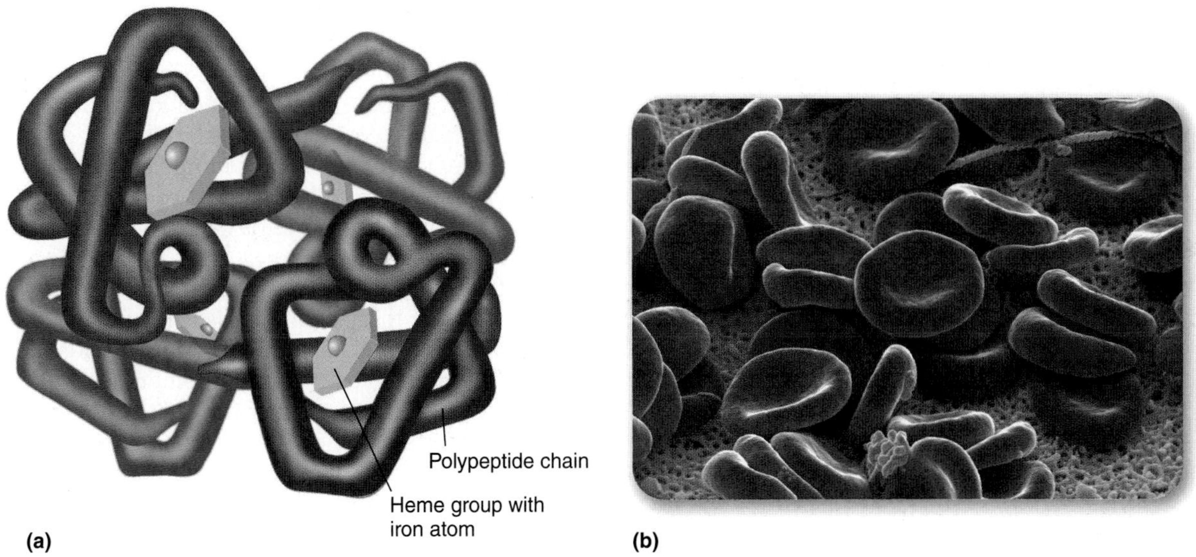

Figure 6.7 Protein shape determines function. **(a)** Hemoglobin, the protein that forms red blood cells, is globular in shape. **(b)** The globular shape of hemoglobin results in red blood cells being shaped like flattened discs.

is helpful. For instance, denaturation of proteins during the digestive process allows for their breakdown into amino acids and the absorption of these amino acids from the digestive tract into the bloodstream.

RECAP **Amino acids bind together to form proteins. Genes regulate the amino acid sequence, and thus the structure, of all proteins. The shape of a protein determines its function. When a protein is denatured by damaging substances, such as heat and acids, it loses its shape and its function.**

Protein Synthesis Can Be Limited by Missing Amino Acids

For protein synthesis to occur, all essential amino acids must be available to the cell. If this is not the case, the amino acid that is missing or in the smallest supply is called the **limiting amino acid.** Without the proper combination and quantity of essential amino acids, protein synthesis slows to the point at which proteins cannot be generated. For instance, the protein hemoglobin contains the essential amino acid histidine. If we do not consume enough histidine, it becomes the limiting amino acid in hemoglobin production. As no other amino acid can be substituted, our bodies become unable to make adequate hemoglobin, and we lose the ability to transport oxygen to our cells.

Inadequate energy consumption also limits protein synthesis. If there is not enough energy available from our diets, our bodies will use any accessible proteins for energy, thus preventing them from being used to build new proteins.

A protein that does not contain all of the essential amino acids in sufficient quantities to support growth and health is called an **incomplete** (*low-quality*) **protein.** Proteins that have all nine of the essential amino acids are considered **complete** (*high-quality*) **proteins.** The most complete protein sources are foods derived from animals and include egg whites, meat, poultry, fish, and milk. Soybeans are the most complete source of plant protein. In general, the typical American diet is very high in complete proteins, as we eat proteins from a variety of food sources.

Protein Synthesis Can Be Enhanced by Mutual Supplementation

Many people believe that we must consume meat or dairy products to obtain complete proteins. Not true! Consider a meal of beans and rice. Beans are low in the amino acids methionine and cysteine but have adequate amounts of isoleucine and lysine. Rice is low in isoleucine and lysine but contains sufficient methionine and cysteine. By combining beans and rice, we create a complete protein.

Mutual supplementation is the process of combining two or more incomplete protein sources to make a complete protein. The two foods involved are called complementary foods; these foods provide **complementary proteins** (**Figure 6.8**), which, when combined, provide all nine essential amino acids.

It is not necessary to eat complementary proteins at the same meal. Recall that we maintain a free pool of amino acids in the blood; these amino acids come from food and sloughed-off cells. When we eat one complementary protein, its amino acids join those in the free amino acid pool. These free amino acids can then combine to synthesize complete proteins. However, it is wise to eat complementary-protein foods during the same day, as partially completed proteins cannot be stored and saved for a later time. Mutual supplementation is important for people eating a vegetarian diet, particularly if they consume no animal products whatsoever.

RECAP **When a particular amino acid is limiting, protein synthesis cannot occur. A complete protein provides all nine essential amino acids. Mutual supplementation combines two complementary-protein sources to make a complete protein.**

limiting amino acid The essential amino acid that is missing or in the smallest supply in the amino acid pool and is thus responsible for slowing or halting protein synthesis.

incomplete proteins Foods that do not contain all of the essential amino acids in sufficient amounts to support growth and health.

complete proteins Foods that contain all nine essential amino acids.

mutual supplementation The process of combining two or more incomplete protein sources to make a complete protein.

complementary proteins Two or more foods that together contain all nine essential amino acids necessary for a complete protein. It is not necessary to eat complementary proteins at the same meal.

Food with limiting amino acid	+	Foods high in limiting amino acid	→	Complementary food combination
Legumes: limited in methionine and cysteine	+	**Grains** **Nuts and Seeds**	→	• Red beans and rice • Rice and lentils • Rice and black-eyed peas • Hummus (garbanzo beans and sesame seeds)
Grains: limited in lysine	+	**Legumes**	→	• Peanut butter and bread • Barley and lentil soup • Corn tortilla and beans
Vegetables: limited in lysine, methionine, and cysteine	+	**Legumes** (lysine) **Grains** (methionine and cysteine) **Nuts and Seeds** (methionine and cysteine)	→	• Tofu and broccoli with almonds • Spinach salad with pine nuts and kidney beans
Nuts and Seeds: limited in lysine and isoleucine	+	**Legumes**	→	• Lentil soup with slivered almonds • Sesame seeds with mixed bean salad

Figure 6.8 Complementary food combinations.

Why Do We Need Proteins?

The functions of proteins in the body are so numerous that only a few can be described in detail in this chapter. Note that proteins function most effectively when we also consume adequate amounts of energy as carbohydrates and fat. When there is not enough energy available, the body uses proteins as an energy source, limiting their availability for the functions described in this section.

Proteins Contribute to Cell Growth, Repair, and Maintenance

The proteins in our bodies are dynamic, meaning that they are constantly being broken down, repaired, and replaced. When proteins are broken down, many amino acids are recycled into new proteins. Think about all of the new proteins that are needed to allow an infant to develop and grow into a mature adult.

Even in adulthood, our cells are constantly turning over, as damaged or worn-out cells are broken down and their components are used to create new cells. Our red blood cells live for only 3 to 4 months and then are replaced by new cells that are produced in bone marrow. The cells lining our intestinal tract are replaced every 3 to 6 days. The "old" intestinal cells are treated just like the proteins in food; they are digested and the amino acids absorbed back into the body. The constant turnover of proteins from our diet is essential for such cell growth, repair, and maintenance.

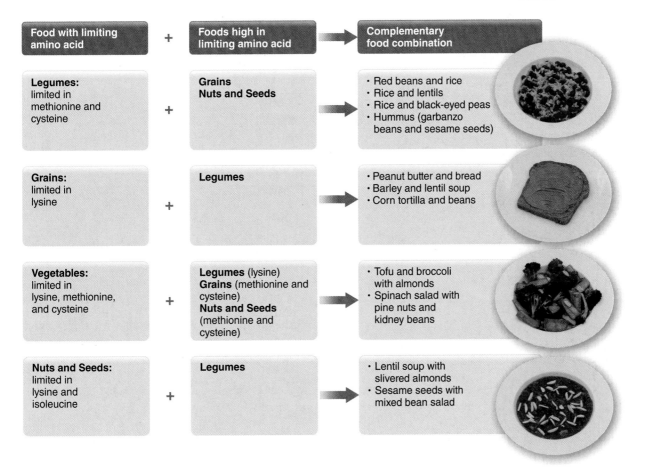

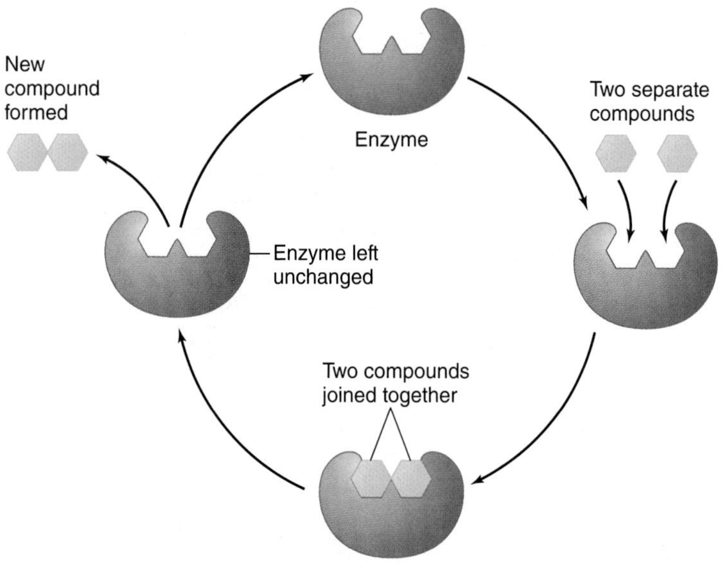

Figure 6.9 Proteins act as enzymes. Enzymes facilitate chemical reactions, such as joining two compounds together.

Proteins Act as Enzymes and Hormones

As you learned in Chapter 3, enzymes are compounds, usually proteins, that speed up chemical reactions, without being changed by the chemical reaction themselves. Enzymes can bind substances together or break them apart and can transform one substance into another. **Figure 6.9** shows how an enzyme can bind two substances together.

Each cell contains thousands of enzymes that facilitate specific cellular reactions. For example, the enzyme phosphofructokinase (PFK) is critical to driving the rate at which we break down glucose and use it for energy during exercise. Without PFK, we would be unable to generate energy at a fast enough rate to allow us to be physically active.

Hormones are substances that act as chemical messengers in the body. Some hormones are made from amino acids, whereas others are made from lipids (see Chapter 5, pages 152–153). Hormones are stored in various glands in the body, which release them in response to changes in the body's environment. They then act on the body's organs and tissues to restore the body to normal conditions. For example, recall from Chapter 4 that insulin, a hormone made from amino acids, acts on cell membranes to facilitate the transport of glucose into cells. Other examples of amino acid–containing hormones are glucagon, which responds to conditions of low blood glucose, and thyroid hormone, which helps control our resting metabolic rate.

Proteins Help Maintain Fluid and Electrolyte Balance

Electrolytes are electrically charged particles that assist in maintaining fluid balance. For our bodies to function properly, fluids and electrolytes must be maintained at healthy levels inside and outside cells and within blood vessels. Proteins attract fluids, and the proteins that are in the bloodstream, in the cells, and in the spaces surrounding the cells work together to keep fluids moving across these spaces in the proper quantities to maintain fluid balance and blood pressure. When protein intake is deficient, the concentration of proteins in the bloodstream is insufficient to draw fluid from the tissues and across the blood vessel walls; fluid then collects in the tissues, causing **edema** (**Figure 6.10**). In addition to being uncomfortable, edema can lead to serious medical problems.

Sodium (Na^+) and potassium (K^+) are examples of common electrolytes. Under normal conditions, Na^+ is more concentrated outside the cell, and K^+ is more concentrated inside the cell. This proper balance of Na^+ and K^+ is accomplished by the action of **transport proteins** located within the cell membrane. **Figure 6.11** shows how these transport proteins work to pump Na^+ outside and K^+ inside of the cell. The conduction of nerve signals and contraction of muscles depend on a proper balance of electrolytes. If protein intake is deficient, we lose our ability to maintain these functions, resulting in potentially fatal changes in the rhythm of the heart. Other consequences of chronically low protein intakes include muscle weakness and spasms, kidney failure, and, if conditions are severe enough, death.

edema A disorder in which fluids build up in the tissue spaces of the body, causing fluid imbalances and a swollen appearance.

transport proteins Protein molecules that help transport substances throughout the body and across cell membranes.

pH Stands for percentage of hydrogen. It is a measure of the acidity—or level of hydrogen—of any solution, including human blood.

Proteins Help Maintain Acid–Base Balance

The body's cellular processes result in the constant production of acids and bases. These substances are transported in the blood to be excreted through the kidneys and the lungs. The human body maintains very tight control over the **pH,** or the

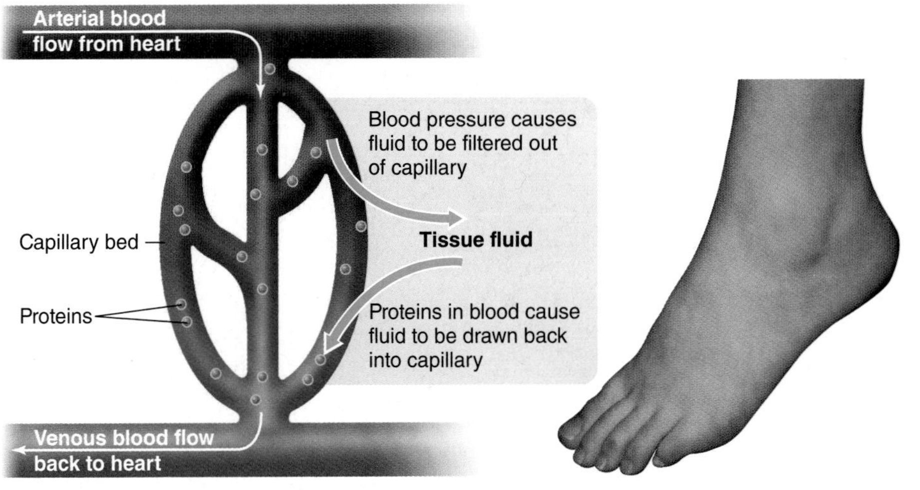
Arterial blood
flow from heart
Blood pressure causes
fluid to be filtered out
of capillary
Capillary bed
Tissue fluid
Proteins
Proteins in blood cause
fluid to be drawn back
into capillary
Venous blood flow
back to heart

(a) Normal fluid balance

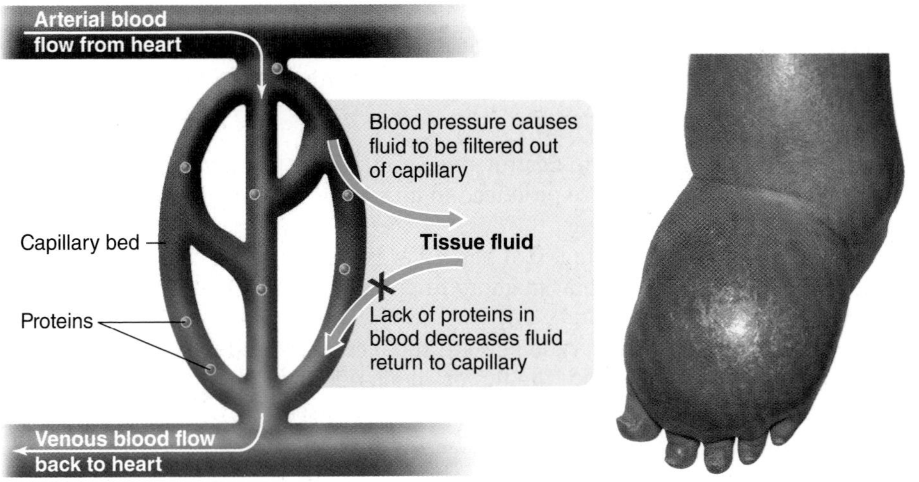
Arterial blood
flow from heart
Blood pressure causes
fluid to be filtered out
of capillary
Capillary bed
Tissue fluid
Proteins
Lack of proteins in
blood decreases fluid
return to capillary
Venous blood flow
back to heart

(b) Edema caused by insufficient protein in bloodstream

Figure 6.10 The role of proteins in maintaining fluid balance. The heartbeat exerts pressure that continually pushes fluids in the bloodstream through the arterial walls and out into the tissue spaces. By the time blood reaches the veins, the pressure of the heartbeat has greatly decreased. In this environment, proteins in the blood are able to draw fluids out of the tissues and back into the bloodstream. **(a)** This healthy (non-swollen) tissue suggests that body fluids in the bloodstream and in the tissue spaces are in balance. **(b)** When the level of proteins in the blood is insufficient to draw fluids out of the tissues, edema can result. This foot with edema is swollen due to fluid imbalance.

acid–base balance, of the blood. The body goes into a state called **acidosis** when the blood becomes too acidic. **Alkalosis** results if the blood becomes too basic (alkaline). Both acidosis and alkalosis can be caused by respiratory or metabolic problems. Acidosis and alkalosis can cause coma and death by denaturing body proteins.

Proteins are excellent **buffers,** meaning that they help maintain proper acid–base balance. Acids contain hydrogen ions, which are positively charged. The side chains of proteins have negative charges that attract the hydrogen ions and neutralize their detrimental effects on the body. Proteins can release the hydrogen ions when the blood becomes too basic. By buffering acids and bases, proteins maintain acid–base balance and blood pH.

Proteins Help Maintain a Strong Immune System

Antibodies are special proteins that are critical components of the immune system. When a foreign substance attacks the body, the immune system produces antibodies to defend against it. Bacteria, viruses, toxins, and allergens (substances that cause allergic reactions) are examples of antigens that can trigger antibody production. (An *antigen* is any substance—but typically a protein—that our bodies recognize as foreign and that triggers an immune response.)

acidosis A disorder in which the blood becomes acidic; that is, the level of hydrogen in the blood is excessive. It can be caused by respiratory or metabolic problems.

alkalosis A disorder in which the blood becomes basic; that is, the level of hydrogen in the blood is deficient. It can be caused by respiratory or metabolic problems.

buffers Proteins that help maintain proper acid–base balance by attaching to, or releasing, hydrogen ions as conditions change in the body.

antibodies Defensive proteins of the immune system. Their production is prompted by the presence of bacteria, viruses, toxins, allergens, and so on.

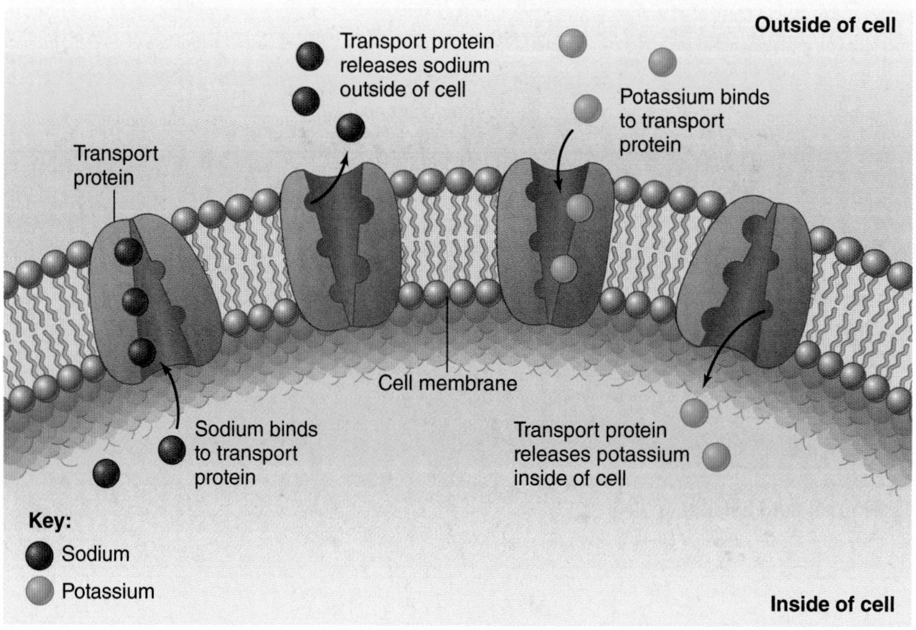

Figure 6.11 Transport proteins help maintain electrolyte balance. Transport proteins in the cell membrane pick up potassium and sodium and transport them across the cell membrane.

Each antibody is designed to destroy one specific invader. When that substance invades the body, antibodies are produced to attack and destroy the specific antigen. Once antibodies have been made, the body "remembers" this process and can respond more quickly the next time that particular invader appears. *Immunity* refers to the development of the molecular memory to produce antibodies quickly upon subsequent invasions.

Adequate protein is necessary to support the increased production of antibodies that occurs in response to a cold, the flu, or an allergic reaction. If we do not consume enough protein, our resistance to illnesses and disease is weakened. On the other hand, eating more protein than we need does not improve immune function.

Proteins Serve as an Energy Source

The body's primary energy sources are carbohydrate and fat. Remember that both carbohydrate and fat have specialized storage forms that can be used for energy—glycogen for carbohydrate and triglycerides for fat. Proteins do not have a specialized storage form for energy. This means that, when proteins need to be used for energy, they are taken from the blood and body tissues, such as the liver and skeletal muscle. In healthy people, proteins contribute very little to energy needs. Because we are efficient at recycling amino acids, protein needs are relatively low as compared to needs for carbohydrate and fat.

To use proteins for energy, the liver removes the amine group from the amino acids in a process called **deamination.** The nitrogen bonds with hydrogen, creating ammonia, which is quickly converted to *urea*. The urea is then transported to the kidneys, where it is excreted in the urine. The remaining fragments of the amino acid contain carbon, hydrogen, and oxygen. The body can use these fragments to generate energy or to build carbohydrates. Certain amino acids can be converted into glucose via gluconeogenesis. This is a critical process during times of low carbohydrate intake or starvation. Fat cannot be converted into glucose, but body proteins can be broken down and converted into glucose to provide needed energy to the brain.

deamination The process by which an amine group is removed from an amino acid. The nitrogen is then transported to the kidneys for excretion in the urine, while the carbon and other components are metabolized for energy or used to make other compounds.

To protect the proteins in our body tissues, it is important that we regularly eat an adequate amount of carbohydrate and fat to provide energy. We also need to consume enough dietary protein to perform the required work without using up the proteins that already are playing an active role in our bodies. Unfortunately, our bodies cannot store excess dietary protein. As a consequence, eating too much protein results in the removal and excretion of the nitrogen in the urine and the use of the remaining components for energy. Any remaining components not used for energy can be converted and stored as body fat.

RECAP **Proteins serve many important functions, including (1) enabling the growth, repair, and maintenance of body tissues; (2) acting as enzymes and hormones; (3) maintaining fluid and electrolyte balance; (4) maintaining acid–base balance; (5) making antibodies, which strengthen our immune system; and (6) providing energy when carbohydrate and fat intake are inadequate. Proteins function best when we also consume adequate amounts of carbohydrate and fat.**

How Do Our Bodies Break Down Proteins?

Our bodies do not directly use proteins from the diet to make the proteins we need. Dietary proteins are first digested and broken into smaller particles, such as amino acids, dipeptides, and tripeptides, so that they can be absorbed and transported to the cells. In this section, we will review how proteins are digested and absorbed. As you read about each step in this process, refer to **Figure 6.12** for a visual tour through the digestive system.

Stomach Acids and Enzymes Break Proteins into Short Polypeptides

Virtually no enzymatic digestion of proteins occurs in the mouth. As shown in step 1 in Figure 6.12, proteins in food are chewed, crushed, and moistened with saliva to ease swallowing and to increase the surface area of the protein for more efficient digestion. There is no further digestive action on proteins in the mouth.

When proteins reach the stomach, *hydrochloric acid* denatures the protein strands (Figure 6.12, step 2). It also converts the inactive enzyme *pepsinogen* into its active form, **pepsin.** Although pepsin is itself a protein, it is not denatured by the acid in the stomach because it has evolved to work optimally in an acidic environment. The hormone *gastrin* controls both the production of hydrochloric acid and the release of pepsin; thinking about food or actually chewing food stimulates the gastrin-producing cells located in the stomach. Pepsin begins breaking proteins into single amino acids and shorter polypeptides; these amino acids and polypeptides then travel to the small intestine for further digestion and absorption.

Enzymes in the Small Intestine Break Polypeptides into Single Amino Acids

As the polypeptides reach the small intestine, the pancreas and the small intestine secrete enzymes that digest them into oligopeptides, tripeptides, dipeptides, and single amino acids (Figure 6.12, step 3). The enzymes that digest proteins in the small intestine are called **proteases.**

The cells in the wall of the small intestine then absorb the single amino acids, dipeptides, and tripeptides. Enzymes in the intestinal cells break the dipeptides and tripeptides into single amino acids. The amino acids are then transported via the portal vein into the liver. Once in the liver, amino acids may be converted to glucose or fat, combined to build new proteins, used for energy, or released into the bloodstream and transported to other cells as needed (Figure 6.12, step 4).

pepsin An enzyme in the stomach that begins the breakdown of proteins into shorter polypeptide chains and single amino acids.

proteases Enzymes that continue the breakdown of polypeptides in the small intestine.

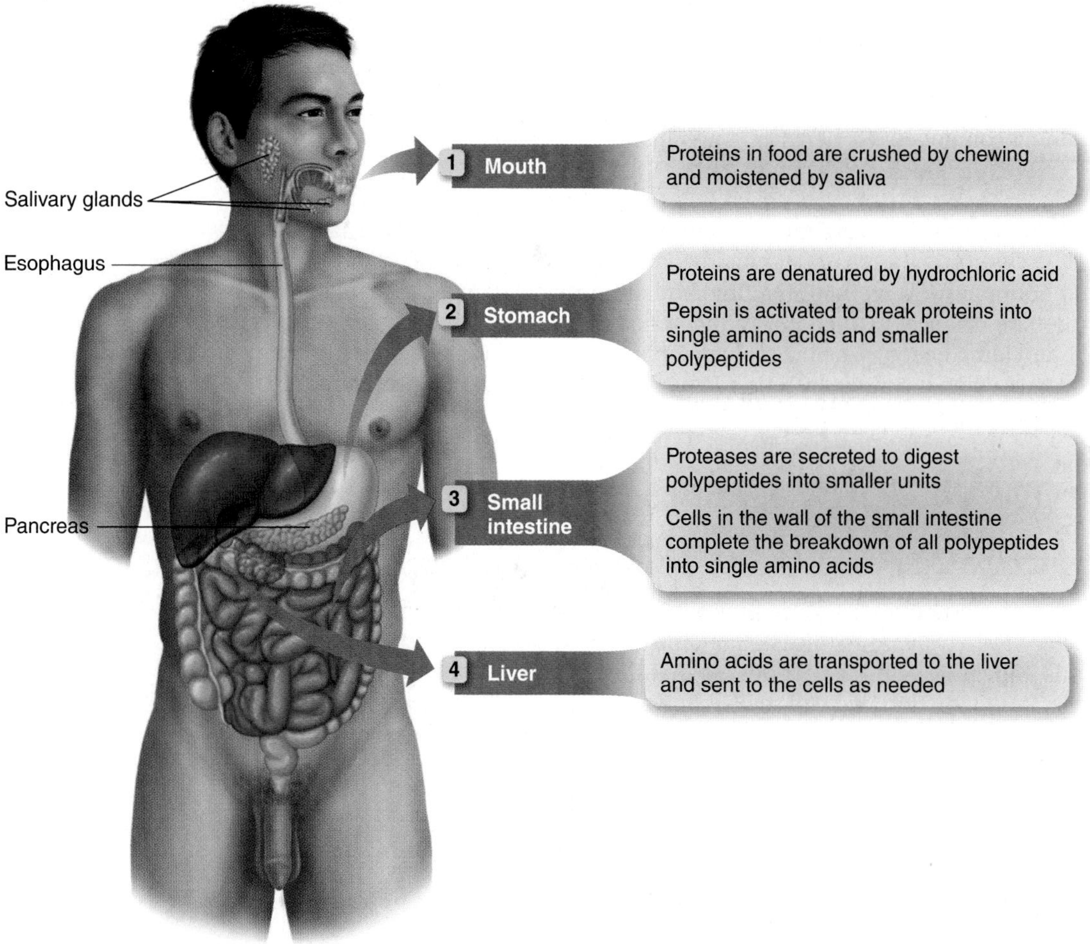
Salivary glands
Esophagus
Pancreas
1 Mouth
Proteins in food are crushed by chewing and moistened by saliva
2 Stomach
Proteins are denatured by hydrochloric acid
Pepsin is activated to break proteins into single amino acids and smaller polypeptides
3 Small intestine
Proteases are secreted to digest polypeptides into smaller units
Cells in the wall of the small intestine complete the breakdown of all polypeptides into single amino acids
4 Liver
Amino acids are transported to the liver and sent to the cells as needed

Figure 6.12 The process of protein digestion.

The cells of the small intestine have different sites that specialize in transporting certain types of amino acids, dipeptides, and tripeptides. This fact has implications for users of amino acid supplements. When very large doses of single amino acids are taken on an empty stomach, they typically compete for the same absorption sites. This competition can block the absorption of other amino acids, causing an imbalance of amino acids and leading to various amino acid deficiencies. Some people believe that this is why it is not beneficial to consume individual amino acid supplements. In reality, people rarely take very large doses of single amino acids on an empty stomach. The primary reason people should not take single amino acids is that the amount taken is usually so small that they don't have any beneficial effect. For more information on amino acid supplements, see Chapter 12.

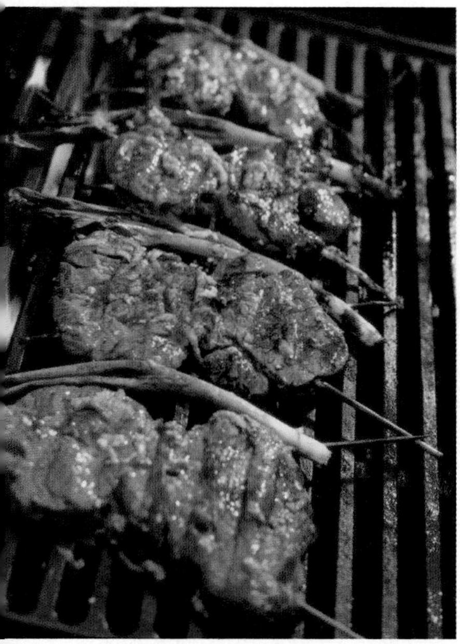

Meats are highly digestible sources of dietary protein.

Protein Digestibility Affects Protein Quality

Earlier in this chapter, we discussed how various protein sources differ in quality of protein. The quantity of essential amino acids in a protein determines its quality: higher-protein-quality foods are those that contain more of the essential amino acids in sufficient quantities needed to build proteins, and lower-quality-protein foods contain fewer essential amino acids. Another factor in protein quality is *digestibility,* or how well our bodies can digest a protein. Animal protein sources, such as meat and dairy products, are highly digestible, as are many soy products; we can absorb more than 90% of the amino acids in these protein sources. Legumes are also highly digestible (about 70% to 80%). Grains and many vegetable proteins are less digestible, ranging from 60% to 90%.

RECAP **In the stomach, hydrochloric acid denatures proteins and converts pepsinogen to pepsin; pepsin breaks proteins into smaller polypeptides and individual amino acids. In the small intestine, proteases break polypeptides into smaller fragments and single amino acids. The cells in the wall of the small intestine break the smaller peptide fragments into single amino acids, which are then transported to the liver for distribution to our cells. Protein digestibility as well as provision of essential amino acids influence protein quality.**

How Much Protein Should We Eat?

Consuming adequate protein is a major concern of many people. In fact, one of the most common concerns among active people and athletes is that their diets are deficient in protein (see the Nutrition Myth or Fact? box below for a discussion of this topic). This concern about dietary protein is generally unnecessary, as we can easily consume the protein our bodies need by eating an adequate and varied diet.

Nitrogen Balance Is a Method Used to Determine Protein Needs

A highly specialized *nitrogen balance* procedure is used to determine a person's protein needs. Nitrogen is excreted through the body's processes of recycling or using proteins; thus, the balance can be used to estimate whether protein intake is adequate to meet protein needs.

Typically performed only in experimental laboratories, the nitrogen balance procedure involves measuring both nitrogen intake and nitrogen excretion over a 2-week

NUTRITION MYTH OR FACT?

Do Athletes Need More Protein than Inactive People?

At one time, it was believed that the Recommended Dietary Allowance (RDA) for protein, which is 0.8 g per kg body weight, was sufficient for both inactive people and athletes. Recent studies, however, show that athletes' protein needs are higher.

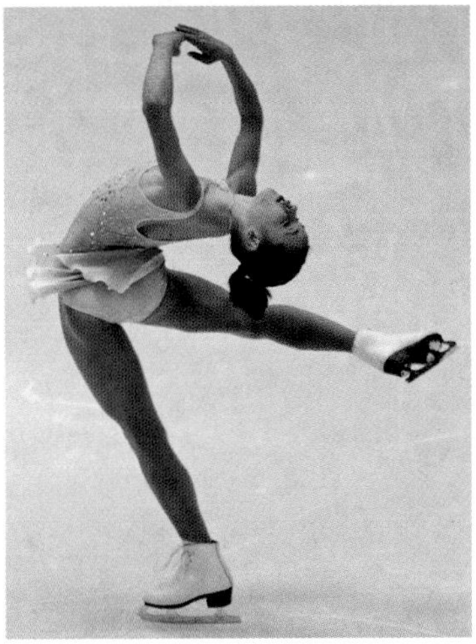

Some athletes who persistently diet are at risk for low protein intake.

Why do athletes need more protein? Regular exercise increases the transport of oxygen to body tissues, requiring changes in the oxygen-carrying capacity of the blood. To carry more oxygen, we need to produce more of the protein that carries oxygen in the blood (i.e., hemoglobin). During intense exercise, we use a small amount of protein directly for energy. We also use protein to make glucose to maintain adequate blood glucose levels and to prevent hypoglycemia (low blood sugar) during exercise. Regular exercise stimulates tissue growth and causes tissue damage, which must be repaired by additional proteins. Strength athletes (such as bodybuilders and weightlifters) need 1.8 to 2 times more protein than the current RDA, and endurance athletes (such as distance runners and triathletes) need 1.5 to 1.75 times more protein than the current RDA. Later in this chapter, we will calculate the protein needs for inactive and active people.

If you're active, does this mean you should add more protein to your diet? Not necessarily. Contrary to popular belief, most Americans, including inactive people *and* athletes, already consume more than twice the RDA for protein. For healthy individuals, evidence does not support eating more than two times the RDA for protein to increase strength, build muscle, or improve athletic performance. In fact, eating more protein as food or supplements or taking individual amino acid supplements does not cause muscles to become bigger or stronger. Only regular strength training can achieve these goals. By eating a balanced diet and consuming a variety of foods, both inactive and active people can easily meet their protein requirements.

period. A standardized diet, the nitrogen content of which has been measured and recorded, is fed to the study participant. The person is required to consume all of the foods provided. Because the majority of nitrogen is excreted in the urine and feces, laboratory technicians directly measure the nitrogen content of the subject's urine and fecal samples. Small amounts of nitrogen are excreted in the skin, hair, and body fluids such as mucus and semen, but, because of the complexity of collecting nitrogen excreted via these routes, the measurements are estimated. Then, technicians add the estimated nitrogen losses to the nitrogen measured in the subject's urine and feces. Nitrogen balance is then calculated as the difference between nitrogen intake and nitrogen excretion.

People who consume more nitrogen than is excreted are considered to be in positive nitrogen balance **(Figure 6.13)**. This state indicates that the body is retaining or

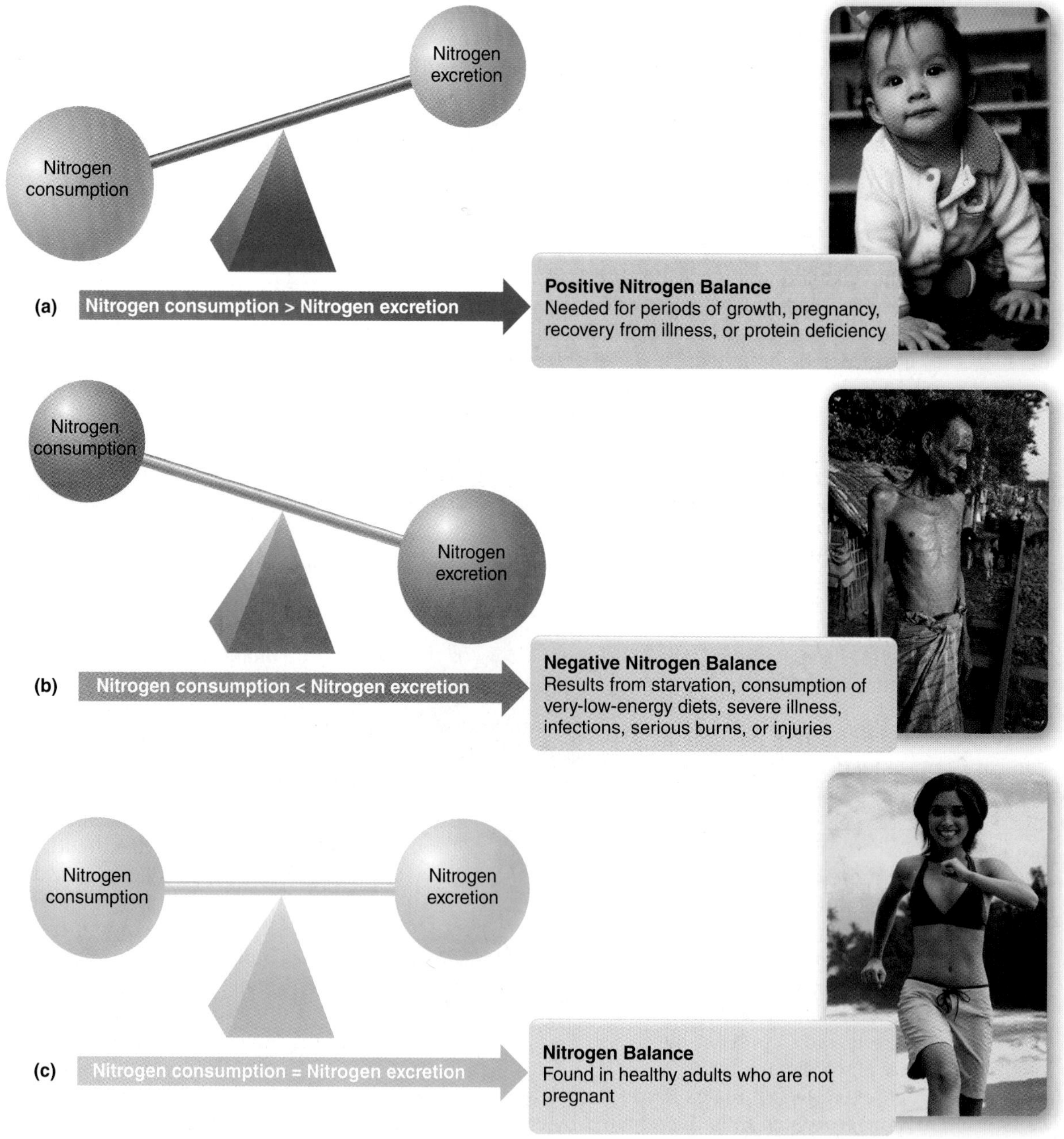
Nitrogen excretion
Nitrogen consumption
(a)
Nitrogen consumption > Nitrogen excretion
Positive Nitrogen Balance
Needed for periods of growth, pregnancy, recovery from illness, or protein deficiency
Nitrogen consumption
Nitrogen excretion
(b)
Nitrogen consumption < Nitrogen excretion
Negative Nitrogen Balance
Results from starvation, consumption of very-low-energy diets, severe illness, infections, serious burns, or injuries
Nitrogen consumption
Nitrogen excretion
(c)
Nitrogen consumption = Nitrogen excretion
Nitrogen Balance
Found in healthy adults who are not pregnant

Figure 6.13 Nitrogen balance describes the relationship between how much nitrogen (or protein) we consume and excrete each day. **(a)** Positive nitrogen balance occurs when nitrogen consumption is greater than excretion. **(b)** Negative nitrogen balance occurs when nitrogen consumption is less than excretion. **(c)** Nitrogen balance is maintained when nitrogen consumption equals excretion.

adding protein, and it occurs during periods of growth, pregnancy, or recovery from illness or a protein deficiency. People who excrete more nitrogen than they consume are in negative nitrogen balance. This situation indicates that the body is losing protein, and it occurs during starvation or when people are consuming very-low-energy diets. This is because, when energy intake is too low to meet energy demands over a prolonged period of time, the body metabolizes body proteins for energy. The nitrogen from these proteins is excreted in the urine and feces. Negative nitrogen balance also occurs during severe illness, infections, high fever, serious burns, or injuries that cause significant blood loss. People in these situations require increased dietary protein. A person is in nitrogen balance when nitrogen intake equals nitrogen excretion. This indicates that protein intake is sufficient to cover protein needs. Healthy adults who are not pregnant are in nitrogen balance.

TABLE 6.2 Recommended Protein Intakes

Group	Protein Intake (grams per kilogram* body weight per day)
Most adults†	0.8
Nonvegetarian endurance athletes‡	1.2 to 1.4
Nonvegetarian strength athletes‡	1.2 to 1.7
Vegetarian endurance athletes‡	1.3 to 1.5
Vegetarian strength athletes‡	1.3 to 1.8

*To convert body weight to kilograms, divide weight in pounds by 2.2.
Weight (lb)/2.2 = Weight (kg)
Weight (kg) × protein recommendation (g/kg body weight/day) = protein intake (g/day)
†Data from Food and Nutrition Board, Institute of Medicine. 2002. *Dietary Reference Intakes for Energy, Carbohydrate, Fiber, Fat, Fatty Acids, Cholesterol, Protein, and Amino Acids (Macronutrients)*, pp. 465–608. Washington, DC: National Academies Press.
‡Data from American College of Sports Medicine, American Dietetic Association, and Dietitians of Canada. 2009. Joint Position Statement. Nutrition and athletic performance. *Med. Sci. Sports Exerc.* 41(3):709–731.

Recommended Dietary Allowance for Protein

How much protein should we eat? The RDA for sedentary people is 0.8 g per kg body weight per day. The recommended percentage of energy that should come from protein is 10% to 35% of total energy intake. Protein needs are higher for children, adolescents, and pregnant/lactating women because more protein is needed during times of growth and development (see Chapters 14 and 15 for details on protein needs during these portions of the life cycle). Protein needs can also be higher for active people and for vegetarians.

Table 6.2 lists the daily recommendations for protein for a variety of lifestyles. How can we convert this recommendation into total grams of protein for the day? In the You Do the Math box, let's calculate Theo's RDA for protein.

Is it possible for Theo to eat this much protein each day? It may surprise you to discover that most Americans eat 1.5 to 2 times the RDA for protein without any effort!

YOU DO THE MATH

Calculating Your Protein Needs

Theo wants to know how much protein he needs each day. During the off-season, he works out three times a week at a gym and practices basketball with friends every Friday night. He is not a vegetarian. Although Theo exercises regularly, he does not qualify as an endurance athlete or as a strength athlete. At this level of physical activity, Theo's RDA for protein probably ranges from the RDA of 0.8 up to 1.0 g per kg body weight per day. To calculate the total number of grams of protein Theo should eat each day:

1. Convert Theo's weight from pounds to kilograms. Theo presently weighs 200 pounds. To convert this value to kilograms, divide by 2.2:

$$200 \text{ pounds} \div 2.2 \text{ pounds/kg} = 91 \text{ kg}$$

2. Multiply Theo's weight in kilograms by his RDA for protein:

$$91 \text{ kg} \times 0.8 \text{ g/kg} = 72.8 \text{ grams of protein per day}$$
$$91 \text{ kg} \times 1.0 \text{ g/kg} = 91 \text{ grams of protein per day}$$

What happens during basketball season, when Theo practices or has games 5 or 6 days a week? This will probably raise his protein needs to approximately 1.0 to 1.2 g per kg body weight per day. How much more protein should he eat?

$$91 \text{ kg} \times 1.2 \text{ g/kg} = 109.2 \text{ grams of protein per day}$$

Now calculate your recommended protein intake based on your activity level.

Most Americans Meet or Exceed the RDA for Protein

Surveys indicate that Americans eat 15–17% of their total daily energy intake as protein.[3–5] In these studies, women reported eating about 65 to 70 g of protein each day, whereas men consumed 88 to 110 g per day. Putting these values into perspective, let's assume that the average man weighs 75 kg (165 pounds) and the average woman weighs 65 kg (143 pounds). Their protein requirements (assuming they are not athletes or vegetarians) are 60 g and 52 g per day, respectively. As you can see, most adults in the United States appear to have no problems meeting their protein needs each day.

What are the typical protein intakes of active people? Research indicates that the self-reported intake of athletes participating in a variety of sports can well exceed current recommendations.[6] For instance, the protein intake for some female distance runners is 1.2 g per kg of body weight per day, accounting for 15% of their total daily energy intake. In addition, some male bodybuilders consume 3 g per kg of body weight per day, accounting for almost 38% of their total daily intake! However, there are certain groups of athletes who are at risk for low protein intakes. Athletes who consume inadequate energy and limit food choices, such as some distance runners, figure skaters, female gymnasts, and wrestlers who are dieting, are all at risk for low protein intakes. Unlike people who consume adequate energy, individuals who are restricting their total energy intake (kilocalories) need to pay close attention to their protein intake.

Protein: Much More Than Meat!

Table 6.3 compares the protein content of a variety of foods. Although some people think that the only good sources of protein are meats (beef, pork, poultry, seafood), many other foods are rich in proteins. These include dairy products (milk, cheese, yogurt, etc.), eggs, legumes (including soy products), whole grains, and nuts. Fruits and many vegetables are not particularly high in protein; however, these foods provide fiber and many vitamins and minerals and are excellent sources of carbohydrates. Thus, eating them can help provide the carbohydrates and energy you need, so that your body can use proteins for building and maintaining tissues.

After reviewing Table 6.3, you might be wondering how much protein you typically eat. See the What About You? feature box on page 204 to find out.

HOT TOPIC

Amino Acid Supplements: Necessity or Waste?

"Amino acid supplements—you can't gain without them!" This is just one of the headlines found in bodybuilding magazines and Internet sites touting amino acid supplements as the key to achieving power, strength, and performance "perfection." Many athletes who read these claims believe that taking amino acid supplements will boost their energy during performance, replace proteins metabolized for energy during exercise, enhance muscle growth and strength, and hasten recovery from intense training or injury. Should you believe the hype?

As noted earlier in this chapter, we use very little protein for energy during exercise, and most Americans already consume more than twice the RDA for protein. Consuming adequate energy and up to two times the RDA for protein in the diet is more than enough to support either strength or endurance exercise training and performance. What about the claims related to muscle-building? Although some research has shown that intravenous infusions of various amino acids in the laboratory can stimulate certain hormones that enhance the building of muscle, there is little evidence that taking individual amino acids or protein supplements orally can build muscle or improve strength.[6] Since these supplements are relatively expensive, getting enough protein via your diet alone will put a lot less strain on your wallet!

TABLE 6.3 Protein Content of Commonly Consumed Foods

Food	Serving Amount	Protein (g)	Food	Serving Amount	Protein (g)
Beef:			*Beans:*		
Ground, lean, baked (15% fat)	3 oz	22	Refried	1/2 cup	7
Prime rib, broiled (1/8-in. fat)	3 oz	18	Kidney, red	1/2 cup	7.7
Top sirloin, broiled (1/8-in. fat)	3 oz	23	Black	1/2 cup	7
Poultry:			*Nuts:*		
Chicken breast, broiled, no skin (bone removed)	1/2 breast	29	Peanuts, dry roasted	1 oz	6.7
Chicken thigh, bone and skin removed	1 thigh	13.5	Peanut butter, creamy	2 tbsp.	8
Turkey breast, roasted, Louis Rich	3 oz	15	Almonds, blanched	1 oz	6
Seafood:			*Cereals, Grains, and Breads:*		
Cod, cooked	3 oz	19	Oatmeal, quick instant	1 cup	5.4
Salmon, Chinook, baked	3 oz	22	Cheerios	1 cup	3
Shrimp, steamed	3 oz	18	Grape-Nuts	1/2 cup	6
Tuna, in water, drained	3 oz	22	Raisin Bran	1 cup	5
Pork:			Brown rice, cooked	1 cup	5
Pork loin chop, broiled	3 oz	25	Whole-wheat bread	1 slice	2.7
Ham, roasted, lean	3 oz	20	Bagel, 3 1/2 -in.-diameter	1 each	7
Dairy:			*Vegetables:*		
Whole milk (3.3% fat)	8 fl. oz	7.9	Carrots, raw (7.5 × 1 1/8 in.)	1 each	0.7
1% milk	8 fl. oz	8.5	Broccoli, raw, chopped	1 cup	2.6
Skim milk	8 fl. oz	8.8	Collards, cooked from frozen	1 cup	5
Low-fat, plain yogurt	8 fl. oz	13	Spinach, raw	1 cup	0.9
American cheese, processed	1 oz	6			
Cottage cheese, low-fat (2%)	1 cup	27			
Soy Products:					
Tofu	3.3 oz	7			
Tempeh, cooked	3.3 oz	18			
Soy milk beverage	1 cup	7			

Data from Values obtained from U.S. Department of Agriculture, Agricultural Research Service. 2009. USDA National Nutrient Database for Standard Reference, Release 22. Nutrient Data Laboratory Home Page, www.ars.usda.gov/ba/bhnrc/ndl.

Legumes

Legumes include foods such as soybeans, kidney beans, pinto beans, black beans, garbanzo beans (chickpeas), lentils, green peas, black-eyed peas, and lima beans. Would you be surprised to learn that the quality of the protein in some of these legumes is almost equal to that of meat? It's true! The quality of soybean protein is almost identical to that of meat and is available as soy milk, tofu, textured vegetable protein, and tempeh, a firm cake that is made by cooking and fermenting whole soybeans. The protein quality of other legumes is also relatively high. In addition to being excellent sources of protein, legumes are high in fiber, iron, calcium, and many of the B-vitamins. They are also low in saturated fat and cholesterol. Eating legumes regularly, including foods made from soybeans, may help reduce the risk for heart disease by lowering blood cholesterol levels. Diets high in legumes and soy products are also associated with lower rates of some cancers. Legumes are not nutritionally complete, however, as they do not contain vitamins B_{12}, C, or A. They're also deficient in methionine, an essential amino acid; however, combining them with grains, nuts, or seeds gives you a complete protein.

Considering their nutrient profile, satiety value, and good taste, it's no wonder that many experts consider legumes an almost perfect food. From main dishes to snacks, here are some simple ways to add legumes to your daily diet.

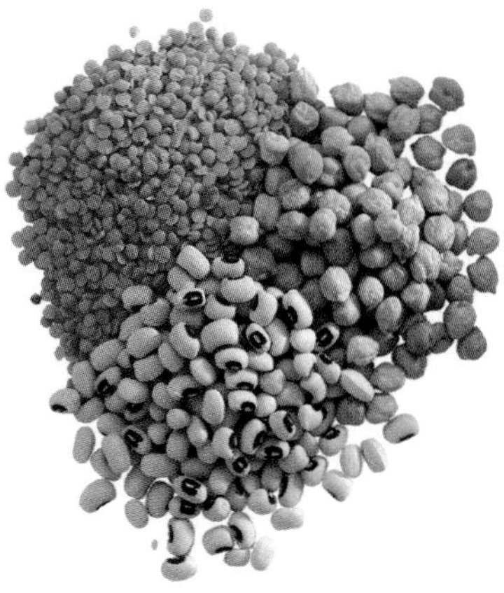

▲ The quality of the protein in some legumes is almost equal to that of meat.

Nuts

Nuts are another healthful high-protein food. In the past, the high fat and energy content of nuts was assumed to be harmful, and people were advised to eat nuts only

What About You?

How Much Protein Do You Eat?

One way to find out if your diet contains enough protein is to keep a food diary. Record everything you eat and drink for at least 3 days, and the grams of protein each item provides. To determine the grams of protein, for packaged foods, use the Nutrition Facts Panel, and make sure to adjust for the amount you actually consume. For products without labels, check Table 6.3 on page 203, or use the diet analysis tools that accompany this text. There is also a U.S. Department of Agriculture website that lists the energy and nutrient content of thousands of foods (go to www.ars.usda.gov/ba/bhnrc/ndl).

Below is an example, using Theo's food choices for 1 day. Do you think he's meeting his protein needs?

As calculated in the You Do the Math box on page 201, Theo's RDA is 72.8 to 91 g of protein. He is consuming 2 1/2 to 3 times that amount! You can see that he does not need to use amino acid or protein supplements, since he has more than adequate amounts of protein to build lean tissue. Now calculate your own protein intake. Are you getting enough protein each day?

Foods Consumed	Protein Content (g)
Breakfast:	
Brewed coffee (2 cups) with 2 tbsp. cream	1
1 large bagel (5-in.-diameter)	10
Low-fat cream cheese (1.5 oz)	4.5
Mid-morning snack:	
Cola beverage (32 fl. oz)	0
Low-fat strawberry yogurt (1 cup)	10
Snackwells Apple Cinnamon Bars (2)	2
Lunch:	
Ham and cheese sandwich:	
Whole-wheat bread (2 slices)	4
Mayonnaise (1.5 tbsp.)	1
Lean ham (4 oz)	24
Swiss cheese (2 oz)	16
Iceberg lettuce (2 leaves)	0.5
Sliced tomato (3 slices)	0.5
Banana (1 large)	1
Triscuit crackers (20 crackers)	7
Bottled water (20 fl. oz)	0

Foods Consumed	Protein Content (g)
Afternoon snack:	
Dry roasted peanuts (1 oz)	7
2% low-fat milk (1 cup)	8
Dinner:	
Cheeseburger:	
Broiled ground beef (1/2 lb cooked)	64
American cheese (1 oz)	6
Seeded bun (1 large)	6
Ketchup (2 tbsp.)	1
Mustard (1 tbsp.)	1
Shredded lettuce (1/2 cup)	0.5
Sliced tomato (3 slices)	0.5
French fries (2- to 3-in. strips; 30 fries)	6
Baked beans (2 cups)	28
2% low-fat milk (1 cup)	8
Evening snack:	
Chocolate chip cookies (4 3-in.-diameter cookies)	3
2% low-fat milk (1 cup)	8
Total Protein Intake for the Day:	**228.5 g**

occasionally and in very small amounts. The results from recent epidemiological studies have helped to substantially change the way nutrition experts view nuts. These studies show that consuming about 2 to 5 oz of nuts per week significantly reduces people's risk for cardiovascular disease.[7–9] Although the exact mechanism for the reduction in cardiovascular disease risk with increased nut intake is not known, nuts contain many nutrients and other substances that are associated with health benefits, including fiber, unsaturated fats, potassium, folate, and plant sterols that inhibit cholesterol absorption.

"New" Foods

A new source of non-meat protein that is available on the market is *quorn*, a protein product derived from fermented fungus. It is mixed with a variety of other foods to produce various types of meat substitutes. Other "new" foods high in protein include some very ancient grains! For instance, you may have heard of pastas and other products made with quinoa (pronounced keen-wah), a plant so essential to the diet of the ancient Incas that they considered it sacred. No wonder: quinoa, cooked much like rice, provides 8 g of protein in a 1-cup serving. It's highly digestible and unlike many more familiar grains, provides all nine essential amino acids. A similar grain, called amaranth, also provides complete protein. Teff, millet, and sorghum are grains long cultivated in Africa as rich sources of protein. They are now widely available in the United States. Although these three grains are low in the essential amino acid lysine, combining them with legumes produces a complete-protein meal.

With such a wide variety of protein sources to choose from, it's easy to eat right all day! See the Eating Right All Day feature for some simple high-protein menu choices that are low in saturated fat and high in nutrients and phytochemicals.

QUICK TIPS

Adding Legumes to Your Daily Diet

Breakfast

✓ Instead of cereal, eggs, or a muffin, microwave a frozen bean burrito for a quick, portable breakfast.

✓ Make your pancakes with soy milk, or pour soy milk on your cereal.

✓ If you normally have a side of bacon, ham, or sausage with your eggs, have a side of black beans instead.

Lunch and Dinner

✓ Try a sandwich made with hummus (a garbanzo bean spread), cucumbers, tomato, avocado, and/or lettuce on whole-wheat bread or in a whole-wheat pocket.

✓ Use deli "meats" made with soy in your sandwich. Also try soy hot dogs, burgers, and "chicken" nuggets.

✓ Add garbanzo beans, kidney beans, or fresh peas to tossed salads, or make a three-bean salad with kidney beans, green beans, and garbanzo beans.

✓ Make a side dish using legumes such as peas with pearl onions, or succotash (lima beans, corn, and tomatoes), or home-made chili with kidney beans and tofu instead of meat.

✓ Make black bean soup, lentil soup, pea soup, minestrone soup, or a batch of dal (a type of yellow lentil used in Indian cuisine) and serve over brown rice. Top with plain yogurt, a traditional accompaniment in many Asian cuisines.

✓ Use soy "crumbles" in any recipe calling for ground beef.

✓ Make burritos with black or pinto beans instead of shredded meat.

✓ To stir-fried vegetables, add cubes of tofu or strips of tempeh.

✓ Make a "meatloaf" using cooked, mashed lentils instead of ground beef.

✓ For fast food at home, keep canned beans on hand. Serve over rice with a salad for a complete and hearty meal.

Snacks

✓ Instead of potato chips or pretzels, try one of the new bean chips.

✓ Dip fresh vegetables in bean dip.

✓ Serve hummus on wedges of pita bread.

✓ Add roasted soy "nuts" to your trail mix.

✓ Keep frozen tofu desserts, such as tofu ice cream, in your freezer.

RECAP **The RDA for protein for most nonpregnant, nonlactating, nonvegetarian adults is 0.8 g per kg body weight. Children, pregnant women, nursing mothers, vegetarians, and active people need slightly more. Most people who eat enough kilocalories and carbohydrates have no problem meeting their RDA for protein. Good sources of protein include meats, eggs, dairy products, legumes, whole grains, and nuts.**

Can a Vegetarian Diet Provide Adequate Protein?

Vegetarianism is the practice of restricting the diet to food substances of plant origin, including vegetables, fruits, grains, and nuts. As stated in the introduction, approximately 6 to 8 million adults in the United States are vegetarians; of these, about 2 to

vegetarianism The practice of restricting the diet to food substances of plant origin, including vegetables, fruits, grains, and nuts.

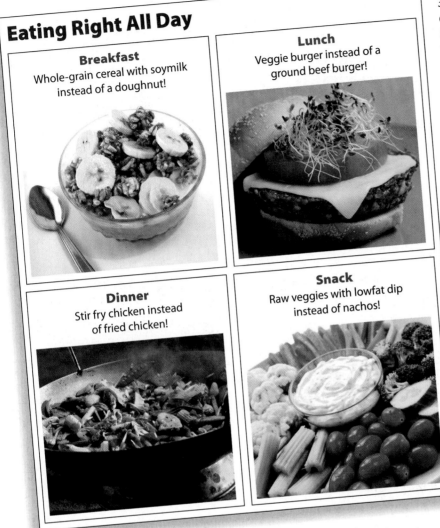

Eating Right All Day

Breakfast
Whole-grain cereal with soymilk instead of a doughnut!

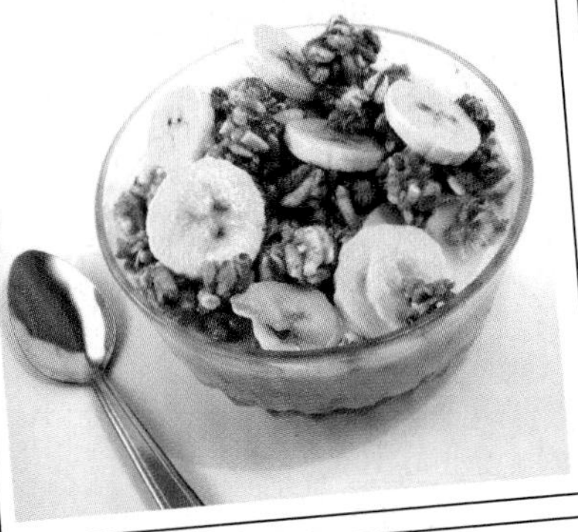

Lunch
Veggie burger instead of a ground beef burger!

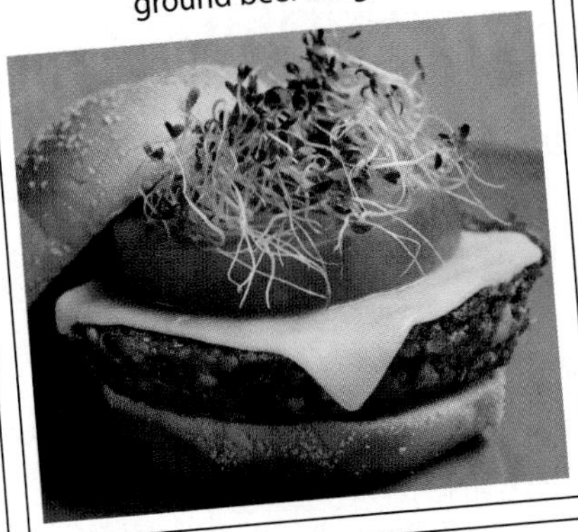

Dinner
Stir fry chicken instead of fried chicken!

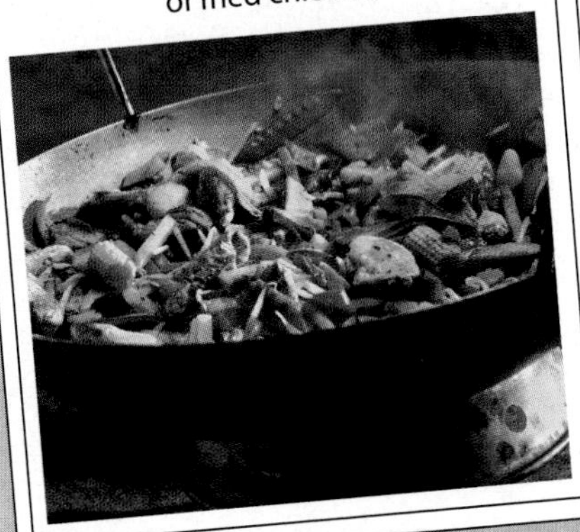

Snack
Raw veggies with lowfat dip instead of nachos!

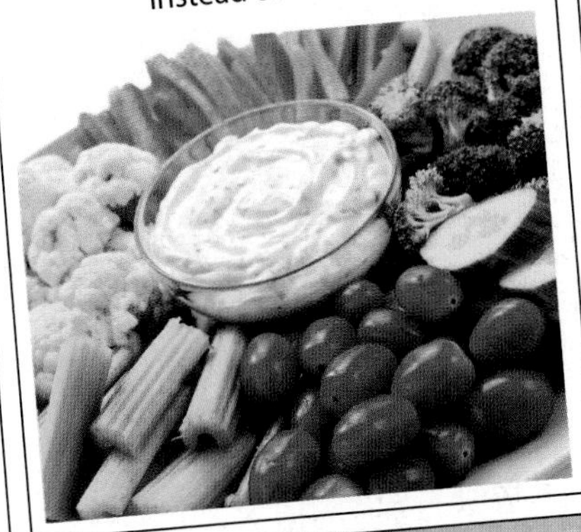

3 million are vegans, people who do not eat any kind of animal product, including dairy foods and eggs.[1] Many vegetarians are college students; moving away from home and taking responsibility for one's eating habits appears to influence some young adults to try vegetarianism as a lifestyle choice.

Types of Vegetarian Diets

There are almost as many types of vegetarian diets as there are vegetarians. Some people who consider themselves vegetarians regularly eat poultry and fish. Others avoid the flesh of animals but consume eggs, milk, and cheese liberally. Still others strictly avoid all products of animal origin, including milk and eggs, and even by-products such as candies and puddings made with gelatin. A type of "vegetarian" diet receiving significant media attention recently is the *flexitarian* diet: Flexitarians are considered semivegetarians who eat mostly plant foods, eggs, and dairy but occasionally eat red meat, poultry, and/or fish.

Table 6.4 identifies the various types of vegetarian diets, ranging from the most inclusive to the most restrictive. Notice that, the more restrictive the diet, the more challenging it becomes to achieve an adequate protein intake.

Why Do People Become Vegetarians?

When discussing vegetarianism, one of the most often asked questions is why people would make this food choice. The most common responses are included here.

Religious, Ethical, and Food-Safety Reasons

Some make the choice for religious or spiritual reasons. Several religions prohibit or restrict the consumption of animal flesh; however, generalizations can be misleading. For example, while certain sects within Hinduism forbid the consumption of meat, perusing the menu at any Indian restaurant will reveal that many other Hindus regularly consume small quantities of meat, poultry, and fish. Many Buddhists are vegetarians, as are some Christians, including Seventh-Day Adventists.

Many vegetarians are guided by their personal philosophy to choose vegetarianism. These people feel that it is morally and ethically wrong to consume animals and any products from animals (such as dairy or egg products) because they view the practices in the modern animal industries as inhumane. They may consume milk and eggs but choose to purchase them only from family farms where animals are treated humanely.

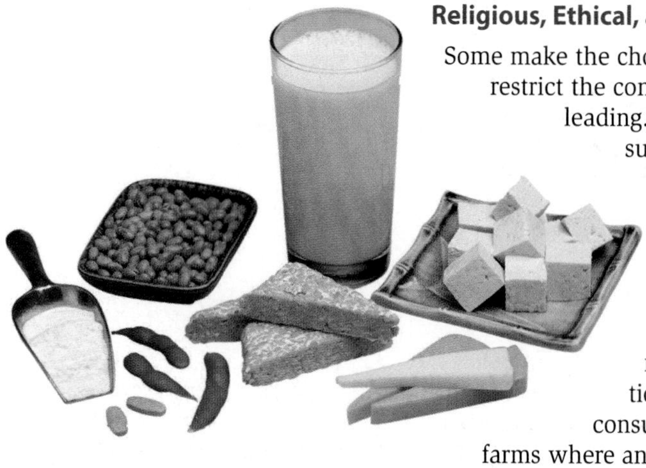

▲ Soy products are a good source of dietary protein.

There is also a great deal of concern about meat handling practices, as contaminated meat has found its way into our food supply. For example, several outbreaks of

TABLE 6.4 Terms and Definitions of a Vegetarian Diet

Type of Diet	Foods Consumed	Comments
Semivegetarian (also called partial vegetarian or flexitarian)	Vegetables, grains, nuts, fruits, legumes; sometimes seafood, poultry, eggs, and dairy products	Typically excludes or limit red meat; may also avoid other meats
Pescovegetarian	Similar to semivegetarian but excludes poultry	*Pesco* means "fish," the only animal source of protein in this diet
Lacto-ovo-vegetarian	Vegetables, grains, nuts, fruits, legumes, dairy products (*lacto*) and eggs (*ovo*)	Excludes animal flesh and seafood
Lacto-vegetarian	Similar to lacto-ovo-vegetarian but excludes eggs	Relies on milk and cheese for animal sources of protein
Ovovegetarian	Vegetables, grains, nuts, fruits, legumes, and eggs	Excludes dairy, flesh, and seafood products
Vegan (also called strict vegetarian)	Only plant-based foods (vegetables, grains, nuts, seeds, fruits, legumes)	May not provide adequate vitamin B_{12}, zinc, iron, or calcium
Macrobiotic diet	Vegan-type of diet; becomes progressively more strict until almost all foods are eliminated; at the extreme, only brown rice and small amounts of water or herbal tea are consumed	Taken to the extreme, can cause malnutrition and death
Fruitarian	Only raw or dried fruit, seeds, nuts, honey, and vegetable oil	Very restrictive diet; deficient in protein, calcium, zinc, iron, vitamin B_{12}, riboflavin, and other nutrients

severe illness, sometimes resulting in permanent disability and even death, have been traced to hamburgers served at fast-food restaurants, as well as ground beef sold in markets and consumed at home. A concern surrounding beef that has taken Europe by storm is the outbreak of *mad cow disease*. See the Nutrition Myth or Fact? box in Chapter 13 for a look at mad cow disease and its impact in the United States and other countries.

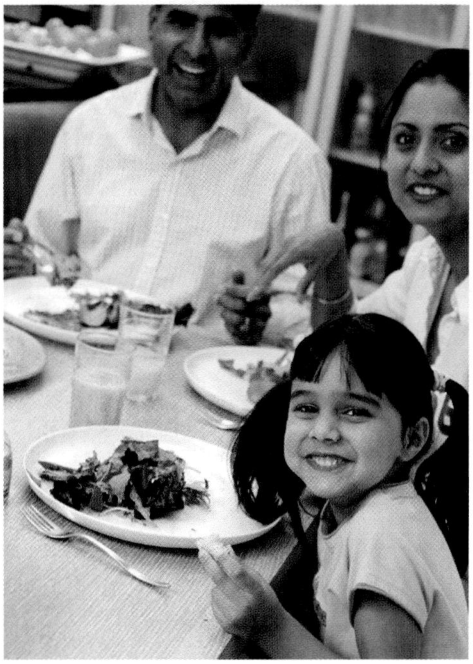

People who follow certain sects of Hinduism refrain from eating meat.

Ecological Benefits

Many people choose vegetarianism because of their concerns about the effect of meat industries on the global environment. Due to the high demand for meat in developed nations, meat production has evolved from small family farming operations to the larger system of agribusiness. Critics point to the environmental costs of agribusiness, including massive uses of water and grain to feed animals, methane gases and other wastes produced by animals themselves, and increased land use to support livestock. For an in-depth discussion of this complex and often emotionally charged topic, see the Nutrition Debate box, Meat Consumption and Global Warming: Tofu to the Rescue? later in this chapter on page 213.

Health Benefits

Still others practice vegetarianism because of its health benefits. Research over several years has consistently shown that a varied and balanced vegetarian diet can reduce the risk for many chronic diseases. Its health benefits include the following:[10]

- Reduced intake of fat and total energy, which reduces the risk for obesity. This may in turn lower a person's risk for type 2 diabetes.
- Lower blood pressure, which may be due to a higher intake of fruits and vegetables. People who eat vegetarian diets tend to be nonsmokers, drink little or no alcohol, and exercise more regularly, which are also factors known to reduce blood pressure and help maintain a healthy body weight.
- Reduced risk for heart disease, which may be due to lower saturated fat intake and a higher consumption of *antioxidants* that are found in plant-based foods. Antioxidants, discussed in detail in Chapter 8, are substances that can protect our cells from damage. They are abundant in fruits and vegetables.
- Fewer digestive problems such as constipation and diverticular disease, perhaps due to the higher fiber content of vegetarian diets. Diverticular disease, discussed

in Chapter 4, occurs when the wall of the bowel (large intestine) pouches and becomes inflamed.

- Reduced risk for some cancers. Research shows that vegetarians may have lower rates of cancer, particularly colon cancer.[10] Many components of a vegetarian diet might contribute to reducing cancer risks, including higher fiber and antioxidant intakes, lower dietary fat intake, lower consumption of **carcinogens** (cancer-causing agents) that are formed when cooking meat, and higher consumption of soy protein, which may have anticancer properties.[10]
- Reduced risk for kidney disease, kidney stones, and gallstones. The lower protein contents of vegetarian diets, plus the higher intake of legumes and vegetable proteins (such as soy), may be protective against these conditions.

What Are the Challenges of a Vegetarian Diet?

Although a vegetarian diet can be healthful, it also presents many challenges. Limiting the consumption of flesh and dairy products introduces the potential for inadequate intakes of certain nutrients, especially for people consuming a vegan, macrobiotic, or fruitarian diet. **Table 6.5** lists the nutrients that can be deficient in a vegan-type diet plan and describes good non-animal sources that can provide these nutrients. Vegetarians who consume dairy and/or egg products obtain these nutrients more easily.

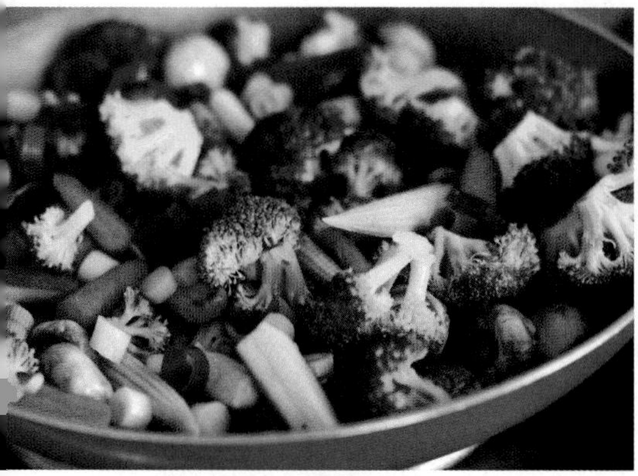

▲ A well-balanced vegetarian diet can provide adequate protein and other nutrients.

Research indicates that a sign of disordered eating in some college females is the switch to a vegetarian diet.[11] Instead of eating a healthy variety of non-animal foods, people struggling with this problem may use vegetarianism as an excuse to restrict many foods from their diets.

Can a vegetarian diet provide enough protein? Because high-quality non-meat protein sources are quite easy to obtain in developed countries, a well-balanced vegetarian diet can provide adequate protein. In fact, the American Dietetic Association and Dietitians of Canada endorse an appropriately planned vegetarian diet as healthful, nutritionally adequate, and beneficial in reducing and preventing various diseases.[10] As you can see, the emphasis is on a *balanced* and *adequate* vegetarian diet; thus, it is important for vegetarians to consume soy products, eat complementary proteins, and obtain enough energy from other macronutrients to spare protein from being used as an energy source. Although the digestibility of a vegetarian diet is potentially lower than that of an animal-based diet, there is no separate protein recommendation for vegetarians who consume complementary plant proteins.[12]

TABLE 6.5 Nutrients of Concern in a Vegan Diet

Nutrient	Functions	Non-Meat/Non-Dairy Food Sources
Vitamin B_{12}	Assists with DNA synthesis; protection and growth of nerve fibers	Vitamin B_{12}–fortified cereals, yeast, soy products, and other meat analogs; vitamin B_{12} supplements
Vitamin D	Promotes bone growth	Vitamin D–fortified cereals, margarines, and soy products; adequate exposure to sunlight; supplementation may be necessary for those who do not get adequate exposure to sunlight
Riboflavin (vitamin B_2)	Promotes release of energy; supports normal vision and skin health	Whole and enriched grains, green leafy vegetables, mushrooms, beans, nuts, and seeds
Iron	Assists with oxygen transport; involved in making amino acids and hormones	Whole-grain products, prune juice, dried fruits, beans, nuts, seeds, and leafy vegetables (such as spinach)
Calcium	Maintains bone health; assists with muscle contraction, blood pressure, and nerve transmission	Fortified soy milk and tofu, almonds, dry beans, leafy vegetables, calcium-fortified juices, and fortified breakfast cereals
Zinc	Assists with DNA and RNA synthesis, immune function, and growth	Whole-grain products, wheat germ, beans, nuts, and seeds

carcinogens Cancer-causing agents, such as certain pesticides, industrial chemicals, and pollutants.

In certain populations, micronutrient supplements can play an important role in promoting good health. These include pregnant women, children with poor eating habits, and people with certain illnesses.

Can Micronutrients Really Prevent or Treat Disease?

Nutritionists and other healthcare professionals clearly accept the role that dietary fat plays in the prevention and treatment of coronary heart disease. The relationship between total carbohydrate intake and the management of diabetes is also firmly established. Less clear, however, are the links between individual vitamins and minerals and certain chronic diseases.

A number of research studies have suggested, but not proven, links between the following vitamins and disease states. In each case, adequate intake of the nutrient has been associated with lower disease risk.

- Vitamin C and cataracts
- Vitamin D and colon cancer
- Vitamin E and complications of diabetes
- Vitamin K and osteoporosis

Other studies have examined relationships between minerals and chronic diseases. Again, in each case, the nutrient seems to be protective against the disease listed.

- Calcium and high blood pressure (hypertension)
- Chromium and type 2 diabetes in older adults
- Magnesium and muscle wasting (sarcopenia) in older adults
- Selenium and certain types of cancer

As consumers, it is important to critically evaluate any claims that are made regarding the protective or disease-preventing ability of a specific vitamin or mineral. Supplements that provide megadoses of micronutrients are potentially harmful, and vitamin/mineral therapies should never replace more traditional, proven methods of disease treatment. Current, reputable information can provide updates as the research into micronutrients continues.

Do More Essential Micronutrients Exist?

Nutrition researchers continue to explore the potential of a variety of substances to qualify as essential micronutrients. Vitamin-like factors, such as carnitine, and trace minerals, such as boron, nickel, and silicon, seem to have beneficial roles in human health, yet additional information is needed in order to fully define their metabolic roles. Until more research is done, we cannot classify such substances as essential micronutrients.

Another subject of controversy is the question "What is the appropriate intake of each micronutrient?" Contemporary research suggests that the answer to this question is to be found in each individual's genetic profile. As you learned in the Nutrition Debate in Chapter 1, the science of *nutrigenomics* blends the study of human nutrition with that of genetics. It is becoming clear that some individuals, for example, require much higher intakes of folate in order to achieve optimal health. Researchers have identified a specific genetic variation in a subset of the population that increases their need for dietary folate.[5] Future studies may identify other examples of how a person's genetic profile influences his or her individual need for vitamins and minerals.

As explained in Chapter 1, the DRI Committees rely on Adequate Intake (AI) guidelines to suggest appropriate nutrient intake levels when research has not clearly defined an Estimated Average Requirement (EAR). As the science of nutrition continues to evolve, the next 50 years will be an exciting time for micronutrient research. Who knows? Within a few decades, we all might have personalized micronutrient prescriptions matched to our gender, age, and DNA!

NutriTools

Check out the companion website at www.pearsonhighered.com/thompsonmanore, or use MyNutritionLab, to access interactive animations including:

- Know Your Calcium Sources
- Know Your Iron Sources
- Let's Go to Lunch! Vitamins
- Let's Go to Lunch! Minerals
- Nutrients: Vitamin or Mineral?

Web Resources

www.fda.gov
U.S. Food and Drug Administration

Locate information on how to evaluate dietary supplements.

www.ars.usda.gov/ba/bhnrc/ndl
Nutrient Data Laboratory Home Page

Find information on food sources of selected vitamins and minerals.

www.nal.usda.gov/fnic
The Food and Nutrition Information Center

Obtain information on vitamin and mineral supplements.

www.dietary-supplements.info.nih.gov
Office of Dietary Supplements

Locate summaries of current research results and helpful information about the use of dietary supplements.

www.lpi.oregonstate.edu
Linus Pauling Institute of Oregon State University

Find up-to-date information on vitamins and minerals that promote health and lower disease risk.

7 Nutrients Involved in Fluid and Electrolyte Balance

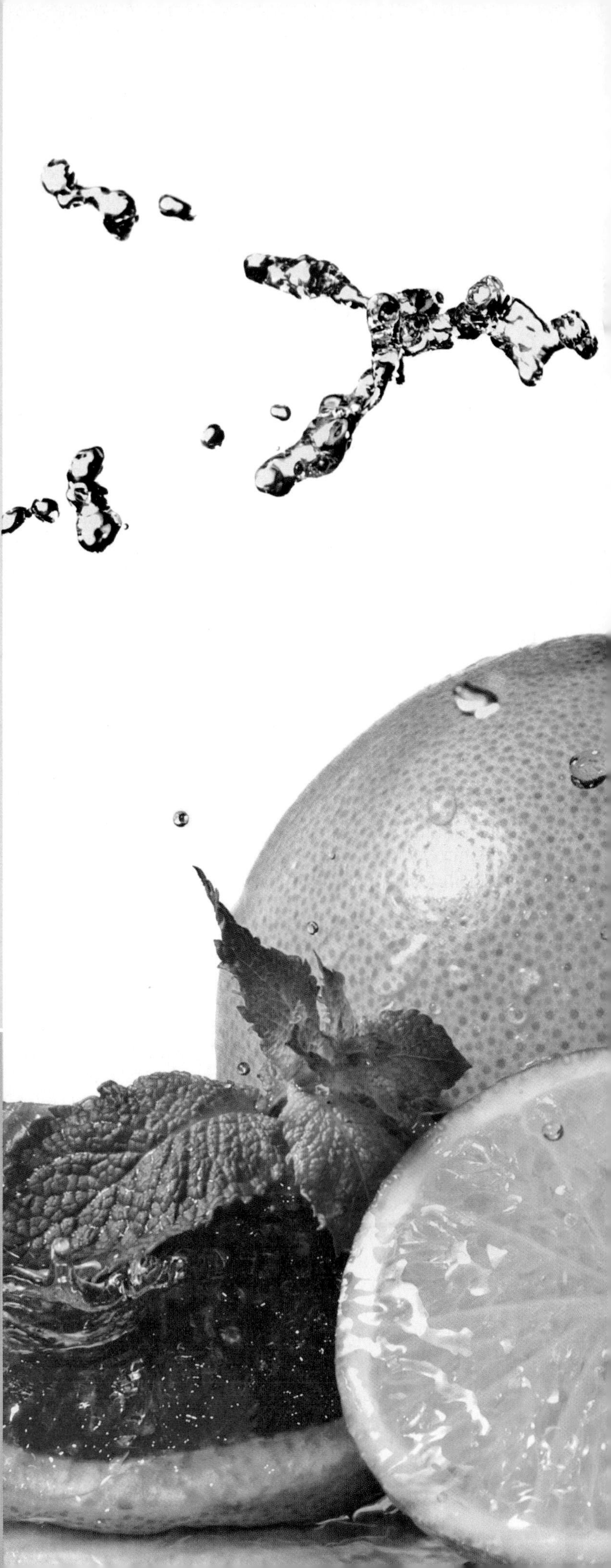

CHAPTER OBJECTIVES

After reading this chapter you will be able to:

1. **Identify four nutrients that function as electrolytes in our body, p. 229.**
2. **List three functions of water in our body, pp. 230–231.**
3. **Describe how electrolytes assist in the regulation of healthful fluid balance, pp. 231–233.**
4. **Discuss the physical changes that trigger our thirst mechanism, p. 234.**
5. **Describe the sources of fluid intake and output in our body, pp. 234–235.**
6. **Compare and contrast hypernatremia and hyponatremia, pp. 241–242.**

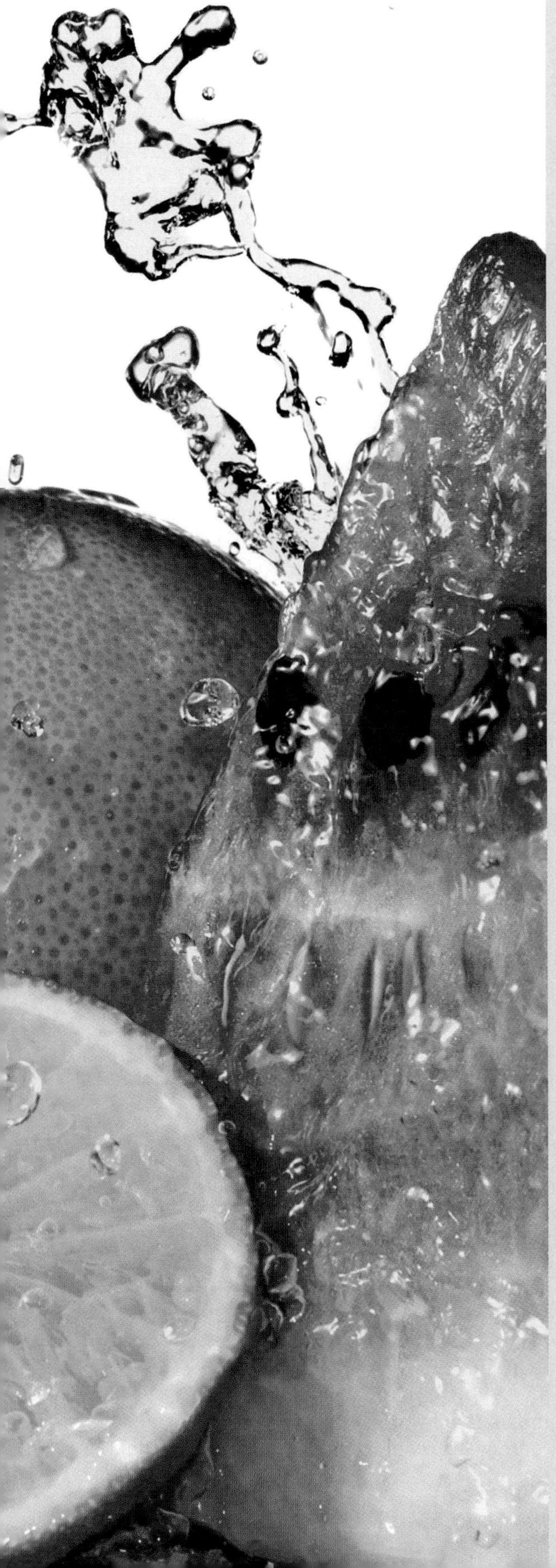

Test Yourself

1. **T F Caffeine is a powerful diuretic, causing the body to lose excessive fluid in the urine.**
2. **T F Sodium is an unhealthful nutrient, and we should avoid consuming it in our diet.**
3. **T F Drinking until we are no longer thirsty always ensures that we are properly hydrated.**

Test Yourself answers can be found at the end of the chapter.

In April of 2002, Cynthia Lucero, a healthy 28-year-old woman who had just completed her doctoral dissertation, was running the Boston Marathon. Although not a professional athlete, Cynthia was running in her second marathon, and in the words of her coach, she had been "diligent" in her training. While her parents, who had traveled from Ecuador, waited at the finish line, friends in the crowd watched as Cynthia steadily completed mile after mile, drinking large amounts of fluid as she progressed through the course. They described her as looking strong as she jogged up Heartbreak Hill, about 6 miles from the finish. But then she began to falter. One of her friends ran to her side and asked if she was okay. Cynthia replied that she felt dehydrated and rubber-legged; then she fell to the pavement. She was rushed to nearby Brigham and Women's Hospital, but by the time she got there, she was in an irreversible coma. The official cause of her death was hyponatremia, commonly called "low blood sodium." According to a study involving the 488 runners in that 2002 Boston Marathon, 13% had hyponatremia by the end of the race.[1] Hyponatremia continues to cause illness and death in runners, triathletes, and even hikers.

What is hyponatremia, and how does it differ from dehydration? Are you at risk for either condition? Do sport beverages offer any protection against these types of fluid imbalances? If at the start of football practice on a hot, humid afternoon, a friend confided to you that he had been on a drinking binge the night before, what would you say to him? Would you urge him to tell his coach, and if so, why?

In this chapter, we'll explore the role of fluids and electrolytes in keeping the body properly hydrated and maintaining

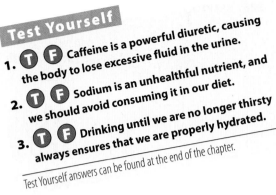

the functions of nerves and muscles. Immediately following this chapter, we take an ***In Depth*** look at some disorders that occur when fluids and electrolytes are out of balance.

What Are Fluids and Electrolytes, and What Are Their Functions?

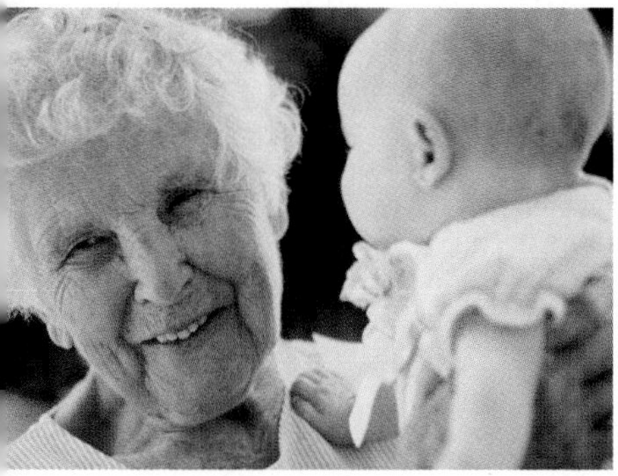

As we age, our body water content decreases: approximately 75% of an infant's body weight is composed of water, while an elderly adult's body weight is only 50% water (or less).

Of course, you know that orange juice, blood, and shampoo are all fluids, but what makes them so? A **fluid** is characterized by its ability to move freely, adapting to the shape of the container that holds it. This might not seem very important, but as you'll learn in this chapter, the fluid composition of your cells and tissues is critical to your body's ability to function.

Body Fluid Is the Liquid Portion of Our Cells and Tissues

Between 50% and 70% of a healthy adult's body weight is fluid. When we cut a finger, we can see some of this fluid dripping out as blood, but the fluid in the bloodstream can't account for such a large percentage. So where is all this fluid hiding?

About two-thirds of an adult's body fluid is held within the walls of cells and is therefore called **intracellular fluid** (**Figure 7.1a**). Every cell in our body contains fluid. When our cells lose their fluid, they quickly shrink and die. On the other hand, when cells take in too much fluid, they swell and burst apart. This is why appropriate fluid balance—which we'll discuss throughout this chapter—is so critical to life.

The remaining third of body fluid is referred to as **extracellular fluid** because it flows outside our cells (Figure 7.1a). There are two types of extracellular fluid:

1. *Tissue fluid* (sometimes called *interstitial fluid*) flows between the cells that make up a particular tissue or organ, such as muscle fibers or the liver (Figure 7.1b). Other extracellular fluids, such as cerebrospinal fluid, mucus, and synovial fluid within joints, are also considered tissue fluid.
2. *Intravascular fluid* is found within blood and lymphatic vessels. Plasma is the fluid portion of blood that transports red blood cells through blood vessels. Plasma also contains proteins that are too large to leak out of blood vessels into the surrounding tissue fluid. As you learned in Chapter 6, protein concentration plays a major role in regulating the movement of fluids into and out of the bloodstream (Figure 7.1c).

Not every tissue in our body contains the same amount of fluid. Lean tissues, such as muscle, are more than 70% fluid by weight, whereas fat tissue is only between 10% and 20% fluid. This is not surprising, considering the water-repellant nature of lipids (see Chapter 5).

Body fluid levels also vary according to gender and age. Compared to females, males have more lean tissue and thus a higher percentage of body weight as fluid. The amount of body fluid as a percentage of total weight decreases with age. About 75% of an infant's body weight is water, whereas the total body water of an elderly person is generally less than 50% of body weight. This decrease in total body water is the result of the loss of lean tissue that typically occurs as people age.

fluid A substance composed of molecules that move past one another freely. Fluids are characterized by their ability to conform to the shape of whatever container holds them.

intracellular fluid The fluid held at any given time within the walls of the body's cells.

extracellular fluid The fluid outside the body's cells, either in the body's tissues or as the liquid portion of blood, called *plasma*.

Body Fluid Is Composed of Water and Salts Called Electrolytes

Water is made up of molecules consisting of two hydrogen atoms bound to one oxygen atom (H_2O). You might think that pure water would be healthful, but we would

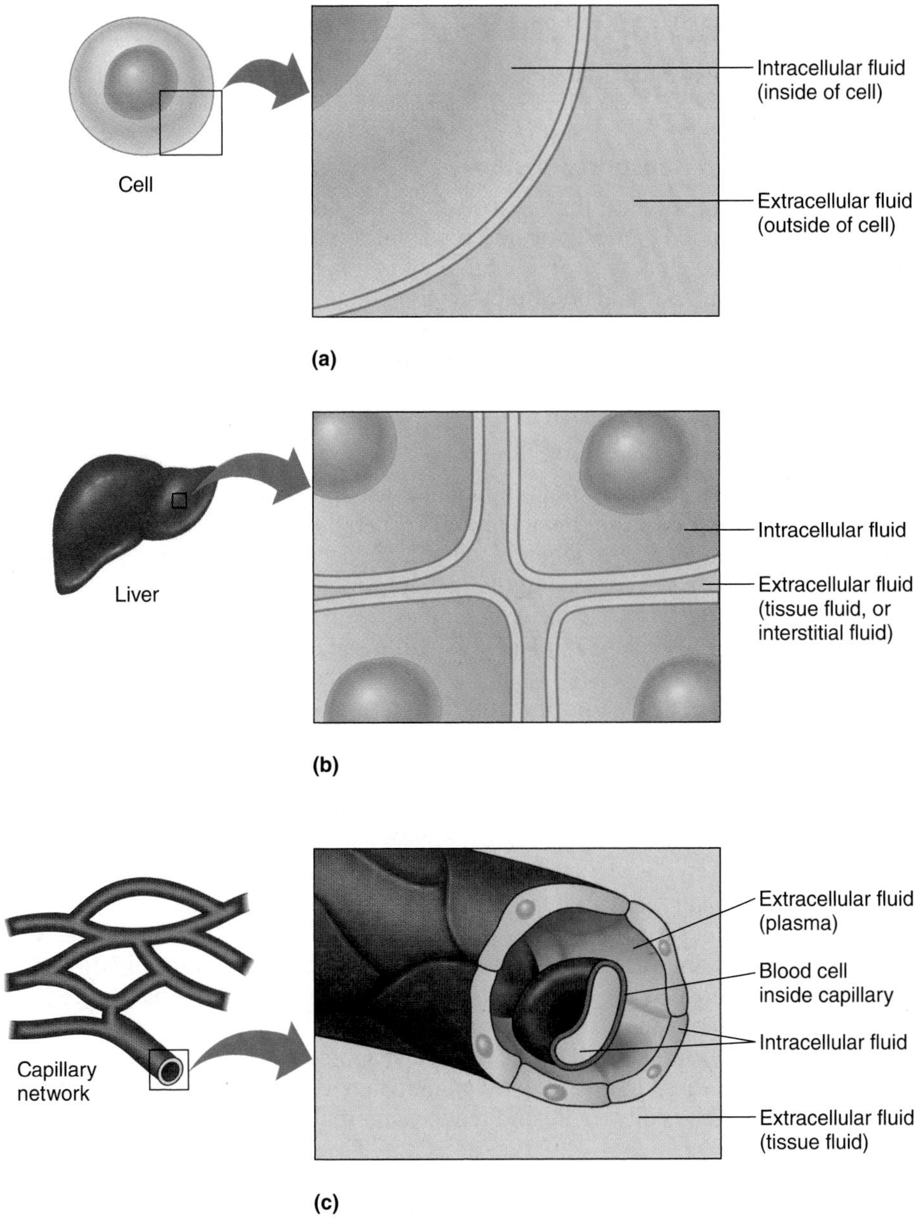

Figure 7.1 The components of body fluid. **(a)** Intracellular fluid is contained inside the cells that make up our body tissues. **(b)** Extracellular fluid is external to cells. Tissue fluid is external to tissue cells. **(c)** Another form of extracellular fluid is intravascular fluid—that is, fluid contained within vessels. Plasma is the fluid in blood vessels and is external to blood cells.

quickly die if our cell and tissue fluids contained only pure water. Instead, within the body fluids are a variety of dissolved substances (called *solutes*) critical to life. These include four major minerals: sodium, potassium, chloride, and phosphorus. We consume these minerals in compounds called *salts,* including table salt, which is made of sodium and chloride.

These mineral salts are called **electrolytes,** because when they dissolve in water, the two component minerals separate and form charged particles called **ions,** which are capable of carrying an electrical current. The electrical charge, which can be positive or negative, is the "spark" that stimulates nerves and causes muscles to contract, making electrolytes critical to body functioning.

Of the four major minerals just mentioned, sodium (Na^+) and potassium (K^+) are positively charged, whereas chloride (Cl^{2-}) and phosphorus (in the form of hydrogen phosphate, or HPO_4^{2-}) are negatively charged. In the intracellular fluid, potassium and phosphate predominate. In the extracellular fluid, sodium and chloride predominate. There is a slight difference in electrical charge on either side of the cell's membrane that is needed in order for the cell to perform its normal functions.

electrolyte A substance that disassociates in solution into positively and negatively charged ions and is thus capable of carrying an electrical current.

ion An electrically charged particle, either positively or negatively charged.

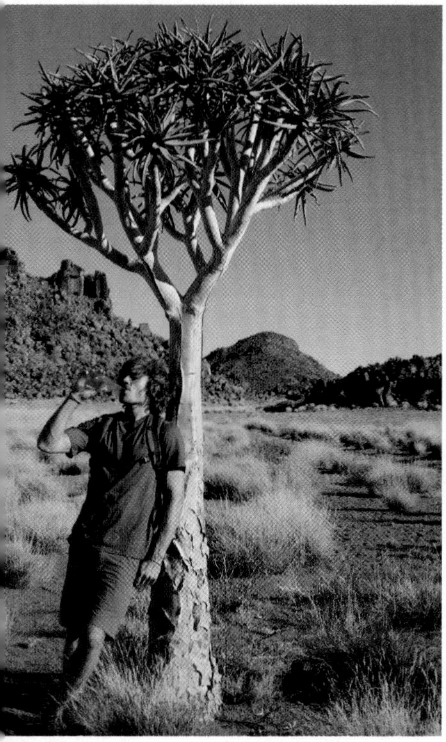

A hiker must consume adequate amounts of water to prevent heat illness in hot and dry environments.

Fluids Serve Many Critical Functions

Water not only quenches our thirst; it also performs a number of functions that are critical to sustain life.

Fluids Dissolve and Transport Substances

Water is an excellent **solvent;** that is, it's capable of dissolving a wide variety of substances. Since blood is mostly water, it's able to transport a variety of solutes—such as amino acids, glucose, water-soluble vitamins, minerals, and medications—to body cells. In contrast, fats do not dissolve in water. To overcome this chemical incompatibility, lipids and fat-soluble vitamins are either attached to or surrounded by water-soluble proteins, so that they, too, can be transported in the blood to the cells.

Fluids Account for Blood Volume

Blood volume is the amount of fluid in blood; thus, appropriate fluid levels are essential to maintaining healthful blood volume. When blood volume rises inappropriately, blood pressure increases; when blood volume decreases inappropriately, blood pressure decreases. As you learned in the ***In Depth*** following Chapter 5, high blood pressure is an important risk factor for heart disease and stroke. In contrast, low blood pressure can cause people to feel tired, confused, or dizzy.

Fluids Help Maintain Body Temperature

Just as overheating is disastrous to a car engine, a high internal temperature can cause our body to stop functioning. Fluids are vital to the body's ability to maintain its temperature within a safe range. Two factors account for the ability of fluids to keep us cool. First, water has a relatively high capacity for heat: in other words, it takes a lot of energy to raise its temperature. Since the body contains a lot of water, only prolonged exposure to high heat can increase body temperature.

Second, body fluids are our primary coolant. When heat needs to be released from the body, there is an increase in the flow of blood from the warm body core to the vessels lying just under the skin. This action transports heat from the body core out to the periphery, where it can be released from the skin. At the same time, sweat glands secrete more sweat from the skin. As this sweat evaporates off of the skin's surface, heat is released and the skin and underlying blood are cooled **(Figure 7.2)**. This cooler blood flows back to the body's core and reduces internal body temperature.

solvent A substance that is capable of mixing with and breaking apart a variety of compounds. Water is an excellent solvent.

blood volume The amount of fluid in blood.

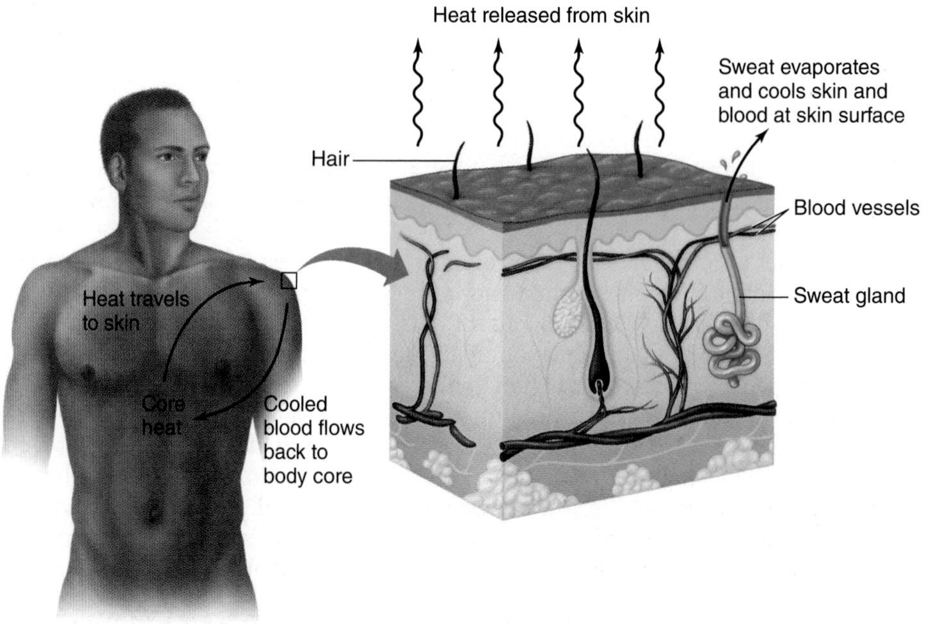

Figure 7.2 Evaporative cooling occurs when heat is transported from the body core through the bloodstream to the surface of the skin. The water evaporates into the air and carries away heat. This cools the blood, which circulates back to the body core, reducing body temperature.

Fluids Protect and Lubricate Our Tissues

Water is a major part of the fluids that protect and lubricate tissues. The cerebrospinal fluid that surrounds the brain and spinal cord protects them from damage, and a fetus in a mother's womb is protected by amniotic fluid. Synovial fluid lubricates joints, and tears cleanse and lubricate the eyes. Saliva moistens the food we eat and the mucus lining the walls of the GI tract eases the movement of food through the stomach and intestines. Finally, pleural fluid covering the lungs allows their friction-free expansion and retraction within the chest cavity.

RECAP **Our body fluids consists of water plus a variety of dissolved substances, including electrically charged minerals called electrolytes. Water serves many important functions in our body, including dissolving and transporting substances, accounting for blood volume, regulating body temperature, and protecting and lubricating body tissues.**

Electrolytes Support Many Body Functions

Now that you know why fluid is so essential to the body's functioning, we're ready to explore the critical roles of the electrolytes.

Electrolytes Help Regulate Fluid Balance

Cell membranes are *permeable* to water, meaning water flows easily through them. Cells cannot voluntarily regulate this flow of water and thus have no active control over the balance of fluid between the intracellular and extracellular environments. In contrast, cell membranes are *not* freely permeable to electrolytes. Sodium, potassium, and the other electrolytes stay where they are, either inside or outside a cell, unless they are actively transported across the cell membrane by special transport proteins. So how do electrolytes help cells maintain their fluid balance? To answer this question, a short review of chemistry is needed.

Imagine that you have a special filter with the same properties as cell membranes; in other words, this filter is freely permeable to water but not permeable to electrolytes. Now imagine that you insert this filter into a glass of pure distilled water to divide the glass into two separate chambers (**Figure 7.3a**). Of course, the water levels on both sides of the filter would be identical, because the filter is freely permeable to water. Now imagine that you add a teaspoon of salt (which contains the electrolytes

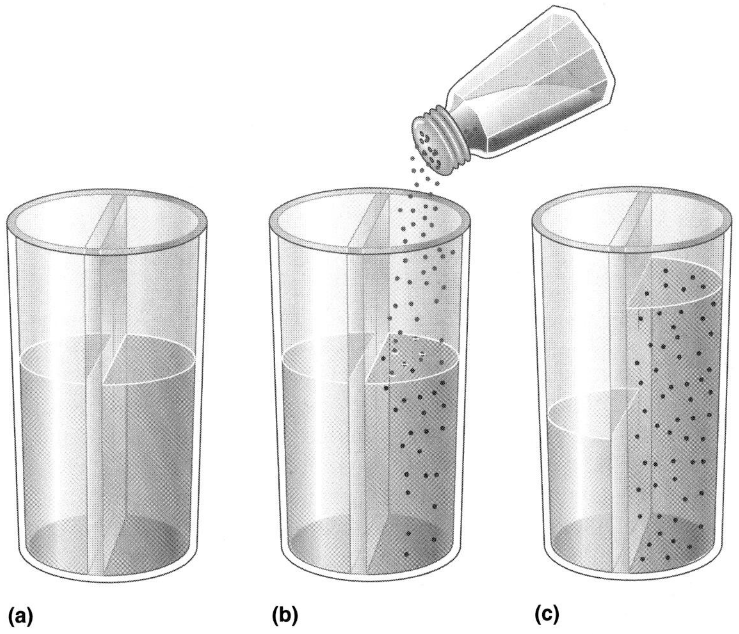

Figure 7.3 Osmosis. **(a)** A filter that is freely permeable to water is placed in a glass of pure water. **(b)** Salt is added to only one side of the glass. **(c)** Drawn by the high concentration of electrolytes, pure water flows to the "salt water" side of the filter. This flow of water into the concentrated solution will continue until the concentration of electrolytes on both sides of the membrane is equal.

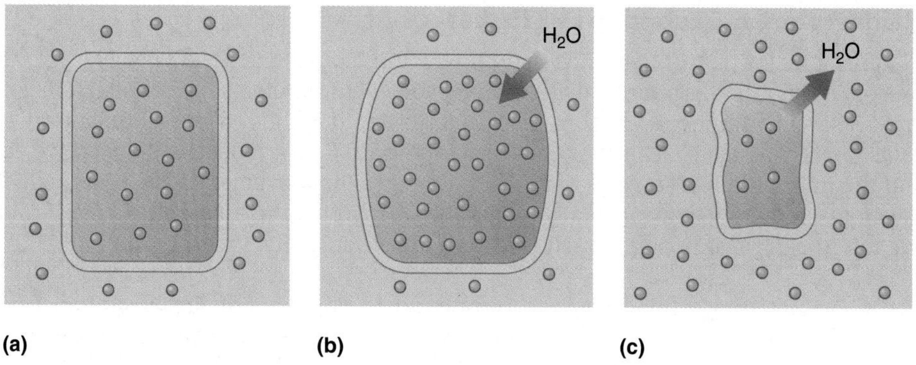

Figure 7.4 The health of our body's cells depends on maintaining the proper balance of fluids and electrolytes on both sides of the cell membrane. **(a)** The concentration of electrolytes is the same on both sides of the cell membrane. **(b)** The concentration of electrolytes is much greater inside the cell, drawing water into the cell and making it swell. **(c)** The concentration of electrolytes is much greater outside the cell, drawing water out of the cell and making it shrink.

sodium and chloride) to the water on only one side of the filter (Figure 7.3b). Immediately, you would see the water on the "pure water" side of the glass begin to flow through the filter to the "salt water" side of the glass (Figure 7.3c). Why would this movement of water occur? It is because water always moves from areas where solutes, such as sodium and chloride, are low in concentration to areas where they are high in concentration. To put it another way, solutes *attract* water toward areas where they are more concentrated. This movement of water toward solutes, called **osmosis,** continues until the concentration of solutes is equal on both sides of the cell membrane.

Osmosis provides the body a mechanism for controlling the movement of fluid into and out of cells. As we saw in Chapter 6, cells can regulate the balance of fluids between their internal and extracellular environments by using special transport proteins to actively pump electrolytes across their membranes (see Chapter 6, Figure 6.11). The health of the body's cells depends on maintaining an appropriate balance of fluid and electrolytes between the intracellular and extracellular environments **(Figure 7.4a)**. If the concentration of electrolytes is much higher inside cells as compared to outside, water will flow into the cells in such large amounts that the cells can burst (Figure 7.4b). On the other hand, if the extracellular environment contains too high a concentration of electrolytes, water flows out of the cells, and they can dry up (Figure 7.4c).

Electrolytes Enable Our Nerves to Respond to Stimuli

In addition to their role in maintaining fluid balance, electrolytes are critical in allowing our nerves to respond to stimuli. Nerve impulses are initiated at the membrane of a nerve cell in response to a stimulus—for example, the touch of a hand or the clanging of a bell. Stimuli prompt changes in membranes that allow an influx of sodium into the nerve cell, causing the cell to become slightly less negatively charged. This is called *depolarization.* If enough sodium enters the cell, an electrical impulse is generated along the cell membrane **(Figure 7.5)**. Once this impulse has been transmitted, the cell membrane returns to its normal electrical state through the release of potassium to the outside of the cell. This return to the initial electrical state is termed *repolarization.* Thus, both sodium and potassium play critical roles in ensuring that nerve impulses are generated, transmitted, and completed.

Electrolytes Signal Our Muscles to Contract

Muscles contract in response to a series of complex physiological changes that will not be described in detail here. Simply stated, muscle contraction occurs in response to stimulation of nerve cells. As described previously, sodium and potassium play a key role in the generation of nerve impulses, or electrical signals. When a muscle fiber is stimulated by an electrical signal, changes occur in the cell membrane that lead to an increased flow of calcium into the muscle from the extracellular space. This movement of calcium into the muscle provides the stimulus for muscle contraction. The muscles relax after a contraction once the electrical signal is complete and calcium has been pumped out of the muscle cell.

Certain illnesses can threaten the delicate balance of fluid inside and outside the cells and impair the function of nerves and muscles. You may have heard of someone

osmosis The movement of water (or any solvent) through a semipermeable membrane from an area where solutes are less concentrated to areas where solutes are highly concentrated.

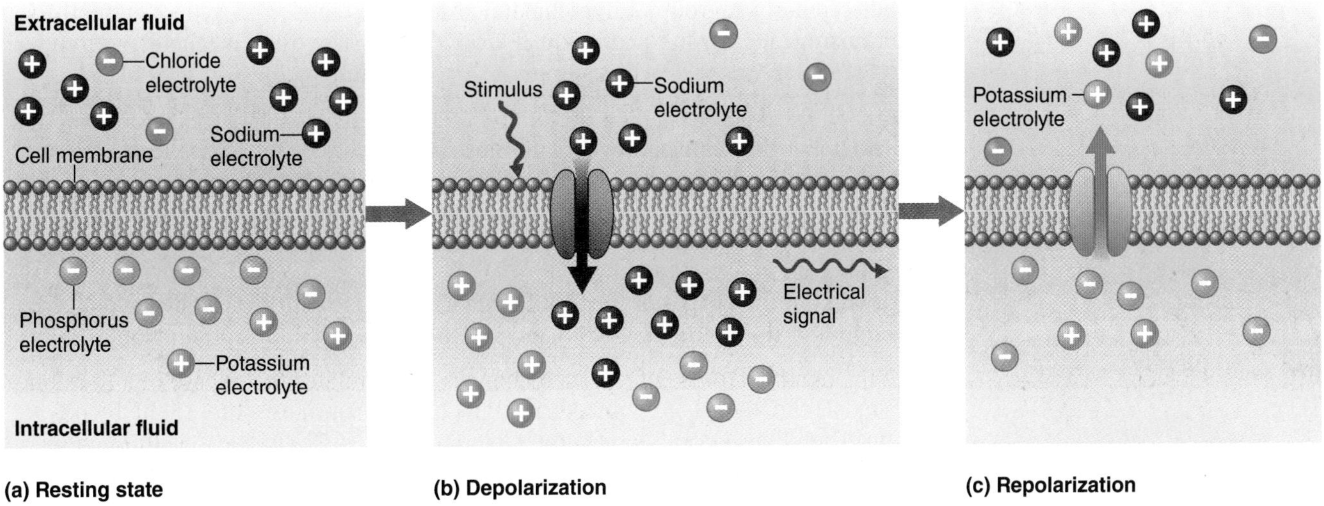

Figure 7.5 The role of electrolytes in conduction of a nerve impulse. **(a)** In the resting state, the intracellular fluid has slightly more electrolytes with a negative charge. **(b)** A stimulus causes changes to occur that prompt the influx of sodium into the interior of the cell. Sodium has a positive charge, so when this happens, the charge inside the cell becomes slightly positive. This is called depolarization. If enough sodium enters the cell, an electrical signal is transmitted to adjacent regions of the cell membrane. **(c)** Release of potassium to the exterior of the cell allows the first portion of the membrane almost immediately to return to the resting state. This is called repolarization.

being hospitalized because of excessive diarrhea and/or vomiting. When this happens, the body loses a great deal of fluid from the intestinal tract and extracellular environment. This large fluid loss causes the extracellular electrolyte concentration to become very high. In response, a great deal of intracellular fluid flows out of the cells (see Figure 7.4c). This imbalance in fluid and electrolytes changes the flow of electrical impulses through the nerve and muscle cells of the heart, causing an irregular heart rate, which can eventually lead to death if left untreated. Food poisoning and eating disorders involving repeated vomiting and diarrhea can also result in death from life-threatening fluid and electrolyte imbalances.

RECAP **Electrolytes help regulate fluid balance by controlling the movement of fluid into and out of cells. Electrolytes, specifically sodium and potassium, play a key role in generating nerve impulses in response to stimuli. Calcium is an electrolyte that stimulates muscle contraction.**

How Does Our Body Maintain Fluid Balance?

The proper balance of fluid is maintained in the body by a series of mechanisms that prompt us to drink and retain fluid when we are dehydrated and to excrete fluid as urine when we consume more than we need.

Our Thirst Mechanism Prompts Us to Drink Fluids

Imagine that, at lunch, you ate a ham sandwich and a bag of salted potato chips. Now it's almost time for your afternoon seminar to end and you are very thirsty. The last 5 minutes of class are a torment, and when the instructor ends the session you dash to the nearest drinking fountain. What prompted you to suddenly feel so thirsty?

The body's command center for fluid intake is in the hypothalamus, part of the forebrain. Recall from Chapter 3 that a cluster of cells in the hypothalamus triggers hunger. Similarly, a group of hypothalamic cells, collectively referred to as the **thirst mechanism,** causes you to consciously desire fluids. The thirst mechanism prompts us to feel thirsty whenever it is stimulated by the following:

- An increased concentration of salt and other dissolved substances in our blood. Remember that ham sandwich and those potato chips? Both these foods are salty, and eating them increased the blood's sodium concentration.
- A reduction in blood volume and blood pressure. This can occur when fluids are lost because of profuse sweating, blood loss, vomiting, or diarrhea, or simply when fluid intake is too low.
- Dryness in the tissues of the mouth and throat. Tissue dryness reflects a lower amount of fluid in the bloodstream, which causes a reduced production of saliva.

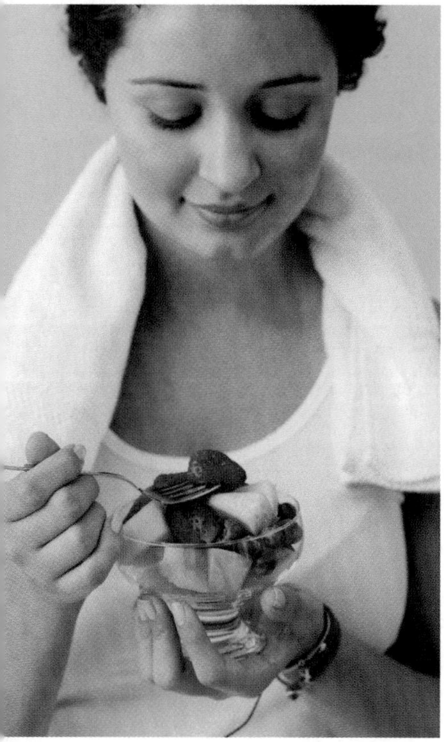

Fruits and vegetables are delicious sources of water.

Once the hypothalamus detects such changes, it stimulates the release of a hormone that signals the kidneys to reduce urine flow and return more water to the bloodstream. The kidneys also secrete an enzyme that triggers blood vessels throughout the body to constrict, helping it retain water. Water is drawn out of the salivary glands in an attempt to further dilute the concentration of blood solutes; this causes the mouth and throat to become even drier. Together, these mechanisms prevent a further loss of body fluid and help the body avoid dehydration.

Although the thirst mechanism can trigger an increase in fluid intake, this mechanism alone is not always sufficient: people tend to drink until they are no longer thirsty, but the amount of fluid they consume may not be enough to achieve fluid balance. This is particularly true when body water is lost rapidly, such as during intense exercise in the heat. Because the thirst mechanism has some limitations, it is important to drink regularly throughout the day and not wait to drink until you become thirsty, especially if you are active.

We Gain Fluids by Consuming Beverages and Foods and Through Metabolism

We obtain the fluid we need each day from three primary sources: beverages, foods, and the body's production of metabolic water. Of course, you know that beverages are mostly water, but it isn't as easy to see the water content in the foods we eat. For example, iceberg lettuce is almost 99% water, and even almonds contain a small amount of water (**Figure 7.6**).

Metabolic water is the water formed from the body's metabolic reactions. This water contributes about 10–14% of the water the body needs each day.

We Lose Fluids Through Urine, Sweat, Evaporation, Exhalation, and Feces

We can perceive—or sense—water loss through urine output and sweating, so we refer to this as **sensible water loss.** Most of the water we consume is excreted through the kidneys in the form of urine. When we consume more water than we need, the kidneys process and excrete the excess in the form of dilute urine.

The second type of sensible water loss is via sweat. Our sweat glands produce more sweat during exercise or when we are in a hot environment. The evaporation of sweat from the skin releases heat, which cools the skin and reduces the body's core temperature.

Water is continuously evaporated from the skin, even when a person is not visibly sweating, and water is continuously exhaled from the lungs during breathing. Water loss through these routes is known as **insensible water loss,** as we do not perceive it. Under normal resting conditions, insensible water loss is less than 1 liter (L) of fluid each day; during heavy exercise or in hot weather, a person can lose up to 2 L of water per hour from insensible water loss.

Under normal conditions, only about 150 to 200 ml of water is lost each day in feces. The gastrointestinal tract typically absorbs much of the fluid that passes through it each day.

thirst mechanism A cluster of nerve cells in the hypothalamus that stimulate our conscious desire to drink fluids in response to an increase in the concentration of salt in our blood or a decrease in blood pressure and blood volume.

metabolic water The water formed as a by-product of our body's metabolic reactions.

sensible water loss Water loss that is noticed by a person, such as through urine output and visible sweating.

insensible water loss The loss of water not noticeable by a person, such as through evaporation from the skin and exhalation from the lungs during breathing.

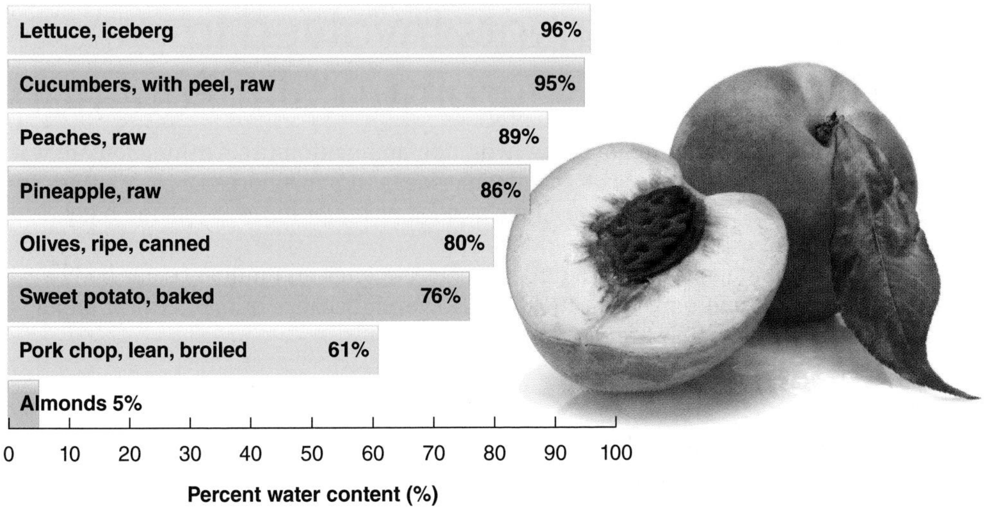

Figure 7.6 Water content of different foods. Much of your daily water intake comes from the foods you eat.

Data from U.S. Department of Agriculture, Agricultural Research Service. 2009. USDA Nutrient Database for Standard Reference, Release 22. Nutrient Data Laboratory Home Page. www.ars.usda.gov/ba/bhnrc/ndl.

In addition to these five avenues of regular fluid loss, certain situations can cause a significant loss of fluid from our body:

- Illnesses that involve fever, coughing, vomiting, diarrhea, and a runny nose significantly increase fluid loss. For instance, when someone suffers from extreme diarrhea, water loss via bowel elimination alone can be as high as several liters per day. This is one reason that doctors advise people to drink plenty of fluids when they are ill.
- Traumatic injury, internal bleeding, blood donation, and surgery also increase loss of fluid because of the blood loss involved.
- Exercise increases fluid loss via sweat and respiration; although urine production typically decreases during exercise, fluid losses increase through the skin and lungs.
- Certain environmental conditions increase fluid loss. One of these is low humidity, such as in a desert or an airplane. When the water content of the environment is low, water from the body more easily evaporates into the surrounding dry air. High altitudes increase fluid loss, because we breathe faster to compensate for the lower oxygen pressure. This results in greater fluid loss via the lungs. Hot and cold environments also increase fluid loss. We've mentioned sensible losses from sweating in the heat, but cold temperatures can trigger hormonal changes that also increase fluid loss.
- Pregnancy increases fluid loss for the mother because fluids are continually diverted to the fetus and amniotic fluid.
- Breastfeeding requires a tremendous increase in fluid intake to make up for the loss of fluid as breast milk.
- Consumption of **diuretics**—substances that increase fluid loss via the urine—can result in dangerously excessive fluid loss. Diuretics include certain prescription medications, alcohol, and many over-the-counter weight-loss remedies. In the past, it was believed that caffeine acted as a diuretic, but recent research suggests that caffeinated drinks do not significantly influence fluid status in healthy adults.

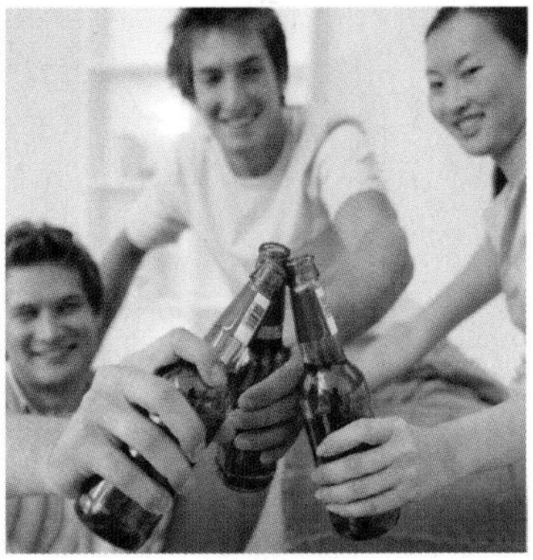

Drinking beverages that contain alcohol causes an increase in water loss, because alcohol is a diuretic.

RECAP **A healthy fluid level is maintained by balancing intake and excretion. The primary sources of fluids are water and other beverages, foods, and the production of metabolic water in the body. Fluid losses occur through urination, sweating, the feces, exhalation from the lungs, and insensible evaporation from the skin.**

diuretic A substance that increases fluid loss via the urine. Common diuretics include alcohol, some prescription medications, and many over-the-counter weight-loss pills.

A Profile of Nutrients Involved in Hydration and Neuromuscular Function

The nutrients involved in maintaining hydration and neuromuscular function are water and the minerals sodium, potassium, chloride, and phosphorus (**Table 7.1**). As discussed in Chapter 1, these minerals are classified as *major minerals,* as the body needs more than 100 mg of each per day.

Calcium and magnesium also function as electrolytes and influence our body's fluid balance and neuromuscular function. However, because of their critical importance to bone health, they are discussed in Chapter 9.

Water

Water is essential for life. Although we can live weeks without food, we can survive only a few days without water, depending on the environmental temperature. The human body does not have the capacity to store water, so we must continuously replace the water lost each day.

How Much Water Should We Drink?

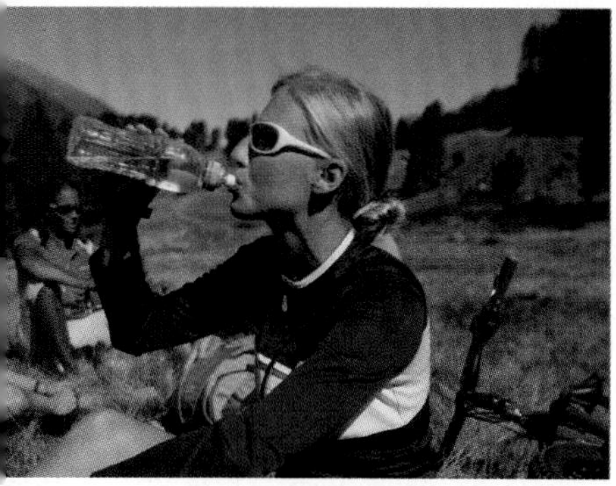

Vigorous exercise causes significant water loss, which must be replenished to optimize performance and health.

Our need for water varies greatly, depending on our age, body size, health status, physical activity level, and exposure to environmental conditions. It is important to pay attention to how much our need for water changes under various conditions, so that we can avoid dehydration.

Fluid requirements are very individualized. For example, a highly active male athlete training in a hot environment may require up to 10 liters (L) of fluid per day to maintain a healthy fluid balance, while an inactive, petite woman who lives in a mild climate and works in a temperature-controlled office building may only require about 3 L of fluid per day.

The DRI for adult men aged 19 to 50 years is 3.7 L of total water per day. This includes approximately 3.0 L (13 cups) as beverages, including water. The DRI for adult women aged 19 to 50 years is 2.7 L of total water per day, including about 2.2 L (9 cups) as beverages.[2]

Figure 7.7 shows the amount and sources of water intake and output for a woman expending 2,500 kcal per day. Based on current recommendations, this woman needs about 3,000 ml (3 L) of fluid per day. As shown,

- Water from metabolism provides 300 ml of water.
- The foods she eats provide her with an additional 500 ml of water each day.
- The beverages she drinks provide the remainder of the water she needs, which is equal to 2,200 ml.

An 8-oz glass of fluid is equal to 240 ml. In this example, the woman would need to drink nine glasses of fluid to meet her needs. You may have read or heard that drinking eight glasses of fluid each day is recommended for most people. Remember, however, that this recommendation is a general guideline. You may need to drink a different amount to meet your individual fluid needs.

TABLE 7.1 Overview of Nutrients Involved in Hydration and Neuromuscular Function

To see the full profile of nutrients involved in hydration and neuromusclar function, see ***In Depth,*** Vitamins and Minerals: Micronutrients with Macro Powers, pages 216–225.

Nutrient	Recommended Intake
Sodium	1.5 g/day*
Potassium	4.7 g/day*
Chloride	2.3 g/day*
Phosphorus	700 mg/day†

*Adequate Intake (AI).
†Recommended Dietary Allowance (RDA).

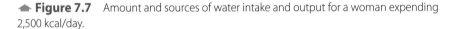

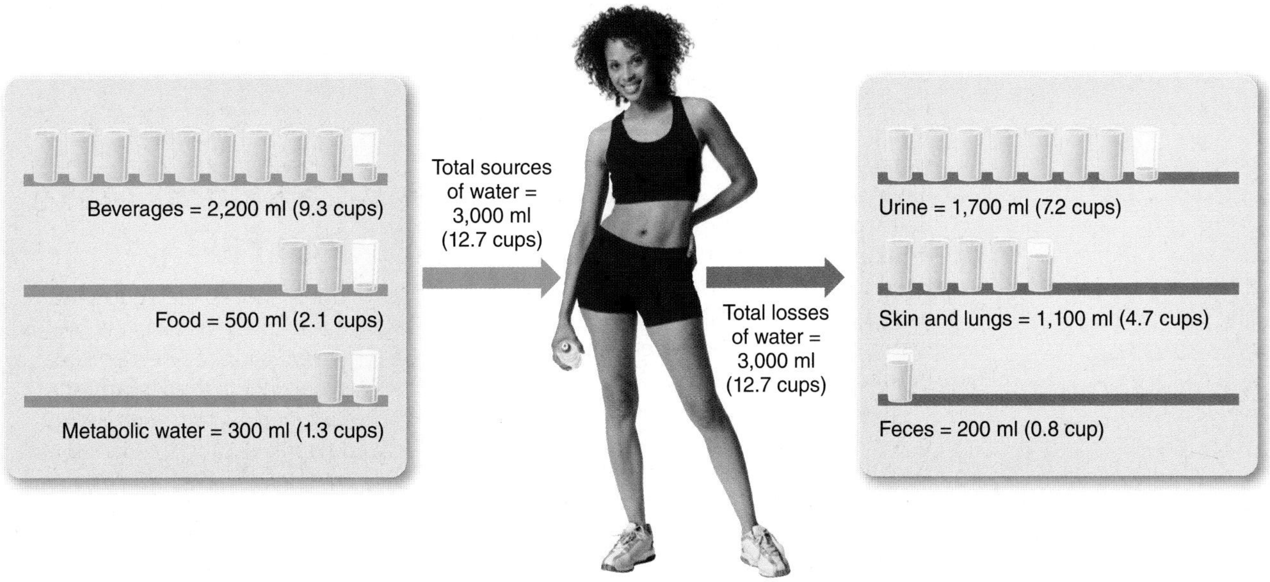

Figure 7.7 Amount and sources of water intake and output for a woman expending 2,500 kcal/day.

Athletes and other people who are active, especially those working in very hot environments, may require more fluid than the current recommendations. The amount of sweat lost during exercise is very individualized and depends on body size, exercise intensity, level of personal fitness, environmental temperature, and humidity. A recent study reported that professional football players lose almost 7 liters of sweat per day when practicing in a hot, humid environment.[3] Thus, these individuals need to drink more to replace the fluid they lose. Sodium is the major electrolyte lost in sweat; some potassium and small amounts of minerals such as iron and calcium are also lost in sweat.

Because of their high fluid and electrolyte losses during exercise, some athletes drink sports beverages instead of plain water to help them maintain fluid balance. Recently, sports beverages have also become popular with recreationally active people and non-athletes. Is it really necessary for people to consume these beverages if they are not highly active? See the Nutrition Debate on sports beverages on page 247 to learn whether they are right for recreationally active people and non-athletes.

Sources of Drinking Water

Millions of Americans routinely consume the tap water found in homes and public places, which generally comes from two sources: surface water and groundwater. *Surface water* comes from lakes, rivers, and reservoirs. *Groundwater* comes from underground rock formations called *aquifers.* Many people who live in rural areas depend on groundwater pumped from a well as their water source. The most common chemical used to treat and purify public water supplies is *chlorine,* which is effective in killing many microorganisms. Water treatment plants also routinely check water supplies for hazardous chemicals, minerals, and other contaminants. Because of these efforts, the United States has one of the safest water systems in the world.

The Environmental Protection Agency (EPA) sets and monitors the standards for public water systems. Local water regulatory agencies, such as cities and counties, must provide an annual report on specific water contaminants to all households served by that agency. The EPA does not monitor water from private wells, but it publishes recommendations for well owners to help them maintain a safe water supply. For more information on drinking water safety, go to the EPA website (see Web Resources at the end of this chapter).

Over the past 20 years, there has been a major shift away from the use of tap water to the consumption of bottled water. Americans now drink about 9 billion gallons of bottled water each year.[4] The meteoric rise in bottled water production and consumption is most likely due to the convenience of drinking bottled water, the health messages related to drinking more water, and the public's fears related to the safety of tap water. Recent environmental concerns related to the disposal of water bottles has, however, slowed the use of bottled water.

The Food and Drug Administration (FDA) is responsible for the regulation of bottled water. As with tap water, bottled water is taken from either surface water or groundwater sources. But it is often treated and filtered differently. Although this treatment may make bottled water taste better than tap water, it doesn't necessarily make it any safer to drink. Also, although some types of bottled water contain more minerals than tap water, there are no other additional nutritional benefits of drinking bottled water. For more information on bottled water, go to www.bottledwater.org.

How pure is your favorite bottled water? Follow the steps in the What About You? box on page 239 to find out!

Many types of bottled water are available in the United States. Carbonated water (seltzer water) contains carbon dioxide gas that either occurs naturally or is added to the water. Mineral waters contain various levels of minerals and offer a unique taste. Some brands, however, contain high amounts of sodium and should be avoided by people who are trying to reduce their sodium intake. Distilled water is mineral-free but has a "flat" taste.

HOT TOPIC

Can Fluids Make You Fat?

Until about 50 years ago, beverage choices were limited. But the introduction of a new, cheap sweetener derived from corn, *high-fructose corn syrup* (see Chapter 4), caused soda and other sweetened beverages to flood the market. Today, Americans take in approximately 21% of their Calories from beverages, mostly in the form of sweetened soft drinks and fruit juices. Recently, sweetened bottled waters, bottled teas, and specialty coffee drinks have contributed to the problem: a coffee mocha at one national chain of cafes provides 350 Calories, which is 17.5% of an average adult's total daily Calorie needs.

It's not surprising, then, that many (although not all!) researchers believe that Calories from such beverages have contributed significantly to the rise in caloric intake among Americans since the late 1970s. That's because beverages with a high Calorie content appear to do little to curb appetite, so people may not compensate for the extra Calories they drink by eating less.[5]

What Happens If We Drink Too Much Water?

Drinking too much water and becoming overhydrated is very rare, but it can occur. Certain illnesses can cause excessive reabsorption, or retention, of water by the kidneys. When this occurs, overhydration and dilution of blood sodium result. As described in the chapter-opening story, marathon runners and other endurance athletes can overhydrate and dangerously dilute their blood sodium concentration. This condition, called *hyponatremia*, is discussed in more detail shortly.

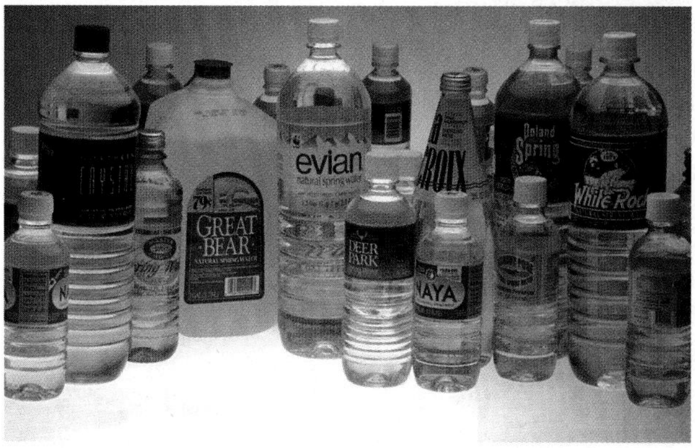

Numerous varieties of drinking water are available to consumers.

What Happens If We Don't Drink Enough Water?

Dehydration results when we do not drink enough water or are unable to retain the water we consume. It is one of the leading causes of death around the world. Dehydration is generally due to some form of illness or gastrointestinal infection that causes diarrhea and vomiting. The impact of dehydration on health is discussed ***In Depth*** immediately following this chapter.

What About You?

How Pure Is Your Favorite Bottled Water?

The next time you reach for a bottle of water, check the label. To find out how pure it is, consider the following factors:

1. Find out where it comes from. If no location is identified, even a bottle labeled "spring water" may actually contain tap water with minerals added to improve the taste. What you're looking for are the words "Bottled at the source." Water that comes from a protected groundwater source is less likely to have contaminants, such as disease-causing microbes. If the label doesn't identify the water's source, it should at least provide contact information, such as a phone number or website of the bottled water company, so that you can track down the source.

2. Find out how the water in the bottle has been treated. There are several ways of treating water, but what you're looking for is either of the following two methods, which have been proven to be effective against the most common waterborne disease-causing microorganisms:

- *Micron filtration* is a process whereby water is filtered through screens with various-sized microscopic holes. High-quality micron filtration can eliminate most chemical contaminants and microbes.
- *Reverse osmosis* is a process often referred to as *ultrafiltration* because it uses a membrane with microscopic openings that allow water to pass through but not larger compounds. Reverse osmosis membranes also utilize electrical charges to reject harmful chemicals.

If the label on your bottle of water says that the water was purified using any of the following methods, you might want to consider switching brands: filtered, carbon-filtered, particle-filtered, ozonated or ozone-treated, ultraviolet light, ion exchange, or deionized. These methods have not been proven to be effective against the most common waterborne disease-causing microorganisms.

3. Check the nutrient content on the label. Ideally, water should be high in magnesium (at least 20 mg per 8 fl. oz serving) and calcium but low in sodium (less than 5 mg per 8 fl. oz serving). Avoid bottled waters with sweeteners, as their "empty Calories" can contribute significantly to your energy intake. These products are often promoted as healthful beverage choices, with names including words such as *vitamins*, *herbs*, *nature*, and *life*, but they are essentially "liquid candy." Check the Nutrition Facts Panel and don't be fooled!

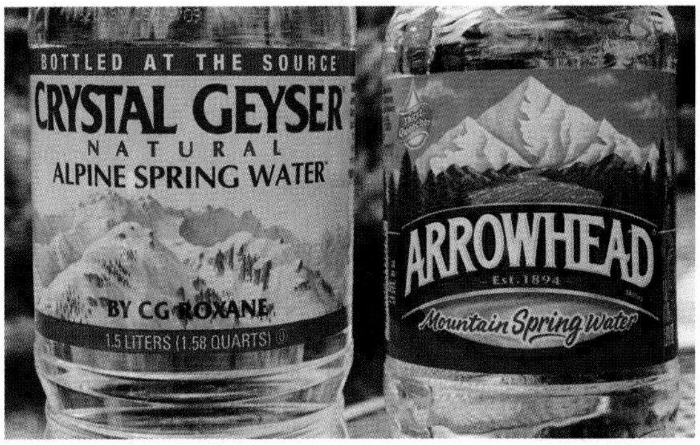

Can you tell where the water in each bottle comes from?

NUTRI-CASE JUDY

"I've heard about how important it is to drink at least 8 cups of fluid a day. At first that seemed like an awful lot, but after keeping track of what I drank yesterday, I figured I'm good. I had a mug of coffee when I first got up, a can of soda on my way to work, a coffee mocha on my morning break, another soda with lunch, and a bottle of Gatorade in the afternoon. On my way home, I stopped to pick up a pizza, and they were offering a free 22-ounce bottle of soda, so I went for it. I'm not sure what all that adds up to, but I know it's more than 8 cups. It's not as hard as I thought to get enough fluid!"

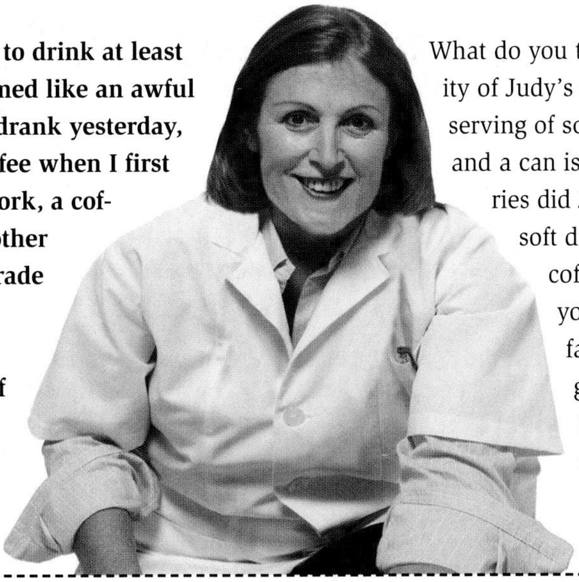

What do you think of the nutritional quality of Judy's fluid choices? If one 8-ounce serving of soda provides about 100 kcal, and a can is 12 ounces, how many Calories did Judy consume just from her soft drinks? And what about that coffee mocha? Given what you've learned about Judy so far in this text, could you suggest some other beverages that might be smarter choices for her?

RECAP Fluid intake needs are highly variable and depend on body size, age, physical activity, health status, and environmental conditions. Drinking too much water can lead to overhydration and dilution of blood sodium. Drinking too little water leads to dehydration, one of the leading causes of death around the world.

Sodium

Over the last 20 years, researchers have linked high sodium intake to an increased risk for high blood pressure among some groups of individuals. Because of this link, many people have come to believe that sodium is harmful to the body. This oversimplification, however, is just not true: sodium is a valuable nutrient that is essential for survival.

Functions of Sodium

Sodium has a variety of functions. As discussed earlier in this chapter, it is the major positively charged electrolyte in the extracellular fluid. Its exchange with potassium across cell membranes allows cells to maintain proper fluid balance, blood pressure, and acid–base balance.

Sodium also assists with the transmission of nerve signals and aids in muscle contraction. To review, the release of sodium from inside to outside the cell stimulates the spread of nerve signals within nervous tissue. The stimulation of muscles by nerve impulses provides the impetus for muscle contraction.

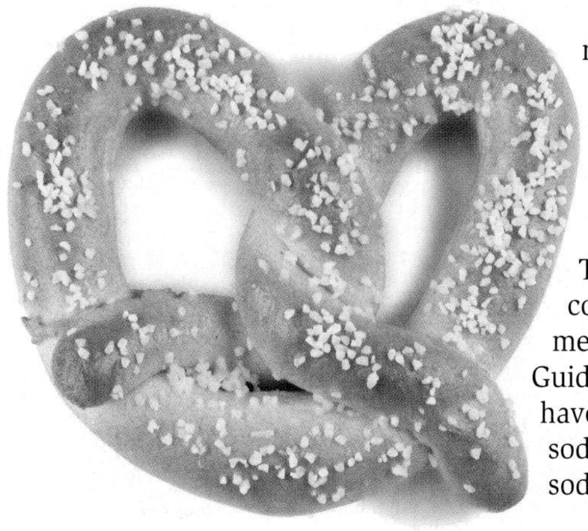

Many popular snack foods are high in sodium.

How Much Sodium Should We Consume?

The AI for sodium is listed in Table 7.1. Most people in the United States consume two to four times the AI daily. Several health organizations recommend a daily sodium intake of no more than 2.3 g per day. The 2010 Dietary Guidelines for Americans specifically recommend that African Americans (who have a higher risk of hypertension, especially when consuming too much sodium) and all persons who already have hypertension limit their daily sodium intake to no more than 1.5 g.[6]

Beyond Table Salt: Sneaky Sources of Sodium

Sodium is found naturally in many whole foods, but most dietary sodium comes from processed foods and restaurant foods, which typically contain large amounts of added sodium. Try to guess which of the following foods contains the most sodium: 1 cup of tomato juice, 1 oz of potato chips, or 4 saltine crackers. Now look at **Table 7.2**

TABLE 7.2 High-Sodium Foods and Lower-Sodium Alternatives

High-Sodium Food	Sodium (mg)	Lower-Sodium Food	Sodium (mg)
Dill pickle (1 large, 4 in.)	1,731	Low-sodium dill pickle (1 large, 4 in.)	23
Ham, cured, roasted (3 oz)	1,023	Pork, loin roast (3 oz)	54
Turkey pastrami (3 oz)	915	Roasted turkey, cooked (3 oz)	54
Tomato juice, regular (1 cup)	877	Tomato juice, lower sodium (1 cup)	24
Macaroni and cheese (1 cup)	800	Spanish rice (1 cup)	5
Ramen noodle soup (chicken flavor) (1 package [85 g])	1,960	Ramen noodle soup made with sodium-free chicken bouillon (1 cup)	0
Teriyaki chicken (1 cup)	3,210	Stir-fried pork/rice/vegetables (1 cup)	575
Tomato sauce, canned (1/2 cup)	741	Fresh tomato (1 medium)	11
Creamed corn, canned (1 cup)	730	Cooked corn, fresh (1 cup)	28
Tomato soup, canned (1 cup)	695	Lower-sodium tomato soup, canned (1 cup)	480
Potato chips, salted (1 oz)	168	Baked potato, unsalted (1 medium)	14
Saltine crackers (4 crackers)	156	Saltine crackers, unsalted (4 crackers)	100

Data from U.S. Department of Agriculture. 2009. USDA Nutrient Database for Standard Reference, Release 22. Nutrient Data Laboratory Home Page. www.ars.usda.gov/ba/bhnrc/ndl.

NUTRI-CASE GUSTAVO

"Something is going on with me this week. Every day, at work, I've been feeling weak and like I'm going to be sick to my stomach. It's been really hot, over a hundred degrees out in the fields, but I'm used to that, and besides, I've been drinking lots of water. It's probably just my high blood pressure acting up again."

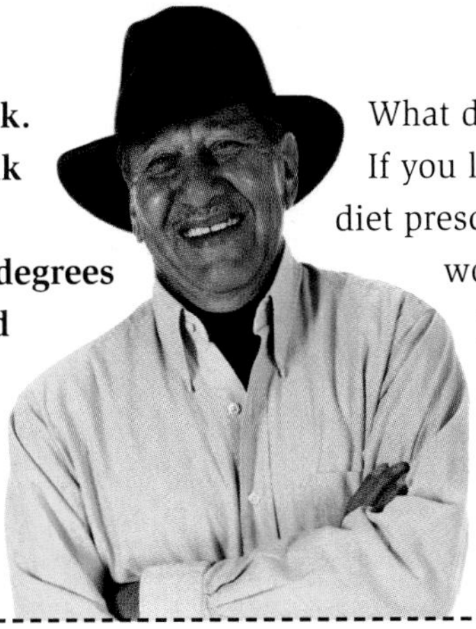

What do you think might be going on with Gustavo? If you learned that he was following a low-sodium diet prescribed to manage his high blood pressure, would this information argue for or against your assumptions, and why? What would you advise Gustavo to do differently at work tomorrow?

tions; in fact, the person is typically sweating heavily. The skin is cool, damp, and pale. While body temperature is above normal, it does not exceed 105°F.

A person with heat exhaustion should be taken indoors or placed in a shaded area and given a sports beverage to drink. Loosen the person's clothing and/or partially remove it, and cool the person off with water from a hose, shower, or bath. If those are not available, have the person hold an ice pack on areas of the body where blood circulating close to the surface can be quickly cooled: the neck, the armpits, and the groin. If symptoms do not subside within 1 hour, seek medical attention. It's critical to treat heat exhaustion promptly and aggressively to prevent it from progressing to heat stroke.

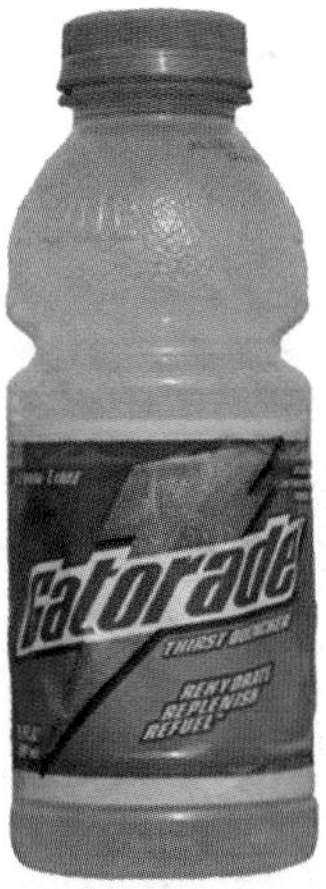

Treatment of heat illnesses includes replacing lost fluids and electrolytes by drinking a sports beverage rather than plain water.

Heat Stroke

Heat stroke is a potentially fatal heat illness characterized by a failure of the body's heat-regulating mechanisms. It should be viewed as a medical emergency. Symptoms include rapid pulse; hyperventilation; high core body temperature (above 105°F); and hallucinations or loss of consciousness. The skin is hot and dry, not sweaty, because the body's normal sweat mechanism has failed.

Anyone who engages in strenuous physical activity in hot weather is vulnerable to heat stroke. As we discussed at the beginning of this essay, National Football League all-star player Korey Stringer died of complications from heat stroke after training for several hours on a hot July morning. The high humidity that day was also a factor, as the body's ability to dissipate heat via evaporation of sweat is extremely limited in a humid environment. In addition, Stringer's tightly fitting uniform, which trapped warm air close to his body, was a factor in his death. His large body size (6'4", 330 pounds) also played a role: the larger the individual and the greater the muscle mass, the more heat the body produces. In addition, excess body fat adds an extra layer of insulation, which makes it even more difficult to dissipate body heat.

Similar deaths have also occurred among high school and collegiate athletes. These deaths have prompted national attention and resulted in strict guidelines requiring regular fluid breaks and the cancellation of training and competition or a change in the time of the event to avoid periods of high heat and humidity.

Any person who is active in a hot environment should stop exercising if dizziness, light-headedness, disorientation, or nausea sets in. Heat stroke can be avoided by maintaining a healthy fluid balance before, during, and after exercise and by avoiding strenuous activity in hot and humid environmental conditions.

If you suspect that someone has heat stroke, provide cooling as quickly and effectively as possible while seeking immediate expert medical care: immerse the person in cool water if possible (keeping the head out of water). Alternatively, wet the person with wet washcloths or a hose and fan the person's body aggressively. If running water is not available, place ice or cold packs on areas of high circulation, such as the neck, armpits, and groin.

Web Resources

www.acsm.org
American College of Sports Medicine

Check out this website for information on heat illness and youth sports.

www.eatright.org
Part of the American Dietetic Association

For general information on dehydration and related content, see this website and its links.

heat stroke A potentially fatal response to high temperature characterized by failure of the body's heat-regulating mechanisms; also commonly called *sunstroke*.

8 Nutrients Involved in Antioxidant Function

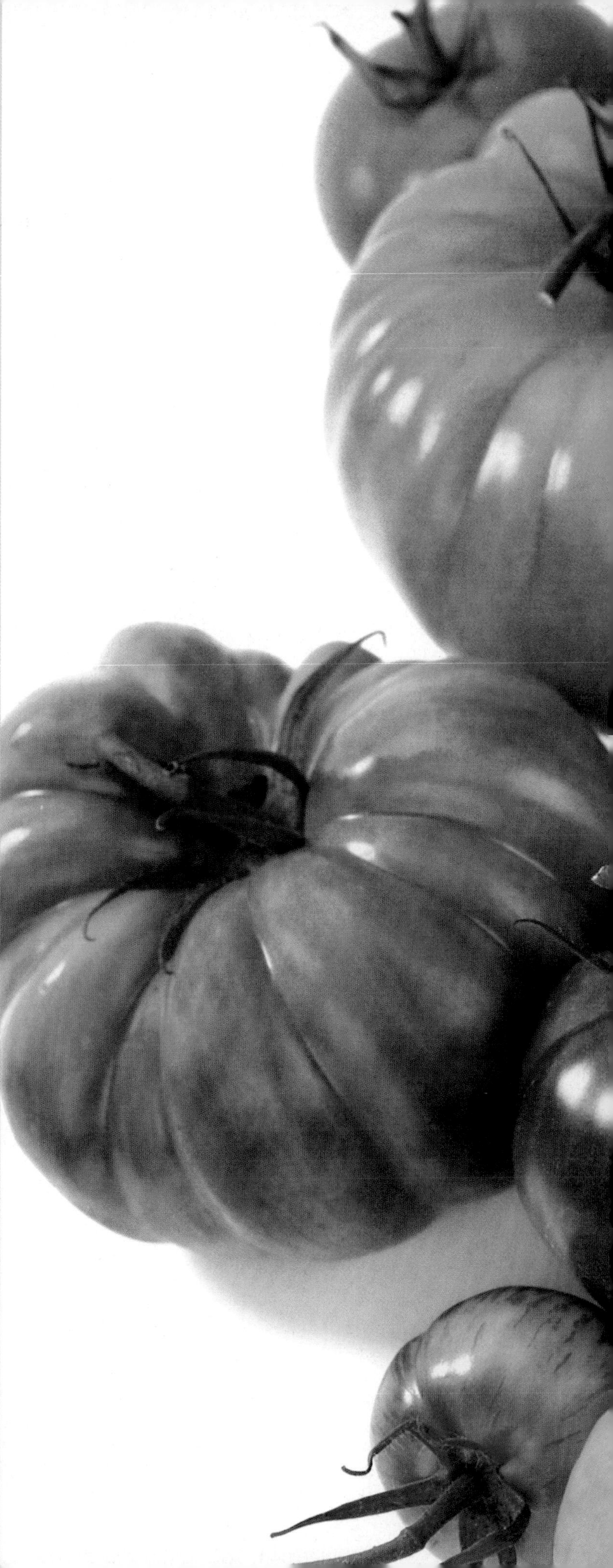

CHAPTER OBJECTIVES

After reading this chapter you will be able to:

1. **Define the term *free radicals* and explain how they can damage cells, pp. 257–259.**
2. **Define the term *antioxidant enzyme systems* and identify the minerals involved in these systems, p. 259.**
3. **Discuss the interrelated roles of vitamins E and C in protecting cells from oxidative damage, pp. 260–266.**
4. **Explain how vitamin C helps maintain bone, skin, tendons, and other tissues, pp. 262–263.**
5. **Describe the relationship between beta-carotene and vitamin A, pp. 267–269.**
6. **Discuss the role of vitamin A in vision, pp. 270, 273–274.**

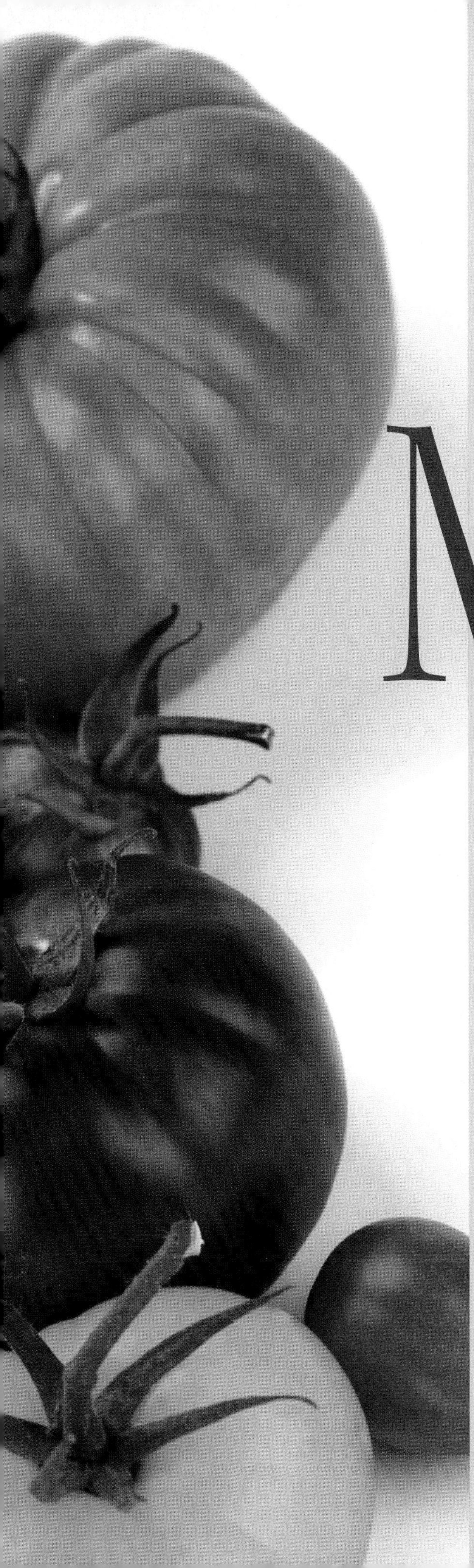

Test Yourself

1. T F Free radicals are a normal by-product of our body functions.
2. T F Taking large doses of vitamin C supplements reduces our risk of suffering from the common cold.
3. T F Eating carrots promotes good vision.

Test Yourself answers can be found at the end of the chapter.

Mika, a first-year student at a university hundreds of miles from home, just opened another care package from her mom. As usual, it contained an assortment of healthful snacks, a box of chamomile tea, and several types of supplements: echinacea extract to ward off colds, powdered papaya for good digestion, and antioxidant vitamins. "Wow, Mika!" her roommate laughed. "Can you let your mom know I'm available for adoption?"

"I guess she just wants me to stay healthy," Mika sighed. She wondered what her mother would think if she ever found out how much junk food Mika had been eating since she'd started college, or that she'd been binge-drinking most weekends, or that she'd been smoking since high school. "Still," Mika reminded herself, "at least I take the vitamins she sends."

What do you think of Mika's current lifestyle? Can a poor diet, binge-drinking, and smoking cause cancer or other health problems, and can the use of dietary supplements provide some protection? What are antioxidant vitamins, and why do you think Mika's mom included a bottle of these in her care package? If your health food store were promoting an antioxidant supplement, would you buy it?

It isn't easy to sort fact from fiction when it comes to antioxidants—especially when they're in the form of supplements. Internet ads and articles in fitness and health magazines tout their benefits, yet some researchers claim that antioxidant supplements don't protect us from diseases and in some cases may even be harmful. In this chapter, you'll learn what antioxidants are and how they work in the body. We'll discuss how antioxidants consumed in foods protect cells from damage that can lead to cancer and cardiovascular disease, and how consuming antioxidants in supplements may work against us. And as we profile each antioxidant nutrient, we'll identify additional roles it plays in protecting and maintaining our health.

What Are Antioxidants, and How Does Our Body Use Them?

Antioxidants are compounds that protect our cells from the damage caused by oxidation. *Anti* means "against," and antioxidants work *against,* or *prevent,* oxidation. Before we can go further in our discussion of antioxidants, we need to learn what oxidation is and how it damages cells.

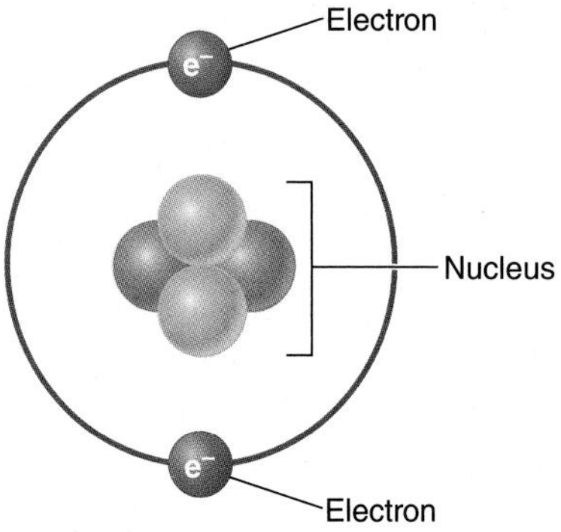

Figure 8.1 An atom consists of a central nucleus and orbiting electrons. The nucleus exerts a positive charge, which keeps the negatively charged electrons in its vicinity. Notice that this atom has an even number of electrons in orbit around the nucleus. This pairing of electrons results in the atom being chemically stable.

Oxidation Is a Chemical Reaction in Which Atoms Lose Electrons

A review of some basic chemistry will help you understand the process of oxidation. In Chapter 3, we said that our body is made up of atoms, tiny units of matter that cannot be broken down by natural means. Hydrogen, carbon, and iron are unique because their atoms are unique. Every atom of carbon, for example, is identical to every other atom of carbon, whether it is present in coal or in cheese. We also said that atoms join together to form molecules, such as saccharides and amino acids, which are the smallest *physical units* of a substance. Some molecules, such as hydrogen gas (H_2), contain only one type of atom—in this case, hydrogen. Most molecules, however, are *compounds*—they contain two or more different types of atoms (such as water, H_2O). Our body is constantly breaking down compounds of food, water, and air into their component atoms, then rearranging these freed atoms to build the different substances our body needs.

Atoms Are Composed of Particles

We just said that atoms cannot be broken down by natural means, but during the 20th century, physicists learned how to split atoms into their components, which they called *particles*. As you can see in **Figure 8.1**, this research revealed that all atoms have a central core, called a **nucleus,** which is positively charged. Orbiting around this nucleus at close to the speed of light are one or more **electrons,** which are negatively charged. The opposite attraction between the positive nucleus and the negative electrons keeps an atom together by making the atom stable, so that its electrons remain with it and do not veer off toward other atoms.

During Metabolism, Atoms Exchange Electrons

As you recall from Chapter 1, the process by which our body breaks down and builds up molecules is called *metabolism*. During metabolism, atoms may lose electrons (**Figure 8.2a**). We call this loss of electrons **oxidation,** because it is fueled by oxygen. Atoms are capable of gaining electrons during metabolism as well. We call

antioxidant A compound that has the ability to prevent or repair the damage caused by oxidation.

nucleus The positively charged, central core of an atom. It is made up of two types of particles—protons and neutrons—bound tightly together. The nucleus of an atom contains essentially all of its atomic mass.

electron A negatively charged particle orbiting the nucleus of an atom.

oxidation A chemical reaction in which molecules of a substance are broken down into their component atoms. During oxidation, the atoms involved lose electrons.

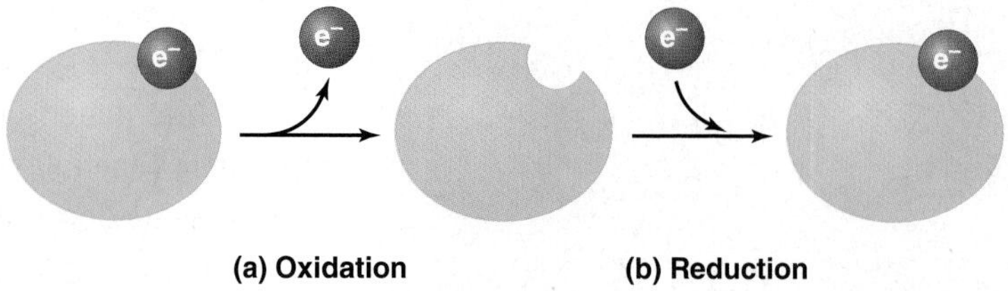

Figure 8.2 The exchange reaction. Exchange reactions consist of two parts. **(a)** During oxidation, atoms *lose* electrons. **(b)** In the second part of the reaction, atoms *gain* electrons, which is called reduction.

this process *reduction* (Figure 8.2b). This loss and gain of electrons typically results in an even exchange of electrons. Scientists call this loss and gain of electrons an *exchange reaction*.

Oxidation Sometimes Results in the Formation of Free Radicals

Stable atoms have an even number of electrons orbiting in pairs at successive distances (called *shells* or *rings*) from the nucleus. When a stable atom loses an electron during oxidation, it is left with an odd number of electrons in its outermost shell. In other words, it now has an *unpaired electron*. In most exchange reactions, unpaired electrons immediately pair up with other unpaired electrons, making newly stabilized atoms, but in some cases, atoms with unpaired electrons in their outermost shell remain unpaired. Such atoms are highly unstable and are called **free radicals.**

Free radicals are formed as a normal by-product of many of our body's fundamental physiologic processes. Still, excessive production of free radicals can cause serious damage to our cells and other body components. Let's look at the most common way they arise. Our body uses oxygen and hydrogen to generate the energy (ATP) it needs (**Figure 8.3**). We are constantly inhaling air into our body, thereby providing the oxygen needed to fuel this reaction. At the same time, we generate the necessary hydrogen as a result of digesting food. As shown in **Figure 8.4**, occasionally during metabolism, oxygen accepts a single electron that was released during this process. When it does so, the oxygen atom becomes an unstable free radical because of the added unpaired electron.

Free radicals are also formed from other physiologic processes, such as when the immune system produces inflammation to fight allergens or infections. Other factors

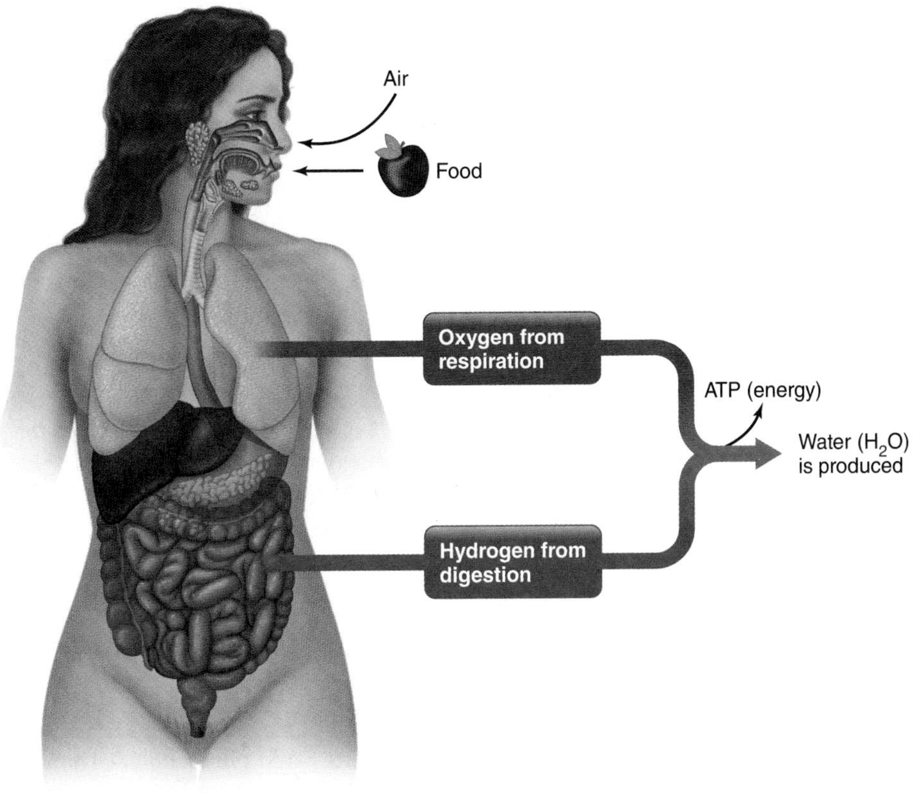

Figure 8.3 Oxygen (O) enters our body when we inhale air. Hydrogen (H) is released through the process of metabolizing food. As a result of exchange reactions during metabolism, electrons are freed to contribute to the production of the energy molecule ATP in body cells. The hydrogen and oxygen then recombine to form water (H_2O).

free radical A highly unstable atom with an unpaired electron in its outermost shell.

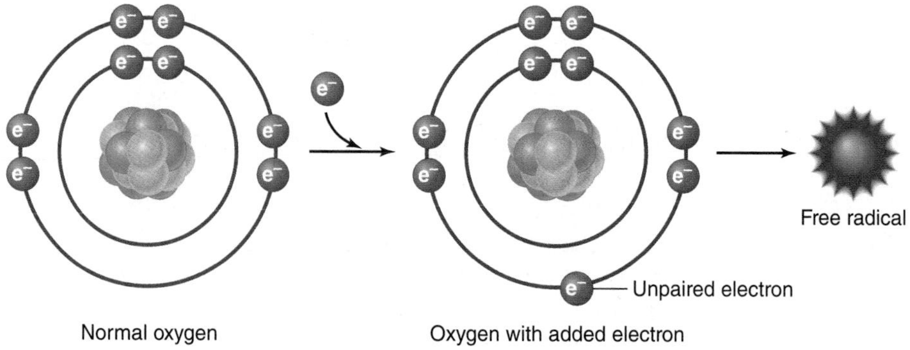

Figure 8.4 Normally, an oxygen atom contains eight electrons. Occasionally, oxygen will accept an unpaired electron during the oxidation process. This acceptance of a single electron causes oxygen to become an unstable atom called a free radical.

that cause free radical formation include exposure to air pollution, ultraviolet (UV) rays from the sun, other types of radiation, tobacco smoke, industrial chemicals, and asbestos. Continual exposure to these factors leads to uncontrollable free radical formation, cell damage, and disease, as discussed next.

Free Radicals Can Destabilize Other Molecules and Damage Our Cells

Why are we concerned with the formation of free radicals? Simply put, it is because of their destabilizing power. If you were to think of paired electrons as a married couple, a free radical would be an extremely seductive outsider. Its unpaired electron exerts a powerful attraction toward all stable atoms and molecules around it. In an attempt to stabilize itself, a free radical will "steal" an electron from these stable neighbors, in turn generating more unstable free radicals. This is a dangerous chain reaction, since the free radicals generated can damage or destroy our cells.

One of the most significant sites of free radical damage is the cell membrane. As shown in **Figure 8.5a**, free radicals that form within the phospholipid bilayer of cell membranes steal electrons from the stable lipid heads. Recall from Chapter 5 that lipids are insoluble in water, so a stable line-up of lipid heads allows cell membranes to keep water out. When these lipid heads are destroyed, the cell membrane can no longer repel water. With the cell membrane's integrity lost, its ability to regulate the movement of fluids and nutrients into and out of the cell is also lost. This loss of cell integrity causes damage to the cell and to all systems affected by the cell.

Other sites of free radical damage include low-density lipoproteins (LDLs), cell proteins, and DNA. Damage to LDLs and cell proteins disrupts the transport of substances into and out of cells and alters cell function, whereas defective DNA results in faulty protein synthesis. These changes can also cause harmful changes (mutations) in cells or prompt cells to die prematurely. Free radicals also promote blood vessel inflammation and the formation of clots, both of which are risk factors for cardiovascular disease (see the ***In Depth*** essay on pages 173–183). Not surprisingly, many diseases are linked with free radical production, including cancer, heart disease, type 2 diabetes, arthritis, cataracts, and kidney, Alzheimer's, and Parkinson's diseases.

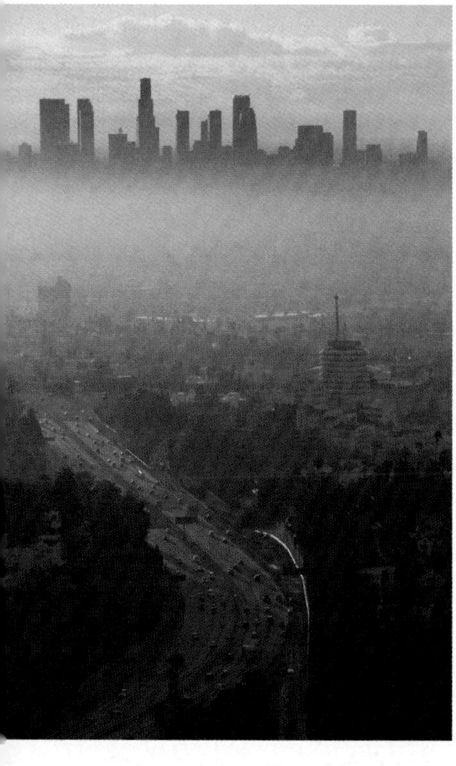

Exposure to pollution from car exhaust and industrial waste increases our production of free radicals.

Antioxidants Work by Stabilizing Free Radicals or Opposing Oxidation

How does our body fight free radicals and repair the damage they cause? These actions are performed by antioxidant vitamins, minerals, and phytochemicals and other compounds. These antioxidants perform their role in three ways:

1. Antioxidant vitamins work independently by donating their electrons or hydrogen atoms to free radicals to stabilize them and reduce the damage caused by oxidation (Figure 8.5b).

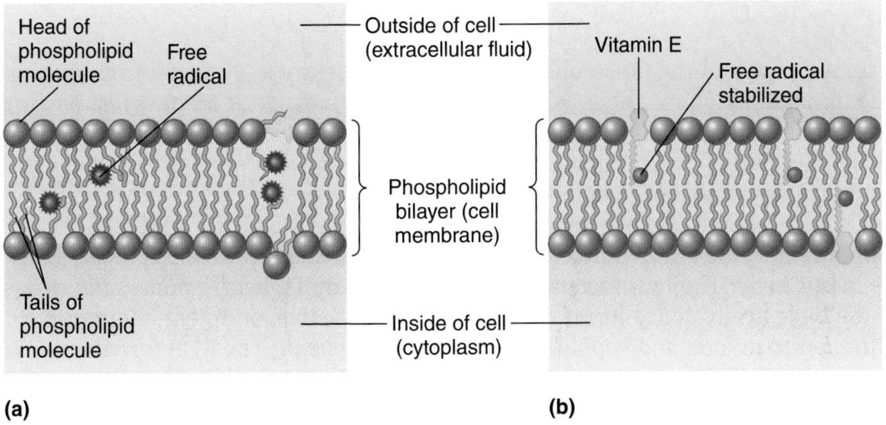

Figure 8.5 **(a)** The formation of free radicals in the lipid portion of our cell membranes can cause a dangerous chain reaction that damages the integrity of the membrane and can cause cell death. **(b)** Vitamin E is stored in the lipid portion of our cell membranes. By donating an electron to free radicals, it protects the lipid molecules in our cell membranes from themselves being oxidized and stops the chain reaction of oxidative damage.

2. Antioxidant minerals, including selenium, copper, iron, zinc, and manganese, act as **cofactors,** substances required to activate enzymes so that they can do their work. These minerals function within complex *antioxidant enzyme systems* that convert free radicals to less damaging substances that are excreted by our body. They also work to break down fatty acids that have become oxidized, thereby destroying the free radicals associated with them. Antioxidant enzyme systems also make more vitamin antioxidants available to fight other free radicals. Examples of these antioxidant enzyme systems are superoxide dismutase, catalase, and glutathione peroxidase.
3. Other compounds, such as beta-carotene and other phytochemicals, help stabilize free radicals and prevent damage to cells and tissues.

In summary, free radical formation is generally kept safely under control by certain vitamins, minerals working within antioxidant enzyme systems, and phytochemicals. Next, we take a look at the specific vitamins and minerals involved. Phytochemicals are discussed ***In Depth*** following Chapter 2.

RECAP **An atom is an infinitely small and unique unit of matter having a nucleus and orbiting electrons. Atoms join together to form molecules. During metabolism, molecules break apart and their atoms gain, lose, or exchange electrons; loss of electrons is called oxidation. Free radicals are highly unstable atoms with an unpaired electron in their outermost shell. A normal by-product of oxidation reactions, they can damage our LDLs, cell proteins, and DNA and are associated with many diseases. Antioxidant vitamins and phytochemicals donate electrons or hydrogen atoms to free radicals to stabilize them and reduce oxidative damage. Antioxidant minerals are part of antioxidant enzyme systems that convert free radicals to less damaging substances.**

TABLE 8.1 Nutrients Involved in Antioxidant Function

To see the full profile of nutrients involved in energy metabolism, turn to ***In Depth,*** Vitamins and Minerals: Micronutrients with Macro Powers, pages 216–225.

Nutrient	Recommended Intake
Vitamin E (fat soluble)	RDA: Women and men = 15 mg alpha-tocopheral
Vitamin C (water soluble)	RDA: Women = 75 mg Men = 90 mg Smokers = 35 mg more per day than RDA
Beta-carotene (fat-soluble provitamin for vitamin A)	None at this time
Vitamin A (fat soluble)	RDA: Women: 700 μg Men: 900 μg
Selenium (trace mineral)	RDA: Women and men = 55 μg

A Profile of Nutrients That Function as Antioxidants

Our body cannot form antioxidants spontaneously. Instead, we must consume them in our diet. Nutrients that appear to have antioxidant properties or are part of our protective antioxidant enzyme systems include vitamins E, C, and A; beta-carotene (a phytochemical that is a precursor to vitamin A); and the mineral selenium **(Table 8.1)**. The minerals copper, iron, zinc, and manganese play a peripheral role in fighting oxidation and are only mentioned in this chapter. Let's review each of these nutrients now and learn more about their functions in the body.

cofactor A mineral or other substance that is needed to allow enzymes to function properly.

Vitamin E

Vitamin E is one of the fat-soluble vitamins; thus, dietary fats carry it from our intestines through the lymphatic system and eventually transport it to our cells. As you remember, our body stores the fat-soluble vitamins: about 90% of the vitamin E in our body is stored in our adipose tissue. The remaining vitamin E is found in cell membranes.

Vitamin E is actually two separate families of compounds, *tocotrienols* and **tocopherols.** None of the different tocotrienol compounds appears to play an active role in our body. The four tocopherol compounds—alpha, beta, gamma, and delta—are the biologically active forms. Of these, the most active, or potent, vitamin E compound found in food and supplements is *alpha-tocopherol.* The RDA for vitamin E is expressed as milligrams of alpha-tocopherol equivalents per day (mg α-tocopherol/day). Food labels and vitamin and mineral supplements may express vitamin E in units of alpha-tocopherol equivalents (α-TE), milligrams, or International Units (IU). For conversion purposes,

- One α-TE is equal to 1 mg of active vitamin E.
- In supplements containing natural sources of vitamin E, 1 IU is equal to 0.67 mg α-TE.
- In supplements containing synthetic sources of vitamin E, 1 IU is equal to 0.45 mg α-TE.

Functions of Vitamin E

The primary function of vitamin E is as an antioxidant: it donates an electron to free radicals, stabilizing them and preventing them from destabilizing other molecules. Once vitamin E is oxidized, it is either excreted from the body or recycled back into active vitamin E through the help of other antioxidant nutrients, such as vitamin C.

Because vitamin E is prevalent in our adipose tissues and cell membranes, its action specifically protects polyunsaturated fatty acids (PUFAs) and other fatty components of our cells and cell membranes from being oxidized (Figure 8.5b). Vitamin E also protects our LDLs from being oxidized, thereby lowering our risk for heart disease. In addition to protecting our PUFAs and LDLs, vitamin E protects the membranes of our red blood cells from oxidation and plays a critical role in protecting the cells of our lungs, which are constantly exposed to oxygen and the potentially damaging effects of oxidation. Vitamin E's role in protecting PUFAs and other fatty components also explains why it is added to many oil-based foods and skincare products—by preventing oxidation in these products, it reduces rancidity and spoilage.

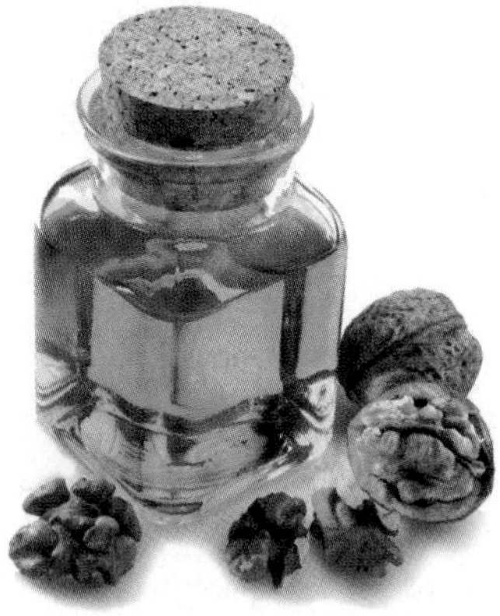

Vegetable oils, nuts, and seeds are good sources of vitamin E.

Vitamin E serves many other roles essential to human health. It is critical for normal fetal and early childhood development of nerves and muscles, as well as for maintenance of their functions. It protects white blood cells and other components of our immune system, thereby helping the body defend against illness and disease. It also improves the absorption of vitamin A if the dietary intake of vitamin A is low.

How Much Vitamin E Should We Consume?

Considering the importance of vitamin E to our health, you might think that you need to consume a huge amount daily. In fact, the RDA is modest: 15 mg alpha-tocopherol per day (see Table 8.1).[1] The Tolerable Upper Intake Level (UL) is 1,000 mg alpha-tocopherol per day. Remember that one of the primary roles of vitamin E is to protect PUFAs from oxidation. Thus, our need for vitamin E increases as we eat more oils and other foods that contain PUFAs. Fortunately, these foods also contain vitamin E, so we typically consume enough vitamin E within them to protect their PUFAs from oxidation.

Vitamin E: The Vegetarian Vitamin

tocopherol The active form of vitamin E in our body.

Vitamin E is widespread in foods from plant sources (**Figure 8.6**). Much of the vitamin E that we consume comes from products such as spreads, salad dressings, and mayonnaise made from vegetable oils, including safflower oil, sunflower oil, canola oil,

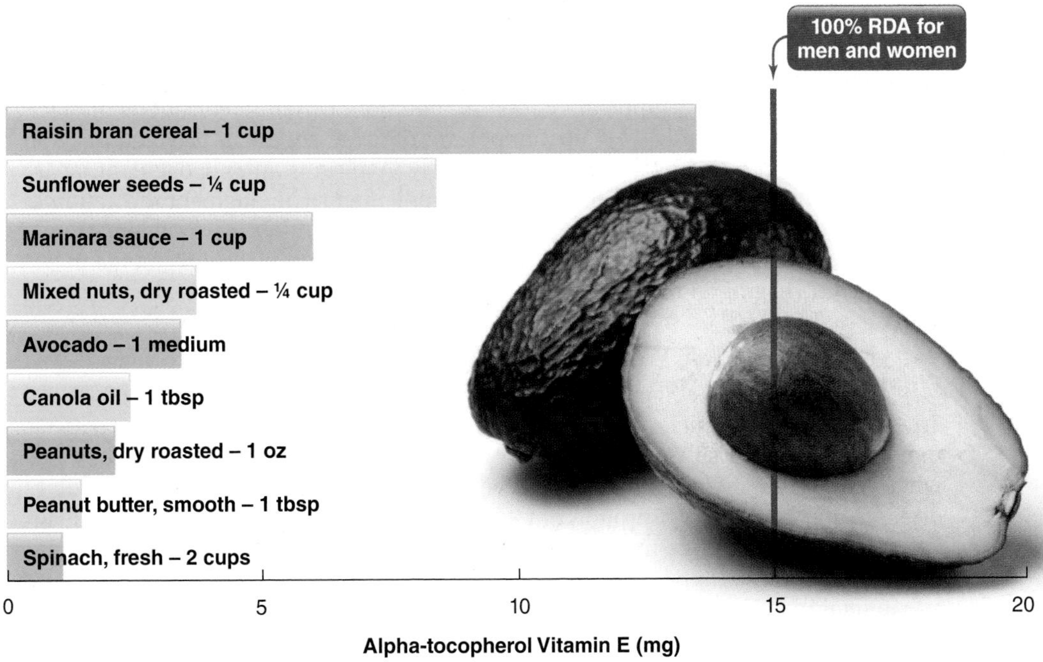

Figure 8.6 Common food sources of vitamin E. The RDA for vitamin E is 15 mg alpha-tocopherol per day for men and women.

Data from U.S. Department of Agriculture, Agricultural Research Service, 2009. USDA Nutrient Database for Standard Reference, Release 22. Nutrient Data Laboratory Home Page, www.ars.usda.gov/ba/bhnrc/ndl.

and soybean oil. Nuts, seeds, soybeans, and some vegetables—including spinach, broccoli, and avocados—also contribute vitamin E to our diet. Although no single fruit or vegetable contains very high amounts of vitamin E, eating the recommended amounts of fruits and vegetables each day will help ensure adequate intake of this nutrient. Cereals are often fortified with vitamin E, and other grain products contribute modest amounts to our diet. Animal and dairy products are poor sources.

Vitamin E is destroyed by exposure to oxygen, metals, ultraviolet light, and heat. Although raw (uncooked) vegetable oils contain vitamin E, heating these oils destroys vitamin E. Thus, fried foods contain little vitamin E. This includes most fast foods. See the Quick Tips above for increasing your intake of vitamin E.

QUICK TIPS

Eating More Vitamin E

- ✓ Eat cereals high in vitamin E for breakfast or as a snack.
- ✓ Add sunflower seeds to salads and trail mixes, or just have them as a snack.
- ✓ Add sliced almonds to salads, granola, and trail mixes to boost vitamin E intake.
- ✓ Pack a peanut butter sandwich for lunch.
- ✓ Eat veggies throughout the day—for snacks, for sides, and in main dishes.
- ✓ When dressing a salad, use vitamin E–rich oils, such as sunflower, safflower, or canola.
- ✓ Enjoy some fresh, homemade guacamole: mash a ripe avocado with a squeeze of lime juice and a sprinkle of garlic salt.

What Happens If We Consume Too Much Vitamin E?

Until recently, standard supplemental doses (one to eighteen times the RDA) of vitamin E were not associated with any adverse health effects. However, a 2005 study found that, among adults 55 years of age or older with vascular disease or diabetes, a daily intake of 268 mg of vitamin E per day (about eighteen times the RDA) for approximately 7 years resulted in a significant increase in heart failure.[2] However, these results have not been confirmed by additional research studies. At this time, it is

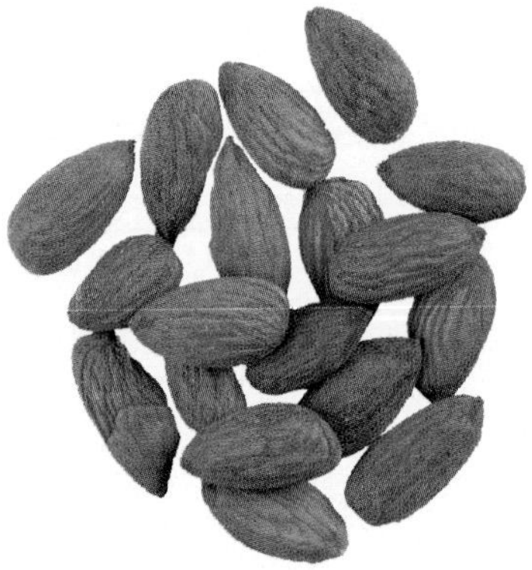

Raw almonds are an appetizing way to help meet your vitamin E needs.

unclear whether these adverse effects are an anomaly or if high supplemental doses of vitamin E may be harmful for certain individuals.

Some individuals report side effects such as nausea, intestinal distress, and diarrhea with vitamin E supplementation. In addition, certain medications interact negatively with vitamin E. The most important of these are the *anticoagulants,* substances that stop blood from clotting excessively. Aspirin is an anticoagulant, as is the prescription drug Coumadin. Vitamin E supplements can augment the action of these substances, causing uncontrollable bleeding. In addition, new evidence suggests that, in some people, long-term use of standard vitamin E supplements may cause hemorrhaging in the brain, leading to a type of stroke called *hemorrhagic stroke.*[3]

What Happens If We Don't Consume Enough Vitamin E?

True vitamin E deficiencies are uncommon in humans. This is primarily because vitamin E is fat soluble, so we typically store adequate amounts in our fatty tissues, even when our current dietary intake is low. Vitamin E deficiencies are usually a result of diseases that cause malabsorption of fat. However, results from the NHANES III survey show that the dietary intake of vitamin E of 27–41% of Americans is low enough that although these individuals probably don't have a true deficiency, they may have suboptimal blood levels of vitamin E, putting them at increased risk for cardiovascular disease.[4]

Despite the rarity of true vitamin E deficiencies, they do occur. One vitamin E deficiency symptom is *erythrocyte hemolysis,* or the rupturing (*lysis*) of red blood cells (*erythrocytes*). The rupturing of our red blood cells leads to *anemia,* a condition in which our red blood cells cannot carry and transport enough oxygen to our tissues, leading to fatigue, weakness, and a diminished ability to perform physical and mental work. We discuss anemia in more detail in Chapter 10. Other symptoms of vitamin E deficiency include loss of muscle coordination and reflexes, leading to impairments in vision, speech, and movement. Vitamin E deficiency can also impair immune function, especially when body stores of the mineral selenium are low.

RECAP **Vitamin E protects our cell membranes from oxidation, enhances immune function, and improves our absorption of vitamin A if dietary intake is low. The RDA for vitamin E is 15 mg alpha-tocopherol per day for men and women. Vitamin E is found primarily in vegetable oils and nuts. Toxicity is uncommon, but taking very high doses can cause excessive bleeding. A genuine deficiency is rare, but symptoms include anemia and impaired vision, speech, and movement.**

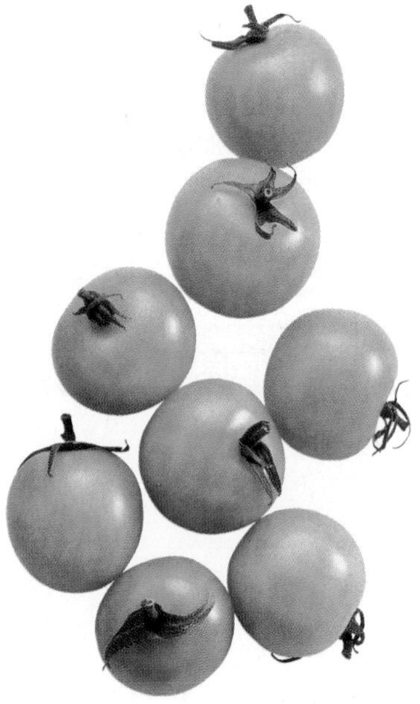

Many fruits, such as these yellow tomatoes, are high in vitamin C.

Vitamin C

Vitamin C is a water-soluble vitamin. We must therefore consume it on a regular basis, as any excess is excreted (primarily in our urine) rather than stored. There are two active forms of vitamin C: ascorbic acid and dehydroascorbic acid. Interestingly, most animals can make their own vitamin C from glucose. Humans and guinea pigs are two groups that cannot synthesize their own vitamin C and must consume it in the diet.

Functions of Vitamin C

Vitamin C is probably most well known for its role in preventing scurvy, a disease that ravaged sailors on long sea voyages centuries ago. In fact, the name *ascorbic acid* is derived from the combined Latin terms *a* (meaning "without") and *scorbic* (meaning "having scurvy"). Scurvy was characterized by bleeding tissues, especially of the gums, and is thought to have caused more than half of the deaths that occurred at sea. During these long voyages, the crew ate all of the fruits and vegetables early in the trip, then had only grain and animal products available until they reached land to resupply. In 1740 in England, Dr. James Lind discovered that citrus fruits can prevent scurvy. This is due to their high vitamin C content. Fifty years after the discovery of the link between citrus fruits and scurvy prevention, the British Navy finally required all ships to provide daily lemon juice rations for each sailor to prevent the onset of scurvy. A century later, sailors were given lime juice rations, earning them the nickname "limeys." It wasn't until 1930 that vitamin C was discovered and identified as a nutrient.

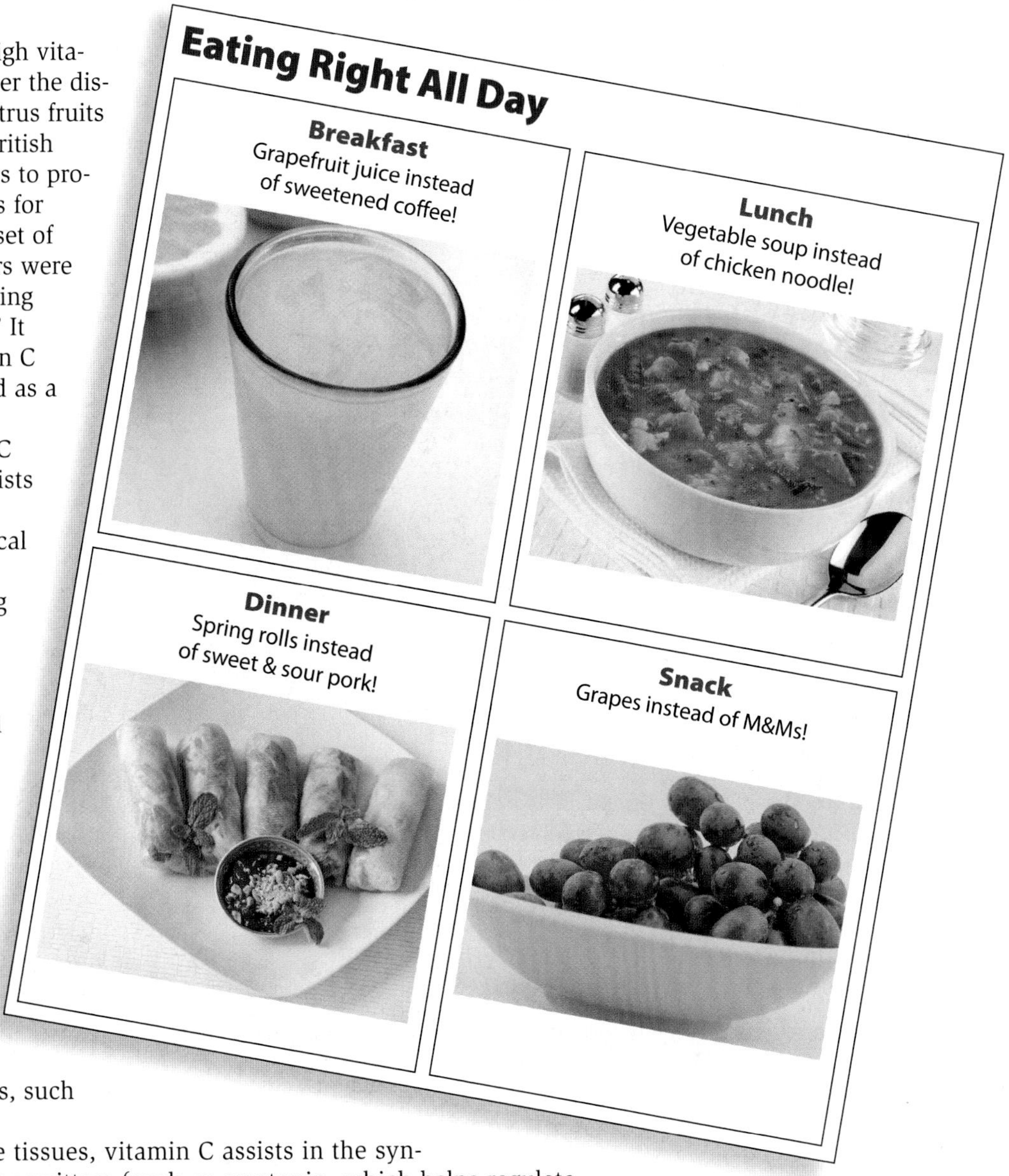
Eating Right All Day
Breakfast
Grapefruit juice instead of sweetened coffee!
Lunch
Vegetable soup instead of chicken noodle!
Dinner
Spring rolls instead of sweet & sour pork!
Snack
Grapes instead of M&Ms!

One reason that vitamin C prevents scurvy is that it assists in the synthesis of **collagen**. Collagen, a protein, is a critical component of all connective tissues in the body, including bone, teeth, skin, tendons, and blood vessels. Collagen assists in preventing bruises, and it ensures proper wound healing, as it is a part of scar tissue and a component of the tissue that mends broken bones. Without adequate vitamin C, the body cannot form collagen, and tissue hemorrhage, or bleeding, occurs. Vitamin C may also be involved in the synthesis of other components of connective tissues, such as elastin and bone matrix.

In addition to connective tissues, vitamin C assists in the synthesis of DNA, bile, neurotransmitters (such as serotonin, which helps regulate mood), and carnitine, which transports long-chain fatty acids from the cytosol into the mitochondria for energy production. Vitamin C also helps ensure that appropriate levels of thyroxine, a hormone produced by the thyroid gland, are produced to support basal metabolic rate and to maintain body temperature. Other hormones that are synthesized with assistance from vitamin C include epinephrine, norepinephrine, and steroid hormones.

Vitamin C also acts as an antioxidant. Because it is water soluble, it is an important antioxidant in the extracellular fluid. Like vitamin E, it donates electrons to free radicals, thus preventing the damage of cells and tissues. It also protects LDL-cholesterol from oxidation, which may reduce the risk for cardiovascular disease. Vitamin C acts as an important antioxidant in the lungs, helping protect us from the damage caused by ozone and cigarette smoke.[5] Vitamin C also regenerates vitamin E after it has been oxidized by donating an electron. This enables vitamin E to continue to protect our cell membranes and other tissues. It also enhances immune function by protecting white blood cells from the oxidative damage that occurs in response to fighting illness and infection. But contrary to popular belief, it is not a miracle cure (see the Nutrition Myth or Fact? box on vitamin C, page 264). In the stomach, vitamin C reduces the formation of *nitrosamines*, cancer-causing agents found in foods such as cured and processed meats. We discuss the role of vitamin C and other antioxidants in preventing some forms of cancer in the ***In Depth*** on pages 281–289.

collagen A protein found in all the connective tissues in our body.

NUTRITION MYTH OR FACT?

Can Vitamin C Prevent the Common Cold?

What do you do when you feel a cold coming on? If you are like many people, you drink a lot of orange juice or take vitamin C supplements to ward it off. Do these tactics really help prevent a cold?

It is well known that vitamin C is important for a healthy immune system. A deficiency of vitamin C can seriously weaken the immune cells' ability to detect and destroy invading microbes, increasing susceptibility to many diseases and illnesses—including the common cold. Many people have taken vitamin C supplements to prevent the common cold, basing their behavior on its actions of enhancing our immune function. Interestingly, scientific studies do not support this action. A recent review of many of the studies of vitamin C and the common cold found that people taking vitamin C regularly in an attempt to ward off the common cold experienced as many colds as people who took a placebo. However, the *duration* of their colds was reduced—by 8% in adults and 13.6% in children.[6] Timing appeared to be important, though: taking vitamin C after the onset of cold symptoms did not reduce either the duration or the severity of the cold. Interestingly, taking vitamin C supplements regularly did reduce the number of colds experienced in marathon runners, skiers, and soldiers participating in exercises done under extreme environmental conditions.

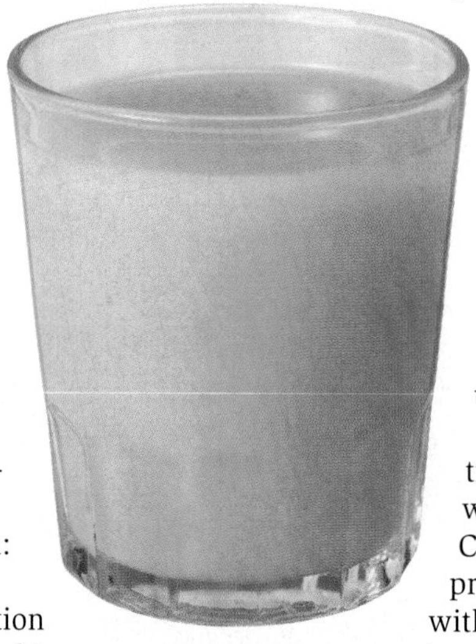

The amount of vitamin C taken in these studies was at least 200 mg per day, with many using doses as high as 4,000 mg per day (more than forty times the RDA), with no harmful effects noted in those studies that reported adverse events.

In summary, it appears that, for most people, taking vitamin C supplements regularly will not prevent colds but may reduce their duration. Consuming a healthful diet that includes excellent sources of vitamin C will also help you maintain a strong immune system. Taking vitamin C after the onset of cold symptoms does not appear to help, so next time you feel a cold coming on, you may want to think twice before taking extra vitamin C.

Vitamin C also enhances the absorption of iron. It is recommended that people with low iron stores consume vitamin C–rich foods along with iron sources to improve absorption of the iron. For people with high iron stores, however, this practice can be dangerous and lead to iron toxicity.

How Much Vitamin C Should We Consume?

Although popular opinion suggests that our need for vitamin C is quite high, we really require amounts that are easily obtained when we eat the recommended amounts of fruits and vegetables daily. The RDA for vitamin C is 90 mg per day for men and 75 mg per day for women (see Table 8.1).[1] The Tolerable Upper Intake Level (UL) is 2,000 mg per day for adults. Smoking increases a person's need for vitamin C; thus, the RDA for smokers is 35 mg more per day than for nonsmokers. This equals 125 mg per day for men and 110 mg per day for women. Other situations that may increase the need for vitamin C include healing from a traumatic injury, surgery, or burns and the use of oral contraceptives among women; there is no consensus on how much extra vitamin C is needed in these circumstances.

Vitamin C: Citrus and More

Fruits and vegetables are the best sources of vitamin C. Because heat and oxygen destroy vitamin C, fresh sources of these foods have the highest content. Cooking foods, especially boiling them, leaches their vitamin C, which is then lost when we strain them. The forms of cooking that are least likely to compromise the vitamin C content of foods are steaming, microwaving, and stir-frying.

As indicated in **Figure 8.7**, many fruits and vegetables are high in vitamin C. Citrus fruits (such as oranges, lemons, and limes), potatoes, strawberries, tomatoes, kiwi fruit, broccoli, spinach and other leafy greens, cabbage, green and red peppers, and cauliflower are excellent sources of vitamin C. Fortified beverages and cereals

Figure 8.7 Common food sources of vitamin C. The RDA for vitamin C is 90 mg/day for men and 75 mg/day for women.

Data from U.S. Department of Agriculture, Agricultural Research Service, 2009. USDA Nutrient Database for Standard Reference, Release 22. Nutrient Data Laboratory Home Page, www.ars.usda.gov/ba/bhnrc/ndl.

QUICK TIPS

Selecting Foods High in Vitamin C

✓ Mix strawberries, kiwi fruit, cantaloupe, and oranges for a tasty fruit salad loaded with vitamin C.

✓ Include tomatoes on salads, wraps, and sandwiches for more vitamin C.

✓ Make your own fresh-squeezed orange or grapefruit juice!

✓ Add your favorite vitamin C–rich fruits, such as strawberries, to smoothies.

✓ Buy ready-to-eat vegetables, such as baby carrots and cherry tomatoes, and toss some in a zip-lock bag to take to school or work.

✓ Put a few slices of romaine lettuce on your sandwich.

✓ Throw a small container of orange slices, fresh pineapple chunks, or berries into your backpack for an afternoon snack.

✓ Store some juice boxes in your freezer to pack with your lunch. They'll thaw slowly, keeping the rest of your lunch cool, and many brands contain a full day's supply of vitamin C in just 6 oz.

✓ Enjoy raw bell peppers with low-fat dip for a crunchy snack.

✓ Serve reduced-salt corn chips with fresh salsa.

✓ Make gazpacho! In a blender, combine 1–3 cups of tomato juice, chunks of green pepper and red onion, a cucumber with seeds removed (no need to peel), the juice of one lime, a garlic clove, a splash each of red-wine vinegar and olive oil, a half teaspoon each of basil and cumin, and salt and pepper to taste. Seed and dice two to three fresh tomatoes and add to blended ingredients. Chill for several hours and serve cold, topped with a dollop of plain yogurt.

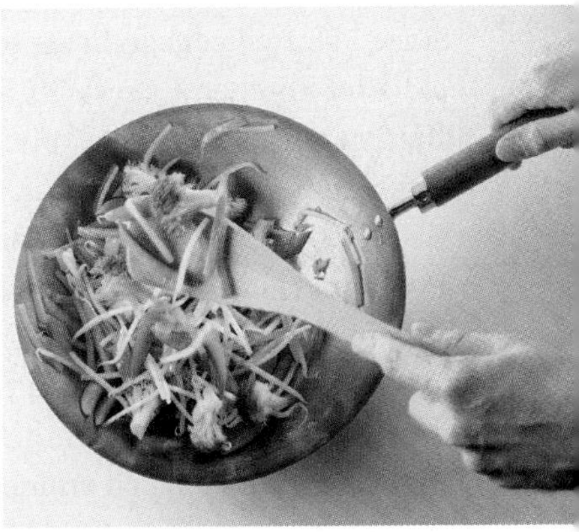

Fresh vegetables are good sources of vitamin C and beta-carotene.

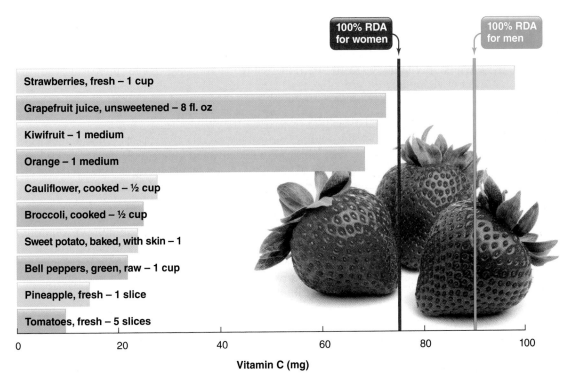

are also good sources. Dairy foods, meats, and nonfortified cereals and grains provide little or no vitamin C. With such a wide variety of foods to choose from, it's easy to eat right all day! See Eating Right All Day for some simple menu choices that are high in vitamin C. In addition, the following are some tips for increasing your intake of vitamin C.

What Happens If We Consume Too Much Vitamin C?

Because vitamin C is water soluble, we usually excrete any excess. Consuming excess amounts in food sources does not lead to toxicity, and only supplements can lead to toxic doses. Taking a **megadose** of vitamin C is not fatally harmful. However, side effects of doses exceeding 2,000 mg/day for a prolonged period include nausea, diarrhea, nosebleeds, and abdominal cramps.

There are rare instances in which consuming even moderately excessive doses of vitamin C can be harmful. As mentioned earlier, vitamin C enhances the absorption of iron. This action is beneficial to people who need to increase iron absorption. It can be harmful, however, to people with a disease called *hemochromatosis,* which causes an excess accumulation of iron in the body. Such iron toxicity can damage our tissues and lead to a heart attack. In people who have preexisting kidney disease, taking excess vitamin C can lead to the formation of kidney stones. This does not appear to occur in healthy individuals.

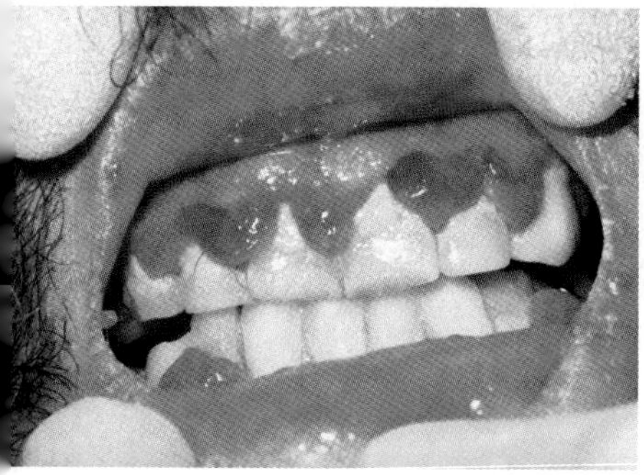

Figure 8.8 Bleeding gums are one symptom of scurvy, the most common vitamin C–deficiency disease.

Critics of vitamin C supplementation claim that taking the supplemental form of the vitamin is "unbalanced" nutrition and leads vitamin C to act as a prooxidant. A **prooxidant,** as you might guess, is a nutrient that promotes oxidation. It does this by pushing the balance of exchange reactions toward oxidation, which promotes the production of free radicals. Although the results of a few studies suggest that vitamin C acts as a prooxidant, these studies were found to be flawed or irrelevant for humans. At the present time, there appears to be no strong scientific evidence that vitamin C, from either food or dietary supplements, acts as a prooxidant in humans.

What Happens If We Don't Consume Enough Vitamin C?

Vitamin C deficiencies are rare in developed countries but can occur in developing countries. Scurvy is the most common vitamin C–deficiency disease. The symptoms of scurvy appear after about 1 month of a vitamin C–deficient diet and include bleeding gums **(Figure 8.8)**, loose teeth, wounds that fail to heal, swollen ankles and wrists, bone pain and fractures, diarrhea, weakness, and depression. Anemia can also result from vitamin C deficiency. The people most at risk are those who eat few fruits and vegetables, including impoverished or homebound individuals, and people who abuse alcohol and drugs.

megadose A dose of a nutrient that is 10 or more times greater than the recommended amount.

prooxidant A nutrient that promotes oxidation and oxidative cell and tissue damage.

NUTRI-CASE HANNAH

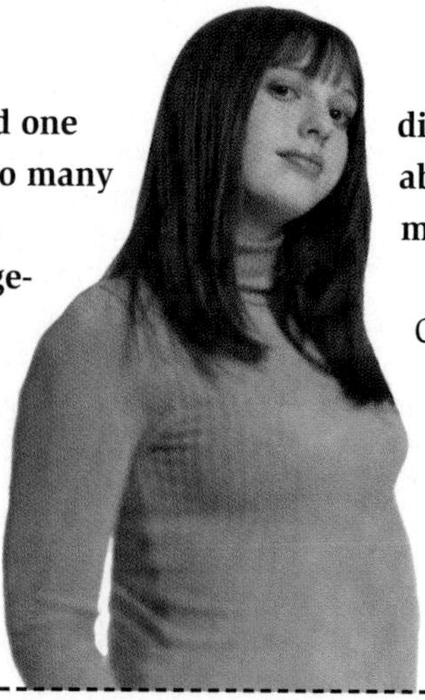

"Since I started college in September, I've had one cold after another. I guess it's being around so many different people every day, plus all the stress. Then a few weeks ago I found this cool orange-tasting vitamin C powder at the health food outlet on campus, and I started mixing it into my orange juice every morning. I guess it's working, because I haven't had a cold since I started using it, but this morning I woke up with stomach cramps and diarrhea, so now I guess I have to worry about a stomach flu. I wish there was a vitamin C powder for that!"

Given what you've learned about the effects of vitamin C supplementation, do you think it is possible that Hannah's vitamin C regimen is doing her more harm than good? Explain.

RECAP Vitamin C scavenges free radicals and regenerates vitamin E after it has been oxidized. It also assists in the synthesis of collagen, hormones, neurotransmitters, and DNA. Vitamin C also enhances iron absorption. The RDA for vitamin C is 90 mg per day for men and 75 mg per day for women. Many fruits and vegetables are high in vitamin C, and our requirements are modest. Toxicity is uncommon; symptoms include nausea, diarrhea, and nosebleeds. Deficiency can result in scurvy or anemia.

Beta-Carotene

Although beta-carotene is not considered an essential nutrient, it is a *provitamin* found in many fruits and vegetables. **Provitamins** are inactive forms of vitamins that the body cannot use until they are converted to their active form. Our body converts beta-carotene to the active form of vitamin A, or *retinol;* thus, beta-carotene is a precursor of retinol. It takes two units of beta-carotene to make one unit of active vitamin A. Not surprisingly, nutritionists express the units of beta-carotene in a food as Retinol Activity Equivalents, or RAE. This measurement tells us how much active vitamin A is available to the body after it has converted the beta-carotene in the food.

Beta-carotene is classified as a **carotenoid,** a class of phytochemicals (see the ***In Depth*** on pages 67–71). As you might guess from their name, carotenoids are a group of plant pigments that are the basis for the orange, red, and deep yellow colors of many fruits and vegetables, including carrots. (Even dark-green leafy vegetables contain plenty of carotenoids, but the green pigment, chlorophyll, masks their color!) Although there are more than 600 carotenoids found in nature, only about 50 are in the typical human diet. The six most common carotenoids found in human blood are alpha-carotene, beta-carotene, beta-cryptoxanthin, lutein, lycopene, and zeaxanthin. Of these, the body can convert only alpha-carotene, beta-carotene, and beta-cryptoxanthin to retinol. These are referred to as *provitamin A carotenoids.* We are just beginning to learn more about how carotenoids function in our body and how they may affect our health.

Functions of Beta-Carotene

Beta-carotene and some other carotenoids are recognized to have antioxidant properties. Like vitamin E, they are fat soluble and fight the harmful effects of oxidation in the lipid portions of our cell membranes and in our LDLs; however, compared to vitamin E, beta-carotene is a relatively weak antioxidant. In fact, other carotenoids, such as lycopene and lutein, may be stronger antioxidants.

Carotenoids play other important roles in our body. Specifically, they

- Enhance our immune system and boost our ability to fight illness and disease.
- Protect our skin from the damage caused by the sun's ultraviolet rays.
- Protect our eyes from damage, preventing or delaying age-related vision impairment.

Carotenoids are also associated with a decreased risk for certain types of cancer. We discuss ***In Depth*** the roles of carotenoids and other antioxidants in cancer on pages 281–289.

How Much Beta-Carotene Should We Consume?

Nutritional scientists do not consider beta-carotene and other carotenoids to be essential nutrients, as they play no known essential roles in our body and are not associated with any deficiency symptoms. Thus, no RDA for these compounds has been established. It has been suggested that consuming 6 to 10 mg of beta-carotene per day from food sources can increase the beta-carotene levels in our blood to amounts that may reduce our risks for some diseases, such as cancer and heart disease.[7] Supplements containing beta-carotene have become very popular,

provitamin An inactive form of a vitamin that the body can convert to an active form. An example is beta-carotene.

carotenoid A fat-soluble plant pigment that the body stores in the liver and adipose tissues. The body is able to convert certain carotenoids to vitamin A.

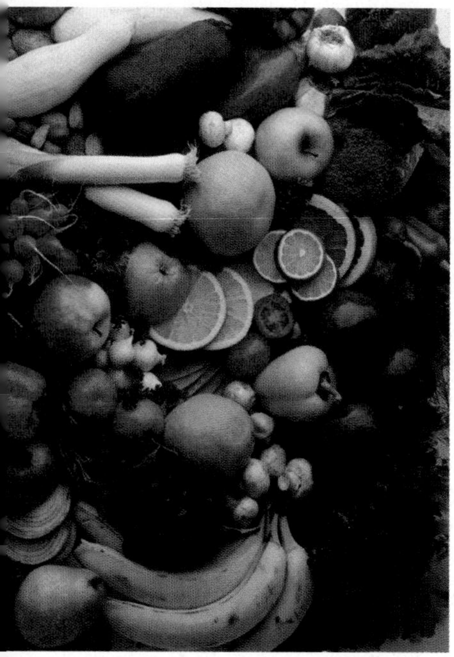

Foods that are high in carotenoids are easy to recognize by their bright colors.

and supplementation studies have prescribed doses of 15 to 30 mg of beta-carotene. Refer to the Nutrition Debate on page 277 to learn more about how antioxidant supplementation, including beta-carotene, may affect your risk for cancer and cardiovascular disease.

Beta-Carotene: Beyond Carrots

Not only carrots, but most vegetables—and fruits—that are red, orange, yellow, or deep green are high in beta-carotene and other carotenoids, such as lutein and lycopene. Tomatoes, sweet potatoes, leafy greens (such as kale and spinach), apricots, cantaloupe, and pumpkin are good sources. Eating the recommended amounts of fruits and vegetables each day ensures an adequate intake of carotenoids. Because of its color, beta-carotene is used as a natural coloring agent for many foods, including margarine, yellow cheddar cheese, cereal, cake mixes, gelatins, and soft drinks. However, these foods are not significant sources of beta-carotene. **Figure 8.9** identifies common foods that are high in beta-carotene.

We generally absorb only between 20% and 40% of the carotenoids present in the foods we eat. In contrast to vitamins E and C, carotenoids are absorbed better from cooked foods. Carotenoids are bound in the cells of plants, and the process of lightly cooking these plants breaks chemical bonds and can rupture cell walls, which humans don't digest. These actions result in more of the carotenoids being released from the plant. For instance, 1 cup of raw carrots contains approximately 10 mg of beta-carotene, whereas the same amount of cooked carrots contains approximately 13 mg.[8] The Quick Tips on the next page suggests ways to increase your intake of beta-carotene.

What Happens If We Consume Too Much Beta-Carotene?

Consuming large amounts of beta-carotene or other carotenoids in foods does not appear to cause toxic symptoms. However, your skin can turn yellow or orange if you consume large amounts of foods that are high in beta-carotene. This condition is referred to as *carotenosis* or *carotenoderma*, and it appears to be both reversible and harmless. Taking beta-carotene supplements is not generally recommended, because we can get adequate amounts of this nutrient by eating more fruits and vegetables, and supplements may be harmful in certain populations.

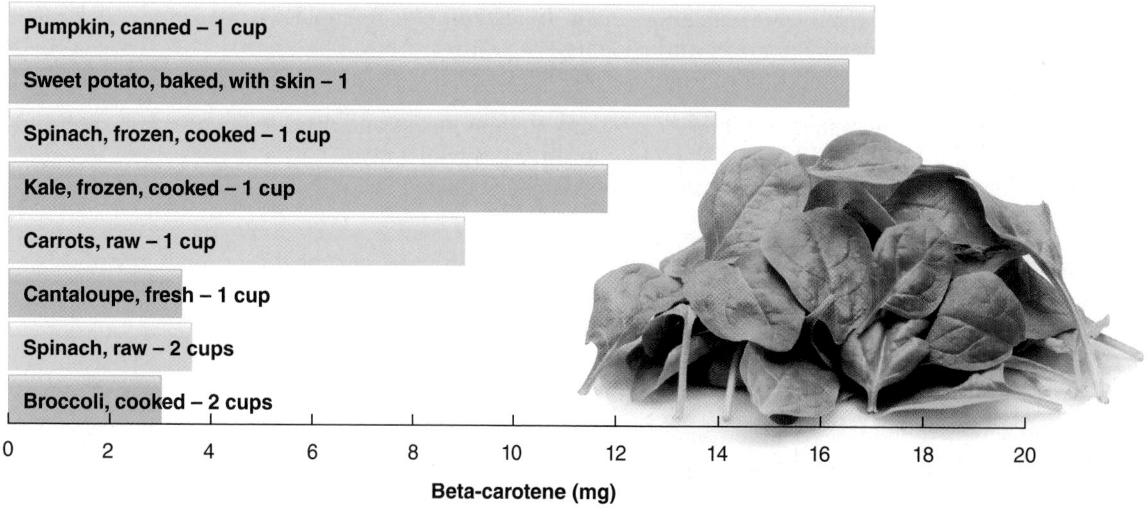

Figure 8.9 Common food sources of beta-carotene. There is no RDA for beta-carotene.

Data from U.S. Department of Agriculture, Agricultural Research Service. USDA—NCC Carotenoid Database for U.S. Foods, 2009. USDA Nutrient Database for Standard Reference, Release 22. Nutrient Data Laboratory Home Page, www.ars.usda.gov/ba/bhnrc/ndl.

QUICK TIPS

Boosting Your Beta-Carotene

✓ Start your day with an orange, grapefruit, a pear, a banana, an apple, or a slice of cantaloupe. All are good sources of beta-carotene.

✓ Pack a zip-lock bag of carrot slices or dried apricots in your lunch.

✓ Instead of french fries, think orange! Slice raw sweet potatoes, toss the slices in olive or canola oil, and bake.

✓ Add veggies to homemade pizza.

✓ Add shredded carrots to cake and muffin batters.

✓ Taking dessert to a potluck? Make a pumpkin pie! It's easy if you use canned pumpkin and follow the recipe on the can.

✓ Go green, too! The next time you have a salad, go for the dark-green leafy vegetables instead of iceberg lettuce.

✓ Add raw spinach or other green leafy vegetables to wraps and sandwiches.

What Happens If We Don't Consume Enough Beta-Carotene?

There are no known deficiency symptoms of beta-carotene or other carotenoids apart from beta-carotene's function as a precursor for vitamin A.

RECAP **Beta-carotene is a carotenoid and a provitamin of vitamin A. It protects the lipid portions of cell membranes and LDL-cholesterol from oxidative damage. It also enhances immune function and protects vision. There is no RDA for beta-carotene. Orange, red, and deep-green fruits and vegetables are good sources of beta-carotene. There are no known toxicity or deficiency symptoms, but yellowing of the skin can occur if too much beta-carotene is consumed.**

Vitamin A: Much More than an Antioxidant Nutrient

As early as AD 30, the Roman writer Aulus Cornelius Celsus described in his medical encyclopedia, *De Medicina,* a condition called night blindness and recommended as a cure the consumption of liver. We now know that night blindness is due to a deficiency of vitamin A, a fat-soluble vitamin stored primarily in the liver of animals. When we consume vitamin A, we store 90% in our liver, and the remainder in our adipose tissue, kidneys, and lungs. Because fat-soluble vitamins cannot dissolve in our blood, they require proteins that can bind with and transport them through the bloodstream to target tissues and cells. *Retinol-binding protein* is one such carrier protein for vitamin A. Retinol-binding protein carries one form of vitamin A, retinol, from the liver to the cells that require it.

There are three active forms of vitamin A in our body: **retinol** is the alcohol form, **retinal** is the aldehyde form, and **retinoic acid** is the acid form. These three forms are collectively referred to as the *retinoids* **(Figure 8.10)**. Of the three, retinol has the starring role in maintaining our body's physiologic functions. Remember from the previous section that beta-carotene is a precursor to vitamin A. When we eat foods that contain beta-carotene, it is converted to retinol in the wall of our small intestine.

The unit of expression for vitamin A is Retinol Activity Equivalents (RAE). You may still see the expression Retinol Equivalents (RE) or International Units (IU) for vitamin A on food labels and dietary supplements. The conversions to RAE from

retinol An active, alcohol form of vitamin A that plays an important role in healthy vision and immune function.

retinal An active, aldehyde form of vitamin A that plays an important role in healthy vision and immune function.

retinoic acid An active, acid form of vitamin A that plays an important role in cell growth and immune function.

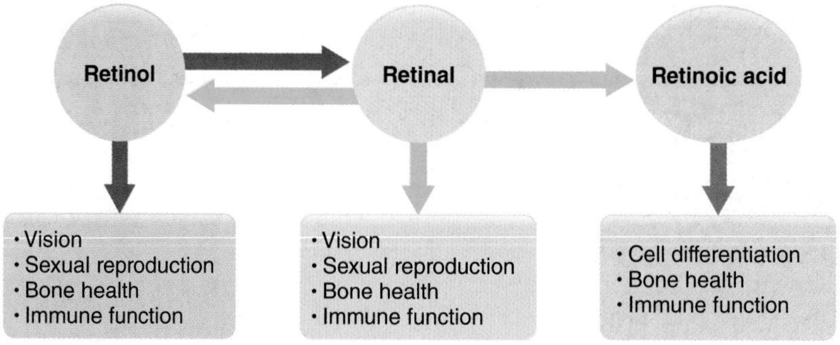

Figure 8.10 The three active forms of vitamin A in our body are retinol, retinal, and retinoic acid. Retinol and retinal can be converted interchangeably; retinoic acid is formed from retinal, and this process is irreversible. Each form of vitamin A contributes to many of our bodily processes.

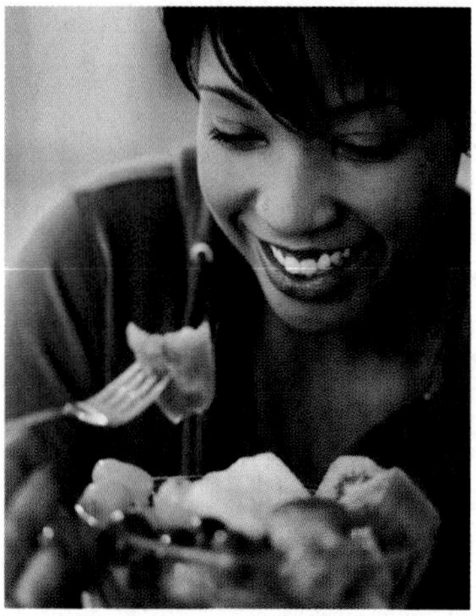

Eating plenty of fruits and vegetables can help prevent vitamin A deficiency.

various forms of retinol are 1 RAE = 1 microgram (μg) retinol, 12 μg beta-carotene, 24 μg alpha-carotene or beta-cryptoxanthin, 1 RE, and 3.3 IU.

Functions of Vitamin A

The known functions of vitamin A are numerous, and researchers speculate that many are still to be discovered.

Vitamin A May Act as an Antioxidant Limited research indicates that vitamin A may act as an antioxidant.[9–11] Like vitamins E and C, it appears to scavenge free radicals and protect our LDLs from oxidation. As you might expect, adequate vitamin A levels in the blood are associated with lower risks for some forms of cancer and heart disease. However, the role of vitamin A as an antioxidant is not strongly established and is still under investigation.

Vitamin A Is Essential to Sight A critical role of vitamin A in our body is certainly in the maintenance of healthy vision. Specifically, vitamin A affects our sight in two ways: it enables us to react to changes in the brightness of light, and it enables us to distinguish between various wavelengths of light—in other words, to see different colors. Let's take a closer look at this process.

Light enters our eyes through the cornea, travels through the lens, and then hits the **retina,** which is a delicate membrane lining the back of the inner eyeball (**Figure 8.11**). You might already have guessed how *retinal* got its name: it is found in—and is integral to—the retina. In the retina, retinal combines with a protein called *opsin* to form **rhodopsin,** a light-sensitive pigment. Rhodopsin is found in the *rod cells,* which are cells that react to dim light and interpret black-and-white images.

When light hits the retina, a reaction occurs in which rhodopsin is split into retinal and opsin. This causes the rod cells to lose their color. It also causes both retinal and opsin to change shape. These changes in turn result in the transmission of a signal to the brain that is interpreted as a black-and-white image. This process goes on continually, allowing our eyes to adjust continuously to subtle changes in our surroundings or in the level of light. Most of the retinal is recycled and combines with opsin to form rhodopsin again. However, some of the retinal is lost with each cycle and must be replaced by retinol from the bloodstream. At the same time, the *cone cells* of the retina, which are effective only in bright light, use retinal to interpret different wavelengths of light as different colors.

In summary, our abilities to adjust to dim light, recover from a bright flash of light, and see in color are all critically dependent on adequate levels of retinal in our eyes.

retina The delicate, light-sensitive membrane lining the inner eyeball and connected to the optic nerve. It contains retinal.

rhodopsin A light-sensitive pigment found in the rod cells that is formed by retinal and opsin.

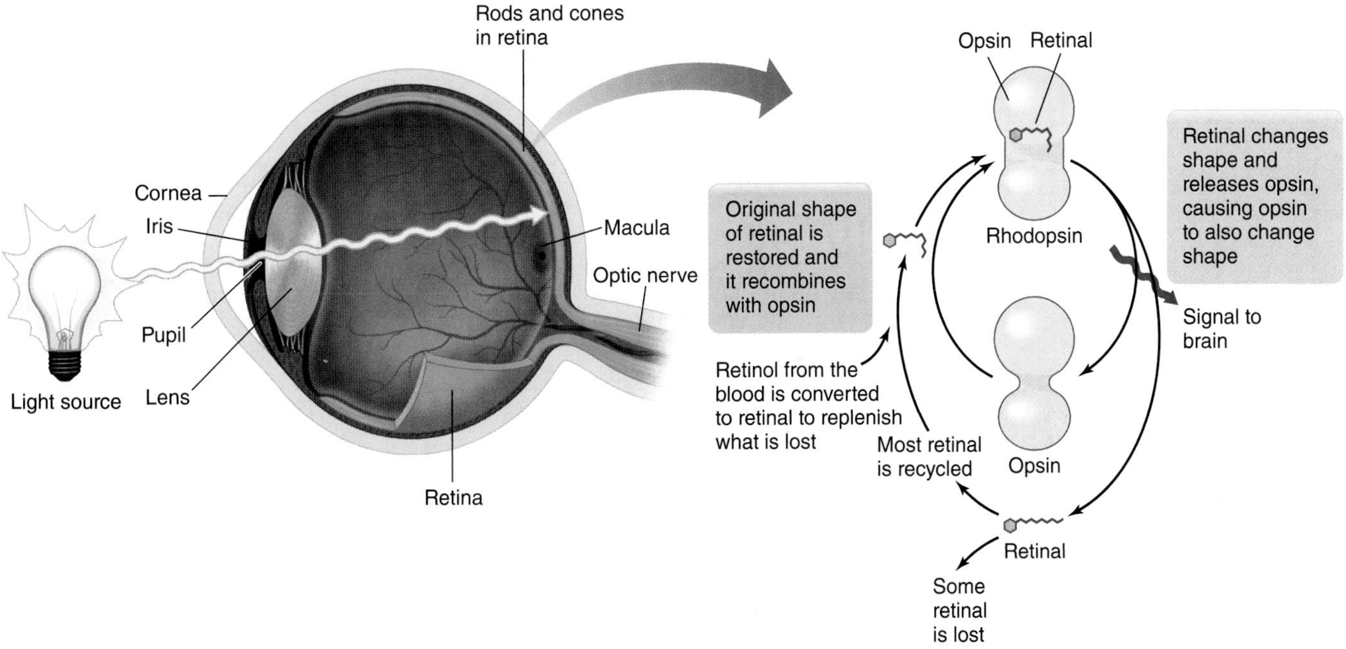

Figure 8.11 Vitamin A is necessary to maintain healthy vision. Light enters the eye through the cornea, travels through the lens, and hits the retina located in the back of the eye. In the rod cells of the retina, retinal is combined with opsin to form rhodopsin. As light hits the rod cells, they lose color, and the components of rhodopsin, retinal and opsin, split and change shape. These changes cause transmission of a signal to the brain that allows us to see.

Vitamin A Contributes to Cell Differentiation Another important role of vitamin A is its contribution to **cell differentiation,** the process by which immature cells develop into highly specialized cells that perform unique functions. Obviously, this process is critical to the development of healthy organs and effectively functioning body systems. For example, specialized cells lining the trachea and bronchi, intestines, stomach, bladder, cornea of the eye, and other organs produce mucus, which lubricates the tissue and helps us propel substances out of our body tissues (for example, when we cough up secretions or empty our bladder). When vitamin A levels are insufficient, these cells fail to differentiate appropriately, and we lose these functions. Vitamin A is also critical to the differentiation of specialized immune cells called *T-lymphocytes*, or *T-cells*, which fight infections. You can now see why vitamin A deficiency can lead to infections and other disorders of the lungs and respiratory tract, urinary tract, vagina, and eyes.

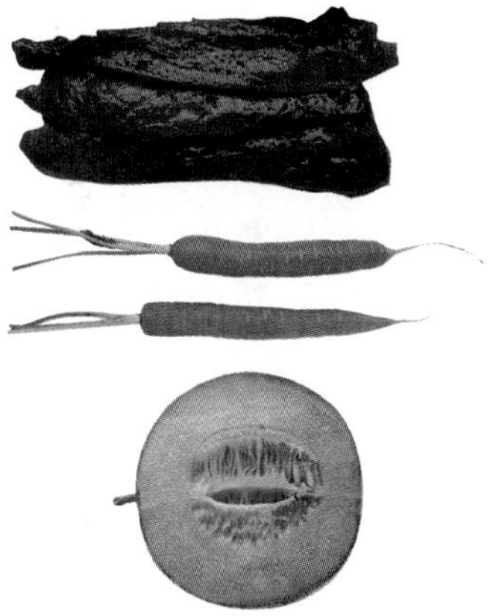

Liver, carrots, and cantaloupe all contain vitamin A.

Other Functions of Vitamin A Vitamin A is involved in reproduction. Although its exact role is unclear, it appears necessary for sperm production in men and for fertilization to occur in women. It also contributes to healthy bone growth by assisting in breaking down old bone, so that new, longer, and stronger bone can develop. As a result of a vitamin A deficiency, children suffer from stunted growth and wasting. Finally, two popular treatments for acne contain derivatives of vitamin A.

How Much Vitamin A Should We Consume?

Vitamin A toxicity can occur readily because it is a fat-soluble vitamin, so it is important to consume only the amount recommended for your gender and age range. The RDA for vitamin A is 900 µg per day for men and 700 µg per day for women (see Table 8.1).[12] The UL is 3,000 µg per day of preformed vitamin A in men and women (including those pregnant and lactating).

cell differentiation The process by which immature, undifferentiated stem cells develop into highly specialized functional cells of discrete organs and tissues.

The most common sources of dietary preformed vitamin A are animal foods, such as beef liver, chicken liver, eggs, and whole-fat dairy products. Vitamin A is also found in fortified reduced-fat milks, margarine, and some breakfast cereals (**Figure 8.12**). The other sources of the vitamin A we consume are foods high in beta-carotene and other carotenoids that can be converted to vitamin A. As discussed earlier in this chapter, dark-green, orange, and deep-yellow fruits and vegetables are good sources of beta-carotene, and thus of vitamin A. Carrots, spinach, mango, cantaloupe, and tomato juice are excellent sources of vitamin A because they contain beta-carotene.

What Happens If We Consume Too Much Vitamin A?

Vitamin A is highly toxic, and toxicity symptoms develop after consuming only three to four times the RDA. Toxicity rarely results from food sources; however, vitamin A supplementation is known to have caused severe illness and even death. In pregnant women, it can cause serious birth defects and spontaneous abortion. Other toxicity symptoms include fatigue, loss of appetite, blurred vision, hair loss, skin disorders, bone and joint pain, abdominal pain, nausea, diarrhea, and damage to the liver and nervous system. If caught in time, many of these symptoms are reversible once vitamin A supplementation is stopped. However, permanent damage can occur to the liver, eyes, and other organs.

What Happens If We Don't Consume Enough Vitamin A?

Night blindness and color blindness can result from vitamin A deficiency. Night blindness is characterized by an inability to adjust to dim light, as well as the failure to regain sight quickly after a bright flash of light (**Figure 8.13**). How severe a problem is night blindness? Although less common among people of developed nations, vitamin A deficiency is a severe public health concern in developing nations. According to the World Health Organization, approximately 250 million preschool children suffer from vitamin A deficiency.[14] Of the children affected, 250,000 to 500,000 become permanently blinded every year. At least half of these children will die within 1 year of losing their sight. Death is due to infections and illnesses, including measles and diarrhea, that are easily treated in wealthier countries. Vitamin A deficiency is also a tragedy for pregnant women in these countries. These women suffer from night blindness, are more likely to transmit HIV to their child if HIV-positive, and run a greater risk for maternal mortality.

night blindness A vitamin A deficiency disorder that results in loss of the ability to see in dim light.

HOT TOPIC

Acne and Vitamin A—Is There a Link?

Search the Internet and you'll find plenty of sites claiming a direct link between vitamin A deficiency and acne, and insisting that vitamin A supplements can successfully treat acne. Should you believe the hype?

In 2006, a study reported an association between low blood levels of vitamin A and the presence of acne: the more severe the acne, the lower the levels of vitamin A.[13] Although these findings may seem suggestive, this study was conducted with a very small number of participants who were not randomly selected. Also, plasma levels of vitamin A were assessed to indicate vitamin A status; however, the Institute of Medicine[12] states that plasma levels of vitamin A are not necessarily an indicator of vitamin A status. To date, these results have not been replicated by other researchers, and there appears to be no evidence that vitamin A deficiency causes acne.

Interestingly, two effective treatments for acne are synthetic derivatives of vitamin A. Retin-A, or tretinoin, is a treatment applied to the skin. Accutane, or isotretinoin, is taken orally. These medications should be used carefully and only under the supervision of a licensed physician.

Contrary to what you might read on the Internet, vitamin A itself has no effect on acne; thus, vitamin A supplements are not recommended in its treatment.

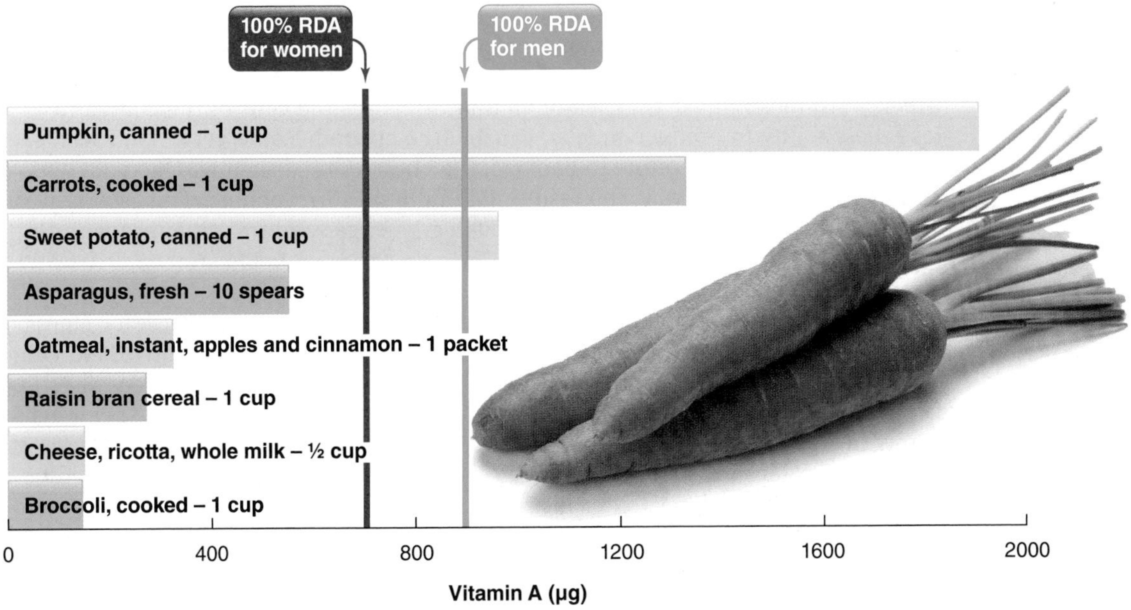

Figure 8.12 Common food sources of vitamin A. The RDA for vitamin A is 900 μg/day for men and 700 μg/day for women.

Data from U.S. Department of Agriculture, Agricultural Research Service, 2009. USDA Nutrient Database for Standard Reference, Release 22. Nutrient Data Laboratory Home Page, www.ars.usda.gov/ba/bhnrc/ndl.

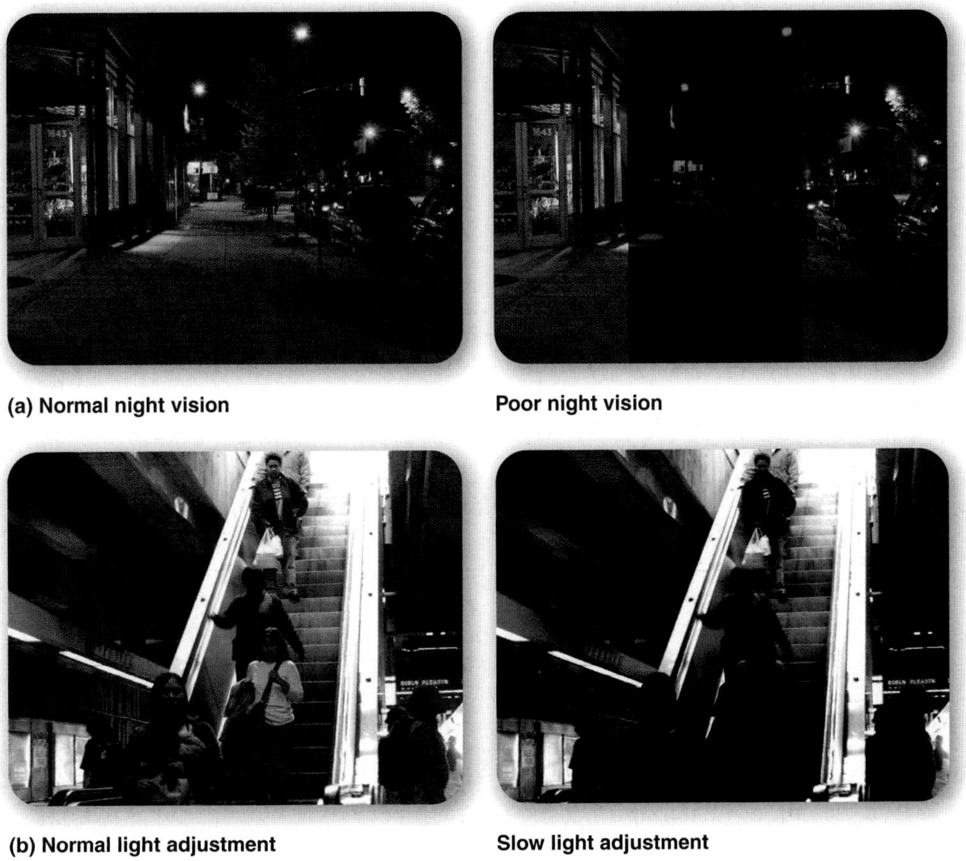

Figure 8.13 A deficiency of vitamin A can result in night blindness. This condition results in **(a)** diminished side vision and overall poor night vision and **(b)** difficulty in adjusting from bright light to dim light.

If vitamin A deficiency progresses, it can result in irreversible blindness due to hardening of the cornea (the transparent membrane covering the front of the eye), a condition called *xerophthalmia*. The prefix of this word, *xero-*, comes from a Greek word meaning "dry." Lack of vitamin A causes the cells of the cornea to lose their ability to produce mucus, causing the eye to become very dry. This leaves the cornea susceptible to damage, infection, and hardening. Once the cornea hardens in this way, the resulting blindness is irreversible. This is why it is critical to catch vitamin A deficiency in its early stages and treat it either with the regular consumption of fruits and vegetables that contain beta-carotene or with vitamin A supplementation.

Other deficiency symptoms include impaired immunity, increased risk for illness and infections, reproductive system disorders, and failure of normal growth. Individuals who are at risk for vitamin A deficiency include elderly people with poor diets, newborn or premature infants (due to low liver stores of vitamin A), young children with inadequate vegetable and fruit intakes, and alcoholics. Any condition that results in fat malabsorption can also lead to vitamin A deficiency. Children with cystic fibrosis; individuals with Crohn's disease, celiac disease, or diseases of the liver, pancreas, or gallbladder; and people who consume large amounts of the fat substitute Olestra are at risk for vitamin A deficiency.

RECAP **The role of vitamin A as an antioxidant is still under investigation. Vitamin A is critical for maintaining our vision. It is also necessary for cell differentiation, reproduction, and growth. The RDA for vitamin A is 900 µg per day for men and 700 µg per day for women. Animal liver, dairy products, and eggs are good animal sources of vitamin A; fruits and vegetables are high in beta-carotene, which our body uses to synthesize vitamin A. Supplementation can be dangerous, as toxicity is reached at levels of only three to four times the RDA. Toxicity symptoms include birth defects, spontaneous abortion, blurred vision, and liver damage. Deficiency symptoms include night blindness, impaired immune function, and growth failure.**

Selenium

Selenium is a trace mineral, and it is found in varying amounts in soil and thus in the food grown there. Keep in mind that although we need only minute amounts of trace minerals, they are just as important to our health as the major minerals.

Functions of Selenium

It is only recently that we have learned about the critical role of selenium as a nutrient in human health. In 1979, Chinese scientists reported an association between a heart disorder called **Keshan disease** and selenium deficiency. This disease occurs in children in the Keshan province of China, where the soil is depleted of selenium. The scientists found that Keshan disease can be prevented with selenium supplementation.

The selenium in our body is contained in amino acids. Two amino acid derivatives contain most of the selenium in our body: *selenomethionine* is the storage form for selenium, while *selenocysteine* is the active form of selenium. Selenium is a critical component of the glutathione peroxidase antioxidant enzyme system mentioned earlier (page 259). Thus, selenium helps spare vitamin E and prevents oxidative damage to our cell membranes.

Like vitamin C, selenium is needed for the production of thyroxine, or thyroid hormone. By this action, selenium is involved in the maintenance of our basal metabolism and body temperature. Selenium appears to play a role in immune function, and poor selenium status is associated with higher rates of some forms of cancer.

Keshan disease A heart disorder caused by selenium deficiency. It was first identified in children in the Keshan province of China.

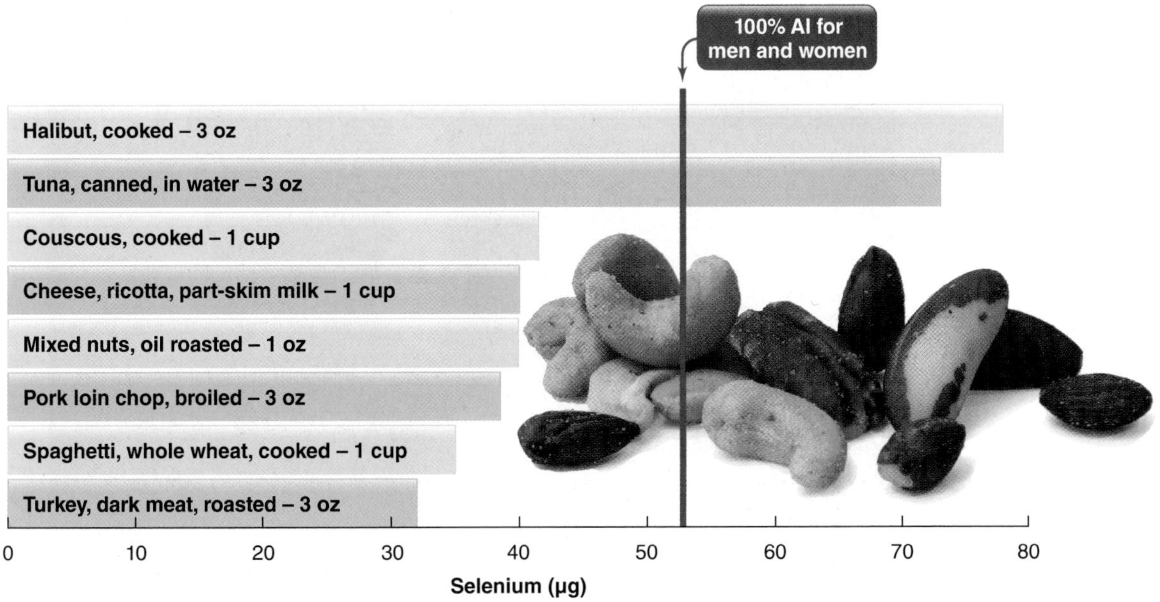

Figure 8.14 Common food sources of selenium. The RDA for selenium is 55 μg/day.
Data from U.S. Department of Agriculture, Agricultural Research Service, 2009. USDA Nutrient Database for Standard Reference, Release 22. Nutrient Data Laboratory Home Page, www.ars.usda.gov/ba/bhnrc/ndl.

How Much Selenium Should We Consume?

The content of selenium in foods is highly variable. As it is a trace mineral, we need only minute amounts to maintain health. The RDA for selenium is 55 μg per day for both men and women (see Table 8.1).[1] The UL is 400 μg per day.

Selenium is present in both animal and plant food sources but in variable amounts. Because it is stored in the tissues of animals, selenium is found in reliably consistent amounts in animal foods. Organ meats, such as liver and kidneys, as well as pork and seafood, are particularly good sources **(Figure 8.14)**.

In contrast, the amount of selenium in plants is dependent on the selenium content of the soil in which the plant is grown. Many companies marketing selenium supplements warn that the agricultural soils in the United States are depleted of selenium and inform us that we need to take selenium supplements. In reality, the selenium content of soil varies greatly across North America, and because we obtain our food from a variety of geographic locations, few people in the United States suffer from selenium deficiency. This is especially true for people who eat even small quantities of meat or seafood.

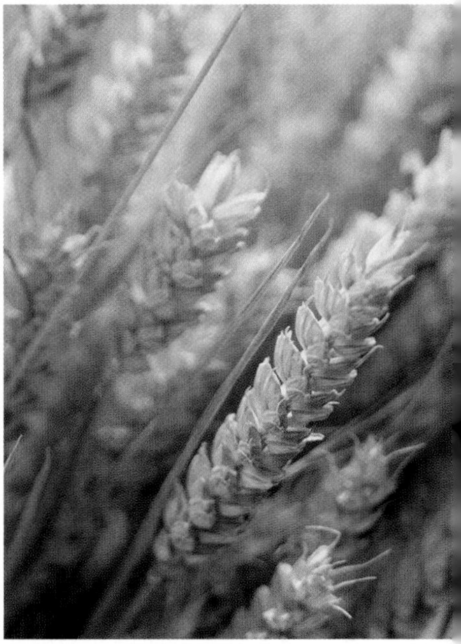

Wheat is a rich source of selenium.

What Happens If We Consume Too Much Selenium?

Selenium toxicity does not result from eating foods high in selenium. However, supplementation can cause toxicity. Toxicity symptoms include brittle hair and nails that can eventually break and fall off. Other symptoms include skin rashes, vomiting, nausea, weakness, and liver disease.

What Happens If We Don't Consume Enough Selenium?

As discussed previously, selenium deficiency is associated with a form of heart disease called Keshan disease. Selenium deficiency does not cause the disease, but selenium is necessary to help the immune system effectively fight the virus that causes the disease. Another deficiency disease is *Kashin-Beck disease*, a deforming arthritis also found in selenium-depleted areas in China and Tibet **(Figure 8.15)**.

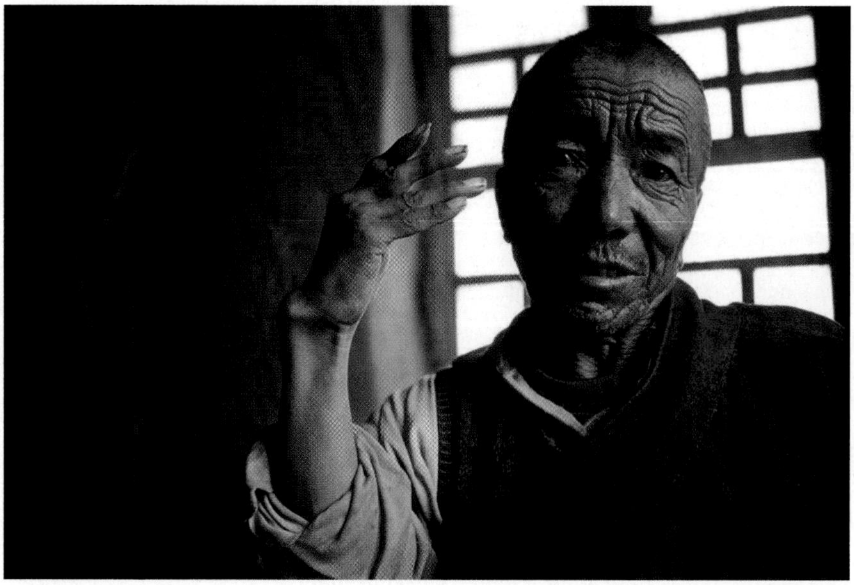

Figure 8.15 Selenium deficiency can lead to deforming arthritis called Kashin-Beck disease.

Other deficiency symptoms include impaired immune responses, increased risk for viral infections, infertility, depression, hostility, impaired cognitive function, and muscle pain and wasting. Deficiencies of both selenium and iodine in pregnant women can cause a form of *cretinism* in the infant (discussed in Chapter 10).

Copper, Iron, Zinc, and Manganese Assist in Antioxidant Function

As discussed earlier, there are numerous antioxidant enzyme systems in our body. Copper, zinc, and manganese are cofactors for the superoxide dismutase antioxidant enzyme system. Iron is a part of the structure of catalase. In addition to their role in protecting against oxidative damage, these minerals play major roles in the optimal functioning of many other enzymes in our body. Copper, iron, and zinc help us maintain the health of our blood, and manganese is an important cofactor in carbohydrate metabolism. The functions, requirements, food sources, and deficiency and toxicity symptoms of these nutrients are discussed in detail in Chapter 10, which focuses on the nutrients involved in energy metabolism and blood health.

RECAP **Selenium is part of the glutathione peroxidase antioxidant enzyme system. It indirectly spares vitamin E from oxidative damage, and it assists with immune function and the production of thyroid hormone. Organ meats, pork, and seafood are good sources of selenium, as are nuts, wheat, and rice. The selenium content of plants is dependent on the amount of selenium in the soil in which they are grown. Toxicity symptoms include brittle hair and nails, vomiting, nausea, and liver cirrhosis. Deficiency symptoms and side effects include Keshan disease, Kashin-Beck disease, impaired immune function, infertility, and muscle wasting. Copper, zinc, and manganese are cofactors for the superoxide dismutase antioxidant enzyme system. Iron is a cofactor for the catalase antioxidant enzyme. These minerals play critical roles in blood health and energy metabolism.**

Nutrition DEBATE

Antioxidants: Food or Supplements?

As you have learned in this chapter, antioxidant nutrients play an important role in reducing free radical damage, which can in turn reduce the risk for chronic diseases such as cancer and cardiovascular disease (CVD). Despite this, research studies on the effects of antioxidant supplements on risks for cancer and CVD show inconsistent results.

The results of the Alpha-Tocopherol Beta-Carotene (ATBC) Cancer Prevention Study and the Beta-Carotene and Retinol Efficacy Trial (CARET) were particularly surprising.[15,16] The ATBC Cancer Prevention Study was conducted in Finland from 1985 to 1993 with the purpose of determining the effects of beta-carotene and vitamin E supplements on the rates of lung cancer and other forms of cancer among male smokers between the ages of 50 and 69 years. Almost 30,000 men participated in the study for an average of 6 years. The participants were given daily a beta-carotene supplement, a vitamin E supplement, a supplement containing both, or a placebo.

Contrary to expectations, the male smokers who took beta-carotene supplements experienced an *increased* number of deaths during the study. More men in this group died of lung cancer, and there were higher rates of prostate and stomach cancers. Also, more men died of CVD. This negative effect appeared to be particularly strong in men who had a higher alcohol intake.

CARET began as a pilot study in the United States in 1985 and included more than 18,000 men and women who were smokers, former smokers, or workers who had been exposed to asbestos. The participants were randomly assigned to take daily supplements of beta-carotene and retinol (vitamin A) or a placebo. After a 4-year follow-up period, the incidence of lung cancer was 28% higher among those taking the beta-carotene and retinol supplement. This significant finding, in addition to the results from the ATBC Cancer Prevention Study, prompted researchers to end the CARET study early and recommend that participants discontinue the supplements.[16]

The reasons that beta-carotene increased lung cancer risk in this population are not clear. However, the results of this study suggest that, for certain people, supplementation with beta-carotene may be harmful.

As with the research conducted on cancer, the studies of antioxidants and CVD show inconsistent results. Two large-scale surveys conducted in the United States show that men and women who eat more fruits and vegetables have a significantly reduced risk of CVD.[17,18] And in the ATBC Cancer Prevention Study, vitamin E was found to lower the number of deaths due to heart disease. However, it had no overall effect on the risk for stroke.[19] In another study, vitamin E had no impact on the risk for CVD in people at high risk for heart attack and stroke.[2] And recently, other large intervention studies conducted in the United States have shown no reductions in major cardiovascular events in men and women taking vitamins E or C.[3,20] Thus, there is growing evidence that antioxidant supplements do not reduce our risk for CVD.

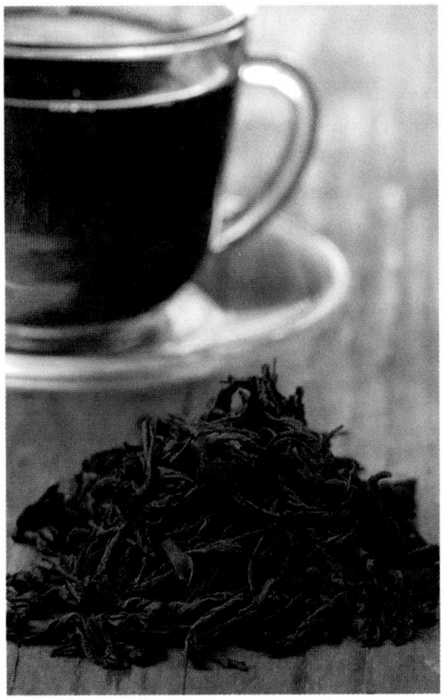

The flavonoids in black tea might reduce the risk for CVD.

Why might foods high in antioxidants be beneficial in reducing our risks for cancer and CVD, whereas supplements are not? It is important to note that other compounds (besides antioxidants) found in fruits, vegetables, and whole grains can reduce our risk for cancer and CVD. Here are just a few examples: dietary fiber has been shown to reduce the risk for colon and rectal cancers, decrease blood pressure, lower total cholesterol levels, and improve blood glucose and insulin levels. Folate, a B-vitamin found in fortified cereals, green leafy vegetables, and some other plant foods, is known to reduce blood levels of the amino acid homocysteine, and a high concentration of homocysteine is a known risk factor for CVD. Flavonoids are a group of phytochemicals found in many plant foods, including black tea. A recent study has shown that individuals who drank more than three cups of black tea per day had a lower rate of heart attacks than non–tea drinkers.[21] Thus, it appears that any number of nutrients and other components in fruits, vegetables, and whole-grain foods may be protective against cancer and CVD. As you can see, there is still much to learn about how people respond to foods high in antioxidant nutrients as compared to antioxidant supplementation.

Chapter Review

Test Yourself ANSWERS

1. True. Free radicals are highly unstable atoms that can destabilize neighboring atoms or molecules and harm our cells; however, they are produced as a normal by-product of human physiology.

2. False. Overall, the research on vitamin C and colds does not show strong evidence that taking vitamin C supplements reduces our risk of suffering from the common cold.

3. True. Carrots are an excellent source of beta-carotene, a precursor for vitamin A, which helps maintain good vision.

Find the Quack

When Bruce and Tina got married, they assumed they'd have no problem becoming parents. But 2 years later, they're still trying. So when Tina comes home from a doctor's appointment and tells Bruce she has some bad news, he doesn't know what to expect. "Bruce," she says, "I know you're not going to like this, but the doctor says you should quit smoking. She says that smoking reduces your sperm count and could be one reason we haven't conceived. And besides, your own doctor has tried to get you to quit because of your high blood pressure." Bruce feels his spirits sink. It's true he has hypertension, and his dad died of a heart attack at age 45. But he's tried to quit smoking before, and the withdrawal symptoms have always been more than he could handle.

That evening he goes onto the Internet and searches under "smoking" and "withdrawal symptoms." He finds a website promoting a supplement called "Quit Calm" that sounds promising, offering relief from the anxiety, sleeplessness, and cravings of nicotine withdrawal. Here's what the site states:

- "Quit Calm offers an all-natural blend of herbs that work together to decrease cravings, eliminate your anxiety, promote your sleep, heal your respiratory tissues, and purge harmful toxins from your body."
- "Ingredients include licorice root, peppermint, ginger, and slippery elm in a proprietary blend that soothes the body's tissues as they recover from nicotine addiction."
- "Independent studies have confirmed the beneficial effects of our patented formula."
- "Take one capsule three times a day 30 minutes before meals."
- "If you order now, a 30-day supply (90 capsules) costs just $29.99. Why wait? Think of all the money you'll be saving by not smoking, and order today!"

1. Bruce finds the statement "Independent studies have confirmed the beneficial effects of our patented formula" reassuring. Do you? Why or why not?
2. Look up licorice root in the "Herbs at a Glance" section of the website of the National Center for Complementary and Alternative Medicine (http://nccam.nih.gov). Would you recommend that Bruce take a supplement containing licorice root? Why or why not?
3. Comment on the advertisement's final bullet urging consumers to "think of all the money you'll be saving by not smoking, and order today!"
4. Instead of a supplements website, where online might Bruce have found reliable help in his quest to quit smoking? What other resources should he consult?

Answers can be found on the companion website at www.pearsonhighered.com/thompsonmanore.

NutriTools Check out the companion website at www.pearsonhighered.com/thompsonmanore, or use MyNutritionLab.com, to access interactive animations, including:

- Nutrients: Vitamin or Mineral?

Review Questions

1. Which of the following is a characteristic of vitamin E?
   a. It enhances the absorption of iron.
   b. It can be manufactured from beta-carotene.
   c. It is a critical component of the glutathione peroxidase system.
   d. It is destroyed by exposure to high heat.
2. Oxidation is best described as a process in which
   a. radiation causes a mutation in a cell's DNA.
   b. an atom loses an electron.
   c. an element loses an atom of oxygen.
   d. a compound loses a molecule of water.
3. Which of the following disorders is linked with the production of free radicals?
   a. cardiovascular disease
   b. carotenosis
   c. ulcers
   d. malaria
4. Which of the following function as a cofactor in antioxidant enzyme systems?
   a. iron
   b. zinc
   c. copper
   d. all of the above
5. Taking daily doses of three to four times the RDA of which of the following nutrients may cause death?
   a. vitamin A
   b. vitamin C
   c. vitamin E
   d. selenium
6. True or false? Tocopherol is the biologically active form of vitamin E in our body.
7. True or false? Free radical formation can occur as a result of normal cellular metabolism.
8. True or false? Vitamin C helps regenerate vitamin A.
9. True or false? Reliable food sources of selenium include beef liver, pork, and seafood.
10. True or false? Pregnant women are advised to consume plenty of beef liver.

Answers to Review Questions can be found at the back of this text, and additional essay questions and answers are located on the companion website at www.pearsonhighered.com/thompsonmanore.

Web Resources

www.who.int
World Health Organization (WHO)

Search for "vitamin A deficiency" to find out more about vitamin A deficiency around the world.

www.cfsan.fda.gov
U.S. Food and Drug Administration (FDA)

This site provides information on how to make informed decisions and evaluate information related to dietary supplements.

www.nal.usda.gov/fnic
The Food and Nutrition Information Center (FNIC)

Click on the Dietary Supplements button to obtain information on vitamin and mineral supplements, including consumer reports and industry regulations.

www.dietary-supplements.info.nih.gov
Office of Dietary Supplements

Go to this site to obtain current research results and reliable information about dietary supplements.

NutriTools

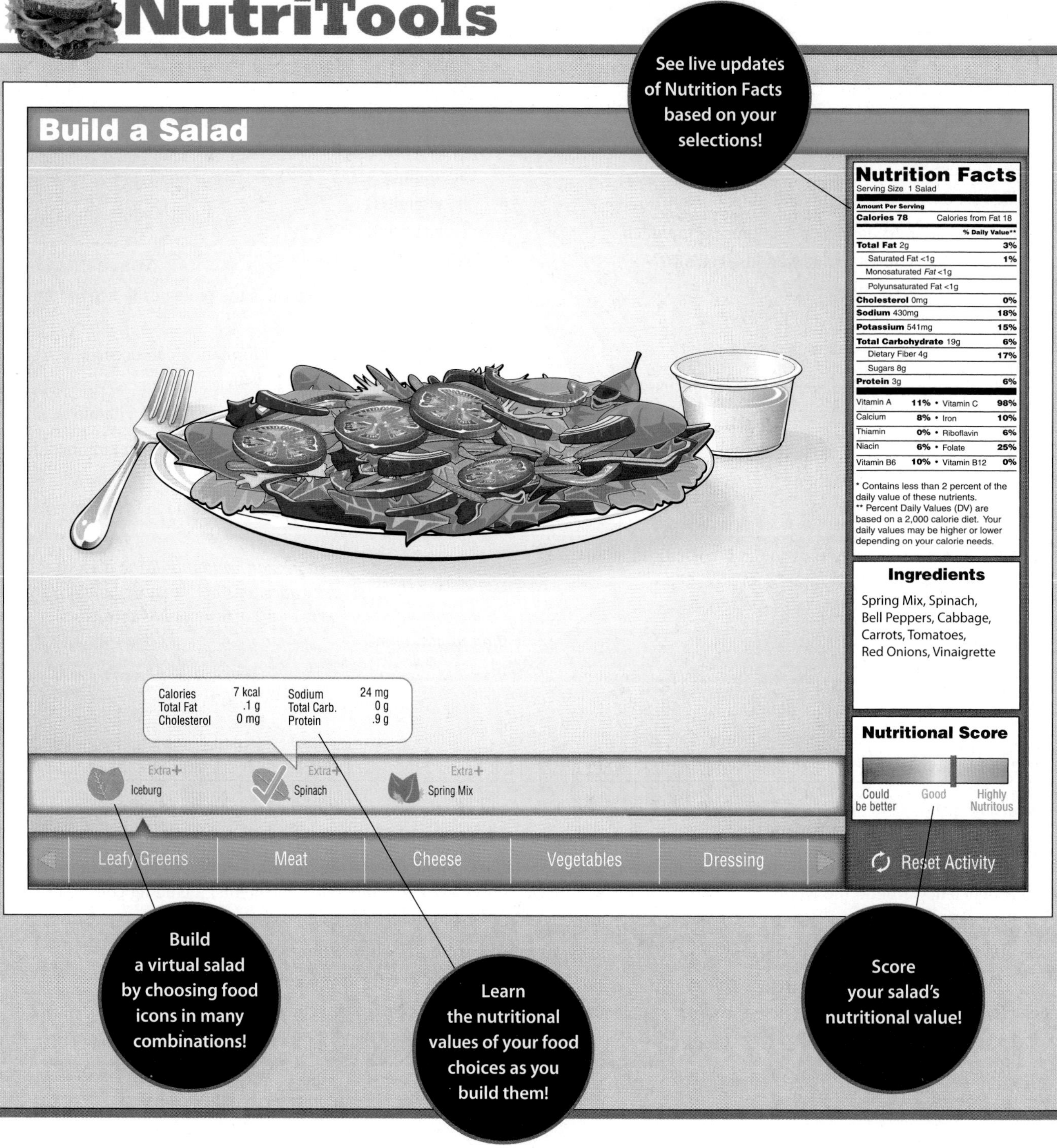

To build your salad, just visit www.pearsonhighered.com/thompsonmanore **or** www.mynutritionlab.com

After building your salad, you should be able to answer these questions:

1. What are some of the best vegetables to select for a highly nutritious salad?
2. How do the types of greens selected for your salad affect its nutritional score?
3. Are your salad toppings making your salad too high in fat? How do you know?
4. Do the kcalories in your salad make it a side dish or a full meal?
5. Which nutrient guidelines are the most challenging in building your salad?

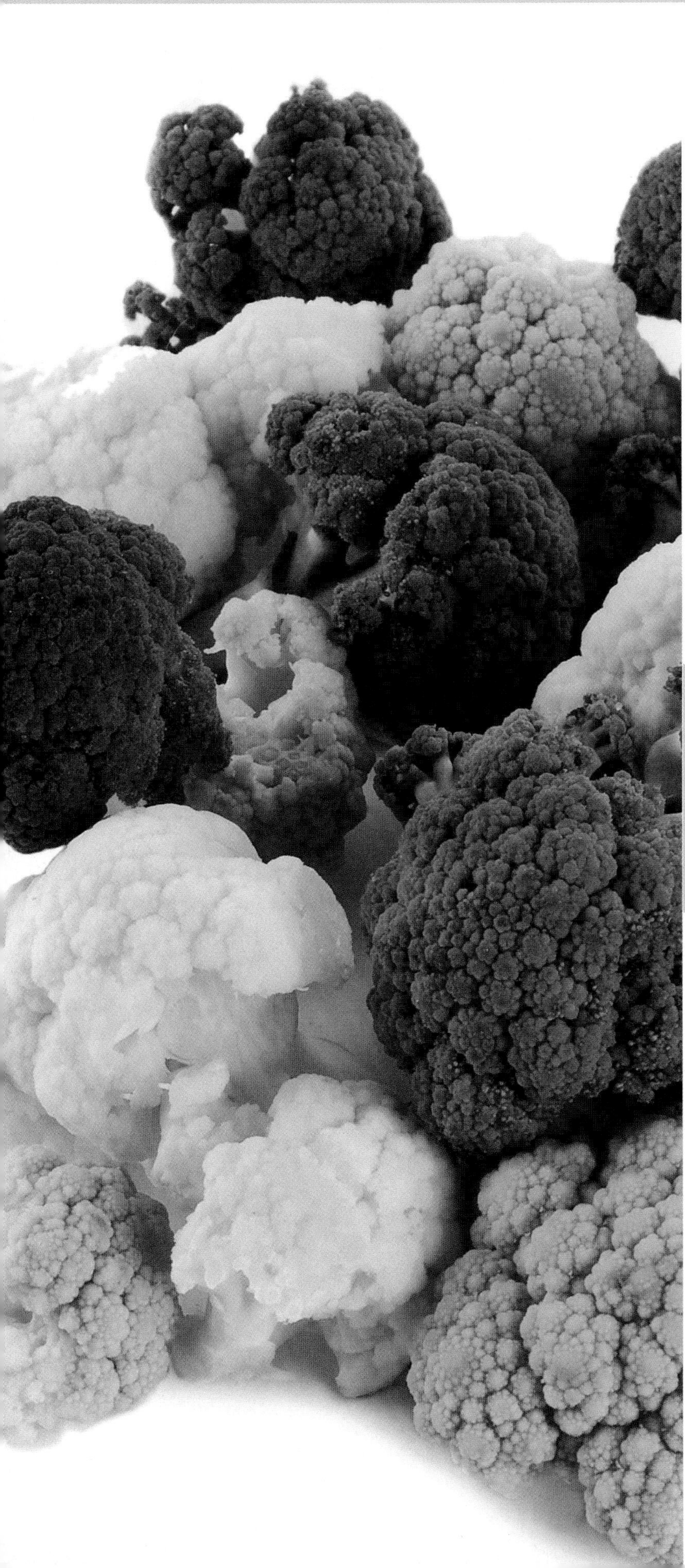

Cancer

WANT TO FIND OUT . . .

- **how your lifestyle can influence your risk for cancer?**
- **about the link between antioxidants and cancer?**
- **if antioxidant supplements can reduce your risk for cancer?**

READ ON.

The American Cancer Society (ACS) estimates that approximately 1,500 Americans die of cancer every day. In the United States, cancer accounts for nearly one out of every four deaths, making it the second most common cause of death in the United States, exceeded only by heart disease.[1]

With such alarming statistics, it's not surprising that television commercials, Internet sites, and health and fitness publications are filled with product claims promising to reduce your risk of developing cancer. Many of these claims tout the benefits of antioxidants. In opposition to these claims, some research evidence suggests that taking antioxidant supplements may actually increase the risk of cancer for certain people (refer back to the Nutrition Debate on page 277). In this *In Depth*, we'll take a closer look at the group of diseases collectively known as cancer. We'll explore how it begins and spreads and identify the factors that most significantly increase our risk. We'll also review what is currently known about the role of antioxidant nutrients in cancer and identify other strategies for reducing your risk.

What Is Cancer?

Before we explore how antioxidants affect the risk for cancer, let's take a closer look at precisely what cancer is and how it spreads. **Cancer** is actually a group of diseases that are all characterized by cells that grow "out of control." By this we mean that cancer cells reproduce spontaneously and independently, and they are not inhibited by the boundaries of tissues and organs. Thus, they can aggressively invade tissues and organs far away from those in which they originally formed.

Most forms of cancer result in one or more **tumors,** which are newly formed masses of undifferentiated cells that are immature and have no physiologic function. Although the word *tumor* sounds frightening, it is important to note that not every tumor is *malignant,* or cancerous. Many are *benign* (not harmful to us) and are made up of cells that will not spread widely.

cancer A group of diseases characterized by cells that reproduce spontaneously and independently and may invade other tissues and organs.

tumor Any newly formed mass of undifferentiated cells.

Cancer Progresses in Three Stages

Figure 1 shows how changes to normal cells prompt a series of other changes that can progress into cancer.

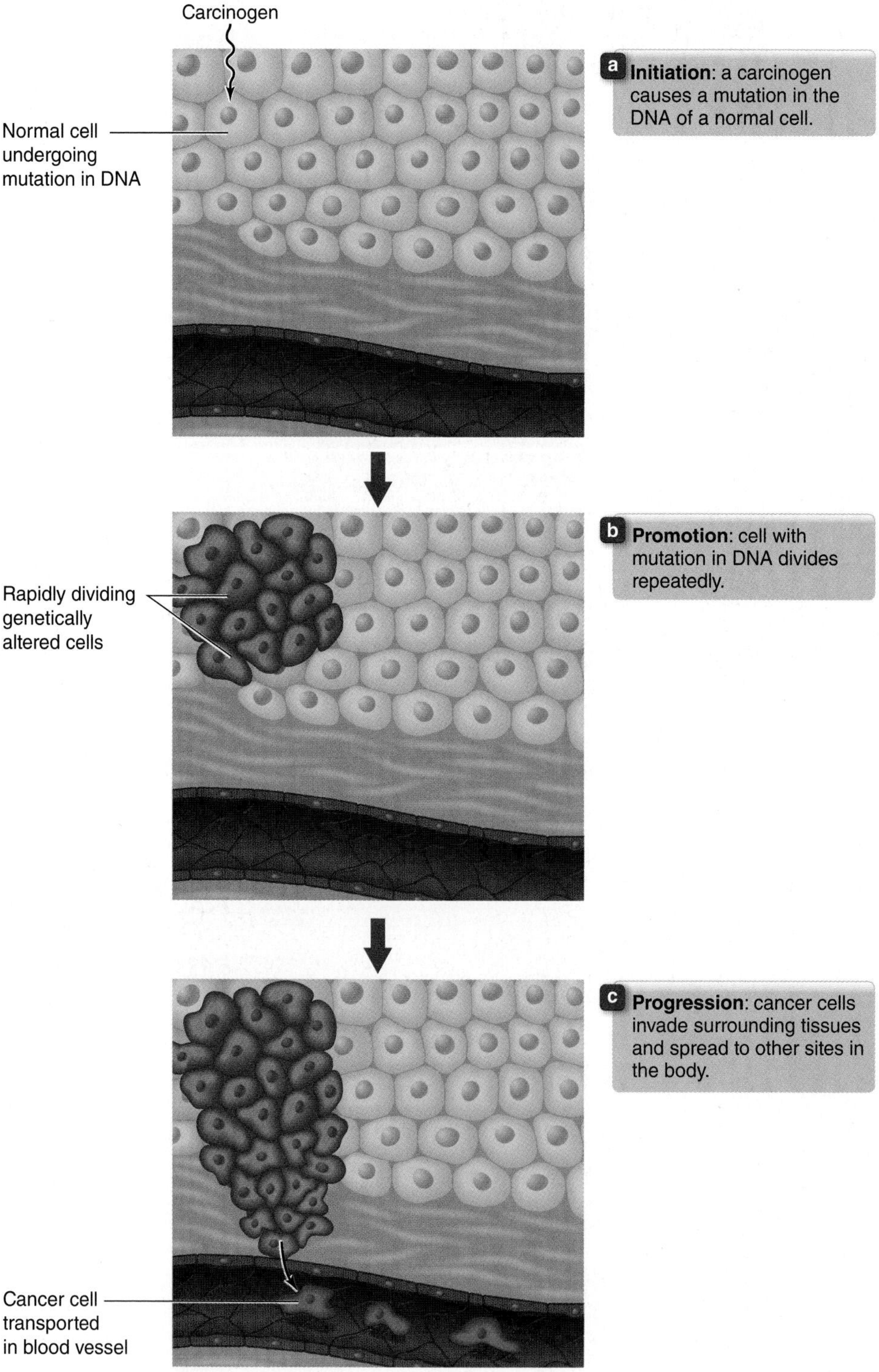

Carcinogen
Normal cell undergoing mutation in DNA
a Initiation: a carcinogen causes a mutation in the DNA of a normal cell.
Rapidly dividing genetically altered cells
b Promotion: cell with mutation in DNA divides repeatedly.
c Progression: cancer cells invade surrounding tissues and spread to other sites in the body.
Cancer cell transported in blood vessel

Figure 1 **(a)** Cancer cells develop as a result of a genetic mutation in the DNA of a normal cell. **(b)** The mutated cell replicates uncontrollably, eventually resulting in a tumor. **(c)** If not destroyed or removed, the cancerous tumor metastasizes and spreads to other parts of the body.

There are three primary stages of cancer development: initiation, promotion, and progression. They occur as follows:

1. *Initiation.* The initiation of cancer occurs when a cell's DNA is *mutated* (changed). This mutation causes permanent changes in the cell.
2. *Promotion.* During this phase, the genetically altered cell is stimulated to divide. A single mutated cell divides in two, and these double to four, and so on. The mutated DNA is locked into each new cell's genetic instructions. Because the enzymes that normally work to repair damaged cells cannot detect alterations in the DNA, the cells can continue to divide uninhibited. Typically, it takes many years for a mutated cell to double repeatedly into a tumor mass large enough to be detectable (about the size of a grape), and promotion is the longest stage in cancer development.[2]
3. *Progression.* During this phase, the cancerous cells reproduce out of control. They grow their own blood vessels, which supply them with blood and nutrients, and invade adjacent tissues. In this early stage of progression, the immune system can sometimes detect these cancerous cells and destroy them. However, if the cells continue to grow, they develop into malignant tumors, disrupting body functioning at their primary site and invading the circulatory and lymphatic systems to *metastasize* (spread) to distant sites in the body.

We noted earlier that cancer is often fatal; however, a majority of people who develop cancer survive. In 2009, the 5-year survival rate for all cancers was 66%. Of course, cancers can be more or less aggressive, some are more readily detectable than others, and some tissues and organs are more vulnerable to cancer. These factors all influence the overall mortality rate associated with different cancers. The type of cancer with the highest mortality rate is lung cancer, with over 150,000 deaths in 2009. Cancer of the colon and/or rectum ranks second (almost 50,000 deaths in 2009), and breast cancer ranks third (just over 40,000 deaths).[3]

A Variety of Factors Influence Cancer Risk

Researchers estimate that about half of all men and one-third of all women will develop cancer during their lifetime.[1] But what factors cause cancer? Are you and your loved ones at risk? The answer depends on several factors, including your family history of cancer, your exposure to environmental agents, and various lifestyle choices.

Heredity can play a role in the development of cancer, because inherited "cancer genes," such as the BRC genes for breast cancer, increase the risk that an individual with those genes will develop cancer. However, only about 5% of all cancers are strongly hereditary.[1] In addition, it's important to bear in mind that a family history of cancer does not guarantee you will get cancer, too. It just means that you are at an increased risk and should take all preventive actions available to you. While some risk factors are out of your control, others are modifiable, which means that you can take positive steps to reduce your risk.

The ACS identifies six modifiable risk factors that have been shown to have the greatest impact on an individual's cancer risk; each is discussed next.[1]

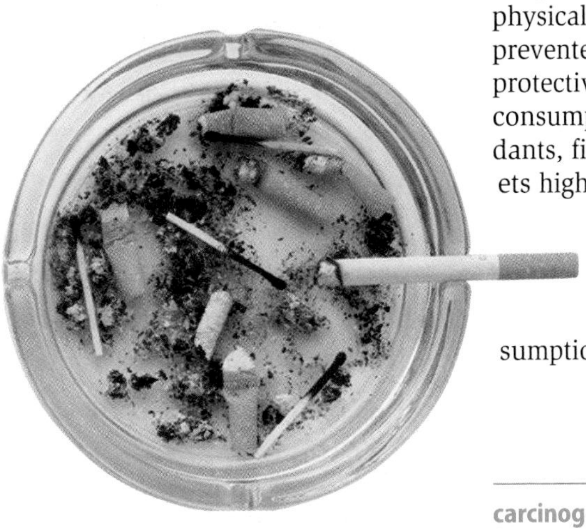

Using tobacco is a risk factor for cancer.

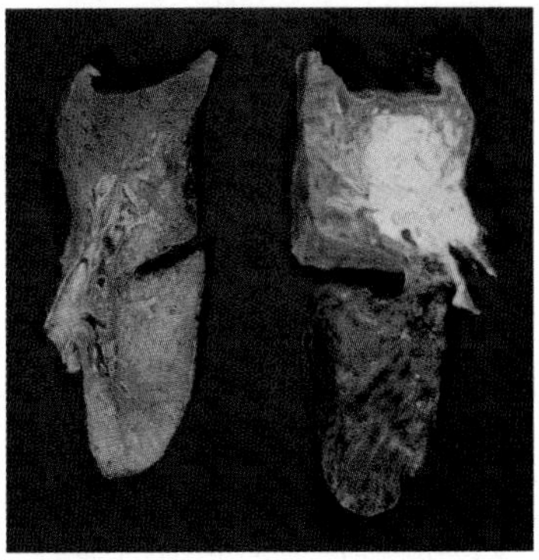

Figure 2 Cigarette smoking significantly increases our risk for lung and other types of cancer. The risk for lung cancer is 22.4 times higher in men who smoke and 12 times higher in women who smoke. **(a)** A normal, healthy lung; **(b)** the lung of a smoker. Notice the deposits of tar as well as the areas of tumor growth.

Tobacco Use

More than 40 compounds in tobacco and tobacco smoke are **carcinogens,** or substances that can cause cancer. Using tobacco increases the risk for cancers of the lung, larynx, mouth, and esophagus and was responsible for about 169,000 deaths in 2009 (**Figure 2**).[1] Smoking can also cause heart disease, stroke, and emphysema. The positive news is that tobacco use is a modifiable risk factor. If you smoke or use smokeless tobacco, you can reduce your risk for cancer considerably by quitting.

Weight, Diet, and Physical Activity

Researchers estimate that one-third of cancer deaths are related to overweight or obesity, poor nutrition, and physical activity and thus could be prevented.[1] Nutritional factors that are protective against cancer include the consumption of foods rich in antioxidants, fiber, and phytochemicals. Diets high in saturated fats and low in fruits and vegetables increase the risk for cancers of the esophagus, colon, breast, and prostate.[4] Consumption of alcohol and compounds

carcinogen Any substance capable of causing the cellular mutations that lead to cancer.

HOT TOPIC

Disorders Linked to Tobacco Use

Many people use smokeless tobacco or smoke cigarettes or cigars. The use of these products can lead to serious health consequences that together reduce life expectancy by more than 13 years in males and 14 years in females.[5] Tobacco use is a risk factor in the development of numerous types of cancers, including lung, larynx, mouth **(Figure 3)**, pharynx, esophagus, bladder, pancreas, uterus, kidney, stomach, and some leukemias. Tobacco use is also a risk factor for heart disease, bronchitis, emphysema, stroke, and erectile dysfunction.

Maternal smoking can cause miscarriage, preterm delivery, stillbirth, infant death, and low birth weight. In addition, smoking causes a variety of other problems, such as the premature wrinkling and coarsening of the skin shown in Figure 3. Smoking also causes bad breath, yellowing of the fingernails and hair, and bad-smelling clothes, hair, and living quarters. Secondhand smoke is another concern, especially for those who live or work with smokers. Nonsmokers who are exposed to secondhand smoke at home or work increase their risk of developing heart disease by 25–30% and increase their risk of developing lung cancer by 20–30%. Research indicates that there is no risk-free level of exposure to secondhand smoke.[6]

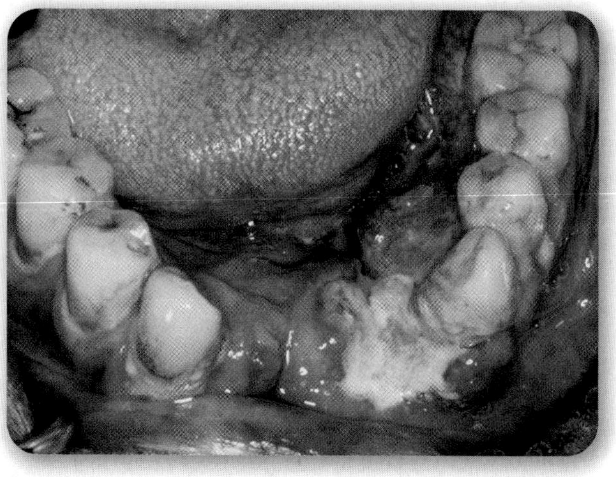

(a)

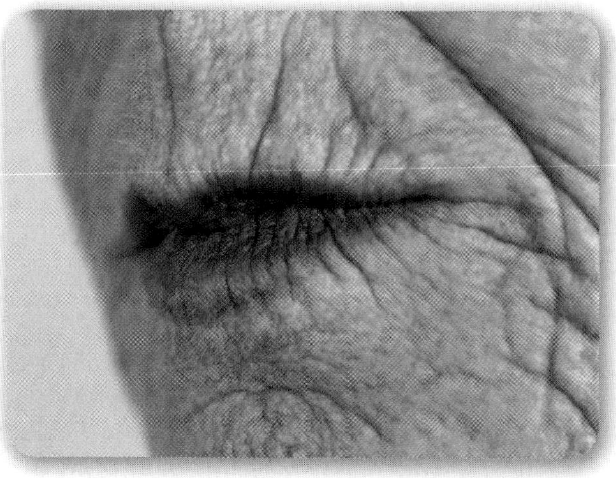

(b)

Figure 3 Effects of tobacco use. In addition to increasing your risk for lung cancer and cardiovascular disease, **(a)** using tobacco increases your risk for mouth cancer, and **(b)** smoking results in premature wrinkling of the skin, especially around the mouth.

found in cured and charbroiled meats can also increase the risk for cancer.

A sedentary lifestyle increases the risk for colon cancer and possibly other forms of cancer.[7] At the same time, a recent review of several studies has found that moderately intense and vigorous physical activity are associated with a 20% to 30% reduction in our overall risk for cancer.[7] A clear protective effect of exercise was found specifically for breast and colon cancers. At this time, we do not know how exercise reduces the overall risk for cancer or for certain types of cancers. However, these findings have prompted the ACS and the National Cancer Institute to promote increased physical activity as a way to reduce our risk for cancer.

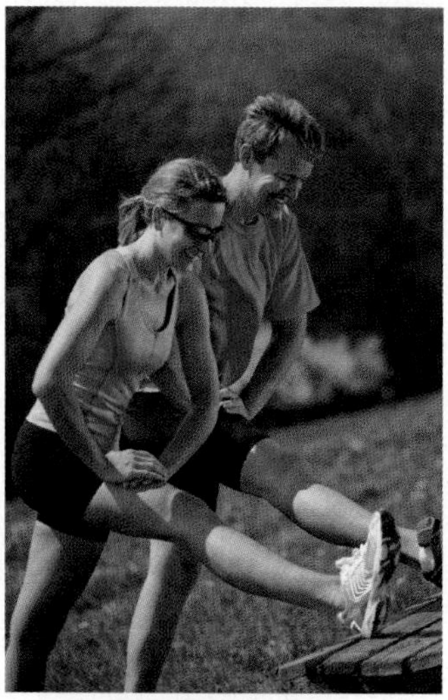

Staying physically active may help reduce the risk for some cancers.

What about you? Are you making dietary and activity choices that help reduce your risk for cancer and other chronic diseases? Check out the What About You? quiz and find out!

Infectious Agents

Infectious agents account for 18% of cancers worldwide. For example, infection of the female cervix with the sexually transmitted virus *Human*

What About You?

Are You Living Smart?

Cancer often seems to strike apparently healthy people "out of the blue." Because genetic and certain environmental factors are beyond your control, you may be wondering how your diet and level of physical activity might be influencing your risk. If so, take the following quiz and see for yourself! Answer each question Yes or No. Then keep reading to see how you can keep living smart!

I eat at least five servings of vegetables and fruits every day.	Yes/No
I eat at least three servings of whole-grain bread, rice, pasta, and cereal every day.	Yes/No
I drink reduced-fat or fat-free milk and yogurt, and I seldom eat high-fat cheeses.	Yes/No
I rarely eat processed and red meat such as bacon, hot dogs, sausage, steak, ground beef, pork, or lamb.	Yes/No
I take it easy on high-Calorie baked goods such as pies, cakes, cookies, sweet rolls, and doughnuts.	Yes/No
I rarely add butter, margarine, oil, sour cream, or mayonnaise to foods when I'm cooking or at the table.	Yes/No
I rarely (less than twice a week) eat fried foods.	Yes/No
I try to maintain a healthful weight.	Yes/No
I get at least 30 minutes of moderate to vigorous physical activity on five or more days of the week.	Yes/No
I usually take the stairs instead of waiting for an elevator.	Yes/No
I try to spend most of my time being active, instead of watching television or sitting at the computer.	Yes/No
I never, or only occasionally, drink alcohol.	Yes/No

How Do You Rate?

Zero to 4 "Yes" answers: Diet Alert!
Your diet is probably too high in fat and too low in plant foods like vegetables, fruits, and grains. You may want to take a look at your eating habits and find ways to make some changes. Trying to watch your intake of saturated fat? See the Quick Tips in Chapter 5 on page 165. Need to increase your vegetables and fruits? See the Quick Tips in Chapter 8 on pages 261, 265, and 269.

5 to 8 "Yes" answers: Not bad! You're Halfway There!
You still have a way to go. Look at your "No" answers to help you decide which areas of your diet need to be improved, or whether your physical activity level should be increased. Check out the Quick Tips on page 288, and see Chapter 12 for ways to increase your level of physical activity.

9 to 12 "Yes" answers: Great Job! You're Living Smart!
Keep up the good habits and keep looking for ways to improve.

Data from American Cancer Society. *Living Smart*. Available at www.cancer.org/downloads/PED/2042_Living_Smart.pdf.

papillomavirus is linked to cervical cancer (**Figure 4**), and infection with the bacterium *Helicobacter pylori* is linked not only to ulcers but also to stomach cancer. Infection with HIV (human immunodeficiency virus) can cause many cancers. As microbial research advances, it is thought that more cancers will be linked to infectious agents.

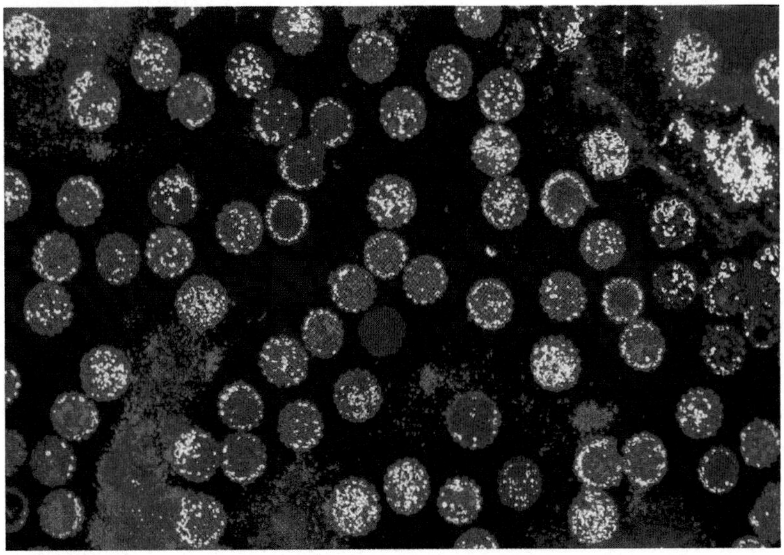

Figure 4 *Human papillomavirus (HPV)* is an infectious agent that can cause cancer.

Ultraviolet Radiation

Skin cancer, the most common form of cancer in the United States, accounts for over half of all cancers diagnosed each year. Most cases of skin cancer are linked to exposure to ultraviolet (UV) rays from the sun and indoor tanning beds. UV rays damage

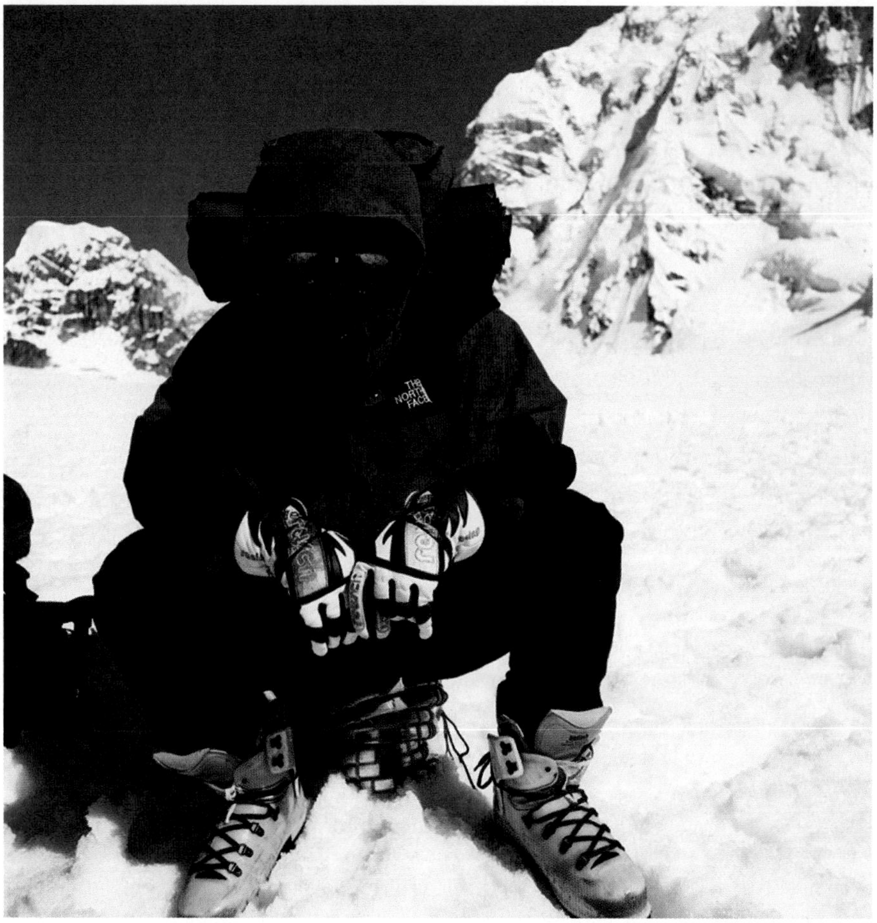

Arctic explorers wear special clothing to protect themselves from the cold as well as the high levels of ultraviolet rays from the sun.

wear sunscreen with at least a 15 sun protection factor (SPF) rating and protective clothing.

Cancer Prompts a Variety of Signs and Symptoms

The signs and symptoms of cancer vary according to the structures affected, how large the tumor is, and how widely it has metastasized. Here, we discuss the most common signs and symptoms that people diagnosed with cancer typically report. However, it's important to bear in mind that these also occur with many other illnesses and even non-illness conditions. Also, having just one or two of these symptoms rarely means that a person has cancer. Still, the ACS suggests that people who experience these symptoms for a long time see their primary healthcare provider.[10]

- *Unexplained weight loss.* Most people with cancer lose weight, so an unexplained weight loss of 10 pounds or more is a hallmark of cancer.

the DNA of immature skin cells, which then reproduce uncontrollably. Research has shown that a person's risk for skin cancer doubles if he or she has had five or more sunburns; however, your risk for skin cancer still increases with UV exposure even if you do not get sunburned.[8] Exposure to tanning beds before age 35 increases by 75% your risk of developing the most invasive form of skin cancer.[9]

Skin cancer includes the non-melanoma cancers (basal cell and squamous cell cancers), which are not typically invasive, and malignant melanoma, which is one of the most deadly of all types of cancer (**Figure 5**). Limiting your exposure to sunlight to no more than 20 minutes between 10 AM and 4 PM can help reduce your risk for skin cancer while allowing your body to synthesize adequate vitamin D. After that,

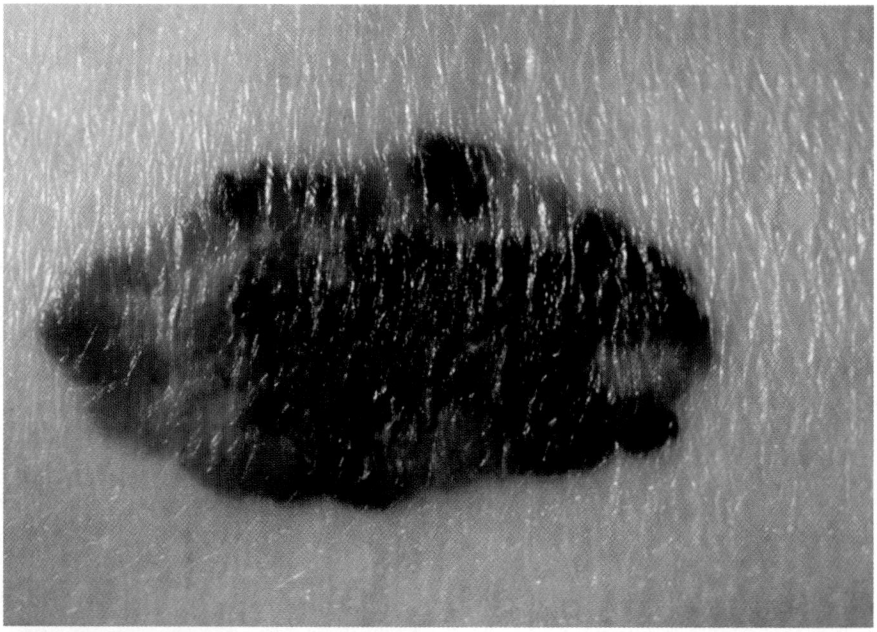

Figure 5 A lesion associated with malignant melanoma is characterized by asymmetry; uneven or blurred borders; mixed shades of tan, brown, black, and sometimes red or blue; and a diameter larger than a pencil eraser (6 mm).

- *Fever.* Fever is very common with cancer, but it often happens when the cancer has metastasized or affects the blood.
- *Fatigue.* Extreme tiredness that isn't relieved with rest may be an important symptom of cancer. The blood loss that occurs with some cancers, such as colon and stomach cancers, can also cause fatigue.
- *Pain.* Headache, back pain, or bone pain can be an early symptom of certain types of cancer.
- *Skin changes.* Along with cancers of the skin, some other cancers can cause skin changes, including a darkened pigmentation, jaundice (yellowish skin tone), redness, excessive hair growth, and itching. Sores that don't heal and recent changes in a wart or mole should also be checked by a healthcare provider.
- *Change in bowel habits or bladder function.* Long-term constipation, diarrhea, painful urination, or the need to pass urine more or less frequently may signal cancer.
- *Indigestion or trouble swallowing.* Although these are most often caused by other disorders, if they persist, they should be evaluated by a healthcare provider.
- *White patches inside the mouth or on the tongue.* Especially in people who smoke or chew tobacco, these are important early signs of oral cancer.
- *Unusual bleeding or discharge.* Blood in the urine or stool, abnormal vaginal bleeding, a bloody discharge from the nipple, and bloody sputum (phlegm) can all occur in early or advanced cancer.
- *Any thickening or lump.* Many cancers can be felt through the skin, especially those involving the breast, testicle, or lymph nodes.
- *Nagging cough or hoarseness.* A cough that doesn't resolve can be a sign of lung cancer, whereas hoarseness can be a sign of cancer of the larynx (voice box) or thyroid gland.

How Is Cancer Treated?

Physicians typically evaluate signs and symptoms of cancer using a variety of blood tests and diagnostic scans, such as ultrasound, CT, and MRI scans. Once a diagnosis is made, the patient is often referred to the care of an oncologist, a physician who specializes in cancer treatment (*onco-* means "tumor").

Cancer treatment varies according to the location of the cancer, the cell type, whether or not it has metastasized, and, if so, how much. Other factors, such as the patient's general health, extent of weight loss, age, and personal preferences, as well as the type, scope, and quality of healthcare insurance coverage, may also come into play. The three major types of cancer treatment are surgery, radiation, and chemotherapy. Surgery is most effective when it can entirely remove the mass. Radiation therapy delivers high-energy x-rays, gamma rays, electron beams, or photons to tumor cells to kill them outright or damage their DNA so that they can no longer reproduce. Chemotherapy is drug therapy, and any of more than 100 different drugs can be combined for different patient needs. For cancers that are localized—that is, confined to a limited area, with no metastasis—surgery may be the only treatment advised. Other cancers may require surgery followed by radiation and/or chemotherapy. Diffuse cancers, such as blood cancers, and tumors in locations that cannot be accessed safely with surgery, such as head and neck tumors, may be considered inoperable, and radiation and/or chemotherapy may be prescribed. In some cases, a large tumor is first radiated, with the goal of shrinking it prior to surgery.

Can Cancer Be Prevented?

Some types of cancer can be prevented. For instance, vaccines, the appropriate use of antibiotics, and behavioral changes can prevent certain cancers known to be caused by infectious agents. Most cancers, however, are multifactorial—we cannot link them to only one cause. This means that there is no way to guarantee that you—or anyone else—won't get cancer. Still, if you consider the population of the United States, about half of all cancer deaths could be prevented if no one used tobacco and everyone took certain key steps to improve his or her health.[11] The ACS advocates four key cancer-prevention behaviors: check, quit, move, and nourish.

Check

Regular screening examinations can allow for the detection and removal of precancerous tissues. For instance, a test called a Pap smear can detect subtle changes in the cells lining a woman's cervix (the entrance to the uterus) that, if allowed to progress, could result in cervical cancer. Women with a Pap smear indicating these changes typically return to their physician for a quick outpatient procedure in which the layer of precancerous cells is removed. Similarly, colonoscopies allow for the detection and removal of precancerous polyps. And regular skin checks allow for suspicious lesions to be removed—and cell samples sent to a lab—to evaluate for skin cancer. Screening can also allow for detection at an early stage, when cancer is most treatable. For example, a mammogram may be able to detect a breast mass that is too small for the woman to feel.

Quit

As we noted earlier, tobacco use is a risk factor in the development of a wide variety of cancers, but all cancers caused by long-term tobacco use are entirely preventable. In fact, about one-third of all cancer deaths could be prevented if everyone followed the ACS recommendation to quit smoking.[1]

Alcohol abuse is also a factor in cancer. Excessive drinking is linked with an increased risk for cancers of

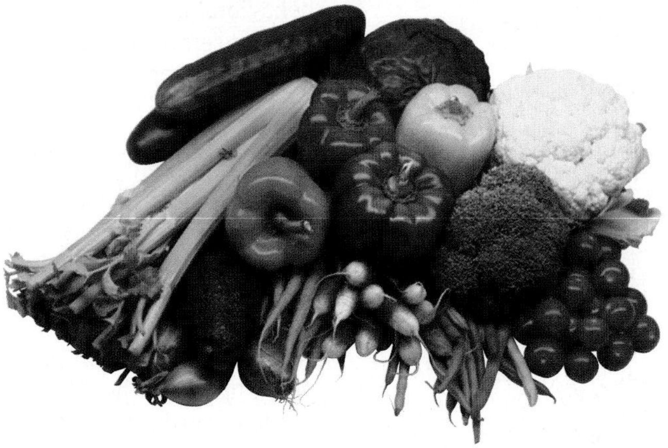

These vegetables provide antioxidant nutrients, fiber, and phytochemicals, all of which reduce the risk for some cancers.

the esophagus, pharynx, and mouth and may increase the risk for cancers of the liver, breast, colon, and rectum. Alcohol may also impair cells' ability to repair damaged DNA, increasing the possibility of cancer initiation.

Move

Regular physical activity can significantly lower your lifetime risk for cancer. The ACS recommends that we engage in at least 30 minutes of moderate to vigorous activity at least 5 days a week. On busy days, try to work in 10 minutes of activity three times a day. For instance, take a walk at lunch; then take a 10-minute exercise break in mid-afternoon. When you get home, cycle for 10 minutes. Short activity sessions like these can quickly add up to 30 minutes.[12]

Nourish

One of the smartest ways to reduce your risk for cancer is to maintain a healthful weight and a healthful diet. See the Quick Tips here for nutrition-related tips.

Antioxidants Play a Role in Preventing Cancer

A large and growing body of evidence suggests that antioxidants play an important role in cancer prevention. But how? The following are some proposed mechanisms:

- Enhancing the immune system, which assists in the destruction and removal of precancerous cells from the body
- Inhibiting the growth of cancer cells and tumors
- Preventing oxidative damage to the cells' DNA by scavenging free radicals and stopping the formation and subsequent chain reaction of oxidized molecules

Eating whole foods that are high in antioxidants—especially fruits, vegetables, and whole grains—is consistently shown to be associated with decreased cancer risk.[13] In addition, populations eating diets low in antioxidant nutrients have a higher risk for cancer. These studies show a strong association between level of dietary antioxidants and cancer risk, but they do not prove cause and effect. Nutrition experts agree that there are important interactions between antioxidant nutrients and other substances in foods, such as fiber and phytochemicals, which work together to reduce the risk for many types of cancers. Studies are now being con-

QUICK TIPS

Reducing Your Cancer Risk

✓ Lose weight or maintain your current healthful weight. Obesity appears to increase the risk for cancers of the breast, colon, prostate, endometrium (the lining of the uterus), cervix, ovary, kidney, gallbladder, liver, pancreas, rectum, and esophagus. The exact links between obesity and increased cancer risk are not clear but may involve hormonal changes associated with fat cells.

✓ Avoid heterocyclic amines in cooked meat. These carcinogenic chemicals are formed when meat is cooked at high temperatures, such as during broiling, barbecuing, and frying.

✓ Avoid nitrites and nitrates in cured meats. These compounds, which are found in some sausages, hams, bacon, and lunch meats, bind with amino acids to form nitrosamines, which are potent carcinogens.

✓ Eat a diet low in saturated fat. Diets high in saturated fat have been associated with increased risk for many cancers, including prostate and breast cancers. However, not all studies support this association.

✓ Eat a diet rich in vegetables and fruits. These foods are high in antioxidants (discussed in more detail shortly) and in fiber, which some studies link to a reduced risk for certain cancers.

✓ Select foods containing phytoestrogens (plant estrogens). These compounds, found in soy-based foods and some vegetables and grains, may decrease the risk for breast, endometrial, and prostate cancers.

✓ Make sure to consume adequate omega-3 fatty acids (see Chapter 5). Consuming foods high in omega-3 fatty acids is associated with reduced rates of breast, colon, and rectal cancers.

NUTRI-CASE GUSTAVO

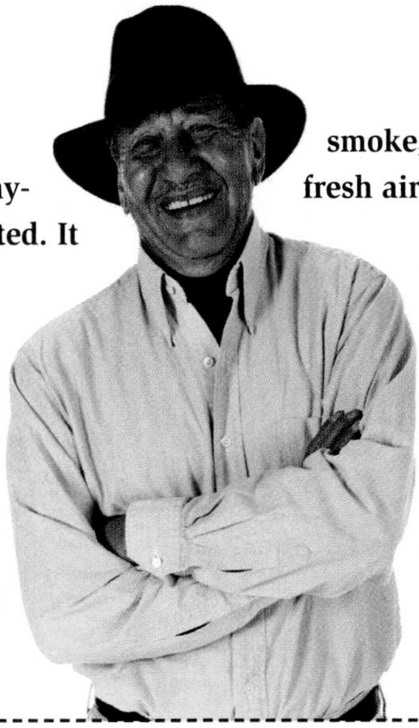

"Last night, there was an actress on TV talking about having colon cancer and saying everybody over age 50 should get tested. It brought back all the memories of my father's cancer, how thin and weak he got before he went to the doctor, so that by the time they found the cancer it had already spread too far. But I don't think I'm at risk. I only eat red meat two or three times a week, and I eat a piece of fruit or a vegetable at every meal. I don't smoke, and I get plenty of exercise, sunshine, and fresh air working in the vineyard."

What lifestyle factors reduce Gustavo's risk for cancer? What factors increase his risk? Would you recommend he increase his consumption of fruits and vegetables? Why or why not? If Gustavo were your father, would you ask him to have the screening test for colon cancer that the actress on television recommended?

ducted to determine whether eating foods high in antioxidants directly causes lower rates of cancer.

As we noted on page 277, the link between taking antioxidant supplements and reducing cancer risk is not clear. Laboratory animal and test tube studies show that the individual nutrients reviewed in this chapter act as antioxidants in various situations. However, supplementation studies in humans do not consistently show benefits of taking antioxidant supplements in the prevention of cancer and other diseases, and some suggest an increased risk.

Why do antioxidant supplements appear to work in some studies and for some cancers but not in others? The human body is very complex, as is the development and progression of the numerous forms of cancer. People differ substantially in their susceptibility and response to carcinogens, as well as to protective factors. These complexities cloud the relationship between nutrition and cancer. In any research study, it is impossible to control all the factors that may increase the risk for cancer. Thus, many unknown factors can affect study outcomes. It has also been speculated that antioxidants taken in supplemental form may act as prooxidants in some situations, whereas antioxidants consumed in foods may be more balanced. Many studies currently being conducted are examining the impact of whole foods and antioxidant supplements on the risk for various forms of cancer. The results of these studies will provide important insights into the link between whole foods, individual nutrients, and cancer.

Web Resources

www.cancer.org
The American Cancer Society

Get recommendations for smoking cessation, nutrition, sun exposure, and physical activity for cancer prevention.

www.cancer.gov
The National Cancer Institute

Learn more about the nutritional factors that can influence your risk for cancer.

9 Nutrients Involved in Bone Health

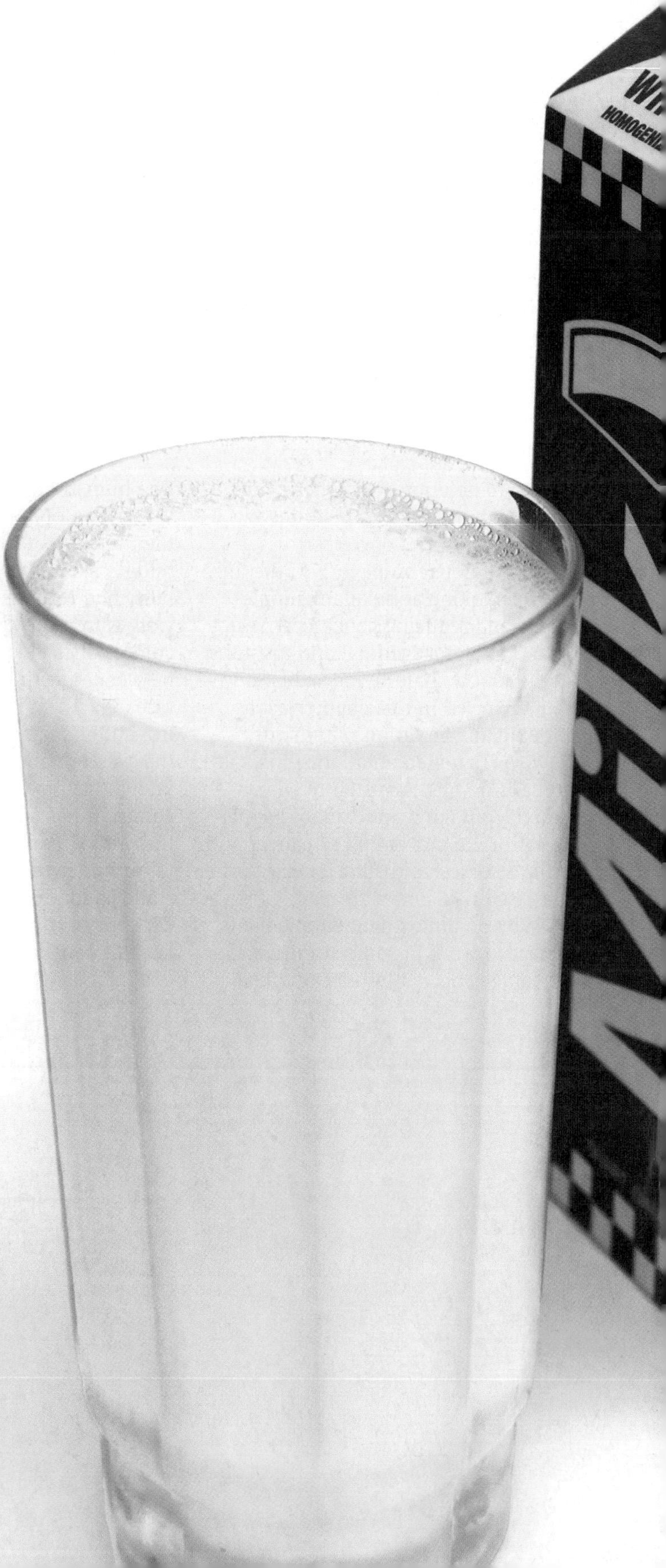

CHAPTER OBJECTIVES

After reading this chapter you will be able to:

1. **Describe the differences between cortical bone and trabecular bone, pp. 292–293.**
2. **Discuss the processes of bone growth, modeling, and remodeling, pp. 293–294.**
3. **List two vitamins and three minerals that play important roles in maintaining bone health, p. 296.**
4. **Identify foods that are good sources of calcium, pp. 298–300.**
5. **Describe how vitamin D assists in regulating blood calcium levels, pp. 302, 306–307.**
6. **Discuss three potential reasons that consumption of soft drinks may be detrimental to bone health, p. 310.**

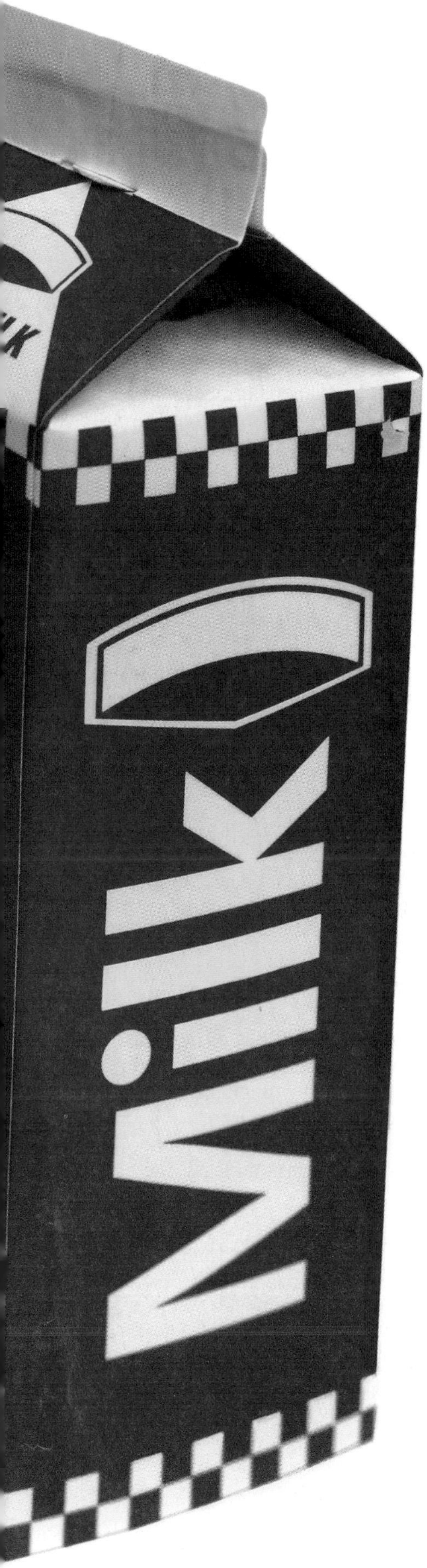

Test Yourself

1. **T F Very few foods—except milk, yogurt, and cheese—provide calcium.**
2. **T F We are capable of making vitamin D within our body by using energy obtained from exposure to sunlight.**
3. **T F Drinking lots of milk can help you lose weight.**

Test Yourself answers can be found at the end of the chapter.

In northern Maine, hockey is the local sport. So what's a poster of NBA star Chris Paul—who plays for the New Orleans Hornets—doing on the cafeteria walls in local schools? Paul is one of many athletes participating in the new "Body by Milk" ad campaign by the Milk Processor Education Program to teach kids about the benefits of drinking milk. On the campaign's TV commercials and website, Paul tells kids that the protein in milk helps build strong muscles and the calcium helps build strong bones.

Is the campaign working? Americans are consuming only about 1.8 cups of dairy (including milk, yogurt, ice cream, and cheese) per day, far short of the recommended 2–3 cups. In addition, the consumption of milk, specifically, plummeted from 31 gallons per person per year in 1970 to 21 gallons in 2005, likely because of competition from soft drinks, bottled waters, and specialty juices, coffees, and teas.[1] This concerns healthcare professionals, because milk is a convenient source of a form of calcium that's easily absorbed by the body, and calcium is required for kids and teens to build dense, compact bones. What's more, milk is fortified with vitamin D and is a good source of phosphorus, two more nutrients critical to bone health.

Still, milk is hardly the only food source of these nutrients. What other foods build bone? And how does bone grow—and break down? We begin this chapter with a quick look at the components and activities of bone tissue. Then we discuss the nutrients, dietary choices, and other lifestyle factors that play a critical role in maintaining bone health.

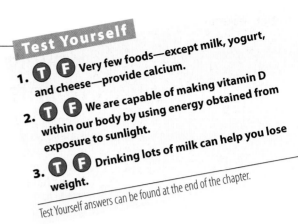

How Does Our Body Maintain Bone Health?

Contrary to what most people think, our skeleton is not an inactive collection of bones that simply holds our body together. Bones are living organs that contain several tissues, including two types of bone tissue, cartilage, and connective tissue. Nerves and blood vessels run within channels in bone tissue, supporting its activities. Bones have many important functions in our body, some of which might surprise you (**Table 9.1**). For instance, did you know that most of your blood cells are formed deep within your bones?

Given the importance of bones, it is critical that we maintain their health. Bone health is achieved through complex interactions among nutrients, hormones, and environmental factors. To better understand these interactions, we first need to learn about how bone structure and the constant activity of bone tissue influence bone health throughout our lifetime.

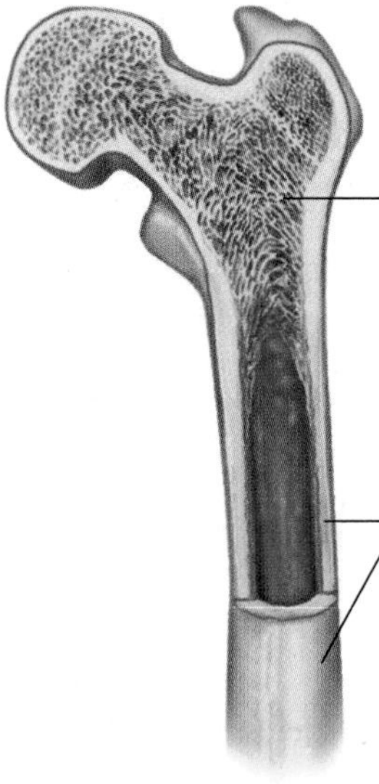

Figure 9.1 The structure of bone. Notice the difference in density between the trabecular (spongy) bone and the cortical (compact) bone.

The Composition of Bone Provides Strength and Flexibility

We tend to think of bones as totally rigid, but if they were, how could we twist and jump our way through a basketball game or even carry an armload of books up a flight of stairs? Our bones need to be both strong and flexible, so that they can resist the compression, stretching, and twisting that occur throughout our daily activities. Fortunately, the composition of bone is ideally suited for its complex job: about 65% of bone tissue is made up of an assortment of minerals (mostly calcium and phosphorus) that provide hardness, but the remaining 35% is a mixture of organic substances that provide strength, durability, and flexibility. The most important of these substances is a fibrous protein called **collagen.** You might be surprised to learn that collagen fibers are actually stronger than steel fibers of similar size! Within our bones, the minerals form tiny crystals (called *hydroxyapatite*) that cluster around the collagen fibers. This design enables bones to bear our weight while responding to our demands for movement.

If you examine a bone very closely, you will notice two distinct types of tissue (**Figure 9.1**): cortical bone and trabecular bone. **Cortical bone,** which is also called **compact bone,** is very dense. It constitutes approximately 80% of our skeleton. The outer surface of all bones is cortical; plus, many small bones of the body, such as the bones of the wrists, hands, and feet, are made entirely of cortical bone. Although cortical bone looks solid to the naked eye, it actually contains many microscopic openings, which serve as passageways for blood vessels and nerves.

In contrast, **trabecular bone** makes up only 20% of our skeleton. It is found within the ends of the long bones (such as the bones of the arms and legs), the

collagen A protein that forms strong fibers in bone and connective tissue.

cortical bone (compact bone) A dense bone tissue that makes up the outer surface of all bones as well as the entirety of most small bones of the body.

trabecular bone (spongy bone) A porous bone tissue that makes up only 20% of our skeleton and is found within the ends of the long bones, inside the spinal vertebrae, inside the flat bones (sternum, ribs, and most bones of the skull), and inside the bones of the pelvis.

TABLE 9.1 Functions of Bone in the Human Body

Functions Related to Structure and Support	Functions Related to Metabolic Processes
Bones provide physical support for organs and body segments.	Bone tissue acts as a storage reservoir for many minerals, including calcium, phosphorus, and fluoride. The body draws upon such deposits when these minerals are needed for various body processes; however, this can reduce bone mass.
Bones protect vital organs; for example, the rib cage protects the lungs, the skull protects the brain, and the vertebrae of the spine protect the spinal cord.	Most blood cells are produced in the bone marrow.
Bones work with muscles and tendons to allow movement—muscles attach to bones via tendons, and their contraction produces movement at the body's joints.	

spinal vertebrae, the sternum (breastbone), the ribs, most bones of the skull, and the pelvis. Trabecular bone is sometimes referred to as **spongy bone** because to the naked eye it looks like a sponge, with cavities and no clear organization. The microscope reveals that trabecular bone is, in fact, aligned in a precise network of columns that protects the bone from stress. You can think of trabecular bone as the scaffolding inside the bone that supports the outer cortical bone.

Cortical and trabecular bone also differ in their rate of turnover—that is, in how quickly the bone tissue is broken down and replenished. Trabecular bone has a faster turnover rate than cortical bone. This makes trabecular bone more sensitive to changes in hormones and nutritional deficiencies. It also accounts for the much higher rate of age-related fractures in the spine and pelvis (including the hip)—both of which contain a significant amount of trabecular bone. Let's investigate how bone turnover influences bone health.

The Constant Activity of Bone Tissue Promotes Bone Health

Our bones develop through a series of three processes: bone growth, bone modeling, and bone remodeling **(Figure 9.2)**. Bone growth and modeling begin during the early months of fetal life, when our skeleton is forming, and continue until early adulthood. Bone remodeling predominates during adulthood; this process helps us maintain a healthy skeleton as we age.

Bone Growth and Modeling Determine the Size and Shape of Our Bones

Through the process of *bone growth*, the size of our bones increases. The first period of rapid bone growth is from birth to age 2, but growth continues in spurts throughout childhood and into adolescence. Most girls reach their adult height by age 14, and boys generally reach adult height by age 17.[1] In the later decades of life, some loss in height usually occurs because of decreased bone density in the spine.

Bone modeling is the process by which the shape of our bones is determined, from the round "pebble" bones that make up our wrists, to the uniquely shaped bones of our face, to the long bones of our arms and legs. Even after bones stop growing in length, they can still increase in thickness if they are stressed by engaging in repetitive exercise, such as weight training, or by being overweight or obese.

Although the size and shape of our bones do not change significantly after puberty, our **bone density,** or the compactness of our bones, continues to develop into early adulthood. *Peak bone density* is the point at which our bones are strongest because they are at their highest density. The following factors are associated with a lower peak bone density:[2–4]

- late pubertal age in boys and late onset of menstruation in girls
- inadequate calcium intake
- low body weight
- physical inactivity during adolescence.

bone density The degree of compactness of bone tissue, reflecting the strength of the bones. *Peak bone density* is the point at which a bone is strongest.

About 90% of a woman's bone density has been built by 17 years of age, whereas the majority of a man's has been built by his twenties. However, male or female,

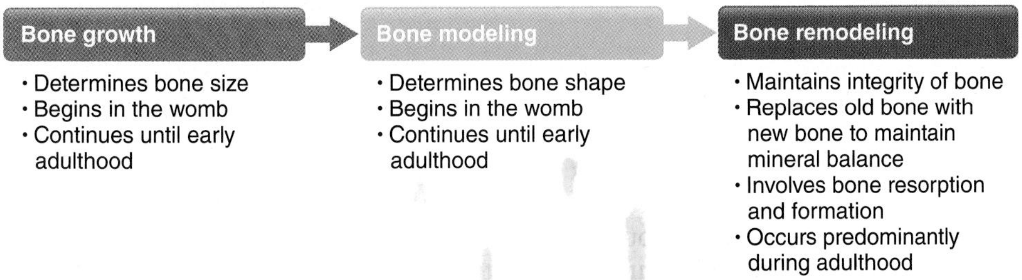

Bone growth
• Determines bone size
• Begins in the womb
• Continues until early adulthood
Bone modeling
• Determines bone shape
• Begins in the womb
• Continues until early adulthood
Bone remodeling
• Maintains integrity of bone
• Replaces old bone with new bone to maintain mineral balance
• Involves bone resorption and formation
• Occurs predominantly during adulthood

Figure 9.2 Bone develops through three processes: bone growth, bone modeling, and bone remodeling.

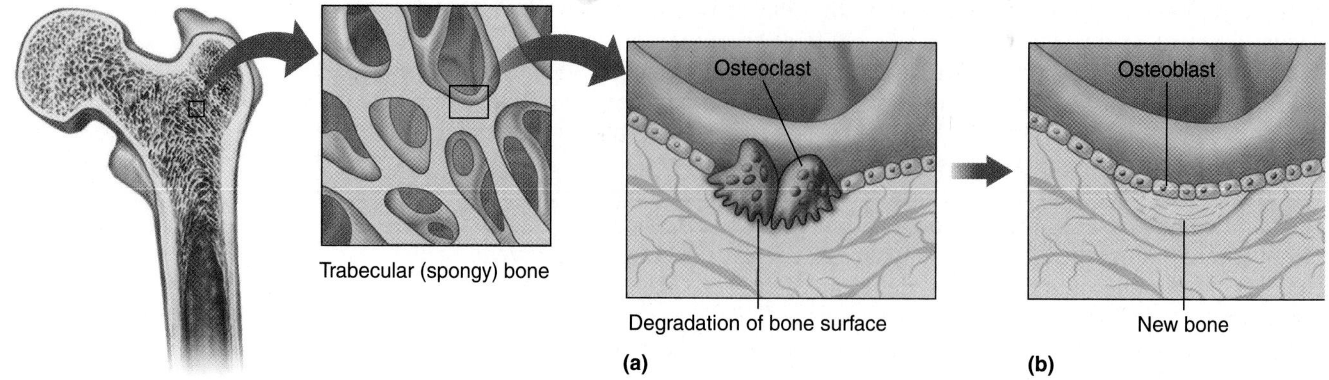

Figure 9.3 Bone remodeling involves resorption and formation. **(a)** Osteoclasts erode the bone surface by degrading its components, including calcium, other minerals, and collagen; these components are then transported to the bloodstream. **(b)** Osteoblasts work to build new bone by filling the pit formed by the resorption process with new bone.

before we reach the age of 30 years, our bodies have reached peak bone mass, and we can no longer significantly add to our bone density. In our thirties, our bone density remains relatively stable, but by age 40, it has begun its irreversible decline.

Bone Remodeling Maintains a Balance Between Breakdown and Repair

Although our bones cannot increase their peak density after our twenties, bone tissue still remains very active throughout adulthood, balancing the breakdown of older bone tissue and the formation of new bone tissue. This bone recycling process is called **remodeling.** Remodeling is also used to repair fractures and to strengthen bone regions that are exposed to higher physical stress. The process of remodeling involves two steps: resorption and formation.

Bone is broken down through a process referred to as **resorption** (Figure 9.3a). During resorption, cells called **osteoclasts** erode the bone surface by secreting enzymes and acids that dig grooves into the bone matrix. Their ruffled surface also acts somewhat like a scrubbing brush to assist in the erosion process. One of the primary reasons the body regularly breaks down bone is to release calcium into the bloodstream. As discussed in more detail later in this chapter, calcium is critical for many physiologic processes, and bone is an important calcium reservoir. The body also breaks down bone that is fractured and needs to be repaired. Resorption at the injury site smooths the rough edges created by the break. Bone may also be broken down in areas away from the fracture site to obtain the minerals that are needed to repair the damage. Regardless of the reason, once bone is broken down, the resulting products are transported into the bloodstream and used for various body functions.

New bone is formed through the action of cells called **osteoblasts,** or "bone builders" (see Figure 9.3b). These cells work to synthesize new bone matrix by laying down the collagen-containing organic component of bone. Within this substance, the hydroxyapatite crystallizes and packs together to create new bone where it is needed.

In young, healthy adults, the processes of bone resorption and formation are equal, so that just as much bone is broken down as is built, maintaining bone mass. Around 40 years of age, bone resorption begins to occur more rapidly than bone formation, and this imbalance results in an overall loss in bone density. Because this affects the vertebrae of the spine, we also tend to lose height as we age. As we will discuss shortly, achieving a high peak bone mass through proper nutrition and exercise when we are young provides us with a stronger skeleton before the loss of bone begins. It can therefore reduce our risk for *osteoporosis,* a disorder characterized by low-density bones that fracture easily. Osteoporosis is discussed ***In Depth*** on pages 318–325.

remodeling The two-step process by which bone tissue is recycled; includes the breakdown of existing bone and the formation of new bone.

resorption The process by which the surface of bone is broken down by cells called osteoclasts.

osteoclasts Cells that erode the surface of bones by secreting enzymes and acids that dig grooves into the bone matrix.

osteoblasts Cells that prompt the formation of new bone matrix by laying down the collagen-containing component of bone, which is then mineralized.

RECAP **Bones are organs that contain metabolically active tissues composed primarily of minerals and a fibrous protein called collagen. Of the two types of bone, cortical bone is more dense; trabecular bone is more porous. Trabecular bone is also more sensitive to hormonal and nutritional factors and turns over more rapidly than cortical bone. The three types of bone activity are growth, modeling, and remodeling. Bones reach their peak bone mass by the late teenage years into the twenties; bone mass begins to decline around age 40.**

How Do We Assess Bone Health?

Over the past 40 years, technological advancements have led to the development of a number of affordable methods for measuring bone health. **Dual energy x-ray absorptiometry (DXA or DEXA)** is considered the most accurate assessment tool for measuring bone density. This method can measure the density of the bone mass over the entire body. Software is also available that provides an estimation of percentage body fat.

The DXA procedure is simple, painless, and noninvasive, and it is considered to be of minimal risk. It takes just 15 to 30 minutes to complete. The person participating in the test remains fully clothed but must remove all jewelry and other metal objects. The participant lies quietly on a table, and bone density is assessed through the use of a very low level of x-ray **(Figure 9.4)**.

DXA is a very important tool in determining a person's risk for osteoporosis. It generates a bone density score, which is compared to the average peak bone density of a healthy 30-year-old. Doctors use this comparison, which is known as a **T-score,** to assess the risk for fracture and determine whether the person has osteoporosis. If bone density is normal, the T-score ranges between +1 and –1 of the value for a healthy 30-year-old. A negative T-score between –1 and –2.5 indicates low bone mass and an increased risk for fractures. If the T-score is more negative than –2.5, the person has osteoporosis.

dual energy x-ray absorptiometry (DXA or DEXA) Currently, the most accurate tool for measuring bone density.

T-score A comparison of an individual's bone density to the average peak bone density of a 30-year-old healthy adult.

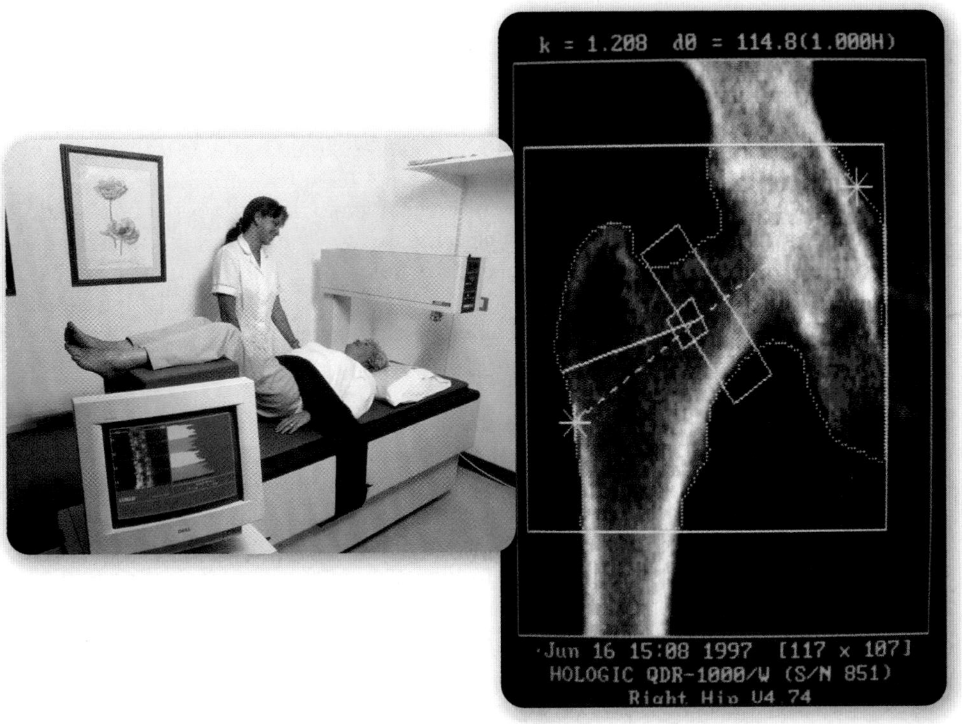

Figure 9.4 Dual energy x-ray absorptiometry is a safe and simple procedure that assesses bone density.

DXA tests are generally recommended for postmenopausal women because they are at highest risk for osteoporosis and fracture. Men and younger women may also be recommended for a DXA test if they have significant risk factors for osteoporosis (see the ***In Depth*** on osteoporosis immediately following this chapter).

Other technologies have been developed to measure bone density. These use ultrasound or different forms of x-ray technology to measure the density of bone in the heel or another more peripheral part of the body. These technologies are frequently used at health fairs because the machines are portable and provide scores faster than the traditional DXA.

RECAP **Dual energy x-ray absorptiometry (DXA or DEXA) is the gold standard measurement of bone mass. It is a simple, painless, and minimal-risk procedure. The result of a DXA is a T-score, which is a comparison of a person's bone density with that of a healthy 30-year-old. A T-score between +1 and −1 is normal; a score between −1 and −2.5 indicates poor bone density; and a score more negative than −2.5 indicates osteoporosis.**

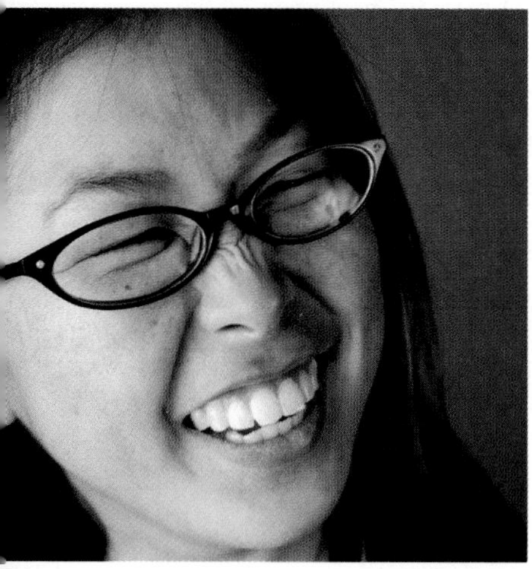

One major role of calcium is to form and maintain bones and teeth.

A Profile of Nutrients That Maintain Bone Health

Calcium is the most recognized nutrient associated with bone health; however, vitamins D and K, phosphorus, magnesium, and fluoride are also essential for strong bones, and the roles of other vitamins, minerals, and phytochemicals are currently being researched.

Calcium

Recall from Chapter 1 that the major minerals are those required in our diet in amounts greater than 100 mg per day. Calcium is by far the most abundant major mineral in our body, constituting about 2% of our entire body weight! Not surprisingly, it plays many critical roles in maintaining overall function and health.

Functions of Calcium

One of the primary functions of calcium is to provide structure to our bones and teeth. About 99% of the calcium found in our body is stored in the hydroxyapatite crystals built up on the collagen foundation of bone. As noted earlier, the combination of crystals and collagen provides both the characteristic hardness of bone and the flexibility needed to support various activities.

The remaining 1% of calcium in our body is found in the blood and soft tissues. Calcium is alkaline, or basic, and plays a critical role in assisting with acid–base balance. We cannot survive for long if our blood calcium level rises above or falls below a very narrow range; therefore, our body maintains the appropriate blood calcium level at all costs.

Figure 9.5 illustrates how various organ systems and hormones work together to maintain blood calcium levels. When blood calcium levels fall (Figure 9.5a), the parathyroid glands are stimulated to produce **parathyroid hormone (PTH).** Also known as parathormone, PTH stimulates the activation of vitamin D. Together, PTH and vitamin D stimulate the kidneys to reabsorb calcium from the bloodstream. They also stimulate osteoclasts to break down bone, releasing more calcium into the bloodstream. In addition, vitamin D increases the absorption of calcium from the intestines. Through these three mechanisms, blood calcium levels increase.

When blood calcium levels are too high, the thyroid gland secretes a hormone called **calcitonin,** which inhibits the actions of vitamin D (Figure 9.5b). Thus, calcitonin prevents the reabsorption of calcium in the kidneys, limits calcium absorption in the intestines, and inhibits the osteoclasts from breaking down bone.

parathyroid hormone (PTH) A hormone secreted by the parathyroid gland when blood calcium levels fall. Also known as parathormone, it increases blood calcium levels by stimulating the activation of vitamin D, increasing reabsorption of calcium from the kidneys, and stimulating osteoclasts to break down bone, which releases more calcium into the bloodstream.

calcitonin A hormone secreted by the thyroid gland when blood calcium levels are too high. Calcitonin inhibits the actions of vitamin D, preventing reabsorption of calcium in the kidneys, limiting calcium absorption in the small intestine, and inhibiting the osteoclasts from breaking down bone.

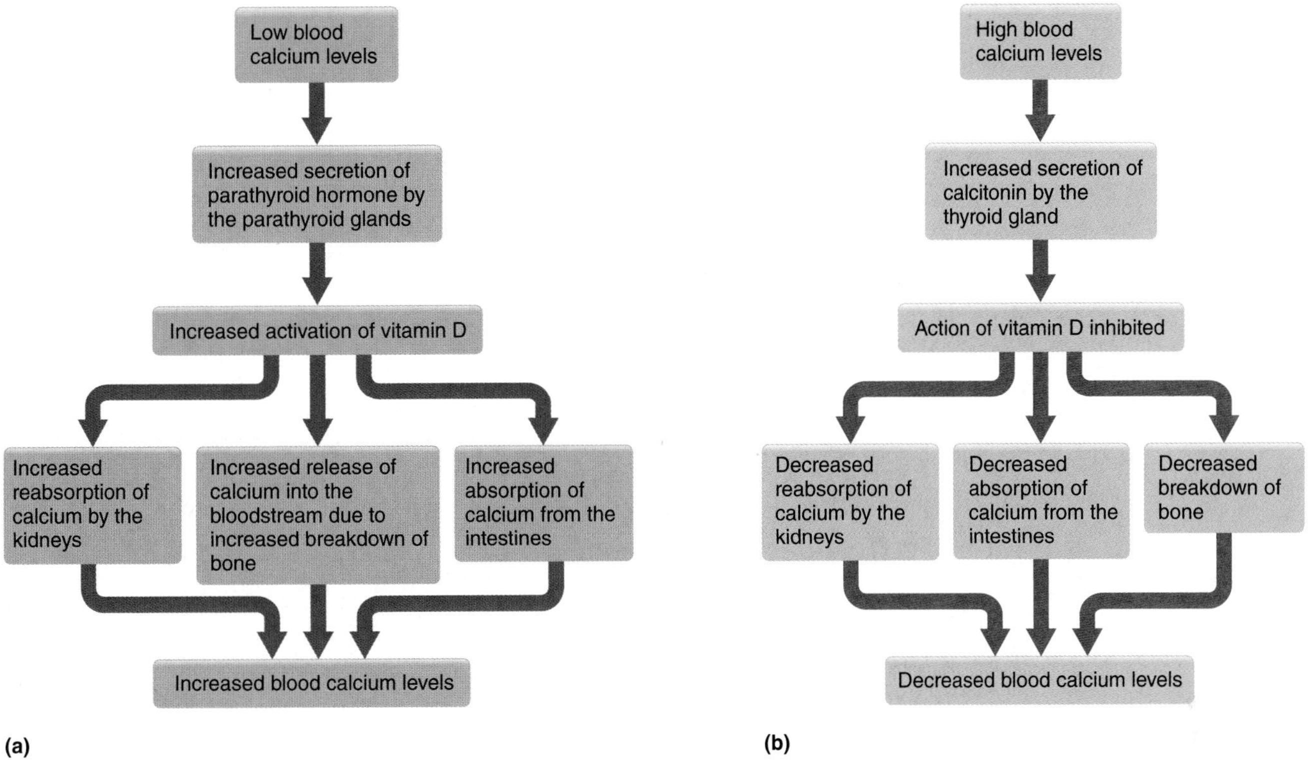

Figure 9.5 Regulation of blood calcium levels by various organs and hormones. **(a)** Low blood calcium levels stimulate the production of parathyroid hormone and activation of vitamin D, which in turn cause an increase in blood calcium levels. **(b)** High blood calcium levels stimulate the secretion of calcitonin, which in turn causes a decrease in blood calcium levels.

As just noted, the body must maintain blood calcium levels within a very narrow range. Thus, when an individual does not consume or absorb enough calcium from the diet, osteoclasts erode bone, so that calcium can be released into the blood. To maintain healthy bone density, we need to consume and absorb enough calcium to balance the calcium taken from our bones.

Calcium is also critical for the normal transmission of nerve impulses. Calcium flows into nerve cells and stimulates the release of molecules called neurotransmitters, which transfer the nerve impulses from one nerve cell (neuron) to another. Without adequate calcium, our nerves' ability to transmit messages is inhibited. Not surprisingly, when blood calcium levels fall dangerously low, a person can experience convulsions.

A fourth role of calcium is to assist in muscle contraction, which is initiated when calcium flows into muscle cells. Conversely, muscles relax when calcium is pumped back outside of muscle cells. If calcium levels are inadequate, normal muscle contraction and relaxation are inhibited, and the person may suffer from twitching and spasms. This is referred to as **calcium tetany.** High levels of blood calcium can cause **calcium rigor,** an inability of muscles to relax, which leads to a hardening or stiffening of the muscles. These problems affect the function not only of skeletal muscles but also of heart muscle and can cause heart failure.

Other functions of calcium include the maintenance of healthy blood pressure, the initiation of blood clotting, and the regulation of various hormones and enzymes.

calcium tetany A condition in which muscles experience twitching and spasms as a result of inadequate blood calcium levels.

calcium rigor A failure of muscles to relax, which leads to a hardening or stiffening of the muscles; caused by high levels of blood calcium.

How Much Calcium Should We Consume?

There are no RDA values for calcium. The Adequate Intake (AI) varies according to age and gender. Adult values are listed in **Table 9.2**. Values for adults over age 70 are higher (1,200 mg/day), and pre-teens and teens have the highest calcium requirements (1,300 mg/day). Many people of all ages fail to consume enough calcium to maintain bone health.

TABLE 9.2 Overview of Nutrients Essential to Bone Health

To see the full profile of nutrients essential to bone health, turn to ***In Depth,*** Vitamins and Minerals: Micronutrients with Macro Powers, pages 216–225.

Nutrient	Recommended Intake
Calcium (major mineral)	Adequate Intake (AI): Women and men aged 19 to 50 years = 1,000 mg/day Women and men aged >50 years = 1,000 to 1,200 mg/day
Vitamin D (fat-soluble vitamin)	AI:* Women and men aged 19 to 50 years = 600 IU/day Women and men aged 50 to 70 years = 600 IU/day Women and men aged >70 years = 800 IU/day
Vitamin K (fat-soluble vitamin)	AI: Women: 90 μg/day Men: 120 μg/day
Phosphorus (major mineral)	Recommended Dietary Allowance (RDA): Women and men = 700 mg/day
Magnesium (major mineral)	RDA: Women aged 19 to 30 years = 310 mg/day Women aged >30 years = 320 mg/day Men aged 19 to 30 years = 400 mg/day Men aged >30 years = 420 mg/day
Fluoride (trace mineral)	AI: Women: 3 mg/day Men: 4 mg/day

**Based on the assumption that a person does not get adequate sun exposure.*

A nutrient's **bioavailability** is the degree to which our body can absorb and use that nutrient. The bioavailability of calcium depends in part on our age and our calcium need. For example, infants, children, and adolescents can absorb more than 60% of the calcium they consume, as calcium needs are very high during these stages of life. In addition, pregnant and lactating women can absorb about 50% of dietary calcium. In contrast, healthy young adults absorb only about 30% of the calcium consumed in the diet. When our calcium needs are high, our body can generally increase its absorption of calcium from the small intestine. Although older adults have a high need for calcium, the ability to absorb calcium diminishes as we age and can be as low as 25%. These variations in bioavailability and absorption capacity were taken into account when calcium recommendations were determined.

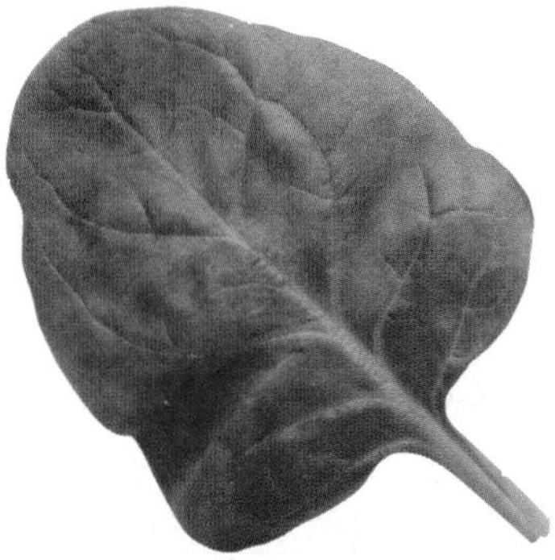

Although spinach contains high levels of calcium, binding factors in the plant prevent much of its absorption.

The bioavailability of calcium also depends on how much calcium we consume throughout the day or at any one time. When our diet is generally high in calcium, absorption of calcium is reduced. In addition, our body cannot absorb more than 500 mg of calcium at any one time, and as the amount of calcium in a single meal or supplement increases up, the fraction that we absorb decreases down. This explains why it is critical to consume calcium-rich foods throughout the day rather than relying on a single, high-dose supplement. Conversely, when dietary intake of calcium is low, the absorption of calcium is increased.

Dietary factors can also affect our absorption of calcium. Binding factors, such as phytates and oxalates, occur naturally in some calcium-rich seeds, nuts, grains, and vegetables, such as spinach and swiss chard. Such factors bind to the calcium in these foods and prevent its absorption from the small intestine. Additionally, consuming calcium with iron, zinc, magnesium, or phosphorus can interfere with the absorption and utilization of all these minerals. Despite these potential interactions, the Institute of Medicine has concluded that there is not sufficient evidence to suggest that these interactions cause deficiencies of calcium or other minerals in healthy individuals.[5]

Finally, because vitamin D is necessary for the absorption of calcium, a lack of vitamin D severely limits the bioavailability of calcium. We'll discuss this and other contributions of vitamin D to bone health shortly.

bioavailability The degree to which our body can absorb and utilize any given nutrient.

Foods Rich in Calcium: Dairy, Greens, and More

Dairy products are among the most common sources of calcium in the U.S. diet. Skim milk, low-fat cheeses, and nonfat yogurt are nutritious sources of calcium **(Figure 9.6)**.

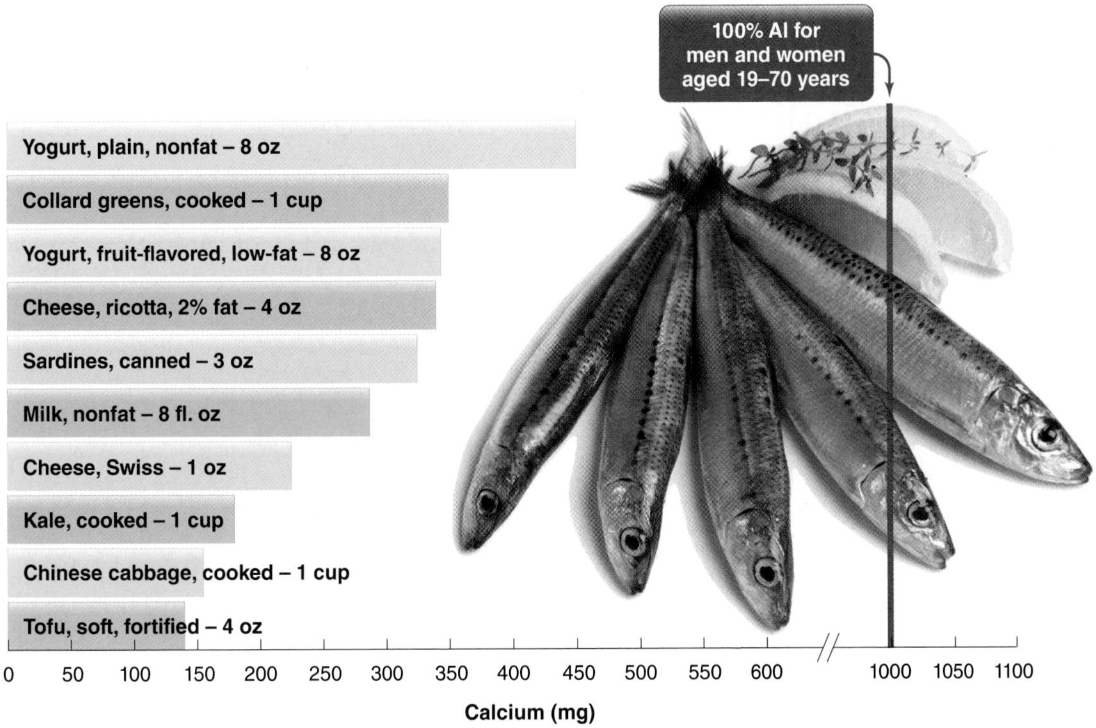

Figure 9.6 Common food sources of calcium. The AI for adult men and women aged 19 to 50 years is 1,000 mg of calcium per day. For men and women older than 70 years of age, the AI increases to 1,200 mg of calcium per day.

Data from U.S. Department of Agriculture, Agricultural Research Service. 2011. USDA Nutrient Database for Standard Reference, Release 23. Nutrient Data Laboratory Home Page. www.ars.usda.gov/ba/bhnrc/ndl.

Ice cream, regular cheese, and whole milk also contain a relatively high amount of calcium, but these foods should be eaten in moderation because of their high fat and energy content. Cottage cheese is one dairy product that is a relatively poor source of calcium, as the processing of this food removes a great deal of the calcium. One cup of low-fat cottage cheese contains approximately 150 mg of calcium, while the same serving of low-fat milk contains almost 300 mg. However calcium-fortified cottage cheese contains 400 mg of calcium.

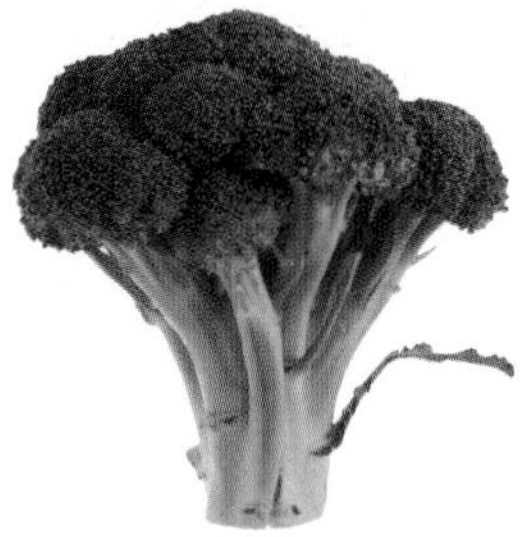

Other good sources of calcium are green leafy vegetables, such as kale, collard greens, turnip greens, broccoli, cauliflower, green cabbage, brussels sprouts, and Chinese cabbage (bok choy). The bioavailability of the calcium in these vegetables is relatively high compared to spinach, as these vegetables contain low levels of oxalates. Many packaged foods are now available fortified with calcium. For example, you can buy calcium-fortified orange juice, soy milk, rice milk, and tofu processed with calcium. Some dairies have even boosted the amount of calcium in their brand of milk!

Figure 9.7 illustrates serving sizes of various calcium-rich foods that contain the same amount of calcium as one glass (8 fl. oz) of skim milk. As you can see from this figure, a wide variety of foods can be consumed each day to contribute to an adequate calcium intake. When you are selecting foods that are good sources of calcium, it is important to remember that we do not absorb 100% of the calcium contained in foods.[6,7] For example, although a serving of milk contains approximately 300 mg of calcium, our body does not actually absorb this entire amount. To learn more about how calcium absorption rates vary for select foods, see the Nutrition Label Activity (page 306).

In general, meats and fish are not good sources of calcium. An exception is canned fish with bones (for example, sardines or salmon),

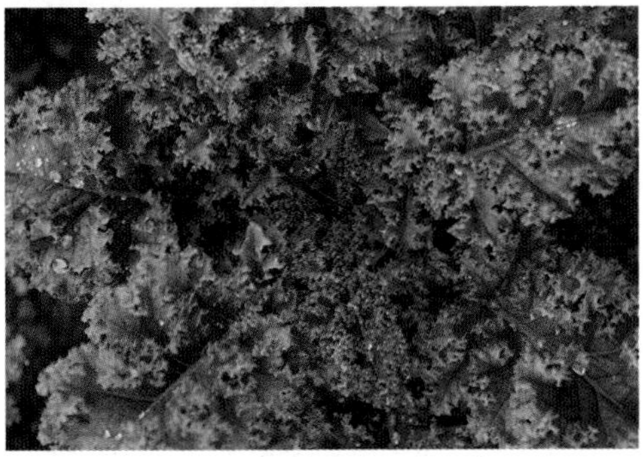

Kale is a good source of calcium.

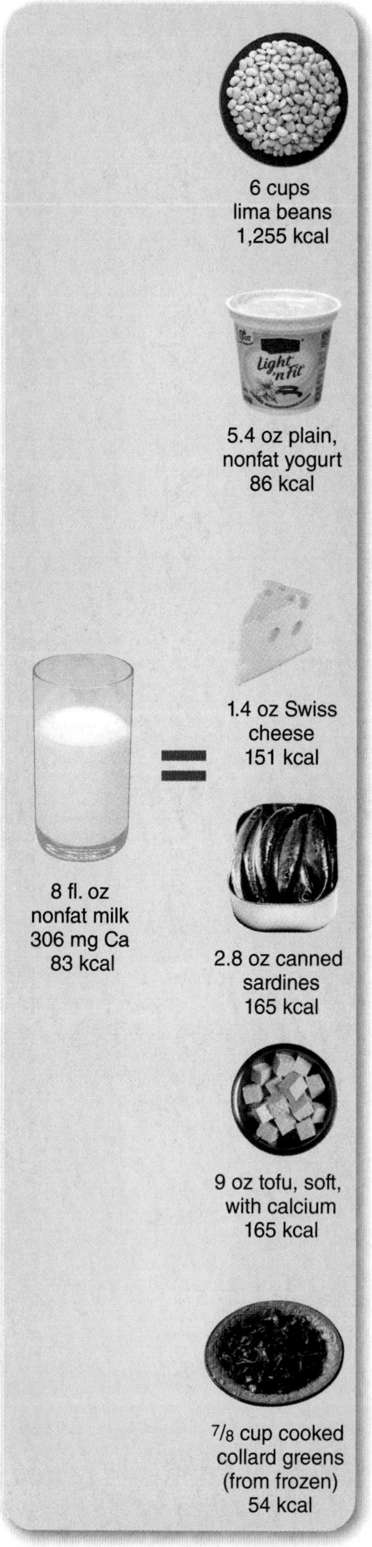

Figure 9.7 Serving sizes and energy content of various foods that contain the same amount of calcium as an 8-fl. oz glass of skim milk.

hypercalcemia A condition marked by an abnormally high concentration of calcium in the blood.

QUICK TIPS

Capitalizing on Calcium

- ✓ At the grocery store, stock up on calcium-fortified juice, soy milk, and rice milk. Look for single-serving portable "juice boxes" with calcium-fortified juice, milk, or chocolate milk.
- ✓ Purchase breakfast cereals and breads that are fortified with calcium.
- ✓ For quick snacks, purchase single-serving cups of yogurt, individually wrapped "cheese sticks," or calcium-fortified protein bars.
- ✓ Keep on hand shredded parmesan or any other hard cheese, and sprinkle it on hot soups, chili, salads, pasta, and other dishes.
- ✓ In any recipe, replace sour cream or mayonnaise with nonfat plain yogurt.
- ✓ Add nonfat dry milk powder to hot cereals, soups, chili, recipes for baked goods, coffee, and hot cocoa. One-third of a cup of nonfat dry milk powder provides the same amount of calcium as a whole cup of nonfat milk.
- ✓ Make a yogurt smoothie by blending nonfat plain or flavored yogurt with fresh or frozen fruit.
- ✓ At your favorite cafe, instead of black coffee, order a skim milk latte. Instead of black tea, order a cup of chai—spiced Indian tea brewed with milk.
- ✓ At home, brew a cup of strong coffee; then add half a cup of warm milk for a café au lait.
- ✓ When eating out, order skim milk instead of a soft drink with your meal.
- ✓ If you do not consume enough dietary calcium, consider taking a calcium supplement. Refer to the ***In Depth*** on osteoporosis following this chapter to learn how to choose a calcium supplement that is right for you.

providing you eat the bones. Fruits (except dried figs) and nonfortified grain products are also poor sources of calcium.

Although many foods in the U.S. diet are good sources of calcium, many Americans do not have adequate intakes because they consume very few dairy-based foods and calcium-rich vegetables. At particular risk are women and young girls. For example, a large national survey conducted by the U.S. Department of Agriculture found that teenage girls consume less than 60% of the recommended amount of calcium.[1]

A variety of quick, simple tools are available on the Internet to help you determine your daily calcium intake. Most of these tools are designed to provide you with an estimated calcium intake score based on the types and amounts of calcium-rich foods you consume. See the Web Resources at the end of this chapter. In addition, following the tips shown above can add more calcium to your bone bank.

As you can see, it's easy to increase your calcium intake by making smart menu choices throughout the day. Eating Right All Day (page 301) shows menu choices high in calcium. Notice that these are also low in fat and Calories.

What Happens If We Consume Too Much Calcium?

In general, consuming too much calcium from foods does not lead to significant toxicity symptoms in healthy individuals. Much of the excess calcium we consume is excreted in the feces. However, an excessive intake of calcium from supplements can lead to health problems.[8] One concern with consuming too much calcium is that it can lead to various mineral imbalances because, as we mentioned earlier, calcium interferes with the absorption of other minerals, including iron, zinc, and magnesium. In some people, the formation of kidney stones is associated with high intakes of calcium, oxalates, protein, and vegetable fiber.[9] However, more studies need to be done to determine whether high intakes of calcium actually cause kidney stones.

Various diseases and metabolic disorders can alter our ability to regulate blood calcium. **Hypercalcemia** is a condition in which our blood calcium levels reach abnormally high concentrations. Hypercalcemia can be caused by cancer and by the

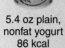

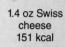

overproduction of parathyroid hormone (PTH). As we noted earlier, PTH stimulates osteoclasts to break down bone and release more calcium into the bloodstream. Symptoms of hypercalcemia include fatigue, loss of appetite, constipation, and mental confusion, and it can lead to coma and possibly death. Hypercalcemia can also result in an accumulation of calcium deposits in the soft tissues, such as the liver and kidneys, causing failure of these organs.

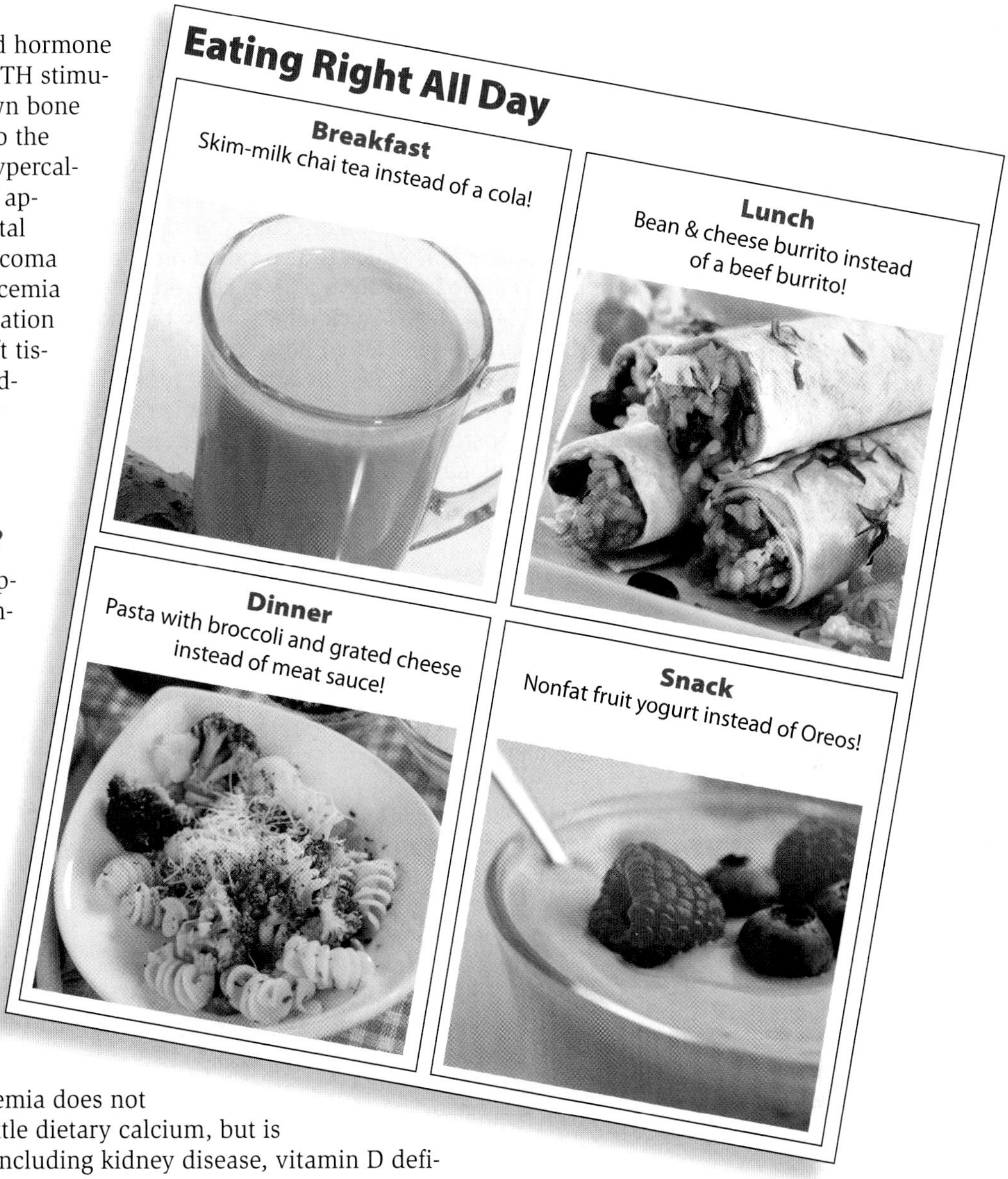

Eating Right All Day
Breakfast
Skim-milk chai tea instead of a cola!
Lunch
Bean & cheese burrito instead of a beef burrito!
Dinner
Pasta with broccoli and grated cheese instead of meat sauce!
Snack
Nonfat fruit yogurt instead of Oreos!

What Happens If We Don't Consume Enough Calcium?

There are no short-term symptoms associated with consuming too little calcium. Even when we do not consume enough dietary calcium, our body continues to tightly regulate blood calcium levels by taking the calcium from bone. A long-term repercussion of inadequate calcium intake is osteoporosis. This disease is discussed ***In Depth*** immediately following this chapter.

Hypocalcemia is an abnormally low level of calcium in the blood. Hypocalcemia does not result from consuming too little dietary calcium, but is caused by various diseases, including kidney disease, vitamin D deficiency, and diseases that inhibit the production of PTH. Symptoms of hypocalcemia include muscle spasms and convulsions.

RECAP **Calcium is the most abundant mineral in the human body and a significant component of our bones. Calcium is necessary for normal nerve and muscle function. Blood calcium is maintained within a very narrow range, and bone calcium is used to maintain normal blood calcium if dietary intake is inadequate. The AI for calcium is highest for pre-teens and teens. Dairy products, canned fish with bones, and some green leafy vegetables are good sources of calcium. The most common long-term effect of inadequate calcium consumption is osteoporosis.**

Vitamin D

Vitamin D is like other fat-soluble vitamins in that we store excess amounts in our liver and adipose tissue. But vitamin D is different from other nutrients in two ways. First, vitamin D does not always need to come from the diet. This is because our body can synthesize vitamin D using energy from exposure to sunlight. However, when we do not get enough sunlight, we must consume vitamin D in our diet. Second, in addition to being a nutrient, vitamin D is considered a *hormone* because it is made in one part of the body, yet it regulates various activities in other parts of the body.

hypocalcemia A condition characterized by an abnormally low concentration of calcium in the blood.

Figure 9.8 illustrates how our body makes vitamin D by converting a cholesterol compound in our skin to the active form of vitamin D that we need to function properly. When the ultraviolet rays of the sun hit our skin, they react with 7-dehydrocholesterol. This cholesterol compound is converted into a precursor of vitamin D, cholecalciferol, which is also called provitamin D_3. This inactive form is then converted to calcidiol in the liver. Calcidiol travels to the kidneys, where it is converted into **calcitriol,** which is considered the primary active form of vitamin D in our body. Calcitriol then circulates to various parts of the body, performing its many functions.

Functions of Vitamin D

As discussed on page 296, vitamin D, PTH, and calcitonin all work together continuously to regulate blood calcium levels, which in turn maintains bone health. They do this by regulating the absorption of calcium and phosphorus from the small intestine, causing more to be absorbed when our needs for them are higher and less when our needs are lower. They also decrease or increase blood calcium levels by signaling the kidneys to excrete more or less calcium in our urine. Finally, vitamin D works with PTH to stimulate osteoclasts to break down bone when calcium is needed elsewhere in the body.

Vitamin D is also necessary for the normal calcification of bone; this means it assists the process by which minerals, such as calcium and phosphorus, are crystallized. Vitamin D may also play a role in decreasing the formation of some cancerous tumors, as it can prevent certain types of cells from growing out of control. Like vitamin A, vitamin D appears to play a role in cell differentiation in various tissues.

How Much Vitamin D Should We Consume?

As for calcium, there is no RDA for vitamin D. The AI is based on the assumption that an individual does not get adequate sun exposure (see Table 9.2). If your exposure to the sun is adequate, then you do not need to consume any vitamin D in your diet. But how do you know whether you are getting enough sun?

Of the many factors that affect your ability to synthesize vitamin D from sunlight, latitude and time of year are the most significant (**Table 9.3**). Individuals living in very sunny climates relatively close to the equator, such as the southern United States and Mexico, may synthesize enough vitamin D from the sun to meet their needs throughout the year—as long as they spend time outdoors. However, vitamin D synthesis from the sun is not possible during most of the winter months for people living in places located at a latitude of more than 40°N or more than 40°S. This is because at these latitudes in winter the sun never rises high enough in the sky to provide the direct sunlight needed. The 40°N latitude runs like a belt across the United States from northern Pennsylvania in the east to northern California in the west (**Figure 9.9**). In addition, entire countries, such as Canada and the United Kingdom, are affected, as are

HOT TOPIC

Can Eating Dairy Foods Help You Lose Weight?

A 2004 research study suggested that a weight-loss diet high in calcium-rich foods may help people lose more weight than if they reduce their energy intake but do not consume enough dietary calcium.[10] This research led to a major advertising campaign by the dairy industry, called the "3-A-Day" campaign. This campaign encourages people who want to lose weight to eat at least 3 servings of dairy foods per day, as study participants who ate calcium-rich foods experienced significantly more weight loss than those who consumed calcium supplements. Interestingly, a 2005 study failed to replicate these findings.[11]

Now the United States Department of Agriculture is conducting its own research into this topic. The study will attempt to determine whether eating various amounts of low-fat dairy foods as part of daily meals and snacks can enhance weight and fat loss in obese adults.[12] We may not know the results of this study for a few more years. Until then, the question of whether eating foods high in dietary calcium can enhance weight loss remains unanswered.

calcitriol The primary active form of vitamin D in the body.

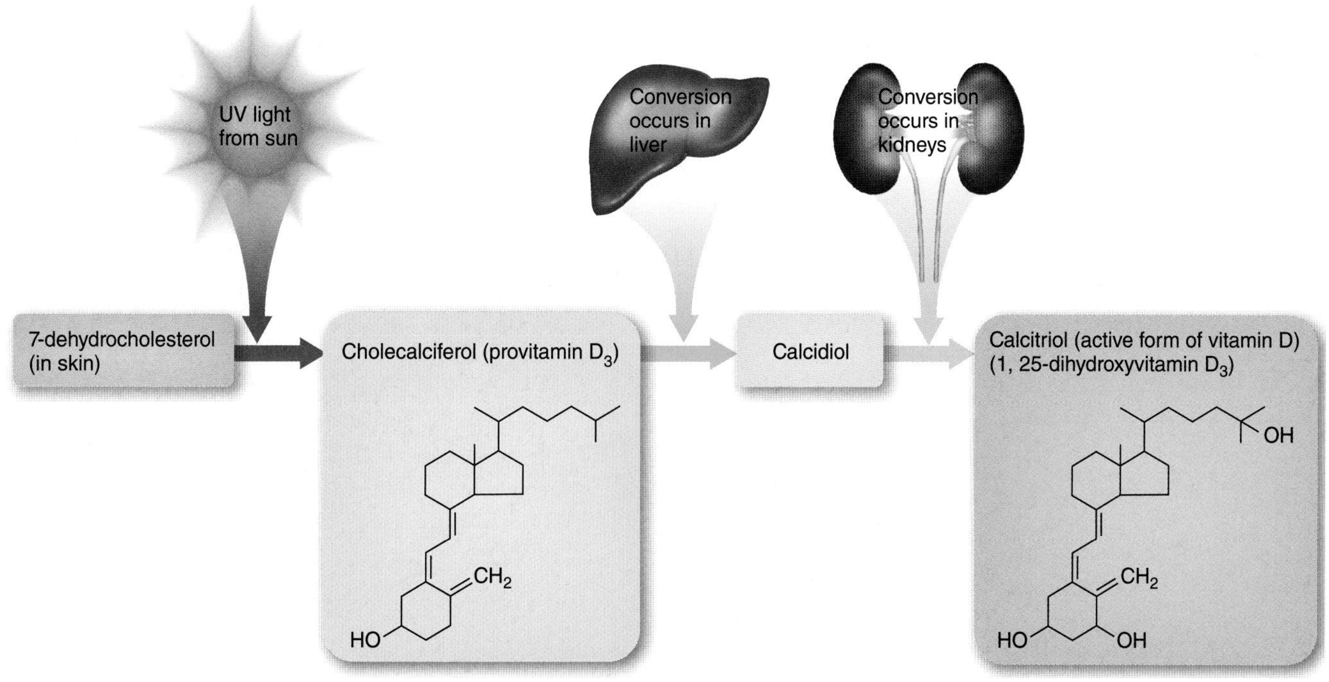

Figure 9.8 The process of converting sunlight into vitamin D in our skin. When the ultraviolet rays of the sun hit our skin, they react with 7-dehydrocholesterol. This compound is converted to cholecalciferol, an inactive form of vitamin D also called provitamin D_3. Cholecalciferol is then converted to calcidiol in the liver. Calcidiol travels to the kidneys, where it is converted into calcitriol, which is considered the primary active form of vitamin D in our body.

countries in the far southern hemisphere. Thus, many people around the world need to consume vitamin D in their diets, particularly during the winter months.

Other factors influencing vitamin D synthesis are time of day, skin color, age, and obesity status:

- More vitamin D can be synthesized when the sun's rays are strongest, generally between 9 AM and 3 PM. Vitamin D synthesis is severely limited or may be nonexistent on overcast days.
- Darker skin contains more melanin pigment, which reduces the penetration of sunlight. Thus, people with dark skin have a more difficult time synthesizing vitamin D from the sun than do light-skinned people.

TABLE 9.3 Factors Affecting Sunlight-Mediated Synthesis of Vitamin D in the Skin

Factors That Enhance Synthesis of Vitamin D	Factors That Inhibit Synthesis of Vitamin D
Season—Most vitamin D is produced during summer months, particularly June and July	Season—Exposure in winter months (October through February) results in little or no vitamin D production
Latitude—Locations closer to the equator get more sunlight throughout the year	Latitude—Locations that are more north of 40°N and more south than 40°S get inadequate sun
Time of day—Generally, between the hours of 9:00 AM and 3:00 PM (dependent on latitude and time of year)	Time of day—Early morning, late afternoon, and evening hours
Age—Younger	Age—Older, due to reduced skin thickness with age
Limited or no use of sunscreen	Use of sunscreen with SPF 8 or greater
Sunny weather	Cloudy weather
Exposed skin	Protective clothing
Lighter skin pigmentation	Darker skin pigmentation
	Obesity—May negatively affect metabolism and storage of vitamin D
	Glass and plastics—Windows and other barriers made of glass or plastic (such as Plexiglas) block the sun's rays

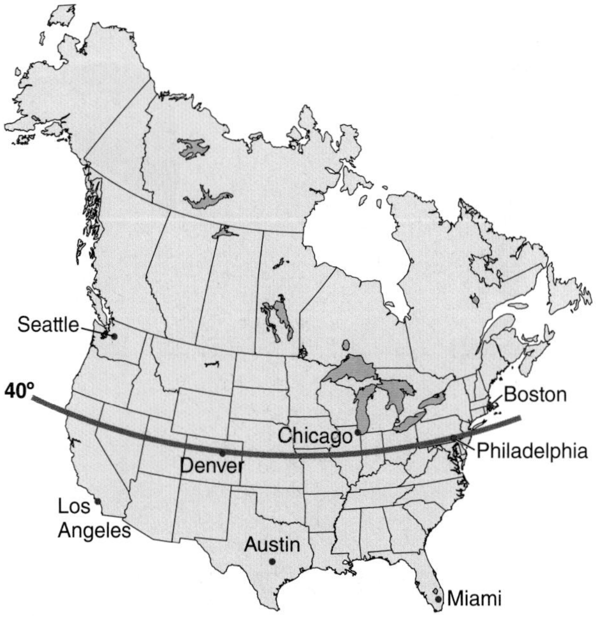

Figure 9.9 This map illustrates the geographical location of 40° latitude in the United States. In southern cities below 40° latitude, such as Los Angeles, Austin, and Miami, the sunlight is strong enough to allow for vitamin D synthesis throughout the year. In northern cities above 40° latitude, such as Seattle, Chicago, and Boston, the sunlight is too weak from about mid-October to mid-March to allow for adequate vitamin D synthesis.

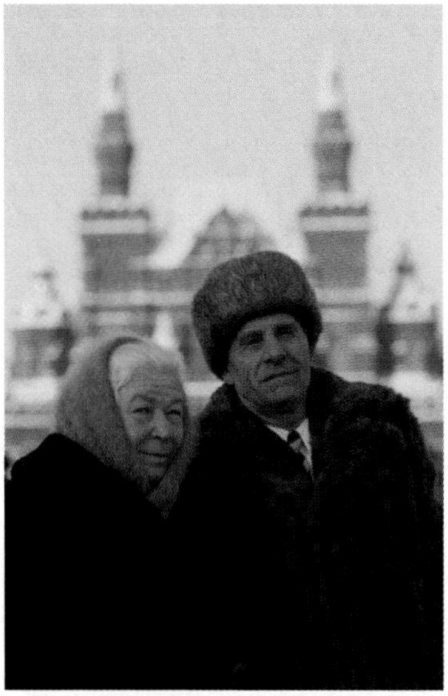

Vitamin D synthesis from the sun is not possible during most of the winter months for people living in high latitudes. Therefore, many people need to consume vitamin D in their diet, particularly during the winter.

- People 65 years of age or older experience a fourfold decrease in their capacity to synthesize vitamin D from the sun.[13,14]
- Obesity is associated with lower levels of circulating vitamin D, possibly because of lower bioavailability of cholecalciferol from adipose tissue, decreased exposure to sunlight due to limited mobility or time spent outdoors with skin exposed, and alterations in vitamin D metabolism in the liver.[15,16]

Wearing protective clothing and sunscreen (with an SPF greater than 8) limits sun exposure, so it is suggested that we expose our hands, face, and arms to the sun two or three times per week for a period of time that is one-third to one-half of the amount needed to get sunburned.[17] This means that, if you normally sunburn in 1 hour, you should expose yourself to the sun for 20 to 30 minutes two or three times per week to synthesize adequate amounts of vitamin D. Again, this guideline does not apply to people living in more northern climates during the winter months; they can get enough vitamin D only by consuming it in their diet.

Recent evidence suggests that the current AI for vitamin D is not sufficient to maintain optimal bone health and reduce the risks for diseases such as cancer; the controversy surrounding the current recommendations for vitamin D are discussed in more detail in the Nutrition Debate at the end of this chapter. What about you? Do you think you're getting enough vitamin D each day? To find out, take the quiz in the What About You? box on page 305.

Vitamin D: Fish, Fortified Foods, Supplements, or Sunlight

There are many forms of vitamin D, but only two can be converted into calcitriol. Vitamin D_2, also called *ergocalciferol,* is found exclusively in plant foods, whereas vitamin D_3, or *cholecalciferol,* is found in animal foods. Recall that cholecalciferol is also the form of vitamin D we synthesize from the sun.

Most foods naturally contain very little vitamin D. The few exceptions are cod liver oil and fatty fish (such as salmon, mackerel, and sardines), foods that few Americans consume in adequate amounts. Eggs, butter, some margarines, and liver also provide small amounts of vitamin D, but we would have to eat very large amounts to consume enough vitamin D.

What About You?

Are You Getting Enough Vitamin D?

After reading this section, you may wonder whether you're getting enough vitamin D to keep your tissues healthy and strong. Take the following simple quiz to find out. For each question, circle either Yes or No:

I live south of 40° latitude (see Figure 9.10) and expose my bare arms and face to sunlight (without sunscreen) for at least a few minutes two or three times per week all year.	Yes/No
I consume a multivitamin supplement or vitamin D supplement that provides at least 5 μg or 200 IU per day.	Yes/No
I consume a diet high in fatty fish, fortified milk, and/or fortified cereals that provides at least 5 μg or 200 IU per day.	Yes/No

If you answered No to all three of these questions, you are at high risk for vitamin D deficiency. You are probably getting enough vitamin D if you answered Yes to at least one of them. However, notice that, if you rely on sun exposure for your vitamin D, you must make sure that you expose your bare skin to sunlight for an adequate length of time. What's adequate varies for each person: the darker your skin tone, the more time you need in the sun. A general guideline is to expose your skin for a period of time that is one-third to one-half the amount of time in which you would get sunburned. This means that, if you normally sunburn in 1 hour, you should get 30 minutes of sun two or three times a week. Expose your skin when the sun is high in the sky (generally between the hours of 9 AM and 3 PM). Put on sunscreen only *after* your skin has had its daily dose of sunlight.[18–20]

Remember: if you live in the northern United States or Canada, you cannot get adequate sun exposure to synthesize vitamin D from approximately October through February, no matter how long you expose your bare skin to the sun. So, if you are not regularly consuming fortified foods, fatty fish, or cod liver oil, you need to supplement vitamin D during those months.

Thus, the primary source of vitamin D in the diet is from fortified foods such as milk **(Figure 9.10)**. In the United States, milk is fortified with 10 μg of vitamin D per quart. Because earlier studies examining the actual vitamin D content of fortified milk found that the amount of vitamin D varied widely, the USDA now monitors dairies to make sure they meet the mandated vitamin D fortification guidelines.

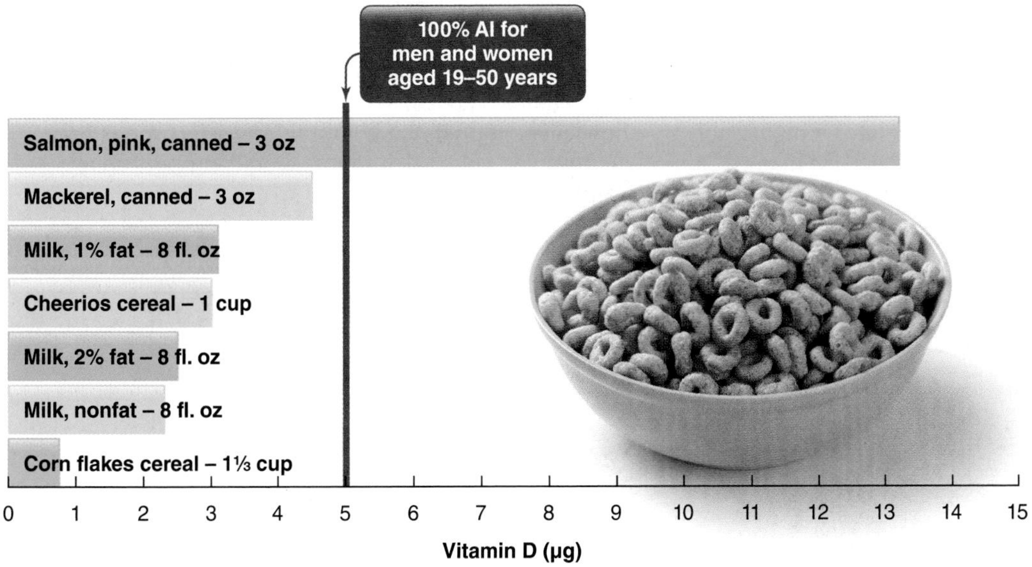

Figure 9.10 Common food sources of vitamin D. For men and women aged 19 to 50 years. The previous AI for vitamin D was 5 μg per day, as reflected in this graph. See Table 9.2 for the 2011 vitamin D recommendations.

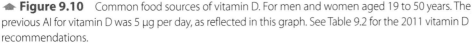

Data from U.S. Department of Agriculture, Agricultural Research Service. 2009. USDA Nutrient Database for Standard Reference, Release 22. Nutrient Data Laboratory Home Page. www.ars.usda.gov/ba/bhnrc/ndl.

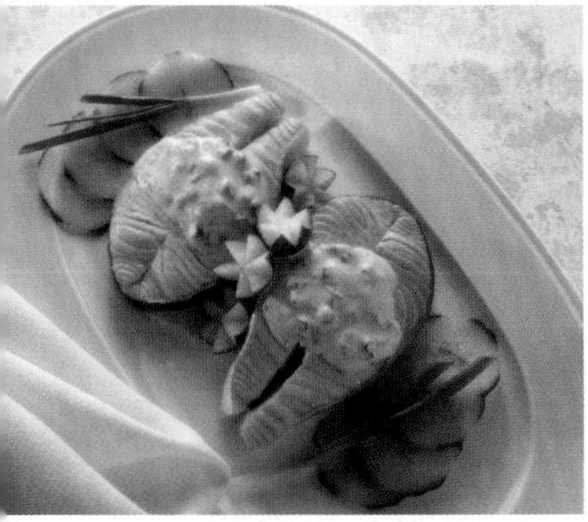

Fatty fish contain vitamin D.

Certain fortified cereals, fortified soy and rice milks, and even some brands of fortified orange juice also provide vitamin D. Since plants naturally contain very little vitamin D, vegans need to obtain their vitamin D from these kinds of fortified foods, from sun exposure, or from supplements. When reading the labels of fortified foods and supplements, you will see the amount of vitamin D expressed in units of either μg or IU. For conversion purposes, 1 μg of vitamin D is equal to 40 IU of vitamin D.

What Happens If We Consume Too Much Vitamin D?

We cannot get too much vitamin D from sun exposure, as our skin has the ability to limit its production. As just noted, foods contain little natural vitamin D. Thus, the only way we can consume too much vitamin D is through supplementation.

NUTRITION LABEL ACTIVITY

How Much Calcium Am I Really Consuming?

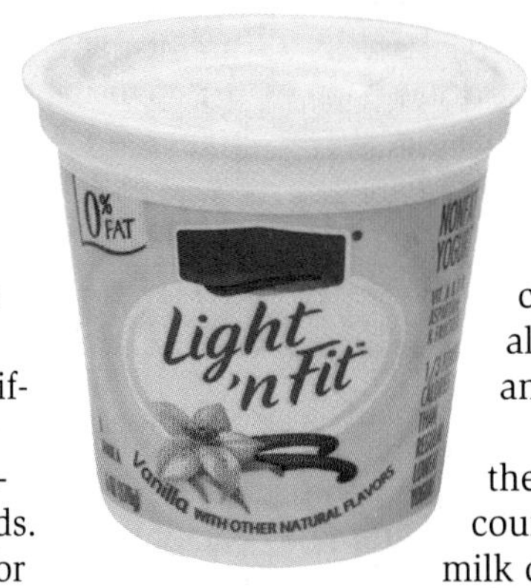

As you have learned in this chapter, we do not absorb 100% of the calcium contained in foods. This is particularly true for individuals who eat lots of foods high in fiber, oxalates, and phytates, such as whole grains and certain vegetables. So if you want to design an eating plan that contains adequate calcium, it's important to understand how the rate of calcium absorption differs for the foods you include.

Unfortunately, the absorption rate of calcium has not been determined for most foods. However, estimates have been established for some common foods that are considered good sources of calcium. The following table shows some of these foods, their calcium content per serving, the calcium absorption rate, and the estimated amount of calcium absorbed from each food.

As you can see from this table, many dairy products have a similar calcium absorption rate, just over 30%. Interestingly, many green leafy vegetables have a higher absorption rate of around 60%; however, because many times a serving of these foods contains less calcium than dairy foods, you would have to eat more vegetables to get the same calcium as you would from a standard serving of dairy foods. Note the relatively low calcium absorption rate for spinach, even though it contains a relatively high amount of calcium. This is due to the high levels of oxalates in spinach, which bind with calcium and reduce its bioavailability.

Remember that the DRIs for calcium take these differences in absorption rate into account. Thus, the 300 mg of calcium in a glass of milk counts as 300 mg toward your daily calcium goal. In general, you can trust that dairy products such as milk and yogurt (but not cottage cheese) are good, absorbable sources of calcium, as are most dark green leafy vegetables. Other dietary sources of calcium with good absorption rates are calcium-fortified orange juice, soy milk and rice milk, tofu processed with calcium, and fortified breakfast cereals, such as Total.[6] Armed with this knowledge, you will be better able to select foods that can optimize your calcium intake and support bone health.

Food	Serving Size	Calcium per Serving (mg)*	Absorption Rate (%)†	Estimated Amount of Calcium Absorbed (mg)
Yogurt, plain skim milk	8 fl. oz	452	32	145
Milk, skim	1 cup	306	32	98
Milk, 2%	1 cup	285	32	91
Kale, frozen, cooked	1 cup	179	59	106
Turnip greens, boiled	1 cup	197	52	103
Broccoli, frozen, chopped, cooked	1 cup	61	61	37
Cauliflower, boiled	1 cup	20	69	14
Spinach, frozen, cooked	1 cup	291	5	14

*Data from U.S. Department of Agriculture, Agricultural Research Service. 2009. USDA National Nutrient Database for Standard Reference, Release 22. www.ars.usda.gov/ba/bhnrc/ndl.
†Data from Weaver, C. M., W. R. Proulx, and R. Heaney. 1999. Choices for achieving adequate dietary calcium with a vegetarian diet. *Am. J. Clin. Nutr.* 70(suppl.):543S–548S; Weaver, C. M., and K. L. Plawecki. 1994. Dietary calcium: adequacy of a vegetarian diet. *Am. J. Clin. Nutr.* 59(suppl.):1238S–1241S.

Consuming too much vitamin D causes hypercalcemia, or high blood calcium concentrations. As discussed in the section on calcium, symptoms of hypercalcemia include weakness, loss of appetite, constipation, mental confusion, vomiting, excessive urine output, and extreme thirst. Hypercalcemia also leads to the formation of calcium deposits in soft tissues, such as the kidneys, liver, and heart. In addition, toxic levels of vitamin D lead to increased bone loss because calcium is then pulled from the bones and excreted more readily from the kidneys.

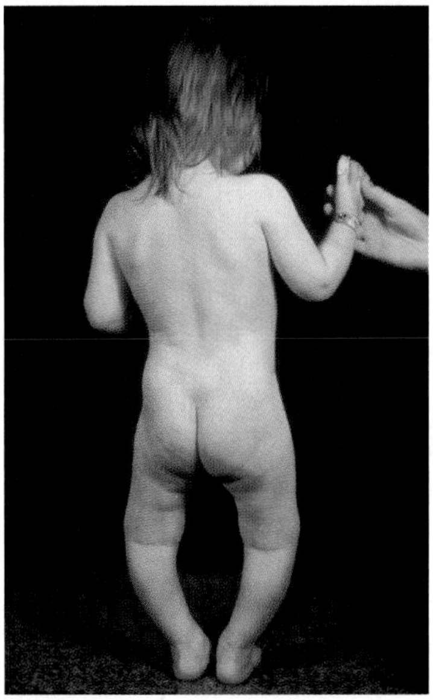

Figure 9.11 A vitamin D deficiency causes a bone-deforming disease in children called rickets.

What Happens If We Don't Consume Enough Vitamin D?

The primary deficiency associated with inadequate vitamin D is loss of bone mass. In fact, when vitamin D levels are inadequate, our small intestine can absorb only 10–15% of the calcium we consume. Vitamin D deficiencies occur most often in individuals who have diseases that cause intestinal malabsorption of fat and thus the fat-soluble vitamins. People with liver disease, kidney disease, Crohn's disease, celiac disease, cystic fibrosis, or Whipple's disease may suffer from vitamin D deficiency and require supplements.

Vitamin D–deficiency disease in children, called **rickets,** is caused by inadequate mineralization or demineralization of the skeleton. The classic sign of rickets is deformity of the skeleton, such as bowed legs and knocked knees (**Figure 9.11**). However, severe cases can be fatal. Rickets is not common in the United States because of the fortification of milk products with vitamin D, but children with illnesses that cause fat malabsorption or who drink no milk and get limited sun exposure are at increased risk. A recent review of reported cases of rickets among children in the United States found that approximately 83% were African American and that 95% had been breast-fed.[21,22] Breast milk contains very little vitamin D, and fewer than 5% of the breast-fed children were reported to have received vitamin D supplementation. Thus, rickets appears to occur more commonly in children with darker skin (their need for adequate sun exposure is higher than that of light-skinned children) and in breast-fed children who do not receive adequate vitamin D supplementation. In addition, rickets is still a significant nutritional problem for children outside of the United States.

Vitamin D–deficiency disease in adults is called **osteomalacia,** a term meaning "soft bones." With osteomalacia, bones become weak and prone to fractures. Osteoporosis, discussed ***In Depth*** on pages 318–325, can also result from a vitamin D deficiency.

Vitamin D deficiencies have recently been found to be more common among American adults than previously thought. This may be partly due to jobs and lifestyle choices that keep people indoors for most of the day. Not surprisingly, the population at greatest risk is older institutionalized individuals who get little or no sun exposure.

rickets A vitamin D–deficiency disease in children. Signs include deformities of the skeleton, such as bowed legs and knocked knees. Severe rickets can be fatal.

osteomalacia A vitamin D–deficiency disease in adults, in which bones become weak and prone to fractures.

NUTRI-CASE THEO

"The health center here on campus is running a study on vitamin D levels among students, and the instructor in my nutrition class invited everybody to participate. I don't think I need to be worried about it, though, 'cause I exercise outdoors a lot—at least, whenever Wisconsin weather allows it! It's true I don't drink much milk, and I hate fish, but otherwise I eat right, and besides, I'm a guy, so I don't have to worry about my bone density."

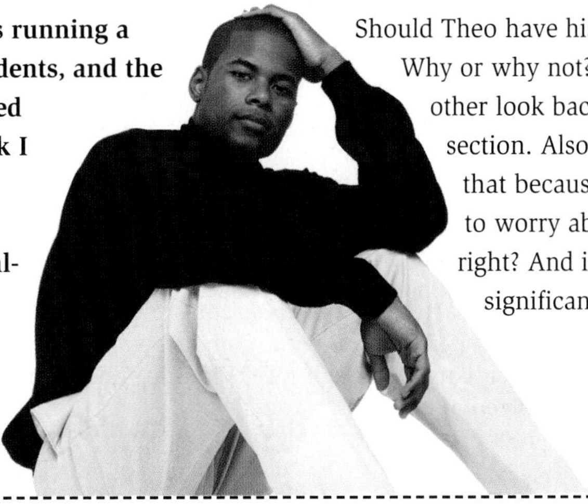

Should Theo have his vitamin D levels checked? Why or why not? Before you answer, take another look back at the information in this section. Also, consider Theo's assertion that because he is male he doesn't have to worry about his bone density. Is he right? And is calcium regulation the only significant role of vitamin D?

Various medications can also alter the metabolism and activity of vitamin D. For instance, glucocorticoids, which are medications used to reduce inflammation, can cause bone loss by inhibiting our ability to absorb calcium through the actions of vitamin D. Antiseizure medications, such as phenobarbital and Dilantin, alter vitamin D metabolism. Thus, people who are taking such medications may need to increase their vitamin D intake.

RECAP **Vitamin D is a fat-soluble vitamin and a hormone. It can be made in the skin using energy from sunlight. Vitamin D regulates blood calcium levels and maintains bone health. Foods contain little vitamin D, with fortified milk being the primary source. Vitamin D toxicity causes hypercalcemia. Vitamin D deficiency can result in osteoporosis; rickets is vitamin D deficiency in children, whereas osteomalacia is vitamin D deficiency in adults.**

Vitamin K

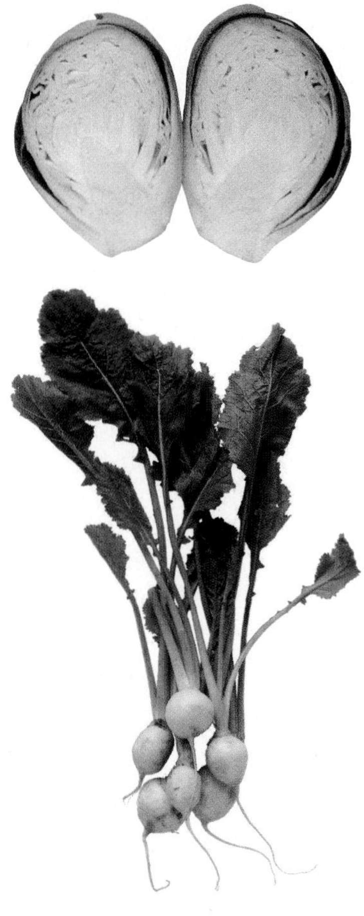

▲ Green leafy vegetables, including brussels sprouts and turnip greens, are good sources of vitamin K.

Vitamin K, a fat-soluble vitamin stored primarily in the liver, is actually a family of compounds known as quinones. *Phylloquinone,* which is the primary dietary form of vitamin K, is also the form found in plants; *menaquinone* is the animal form of vitamin K produced by bacteria in the large intestine.

The primary function of vitamin K is to assist in the production of *prothrombin,* a protein that plays a critical role in blood clotting. This is discussed in more detail in Chapter 10. Vitamin K also assists in the production of *osteocalcin,* a protein associated with bone turnover.

We can obtain vitamin K from our diet, and we absorb the vitamin K produced by bacteria in our large intestine. These two sources usually provide adequate amounts of this nutrient to maintain health, and there is no RDA or UL for vitamin K. AI recommendations are listed in Table 9.2.

Only a few foods contribute substantially to our dietary intake of vitamin K. Green leafy vegetables, including kale, spinach, collard greens, turnip greens, and lettuce, are good sources, as are broccoli, brussels sprouts, and cabbage. Vegetable oils, such as soybean oil and canola oil, are also good sources. **Figure 9.12** identifies the amount of vitamin K in micrograms per serving for these foods.

Based on our current knowledge, for healthy individuals there appear to be no side effects associated with consuming large amounts of vitamin K.[23] This appears to be true for both supplements and food sources.

Vitamin K deficiency is associated with a reduced ability to form blood clots, leading to excessive bleeding; however, primary vitamin K deficiency is rare in humans. People with diseases that cause malabsorption of fat, such as celiac disease, Crohn's disease, and cystic fibrosis, can suffer secondarily from a deficiency of vitamin K. Newborns are typically given an injection of vitamin K at birth, as they lack the intestinal bacteria necessary to produce this nutrient.

The impact of vitamin K deficiency on bone health is controversial. A recent study of vitamin K intake and a risk for hip fractures found that women who consumed the least amount of vitamin K had a higher risk for bone fractures than women who consumed relatively more vitamin K. Despite the results of this study, there is not enough scientific evidence to support the contention that vitamin K deficiency leads to osteoporosis.[23] In fact, there is no significant impact on overall bone density in people who take anticoagulant medications that result in a relative state of vitamin K deficiency.

RECAP **Vitamin K is a fat-soluble vitamin and coenzyme that is important for blood clotting and bone metabolism. We obtain vitamin K largely from bacteria in our large intestine. Green leafy vegetables and vegetable oils contain vitamin K. There are no known toxicity symptoms for vitamin K in healthy individuals. Although rare, Vitamin K deficiency is rare and may lead to excessive bleeding.**

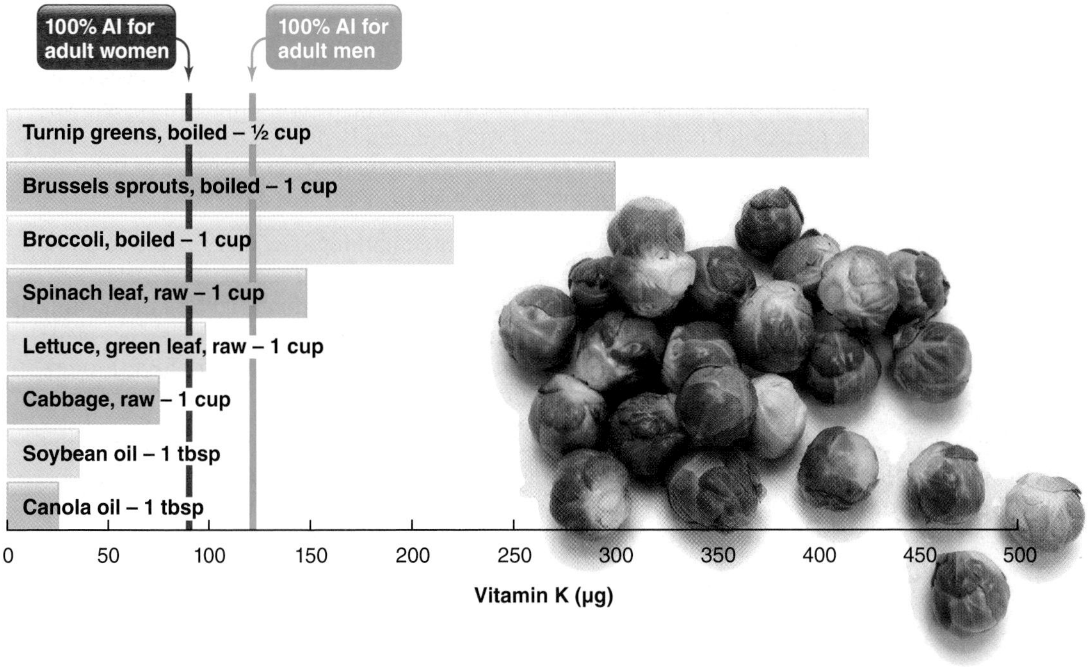

Figure 9.12 Common food sources of vitamin K. The AIs for adult men and women are 120 μg per day and 90 μg per day, respectively.

Data from U.S. Department of Agriculture, Agricultural Research Service. 2009. USDA Nutrient Database for Standard Reference, Release 22. Nutrient Data Laboratory Home Page. www.ars.usda.gov/ba/bhnrc/ndl.

Phosphorus

As discussed in Chapter 7, phosphorus is the major intracellular negatively charged electrolyte. In our body, phosphorus is most commonly found combined with oxygen in the form of phosphate (PO_4^{3-}). Phosphorus is an essential constituent of all cells and is found in both plants and animals.

Functions of Phosphorus

Phosphorus plays a critical role in bone formation, as it is a part of the mineral complex of bone. As discussed earlier in this chapter, calcium and phosphorus crystallize to form hydroxyapatite crystals, which provide the hardness of bone. About 85% of our body's phosphorus is stored in our bones, with the rest stored in soft tissues, such as muscles and organs.

The role of phosphorus in maintaining proper fluid balance was examined in detail in Chapter 7. Phosphorus also helps activate and deactivate enzymes, and it is a component of lipoproteins, cell membranes, DNA and RNA, and several energy molecules, including adenosine triphosphate (ATP).

How Much Phosphorus Should We Consume?

The details of phosphorus recommendations, food sources, and deficiency and toxicity symptoms were discussed in Chapter 7. The RDA for phosphorus is listed in Table 9.2. In general, phosphorus is widespread in many foods and is found in high amounts in foods that contain protein. Milk, meats, and eggs are good sources. See Figure 7.9 (page 246) for a review of the phosphorus content of various foods.

Phosphorus is also found in many processed foods as a food additive, where it enhances smoothness, binding, and moisture retention. Moreover, in the form of phosphoric acid, it is added to soft drinks to give them a sharper, or more tart, flavor and to slow the growth of molds and bacteria. Our society has increased its consumption

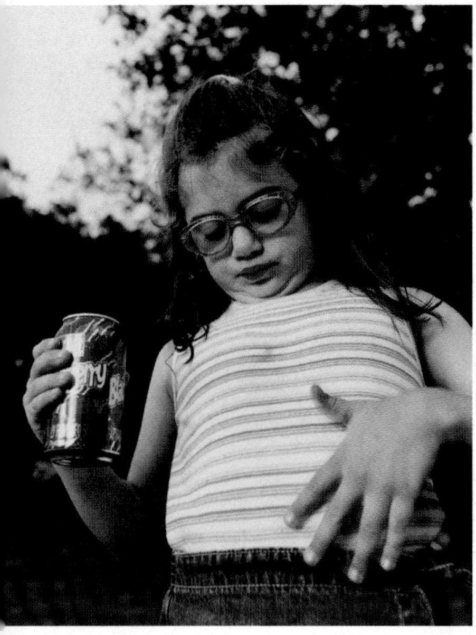

Phosphorus, in the form of phosphoric acid, is a major component of soft drinks.

of processed foods and soft drinks substantially over the past 30 years, resulting in an estimated 10–15% increase in phosphorus consumption.[5]

Nutrition and medical professionals have become increasingly concerned that heavy consumption of soft drinks may be detrimental to bone health. Studies have shown that consuming soft drinks is associated with reduced bone mass or an increased risk for fractures in both youth and adults.[24–26] Researchers have proposed three theories to explain why the consumption of soft drinks may be detrimental to bone health:

- Consuming soft drinks in place of calcium-containing beverages, such as milk, leads to a deficient intake of calcium.
- The phosphoric acid content of soft drinks causes an increased loss of calcium because calcium is drawn from bone into the blood to neutralize the excess acid.
- The caffeine found in many soft drinks causes increased calcium loss through the urine.

A recent study evaluating these factors concluded that the most likely explanation for the link between soft drink consumption and poor bone health is the *milk-displacement effect;* that is, soft drinks take the place of milk in our diet, depriving us of calcium and vitamin D.[27]

What Happens If We Consume Too Much Phosphorus?

As discussed in Chapter 7, people with kidney disease and those who take too many vitamin D supplements or too many phosphorus-containing antacids can suffer from high blood phosphorus levels. Severely high levels of blood phosphorus can cause muscle spasms and convulsions.

What Happens If We Don't Consume Enough Phosphorus?

Phosphorus deficiencies are rare but can occur in people who abuse alcohol, in premature infants, and in elderly people with poor diets. People with vitamin D deficiency, people with hyperparathyroidism (oversecretion of parathyroid hormone), and those who overuse antacids that bind with phosphorus may also have low blood phosphorus levels.

RECAP **Phosphorus is the major negatively charged electrolyte inside of the cell. It helps maintain fluid balance and bone health. It also assists in regulating chemical reactions, and it is a primary component of ATP, DNA, and RNA. Phosphorus is commonly found in high-protein foods. Excess phosphorus can lead to muscle spasms and convulsions, whereas phosphorus deficiencies are rare.**

Magnesium

Magnesium is a major mineral. Our total body magnesium content is approximately 25 g. About 50–60% of our body's magnesium is found in our bones, with the rest located in our soft tissues.

Functions of Magnesium

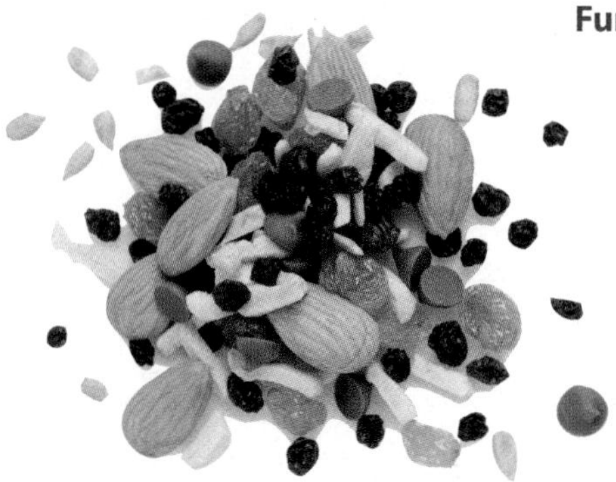

Trail mix with chocolate chips, nuts, and seeds is one common food source of magnesium.

Magnesium is one of the minerals that make up the structure of bone. It is also important in the regulation of bone and mineral status. Specifically, magnesium influences the formation of hydroxyapatite crystals through its regulation of calcium balance and its interactions with vitamin D and parathyroid hormone.

Magnesium is a critical *cofactor* for more than 300 enzyme systems. Recall from Chapter 8 that a cofactor is a compound that is needed for an enzyme to be active. Magnesium is necessary for the production of ATP, and it plays an important role in DNA and protein synthesis and repair. Magnesium supplementation has been shown to improve insulin sensitivity, and there is epidemiological evidence that a high magnesium intake is associated with a decrease in the risk for colorectal cancer.[28,29] Magnesium supports normal vitamin D metabolism and action and is necessary for normal muscle contraction and blood clotting.

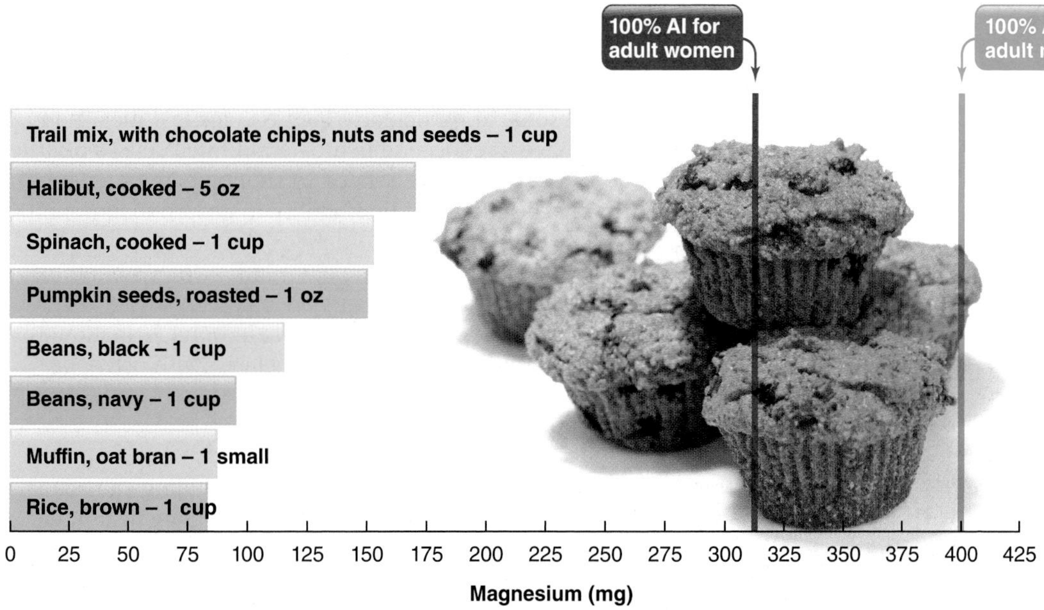

Figure 9.13 Common food sources of magnesium. For adult men 19 to 30 years of age, the RDA for magnesium is 400 mg per day; the RDA increases to 420 mg per day for men 31 years of age and older. For adult women 19 to 30 years of age, the RDA for magnesium is 310 mg per day; this value increases to 320 mg per day for women 31 years of age and older.

Data from U.S. Department of Agriculture, Agricultural Research Service. 2009. USDA Nutrient Database for Standard Reference, Release 22. Nutrient Data Laboratory Home Page. www.ars.usda.gov/ba/bhnrc/ndl.

How Much Magnesium Should We Consume?

As magnesium is found in a wide variety of foods, people who are adequately nourished generally consume enough magnesium in their diet. The RDA for magnesium is identified in Table 9.2. There is no UL for magnesium for food and water; the UL for magnesium from pharmacologic sources is 350 mg per day.

Magnesium is found in green leafy vegetables, such as spinach. It is also found in whole grains, seeds, and nuts. Other good food sources of magnesium include seafood, beans, and some dairy products. Refined and processed foods are low in magnesium. **Figure 9.13** shows many foods that are good sources of magnesium.

The magnesium content of drinking water varies considerably. The "harder" the water, the higher its content of magnesium. This variability makes it impossible to estimate how much our drinking water may contribute to the magnesium content of our diet.

The ability of the small intestine to absorb magnesium is reduced when one consumes a diet that is extremely high in fiber and phytates, because these substances bind with magnesium. Even though seeds and nuts are relatively high in fiber, they are excellent sources of absorbable magnesium. Overall, our absorption of magnesium should be sufficient if we consume the recommended amount of fiber each day (20–35 g per day). In contrast, higher dietary protein intakes enhance the absorption and retention of magnesium.

What Happens If We Consume Too Much Magnesium?

There are no known toxicity symptoms related to consuming excess magnesium in the diet. The toxicity symptoms that result from pharmacologic overuse of magnesium include diarrhea, nausea, and abdominal cramps. In extreme cases, large doses can result in acid–base imbalances, massive dehydration, cardiac arrest, and death. High blood magnesium levels, or **hypermagnesemia,** occur in individuals with impaired kidney function who consume large amounts of nondietary magnesium, such as antacids. Side effects include the impairment of nerve, muscle, and heart function.

hypermagnesemia A condition marked by an abnormally high concentration of magnesium in the blood.

What Happens If We Don't Consume Enough Magnesium?

Hypomagnesemia, or low blood magnesium, results from magnesium deficiency. This condition may develop secondary to kidney disease, chronic diarrhea, or chronic alcohol abuse. Elderly people seem to be at particularly high risk for low dietary intakes of magnesium because they have a reduced appetite and blunted senses of taste and smell. In addition, the elderly face challenges related to shopping and preparing meals that contain foods high in magnesium, and their ability to absorb magnesium is reduced.

Low blood calcium levels are a side effect of hypomagnesemia. Other symptoms of magnesium deficiency include muscle cramps, spasms or seizures, nausea, weakness, irritability, and confusion. Considering magnesium's role in bone formation, it is not surprising that long-term magnesium deficiency is associated with osteoporosis. Magnesium deficiency is also associated with many other chronic diseases, including heart disease, high blood pressure, and type 2 diabetes.[5]

RECAP **Magnesium is a major mineral found in fresh foods, including spinach, nuts, seeds, whole grains, and meats. It is important for bone health, energy production, and muscle function. The RDA for magnesium varies with age and gender. Hypermagnesemia can result in diarrhea, muscle cramps, and cardiac arrest. Hypomagnesemia causes hypocalcemia, muscle cramps, spasms, and weakness. Magnesium deficiencies are also associated with osteoporosis, heart disease, high blood pressure, and type 2 diabetes.**

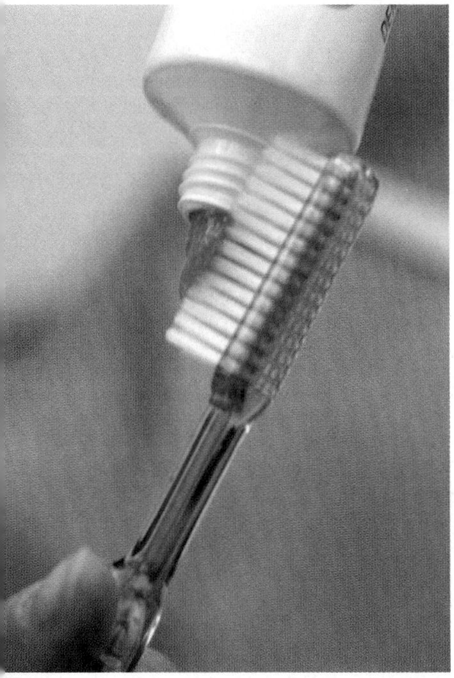

Fluoride is readily available in many communities in the United States through fluoridated water and dental products.

Fluoride

Fluoride. a trace mineral, is the ionic form of the element fluorine. As discussed in Chapter 1, trace minerals are minerals that our body needs in amounts less than 100 mg per day; the amount of trace minerals in our body is less than 5 g. About 99% of the fluoride in our body is stored in our teeth and bones.

Functions of Fluoride

Fluoride assists in the development and maintenance of our teeth and bones. During the development of both our baby and permanent teeth, fluoride combines with calcium and phosphorus to form *fluorohydroxyapatite,* which is more resistant to destruction by acids and bacteria than is hydroxyapatite. Even after all of our permanent teeth are in, treating them with fluoride, whether at the dentist's office or with fluoridated toothpaste, gives them more protection against dental caries (cavities) than teeth that have not been treated. That's because fluoride enhances tooth mineralization, decreases and reverses tooth demineralization, and inhibits the metabolism of the acid-producing bacteria that cause tooth decay.

Fluoride also stimulates new bone growth, and it is being researched as a potential treatment for osteoporosis, both alone and in combination with other medications.[32–34] While early results are promising, more research needs to be conducted to determine if fluoride is an effective treatment for osteoporosis.[30–33]

How Much Fluoride Should We Consume?

Our need for fluoride is relatively small. The AI for fluoride is listed in Table 9.2. The UL is 2.2 mg per day for children aged 4 to 8 years; the UL for everyone older than 8 years of age is 10 mg per day.

hypomagnesemia A condition characterized by an abnormally low concentration of magnesium in the blood.

Fluoride is readily available in many communities in the United States through fluoridated water and dental products. Fluoride is absorbed directly in the mouth into the teeth and gums, and it can be absorbed from the gastrointestinal tract once it is ingested. In the early 1990s, there was considerable concern that our intake of fluoride was too high due to the consumption of fluoridated water and fluoride-containing toothpastes and mouthwashes; it was speculated that this high intake could be contributing to an increased risk for cancer, bone fractures, kidney and other organ damage, infertility, and Alzheimer's disease. After reviewing the potential health hazards of fluoride, the U.S. Department of Health and Human Services found that there is no reliable scientific evidence available to indicate that fluoride increases our risk for these illnesses.[34]

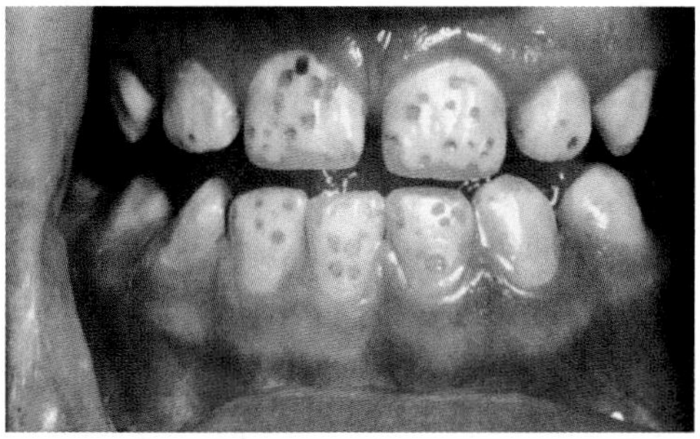

Figure 9.14 Consuming too much fluoride causes fluorosis, leading to staining and pitting of the teeth.

There are concerns that individuals who consume bottled water exclusively may be getting too little fluoride and increasing their risk for dental caries, as most bottled waters do not contain fluoride. However, these individuals may still consume fluoride through other beverages that contain fluoridated water and through fluoridated dental products. Toothpastes and mouthwashes that contain fluoride are widely marketed and used by the majority of consumers in the United States, and these products can contribute as much if not more fluoride to our diet than fluoridated water. Fluoride supplements are available only by prescription, and they are generally given only to children who do not have access to fluoridated water. Incidentally, tea is a good source of fluoride: one 8-oz cup provides about 20–25% of the AI.

What Happens If We Consume Too Much Fluoride?

Consuming too much fluoride increases the protein content of tooth enamel, resulting in a condition called **fluorosis.** Because increased protein makes the enamel more porous, the teeth become stained and pitted (**Figure 9.14**). Teeth seem to be at highest risk for fluorosis during the first 8 years of life, when the permanent teeth are developing. To reduce the risk for fluorosis, children should not swallow oral care products that are meant for topical use only, and children under the age of 6 years should be supervised while using fluoride-containing products.[34] Mild fluorosis generally causes white patches on the teeth, and it has no effect on tooth function. Although moderate and severe fluorosis cause greater discoloration of the teeth, there appears to be no adverse effect on tooth function.[5]

Excess consumption of fluoride can also cause fluorosis of our skeleton. Mild skeletal fluorosis results in an increased bone mass and stiffness and pain in the joints. Moderate and severe skeletal fluorosis can be crippling, but it is extremely rare in the United States, with only five confirmed cases in the last 35 years.[5]

What Happens If We Don't Consume Enough Fluoride?

The primary result of fluoride deficiency is dental caries. Adequate fluoride intake appears necessary at an early age and throughout our adult life to reduce our risk for tooth decay. Inadequate fluoride intake may also be associated with lower bone density, but there is not enough research available to support the widespread use of fluoride to prevent osteoporosis. Studies are being done to determine the role fluoride might play in reducing our risk for osteoporosis and fractures.

RECAP **Fluoride is a trace mineral whose primary function is to support the health of teeth and bones. Primary sources of fluoride are fluoridated dental products and fluoridated water. Fluoride toxicity causes fluorosis of the teeth and skeleton, while fluoride deficiency causes an increase in tooth decay.**

fluorosis A condition marked by staining and pitting of the teeth; caused by an abnormally high intake of fluoride.

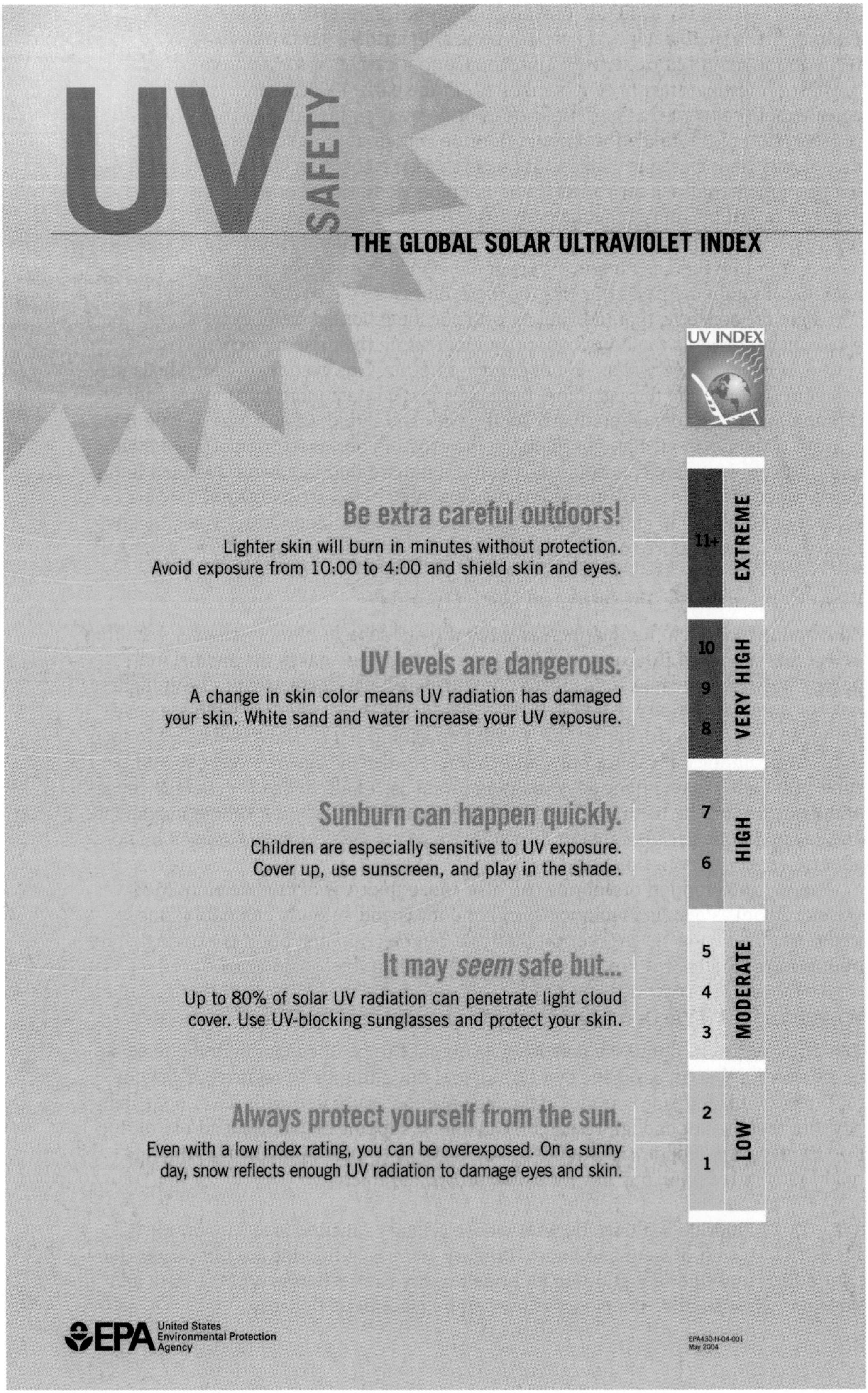

The Environmental Protection Agency is just one of many public health agencies that warn Americans about the danger of exposure to even low levels of sun.

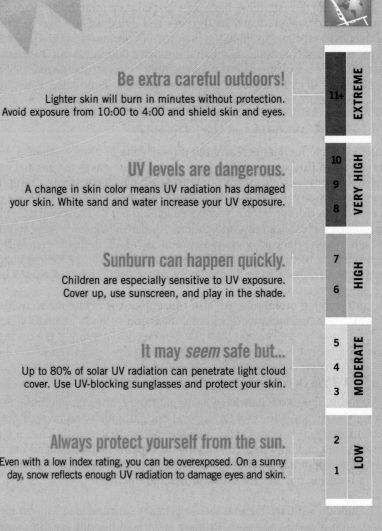

Nutrition DEBATE

Vitamin D Deficiency: Why the Surge, and What Can Be Done?

No doubt about it: unless you live at a latitude within 40° of the equator and spend time outdoors without sunscreen, it's tough to get enough vitamin D. That's because, as you learned in this chapter, there are very few natural food sources of vitamin D, and even fortified food sources are limited to milk and a handful of other products. But if meeting the Institute of Medicine's current AI for vitamin D is already posing a challenge to many Americans, why are some researchers calling for an even higher intake recommendation?

Measurements of vitamin D status in a variety of population studies in recent years have led to a growing concern about widespread vitamin D deficiency and its associated diseases, including rickets in children and osteomalacia and osteoporosis in adults. Recent data from the National Health and Examination Survey (NHANES) indicate that, from 1994 to 2004, the prevalence of vitamin D deficiency in U.S. adults almost doubled, with over 90% of people with darker-pigmented skin (African Americans and Latinos) estimated to be vitamin D deficient.[35] In addition, since the Institute of Medicine set its vitamin D recommendations in 1997, new information has been published about vitamin D metabolism and its potential role in reducing the risks for diseases such as type 1 diabetes, some cancers, multiple sclerosis, and metabolic syndrome.[36,37] These discussions have resulted in some nutrition and bone health experts calling for a full review of the recent research on vitamin D and a reevaluation of the current recommendations.[38]

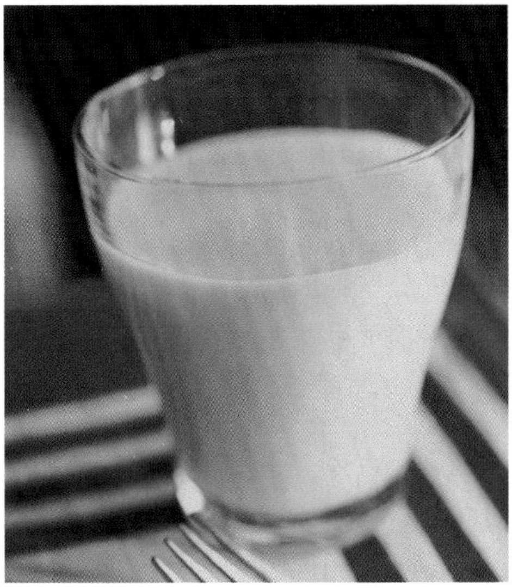

What is contributing to this dramatic increase in vitamin D insufficiency among Americans, and what can we do about it? Researchers have proposed the following three factors:[37,39]

- a downward trend in the consumption of vitamin D–fortified milk products
- a significant increase in sun avoidance and the use of sun protection products
- an increased rate of obesity, as obesity appears to alter the metabolism and storage of vitamin D such that vitamin D deficiency is more likely to occur

To address the first factor, people can increase their intake of vitamin D–fortified milk products; however, it is difficult to meet even the current AI from consumption of milk alone. For instance, children and teens would have to drink a full quart each day to meet the recommendation![40] As a result, the use of vitamin D supplements is gaining wide support. Many healthcare providers now recommend that most children and adolescents who do not or cannot get adequate sun exposure should take a supplement that provides up to 400 IU of vitamin D per day. Whether adults should consume a vitamin D supplement is currently under review by the Food and Nutrition Board, and its decision is expected to be published in the near future. Supplementation with vitamin D is efficient, inexpensive, and effective. Used correctly, it is also very safe. Although vitamin D toxicity is rare, supplementation should be monitored to ensure both a safe and an adequate intake.

What about the second factor—lack of sufficient exposure to sunlight? Responsible, safe exposure to sunlight offers many advantages: it will never lead to vitamin D toxicity, it is easy and virtually cost-free, and sun exposure may offer benefits beyond that of improved vitamin D status.[41] That's why many healthcare professionals advocate moderate sun exposure. They suggest that public health authorities soften the "sun avoidance" campaigns of recent years (see the accompanying figure); they would like to see "well-balanced" recommendations that promote brief (15 minutes or so) periods of sun exposure without sunscreen or sun-blocking clothing two or three times a week, with avoidance of mid-day sun during summer months.[42]

To address the third factor in vitamin D deficiency—obesity—the only solution is to maintain a healthful weight. That means losing weight if you are overweight or obese. By doing so, you'll reduce your risk not only for vitamin D deficiency but also for cardiovascular disease, type 2 diabetes, and many forms of cancer.

Thus, although vitamin D deficiency is becoming a public health issue in the United States, there appear to be a number of strategies you can use to maintain a healthy vitamin D status.

Chapter Review

Test Yourself ANSWERS

1. False. There are many good sources of calcium besides milk, yogurt, and cheese, including calcium-fortified juices, soy/rice beverages, and green leafy vegetables, such as kale, broccoli, and collard greens.

2. True. Our body can convert a cholesterol compound in our skin into vitamin D.

3. False. There is no clear, decisive evidence that consuming dairy products high in calcium, such as milk and yogurt, can result in weight loss.

Find the Quack

Wyn just got some bad news: her mom phoned to say that a DXA scan ordered by her physician shows that she has osteoporosis. Wyn decides to go online to see if she can learn more about osteoporosis. When she discovers the importance of calcium and vitamin D, she searches on "calcium supplements." That's when she finds a site promoting "a unique form of calcium from Pacific sea coral." She reads that this form of "coral calcium" is derived from remnants of coral that have broken off from coral reefs and are mined from ocean beds. The manufacturer makes the following claims for coral calcium:

- "Coral calcium is absorbed into the body within 20 minutes, rather than within 6–8 hours, like other calcium supplements."
- "The calcium carbonate in coral calcium is 100% absorbable, whereas the calcium in milk is only 17% absorbable."
- "The most important daily habits people can adopt to preserve their health are to consume coral calcium and get a minimum of 2 hours of sunlight on their face, without sunscreen."
- "Calcium deficiency not only causes osteoporosis but also makes the body acidic and leads to a host of other diseases, including heart disease, multiple sclerosis, and cancer. People who live on the Japanese island of Okinawa never experience cancer because there is coral calcium in their drinking water, which keeps their body alkaline and cancels out disease-causing acids."
- "Coral calcium is only $19.95 for a 30-day supply."

1. Recall what you learned about digestion in Chapter 3. Do you think it is likely that coral calcium is absorbed into the body within 20 minutes? Why or why not?
2. Do you accept the claim that the calcium in milk is 17% absorbable but the calcium carbonate in coral calcium is 100% absorbable? Why or why not? If necessary, review the information on calcium absorption in this chapter.
3. Comment on the statement "The most important daily habits people can adopt to preserve their health are to consume coral calcium and get a minimum of 2 hours of sunlight on their face, without sunscreen."
4. Comment on the statement that calcium deficiency causes a host of diseases, such as heart disease, multiple sclerosis, and cancer, and that Okinawans "never experience cancer because there is coral calcium in their drinking water, which keeps their body alkaline and cancels out disease-causing acids."

Answers can be found on the companion website, at www.pearsonhighered.com/thompsonmanore.

NutriTools

Check out the companion website at www.pearsonhighered.com/thompsonmanore, or use MyNutritionLab.com, to access interactive animations, including:

- Vitamin Functionality
- Mineral Functionality

Review Questions

1. Hydroxyapatite crystals are predominantly made up of
   a. calcium and phosphorus.
   b. hydrogen, oxygen, and titanium.
   c. calcium and vitamin D.
   d. calcium and magnesium.
2. On a DXA test, a T-score of +1.0 indicates that the patient
   a. has osteoporosis.
   b. is at greater risk for fractures than an average, healthy 30-year-old.
   c. has normal bone density as compared to an average, healthy 30-year-old.
   d. has slightly lower bone density than an average, healthy person of the same age.
3. Which of the following statements about trabecular bone is true?
   a. It accounts for about 80% of our skeleton.
   b. It forms the core of almost all the bones of our skeleton.
   c. It is also called compact bone.
   d. It provides the scaffolding for cortical bone.
4. Which of the following individuals is most likely to require vitamin D supplements?
   a. a dark-skinned child living and playing outdoors in Hawaii
   b. a fair-skinned construction worker living in Florida
   c. a fair-skinned retired teacher living in a nursing home in Ohio
   d. None of the above individuals is likely to require vitamin D supplements.
5. Calcium is necessary for several body functions, including
   a. demineralization of bone, nerve transmission, and immune responses.
   b. cartilage structure, nerve transmission, and muscle contraction.
   c. structure of bone, nerve, and muscle tissue; immune responses; and muscle contraction.
   d. structure of bone, nerve transmission, and muscle contraction.
6. True or false? The process by which bone is formed through the action of osteoblasts and resorbed through the action of osteoclasts is called remodeling.
7. True or false? The amount of calcium we absorb depends on our age, our calcium intake, the types of calcium-rich foods we eat, and our body's supply of vitamin D.
8. True or false? Our body absorbs vitamin D from sunlight.
9. True or false? Magnesium is a trace mineral.
10. True or false? Fluoride inhibits the reproduction of acid-producing bacteria in the mouth.

Answers to Review Questions can be found at the back of this text, and additional essay questions and answers are located on the companion website at www.pearsonhighered.com/thompsonmanore.

Web Resources

www.dairycouncilofca.org/Tools/CalciumQuiz
Dairy Council of California's Calcium Quiz

Use this online interactive quiz to estimate your calcium intake.

www.nlm.nih.gov/medlineplus
MEDLINE Plus Health Information

Search for rickets or osteomalacia to learn more about these vitamin D–deficiency diseases.

www.ada.org
American Dental Association

Look under "Your Oral Health" to learn more about the fluoridation of community water supplies and the use of fluoride-containing products.

Osteoporosis

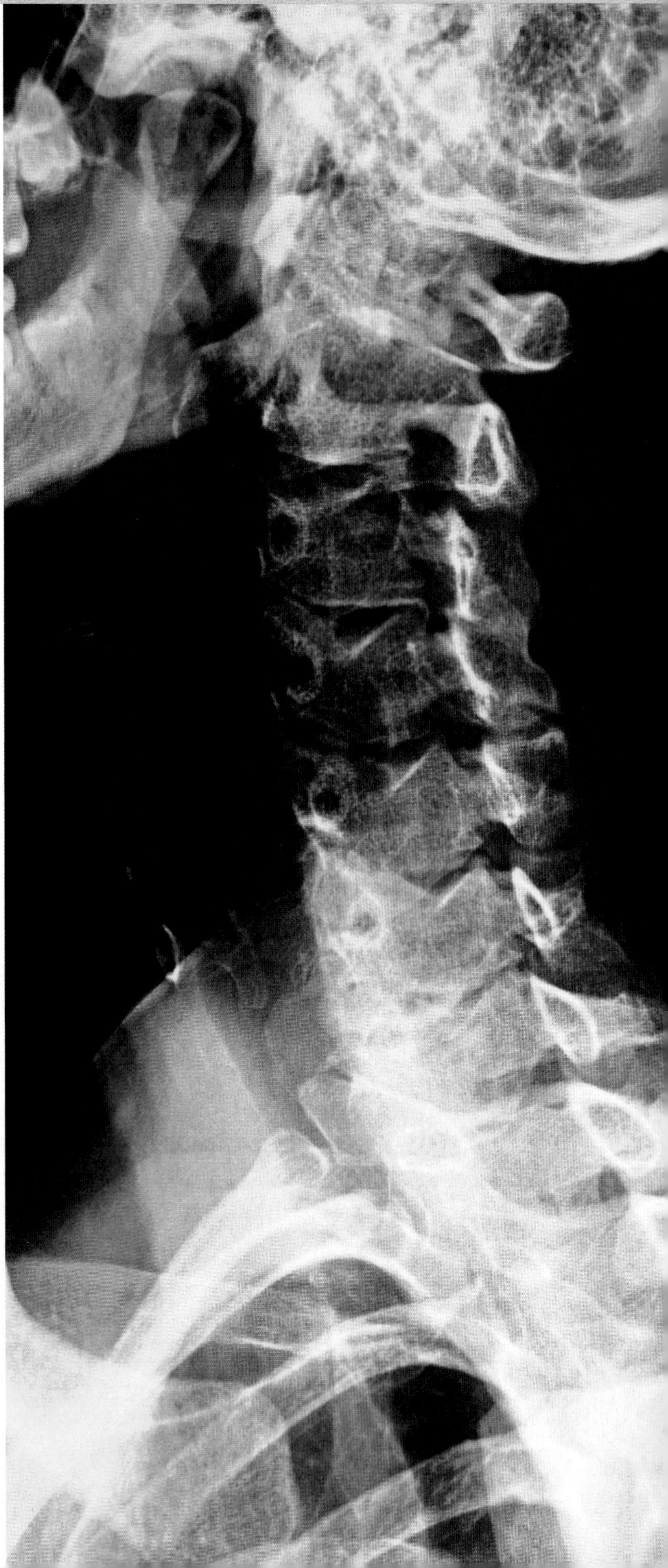

WANT TO FIND OUT...

- **how a bone can break spontaneously—without any trauma at all?**
- **about the link between what you eat when you're young and your risk for osteoporosis later?**
- **if calcium supplements can reduce your risk for osteoporosis?**

READ ON.

As a young woman, Erika Goodman leapt across the stage in leading roles with the Joffrey Ballet, one of the premier dance companies in the world. But at the age of 59, she died after falling in her Manhattan apartment. Goodman had a disease called *osteoporosis,* which means "porous bone." As we noted in Chapter 9, the less dense the bone, the more likely it is to break; in fact, osteoporosis can cause bones to break during even minor weight-bearing activities, such as carrying groceries. In advanced cases, bones in the hip and spine can fracture spontaneously, merely from the effort of holding the body erect.

In this *In Depth*, we'll take a closer look at the disease of osteoporosis. We'll explore the impact of osteoporosis on a person's health and longevity and identify the factors that most significantly increase our risk. We'll also review what is currently known about the role of prescription medications in treating osteoporosis and identify other strategies for reducing your risk.

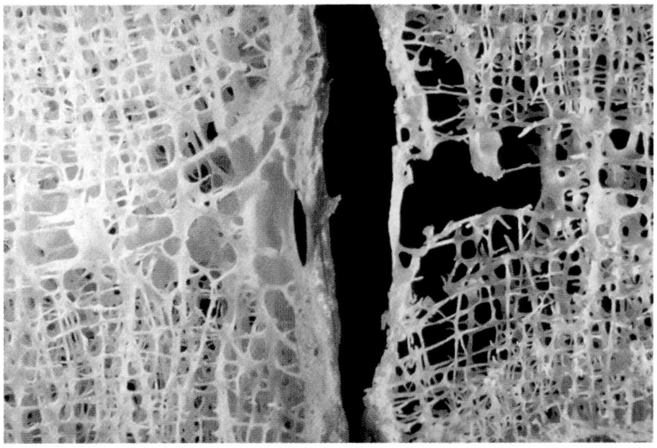

Figure 1 The vertebrae of a person with osteoporosis (right) are thinner and more collapsed than the vertebrae of a healthy person (left), in which the bone is more dense and uniform.

What Is Osteoporosis?

Of the many disorders associated with poor bone health, the most prevalent in the United States is **osteoporosis,** a disease characterized by low bone mass. The bone tissue of a person with osteoporosis deteriorates over time, becoming thinner and more porous than that of a person with healthy bone. These structural changes weaken the bone, leading to a significantly reduced ability of the bone to bear weight (**Figure 1**). This greatly increases the person's risk for a fracture (a broken bone). In the United States, more than 2 million fractures each year are attributed to osteoporosis.[1]

Since the hip and the vertebrae of the spinal column are common sites of osteoporosis, it's not surprising that osteoporosis is the single most common cause of fractures of the hip and spine in older adults (**Figure 2**). These fractures are extremely painful and can be debilitating, with many individuals requiring nursing home care. In addition, they increase the person's risk for infection and other related illnesses that can lead to premature death. In fact, about 20% of older adults who suffer a hip fracture die within 1 year after the fracture occurs, and because men are typically older at the time of fracture, death rates are higher for men than for women.[2]

Osteoporosis of the spine also causes a generalized loss of height, which can be both disfiguring and painful: gradual compression fractures in the vertebrae of the upper back lead to a shortening and hunching of the spine called *kyphosis,* commonly referred to as *dowager's hump* (**Figure 3**). Moreover, back pain from collapsed or fractured vertebrae can be severe. However, especially in the early stages, osteoporosis can be a silent disease: the person may have no awareness of the condition until a fracture occurs.

Osteoporosis is a common disease: worldwide, one in three women and one in five men over the age of 50 are affected. In the United States, more than 10 million people have been diagnosed, and half of all women and one in four men over the age of 50 will suffer an osteoporosis-related fracture in their lifetime.[1,2]

osteoporosis A disease characterized by low bone mass and deterioration of bone tissue, leading to increased bone fragility and fracture risk.

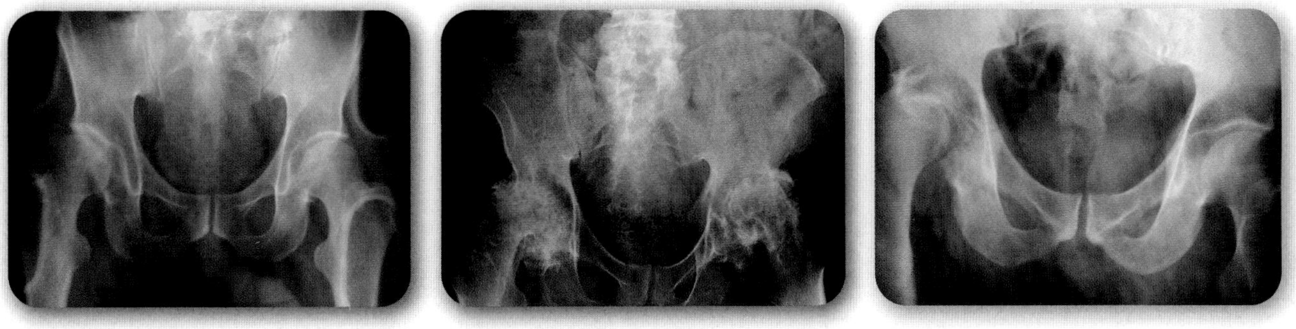

(a) Healthy hip bone **(b) Osteoporotic hip bone** **(c) Fractured hip bone**

Figure 2 These x-rays reveal the progression of osteoporosis in hip bones. **(a)** Healthy bone. **(b)** A hip bone weakened by osteoporosis. **(c)** An osteoporotic bone that has fractured.

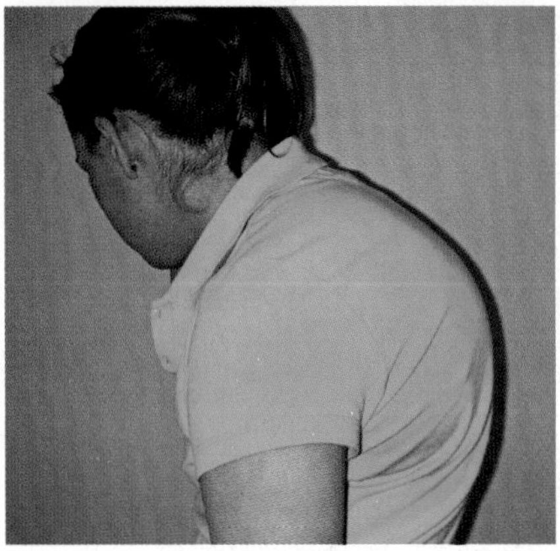

Figure 3 Osteoporosis of the spine causes kyphosis, marked by shortening and hunching of the spine.

What Influences Osteoporosis Risk?

The factors that influence the risk for osteoporosis are age, gender, genetics, nutrition, and physical activity (**Table 1**). Let's review these factors and identify lifestyle changes that reduce the risk for osteoporosis.

Aging Increases Osteoporosis Risk

Because bone density declines with age, low bone mass and osteoporosis are significant health concerns for older adults. The prevalence of osteoporosis and low bone mass are predicted to increase in the United States during the next 20 years, primarily because of increased longevity; as the U.S. population ages, more people will live long enough to suffer from osteoporosis.

Hormonal changes that occur with aging have a significant impact on bone loss. Average bone loss is approximately 0.3–0.5% per year after 30 years of age; however, during menopause in women, levels of the hormone estrogen decrease dramatically and cause bone loss to increase to about 3% per year during the first 5 years of menopause. Both estrogen and testosterone play important roles in promoting the deposition of new bone and limiting the activity of osteoclasts. Thus, men can also suffer from osteoporosis, caused by age-related decreases in testosterone. In addition, reduced levels of physical activity in older people and a decreased ability to metabolize vitamin D with age exacerbate the hormone-related bone loss.

Gender and Genetics Affect Osteoporosis Risk

Approximately 80% of Americans with osteoporosis are women. There are three primary reasons for this:

- Women have a lower absolute bone density than men. From birth through puberty, bone mass is the same in girls as in boys. But during puberty, bone mass increases more in boys, probably because of their prolonged period of accelerated growth. This means that, when bone loss begins around age 40, women have less bone stored in their skeleton; thus, the loss of bone that occurs with aging causes osteoporosis sooner and to a greater extent in women.
- The hormonal changes that occur in men as they age do not have as dramatic an effect on bone density as those in women.
- On average, women live longer than men, and because risk increases with age, more elderly women suffer from this disease.

A secondary factor that is gender-specific is the social pressure on girls to be thin. Extreme dieting is particularly harmful in adolescence, when bone mass is building and an adequate consumption of calcium and other nutrients is critical. In many girls, weight loss causes both a loss of estrogen and reduced weight-bearing stress on the bones. In contrast, men experience pressure to "bulk up," typically by lifting weights. This puts healthful stress on the bones, resulting in increased density.

Some individuals have a family history of osteoporosis, which increases their risk for this disease. Particularly at risk are Caucasian women of low body weight who have a first-degree relative (such as a mother or sister) with osteoporosis. Asian women are at higher risk than other non-Caucasian groups. Although we cannot change our gender or genetics, we can modify the lifestyle factors that affect our risk for osteoporosis.

Tobacco, Alcohol, and Caffeine Influence Osteoporosis Risk

Cigarette smoking is known to decrease bone density because of its effects on the hormones that influence bone formation and resorption. For this reason, cigarette smoking increases the risk for osteoporosis and resulting fractures.

TABLE 1 Risk Factors for Osteoporosis

Modifiable Risk Factors	Nonmodifiable Risk Factors
Smoking	Older age (elderly)
Low body weight	Caucasian or Asian race
Low calcium intake	History of fractures as an adult
Low sun exposure	Family history of osteoporosis
Alcohol abuse	Gender (female)
History of amenorrhea (failure to menstruate) in women with inadequate nutrition	History of amenorrhea (failure to menstruate) in women with no recognizable cause
Estrogen deficiency (females)	
Testosterone deficiency (males)	
Repeated falls	
Sedentary lifestyle	

Data from J. J. Milott et al. Osteoporosis: Evaluation and Treatment. *Comp. Ther.* 2000. 26:183–189.© 2000. Reprinted with permission from Springer Science and Business Media.

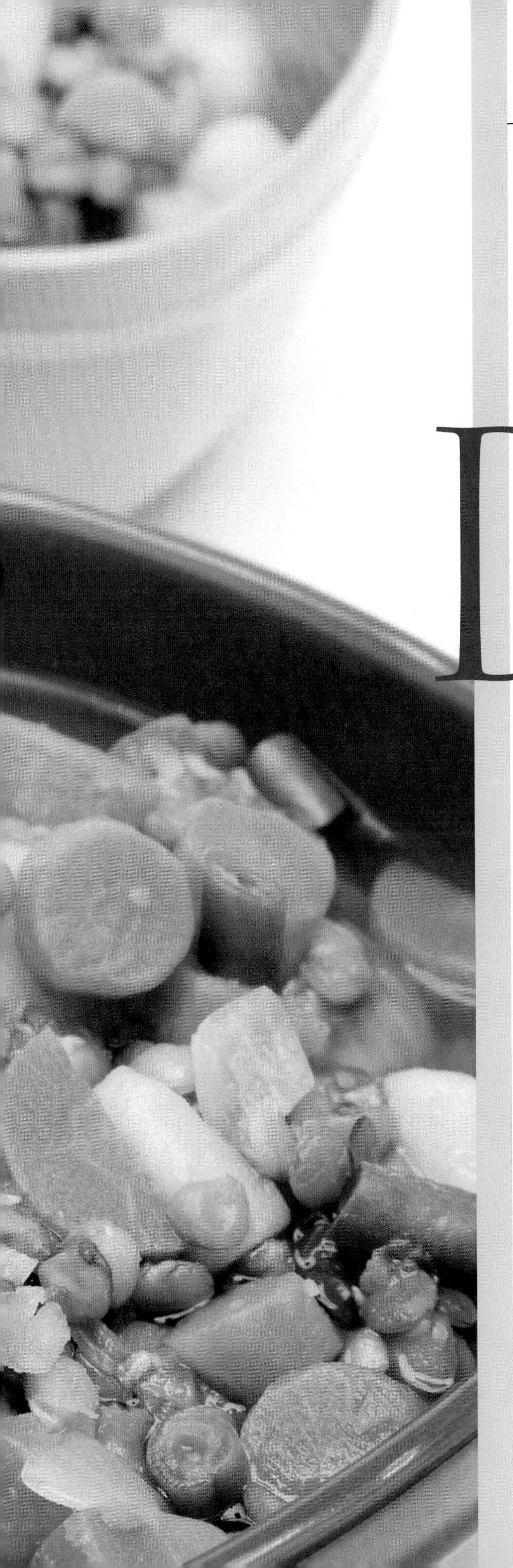

Test Yourself

1. T F The B-vitamins are an important source of energy for our body.
2. T F People consuming a vegan diet are at greater risk for micronutrient deficiencies than are people who eat foods of animal origin.
3. T F Iron deficiency is the most common nutrient deficiency in the world.

Test Yourself answers can be found at the end of the chapter.

Dr. Leslie Bernstein looked in astonishment at the 80-year-old man in his office. A leading gastroenterologist and professor of medicine at Albert Einstein College of Medicine in New York City, he had admired Pop Katz for years as one of his most healthy patients, a strict vegetarian and athlete who just weeks before had been going on 3-mile runs as if he were 40 years younger. Now he could barely stand. He was confused, cried easily, was wandering away from the house partially clothed, and had lost control of his bladder. Tests showed that he was not suffering from Alzheimer's disease, had not had a stroke, did not have a tumor or an infection, and had no evidence of exposure to pesticides, metals, drugs, or other toxins. Blood tests were normal, except that his red blood cells were slightly enlarged. Bernstein consulted with a neurologist, who diagnosed "rapidly progressive dementia of unknown origin."

Bernstein was unconvinced: "In a matter of weeks, a man who hadn't been sick for 80 years suddenly became demented. 'Holy smoke!' I thought, 'I'm an idiot! The man's been a vegetarian for 38 years. No meat. No fish. No eggs. No milk. He hasn't had any animal protein for decades. He has to be B_{12} deficient!'" Bernstein immediately tested Katz's blood, then gave him an injection of B_{12}. The blood test confirmed Bernstein's hunch: the level of B_{12} in Katz's blood was too low to measure. The morning after his injection, Katz could sit up without help. Within a week of continuing treatment, he could read, play card games, and hold his own in conversations. Unfortunately, the delay in diagnosis left some permanent neurologic damage, including alterations in his personality and an inability to concentrate. Bernstein notes, "A diet free of animal protein can be healthful and safe, but it should be supplemented periodically with B_{12} by mouth or by injection."[1]

It was not until 1906—when the English biochemist F. G. Hopkins discovered what he called *accessory factors*—that scientists began to appreciate the many critical roles of micronutrients in maintaining human health. Vitamin B_{12}, for instance, was not isolated until 1948! In Chapters 7 through 9, we explored several key roles of vitamins and minerals, including regulation of fluids and nerve-impulse transmission, protection against the damage caused by oxidation, and maintenance of healthy bones. In this chapter, we conclude our exploration of the micronutrients with a discussion of two final roles: their contribution to the metabolism of carbohydrates, fats, and proteins and their role in the formation and maintenance of our blood.

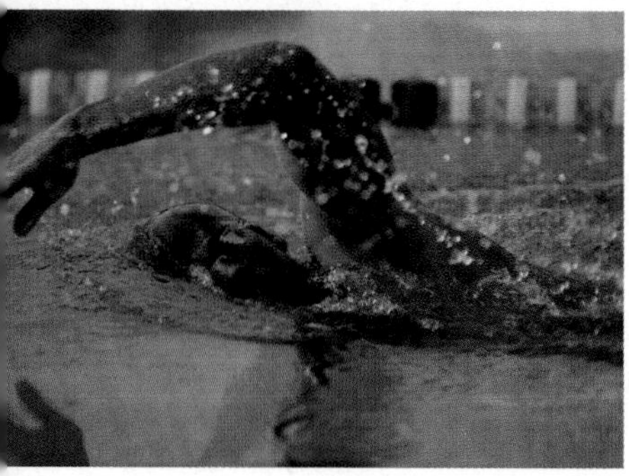

Vitamins do not provide energy directly, but the B-vitamins help our body create the energy we need from the foods we eat.

How Does Our Body Regulate Energy Metabolism?

We explored the digestion and metabolism of carbohydrates, fats, and proteins in Chapters 3 through 6 of this text. In those chapters, you learned that the regulation of energy metabolism is a complex process involving numerous biological substances and chemical pathways. Here, we describe how the micronutrients we consume in our diet assist us in generating energy from the carbohydrates, fats, and proteins we eat along with them.

Our Body Requires Vitamins and Minerals to Produce Energy

Although vitamins and minerals do not directly provide energy, we are unable to generate energy from the macronutrients without them. The B-vitamins are particularly important in assisting us with energy metabolism. They include thiamin, riboflavin, vitamin B_6, niacin, folate, vitamin B_{12}, pantothenic acid, and biotin.

The primary role of the B-vitamins is to act as coenzymes. Recall that an *enzyme* is a protein that accelerates the rate of chemical reactions but is not used up or changed during the reaction. A **coenzyme** is a molecule that combines with an enzyme to activate it and help it do its job. **Figure 10.1** illustrates how coenzymes work.

coenzyme A molecule that combines with an enzyme to activate it and help it do its job.

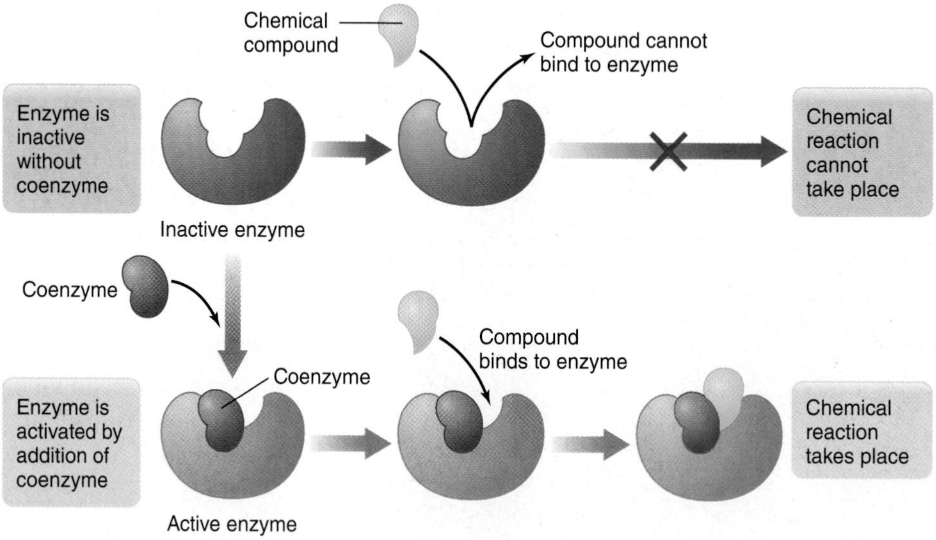

Figure 10.1 Coenzymes combine with enzymes to activate them, ensuring that the chemical reactions that depend on these enzymes can occur.

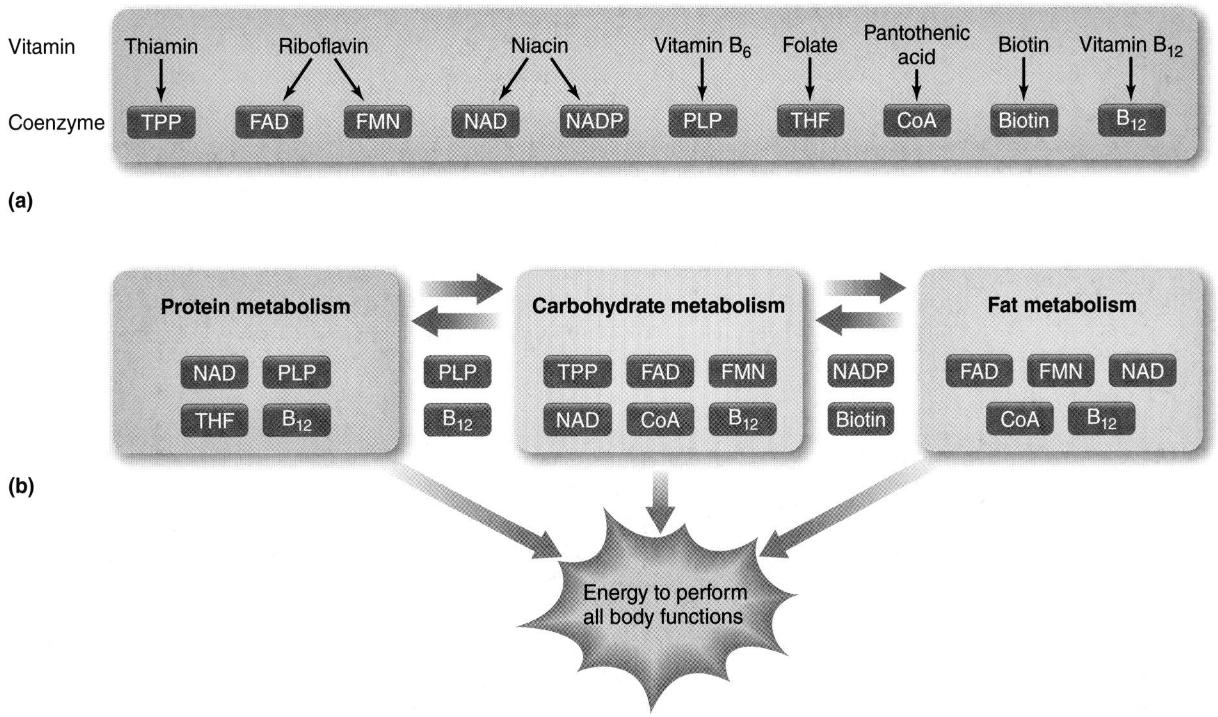

Figure 10.2 The B-vitamins play many important roles in the reactions involved in energy metabolism. **(a)** B-vitamins and the coenzymes they are a part of. **(b)** This chart illustrates many of the coenzymes essential for various metabolic functions; however, this is only a small sample of the thousands of roles that the B-vitamins serve in our body.

Without coenzymes, we would be unable to produce the energy necessary for sustaining life and supporting daily activities.

Figure 10.2 provides an overview of how some of the B-vitamins act as coenzymes to promote energy metabolism. For instance, thiamin is part of the coenzyme thiamin pyrophosphate, or TPP, which assists in the breakdown of glucose. Riboflavin is a part of two coenzymes, flavin mononucleotide (FMN) and flavin adenine dinucleotide (FAD), which help break down both glucose and fatty acids. The specific functions of each B-vitamin are described in detail shortly.

Some Micronutrients Assist with Nutrient Transport and Hormone Production

Some micronutrients promote energy metabolism by facilitating the transport of nutrients into the cells. For instance, the mineral chromium helps improve glucose uptake into cells. Other micronutrients assist in the production of hormones that regulate metabolic processes; the mineral iodine, for example, is necessary for the synthesis of thyroid hormones, which regulate our metabolic rate and promote growth and development. The details of these processes and their related nutrients are discussed in the following section.

RECAP **Vitamins and minerals are not direct sources of energy, but they help generate energy from carbohydrates, fats, and proteins. Acting as coenzymes, nutrients such as the B-vitamins assist enzymes in metabolizing nutrients to produce energy. Minerals such as chromium and iodine assist with nutrient uptake into the cells and with regulating energy production and cell growth.**

A Profile of Nutrients Involved in Energy Metabolism

Thiamin (vitamin B_1), riboflavin (vitamin B_2), niacin (nicotinamide and nicotinic acid), vitamin B_6 (pyridoxine), folate (folic acid), vitamin B_{12} (cobalamin), pantothenic acid, and biotin are the nutrients identified as the B-vitamins. Other nutrients involved in energy metabolism include a vitamin-like substance called choline and the minerals iodine, chromium, manganese, and sulfur. In this section, we discuss the functions, food sources, toxicity, and deficiency symptoms for these vitamins and minerals. For a list of recommended intakes, see **Table 10.1**.

TABLE 10.1 Overview of Nutrients Involved in Energy Metabolism

To see the full profile of nutrients involved in energy metabolism, turn to ***In Depth,*** Vitamins and Minerals: Micronutrients with Macro Powers, following Chapter 6, pages 216–225.

Nutrient	Recommended Intake
Thiamin (vitamin B_1)	RDA for 19 years and older: Women = 1.1 mg/day Men = 1.2 mg/day
Riboflavin (vitamin B_2)	RDA for 19 years and older: Women = 1.1 mg/day Men = 1.3 mg/day
Niacin (nicotinamide and nicotinic acid)	RDA for 19 years and older: Women = 14 mg/day Men = 16 mg/day
Vitamin B_6 (pyridoxine)	RDA for 19 to 50 years of age: Women and men = 1.3 mg/day RDA for 51 years and older: Women = 1.5 mg/day Men = 1.7 mg/day
Folate (folic acid)	RDA for 19 years and older: Women and men = 400 µg/day
Vitamin B_{12} (cobalamin)	RDA for 19 years and older: Women and men = 2.4 µg/day
Pantothenic acid	AI for 19 years and older: Women and men = 5 mg/day
Biotin	AI for 19 years and older: Women and men = 30 µg/day
Choline	AI for 19 years and older: Women = 425 mg/day Men = 550 mg/day
Iodine	RDA for 19 years and older: Women and men = 150 µg/day
Chromium	RDA for 19 to 50 years of age: Women = 25 µg/day Men = 35 µg/day RDA for 51 years and older: Women = 20 µg/day Men = 30 µg/day
Manganese	AI for 19 years and older: Women = 1.8 mg/day Men = 2.3 mg/day

Thiamin (Vitamin B_1)

Thiamin deficiency results in a disease called **beriberi.** The symptoms, which include paralysis of the lower limbs, have been described throughout recorded history. But it was not until the 19th century, when steam-powered mills began removing the outer shell of grains, especially rice, that the disease became widespread, especially in Southeast Asia. At the time, it was thought that milling grain improved the quality of the grain and made it more acceptable to consumers. What wasn't known was that the outer layer of the grain contained the highest concentrations of B-vitamins, especially thiamin.[2] Thus, most of the B-vitamins were being removed and discarded as the grain was milled or the rice polished. In 1885, Dr. Kanehiro Takaki, a Japanese naval surgeon, discovered that he could prevent beriberi by improving the quality of the diets of seamen. Then in 1906, Dr. Christiaan Eijkman, a Dutch physician living in Java, and his colleague, Dr. Gerrit Grijns, described how they could produce beriberi in chickens or pigeons by feeding them polished rice and could cure them by feeding back the rice bran that was removed during polishing.[2,3] In 1911, Polish chemist Casimir Funk was able to isolate the water-soluble nitrogen-containing compound in rice bran that was responsible for the cure. He referred to this compound as a "vital amine" and called it thiamin. Because it was the first B-vitamin discovered, it is designated vitamin B_1.[2]

Thiamin is part of the coenzyme thiamin pyrophosphate, or TPP. As a part of TPP, thiamin plays a critical role in the breakdown of glucose for energy and acts as a coenzyme in the metabolism of the essential amino acids leucine, isoleucine, and valine, also referred to as the *branched-chain amino acids*. These amino acids are metabolized primarily in the muscle and can be used to produce glucose if necessary. TPP also assists in producing DNA and RNA and plays a role in the synthesis of *neurotransmitters*, chemicals important in the transmission of messages throughout the nervous system.

Good food sources of thiamin include enriched cereals and grains, whole-grain products, wheat germ and yeast extracts, ready-to-eat cereals, ham and other pork products, organ meats of most animals, and some green vegetables, including peas, asparagus, and okra **(Figure 10.3)**. Overall, whole grains are some of the best sources

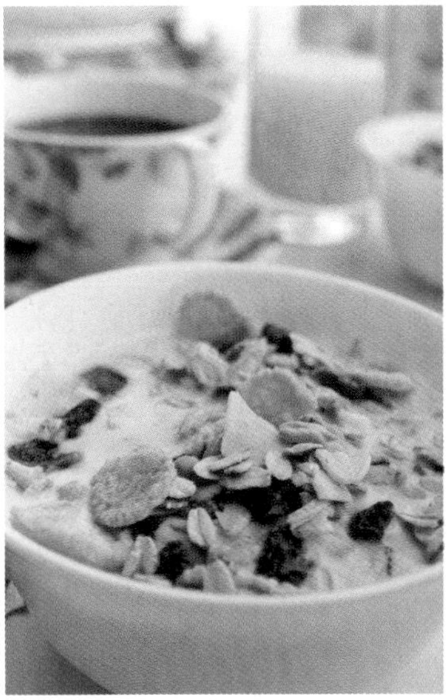

Ready-to-eat cereals are a good source of thiamin and other B-vitamins.

beriberi A disease of muscle wasting and nerve damage caused by thiamin deficiency.

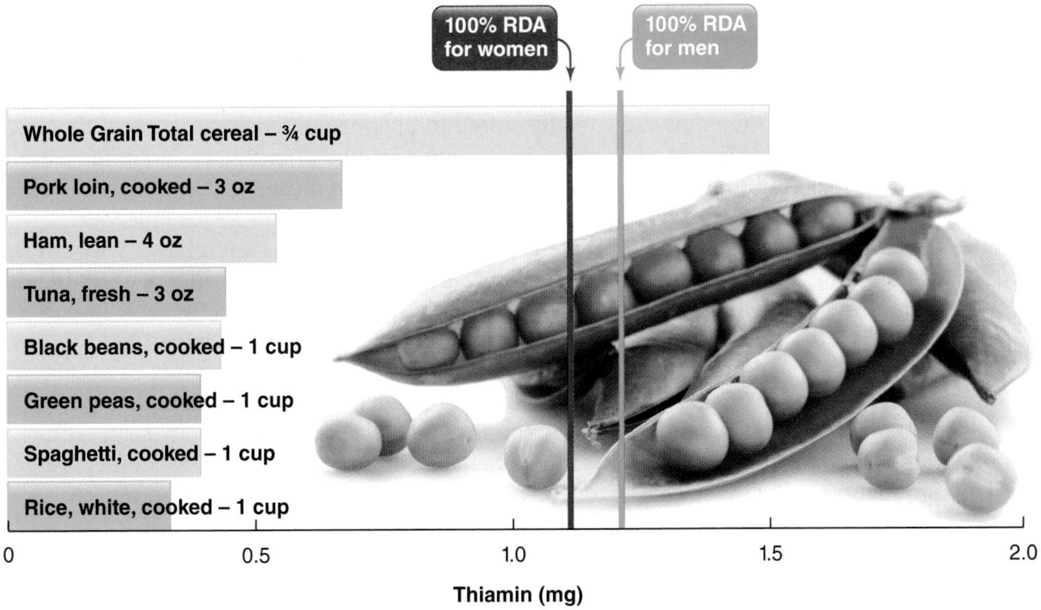

Figure 10.3 Common food sources of thiamin. The RDA for thiamin is 1.2 mg/day for men and 1.1 mg/day for women 19 years and older.

Data from U.S. Department of Agriculture, Agricultural Research Service. 2009. USDA Nutrient Database for Standard Reference, Release 22. Nutrient Data Laboratory Home Page. www.ars.usda.govba/bhnrc/ndl.

of thiamin, while more processed foods, such as refined sugars and fats, are the lowest sources. Unless milled grains are fortified (that is, the thiamin is added back), they are poor sources.

Because thiamin is involved in energy-generating processes, the symptoms of beriberi include a combination of fatigue, apathy, muscle weakness, and detriments in cognitive function. The body's inability to metabolize energy or synthesize neurotransmitters also leads to muscle wasting, nerve damage, and the characteristic paralysis; in later stages, patients may be unable to move at all. The heart muscle may also be affected, and the patient may die of heart failure.

Beriberi is seen in countries in which unenriched, processed grains are a primary food source; for instance, beriberi was widespread in China when rice was processed and refined, and it still occurs in refugee camps and other settlements dependent on poor-quality food supplies. Beriberi is also seen in industrialized countries in people with heavy alcohol consumption and limited food intake. Chronic alcohol abuse is associated with a host of neurologic symptoms, collectively called Wernicke-Korsakoff syndrome, in which thiamin intake is decreased and absorption and utilization impaired.[2] Although thiamin supplementation has been the treatment of choice for beriberi for nearly 100 years, there is still uncertainty about the appropriate dose and duration of supplementation.[4] There are no known adverse effects from consuming excess amounts of thiamin.

Riboflavin (Vitamin B_2)

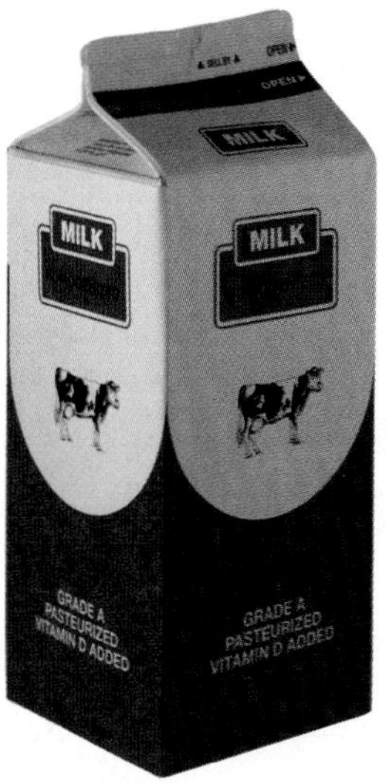

Milk is a good source of riboflavin and is stored in opaque containers to prevent the destruction of riboflavin by light.

The theory that there might be more than one vitamin in rice bran was first proposed in the early 1900s after researchers noticed that rats fed diets of polished rice had poor growth.[3] Finally, in 1917 researchers found that there were at least two vitamins in the extracts of rice polishing, one that cured beriberi and another that stimulated growth. The latter substance was first called vitamin B_2 and then named riboflavin for its ribose-like side chain and the yellow color it produced in water (*flavus* means "yellow" in Latin).[5]

Riboflavin is an important component of coenzymes that are involved in chemical reactions occurring within the energy-producing metabolic pathways. These coenzymes, flavin mononucleotide (FMN) and flavin adenine dinucleotide (FAD), are involved in the metabolism of carbohydrates and fat. Riboflavin is also a part of the antioxidant enzyme glutathione peroxidase, thus assisting in the fight against oxidative damage.

Milk is a good source of riboflavin; however, riboflavin is destroyed when it is exposed to light. Thus, milk is generally stored in opaque containers to prevent the destruction of riboflavin. In the United States, meat and meat products, including poultry, fish, and milk and other dairy products, are the most significant sources of dietary riboflavin.[6] However, green vegetables, such as broccoli, asparagus, and spinach, are also good sources. Finally, although whole grains are relatively low in riboflavin, fortification and enrichment of grains have increased the intake of riboflavin from these sources, especially ready-to-eat cereals and energy bars, which can provide 25–100% of the Daily Value (DV) for riboflavin in 1 serving **(Figure 10.4)**.

There are no known adverse effects from consuming excess amounts of riboflavin. Because coenzymes derived from riboflavin are so widely distributed in metabolism, riboflavin deficiency, referred to as **ariboflavinosis,** lacks the specificity seen with other vitamins. However, riboflavin deficiency can have profound effects on energy production, which result in "nondescript" symptoms such as fatigue and muscle weakness. More advanced riboflavin deficiency can result in lips that are dry and scaly, inflammation and ulcers of the mucous membranes of the mouth and throat, irritated patches on the skin, changes in the cornea, anemia, and in some cases personality changes.[6] It is now known that cataract formation can be decreased by higher riboflavin intakes.[7] In addition, riboflavin is important in the metabolism of four other vitamins: folic acid, vitamin B_6, vitamin K, and niacin.[6] Thus, a deficiency in riboflavin can affect a number of body systems.

ariboflavinosis A condition caused by riboflavin deficiency.

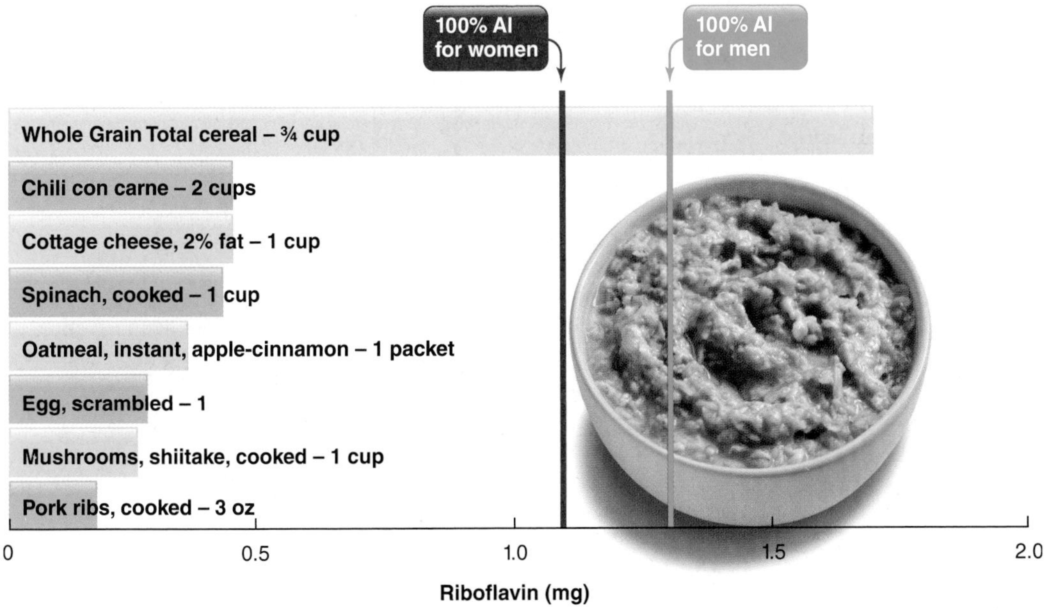

Figure 10.4 Common food sources of riboflavin. The RDA for riboflavin is 1.3 mg/day for men and 1.1 mg/day for women 19 years and older.

Data from U.S. Department of Agriculture, Agricultural Research Service, 2009, USDA Nutrient Database for Standard Reference, Release 22. Nutrient Data Laboratory Home Page, www.ars.usda.gov/ba/bhnrc/ndl.

Niacin

Pellagra, the deficiency of niacin, was first described in the 1700s in northern Spain but was also seen widely across the United States, Western and Eastern Europe, and the Middle East, where corn or maize was the dietary staple.[3] The term *pellagra* literally means "raw skin."[8] The four characteristic symptoms—dermatitis, diarrhea, dementia, and death—are referred to as the *four Ds*. Individuals who develop the disease first complain of inflammation and soreness in the mouth, followed by red, raw skin (dermatitis) on areas exposed to sunlight. The disease then progresses to the digestive and nervous systems. The symptoms of this stage of the disease are diarrhea, vomiting, and dementia. At the present time, pellagra is rarely seen in industrialized countries, except in cases of chronic alcoholism. Pellagra is still found in impoverished areas of some developing nations. (For more information on pellagra, see the Nutrition Myth or Fact? box in chapter 1 on page 5.)

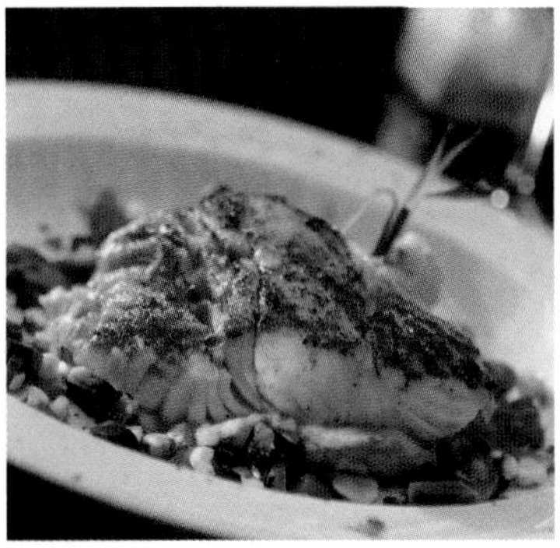

Halibut is a good source of niacin.

Corn-based diets are low in niacin and the amino acid tryptophan, which can be converted to niacin in the body. The term *niacin* actually refers to two compounds, nicotinamide and nicotinic acid, which are converted to active coenzymes that assist in the metabolism of carbohydrates and fatty acids for energy. Niacin also plays an important role in DNA replication and repair and in the process of cell differentiation. Thus, it is not surprising that a deficiency of niacin can disrupt so many systems in the body.

Niacin is widely distributed in foods, with good sources being yeast, meats (including fish and poultry), cereals, legumes, and seeds **(Figure 10.5)**. Other foods such as milk, leafy vegetables, coffee, and tea can also add appreciable amounts of niacin to the diet.[8] As with riboflavin, enriched or fortified breads, ready-to-eat cereals, and energy bars frequently provide 25–100% of the Daily Value for niacin.

Niacin can cause toxicity symptoms when taken in supplement form. These symptoms include *flushing,* which is defined as burning, tingling, and itching sensations accompanied by a reddened flush primarily on the face, arms, and chest. Liver damage, glucose intolerance, blurred vision, and edema of the eyes can be seen with very large doses of niacin taken over long periods of time.

pellagra A disease that results from severe niacin deficiency.

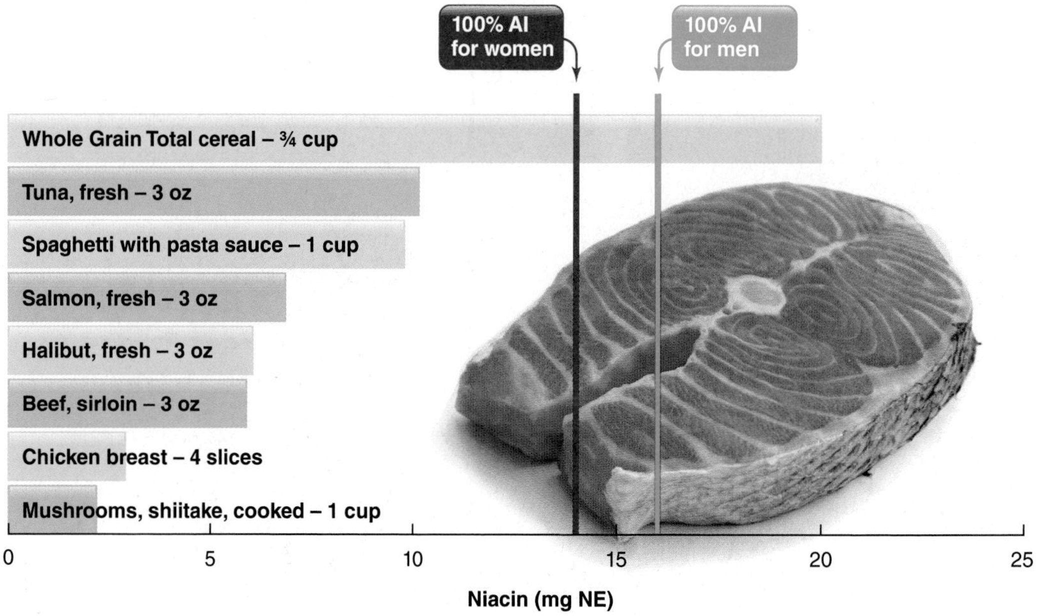

Figure 10.5 Common food sources of niacin. The RDA for niacin is 16 mg niacin equivalents (NE)/day for men and 14 mg NE/day for women 19 years and older.
Data from U.S. Department of Agriculture, Agricultural Research Service, 2009, USDA Nutrient Database for Standard Reference, Release 22. Nutrient Data Laboratory Home Page, www.ars.usda.gov/ba/bhnrc/ndl.

RECAP The B-vitamins include thiamin, riboflavin, niacin, vitamin B_6 (pyridoxine), folate, vitamin B_{12} (cobalamin), pantothenic acid, and biotin. Thiamin plays critical roles in the metabolism of glucose and the branched-chain amino acids. Whole grains are good sources. Thiamin-deficiency disease is called beriberi. Riboflavin is an important coenzyme involved in the metabolism of carbohydrates and fat. Milk, meats, and green vegetables are good sources. Riboflavin-deficiency disease is called ariboflavinosis. Niacin assists in the metabolism of carbohydrates and fatty acids. It also plays an important role in DNA replication and repair and in cell differentiation. Corn-based diets can be low in niacin and can result in the deficiency disease pellagra.

Vitamin B_6 (Pyridoxine)

Researchers discovered vitamin B_6 by ruling out a deficiency of other B-vitamins as the cause of a scaly dermatitis in rats.[3] They then discovered that B_6 deficiency was associated with convulsions in birds and later that infants fed formulas lacking B_6 also had convulsions and dermatitis.[9]

Functions of Vitamin B_6

The term *vitamin B_6* can actually refer to any of six related compounds: pyridoxine (PN), pyridoxal (PL), pyridoxamine (PM), and the phosphate forms of these three compounds. A coenzyme for more than 100 enzymes, vitamin B_6 is involved in many metabolic processes within the body, including the following:

- Amino acid metabolism. Vitamin B_6 is important for the metabolism of amino acids because it plays a critical role in transamination, which is a key process in making nonessential amino acids (see Chapter 6). Without adequate vitamin B_6, all amino acids become essential, as our body cannot make them in sufficient quantities.
- Neurotransmitter synthesis. Vitamin B_6 is a cofactor for enzymes involved in the synthesis of several neurotransmitters, which is also a transamination process. Because of this, vitamin B_6 is important in cognitive function and normal brain

activity. Abnormal brain waves have been observed in both infants and adults in vitamin B_6–deficient states.[10]

- Carbohydrate metabolism. Vitamin B_6 is a coenzyme for an enzyme that breaks down stored glycogen to glucose. Thus, vitamin B_6 plays an important role in maintaining blood glucose during exercise. It is also important for the conversion of amino acids to glucose.
- Heme synthesis. The synthesis of heme, required for the production of hemoglobin and thus the transport of oxygen, requires vitamin B_6. Chronic vitamin B_6 deficiency can lead to small red blood cells with inadequate amounts of hemoglobin.[10]
- Immune function. Vitamin B_6 plays a role in maintaining the health and activity of lymphocytes and in producing adequate levels of antibodies in response to an immune challenge. The depression of immune function seen in vitamin B_6 deficiency may also be due to a reduction in the vitamin B_6–dependent enzymes involved in DNA synthesis.
- Metabolism of other nutrients. Vitamin B_6 also plays a role in the metabolism of other nutrients, including niacin, folate, and carnitine.[10]
- Reduction of cardiovascular disease (CVD) risk. As discussed later in this chapter, high blood levels of homocysteine are considered an independent risk factor for CVD.[11] **Homocysteine** is a metabolic by-product of the metabolism of methionine, an essential amino acid. The enzymes involved in homocysteine metabolism require three key vitamins: folate, vitamin B_6, and vitamin B_{12}.[12] If they are not available to completely metabolize methoinine, blood levels of homocysteine increase. Adequate intakes of folate, vitamin B_6, and vitamin B_{12} can help keep blood levels of homocysteine low.

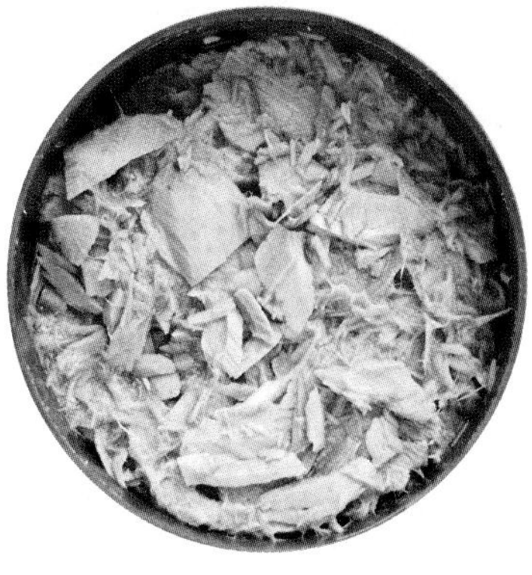

Tuna is a good source of vitamin B_6.

homocysteine An amino acid that requires adequate levels of folate, vitamin B_6, and vitamin B_{12} for its metabolism. High levels of homocysteine in the blood are associated with an increased risk for vascular diseases, such as cardiovascular disease.

How Much Vitamin B_6 Should We Consume?

The recommended intakes for vitamin B_6 are listed in Table 10.1. Rich sources of vitamin B_6 are meats, fish, poultry, eggs, dairy products, and peanut butter **(Figure 10.6)**. Many vegetables, such as asparagus, potatoes, and carrots; fruits, especially bananas; and whole-grain cereals are also good sources of vitamin B_6. As with the other B-vitamins

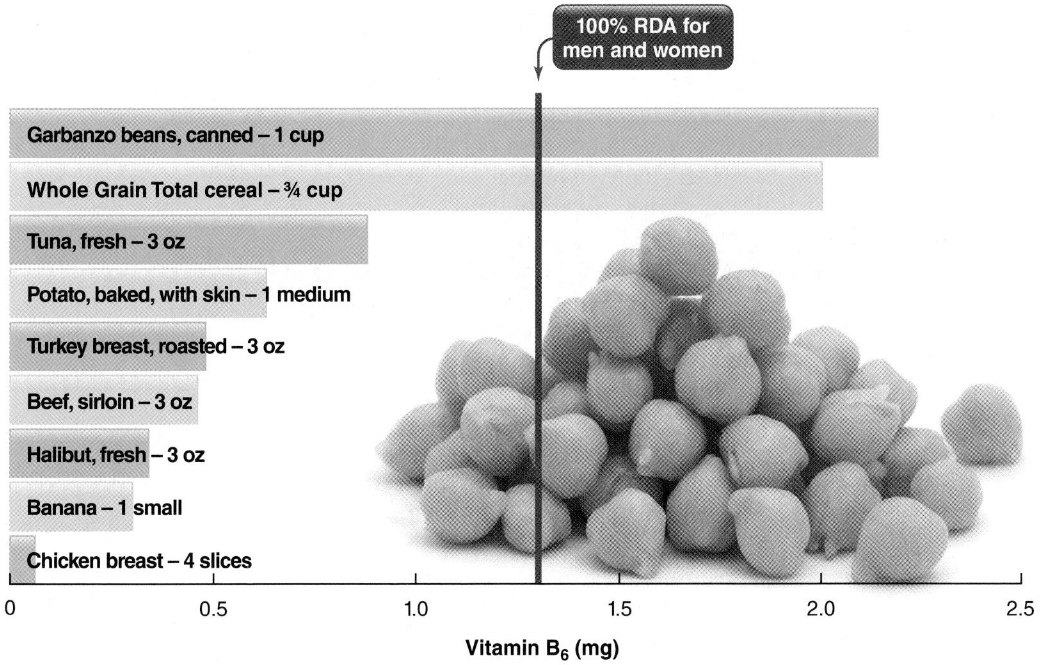

Figure 10.6 Common food sources of vitamin B_6. The RDA for vitamin B_6 is 1.3 mg/day for men and women 19–50 years.

Data from U.S. Department of Agriculture, Agricultural Research Service, 2009, USDA Nutrient Database for Standard Reference, Release 22. Nutrient Data Laboratory Home Page, www.ars.usda.gov/ba/bhnrc/ndl.

discussed in this chapter, fortified or enriched grains, cereals, and energy bars can provide 25–100% of the Daily Value in 1 serving. Little vitamin B_6 is lost in the storage or handling of foods, except the milling of grains; however, vitamin B_6 is sensitive to both heat and light, so it can easily be lost in cooking.

Vitamin B_6 supplements have been used to treat conditions such as premenstrual syndrome (PMS) and carpal tunnel syndrome. You need to use caution, however, when using such supplements. Whereas consuming excess vitamin B_6 from food sources does not cause toxicity, excess B_6 from supplementing can result in nerve damage and lesions of the skin. A condition called *sensory neuropathy* (damage to the sensory nerves) has been documented in individuals taking high-dose B_6 supplements. The symptoms of sensory neuropathy include numbness and tingling involving the face, neck, hands, and feet, with difficulty manipulating objects and walking.

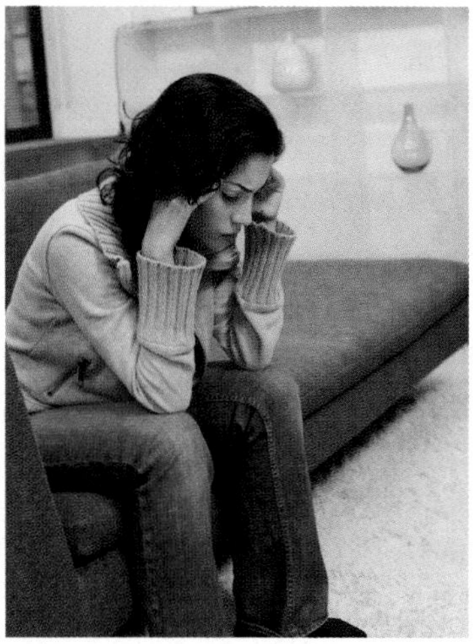

Headaches, anxiety, irritability, tension, and depression are common symptoms of PMS.

The symptoms of vitamin B_6 deficiency include anemia, convulsions, depression, confusion, and inflamed, irritated patches on the skin. Deficiency of vitamin B_6 has also been associated with a decreased ability to metabolize the amino acid methionine and a resultant increased risk for cardiovascular, cerebrovascular, and peripheral vascular disease. This condition also occurs with a deficiency of folate and vitamin B_{12}, and is discussed in more detail in the next section.

Folate

Reports of the symptoms we now recognize as folate deficiency go back two centuries.[13] By the late 1800s, a disorder associated with large red blood cells had been characterized, but it wasn't until the 1930s that researchers understood that the condition is related to diet. It took another 40 years before researchers more fully understood the relationship between this blood abnormality and a deficiency of folate, a substance found in many foods, especially leafy green vegetables. The name *folate* originated from the fact the vitamin is abundant in "foliage."[13]

Functions of Folate

Folate-requiring reactions in the body are collectively called *1-C metabolism*. This means folate is involved in adding "one-carbon units" to other organic compounds during the synthesis of new compounds or the modification of existing ones. Thus, the most basic cellular functions, such as the synthesis of DNA, require folate. The following are some of these functions:

- Nucleotide synthesis. Folate is required for the synthesis of nitrogen-containing

HOT TOPIC

B_6 for PMS? Think Twice!

Perform an Internet search for treatments for premenstrual syndrome (PMS) and you are likely to find many recommendations for supplementing with high doses of vitamin B_6. In addition, almost any PMS supplement sold in a pharmacy or health food store will contain 50 to 200 mg of vitamin B_6 per capsule or tablet, with the recommendation that the consumer take at least two capsules per day. The UL of vitamin B_6 is 100 mg/day, and high doses of vitamin B_6 over an extended period of time can cause neurologic disorders, including numbness, tingling, and a loss of motor function, such as inability to walk. Considering these serious adverse effects, is there any research to support recommending high levels of vitamin B_6 for PMS? Do the benefits of supplementing outweigh the risks for toxicity?

To date, nine randomized clinical trials have tested whether vitamin B_6 supplementation improves PMS symptoms. A review of these nine trials, which included 940 subjects, concluded that "there was insufficient evidence of high enough quality to give a confident recommendation for using vitamin B_6 in the treatment of PMS."[14] Many of the studies showed improvement in only some of the symptoms of PMS, such as anxiety and food cravings, but not headaches and depression. Also, the level of treatment in the studies varied from 50 to 600 mg/day of vitamin B_6. Thus, although some studies suggest a benefit, the evidence is not convincing, so before you start taking a supplement that could cause serious side effects, check with your doctor.[14–17]

NUTRITION MYTH OR FACT?

Can Chromium Supplements Enhance Body Composition?

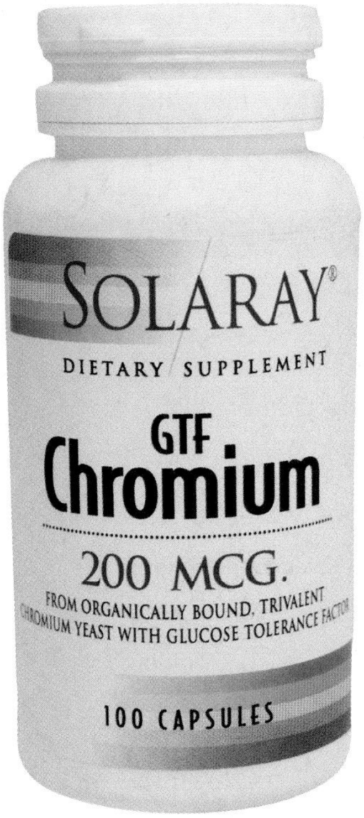

Because athletes are always looking for a competitive edge, a multitude of supplements are marketed and sold to enhance exercise performance and body composition. Chromium supplements, predominantly in the form of chromium picolinate, are popular with bodybuilders and weight lifters. This popularity stems from the claims that chromium increases muscle mass and muscle strength and decreases body fat.

An early study of chromium supplementation was promising, in that chromium use in both untrained men and football players was found to decrease body fat and increase muscle mass.[27] These findings caused a surge in the popularity of chromium supplements and motivated many scientists across the United States to test the reproducibility of these early findings. The next study of chromium supplementation found no effects of chromium on muscle mass, body fat, or muscle strength.[28]

These contradictory reports led experts to closely examine the two studies and to design more sophisticated studies to assess the effect of chromium on body composition. There were a number of flaws in the methodology of these early studies. One major concern was that the chromium status of the research participants prior to the study was not measured or controlled. It is possible that the participants were deficient in chromium; this deficiency could have caused a more positive reaction to chromium than would be expected in people with normal chromium status.

A second major concern was that body composition was measured in these studies using the skinfold technique, in which calipers are used to measure the thickness of the skin and fat at various sites on the body. While this method gives a good general estimate of body fat in young, lean, healthy people, it is not sensitive to small changes in muscle mass. Thus, subsequent studies of chromium used more sophisticated methods of measuring body composition.

The results of research studies conducted over the past 15 years consistently show that chromium supplementation has no effect on muscle mass, body fat, or muscle strength in a variety of groups, including untrained college males and females, obese females, collegiate wrestlers, and older men and women.[29–37] Despite the overwhelming evidence to the contrary, many supplement companies still claim that chromium supplements enhance strength and muscle mass and reduce body fat. These claims result in millions of dollars of sales of supplements to consumers each year. Armed with this information, you can avoid being fooled by such an expensive nutrition myth.

The recommended intakes for manganese are listed in Table 10.1. Manganese requirements are easily met, as this mineral is widespread in foods and is readily available in a varied diet. Whole-grain foods, such as oat bran, wheat flour, whole-wheat spaghetti, and brown rice, are good sources of manganese (**Figure 10.11**). Other good sources include pineapple, pine nuts, okra, spinach, and raspberries.

Manganese toxicity can occur in occupational environments in which people inhale manganese dust; it can also result from drinking water high in manganese. Toxicity results in impairment of the neuromuscular system, causing symptoms similar to those seen in Parkinson's disease, such as muscle spasms and tremors. Manganese deficiency is rare in humans. Symptoms of manganese deficiency include impaired growth and reproductive function, reduced bone density and impaired skeletal growth, impaired glucose and lipid metabolism, and skin rash.

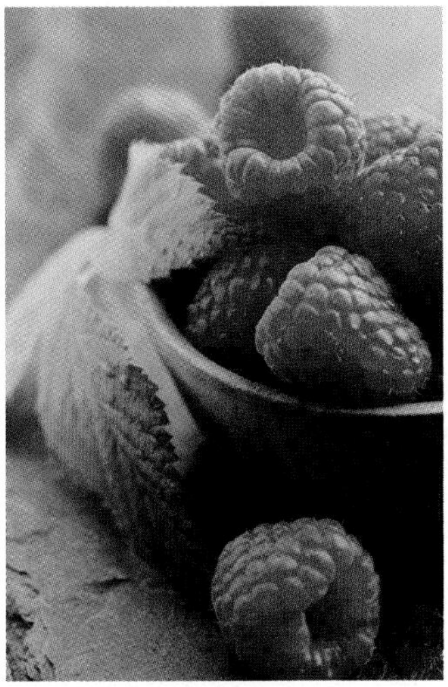

Raspberries are one of the many foods that contain manganese.

Sulfur

Sulfur is a major mineral and a component of the B-vitamins thiamin and biotin. In addition, as part of the amino acids methionine and cysteine, sulfur helps stabilize the three-dimensional shapes of proteins. The liver requires sulfur to assist in the

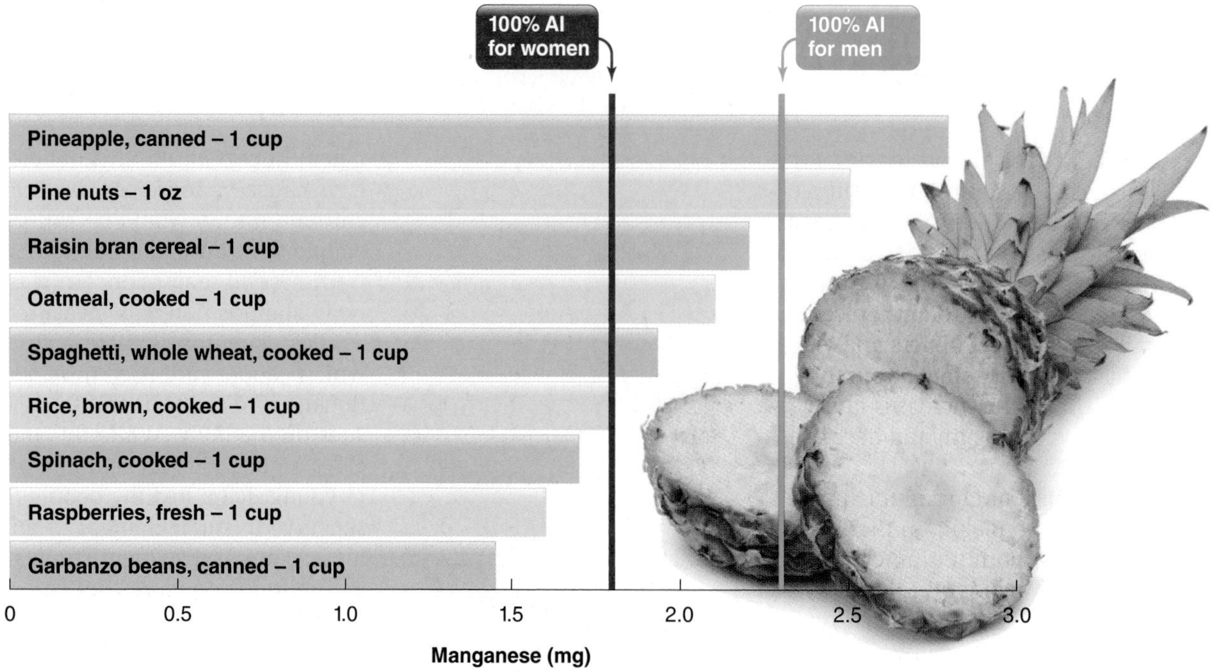

Figure 10.11 Common food sources of manganese. The AI for manganese is 2.3 mg/day for men and 1.8 mg/day for women.
Data from U.S. Department of Agriculture, Agricultural Research Service, 2009, USDA Nutrient Database for Standard Reference, Release 22. Nutrient Data Laboratory Home Page, www.ars.usda.gov/ba/bhnrc/ndl.

detoxification of alcohol and various drugs, and sulfur helps the body maintain acid–base balance.

We are able to synthesize ample sulfur from the protein-containing foods we eat; as a result, we do not need to consume sulfur in the diet, and there is no DRI for sulfur. There are no known toxicity or deficiency symptoms associated with sulfur.

RECAP **Choline is a vitamin-like substance that assists in homocysteine metabolism and the production of acetylcholine. Iodine is necessary for the synthesis of thyroid hormones, which regulate metabolic rate and body temperature. Chromium promotes glucose transport, metabolism of RNA and DNA, and immune function and growth. Manganese is involved in energy metabolism, urea formation, synthesis of bone and cartilage, and protection against free radicals. Sulfur is part of thiamin and biotin and the amino acids methionine and cysteine.**

What Is the Role of Blood in Maintaining Health?

Blood is critical to maintaining life, as it transports virtually everything in our body. No matter how efficiently we metabolize carbohydrates, fats, and proteins, without healthy blood to transport those nutrients to our cells, we could not survive. In addition to transporting nutrients and oxygen, blood removes the waste products generated from metabolism, so that they can be properly excreted. Our health and our ability to perform daily activities are compromised if the quantity and quality of our blood are diminished.

Blood is actually a tissue, the only fluid tissue in our body. It has four components (Figure 10.12). **Erythrocytes,** or red blood cells, are the cells that transport oxygen. **Leukocytes,** or white blood cells, are the key to our immune function and protect us from infection and illness. **Platelets** are cell fragments that assist in the formation of blood clots and help stop bleeding. **Plasma** is the fluid portion of the

erythrocytes The red blood cells, which are the cells that transport oxygen in our blood.

leukocytes The white blood cells, which protect us from infection and illness.

platelets Cell fragments that assist in the formation of blood clots and help stop bleeding.

plasma The fluid portion of the blood; needed to maintain adequate blood volume, so that the blood can flow easily throughout our body.

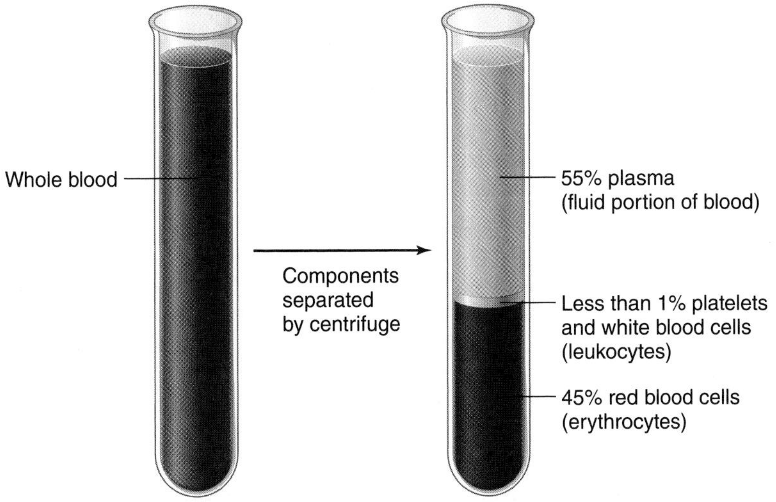

Figure 10.12 Blood has four components, which are visible when the blood is drawn into a test tube and spun in a centrifuge. The bottom layer is the erythrocytes, or red blood cells. The milky layer above the erythrocytes contains the leukocytes and platelets. The yellow fluid on top is the plasma.

blood, and it is needed to maintain adequate blood volume, so that the blood can flow easily throughout our blood vessels.

Certain micronutrients play important roles in the maintenance of blood health through their actions as cofactors, coenzymes, and regulators of oxygen transport. These nutrients are discussed in detail in the following section.

A Profile of Nutrients That Maintain Healthy Blood

The nutrients recognized as playing a critical role in maintaining blood health are vitamin K, iron, zinc, and copper. Folate and vitamin B_{12}, already discussed, are also essential for blood health. A list of recommended intakes of these nutrients is provided in **Table 10.2**.

Vitamin K

Vitamin K is a fat-soluble vitamin important for both bone and blood health. The role of vitamin K in the synthesis of proteins involved in maintaining bone density was discussed in detail on page 308 in Chapter 9. In addition, vitamin K acts as a coenzyme that assists in the synthesis of a number of proteins that are involved in the coagulation of blood, including *prothrombin* and the *procoagulants, factors VII, IX,* and *X*. Without adequate vitamin K, blood does not clot properly: clotting time can be delayed, or clotting may even fail to occur. The failure of blood to clot can lead to increased bleeding from even minor wounds, as well as internal hemorrhaging.

Our needs for vitamin K are relatively small, but intakes of this nutrient in the United States are highly variable because vitamin K is found in few foods.[38] Green, leafy vegetables are good sources, as are soybean and canola oils. The recommended intakes for vitamin K are listed in Table 10.2. There is no upper limit (UL) established for vitamin K at this time.[39] Healthful intestinal bacteria produce vitamin K in our large intestine, providing us with an important non-dietary source of vitamin K.

TABLE 10.2 Overview of Nutrients Essential to Blood Health

To see the full profile of nutrients essential to bone health, turn to ***In Depth,*** Vitamins and Minerals: Micronutrients with Macro Powers, following Chapter 6, pages 216–225.

Nutrient	Recommended Intake (RDA or AI and UL)
Iron	RDA: Women 19 to 50 years = 18 mg/day Men 19 to 50 years = 8 mg/day UL = 45 mg/day
Zinc	RDA: Women 19 to 50 years = 8 mg/day Men 19 to 50 years =11 mg/day UL = 40 mg/day
Copper	RDA for all people 19 to 50 years = 90 μg/day UL = 10,000 μg/day
Vitamin K	AI: Women 19 to 50 years = 90 μg/day Men 19 to 50 years = 120 μg/day UL = none determined
Folate (folic acid)	RDA for all people 19 to 50 years = 400 μg/day UL = 1,000 μg/day
Vitamin B_{12} (cyanocobalamin)	RDA for all people 19 to 50 years = 2.4 μg/day UL = not determined (ND)

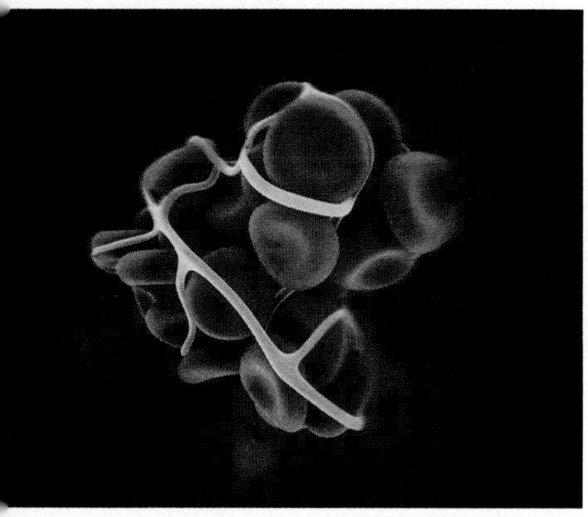

Without enough vitamin K, our blood will not clot properly.

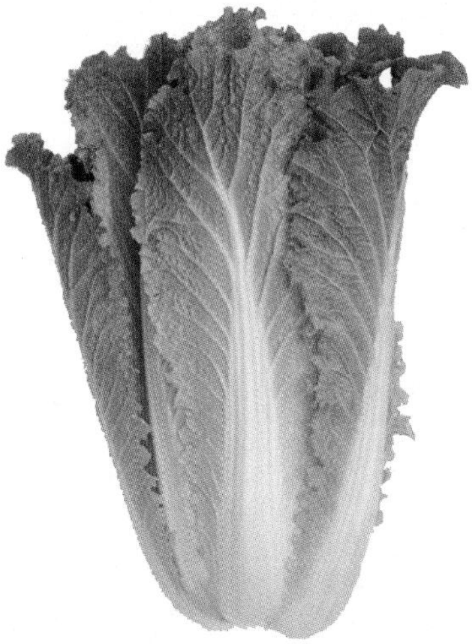

Green, leafy vegetables are a good source of vitamin K.

There are no known side effects associated with consuming large amounts of vitamin K from supplements or from food.[39] In the past, a synthetic form of vitamin K was used for therapeutic purposes and was shown to cause liver damage; this form is no longer used.

Vitamin K deficiency inhibits our ability to form blood clots, resulting in excessive bleeding and even severe hemorrhaging in some cases. Although vitamin K deficiency is rare in humans, people with diseases that cause malabsorption of fat, such as celiac disease, Crohn's disease, and cystic fibrosis, can suffer secondarily from a deficiency of vitamin K. Newborns are typically given an injection of vitamin K at birth, as they lack the intestinal bacteria necessary to produce this nutrient.

As discussed in Chapter 9, the impact of vitamin K deficiency on bone health is controversial. Although a recent study found that low intakes of vitamin K were associated with a higher risk for bone fractures in women, there is not enough scientific evidence to strongly illustrate that vitamin K deficiency causes osteoporosis.[39,40]

RECAP **Blood is a fluid tissue composed of erythrocytes, leukocytes, plasma, and platelets. It transports nutrients and oxygen to our cells to support life and removes the waste products generated from metabolism. Vitamin K is a fat-soluble vitamin and coenzyme that is important for blood clotting and bone metabolism. Bacteria manufacture vitamin K in our large intestine.**

Iron

With few exceptions, iron is important for every known living organism. It is essential to cells but can be toxic in high doses. Thus, the body needs to regulate iron levels carefully to be sure adequate iron is supplied to cover the essential functioning of biological processes but prevent excess accumulation. Thus, iron is a trace mineral that is needed in very small amounts in our diets. Despite our relatively small need for iron, iron deficiency is the most common nutrient deficiency in the world.

Functions of Iron

Iron is a component of four primary iron-containing protein groups that carry out a number of important functions within the body. Two of these groups are oxygen-carrying proteins: hemoglobin and myoglobin. Almost two-thirds of all the iron in our body is found in **hemoglobin,** the oxygen-carrying protein in our red blood cells. As shown in **Figure 10.13**, the hemoglobin molecule consists of four polypeptide chains studded with four iron-containing **heme** groups. You know that we cannot survive for more than a few minutes without oxygen. Thus, hemoglobin's ability to transport oxygen throughout the body is absolutely critical to life. To carry oxygen, hemoglobin depends on the iron in its heme groups. Iron is able to bind with and release atoms such as oxygen, nitrogen, and sulfur very easily. It does this by transferring electrons to and from the other atoms as it moves between various oxidation states. In the bloodstream, iron acts as a shuttle, picking up oxygen from the environment, binding it during its transport in the bloodstream, and then dropping it off again in our tissues. Iron is also a component of **myoglobin,** a protein similar to hemoglobin but found in muscle cells. As a part of myoglobin, iron assists in the transport of oxygen into muscle cells.

Iron is also found in a number of enzymes involved in energy production. Iron-requiring enzymes called *cytochromes* are electron carriers within the metabolic pathways that result in the production of energy from carbohydrates, fats, and proteins. In the mitochondria alone, there are more than twelve of these iron-requiring enzymes that help produce energy.[41] Iron is also critical to the function of certain enzymes important to some immune cells and their communication pathways; thus, iron is required for humans to mount an effective immune response to pathogens.[41] Finally, as you learned in Chapter 8, iron is a part of the antioxidant enzyme system that assists in fighting free radicals. Interestingly, excess iron can also act as a prooxidant and promote the production of free radicals.

hemoglobin The oxygen-carrying protein found in our red blood cells; almost two-thirds of all the iron in our body is found in hemoglobin.

heme The iron-containing molecule found in hemoglobin.

myoglobin An iron-containing protein similar to hemoglobin except that it is found in muscle cells.

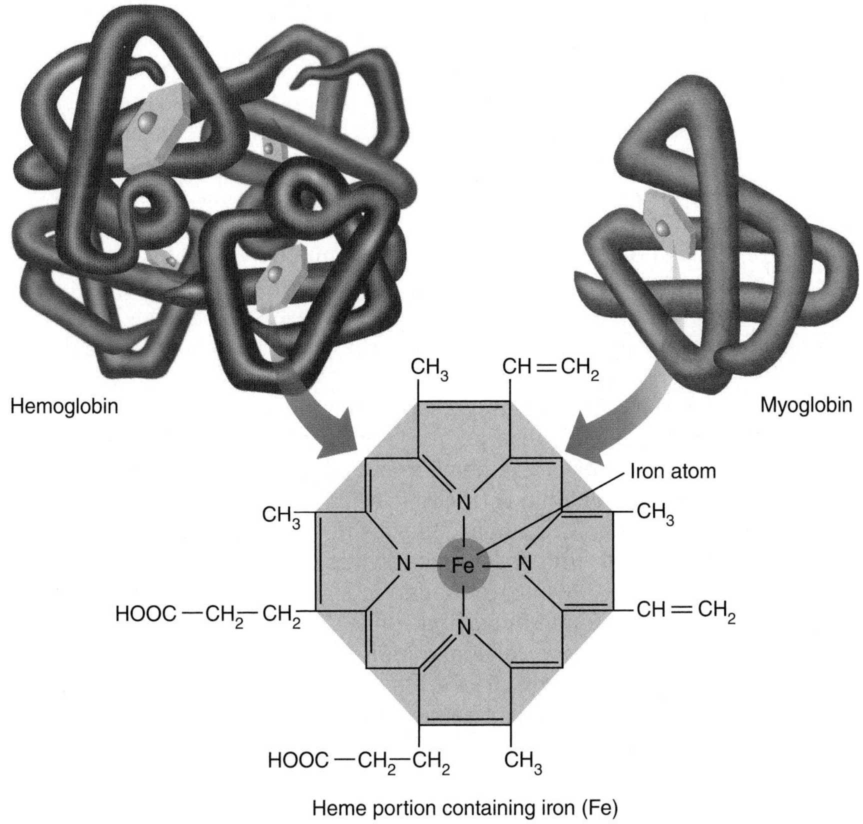

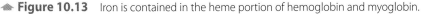

Figure 10.13 Iron is contained in the heme portion of hemoglobin and myoglobin.

Research over the last 30 years has also documented the importance of iron in neuromuscular functions. Like vitamin B_{12}, iron is required for maintenance of the myelin sheath covering nerve fibers; as noted earlier, without adequate myelin, conduction of nerve impulses is slowed. Iron is also needed for the production of neurotransmitters, including serotonin, norepinephrine, and dopamine. Moreover, iron is important for muscle function. Individuals who have poor iron status complain of lethargy, apathy, and listlessness, which may be independent of iron's role in oxygen delivery. Some of these complaints might be due to the impact of iron deficiency on the brain or on fuel metabolism.

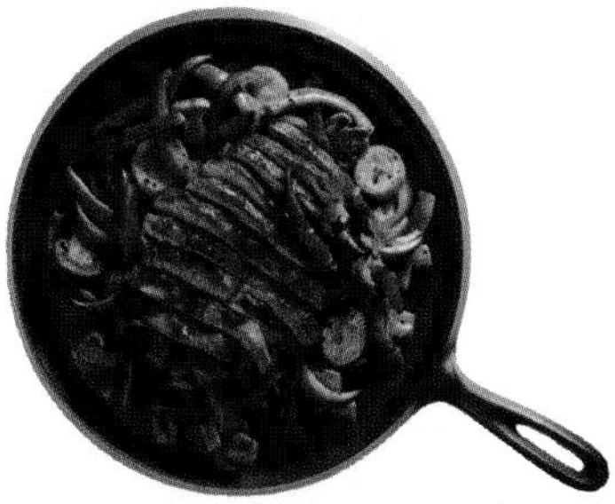

Cooking foods in cast-iron pans significantly increases their iron content.

How Is Iron Absorbed?

Our body contains relatively little iron; men have less than 4 g of iron in their body, while women have just over 2 g. Our body is capable of storing excess iron in two storage forms, **ferritin** and **hemosiderin.** The most common areas of iron storage in our body are the liver, bone marrow, intestinal mucosa, and spleen. Because iron is so important for life, our body recycles the iron lost when aging cells are broken down, especially cells high in iron, such as red blood cells. The liver and spleen are responsible for breaking down old red blood cells and recycling the components, including the iron. This iron-recycling program reduces the body's reliance on dietary iron. Each day, about 85% of the iron released from hemoglobin breakdown is reused by the body.

Our ability to absorb iron from the diet is influenced by a number of factors, including iron status, stomach acid content, the amount and type of iron in the foods we eat, and the presence of dietary factors that can either enhance or inhibit the absorption of iron. Absorption of iron is highest when our iron stores are low. Thus, people who have poor iron status, such as those with iron deficiency, pregnant women, and people who have recently experienced blood loss (including menstruation), have the highest iron absorption rates. In addition, adequate amounts of

ferritin A storage form of iron in our body, found primarily in the intestinal mucosa, spleen, bone marrow, and liver.

hemosiderin A storage form of iron in our body, found primarily in the intestinal mucosa, spleen, bone marrow, and liver.

stomach acid are necessary for iron absorption. People with low levels of stomach acid, including many older adults, have a decreased ability to absorb iron.

The total amount of iron in your diet influences your absorption rate. People who consume low levels of dietary iron absorb more iron from their foods than those with higher dietary iron intakes. Our body can also detect when iron stores are high; when this occurs, less iron is absorbed from food.

The type of iron in the foods you eat is a major factor influencing your iron absorption. Two types of iron are found in foods: heme iron and non-heme iron. **Heme iron** is a part of hemoglobin and myoglobin and is found only in animal-based foods, such as meat, fish, and poultry. **Non-heme iron** is the form of iron that is not a part of hemoglobin or myoglobin. It is found in both plant-based and animal-based foods. Heme iron is much more absorbable than non-heme iron. Since the iron in animal-based foods is about 40% heme iron and 60% non-heme iron, animal-based foods are good sources of absorbable iron. Meat, fish, and poultry also contain a special **meat factor,** which enhances the absorption of non-heme iron. In contrast, all of the iron found in plant-based foods is non-heme iron, and no absorption-enhancing factor is present. However, any vitamin C (ascorbic acid) in the food itself or in an accompanying food or beverage will enhance the absorption of non-heme iron.

Dietary factors that impair iron absorption include phytates, polyphenols, vegetable proteins, and calcium. Phytates are found in legumes, rice, and whole grains. Polyphenols include tannins found in tea and coffee, and they are present in oregano and red wine. Soybean protein and calcium inhibit iron absorption. Because of the variability of iron absorption as a result of these dietary factors, it is estimated that the bioavailability of iron from a vegan diet is approximately 10%, while it averages 18% for a mixed Western diet.[39]

How Much Iron Should We Consume?

The variability of iron availability from food sources was taken into consideration when estimating dietary recommendations for iron, which are listed in Table 10.2. Notice that the higher iron requirement for younger women is due to the excess iron and blood lost during menstruation.

A number of special circumstances can significantly affect iron requirements. These are identified in **Table 10.3**.

Finding Iron-Rich Foods

Good food sources of heme iron are meats, poultry, and fish **(Figure 10.14)**. Clams, oysters, and beef liver are particularly good sources. Many breakfast cereals and breads are enriched with iron; although this iron is the non-heme type and less absorbable, it is still significant because these foods are a major part of the U.S. diet. Some vegetables and legumes are also good sources of iron, and the absorption of their non-heme iron can be enhanced by eating them with even a small amount of meat, fish, or poultry, or with vitamin C–rich foods, such as citrus foods, red and green peppers, and broccoli.

Another way to increase your iron intake is to make smart menu choices throughout the day. The Eating Right All Day feature (page 353) shows menu choices high in iron. Some of these choices provide heme iron, whereas others are combination foods. For instance, the orange juice helps improve the absorption of the non-heme iron in the enriched bread. And see the Quick Tips on page 352 for other iron food sources.

What Happens If We Consume Too Much Iron?

Accidental iron overdose is the most common cause of poisoning deaths in children younger than 6 years of age in the United States.[42] It is important for parents to take the same precautions with dietary supplements as they would with other drugs, keeping them in a locked cabinet or well out of reach of children. Symptoms of iron toxicity include nausea, vomiting, diarrhea, dizziness, confusion, and rapid heartbeat. If iron toxicity is not treated quickly, significant damage to the heart, central nervous system, liver, and kidneys can result in death.

Adults who take iron supplements even at prescribed doses commonly experience constipation. Taking vitamin C with the iron supplement not only enhances absorp-

heme iron Iron that is a part of hemoglobin and myoglobin; found only in animal-based foods, such as meat, fish, and poultry.

non-heme iron The form of iron that is not a part of hemoglobin or myoglobin; found in animal- and plant-based foods.

meat factor A special factor found in meat, fish, and poultry that enhances the absorption of non-heme iron.

TABLE 10.3 Special Circumstances Affecting Iron Status

Circumstances That Improve Iron Status	Circumstances That Diminish Iron Status
• Use of oral contraceptives: use of oral contraceptives reduces menstrual blood loss in women. • Breastfeeding: breastfeeding delays resumption of menstruation in new mothers, so it reduces menstrual blood loss. It is therefore an important health measure, especially in developing nations. • Consumption of iron-containing foods and supplements.	• Use of hormone replacement therapy: use of hormone replacement therapy in postmenopausal women can cause uterine bleeding, increasing iron requirements. • Eating a vegetarian diet: vegetarian diets, particularly vegan diets, contain no sources of heme iron or meat factor. Due to the low absorbability of non-heme iron, vegetarians have iron requirements that are 1.8 times higher than those of nonvegetarians. • Intestinal parasitic infection: approximately 1 billion people suffer from intestinal parasitic infection. Many of these parasites cause intestinal bleeding and occur in countries in which iron intakes are inadequate. Iron-deficiency anemia is common in people with intestinal parasitic infection. • Blood donation: blood donors have lower iron stores than nondonors; people who donate frequently, particularly premenopausal women, may require iron supplementation to counter the iron losses that occur with blood donation. • Intense endurance exercise training: people engaging in intense endurance exercise appear to be at risk for poor iron status due to many factors, including suboptimal iron intake and increased iron loss in sweat and increased fecal losses.

Data from "Dietary Reference Intakes for Vitamin A, Vitamin K, Arsenic, Boron, Chromium, Copper, Iodine, Manganese, Molybdenum, Nickel, Silicon, Vanadium, and Zinc," © 2002 by the National Academy of Sciences. Reprinted by permission.

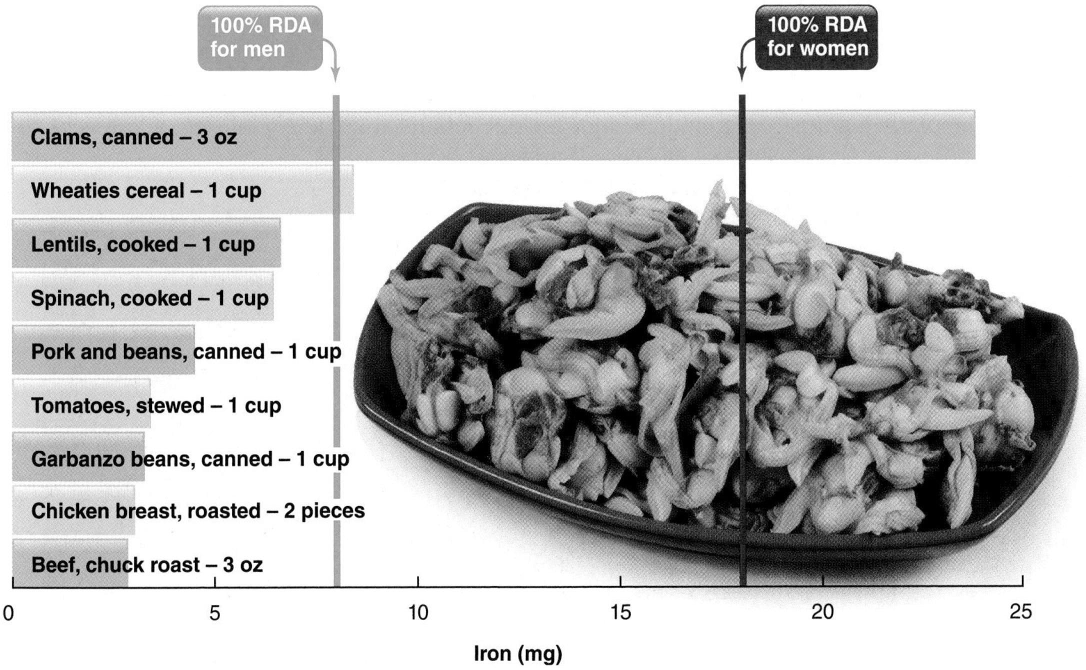

Figure 10.14 Common food sources of iron. The RDA for iron is 8 mg/day for men and 18 mg/day for women aged 19 to 50 years.

Data from U.S. Department of Agriculture, Agricultural Research Service, 2009, USDA Nutrient Database for Standard Reference, Release 22. Nutrient Data Laboratory Home Page, www.ars.usda.gov/ba/bhnrc/ndl.

QUICK TIPS

Increasing Your Iron Intake

✓ Shop for iron-fortified breads and breakfast cereals. Check the Nutrition Facts Panel!

✓ Consume a food or beverage that is high in vitamin C along with plant or animal sources of iron. For instance, drink a glass of orange juice with your morning toast to increase the absorption of the non-heme iron in the bread. Or add chopped tomatoes to beans or lentils. Or sprinkle lemon juice on fish.

✓ Add small amounts of meat, poultry, or fish to baked beans, vegetable soups, stir-fried vegetables, or salads to enhance the absorption of the non-heme iron in the plant-based foods.

✓ Cook foods in cast-iron pans to significantly increase the iron content of foods: the iron in the pan will be absorbed into the food during the cooking process.

✓ Avoid drinking red wine, coffee, or tea when eating iron-rich foods, as the polyphenols in these beverages will reduce iron absorption.

✓ Avoid drinking cow's milk or soy milk with iron-rich foods, as both calcium and soybean protein inhibit iron absorption.

✓ Avoid taking calcium supplements or zinc supplements with iron-rich foods, as these minerals decrease iron absorption.

tion but also can help reduce constipation. Other gastrointestinal symptoms include nausea, vomiting, and diarrhea. As introduced in Chapter 8, some individuals suffer from a hereditary disorder called hemochromatosis. This disorder affects between 1 in 200 and 1 in 400 individuals of northern European descent.[43] Hemochromatosis is characterized by excessive absorption of dietary iron and altered iron storage. The accumulation of iron in these individuals over many years causes cirrhosis of the liver, liver cancer, heart attack and heart failure, diabetes, and arthritis. Men are more at risk for this disease than women due to the higher losses of iron in women through menstruation. Treatment includes reducing dietary intake of iron, avoiding high intakes of vitamin C, and withdrawing blood occasionally.

What Happens If We Don't Consume Enough Iron?

Iron deficiency is the most common nutrient deficiency in the world. People at particularly high risk for iron deficiency include infants and young children, adolescent girls, premenopausal women, and pregnant women.

Iron deficiency progresses through three stages (**Figure 10.15**). The first stage of iron deficiency causes a decrease in iron *stores*, resulting in reduced levels of ferritin.

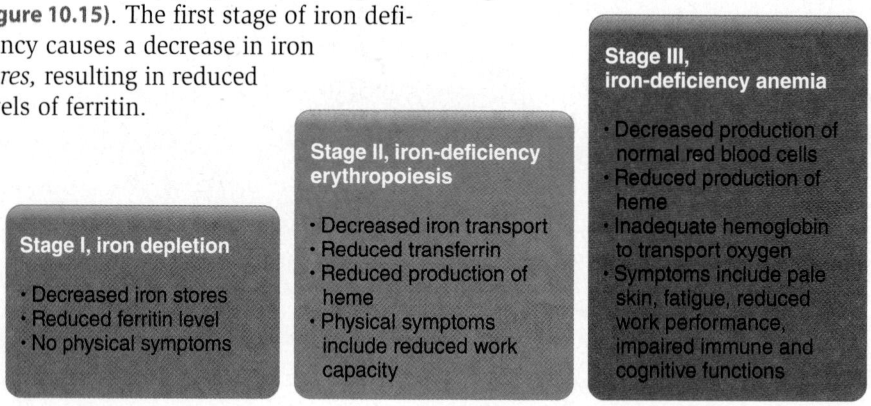
Stage I, iron depletion
· Decreased iron stores
· Reduced ferritin level
· No physical symptoms
Stage II, iron-deficiency erythropoiesis
· Decreased iron transport
· Reduced transferrin
· Reduced production of heme
· Physical symptoms include reduced work capacity
Stage III, iron-deficiency anemia
· Decreased production of normal red blood cells
· Reduced production of heme
· Inadequate hemoglobin to transport oxygen
· Symptoms include pale skin, fatigue, reduced work performance, impaired immune and cognitive functions

Figure 10.15 Iron deficiency passes through three stages. The first stage is identified by decreased iron stores, or reduced ferritin levels. The second stage is identified by decreased iron transport, or a reduction in transferrin. The final stage of iron deficiency is iron-deficiency anemia, which is identified by decreased production of normal, healthy red blood cells and inadequate hemoglobin levels.

transferrin The transport protein for iron.

iron-deficiency anemia A form of anemia that results from severe iron deficiency.

During this first stage, there are generally no physical symptoms because hemoglobin levels are not yet affected. The second stage of iron deficiency causes a decrease in the *transport* of iron. This manifests as a reduction in the transport protein for iron, called **transferrin.** The production of heme also starts to decline during this stage, leading to symptoms of reduced work capacity. During the third and final stage of iron deficiency, **iron-deficiency anemia** results.

In iron-deficiency anemia, the production of normal, healthy red blood cells decreases. Red blood cells that are produced are smaller than normal and do not contain enough hemoglobin to transport adequate oxygen or to allow the proper transfer of electrons to produce energy. This type of anemia is often referred to as *microcytic anemia* (*micro,* meaning "small," and *cyte,* meaning "cell"). As normal cellular death occurs over time, more and more healthy red blood cells are replaced by these deficient cells, and the classic symptoms of oxygen and energy deprivation develop. These symptoms include impaired work performance, general fatigue, pale skin, depressed immune

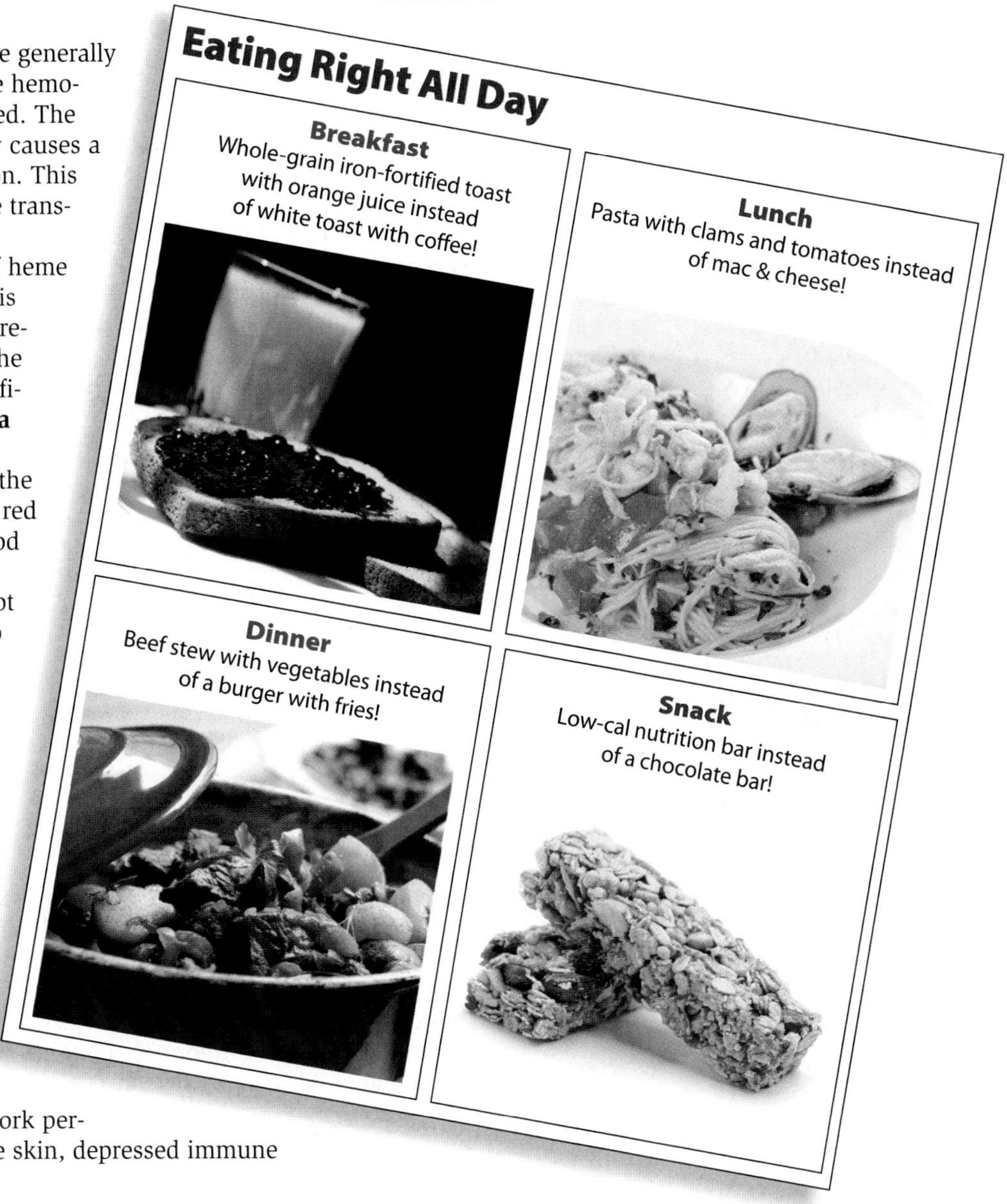
Eating Right All Day
Breakfast
Whole-grain iron-fortified toast with orange juice instead of white toast with coffee!
Lunch
Pasta with clams and tomatoes instead of mac & cheese!
Dinner
Beef stew with vegetables instead of a burger with fries!
Snack
Low-cal nutrition bar instead of a chocolate bar!

NUTRI-CASE LIZ

"It was really hard spending last summer with my parents, because we kept arguing over food! Even though I'd told them that I'm a vegetarian, they kept serving meals with meat! Then they'd get mad when I'd fix myself a hummus sandwich! When it was my turn to cook, I made lentils with brown rice, whole-wheat pasta primavera, vegetarian curries, and lots of other yummy meals, but my dad kept insisting, "You have to eat meat or you won't get enough iron!" I told him that plant foods have lots of iron, but he wouldn't listen. Was I ever glad to get back onto campus this fall!"

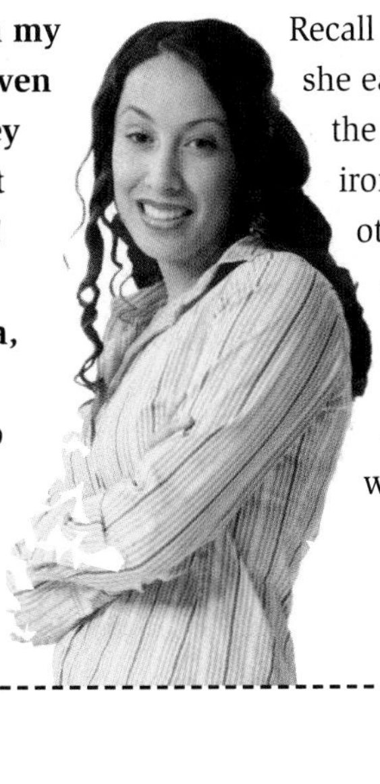

Recall that Liz is a ballet dancer who trains daily. If she eats a vegetarian diet including meals such as the ones she describes here, will she be at risk for iron deficiency? Why or why not? Are there any other micronutrients that might be low in Liz's diet because she avoids meat? If so, what are they? Overall, will Liz get enough energy to support her high level of physical activity on a vegetarian diet? How would she know if she were low energy?

function, impaired cognitive and nerve function, and impaired memory. Pregnant women with severe anemia are at higher risk for low-birth-weight infants, premature delivery, and increased infant mortality.

RECAP Iron is a trace mineral that, as part of the hemoglobin protein, plays a major role in the transportation of oxygen in our blood. Iron is also a coenzyme in many metabolic pathways involved in energy production. Meat, fish, and poultry are good sources of heme iron, which is more absorbable than non-heme iron. Toxicity symptoms for iron range from nausea and vomiting to organ damage and potentially death. If left untreated, iron deficiency eventually leads to iron-deficiency anemia.

Zinc

Zinc is a trace mineral that acts as a cofactor for approximately a hundred different enzymes. It thereby plays an important role in many physiologic processes in nearly every body system.

Functions of Zinc

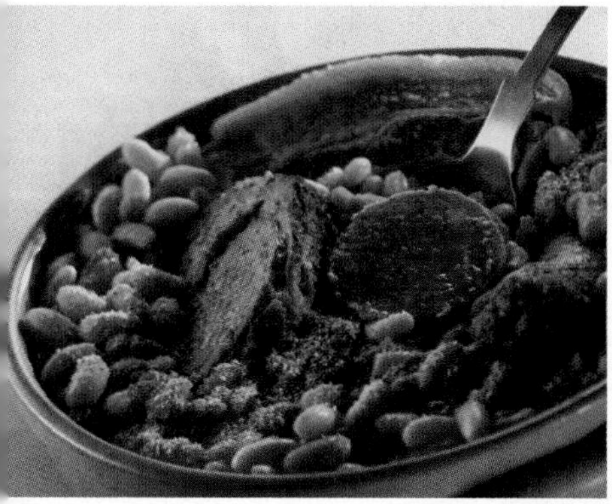

Zinc can be found in pork and beans.

As a cofactor, zinc assists in the production of hemoglobin, indirectly supporting the adequate transport of oxygen to our cells. Zinc is also part of the superoxide dismutase antioxidant enzyme system and thus helps fight the oxidative damage caused by free radicals. It assists enzymes in generating energy from carbohydrates, fats, and protein and in activating vitamin A in the retina of the eye.

Zinc also plays a role in facilitating the folding of proteins into biologically active molecules used in gene regulation. Thus, it is critical for cell replication and normal growth. In fact, zinc deficiency was discovered in the early 1960s, when researchers were trying to determine the cause of severe growth retardation, anemia, and poorly developed testicles in a group of Middle Eastern men. These symptoms of zinc deficiency illustrate its critical role in normal growth and sexual maturation.

Zinc is vital for the proper development and functioning of the immune system. In fact, zinc has received so much attention for its contribution to immune system health that zinc lozenges have been formulated to fight the common cold. The Nutrition Debate at the end of this chapter explores the question of whether or not these lozenges are effective.

How Much Zinc Should We Consume?

As with iron, our need for zinc is relatively small, but our intakes are variable and absorption is influenced by a number of factors. Overall, zinc absorption is similar to that of iron, ranging from 10% to 35% of dietary zinc. People with poor zinc status absorb more zinc than individuals with optimal zinc status, and zinc absorption increases during times of growth, sexual development, and pregnancy.

Several dietary factors influence zinc absorption. High non-heme iron intakes can inhibit zinc absorption, which is a primary concern with iron supplements (which are non-heme), particularly during pregnancy and lactation. High intakes of heme iron appear to have no effect on zinc absorption. The phytates and fiber found in whole grains and beans strongly inhibit zinc absorption. In contrast, dietary protein, especially animal-based protein, enhances zinc absorption. It's not surprising, then, that the primary cause of the zinc deficiency in the Middle Eastern men just mentioned was their low consumption of meat and high consumption of beans and unleavened breads (also called *flat breads*). In leavening bread, the baker adds yeast to the dough. This not only makes the bread rise but also helps reduce the phytate content of the bread.

The recommended intakes for zinc are listed in Table 10.2. Good food sources of zinc include red meats, some seafood, whole grains, and enriched grains and cereals. The dark meat of poultry has a higher content of zinc than white meat. As zinc is significantly more absorbable from animal-based foods, zinc deficiency is a concern for

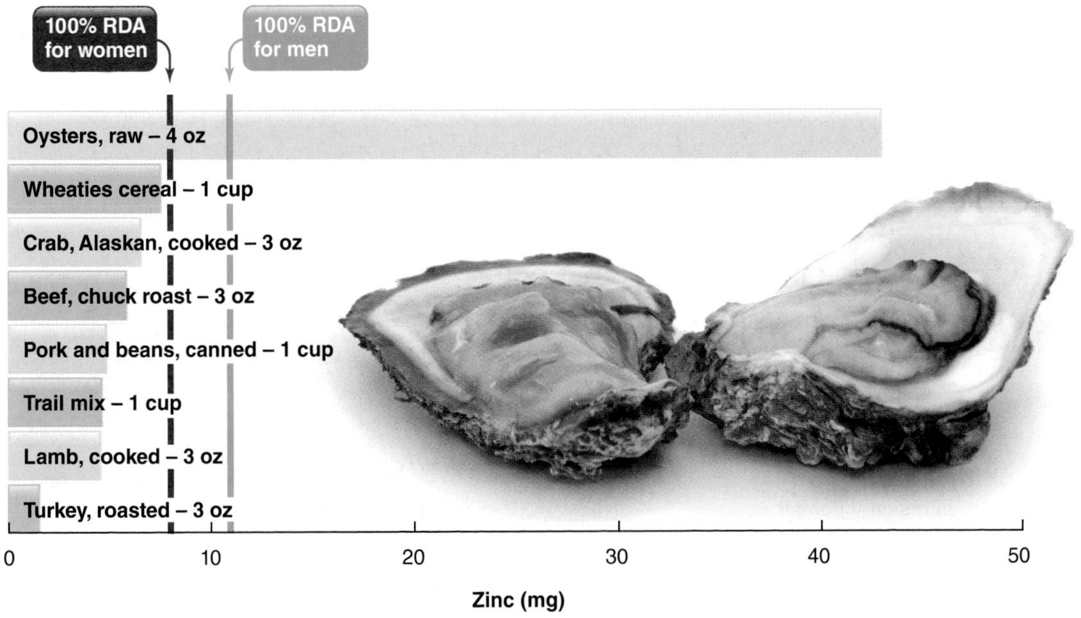

Figure 10.16 Common food sources of zinc. The RDA for zinc is 11 mg/day for men and 8 mg/day for women.
Data from U.S. Department of Agriculture, Agricultural Research Service, 2009, USDA Nutrient Database for Standard Reference, Release 22. Nutrient Data Laboratory Home Page, www.ars.usda.gov/ba/bhnrc/ndl.

people eating a vegan diet. **Figure 10.16** shows various foods that are relatively high in zinc.

What Happens If We Consume Too Much Zinc?

Eating high amounts of dietary zinc does not appear to lead to toxicity. Zinc toxicity can occur from consuming zinc in supplement form and in fortified foods. Toxicity symptoms include intestinal pain and cramps, nausea, vomiting, loss of appetite, diarrhea, and headaches. Excessive zinc supplementation has also been shown to depress immune function and decrease high-density lipoprotein concentrations. High intakes of zinc can also reduce copper status, as zinc absorption interferes with the absorption of copper.

What Happens If We Don't Consume Enough Zinc?

Zinc deficiency is uncommon in the United States but occurs more often in countries in which people consume predominantly grain-based foods. Symptoms of zinc deficiency include growth retardation, diarrhea, delayed sexual maturation and impotence, eye and skin lesions, hair loss, and impaired appetite. As zinc is critical to a healthy immune system, zinc deficiency also results in increased incidence of infections and illnesses.

Copper

Copper is a trace mineral that functions as a cofactor in many physiologic reactions. It functions as a cofactor in the metabolic pathways that produce energy, in the production of the connective tissues collagen and elastin, and as part of the superoxide dismutase enzyme system that fights the damage caused by free radicals. Copper is a component of *ceruloplasmin,* a protein that is critical for the proper transport of iron. If ceruloplasmin levels are inadequate, iron accumulation results, causing symptoms similar to those described with the genetic disorder hemochromatosis (page 352). Copper is also necessary for the regulation of certain neurotransmitters important to brain function.

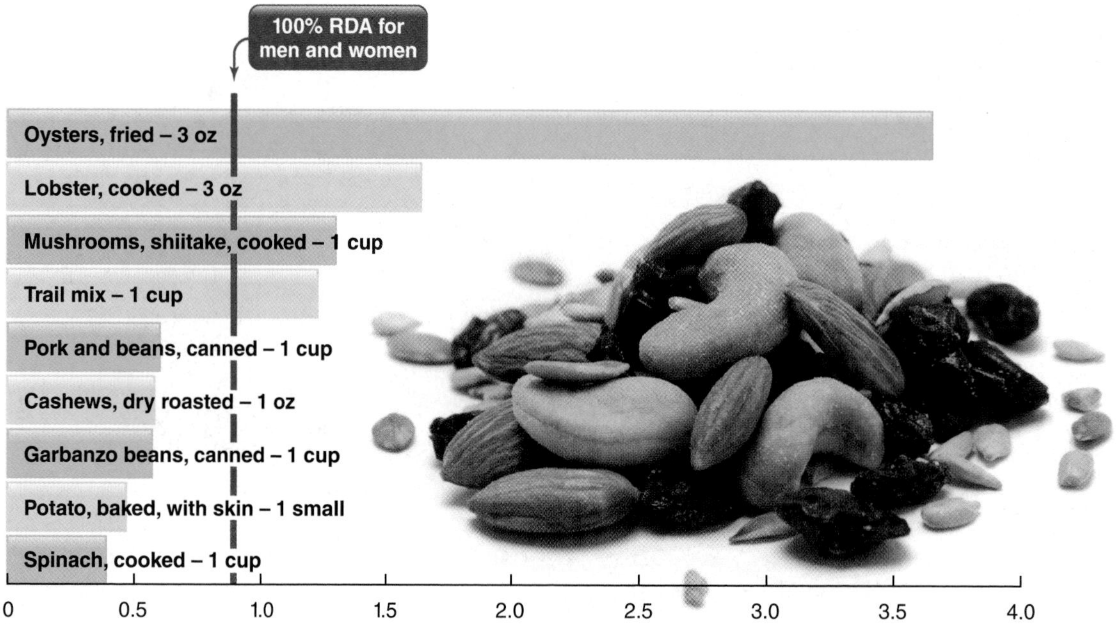

Figure 10.17 Common food sources of copper. The RDA for copper is 900 μg/day for men and women.

Data from U.S. Department of Agriculture, Agricultural Research Service, 2009, USDA Nutrient Database for Standard Reference, Release 22. Nutrient Data Laboratory Home Page, www.ars.usda.gov/ba/bhnrc/ndl.

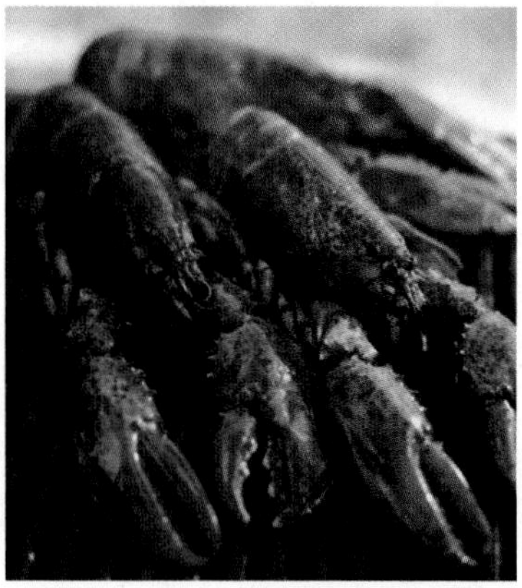

Lobster is a food that contains copper.

As you can see in Table 10.2, our need for copper is small. Copper is widely distributed in foods, and people who eat a varied diet can easily meet their requirements. Good food sources of copper include organ meats, seafood, nuts, and seeds. Whole-grain foods are also relatively good sources. **Figure 10.17** identifies some foods relatively high in copper.

As we saw with iron and zinc, people with low dietary copper intakes absorb more copper than people with high dietary intakes. Also recall that high zinc intakes can reduce copper absorption and, subsequently, copper status. In fact, zinc supplementation is used to treat a rare disorder called Wilson's disease, in which copper toxicity occurs. High iron intakes can also interfere with copper absorption in infants.

The long-term effects of copper toxicity are not well studied in humans. Toxicity symptoms include abdominal pain and cramps, nausea, diarrhea, and vomiting. Liver damage occurs in the extreme cases of copper toxicity that occur with Wilson's disease and other health conditions associated with excessive copper levels.

Copper deficiency is rare but can occur in premature infants fed milk-based formulas and in adults fed prolonged formulated diets that are deficient in copper. Deficiency symptoms include anemia, reduced levels of white blood cells, and osteoporosis in infants and growing children.

RECAP Zinc is a trace mineral that is a part of almost a hundred enzymes that impact virtually every body system. It plays a critical role in hemoglobin synthesis, physical growth and sexual maturation, and immune function and assists in fighting oxidative damage. Copper is a trace mineral that functions as a cofactor in the metabolic pathways that produce energy, in the production of connective tissues, and as part of an antioxidant enzyme system. It is also a component of ceruloplasmin, a protein that is critical for the transport of iron.

Nutrition DEBATE

Do Zinc Lozenges Help Fight the Common Cold?

Approximately 1 billion colds occur in the United States each year.[44] Children suffer from six to ten colds each year, and adults average two to four. Although colds are typically benign, they result in significant absenteeism from work and cause discomfort and stress. It is estimated that more than two hundred different viruses can cause a cold. Because of this variety, developing vaccines or other preventive measures for colds is extremely challenging. Thus, finding a cure for the common cold has been at the forefront of modern medicine for many years.

The role of zinc in the health of our immune system is well known, but zinc has also been shown to inhibit the replication of some of the viruses that cause the common cold. These findings have led to speculation that taking zinc supplements may reduce the length and severity of colds.[45,46] Zinc lozenges were formulated as a means of providing potential relief from cold symptoms. These lozenges are readily found in a variety of formulations and dosages in most drugstores.

Does taking zinc in lozenge form actually reduce the length and severity of a cold? During the past 20 years, numerous research studies have been conducted to try to answer this question. Unfortunately, the results of these studies are inconclusive: about half have found that zinc lozenges do reduce the length and severity of a cold, whereas about half have found that zinc lozenges have no effect on cold symptoms or duration.[47] Some reasons that researchers have proposed to explain these different findings include the following:

- Researchers are unable to truly "blind" participants to the treatment. Because zinc lozenges have a unique taste, it may be difficult to keep the research participants uninformed about whether they are getting zinc lozenges or a placebo. Knowing what they are taking could lead participants to report biased results.
- Self-reported symptoms are subject to inaccuracy. Many studies had the research participants self-report changes in symptoms. Such self-reports may be inaccurate and influenced by emotional factors.
- A wide variety of viruses can cause a cold. We noted that more than two hundred different viruses can cause a cold, and it is highly unlikely that zinc can combat all of these. It is possible that people who do not respond favorably to zinc lozenges are suffering from a cold virus that cannot be treated with zinc.
- Zinc dosages and formulations differ. The dosages of zinc consumed, the timing of consumption, and the formulation of the lozenge used differed across studies. For example, it is estimated that, for zinc to be effective, at least 80 mg of zinc should be consumed each day and that people should begin using zinc lozenges within 48 hours of the onset of cold symptoms, yet the studies followed a variety of dosing and timing protocols. Also, different sweeteners and flavorings found in different zinc-lozenge formulations may bind the zinc and inhibit its ability to be absorbed into the body, limiting its effectiveness.
- Supplements may provide excessive zinc and actually impair immune function! The level of zinc noted earlier as the effective dose—80 mg/day—is nearly ten times the RDA and can decrease the absorption of copper and iron if continued for long periods of time. In addition, one experimental study showed that 300 mg/day of supplemental zinc *reduced* immune cell response and *decreased* destruction of bacteria.[48] This amount is about six tablets of a zinc gluconate pill that has 50 mg of elemental zinc.
- Measuring the compliance of test participants can be difficult. Typically, participants need to take one zinc lozenge every 2 to 3 hours while they are awake for the duration of the study, which can last 6 to 10 days. Unless the participants are monitored by research staff, researchers have to rely on the participants to self-report their compliance to the study protocol. Of course, different compliance rates can alter the outcomes of different studies.

Zinc lozenges come in different formulations and dosages.

In short, there is no conclusive evidence supporting or refuting the effectiveness of zinc lozenges in treating the common cold.

One word of caution: if you decide to use zinc lozenges, more is not better. Excessive or prolonged zinc supplementation can reduce immune function and cause other mineral imbalances. Check the label of the product you are using, and do not exceed its recommended dosage or duration of use.

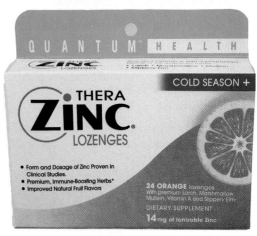

Chapter Review

Test Yourself ANSWERS

1. **False.** B-vitamins do not directly provide energy for our body. However, they play critical roles in ensuring that our body is able to generate energy from carbohydrates, fats, and proteins.

2. **True.** People who consume a vegan diet need to pay particularly close attention to consuming enough vitamin B_{12}, iron, and zinc. In some cases, these individuals may need to take supplements to consume adequate amounts of these nutrients.

3. **True.** This deficiency is particularly common in infants, children, and women of childbearing age.

Find the Quack

Like many college students, Dionna maintains a full course load and works part-time. She also participates in aerobics and yoga classes four afternoons a week, is a member of her college math and chess clubs, and spends Saturday mornings volunteering at a local food bank. With so much going on in her life, she's had to stay up way past midnight almost every night for the past few weeks to finish homework assignments and study for exams. Coming out of aerobics class yesterday, she collapsed onto the bench in the locker room, feeling utterly exhausted. Her friend Addie asked what was wrong and, when Dionna explained, gave her a hug and opened her gym bag. "Here," she said, handing Dionna a bottle of supplements. The label said *Fatigue-Fighting Formula for Women*, and the ingredients list indicated that the supplement provided 100% of the Daily Value for all eight B-vitamins, as well as iron, selenium, chromium, and manganese. "Start taking one of these every day, like I do, and you'll have all the energy you need!"

Dionna took a swig from her water bottle and swallowed a tablet. Then she read the back of the supplement label. It said:

- "If you experience fatigue, muscle weakness, difficulty concentrating, or depression, you may have a deficiency of the vitamins and minerals important in maintaining an adequate level of energy."
- "One tablet a day of *Fatigue-Fighting Formula for Women* may help restore your natural vitality."
- Our average customer rating for this product is five stars! A typical satisfied customer: "I used to feel so exhausted that I could barely drag myself through the days. *Fatigue-Fighting Formula for Women* has given me energy to spare!" —Tasha from Santa Monica.

Dionna asked her friend how much a bottle of the supplement—which included 60 tablets, or a 2-month supply—cost. Addie said that she ordered them online for $23.99 and would be placing another order soon. "Want me to get a bottle for you?"

1. Read carefully the first two bulleted statements from the back of the supplement label. Do these assertions strike you as reasonable, exaggerated, misleading, or entirely false? Explain your answer.
2. What, if any, health concerns might the level of vitamins and minerals in this supplement raise?
3. Tasha from Santa Monica states that the supplement "has given me energy to spare." Comment on the implication of her statement that the micronutrients it provides give us energy.
4. Should Dionna have Addie order a bottle of the supplements for her? Why or why not?

Answers can be found on the companion website, at www.pearsonhighered.com/thompsonmanore.

NutriTools Check out the companion website at www.pearsonhighered.com/thompsonmanore, or use MyNutritionLab.com, to access interactive animations including:

- Vitamin Functionality
- Mineral Functionality

Review Questions

1. The B-vitamins include
   a. niacin, folate, and iodine.
   b. cobalamin, iodine, and chromium.
   c. manganese, riboflavin, and pyridoxine.
   d. thiamin, pantothenic acid, and biotin.
2. The micronutrient most closely associated with blood clotting is
   a. iron.
   b. vitamin K.
   c. zinc.
   d. vitamin B_{12}.
3. Which of the following statements about iron is true?
   a. Iron is stored primarily in the liver, the blood vessel walls, and the heart muscle.
   b. Iron is a component of hemoglobin, myoglobin, and certain enzymes.
   c. Iron is a component of red blood cells, platelets, and plasma.
   d. Excess iron is stored primarily in the form of ferritin, cytochromes, and intrinsic factor.
4. Homocysteine is
   a. a by-product of glycolysis.
   b. a trace mineral.
   c. an amino acid.
   d. a B-vitamin.
5. Which of the following statements about choline is true?
   a. Choline is found exclusively in foods of animal origin.
   b. Choline is a B-vitamin that assists in homocysteine metabolism.
   c. Choline is a neurotransmitter that is involved in muscle movement and memory storage.
   d. Choline is necessary for the synthesis of phospholipids and other components of cell membranes.
6. True or false? Blood has four components: erythrocytes, leukocytes, platelets, and plasma.
7. True or false? There is no DRI for sulfur.
8. True or false? Iron is found only in foods of animal origin.
9. True or false? The best way for a pregnant woman to protect her fetus against neural tube defects is to begin taking a folate supplement as soon as she learns she is pregnant.
10. True or false? Wilson's disease occurs when copper deficiency allows accumulation of iron in the body.

Answers to Review Questions can be found at the back of this text, and additional essay questions and answers are located on the companion website at www.pearsonhighered.com/thompsonmanore.

Web Resources

www.ars.usda.gov
Nutrient Data Laboratory Home Page

Click on Search to find reports listing food sources for selected nutrients.

www.anemia.com
Anemia Lifeline

Visit this site to learn about anemia and its various treatments.

www.unicef.org/nutrition
UNICEF-Nutrition

This site provides information about micronutrient deficiencies in developing countries and the efforts to combat them.

www.thearc.org
The Arc

Search this site for "neural tube defects" and find a wealth of information on the development and prevention of these conditions.

IN DEPTH

Dietary Supplements: Necessity or Waste?

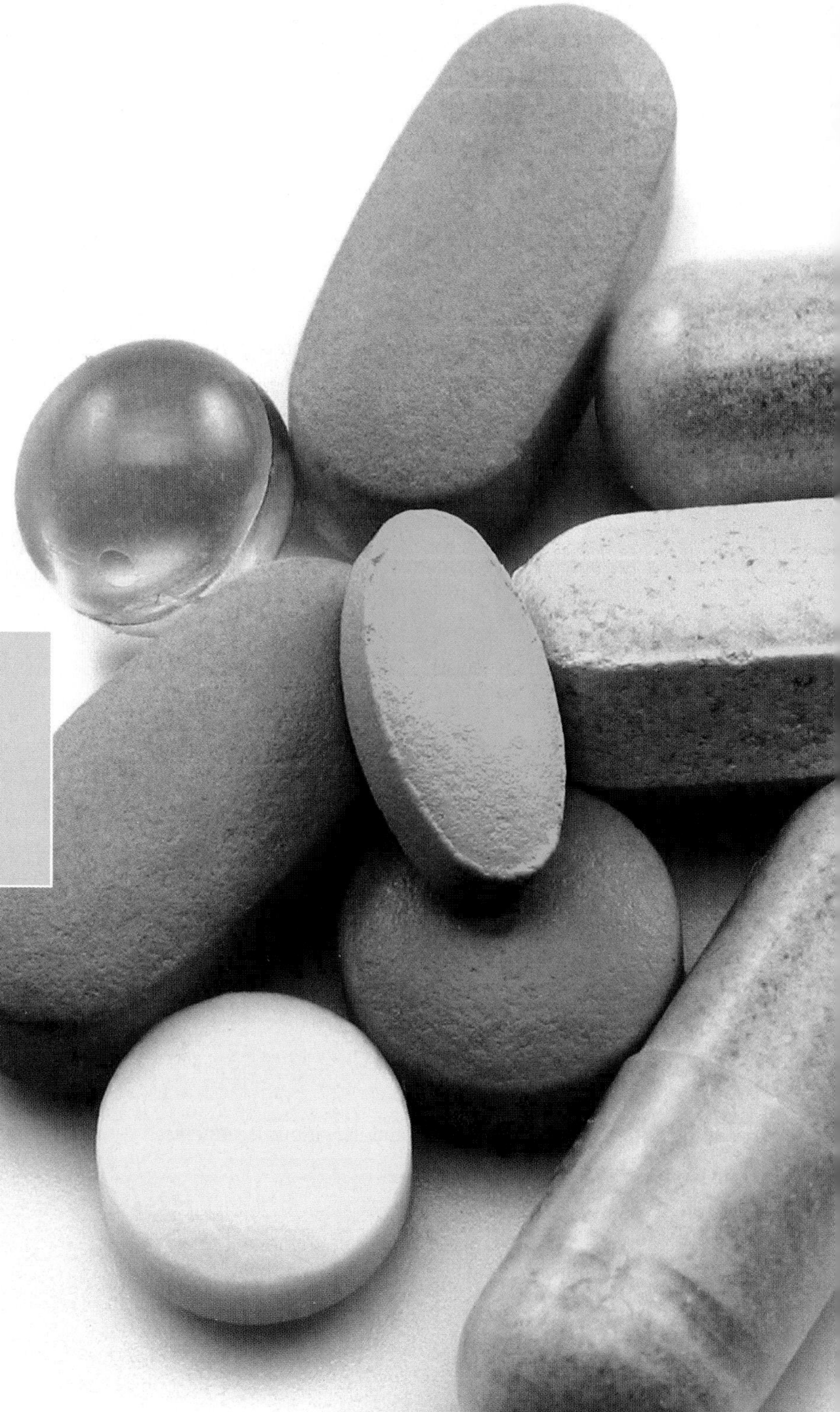

WANT TO FIND OUT. . .

- if dietary supplements are as tightly regulated as drugs?
- how to spot a fraudulent supplement?
- whether or not you should take a multivitamin-mineral supplement?

READ ON.

Marcus has type 2 diabetes and high blood pressure and is worried about his health. He attended a nutrition seminar in which the health benefits of various dietary supplements were touted. After attending this seminar, Marcus was convinced that he needed to take a supplement providing 200–800% of the Daily Value for many vitamins and minerals, as well as an herbal preparation for "heart health." After a few months of taking these supplements on a daily basis, Marcus started to experience headaches, nausea, diarrhea, and tingling in his hands and feet. Although Marcus was not an expert in nutrition, he suspected that he might be experiencing side effects related to nutrient toxicity. He decided to talk to his doctor about the supplements he was taking to determine whether they could be causing his symptoms.

Marcus's story is not unique. The use of dietary supplements in the United States has skyrocketed in recent years. One industry source cites annual sales of supplements in the United States at $25.5 billion.[1] A recent review of national opinion surveys found that a significant number of Americans regularly take dietary supplements, but they do not report the use of these products to their physicians because they feel their physicians have little knowledge of these products and may harbor a bias toward their use.[2] Interestingly, many supplement users state that they would continue to use these products even if scientific studies found them to be ineffective!

Why do so many people take dietary supplements? Many people believe they cannot consume adequate nutrients in their diet, and they take a supplement as extra nutritional insurance. Others have been advised by their healthcare provider to take a supplement to address a given health concern. There are people, like Marcus, who believe that they can use certain supplements to treat their disease. Others use supplements in the hope that they'll enhance their appearance or athletic performance.

Are such uses wise? A waste of money? Dangerous? Who *should* be taking supplements? Here, we explore ***In Depth*** the answers to these questions and more.

What Are Dietary Supplements?

According to the U.S. Food and Drug Administration (FDA), a **dietary supplement** is "a product taken by mouth that contains a 'dietary ingredient' intended to supplement the diet."[3] Supplements may contain vitamins, minerals, herbs or other botanicals, amino acids, enzymes, tissues from animal organs or glands, or a concentrate, a metabolite, a constituent, or an extract. Supplements come in many forms, including pills, capsules, liquids, and powders **(Figure 1)**.

How Are Dietary Supplements Regulated?

As presented in the Dietary Supplement Health and Education Act (DSHEA) of 1994, dietary supplements are categorized within the general group of foods, not drugs. This means that the regulation of supplements is much less rigorous than the regulation of drugs. Currently, the FDA is reconsidering how it regulates food and supplements that are marketed with health claims, but no changes have been finalized at this time. As an informed consumer, you should know that

- Dietary supplements do not need approval from the FDA before they are marketed.

dietary supplement A product taken by mouth that contains a "dietary ingredient" intended to supplement the diet.

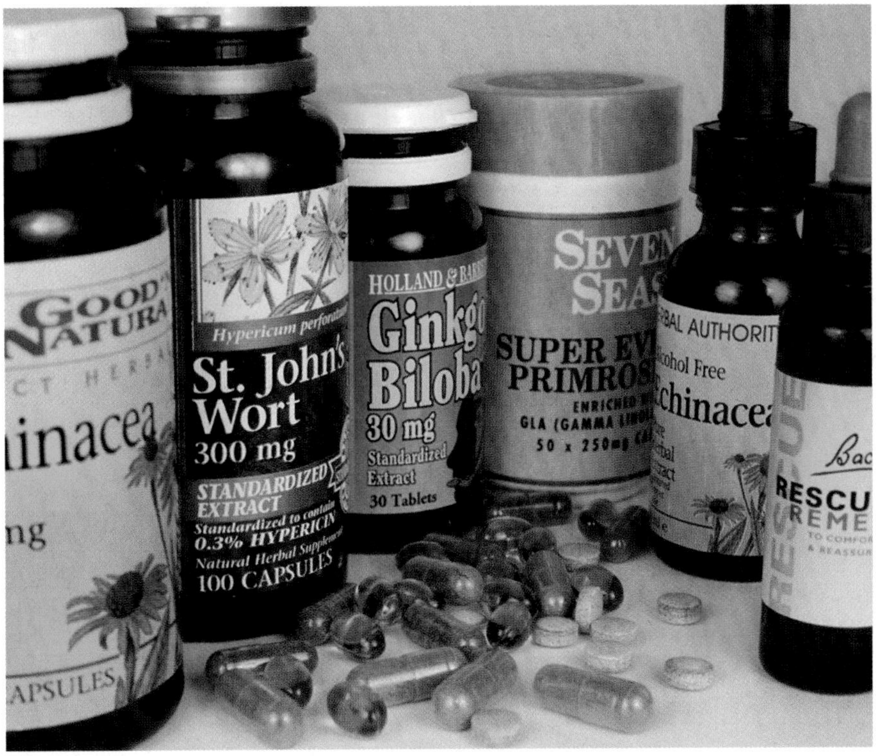

Figure 1 Dietary supplements can be pills, capsules, powders, or liquids and contain micronutrients, amino acids, herbs, or other substances.

- The company that manufactures a supplement is responsible for determining that the supplement is safe; the FDA does not test any supplement for safety prior to marketing.
- Supplement companies do not have to provide the FDA with any evidence that their supplements are safe unless the company is marketing a new dietary ingredient that was not sold in the United States prior to 1994.
- There are at present no federal guidelines on practices to ensure the purity, quality, safety, and composition of dietary supplements.
- There are no rules to limit the serving size or amount of a nutrient in any dietary supplement.
- Once a supplement is marketed, the FDA must prove it unsafe before the product will be removed from the market.

Despite these limitations in supplement regulation, supplement manufacturers are required to follow dietary supplement labeling guidelines. **Figure 2** shows a label from a multivitamin and mineral supplement. As you can see, there are specific requirements for the information that must be included on the supplement label. Federal advertising regulations also require that any claims on the label must be truthful and not misleading and that advertisers must be able to substantiate all label claims. In addition, labels bearing a claim must also include the disclaimer "This statement has not been evaluated by the FDA. This product is not intended to diagnose, cure, or prevent any disease." Any products not meeting these guidelines can be removed from the market.

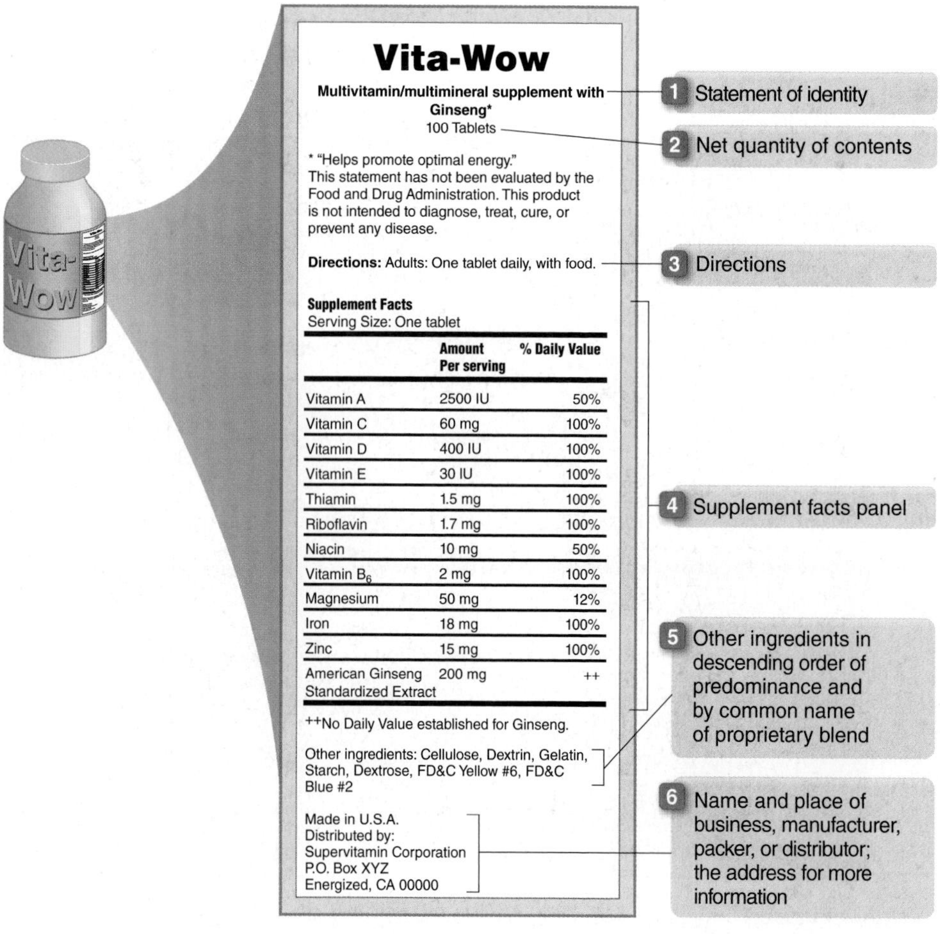
Vita-Wow
Multivitamin/multimineral supplement with Ginseng*
100 Tablets
* "Helps promote optimal energy."
This statement has not been evaluated by the Food and Drug Administration. This product is not intended to diagnose, treat, cure, or prevent any disease.
Directions: Adults: One tablet daily, with food.
Supplement Facts
Serving Size: One tablet
Amount Per serving
% Daily Value
Vitamin A 2500 IU 50%
Vitamin C 60 mg 100%
Vitamin D 400 IU 100%
Vitamin E 30 IU 100%
Thiamin 1.5 mg 100%
Riboflavin 1.7 mg 100%
Niacin 10 mg 50%
Vitamin B6 2 mg 100%
Magnesium 50 mg 12%
Iron 18 mg 100%
Zinc 15 mg 100%
American Ginseng Standardized Extract 200 mg ++
++No Daily Value established for Ginseng.
Other ingredients: Cellulose, Dextrin, Gelatin, Starch, Dextrose, FD&C Yellow #6, FD&C Blue #2
Made in U.S.A.
Distributed by:
Supervitamin Corporation
P.O. Box XYZ
Energized, CA 00000
1 Statement of identity
2 Net quantity of contents
3 Directions
4 Supplement facts panel
5 Other ingredients in descending order of predominance and by common name of proprietary blend
6 Name and place of business, manufacturer, packer, or distributor; the address for more information

Figure 2 A multivitamin-mineral supplement label highlighting the dietary supplement labeling guidelines.

How Can You Avoid Fraudulent or Dangerous Supplements?

Although many of the supplement products sold today are safe, some are not. In addition, some companies are less than forthright about the true content of ingredients in their supplements. How can you avoid purchasing fraudulent or dangerous supplements? The FDA suggests that consumers can practice tips (see Quick Tips on page 363) to protect themselves from fraudulent or dangerous supplements.[4]

Many supplements are also sold over the Internet. Researchers suggest six criteria that can be used to evaluate dietary supplement websites.[5] Keep these criteria in mind each time you consider buying a dietary supplement over the Web:

1. What is the purpose of the website? Is it trying to sell a product or educate the consumer? Keep in mind that the primary purpose of supplement companies is to make money. Look for sites that provide educational information about a specific nutrient or product and that don't just focus on selling the products.
2. Does the site contain accurate information? Accuracy of the information on the website is the most difficult thing for a consumer to determine. Testimonials are *not* reliable and accurate; claims supported by scientific research are most desirable. If what the company claims about its product sounds too good to be true, it probably is.
3. Does the site contain reputable references? References should be from articles published in peer-reviewed scientific journals. References should be complete and contain author

QUICK TIPS

Taking Precautions with Supplements

✓ Look for the U.S. Pharmacopoeia (U.S.P.) symbol or notation on the label. This symbol indicates that the manufacturer followed the standards that the U.S.P. has established for features such as purity, strength, quality, packaging, labeling, and acceptable length of storage.

✓ Consider buying recognized brands of supplements. Although not guaranteed, products made by nationally recognized companies more likely have well-established manufacturing standards.

✓ Do not assume that the word *natural* on the label means that the product is safe. Arsenic, lead, and mercury are all natural substances that can kill you if consumed in large enough quantities.

✓ Do not hesitate to question a company about how it makes its products. Reputable companies have nothing to hide and are more than happy to inform their customers about the safety and quality of their products.

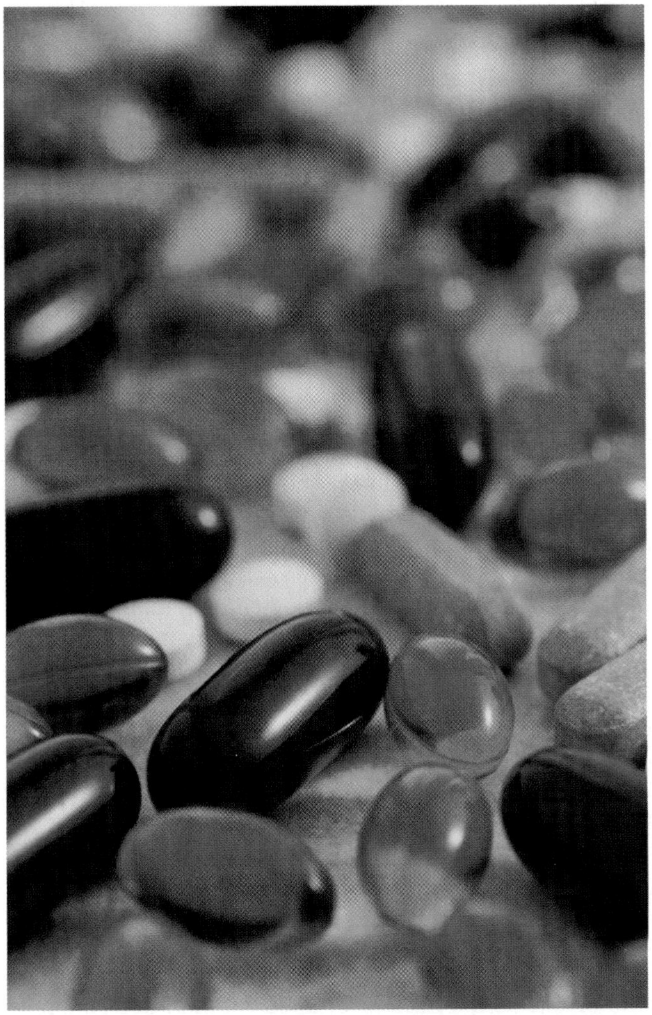

Always research a dietary supplement and its manufacturer before taking it.

names, article title, journal title, date, volume, and page numbers. This information allows the consumer to check original research for the validity of a company's claims about its product. Be cautious of sites that refer to claims that are "proven by research studies" but fail to provide a complete reference.

4. Who owns or sponsors the site? Full disclosure regarding sponsorship and possible sources of bias or conflict of interest should be included in the site's information.
5. Who wrote the information? Websites should clearly identify the author of the article and include the credentials of the author. Recognized experts include individuals with relevant health-related credentials, such as RD, PhD, MD, or MS. Keep in mind that this person is responsible for the information posted in the article but may not be the creator of the website.
6. Is the information current and updated regularly? As information about supplements changes regularly, websites should be updated regularly, and the date should be clearly posted. All websites should also include contact information to allow consumers to ask questions about the information posted.

Are There Special Precautions for Herbal Supplements?

A common saying in India cautions that "A house without ginger is a sick house." Indeed, ginger, echinacea, lavender, and many other herbs have been used by different cultures throughout the world for centuries to promote health and treat discomfort and disease. The National Center for Complementary and Alternative Medicine (NCCAM) defines an **herb** (also

herb A plant or plant part used for its scent, flavor, and/or therapeutic properties (also called a *botanical*).

called a *botanical*) as a plant or plant part used for its scent, flavor, and/or therapeutic properties.[6] As you would suspect, with a definition this broad there are hundreds of different herbs on the market. In 2008, U.S. consumers spent $4.8 billion on herbal and botanical supplements.[1]

It is clear that some herbs are effective medicines, but for what disorders, in what forms, and at what dosages? And are some herbs promoted as medicines ineffective, or even dangerous? To answer these questions about herbs you might be considering, NCCAM evaluates dozens of the most commonly used herbs in "Herbs at a Glance" fact sheets, available at its website. See the Web Resources at the end of this chapter. In addition, NCCAM recommends that you practice the Quick Tips listed earlier for all types of dietary supplements, as well as the following precautions, which are specific to the use of herbs.

The most essential of these precautions is to consult your healthcare provider before using any herbal supplement. Herbs can act the same way as drugs; therefore, they can cause medical problems if not used correctly or if taken in large amounts. In some cases, people have experienced negative effects even though they followed the instructions on a supplement label. It's especially important to check with your healthcare provider if you are taking any prescription medications. Some herbal supplements are known to interact with medications in ways that cause health problems.

It is critical to avoid using herbs if you are pregnant or nursing, unless your physician has approved their use. Some can promote miscarriage or birth defects or can enter breast milk. This caution also applies to treating children with herbal supplements.

Finally, be aware that the active ingredients in many herbs and herbal supplements are not known. There may be dozens, even hundreds, of unknown compounds in an herbal supplement. Also, published analyses of herbal supplements have found differences between what's listed on the label and what's in the bottle. This means you may be taking less—or more—of the supplement than what the label indicates or ingesting substances not mentioned on the label. Some herbal supplements have been found to be contaminated with metals, unlabeled prescription drugs, microorganisms, and other substances. An investigation by the United States Government Accountability Office reported in 2010 that nearly all of the herbal supplements they had tested were found to contain traces of lead and other contaminants.[7] Be aware that the word *standardized, certified,* or *verified* on a label is no guarantee of product quality; in the United States, these terms have no legal definition for supplements.

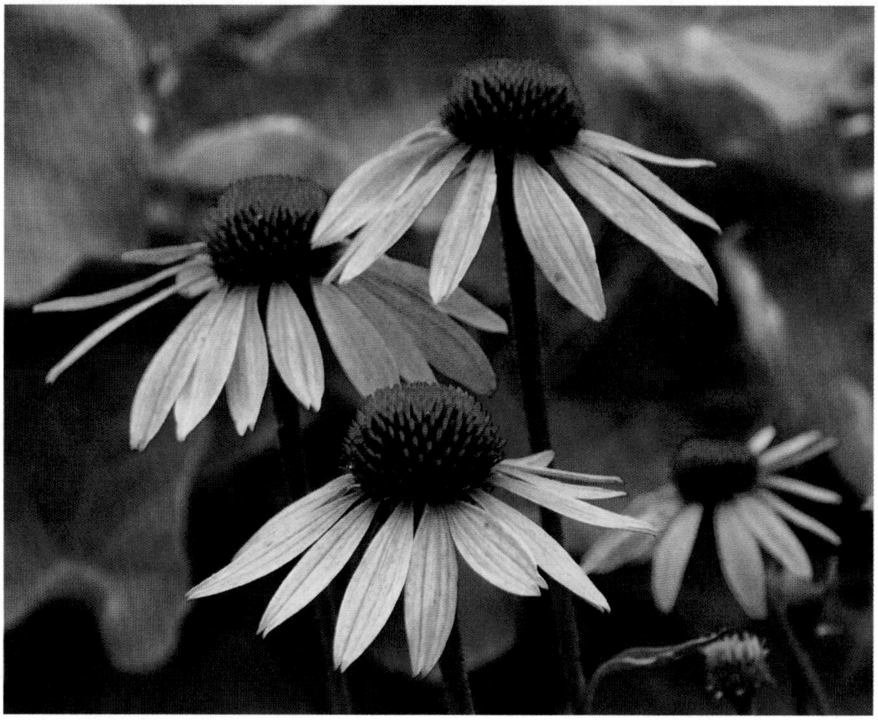

Echinacea, commonly known as purple coneflower, has been used for centuries to prevent colds, flu, and other infections.

Should You Take a Dietary Supplement?

Contrary to what some people believe, the U.S. food supply is not void of nutrients, and all people do not need to supplement their diets all of the time. In fact, we now know that foods contain a diverse combination of compounds that are critical to our health, and vitamin and mineral supplements do not contain the same amount or variety of substances found in foods. Thus, dietary supplements are not substitutes for whole foods. However, nutritional needs change throughout the life span, so you may benefit from taking a supplement at certain times for certain reasons. For instance, if you adopt a vegan diet in your college years, your healthcare provider might prescribe a supplement providing riboflavin, vitamin B_{12}, vitamin D, calcium, iron, and zinc. Animal products are high in these nutrients, so if you eliminate these foods, you might not get enough of these nutrients in the other foods you are eating. Or if you're a member of your college soccer team, your team's sport dietitian might advise taking a supplement specially formulated to provide micronutrients that support intense physical activity.

Dietary supplements include hundreds of thousands of products sold for many purposes, and it is impossible to discuss here all of the various situations in which their use may be advisable. So to simplify this discussion, let's focus on identifying the groups of people who may or may not benefit from taking vitamin and mineral supplements.

Table 1 lists groups of people who may benefit from supplementation. But even if you fall within one of these groups, it's still important to analyze your total diet to determine whether you might need to take the vitamin or mineral supplement indicated. It is also a good idea to check with your healthcare provider or a registered dietitian (RD) before taking any supplements, as supplements can interfere with some prescription and over-the-counter medications.

Of course, many people who do not need to take supplements do so, anyway. The following are instances in which taking vitamin and mineral supplements is unnecessary, or even harmful:

1. Providing fluoride supplements to children who already drink fluoridated water.
2. Taking supplements in the belief that they will cure a disease, such as cancer, diabetes, or heart disease.
3. Taking supplements with certain medications. For instance, people who take the blood-thinning drug Coumadin should not take vitamin E or K supplements, as this can cause excessive bleeding. People who take aspirin daily should check with their physician before taking vitamin E or K supplements, as aspirin also thins the blood.[8]
4. Taking nonprescribed supplements if you have liver or kidney disease. Physicians may prescribe vitamin and mineral supplements for their patients because many nutrients are lost during treatment for these diseases. However, these individuals cannot properly metabolize certain supplements and should not take any that are not prescribed by their physician because of a high risk for toxicity.
5. Taking beta-carotene supplements if you are a smoker. There is evidence that beta-carotene supplementation increases the risk for lung and other cancers in smokers.
6. Taking vitamins and minerals in an attempt to improve physical appearance or athletic performance. There is no evidence that vitamin and mineral supplements enhance appearance or athletic performance in healthy adults who consume a varied diet with adequate energy.
7. Taking supplements to increase your energy level. Vitamin and mineral supplements do not provide energy, because they do not contain fat, carbohydrate, or protein (sources of Calories). Although many vitamins and minerals are necessary for us to produce energy, taking dietary

TABLE 1 Individuals Who May Benefit from Dietary Supplementation

Type of Individual	Specific Supplements That May Help
Newborns	Routinely given a single dose of vitamin K at birth
Infants	Depends on age and nutrition; may need iron, vitamin D, or other nutrients
Children not drinking fluoridated water	Fluoride supplements
Children on strict vegetarian diets	Vitamin B_{12}, iron, zinc, vitamin D (if not exposed to sunlight)
Children with poor eating habits or overweight children on an energy-restricted diet	Multivitamin/multimineral supplement that does not exceed the RDA for the nutrients it contains
Pregnant teenagers	Iron and folic acid; other nutrients may be necessary if diet is very poor
Women who may become pregnant	Multivitamin or multivitamin/multimineral supplement that contains 0.4 mg of folic acid
Pregnant or lactating women	Multivitamin/multimineral supplement that contains iron, folic acid, zinc, copper, calcium, vitamin B_6, vitamin C, and vitamin D
People on prolonged weight-reduction diets	Multivitamin/multimineral supplement
People recovering from serious illness or surgery	Multivitamin/multimineral supplement
People with HIV/AIDS or other wasting diseases; people addicted to drugs or alcohol	Multivitamin/multimineral supplement or single-nutrient supplements
People who do not consume adequate calcium	Calcium supplements: for example, women need to consume 1,300 mg of dietary calcium per day; thus, supplements may be necessary
People whose exposure to sunlight is inadequate to allow synthesis of adequate vitamin D	Vitamin D
People eating a vegan diet	Vitamin B_{12}, riboflavin, calcium, vitamin D, iron, and zinc
People who have had portions of their intestinal tract removed; people who have a malabsorptive disease	Depends on the exact condition; may include various fat-soluble and/or water-soluble vitamins and other nutrients
People with lactose intolerance	Calcium supplements
Elderly people	Multivitamin/multimineral supplement, vitamin B_{12}

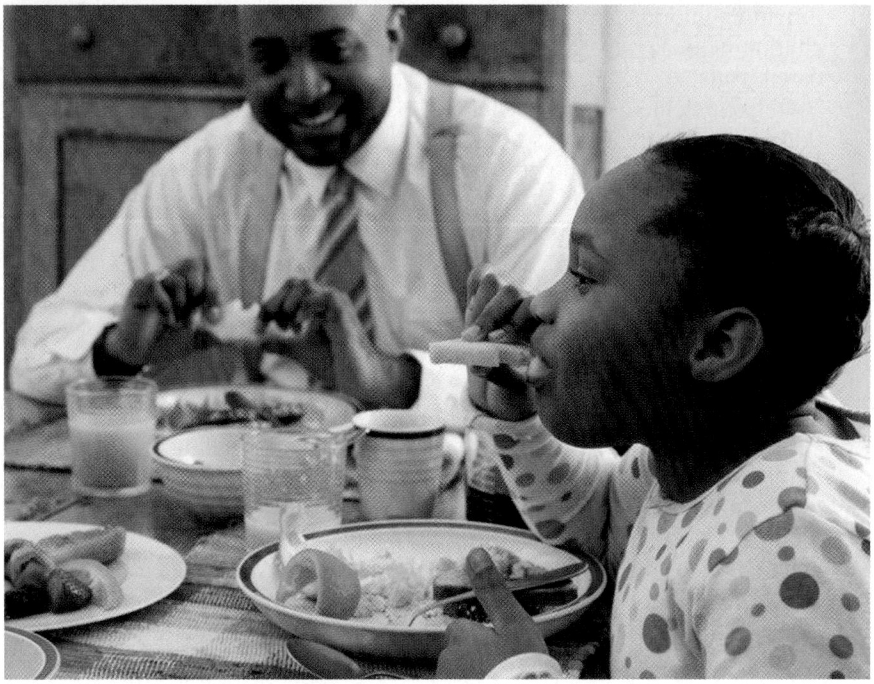

One of the best strategies for maintaining good health is to eat a diet that provides a rich variety of whole foods. If you do that, you probably won't need to take supplements.

supplements in place of eating food will not provide us with the energy necessary to live a healthy and productive life.

8. Taking single-nutrient supplements, unless a qualified healthcare practitioner prescribes a single-nutrient supplement for a diagnosed medical condition (for example, prescribing iron supplements for someone with anemia). These products contain very high amounts of the given nutrient, and taking them can quickly lead to toxicity.

The American Dietetic Association advises that the ideal nutritional strategy for optimizing health is to eat a healthful diet that contains a variety of whole foods.[9] This way, you probably will not need to take vitamin and mineral supplements. And if you do use a supplement, select one that contains no more than 100% of the recommended levels for the nutrients it contains. Avoid taking single-nutrient supplements unless advised to do so by your healthcare practitioner. Finally, avoid taking supplements that contain substances that are known to cause illness or injuries. Some of these substances are listed in **Table 2**.

NUTRI-CASE THEO

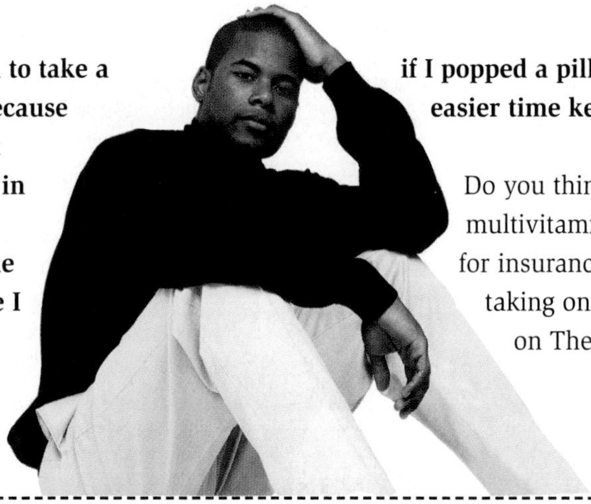

"You know, I never thought I needed to take a multivitamin-mineral supplement because I'm healthy and I eat lots of different kinds of foods. But now I've learned in my nutrition course about what all these vitamins and minerals do in the body, and I'm thinking, heck, maybe I should take one just for insurance. I mean, I use up a lot of fuel playing basketball and working out. Maybe if I popped a pill every day, I'd have an easier time keeping my weight up!"

Do you think Theo should take a multivitamin-mineral supplement "just for insurance"? Why or why not? Would taking one be likely to have any effect on Theo's weight?

TABLE 2 Supplement Ingredients Associated with Illnesses and Injuries

Ingredient	Potential Risks
Herbal Ingredients	
Chaparral	Liver disease
Kava (also known as kava kava)	Severe liver toxicity
Comfrey	Obstruction of blood flow to liver, possible death
Slimming/dieter's teas	Nausea, diarrhea, vomiting, stomach cramps, constipation, fainting, possible death
Ephedra (also known as *ma huang*, Chinese ephedra, and epitonin)	High blood pressure, irregular heartbeat, nerve damage, insomnia, tremors, headaches, seizures, heart attack, stroke, possible death
Germander	Liver disease, possible death
Lobelia	Breathing problems, excessive sweating, rapid heartbeat, low blood pressure, coma, possible death
Magnolia-Stephania preparation	Kidney disease, can lead to permanent kidney failure
Willow bark	Reye's syndrome (a potentially fatal disease that may occur when children take aspirin), allergic reaction in adults
Wormwood	Numbness of legs and arms, loss of intellectual processing, delirium, paralysis
Vitamins and Essential Minerals	
Vitamin A (when taking 25,000 IU or more per day)	Birth defects, bone abnormalities, severe liver disease
Vitamin B_6 (when taking more than 100 mg per day)	Loss of balance, injuries to nerves that alter our touch sensation
Niacin (when taking slow-release doses of 500 mg or more per day, or when taking immediate-release doses of 750 mg or more per day)	Stomach pain; nausea; vomiting; bloating; cramping; diarrhea; liver disease; damage to the muscles, eye, and heart
Selenium (when taking 800 to 1,000 μg per day)	Tissue damage
Other Ingredients	
Germanium (a nonessential mineral)	Kidney damage
L-tryptophan (an amino acid)	Eosinophilia-myalgia syndrome (a potentially fatal blood disorder that causes high fever)

Data from U.S. Food and Drug Administration. 2007. Dietary supplements. Warnings and safety information. Available at http://www.cfsan.fda.gov/~dms/ds-warn.html; and U.S. Food and Drug Administration. 1998. Supplements associated with illnesses and injuries. *FDA Consumer Magazine*, September/October. Available at www.fda.gov/fdac/features/1998/dietchrt.html.

Web Resources

www.dietary-supplements.info.nih.gov
Office of Dietary Supplements

Search this website to find reports evaluating individual supplements you might be considering, as well as general information about the health benefits, safety, and regulation of dietary supplements.

www.cfsan.fda.gov
U.S. Food and Drug Administration (FDA)

This site provides information on how to make informed decisions and evaluate information related to dietary supplements.

www.nal.usda.gov/fnic
The Food and Nutrition Information Center (FNIC)

Click on the Dietary Supplements button to obtain information on vitamin and mineral supplements, including consumer reports and industry regulations.

www.nccam.nih.gov/health/herbsataglance
National Center for Complementary and Alternative Medicine

Click on the name of an herb to find out how it has traditionally been used, the status of current research into its effectiveness and safety, and other information.

11 Achieving and Maintaining a Healthful Body Weight

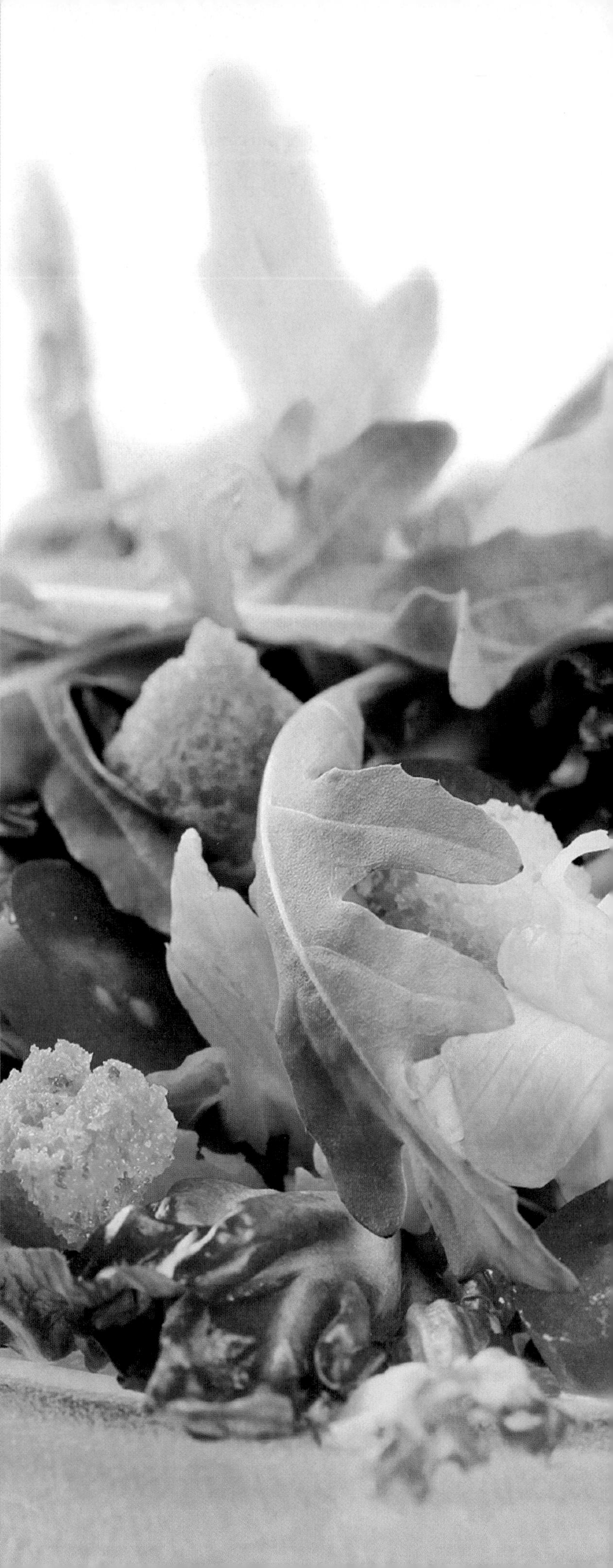

CHAPTER OBJECTIVES

After reading this chapter you will be able to:

1. **Describe what is meant by a healthful weight, p. 370.**
2. **Define the terms *underweight*, *overweight*, *obesity*, and *morbid obesity*, pp. 370–371.**
3. **List at least three methods that can be used to assess your body composition or risk for overweight, pp. 372–374.**
4. **Identify and discuss the three components of energy expenditure, pp. 375–379.**
5. **List and describe at least two theories that link genetic influences to control of body weight, pp. 381–382.**
6. **Discuss at least two societal factors that influence our body weight, pp. 385–387.**
7. **Develop an action plan for healthful weight loss, pp. 390–397.**

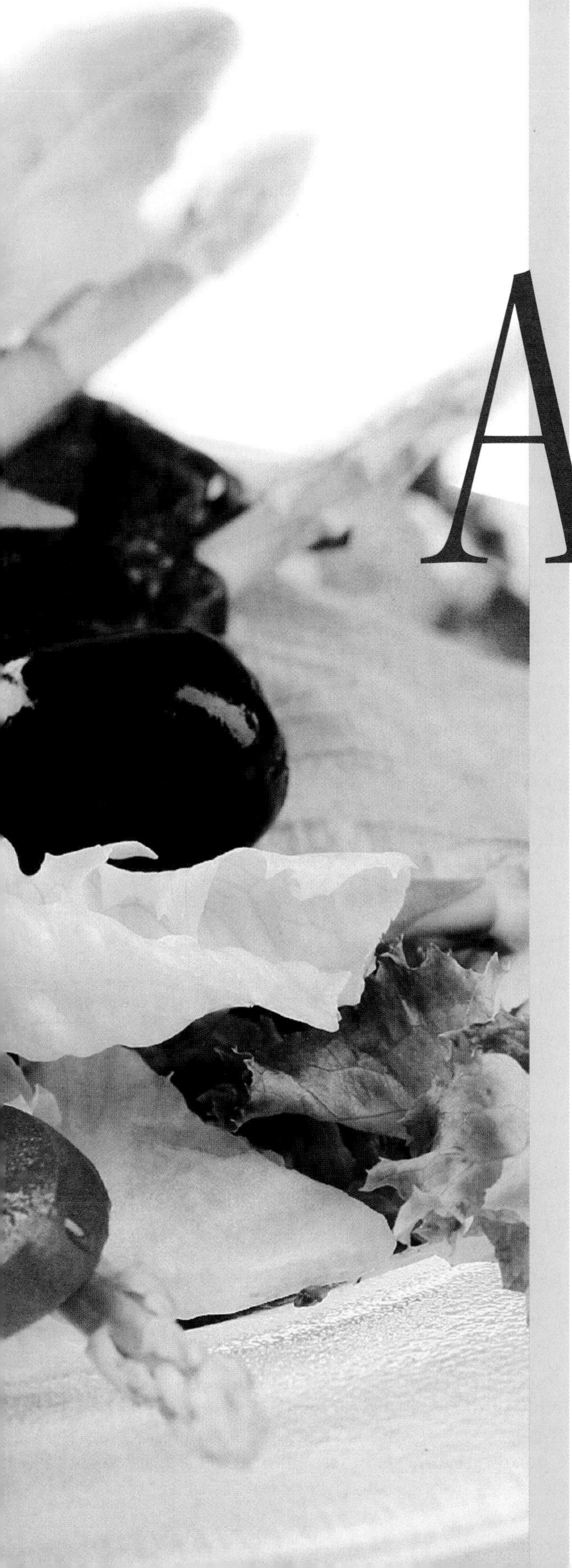

Test Yourself

1. **T F Being underweight can be just as detrimental to our health as being obese.**
2. **T F Getting your body composition measured at the local fitness club will give you an accurate assessment of your body fat level.**
3. **T F Although a majority of Americans are overweight, only about 10% of Americans are obese.**

Test Yourself answers can be found at the end of the chapter.

As a teenager, she won a full athletic scholarship to Syracuse University, where she was honored for her "significant contribution to women's athletics and to the sport of rowing." After graduating, she became a television reporter and anchor for an NBC station in Flagstaff, Arizona. Then she went into modeling, and soon her face smiled out from the covers of fashion magazines, cosmetics ads, even a billboard in Times Square. Now considered a "supermodel," she has her own website, her own clothing line, and even a collection of dolls. *People* magazine has twice selected her as one of the "50 Most Beautiful People," and *Glamour* magazine named her "Woman of the Year." So who is she? Her name is Emme Aronson . . . and, by the way, at 5′11″ tall, her average weight is 190 pounds.

Emme describes herself as "very well-proportioned." She focuses not on maintaining a certain weight but on keeping healthy and fit. A cancer survivor, she follows a nutritious diet and works out regularly. Observing that "we live in a society that is based on the attainment of unrealistic beauty," Emme works hard to get out the message that self-esteem should not be contingent on size. On news programs and talk shows, at high schools and on college campuses, she speaks out against weight-based discrimination and promotes acceptance of body diversity. Citing reports that 80% of women and many men are unhappy with their body, she encourages people of all sizes to celebrate their individuality.[1,2]

Are you happy with your weight, shape, body composition, and fitness? If not, what needs to change—your attitude, your diet, your level of physical activity? What role do diet and physical activity play in maintaining a healthful body weight? How much of your body size and shape is due to genetics?

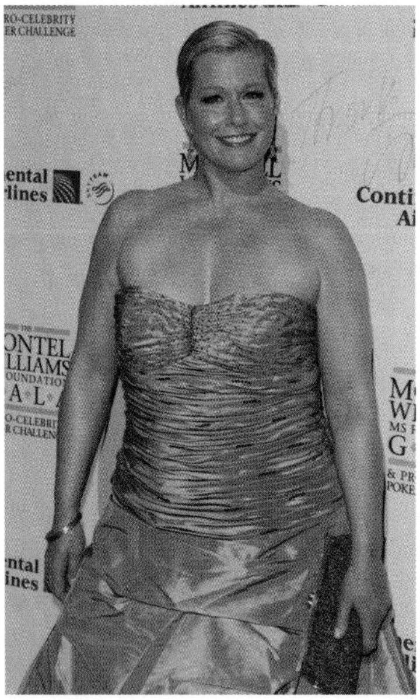

Fashion model Emme's weight is healthful for her.

What influence does society—including food advertising—have on your weight? And if you decide that you do need to lose weight, what's the best way to do it? In this chapter, we'll explore these questions and provide some answers.

How Can You Evaluate Your Body Weight?

As you begin to think about achieving and maintaining a healthful weight, it's important to make sure you understand what a healthful body weight actually is and the various methods you can use to figure out if your own weight is healthful.

Understand What a Healthful Body Weight Really Is

We can define a healthful weight as all of the following:[3]

- A weight that is appropriate for your age and physical development
- A weight that you can achieve and sustain without severely curtailing your food intake or constantly dieting
- A weight that is compatible with normal blood pressure, lipid levels, and glucose tolerance
- A weight that is based on your genetic background and family history of body shape and weight
- A weight that promotes good eating habits and allows you to participate in regular physical activity
- A weight that is acceptable to you

As you can see, a healthful weight is not one at which a person must be extremely thin or overly muscular. In addition, there is no one body type that can be defined as healthful. Thus, achieving a healthful body weight should not be dictated by the latest fad or current societal expectations of what is acceptable.

Various methods are available to help you determine whether you are currently maintaining a healthful body weight. Let's review a few of these methods.

Determine Your Body Mass Index (BMI)

Body mass index (BMI, or *Quetelet's index*) is a commonly used index representing the ratio of a person's body weight to the square of his or her height. You can calculate your BMI using the following equation:

$$\text{BMI (kg/m}^2) = \text{weight (kg)} / \text{height (m)}^2$$

For those less familiar with the metric system, there is an equation to calculate BMI using weight in pounds and height in inches:

$$\text{BMI (kg/m}^2) = [\text{weight (lb)} / \text{height (in.)}^2] \times 703$$

A less exact but practical method is to use the graph in **Figure 11.1**, which shows approximate BMIs for your height and weight and whether your BMI is in a healthful range. You can also calculate your BMI on the Internet using the BMI calculator found at www.nhlbisupport.com/bmi.

Why Is BMI Important?

Your body mass index provides an important clue to your overall health. Physicians, nutritionists, and other scientists define **underweight** as having too little body fat to maintain health, causing a person to have a weight that is below an acceptably defined standard for a given height. A person having a BMI less than 18.5 kg/m^2 is considered underweight. Normal weight ranges from 18.5 to 24.9 kg/m^2. **Overweight** is

body mass index (BMI) A measurement representing the ratio of a person's body weight to his or her height.

underweight Having too little body fat to maintain health, causing a person to weight less than an acceptably defined standard for a given height.

overweight Having a moderate amount of excess body fat, resulting in a person weighing more than an accepted standard for a given height, but not considered obese.

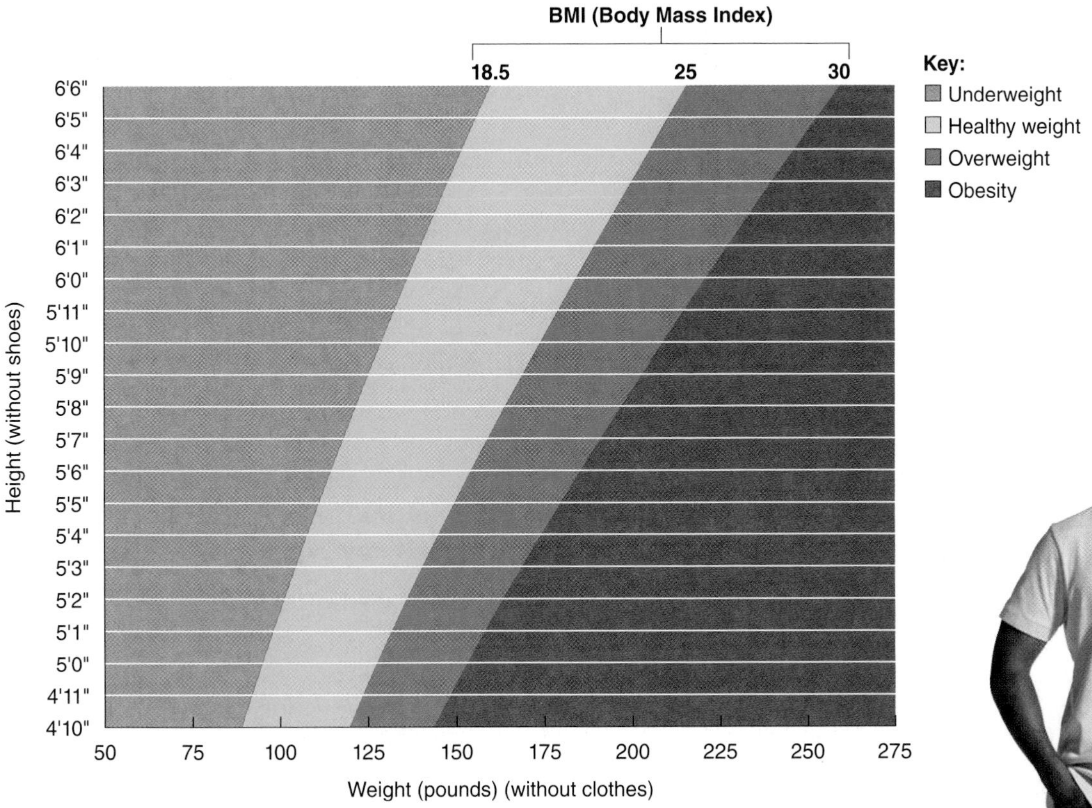

Figure 11.1 Measure your body mass index (BMI) using this graph. To determine your BMI, find the value for your height on the left and follow this line to the right until it intersects with the value for your weight on the bottom axis. The area on the graph where these two lines intersect is your BMI.

defined as having a moderate amount of excess body fat, resulting in a person having a weight that is greater than some accepted standard for a given height but is not considered obese. Having a BMI between 25 and 29.9 kg/m^2 indicates that a person is overweight. **Obesity** is defined as having an excess of body fat that adversely affects health, resulting in a person having a weight that is substantially greater than some accepted standard for a given height. A BMI value between 30 and 39.9 kg/m^2 is consistent with obesity. People can also suffer from **morbid obesity,** defined as a BMI greater than or equal to 40 kg/m^2; in this case, the person's body weight exceeds 100% of normal, putting him or her at very high risk for serious health consequences.

Research studies show that a person's risk for type 2 diabetes, high blood pressure, heart disease, and many other diseases increases significantly when BMI is above a value of 30. On the other hand, being underweight and having a very low BMI, below 18.5, are also associated with an increased risk for health problems.

Figure 11.2 shows how the *mortality rate,* or death rate, from all diseases increases significantly with a BMI value below 18.5 kg/m^2 or above 30 kg/m^2. Having a BMI value within the healthful range means that your risk of dying prematurely is within the expected average. If your BMI value falls outside this range, either higher or lower, your risk of dying prematurely is greater than the average risk. For example, people with a BMI equal to or greater than 30 kg/m^2 have a risk of dying prematurely that is 50–100% higher that of people with a BMI value in the range of 20–25 kg/m^2.

Theo always worries about being too thin, and he wonders if he is underweight. Theo calculates his BMI (see the calculations in the You Do the Math box) and is surprised to find that it is 22 kg/m^2 and falls within the healthy range.

Limitations of BMI

While calculating your BMI can be very helpful in estimating your health risk, this method has a number of limitations that should be taken into consideration. BMI

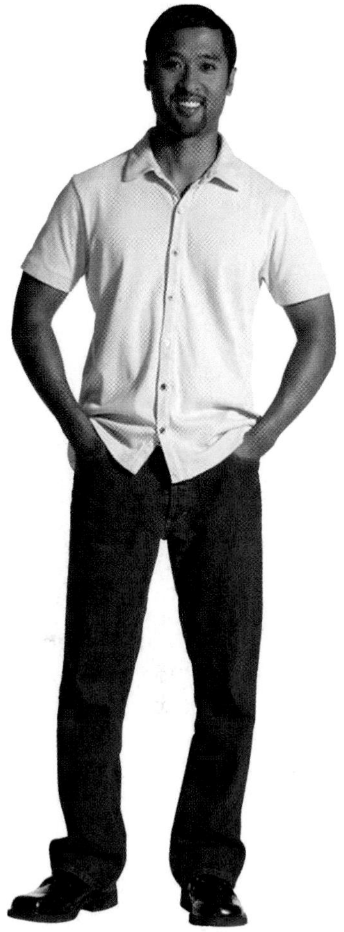

A healthful weight is one that is appropriate for your age, physical development, heredity, and other factors.

obesity Having an excess of body fat that adversely affects health, resulting in a person weighing substantially more than an accepted standard for a given height.

morbid obesity A condition in which a person's body weight exceeds 100% of normal, putting him or her at very high risk for serious health consequences.

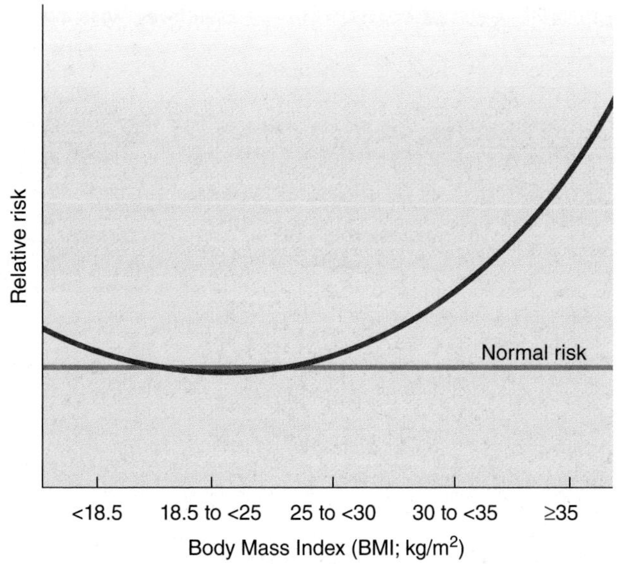

Figure 11.2 Having a body mass index value below 18.5 kg/m^2 or above 30 kg/m^2 is significantly associated with an increased risk for premature mortality.

cannot tell us how much of a person's body mass is composed of fat, nor can it give us an indication of where on the body excess fat is stored. As we'll discuss shortly, upper-body fat stores increase the risk for chronic disease more than fat stores in the lower body. A person's age affects his or her BMI; BMI does not give a fair indication of overweight or obesity in people over the age of 65 years, as the BMI standards are based on data from younger people, and BMI does not accurately reflect the differential rates of bone and muscle loss in older people. BMI also cannot reflect differences in bone and muscle growth in children. Recent research indicates that BMI is more strongly associated with height in young people; thus, taller children are more likely to be identified as overweight or obese, even though they may not have higher levels of body fat.[4]

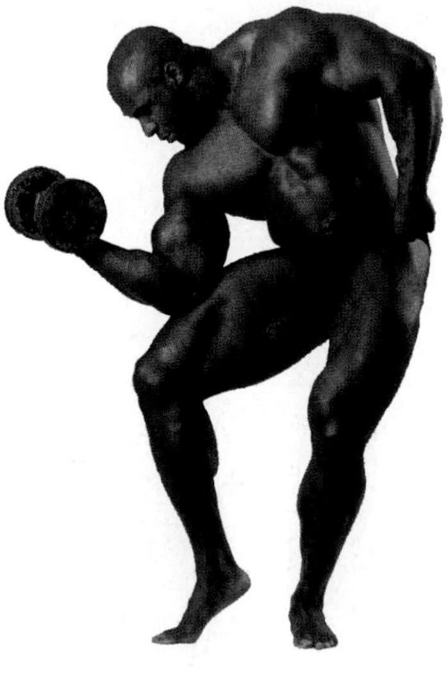

BMI is not an accurate indicator of overweight for certain populations, including heavily muscled people.

BMI also does not take into account physical and metabolic differences between people of different ethnic backgrounds. At the same BMI, people from different ethnic backgrounds will have different levels of body fat. For instance, African American and Polynesian people have less body fat than whites at the same BMI value, while Indonesians, Thais, and Ethiopians have more body fat than whites at the same BMI value.[5] There is also evidence that, even at the same BMI level, Asian, Hispanic, and African American women have a higher risk for diabetes than white women.[6] The same study also found that, when Asian and Hispanic women gained weight, their risk of developing diabetes over a 20-year period was approximately twice as high as it was for white and African American women who gained the same amount of weight.

Finally, BMI is limited when used with people who have a disproportionately higher muscle mass for a given height. People who fall into this category include some athletes and pregnant and lactating women. For example, one of Theo's friends, Randy, is a 23-year-old weight lifter who is 5′7″ and weighs 210 pounds. According to our BMI calculations, Randy's BMI is 32.9, placing him in the obese and high-risk category for many diseases. Is Randy really obese? In cases such as his, an assessment of body composition is necessary.

Measure Your Body Composition

body composition The ratio of a person's body fat to lean body mass.

There are many methods available to assess your **body composition,** or the amount of body fat (or *adipose tissue*) and lean body mass (or *lean tissue*) you have. **Figure 11.3** lists and describes some of the more common methods. It is important

Method		Limitations
Underwater weighing: Considered the most accurate method. Estimates body fat within a 2–3% margin of error. This means that if your underwater weighing test shows you have 20% body fat, this value could be no lower than 17% and no higher than 23%. Used primarily for research purposes.	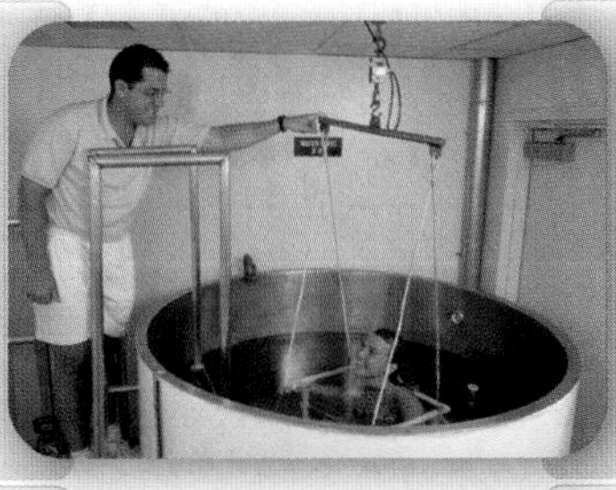	• Must be comfortable in water. • Requires trained technician and specialized equipment. • Does not work well with obese people. • Must abstain from food for at least 8 hours and from exercise for at least 12 hours prior to testing.
Skinfolds: Involves "pinching" a person's fold of skin (with its underlying layer of fat) at various locations of the body. The fold is measured using a specially designed caliper. When performed by a skilled technician, it can estimate body fat with an error of 3–4%. This means that if your skinfold test shows you have 20% body fat, your actual value could be as low as 16% or as high as 24%.	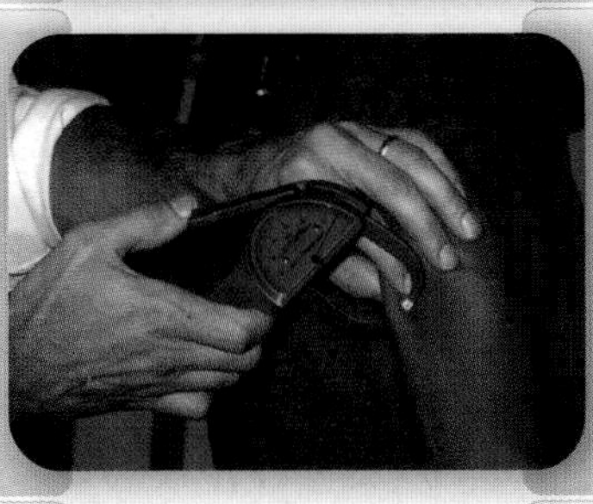	• Less accurate unless technician is well trained. • Proper prediction equation must be used to improve accuracy. • Person being measured may not want to be touched or to expose their skin. • Cannot be used to measure obese people, as their skinfolds are too large for the caliper.
Bioelectrical impedance analysis (BIA): Involves sending a very low level of electrical current through a person's body. As water is a good conductor of electricity and lean body mass is made up of mostly water, the rate at which the electricity is conducted gives an indication of a person's lean body mass and body fat. This method can be done while lying down, with electrodes attached to the feet, hands, and the BIA machine. Hand-held and standing models (which look like bathroom scales) are now available. Under the best of circumstances, BIA can estimate body fat with an error of 3–4%.	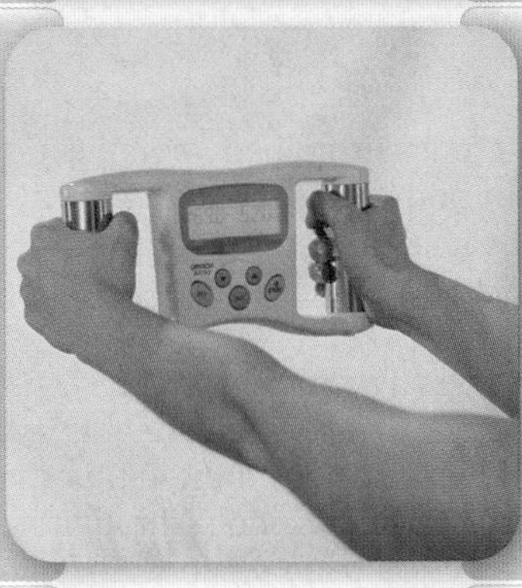	• Less accurate. • Body fluid levels must be normal. • Proper prediction equation must be used to improve accuracy. • Should not eat for 4 hours and should not exercise for 12 hours prior to the test. • No alcohol should be consumed within 48 hours of the test. • Females should not be measured if they are retaining water due to menstrual cycle changes.
Dual-energy x-ray absorptiometry (DXA): The technology is based on using very low level x-rays to differentiate among bone tissue, soft (or lean) tissue, and fat (or adipose) tissue. It involves lying for about 30 minutes on a specialized bed fully clothed, with all metal objects removed. The margin of error for predicting body fat ranges from 2% to 4%.	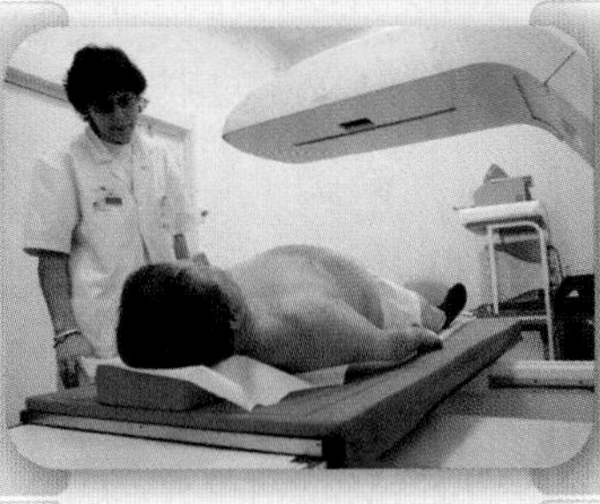	• Expensive; requires trained technician with specialized equipment. • Cannot be used to measure extremely tall, short, or obese people, as they do not fit properly within the scanning area.
Bod Pod: A machine that uses air displacement to measure body composition. This machine is a large, egg-shaped chamber made from fiberglass. The person being measured sits inside wearing a swimsuit. The door is closed and the machine measures how much air is displaced. This value is used to calculate body composition. It appears promising as an easier and equally accurate alternative to underwater weighing in many populations, but it may overestimate body fat in some African-American men.	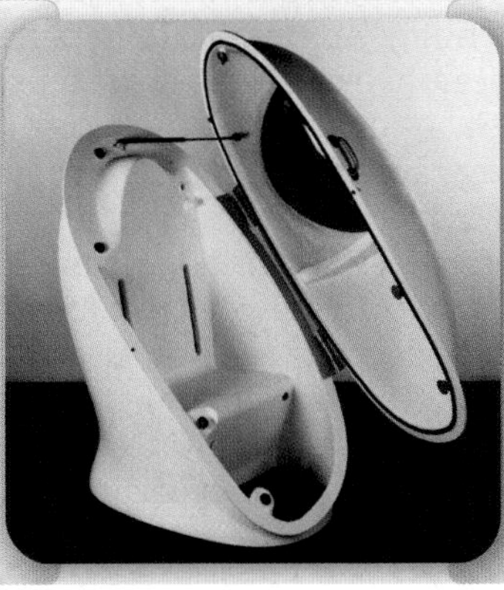	• Expensive. • Less accurate in some populations.

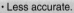

Figure 11.3 Overview of various body composition assessment methods.

YOU DO THE MATH

Calculating Your Body Mass Index

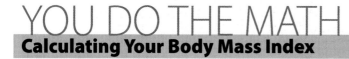

Calculate your personal BMI value based on your height and weight. Let's use Theo's values as an example:

$$\text{BMI} = \text{weight (kg)} / \text{height (m)}^2$$

1. Theo's weight is 200 pounds. To convert his weight to kilograms, divide his weight in pounds by 2.2 pounds per kilogram:

$$200 \text{ lb} / 2.2 \text{ lb per kg} = 90.91 \text{ kg}$$

2. Theo's height is 6 feet 8 inches, or 80 inches. To convert his height to meters, multiply his height in inches by 0.0254 meter per inch:

$$80 \text{ in.} \times 0.0254 \text{ m/in.} = 2.03 \text{ m}$$

3. Find the square of his height in meters:

$$2.03 \text{ m} \times 2.03 \text{ m} = 4.13 \text{ m}^2$$

4. Then, divide his weight in kilograms by his height in meters squared to get his BMI value:

$$90.91 \text{ kg} / 4.13 \text{ m}^2 = 22.01 \text{ kg/m}^2$$

Is Theo underweight, according to this BMI value? As you can see in Figure 11.1, this value shows that he is maintaining a normal, healthful weight!

to remember that measuring body composition provides only an estimate of your body fat and lean body mass, meaning that you cannot measure your exact level of these tissues. Because the range of error of these methods can be from 3% to more than 20%, body composition results should not be used as the only indicator of health status.

Let's return to Randy, whose BMI of 32.9 kg/m^2 places him in the obese category. But is he obese? Randy trains with weights 4 days per week, rides an exercise bike for about 30 minutes per session three times per week, and does not take drugs, smoke cigarettes, or drink alcohol. Through his local gym, Randy contacted a trained technician who assesses body composition. The results of his skinfold measurements show that his body fat is 9%. This value is within the healthful range for men. Randy is an example of a person whose BMI appears to be very high but who is not actually obese.

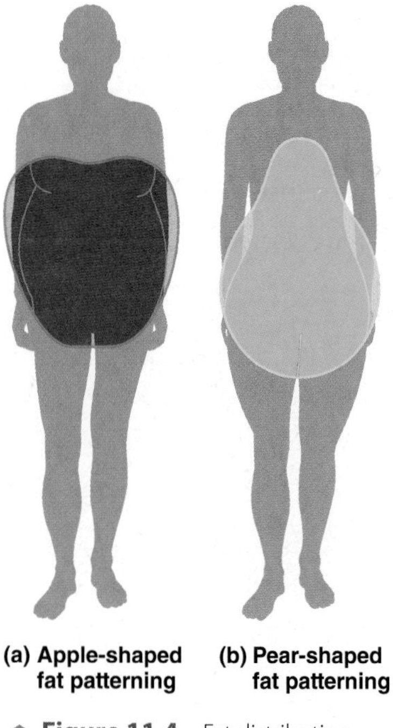

Figure 11.4 Fat distribution patterns. **(a)** An apple-shaped fat distribution pattern increases an individual's risk for many chronic diseases. **(b)** A pear-shaped fat distribution pattern does not seem to be associated with an increased risk for chronic disease.

Assess Your Fat Distribution Patterns

To evaluate the health of your current body weight, it is also helpful to consider the way fat is distributed throughout your body. This is because your fat distribution pattern is known to affect your risk for various diseases. **Figure 11.4** shows two types of fat patterning. *Apple-shaped fat patterning*, or upper-body obesity, is known to significantly increase a person's risk for many chronic diseases, such as type 2 diabetes, heart disease, and high blood pressure. It is thought that the apple-shaped patterning causes problems in the metabolism of fat and carbohydrate, leading to unhealthful changes in blood cholesterol, insulin, glucose, and blood pressure. In contrast, *pear-shaped fat patterning*, or lower-body obesity, does not seem to significantly increase your risk for chronic diseases. Women tend to store fat in their lower body, and men in their abdominal region. In 2004, a study involving more than 10,000 people found that 64% of women are pear-shaped and 38% of men are apple-shaped.[7]

You can use the following three-step method to determine your type of fat patterning:

1. Ask a friend to measure the circumference of your natural waist—that is, the narrowest part of your torso as observed from the front (**Figure 11.5a**).
2. Then, have that friend measure your hip circumference at the maximal width of the buttocks as observed from the side (Figure 11.5b).

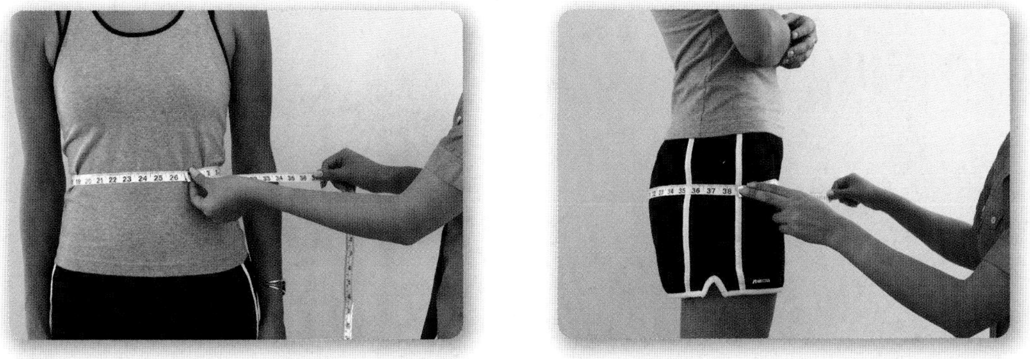

(a) (b)

Figure 11.5 Determining your type of fat patterning. **(a)** Measure the circumference of your natural waist. **(b)** Measure the circumference of your hips at the maximal width of the buttocks as observed from the side. Dividing the waist value by the hip value gives you your waist-to-hip ratio.

3. Then, divide the waist value by the hip value. This measurement is called your *waist-to-hip ratio*. For example, if your natural waist is 30 inches and your hips are 40 inches, then your waist-to-hip ratio is 30 divided by 40, which equals 0.75.

Once you figure out your ratio, how do you interpret it? An increased risk for chronic disease is associated with the following waist-to-hip ratios:

- In men, a ratio higher than 0.90
- In women, a ratio higher than 0.80

These ratios suggest an apple-shaped fat distribution pattern. In addition, waist circumference alone can indicate your risk for chronic disease. For males, your risk of chronic disease is increased if your waist circumference is above 40 inches (102 cm). For females, your risk is increased at measurements above 35 inches (88 cm).

RECAP **Body mass index, body composition, and the waist-to-hip ratio and waist circumference are tools that can help you evaluate the health of your current body weight. None of these methods is completely accurate, but most may be used appropriately as general health indicators.**

What Makes Us Gain and Lose Weight?

Have you ever wondered why some people are thin but others are overweight, even though they seem to eat about the same diet? If so, you're not alone. For hundreds of years, researchers have puzzled over what makes us gain and lose weight. In this section, we'll explore some information and current theories that may shed some light on this question.

We Gain or Lose Weight When Our Energy Intake and Expenditure Are Out of Balance

Fluctuations in body weight are a result of changes in our **energy intake** (the food we eat) and our **energy expenditure** (the amount of energy we expend at rest and during physical activity). This relationship between what we eat and what we do is defined by the energy balance equation:

Energy balance occurs when energy intake = energy expenditure

This means that our energy is balanced when we consume the same amount of energy that we burn each day. **Figure 11.6** shows how our weight changes when we

energy intake The amount of food a person eats; in other words, it is the number of kilocalories consumed.

energy expenditure The energy the body expends to maintain its basic functions and to perform all levels of movement and activity.

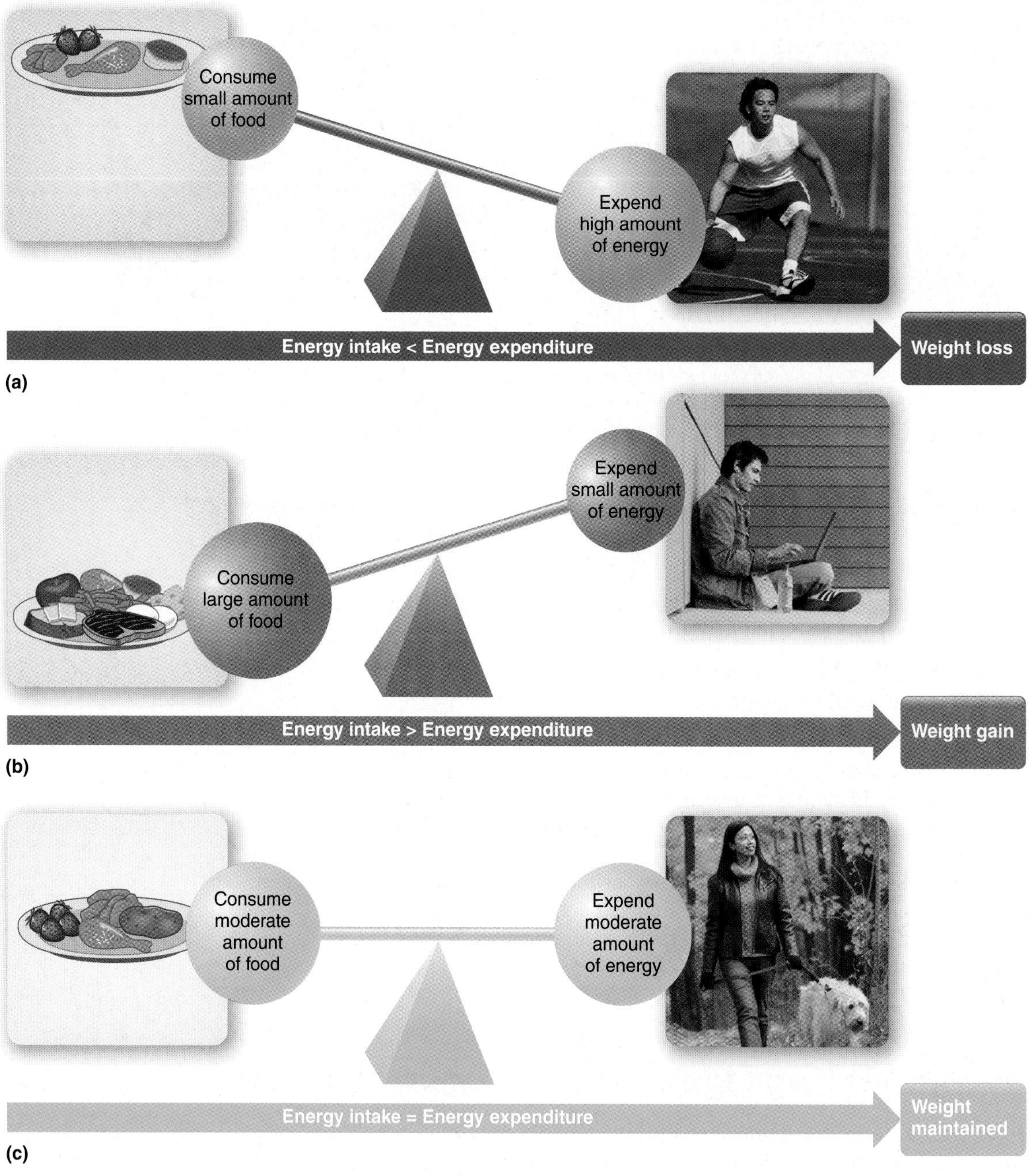

Figure 11.6 Energy balance is the relationship between the food we eat and the energy we burn each day. **(a)** Weight loss occurs when food intake is less than energy output. **(b)** Weight gain occurs when food intake is greater than energy output. **(c)** We maintain our body weight when food intake equals energy output.

change either side of this equation. From this figure, you can see that, in order to lose body weight, we must expend more energy than we consume. In contrast, to gain weight, we must consume more energy than we expend. Finding the proper balance between energy intake and expenditure allows us to maintain a healthful body weight.

Energy Intake Is the Food We Eat Each Day

Energy intake is equal to the amount of energy in the food we eat each day. This value includes all foods and beverages. Daily energy intake is expressed as *kilocalories per day* (*kcal/day,* or *kcal/d*). You can estimate your energy intake by using food composition tables or computerized dietary analysis programs. The energy content of each food is a function of the amount of carbohydrate, fat, protein, and alcohol that each food contains; vitamins and minerals have no energy value, so they contribute zero kilocalories to energy intake.

Remember that the energy value of carbohydrate and protein is 4 kcal/g and the energy value of fat is 9 kcal/g. The energy value of alcohol is 7 kcal/g. By multiplying the energy value (in kcal/g) by the amount of the nutrient (in g), you can calculate how much energy is in a particular food. For instance, 1 cup of quick oatmeal contains 6 g of protein, 25 g of carbohydrate, and 2 g of fat. Using the energy values for each nutrient, you can calculate the total energy content as follows:

$$6 \text{ g protein} \times 4 \text{ kcal/g} = 24 \text{ kcal from protein}$$

$$25 \text{ g carbohydrate} \times 4 \text{ kcal/g} = 100 \text{ kcal from carbohydrate}$$

$$2 \text{ g fat} \times 9 \text{ kcal/g} = 18 \text{ kcal from fat}$$

$$\text{Total kcal for 1 cup oatmeal} = 24 \text{ kcal} + 100 \text{ kcal} + 18 \text{ kcal} = 142 \text{ kcal}$$

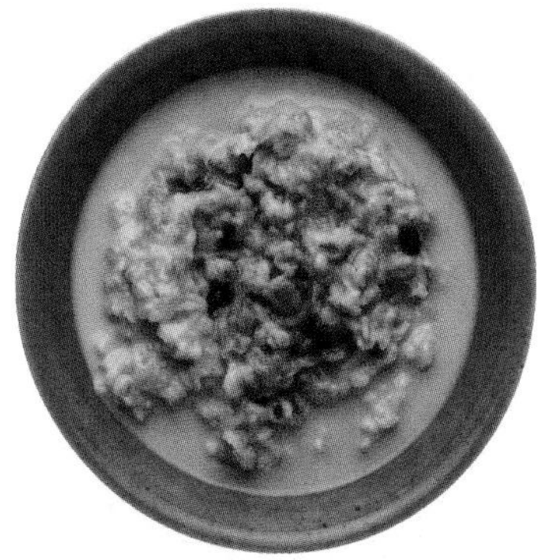

The energy provided by a bowl of oatmeal is derived from its protein, carbohydrate, and fat content.

When someone's total daily energy intake exceeds the amount of energy that person expends, he or she gains weight. An excess intake of approximately 3,500 kcal will result in a gain of 1 pound. Without exercise, this gain will likely be fat.

Energy Expenditure Includes More than Just Physical Activity

Energy expenditure (also known as energy output) is the energy our body expends to maintain its basic functions and to perform all levels of movement and activity. Total 24-hour energy expenditure is calculated by estimating the energy used during rest and as a result of physical activity. There are three components of energy expenditure: basal metabolic rate (BMR), thermic effect of food (TEF), and energy cost of physical activity (**Figure 11.7**).

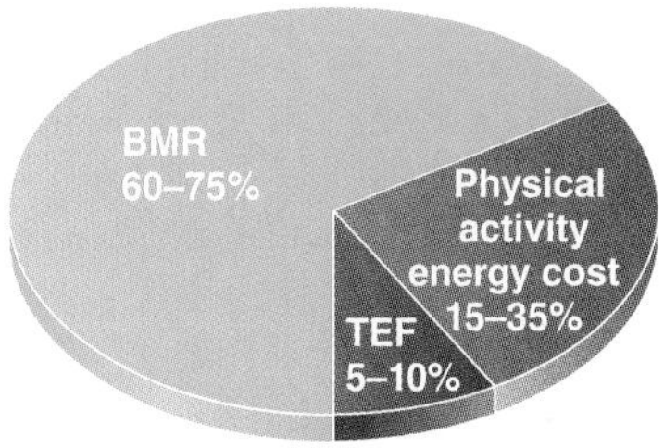

Components of energy expenditure

Figure 11.7 The components of energy expenditure are basal metabolic rate (BMR), the thermic effect of food (TEF), and the energy cost of physical activity. BMR accounts for 60–75% of our total energy output, whereas TEF and physical activity together account for 25–40%.

Our Basal Metabolic Rate Is Our Energy Expenditure at Rest **Basal metabolic rate,** or **BMR,** is the energy we expend just to maintain our body's *basal,* or *resting,* functions. These functions include respiration, circulation, body temperature, synthesis of new cells and tissues, secretion of hormones, and nervous system activity. The majority of our energy output each day (about 60–75%) is a result of our BMR. This means that 60–75% of our energy output goes to fuel the basic activities of staying alive, aside from any physical activity.

BMR varies widely among people. The primary determinant of our BMR is the amount of lean body mass we have. People with a higher lean body mass have a higher BMR, as lean body mass is more metabolically active than body fat. Thus, it takes more energy to support this active tissue. One common assumption is that obese people have a depressed BMR. This is usually not the case. Most studies of obese people show that the amount of energy they expend for every kilogram of lean body mass is similar to that of a non-obese person. In general, people who weigh more also have more lean body mass and consequently have a *higher* BMR. See **Figure 11.8** for an example of how lean body mass can vary for people with different body weights and body fat levels.

BMR decreases with age, approximately 3–5% per decade after age 30. This age-related decrease results partly from hormonal changes, but much of this change is due to the loss of lean body mass resulting from physical inactivity. Thus, a large proportion of this decrease can be prevented with regular physical activity. There are other factors that can affect a person's BMR, and some of these are listed in **Table 11.1**.

How can you estimate the amount of energy you expend for your BMR? Of the many equations that can be used, one of the simplest ways to estimate your BMR is to multiply your body weight in kilograms by 1.0 kcal per kilogram of body weight per hour for men or by 0.9 kcal per kilogram of body weight per hour for women. A little later in this chapter, you'll have an opportunity to calculate your BMR and determine your total daily energy needs.

basal metabolic rate (BMR) The energy the body expends to maintain its fundamental physiologic functions.

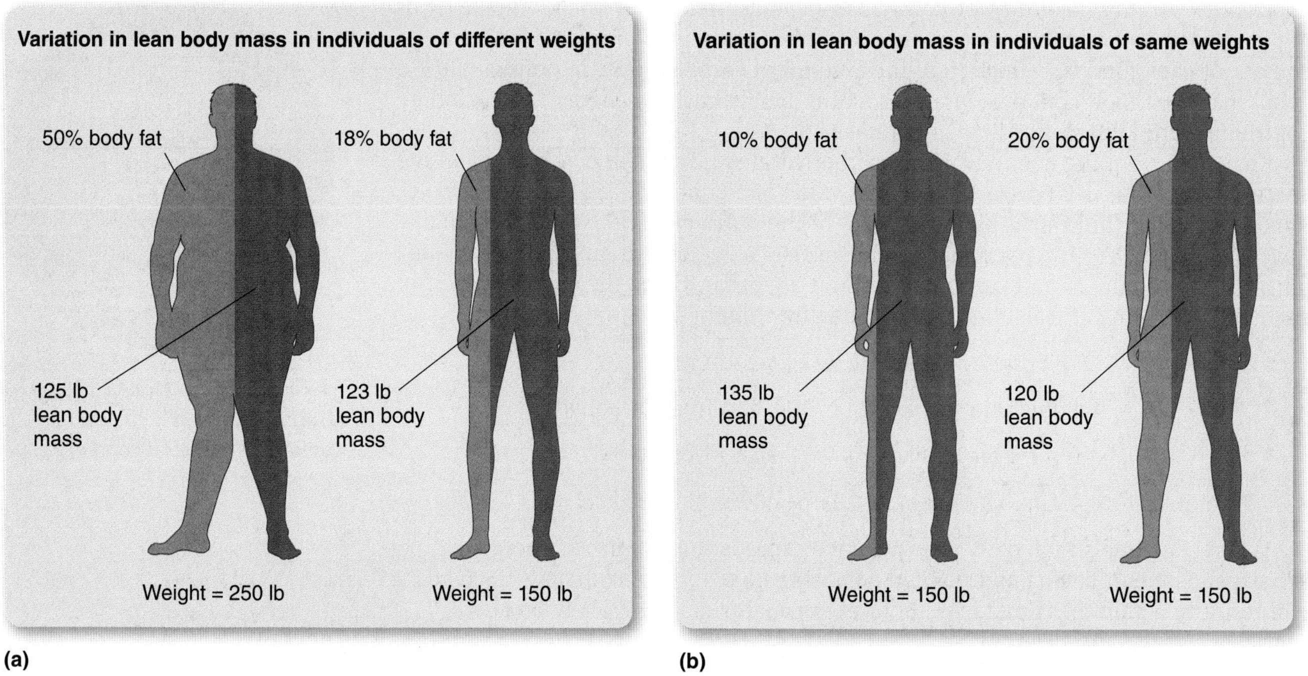

Figure 11.8 Lean body mass varies in people with different body weights and body fat levels. **(a)** The person on the left has greater body weight, body fat, and lean body mass than the person on the right. **(b)** The two people are the same weight, but the person on the right has more body fat and less lean body mass than the person on the left.

TABLE 11.1 Factors Affecting Basal Metabolic Rate (BMR)

Factors That Increase BMR	Factors That Decrease BMR
Higher lean body mass	Lower lean body mass
Greater height (more surface area)	Lower height
Younger age	Older age
Elevated levels of thyroid hormone	Depressed levels of thyroid hormone
Stress, fever, illness	Starvation or fasting
Male gender	Female gender
Pregnancy and lactation	
Certain drugs, such as stimulants, caffeine, and tobacco	

The Thermic Effect of Food Is the Energy Expended to Process Food The **thermic effect of food (TEF)** is the energy we expend as a result of processing the food we eat. A certain amount of energy is needed to digest, absorb, transport, metabolize, and store the nutrients we need. The TEF is equal to about 5–10% of the energy content of a meal, a relatively small amount. Thus, if a meal contains 500 kcal, the thermic effect of processing that meal is about 25–50 kcal. These values apply to eating what is referred to as a mixed diet, or a diet containing a mixture of carbohydrate, fat, and protein. Most of us eat some combination of these nutrients throughout the day. Individually, the processing of each nutrient takes a different amount of energy. While fat requires very little energy to digest, transport, and store in our cells, protein and carbohydrate require relatively more energy to process.

thermic effect of food (TEF) The energy expended as a result of processing food consumed.

energy cost of physical activity The energy that is expended on body movement and muscular work above basal levels.

The Energy Cost of Physical Activity Is Highly Variable The **energy cost of physical activity** represents about 15–35% of our total energy output each day. This is the energy we expend due to any movement or work above basal levels. This includes both

TABLE 11.2 Energy Costs of Various Physical Activities

Activity	Intensity	Energy Cost (kcal/kg body weight/min)
Sitting, knitting/sewing	Light	0.026
Cooking or food preparation (standing or sitting)	Light	0.035
Walking, shopping	Light	0.040
Walking, 2 mph (slow pace)	Light	0.044
Cleaning (dusting, straightening up, vacuuming, changing linen, carrying out trash)	Moderate	0.044
Stretching—hatha yoga	Moderate	0.044
Weight lifting (free weights, Nautilus, or universal type)	Light or moderate	0.052
Bicycling $<$10 mph	Leisure (work or pleasure)	0.070
Walking, 4 mph (brisk pace)	Moderate	0.088
Aerobics	Low impact	0.088
Weight lifting (free weights, Nautilus, or universal type)	Vigorous	0.105
Bicycling, 12 to 13.9 mph	Moderate	0.140
Running, 5 mph (12 minutes per mile)	Moderate	0.140
Running, 6 mph (10 minutes per mile)	Moderate	0.175
Running, 8.6 mph (7 minutes per mile)	Vigorous	0.245

Data from Ainsworth, B. E., W. L. Haskell, M. C. Whitt, M. L. Irwin, A. M. Swartz, S. J. Strath, W. L. O'Brien, D. R. Bassett, Jr., K. H. Schmitz, P. O. Emplaincourt, D. R. Jacobs, Jr., and A. S. Leon. 2000. Compendium of physical activities: an update of activity codes and MET intensities. *Med. Sci. Sports Exerc.* 32:S498–S516. Lippincott, Williams & Wilkins. Reprinted with permission.

lower-intensity activities, such as sitting, standing, and walking, and higher-intensity activities, such as running, skiing, and bicycling. One of the most obvious ways to increase how much energy we expend as a result of physical activity is to do more activities for a longer period of time.

Table 11.2 lists the energy costs for certain activities. As you can see, activities such as running, swimming, and cross-country skiing, which involve moving our larger muscle groups (or more parts of the body), require more energy. The amount of energy we expend during activities is also affected by our body size, the intensity of the activity, and how long we perform the activity. That is why the values in Table 11.2 are expressed as kilocalories of energy per kilogram of body weight per minute.

Using the energy value for running at 6 miles per hour (or a 10-minute-per-mile running pace) for 30 minutes, let's calculate how much energy Theo would expend doing this activity:

- Theo's body weight (in kg) = 200 lb / 2.2 lb/kg = 90.91 kg.
- Energy cost of running at 6 mph = 0.175 kcal/kg body weight/min.
- At Theo's weight, the energy cost of running per minute = 0.175 kcal/kg body weight/min × 90.91 kg = 15.91 kcal/min.
- If Theo runs at this pace for 30 minutes, his total energy output = 15.91 kcal/min × 30 min = 477 kcal.

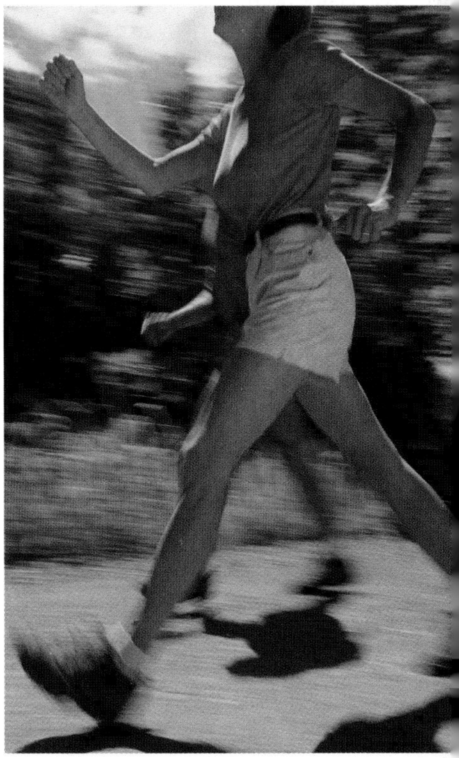

Brisk walking expends energy.

Given everything we've discussed so far, you're probably asking yourself, "How many kilocalories do I need each day to maintain my current weight?" This question is not always easy to answer, as our energy needs fluctuate from day to day according to our activity level, the environmental conditions, and other factors, such as the amount and type of food we eat and our intake of caffeine, which temporarily increase our BMR. However, you can get a general estimate of how much energy your body needs to maintain your present weight. The You Do the Math box on page 380 describes how you can estimate your total daily energy needs.

RECAP **The energy balance equation relates food intake to energy expenditure. Eating more energy than you expend causes weight gain, while eating less energy than you expend causes weight loss. The three components of energy expenditure are basal metabolic rate, the thermic effect of food, and the energy cost of physical activity.**

YOU DO THE MATH

Calculating BMR and Total Daily Energy Needs

You can estimate how much energy you need each day by recording your total food and beverage intake for a defined period of time, such as 3 or 7 days. You can then use a food composition table or computerized dietary assessment program to estimate the amount of energy you eat each day. Assuming that your body weight is stable over this period of time, your average daily energy intake should represent how much energy you need to maintain your present weight.

Unfortunately, many studies of energy intake in humans have shown that dietary records estimating energy needs are not very accurate. Most studies show that people underestimate the amount of energy they eat by 10–30%. Overweight people tend to underestimate by an even higher margin, at the same time overestimating the amount of activity they do. This means that someone who really eats about 2,000 kcal/day may record eating only 1,400–1,800 kcal/day. So one reason many people are confused about their ability to lose weight is that they are eating more than they realize.

A simpler and more accurate way to estimate your total daily energy needs is to calculate your BMR and then add the amount of energy you expend as a result of your activity level. Refer to the following example to learn how to do this. Because the energy cost for the thermic effect of food is very small, you don't need to include it in your calculations.

1. *Calculate your BMR.* If you are a man, you will need to multiply your body weight in kilograms by 1 kcal per kilogram body weight per hour. Assuming you weigh 175 pounds, your body weight in kilograms is 175 lb / 2.2 lb/kg = 79.5 kg. Next, multiply your weight in kilograms by 1 kcal per kilogram body weight per hour:

   $$1 \text{ kcal/kg body weight/hour} \times 79.5 \text{ kg} = 79.5 \text{ kcal/hour}$$

   Calculate your BMR for the total day (24 hours):

   $$79.5 \text{ kcal/hour} \times 24 \text{ hours/day} = 1{,}909 \text{ kcal/day}$$

   (If you are a woman, multiply your body weight in kg by 0.9 kcal/kg body weight/hour.)

2. *Estimate your activity level by selecting the description that most closely fits your general lifestyle.* The energy cost of activities is expressed as a percentage of your BMR. Refer to the values in the following table when estimating your own energy output.

	Men	Women
Sedentary/Inactive Involves mostly sitting, driving, or very low levels of activity	25–40%	25–35%
Lightly Active Involves a lot of sitting; may also involve some walking, moving around, and light lifting	50–70%	40–60%
Moderately Active Involves work plus intentional exercise, such as an hour of walking or cycling 4 or 5 days per week; may have a job requiring some physical labor	65–80%	50–70%
Heavily Active Involves a great deal of physical labor, such as roofing, carpentry work, and/or regular heavy lifting and digging	90–120%	80–100%
Exceptionally Active Involves a lot of physical activities for work and intentional exercise; also applies to athletes who train for many hours each day, such as triathletes and marathon runners or other competitive athletes performing heavy, regular training	130–145%	110–130%

3. *Multiply your BMR by the decimal equivalent of the lower and higher percentage values for your activity level.* Let's use the man referred to in step 1. He is a college student who lives on campus. He walks to classes located throughout campus, carries his book bag, and spends most of his time reading and writing. He does not exercise on a regular basis. His lifestyle would be defined as lightly active, meaning he expends 50–70% of his BMR each day in activities. You want to calculate how much energy he expends at both ends of this activity level. How many kcal does this equal?

   $$1{,}909 \text{ kcal/day} \times 0.50\ (50\%) = 955 \text{ kcal/day}$$
   $$1{,}909 \text{ kcal/day} \times 0.70\ (70\%) = 1{,}336 \text{ kcal/day}$$

   These calculations show that this man expends about 955–1,336 kcal/day doing daily activities.

4. *Calculate total daily energy output by adding together BMR and the energy needed to perform daily activities.* In this man's case, his total daily energy output is

   $$1{,}909 \text{ kcal/day} + 955 \text{ kcal/day} = 2{,}864 \text{ kcal/day}$$

   or

   $$1{,}909 \text{ kcal/day} + 1{,}336 \text{ kcal/day} = 3{,}245 \text{ kcal/day}$$

   Assuming this man is maintaining his present weight, he requires between 2,864 and 3,245 kcal/day to stay in energy balance!

Genetic Factors Affect Body Weight

Our genetic background influences our height, weight, body shape, and metabolic rate. A classic study showed that the body weights of adults who were adopted as children are similar to the weights of their biological parents, not their adoptive parents.[8] **Figure 11.9** shows that about 25% of our body fat is accounted for by genetic influences. Two theories linking genetics with our body weight are the thrifty gene theory and the set-point theory.

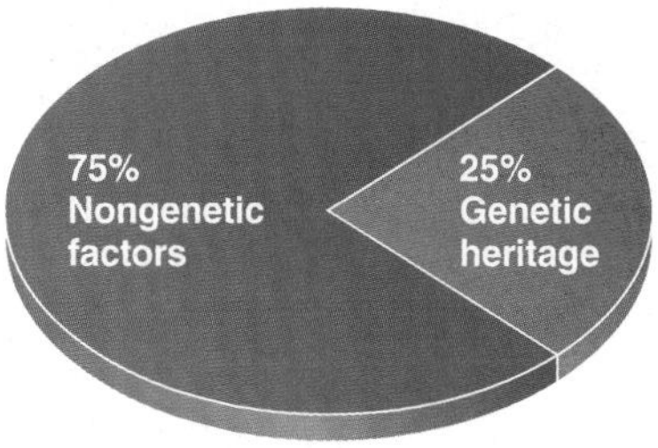

Figure 11.9 Research indicates that about 25% of our body fat is accounted for by our genetic heritage. However, nongenetic factors, such as diet and exercise, play a much larger role.

The Thrifty Gene Theory

The **thrifty gene theory** suggests that some people possess a gene (or genes) that causes them to be energetically thrifty. This means that at rest and even during active times these individuals expend less energy than people who do not possess this gene. The proposed purpose of this gene is to protect a person from starving to death during extreme food shortages. This theory has been applied to some Native American tribes, as these societies were exposed to centuries of feast or famine. Those with a thrifty metabolism survived when little food was available, and this trait was passed on to future generations. Although an actual thrifty gene (or genes) has not yet been identified, researchers continue to study this explanation as a potential cause of obesity.

If this theory were true, think about how people who possessed this thrifty gene would respond to today's environment. Low levels of physical activity, inexpensive food sources that are high in fat and energy, and excessively large serving sizes are the norm in our society. People with a thrifty metabolism would experience a great amount of weight gain, and their body would be more resistant to weight loss. Theoretically, having thrifty genetics would be advantageous during times of minimal food resources; however, this state could lead to very high levels of obesity in times of plenty.

The Set-Point Theory

The **set-point theory** suggests that our body is designed to maintain our weight within a narrow range, or at a "set point." In many cases, our body appears to respond in such a way as to maintain our present weight. When we dramatically reduce our energy intake (such as with fasting or strict diets), our body responds with physiologic changes that cause our BMR to drop. This causes a significant slowing of our energy output. In addition, being physically active while fasting or starving is difficult because we just don't have the energy for it. These two mechanisms of energy conservation may contribute to some of the rebound weight gain many dieters experience after they quit dieting.

Conversely, overeating in some people may cause an increase in BMR and is thought to be associated with an increased thermic effect of food, as well as an increase in spontaneous movements, or fidgeting. This in turn increases energy output and prevents weight gain. These changes may explain how some people fail to gain all of the weight expected from eating excess food. We don't eat exactly the same amount of food each day; some days we overeat, while other days we eat less. When you think about how much our daily energy intake fluctuates (about 20% above and below our average monthly intake), our ability to maintain a certain weight over long periods of time suggests that there is some evidence to support the set-point theory.

Can we change our weight set point? It appears that, when we maintain changes in our diet and activity level over a long period of time, weight change does occur. This is obvious in the case of obesity, since many people become obese during middle adulthood, and they are not able to maintain the lower body weight they had as a younger adult. Also, many people do successfully lose weight and maintain that weight loss over long periods of time. Thus, the set-point theory cannot entirely account for our body's resistance to weight loss.

A classic study on weight gain in twins demonstrated how genetics may affect our tendency to maintain a set point.[9] Twelve pairs of male identical twins volunteered to

thrifty gene theory The theory that some people possess a gene (or genes) that causes them to be energetically thrifty, resulting in their expending less energy at rest and during physical activity.

set-point theory The theory that the body raises or lowers energy expenditure in response to increased or decreased food intake and physical activity. This action maintains an individual's body weight within a narrow range.

stay in a dormitory, where they were supervised 24 hours a day for 120 consecutive days. Researchers measured how much energy each man needed to maintain his body weight at the beginning of the study. For 100 days, the subjects were fed 1,000 kcal more per day than they needed to maintain body weight. Daily physical activity was limited, but each person was allowed to walk outdoors for 30 minutes each day, read, watch television and videos, and play cards and video games. The research staff stayed with these men to ensure that they did not stray from the study protocol.

The average weight gain this group of men experienced was almost 18 pounds. Although they were all overfed enough energy to gain about 26 pounds, the average weight gain was 8 pounds less than expected. These men gained mostly fat but also gained about 6 pounds of lean body mass. Interestingly, there was a very wide range of weight gained. One man gained only about 9.5 pounds, while another man gained more than 29 pounds! Keep in mind that the food these men ate and the activities they performed were tightly controlled.

This study shows that, when people overeat by the same amount of food, they can gain very different amounts of weight and body fat. While each twin gained an amount similar to that of his brother, there was a lot of difference in how each set of twins responded. It is suggested that those who are more resistant to weight gain when they overeat have the ability to increase BMR, store more excess energy as lean body mass instead of fat, and increase spontaneous movements, such as fidgeting. Thus, genetic differences may explain why some people are better able to maintain a certain weight set point.

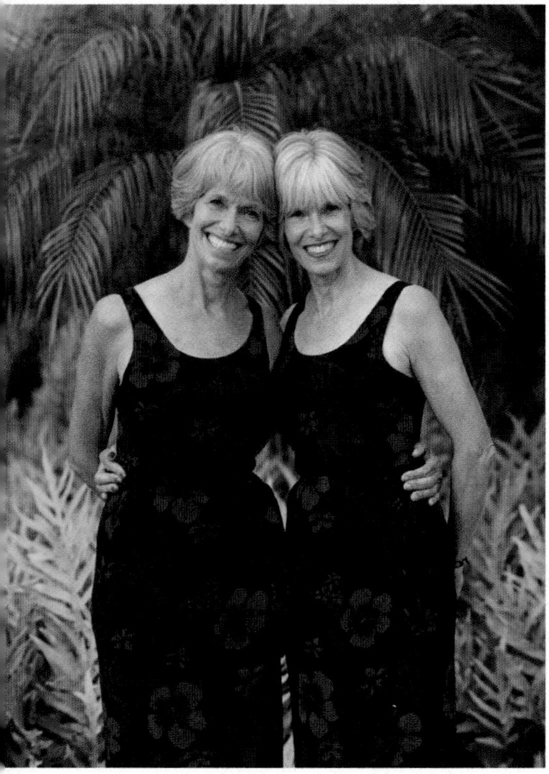

Identical twins tend to maintain a similar weight throughout life.

RECAP **Many factors affect our ability to gain and lose weight. Our genetic background influences our height, weight, body shape, and metabolic rate. The thrifty gene theory suggests that some people possess a thrifty gene, or set of genes, that causes them to expend less energy at rest and during physical activity than people who do not have this gene (or genes). The set-point theory suggests that our body is designed to maintain weight within a narrow range, also called a set point.**

Composition of the Diet Affects Fat Storage

As previously discussed, when we eat more energy than we expend, we gain weight. Most people eat a mixed diet, containing a mix of carbohydrate, fat, and protein. Scientists used to think that people would gain the same amount of weight if they ate too much food of any type, but now there is evidence that, when we overeat dietary fat, we store it much more easily as adipose tissue than we do either carbohydrate or protein.[10] This may be due to the fact that eating fat doesn't cause much of an increase in metabolic rate, and the body stores fat in the form of adipose tissue quite easily. In contrast, when we overeat protein or carbohydrate, our body's initial response is to use this extra food for energy or the building of tissues, with a smaller amount of the excess stored as fat. This does not mean, however, that you can eat as many low-fat foods as you want and not gain weight! Consistently overeating protein or carbohydrate will also lead to weight gain. Instead, maintain a balanced diet combining fat, carbohydrate, and protein, and lower your intake of dietary fat to less than 35% of total energy. This strategy may help reduce your storage of fat energy as adipose tissue.

Physiologic Factors Influence Body Weight

Numerous physiologic factors affect body weight, including hypothalamic regulation of hunger and satiety, specific proteins, and other factors. Together, these contribute to the complexities of weight regulation.

Hunger and Satiety

As introduced in Chapter 3, *hunger* is the innate, physiologic drive or need to eat. Physical signals, such as a growling stomach and light-headedness, indicate when one is hungry. This drive for food is triggered by physiologic changes, such as low blood glucose, that affect chemicals in the brain. The hypothalamus plays an important role in hunger regulation. Special hypothalamic cells referred to as *feeding cells* respond to conditions of low blood glucose, causing hunger and driving a person to eat. Once one has eaten and the body has responded accordingly, other centers in the hypothalamus are triggered, and the desire to eat is reduced. The state reached in which there is no longer a desire to eat is referred to as *satiety.* Some people may have an insufficient satiety mechanism, which prevents them from feeling full after a meal, allowing them to overeat.

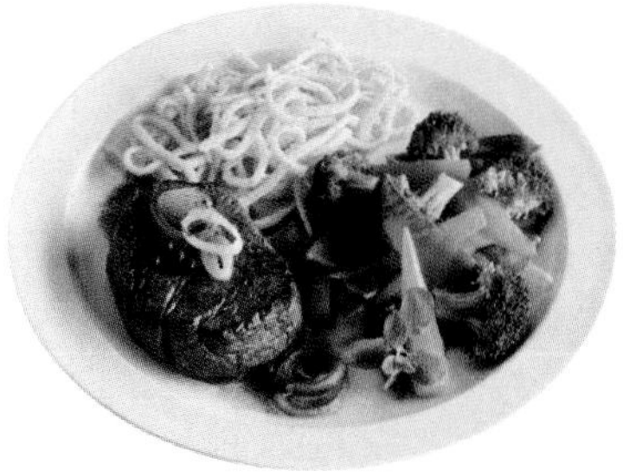

A balanced diet contains protein, carbohydrate, and fat.

Proteins

Leptin is a protein; it is produced by adipose cells and functions as a hormone. First discovered in mice, leptin reduces food intake and causes a decrease in body weight and body fat. A gene called the *ob* gene (obesity gene) codes for the production of leptin. Obese mice were found to have a genetic mutation in the *ob* gene. This mutation reduces the ability of adipose cells to synthesize leptin in sufficient amounts; therefore, food intake increases dramatically, energy output is reduced, and weight gain occurs.

When these findings were first published, a great deal of excitement was generated about how leptin might decrease obesity in humans. Unfortunately, studies have shown that, although obese mice respond positively to leptin injections, obese humans do not. Instead, they tend to have very high amounts of leptin in their body and are insensitive to leptin's effects. In truth, we have just begun to learn about leptin and its role in the human body. Researchers are currently studying leptin's relation to starvation and overeating, and it might be involved in cardiovascular and kidney complications that result from obesity and related diseases.

In addition to leptin, numerous proteins affect the regulation of appetite and storage of body fat. Primary among these is **ghrelin,** a protein synthesized in the stomach. It acts as a hormone and plays an important role in appetite regulation through its actions in the hypothalamus. Ghrelin stimulates appetite and increases food intake. Ghrelin levels increase before a meal and fall within about 1 hour after a meal. This action indicates that ghrelin may be a primary contributor to both hunger and satiety. Ghrelin levels appear to increase after weight loss, and researchers speculate that this factor might explain why people who have lost weight have difficulty keeping it off.[11] We noted earlier that obese people seem to lose their sensitivity to leptin, but this is not true for ghrelin: obese people are just as sensitive to the effects of ghrelin as non-obese people.[12] For this reason, potential mechanisms that can block the actions of ghrelin are currently a prime target of research into the treatment of obesity.

Peptide YY, or **PYY,** is a protein produced in the gastrointestinal tract. It is released after a meal, in amounts proportional to the energy content of the meal. In contrast with ghrelin, PYY decreases appetite and inhibits food intake in animals and humans.[13] Interestingly, obese individuals have lower levels of PYY when they are fasting and show less of an increase in PYY after a meal than non-obese individuals, which suggests that PYY may be important in the manifestation and maintenance of obesity.[14]

Uncoupling proteins have recently become the focus of research into body weight. These proteins are found in the inner membrane of mitochondria, which you may recall from Chapter 3 are organelles present within cells that generate ATP, including skeletal muscle cells and adipose cells. Some research suggests that uncoupling proteins uncouple certain steps in ATP production; when this occurs, the process produces heat instead of ATP. This production of heat increases energy expenditure and results in less storage of excess energy. Thus, a person with more uncoupling proteins or a higher activity of these proteins would be more resistant to weight gain and obesity.

Three forms of uncoupling proteins have been identified: UCP1 is found exclusively in **brown adipose tissue,** a type of adipose tissue that has more mitochondria than white adipose tissue. It is found in significant amounts in animals and newborn humans. It was traditionally thought that adult humans had very little brown adipose tissue. However, recent evidence suggests that humans may have substantially more

leptin A hormone, produced by body fat, that acts to reduce food intake and to decrease body weight and body fat.

ghrelin A protein, synthesized in the stomach, that acts as a hormone and plays an important role in appetite regulation by stimulating appetite.

peptide YY (PYY) A protein, produced in the gastrointestinal tract, that is released after a meal in amounts proportional to the energy content of the meal; it decreases appetite and inhibits food intake.

brown adipose tissue A type of adipose tissue that has more mitochondria than white adipose tissue, and which can increase energy expenditure by uncoupling oxidation from ATP production. It is found in significant amounts in animals and newborn humans.

brown adipose tissue than previously assumed[15] and that people with higher BMI values have lower amounts of brown adipose tissue.[16] These findings suggest a possible role of brown adipose tissue in obesity. Two other uncoupling proteins, UCP2 and UCP3, are known to be important to energy expenditure and resistance to weight gain. These proteins are found in various tissues, including white adipose tissue and skeletal muscle. The roles of brown adipose tissue and uncoupling proteins in human obesity are currently being researched.

Other Physiologic Factors

The following are other physiologic factors known to increase satiety (or decrease food intake):

- The hormones serotonin and cholecystokinin (CCK); serotonin is made from the amino acid tryptophan, and CCK is produced by the intestinal cells and stimulates the gallbladder to secrete bile
- An increase in blood glucose levels, such as that normally seen after the consumption of a meal
- Stomach expansion
- Nutrient absorption from the small intestine

The following are other physiologic factors that can decrease satiety (or increase food intake):

- Beta-endorphins, which are hormones that enhance a sense of pleasure while eating, increasing food intake
- Neuropeptide Y, an amino acid–containing compound produced in the hypothalamus; neuropeptide Y stimulates appetite
- Decreased blood glucose levels, such as the decrease that occurs after an overnight fast

Cultural and Economic Factors Affect Food Choices and Body Weight

Both cultural and economic factors can contribute to obesity. As discussed in detail in Chapter 1, cultural factors (including religious beliefs and learned food preferences) affect our food choices and eating patterns. In addition, the customs of many cultures put food at the center of celebrations of festivals and holidays, and overeating is tacitly encouraged. In addition, because both parents work outside the home in most American families, more people are embracing the "fast-food culture," preferring and almost exclusively choosing highly processed and highly caloric fast foods from restaurants and grocery stores.

Coinciding with these cultural influences on food intake are cultural factors that promote inactivity. These include the shift from manual labor to more sedentary jobs and increased access to labor-saving devices in all areas of our lives. Even seemingly minor changes—such as texting someone in your dorm instead of walking down the hall to chat, or walking through an automated door instead of pushing a door open—add up to a lower expenditure of energy by the end of the day. Research with sedentary ethnic minority women in the United States indicates that other common barriers to increasing physical activity include lack of personal motivation, no physically active role models to emulate, acceptance of larger body size, exercise being considered culturally unacceptable, and fear for personal safety in both rural and urban settings.[17,18] In short, cultural factors influence both food consumption and levels of physical activity and can contribute to weight gain.

Economic status is related to health status, particularly in developed countries, such as the United States: people of lower economic status have higher rates of obesity and related chronic diseases than people with higher incomes.[19] In addition to the impact of one's income on access to healthcare, economic factors strongly impact our food choices and eating behaviors. It is a common belief that healthful foods are expensive, and that only wealthy people can afford to purchase them. While it is true that certain foods considered more healthful, such as organic foods, imported fruits and vegetables, many fish, and leaner selections of some meats, can be costly, does healthful eating always have to be expensive? Refer to the Nutrition Myth or Fact? box on page 386 to learn more about whether a healthful diet can also be an affordable one.

Psychological and Social Factors Influence Behavior and Body Weight

In Chapter 3, we explored the concept that *appetite* can be experienced in the absence of hunger. Appetite may therefore be considered a psychological drive to eat, being stimulated by learned preferences for food and particular situations that promote eating. People may also follow social cues related to the timing and size of meals. Mood can also affect appetite, as some people will eat more or less if they feel depressed or happy. As you can imagine, appetite leads many people to overeat.

Some Social Factors Promote Overeating

Social factors—such as pressure from family and friends to eat the way they do—can encourage people to overeat. For instance, the pressure to overeat on holidays is high, as family members or friends offer extra servings of favorite holiday foods and follow a very large meal with a rich dessert.

Americans also have numerous opportunities to overeat because of easy access throughout the day to foods high in fat and energy. Vending machines selling junk foods are everywhere: at some schools, in business offices, and even at fitness centers. Shopping malls are filled with fast-food restaurants, where inexpensive, large serving sizes are the norm. Food manufacturers are producing products in ever-larger serving sizes, from the Monster Thickburger from Hardee's restaurant to the Enormous Omelet Sandwich from Burger King.[20] Even some foods traditionally considered healthful, such as some brands of peanut butter, yogurt, chicken soup, and milk, are filled with added sugars and other ingredients that are high in energy. This easy access to large servings of high-energy meals and snacks leads many people to consume excess energy.

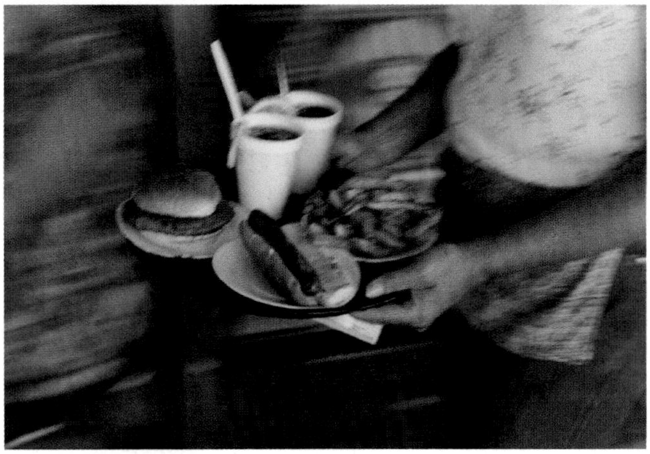

Fast foods may be inexpensive and filling, but they're usually high in saturated fat, salt, and sugar.

Some Social Factors Promote Inactivity

Social factors can also cause people to be less physically active. For instance, we don't even have to spend time or energy preparing food anymore, as everything either is ready to serve or requires just a few minutes to cook in a microwave oven. Other social factors restricting physical activity include living in an unsafe community; watching a lot of television; coping with family, community, and work responsibilities that do not involve physical activity; and living in an area with harsh weather conditions. Many overweight people identify such factors as major barriers to maintaining a healthful body weight, and research seems to confirm their influence.

Certainly, social factors are contributing to decreased physical activity among children. There was a time when children played outdoors regularly and when physical education was offered daily in school. In today's society, many children cannot play outdoors due to safety concerns and a lack of recreational facilities, and few schools have the resources to regularly offer physical education to children.

Another social factor promoting inactivity in both children and adults is the increasing dominance of technology in our choices of entertainment. Instead of participating in sports or gathering for a dance at the community hall, we go to the movies or stay at home watching television, surfing the Internet, and playing with video games and other hand-held devices. By reducing energy expenditure, these behaviors contribute to weight gain. For instance, a study of 11- to 13-year-old schoolchildren found that children who watched more than 2 hours of television per night were more likely to be

NUTRITION MYTH OR FACT?

Does It Cost More to Eat Right?

The shelves of American supermarkets are filled with an abundance of healthful food options: organic meats and produce, exotic fish, out-of-season fresh fruits and vegetables that are flown in from warmer climates, whole-grain breads and cereals. With all of these choices, it would seem easy for anyone to consume healthful foods throughout the year. But a closer look at the prices of these foods suggests that, for many, they simply are not affordable. This raises the question "Does eating right have to be expensive?"

Organic foods are more expensive than non-organic options. However, as we'll explore in detail in Chapter 13, there is little evidence that organic foods are actually more nutritious than non-organic foods. In addition, some of the lowest-cost foods are also some of the most healthful: beans, lentils, and other legumes; seasonal fruits; root vegetables, such as potatoes and winter squashes; frozen fruits and vegetables; and cooking oils high in mono- and polyunsaturated fats. In fact, frozen as well as canned fruits and vegetables are generally just as nutritious as fresh options, and they may be more so, depending on how long the fresh produce has been transported and stored, and how long it has been sitting on the supermarket shelves. Thus, with some knowledge, skills, and focused attention, anyone can eat healthfully on a tight budget.

Here are some tips to help you save money when shopping for healthful foods:

- Buy whole grains, such as cereals, brown rice, and pastas in bulk—they store well for longer periods and provide a good base for meals and snacks.
- Buy frozen vegetables on sale and stock up—these are just as healthful as fresh vegetables and require less preparation.
- If lower-sodium options of canned vegetables are too expensive, buy the less expensive regular option and drain the fluid from the vegetables before cooking.
- Consume smaller amounts of leaner meats—by eating less, you'll not only save money but reduce your total intake of energy and fat.
- Choose frozen fish or canned salmon or tuna packed in water as an alternative to fresh fish.
- Avoid frozen or dehydrated prepared meals. These are usually expensive; high in sodium, saturated fats, and energy; and low in fiber and other important nutrients.
- Buy generic or store brands of foods—be careful to check the labels to ensure the foods are similar in nutrient value to the higher-priced options.
- Cut coupons from local newspapers and magazines, and watch the sale circulars, so that you can stock up on healthful foods you can store.
- Consider cooking more meals at home; you'll have more control over what goes into your meals and will be able to cook larger amounts and freeze leftovers for future meals.

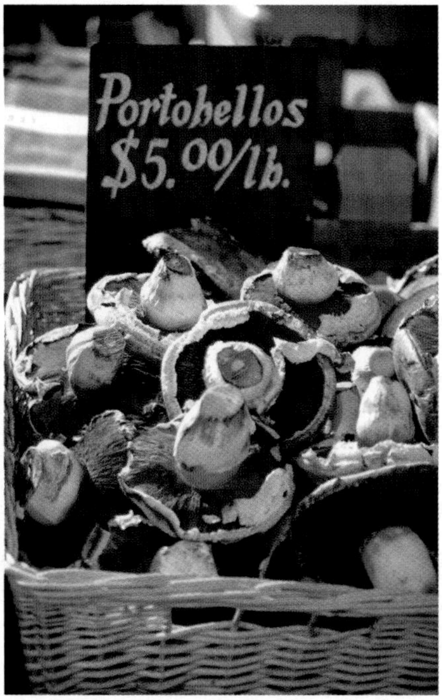

Although specialty foods (such as organic or imported products) can be expensive, lower-cost alternatives can be just as nutritious.

As you can see, eating healthfully does not have to be expensive. However, it helps to become a savvy consumer by reading food labels, comparing prices, and gaining the skills and confidence to cook at home. The information shared throughout this text should help you acquire these skills, so that you can eat healthfully, even on a limited budget!

overweight or obese than children who watched less than 2 hours of television per night. Similarly, adults who reported an increase in television watching of 20 hours per week (approximately 3 hours per day) over a 9-year period had a significant increase in waist circumference, indicating significant weight gain.[21]

Social Pressures Can Promote Underweight

On the other hand, social pressures to maintain a lean body are great enough to encourage many people to undereat or to avoid foods that are perceived as "bad," especially fats. Our society ridicules and often ostracizes overweight people, many of

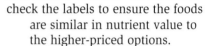

NUTRI-CASE HANNAH

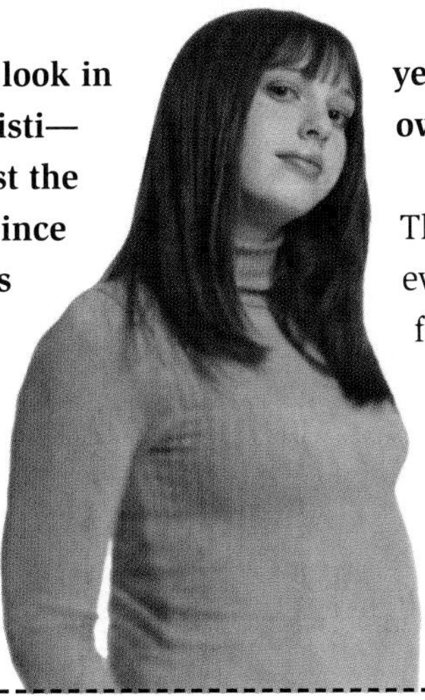

"I wonder what it would be like to be able to look in the mirror and not feel fat. Like my friend Kristi—she's been skinny since we were kids. I'm just the opposite: I've felt bad about my weight ever since I can remember. One of my worst memories is from the YMCA swim camp the summer I was 10 years old. Of course, we had to wear a swimsuit, and the other kids picked on me so bad I'll never forget it. One of the boys called me 'fatso,' and the girls were even meaner, especially when I was changing in the locker room. That was the last year I was in the swim camp, and I haven't owned a swimsuit since."

Think back to your own childhood. Were you ever teased for some personal aspect that you felt unable to change? How might organizations that work with children, such as schools, YMCAs, scout troops, and church-based groups, increase their leaders' awareness of the social stigmatization of overweight children and reduce incidents of teasing, bullying, and other insensitivity?

whom face discrimination in many areas of their lives, including employment. A recent study found that children who are obese are 60% more likely to experience bullying than children of normal weight.[22] Moreover, media images of waiflike fashion models and men in tight jeans with muscular chests and abdomens encourage many people—especially adolescents and young adults—to skip meals, resort to crash diets, and exercise obsessively. Even some people of normal body weight push themselves to achieve an unrealistic and unattainable weight goal, in the process threatening their health and even their lives (see the ***In Depth*** following Chapter 12 for the consequences of disordered eating).

It should be clear that how a person gains, loses, and maintains body weight is a complex matter. Most people who are overweight have tried several weight-loss programs but have been unsuccessful in maintaining long-term weight loss. A significant number of these people have consequently given up all weight-loss attempts. Some even suffer from severe depression related to their body weight. Should we condemn these people as failures and continue to pressure them to lose weight? Should people who are overweight but otherwise healthy (for example, having low blood pressure, cholesterol, triglyceride, and glucose levels) be advised to lose weight? As we continue to search for ways to help people achieve and maintain a healthful body weight, our society must take measures to reduce the social pressures facing people who are overweight or obese.

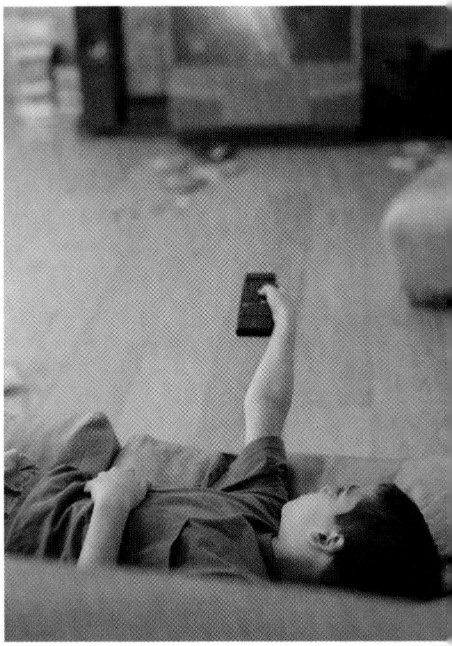

Behaviors learned as a child can affect weight and physical activity patterns.

RECAP **The macronutrient composition of the diet influences the storage of body fat, and physiologic factors, such as hunger, leptin, ghrelin, peptide YY, uncoupling proteins, and various hormones, impact body weight by their effects on satiety, appetite, and energy expenditure. Cultural and economic factors can significantly influence the amounts and types of food we eat. Psychological and social factors influencing weight include the ready availability of large portions of high-energy foods and lack of physical activity. Social pressures on those who are overweight can drive people to use harmful methods to achieve an unrealistic body weight.**

How Can You Achieve and Maintain a Healthful Body Weight?

Now that you understand what constitutes a healthful body weight, how are you feeling about yours? You might decide that you'd like to lose weight, but are you really committed to making the changes required? To find out, check out the What About

You? box starting on page 390. If your results suggest that you are, then take heart. Losing weight and maintaining that weight loss are goals well within your reach using three primary strategies:

- Gradual reduction in energy intake
- Regular and appropriate physical activity
- Application of behavior modification techniques

In this section, we'll first discuss popular diet plans that may or may not incorporate these strategies. We'll then explore how to design a personalized weight-loss program that includes all three of them.

If You Decide to Follow a Popular Diet Plan, Choose One Based on the Three Strategies

If you'd like to lose weight, the information on pages 390–397 will help you to design your own personalized diet plan. If you'd feel more comfortable following an established plan, however, many are available. How can you know whether it is based on sound dietary principles, and whether its promise of long-term weight loss will prove true for *you*? Look to the three strategies just identified: Does the plan promote gradual reductions in energy intake? Does it advocate increased physical activity? Does it include strategies for modifying your eating and activity-related behaviors? Reputable diet plans incorporate all of these strategies. Unfortunately, many dieters are drawn to fad diets, which do not.

Avoid Fad Diets

Beware of fad diets! They are simply what their name implies—fads that do not result in long-term, healthful weight changes. To be precise, fad diets are programs that enjoy short-term popularity and are sold based on a marketing gimmick that appeals to the public's desires and fears. Of the hundreds of such diets on the market today, most will "die" within a year, only to be born again as a "new and improved" fad diet. The goal of the person or company designing and marketing a fad diet is to make money.

How can you tell if the program you are interested in qualifies as a fad diet? Here are some pointers to help you:

- The promoters of the diet claim that the program is new, improved, or based on some new discovery; however, no scientific data are available to support these claims.
- The program is touted for its ability to promote rapid weight loss or body fat loss, usually more than 2 pounds per week, and may claim that weight loss can be achieved with little or no physical exercise.
- The diet includes special foods and supplements, many of which are expensive and/or difficult to find or can be purchased only from the diet promoter. Common recommendations for these diets include avoiding certain foods, eating only a special combination of certain foods, and including "magic" foods in the diet that "burn fat" and "speed up metabolism."
- The diet may include a rigid menu that must be followed daily or may limit participants to eating a few select foods each day. Variety and balance are discouraged, and restriction of certain foods (such as fruits and vegetables) is encouraged.
- Many programs promote supplemental foods and/or nutritional supplements that are described as critical to the success of the diet. They usually include claims that these supplements can cure or prevent a variety of health ailments or that the diet can stop the aging process.

In a world where many of us feel we have to meet a certain physical standard to be attractive and "good enough," these types of diets flourish: it is estimated that we spend more than $33 billion on fad diets each year.[23] Unfortunately, the only people who usually benefit from them are their marketers, who can become very wealthy promoting programs that are highly ineffectual.

Diets Focusing on Macronutrient Composition May or May Not Work for You

It is well recognized that achieving a negative energy balance is the major factor in successful weight loss. The impact of the macronutrient composition of a diet is currently a topic of considerable debate. The three main types of weight-loss diets that have been most seriously and comprehensively researched all encourage increased consumption of certain macronutrients and restrict the consumption of others. Provided here is a brief review of these three main types and their general effects on weight loss and health parameters.[24]

Diets High in Carbohydrate and Moderate in Fat and Protein Balanced high-carbohydrate, moderate-fat and -protein diets typically contain 55–60% of total energy intake as carbohydrate, 20–30% of total energy intake as fat, and 15–20% of energy intake as protein. These diets include Weight Watchers, Jenny Craig, and others that follow the general guidelines of the DASH diet and the Dietary Guidelines. All of these diet plans emphasize that weight loss occurs when energy intake is lower than energy expenditure. The goal is gradual weight loss, or about 1 to 2 lb of body weight per week. Typical energy deficits are between 500 and 1,000 kcal/day. It is recommended that women eat no less than 1,000 to 1,200 kcal/day and that men consume no less than 1,200 to 1,400 kcal/day. Regular physical activity is encouraged.

To date, these types of low-energy diets have been researched more than any others. A substantial amount of high-quality scientific evidence (from randomized controlled trials) indicates that they are effective in decreasing body weight. In addition, the people who lose weight on these diets also decrease their LDL-cholesterol, reduce their blood triglyceride levels, and decrease their blood pressure. The diets are nutritionally adequate if the individual's food choices follow the USDA Food Guide. If the individual's food choices are not varied and balanced, the diet may be low in nutrients such as fiber, zinc, calcium, iron, and vitamin B_{12}. Under these circumstances, supplementation is needed.

Diets Low in Carbohydrate and High in Fat and Protein Low-carbohydrate, high-fat and -protein diets cycle in and out of popularity on a regular basis. By definition, these types of diets generally contain less than 100 g of carbohydrate per day, about 55–65% of total energy intake as fat, and the balance of daily energy intake as protein. Examples of these types of diets are Dr. Atkins' Diet Revolution, the Carbohydrate Addict's Diet, Life Without Bread, Sugar Busters, and Protein Power. These diets minimize the role of restricting total energy intake on weight loss. They instead advise participants to restrict carbohydrate intake, proposing that carbohydrates are addictive and cause significant overeating, insulin surges leading to excessive fat storage, and an overall metabolic imbalance that leads to obesity. The goal is to reduce carbohydrates enough to cause ketosis, which will decrease blood glucose and insulin levels and can reduce appetite.

Countless people claim to have lost substantial weight on these types of diets; however, quality scientific studies of these diets are just beginning to be conducted. The current limited evidence suggests that individuals in both free-living and experimental conditions do lose weight with these diets. In addition, it appears that people who lose weight may also experience positive metabolic changes, such as decreased blood lipid levels, decreased blood pressure, and decreased blood glucose and insulin. However, the amount of weight loss and improvements in metabolic health measured with these diets are no greater than those seen with higher-carbohydrate diets. Our current limited evidence of the effectiveness, along with concerns about long-term compliance,

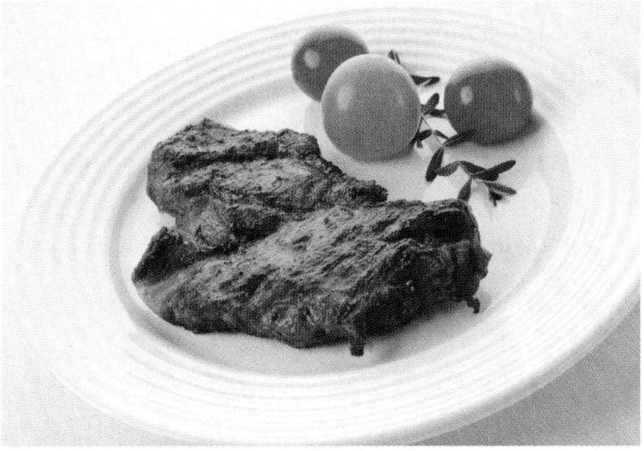

"Low-carb" diets may lead to weight loss, but can be nutritionally inadequate and have negative side effects.

What About You?

Are You Really Ready to Lose Weight?

How well do your attitudes equip you for a weight-loss program? For each question, circle the answer that best describes your attitude. As you complete sections 2–5, tally your score and analyze it according to the scoring guide.

1. Diet History

A. How many times in the last year have you been on a diet?

0 times 1–3 times 4–10 times 11–20 times More than 20

B. What is the most weight you lost on any of these diets?

0 lb 1–5 lb 6–10 lb 11–20 lb More than 20 lb

C. How long did you stay at the new lower weight?

Less than 1 mo 2–3 mo 4–6 mo 6–12 mo Over 1 yr

D. Why do you think you started to regain the weight?

E. Put a check mark by each dieting method you have tried:

____ skipping breakfast
____ skipping lunch or dinner
____ taking over-the-counter appetite suppressants
____ counting Calories
____ cutting out most fats
____ cutting out most carbohydrates
____ increasing regular exercise
____ taking weight-loss supplements
____ cutting out all snacks
____ using meal replacements such as Slim-Fast
____ taking prescription appetite suppressants
____ taking laxatives
____ inducing vomiting
____ other ____________________

2. Readiness to Start a Weight-Loss Program

If you are thinking about starting a weight-loss program, answer questions A–F.

A. How motivated are you to lose weight?

1	**2**	**3**	**4**	**5**
Not at all motivated	Slightly motivated	Somewhat motivated	Quite motivated	Extremely motivated

B. How certain are you that you will stay committed to a weight-loss program long enough to reach your goal?

1	**2**	**3**	**4**	**5**
Not at all certain	Slightly certain	Somewhat certain	Quite certain	Extremely certain

C. Taking into account other stresses in your life (school, work, and relationships), to what extent can you tolerate the effort required to stick to your diet plan?

1	**2**	**3**	**4**	**5**
Cannot commit	Can commit somewhat	Uncertain	Can commit well	Can commit easily

D. Assuming you should lose no more than 1 to 2 pounds per week, have you allotted a realistic amount of time for weight loss?

1	**2**	**3**	**4**	**5**
Very unrealistic	Somewhat unrealistic	Moderately unrealistic	Somewhat realistic	Very realistic

E. While dieting, do you fantasize about eating your favorite foods?

1	**2**	**3**	**4**	**5**
Always	Frequently	Occasionally	Rarely	Never

F. While dieting, do you feel deprived, angry, upset?

1	**2**	**3**	**4**	**5**
Always	Frequently	Occasionally	Rarely	Never

Total your scores from questions A–F and circle your score category.

6 to 16: This may not be a good time for you to start a diet. Inadequate motivation and commitment and unrealistic goals could block your progress. Think about what contributes to your unreadiness. What are some of the factors? Consider changing these factors before undertaking a diet.

17 to 23: You may be nearly ready to begin a program but should think about ways to boost your readiness.

24 to 30: The path is clear—you can decide how to lose weight in a safe, effective way.

3. Hunger, Appetite, and Eating

Think about your hunger and the cues that stimulate your appetite or eating, and then answer questions A–C.

A. When food comes up in conversation or in something you read, do you want to eat, even if you are not hungry?

1	2	3	4	5
Never	Rarely	Occasionally	Frequently	Always

B. How often do you eat for a reason other than physical hunger?

1	2	3	4	5
Never	Rarely	Occasionally	Frequently	Always

C. When your favorite foods are around the house, do you succumb to eating them between meals?

1	2	3	4	5
Never	Rarely	Occasionally	Frequently	Always

Total your scores from questions A–C and circle your score category.

3 to 6: You might occasionally eat more than you should, but it is due more to your own attitudes than to temptation and other environmental cues. Controlling your own attitudes toward hunger and eating may help you.

7 to 9: You may have a moderate tendency to eat just because food is available. Losing weight may be easier for you if you try to resist external cues and eat only when you are physically hungry.

10 to 15: Some or much of your eating may be in response to thinking about food or exposing yourself to temptations to eat. Think of ways to minimize your exposure to temptations so you eat only in response to physical hunger.

4. Controlling Overeating

How good are you at controlling overeating when you are on a diet? Answer questions A–C.

A. A friend talks you into going out to a restaurant for a midday meal instead of eating a brown-bag lunch. As a result, you:

1	2	3	4	5
Would eat much less	Would eat somewhat less	Would make no difference	Would eat somewhat more	Would eat much more

B. You "break" your diet by eating a fattening, "forbidden" food. As a result, for the day, you:

1	2	3	4	5
Would eat much less	Would eat somewhat less	Would make no difference	Would eat somewhat more	Would eat much more

C. You have been following your diet faithfully and decide to test yourself by taking a bite of something you consider a treat. As a result, for the day, you:

1	2	3	4	5
Would eat much less	Would eat somewhat less	Would make no difference	Would eat somewhat more	Would eat much more

Total your scores from questions A–C and circle your score category.

3 to 7: You recover rapidly from mistakes. However, if you frequently alternate between out-of-control eating and very strict dieting, you may have a serious eating problem and should get professional help.

8 to 11: You do not seem to let unplanned eating disrupt your program. This is a flexible, balanced approach.

12 to 15: You may be prone to overeating after an event breaks your control or throws you off track. Your reaction to these problem-causing events could use improvement.

5. Emotional Eating

Consider the effects of your emotions on your eating behaviors, and answer questions A–C.

A. Do you eat more than you would like to when you have negative feelings such as anxiety, depression, anger, or loneliness?

1	2	3	4	5
Never	Rarely	Occasionally	Frequently	Always

B. Do you have trouble controlling your eating when you have positive feelings (i.e., do you celebrate feeling good by eating)?

1	2	3	4	5
Never	Rarely	Occasionally	Frequently	Always

(continued)

C. When you have unpleasant interactions with others in your life or after a difficult day at work, do you eat more than you'd like?

1	2	3	4	5
Never	Rarely	Occasionally	Frequently	Always

Total your scores from questions A–C and circle your score category.

3 to 8: You do not appear to let your emotions affect your eating.

9 to 11: You sometimes eat in response to emotional highs and lows. Monitor this behavior to learn when and why it occurs, and be prepared to find alternative activities to respond to your emotions.

12 to 15: Emotional ups and downs can stimulate your eating. Try to deal with the feelings that trigger the eating and find other ways to express them.

6. Exercise Patterns and Attitudes

Exercise is key for weight loss. Think about your attitudes toward it, and answer questions A–D.

A. How often do you exercise?

1	2	3	4	5
Never	Rarely	Occasionally	Somewhat frequently	Frequently

B. How confident are you that you can exercise regularly?

1	2	3	4	5
Not at all confident	Slightly confident	Somewhat confident	Highly confident	Completely confident

C. When you think about exercise, do you develop a positive or negative picture in your mind?

1	2	3	4	5
Completely negative	Somewhat negative	Neutral	Somewhat positive	Completely positive

D. How certain are you that you can work regular exercise into your daily schedule?

1	2	3	4	5
Not at all certain	Slightly certain	Somewhat certain	Quite certain	Extremely certain

Total your scores from questions A–D and circle your score category.

4 to 10: You're probably not exercising as regularly as you should. Determine whether it is your attitude about exercise or your lifestyle that is blocking your way, then change what you must and put on those walking shoes!

11 to 16: You need to feel more positive about exercise so you can do it more often. Think of ways to be more active that are fun and fit your lifestyle.

17 to 20: The path is clear for you to be active. Now think of ways to get motivated.

Data from "The Diet Readiness Test," in Kelly D. Brownell, "When and How to Diet," *Psychology Today* (June 1989) 41–46.

potential health risks, and side effects, has made these diets controversial. Refer to the Nutrition Debate at the end of this chapter to learn more about these diets.

Low-Fat and Very-Low-Fat Diets Low-fat diets contain 11–19% of total energy as fat, whereas very-low-fat diets contain less than 10% of total energy as fat. Both of these types of diets are high in carbohydrate and moderate in protein. Examples are Dr. Dean Ornish's Program for Reversing Heart Disease and the New Pritikin Program. These diets do not focus on total energy intake but emphasize eating foods higher in complex carbohydrates and fiber. Consumption of sugar and white flour is very limited. The Ornish diet is vegetarian, whereas the Pritikin diet allows 3.5 oz of lean meat per day. Regular physical activity is a key component of these diets.

These programs were not originally designed for weight loss but, rather, were developed to decrease or reverse heart disease. Also, these diets are not popular with consumers, who view them as too restrictive and difficult to follow. Thus, there are limited data on their effects. However, high-quality evidence suggests that people following these diets do lose weight, and some data suggest that these diets may also decrease LDL-cholesterol, triglyceride, glucose, and insulin levels, as well as blood pressure. Few side effects have been reported on these diets; the most common is flatus, which typically decreases over time. Low-fat diets are low in vitamin B_{12}, and very-low-fat diets are low in essential fatty acids, vitamins B_{12} and E, and zinc. Thus, supplementation is needed. These types of diets are not considered safe for people with diabetes who are insulin dependent (either type 1 or type 2) or for people with carbohydrate-malabsorption illnesses.

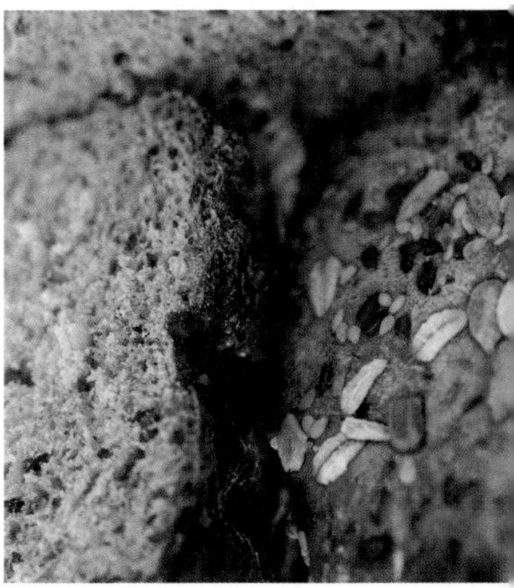

Low-fat and very-low-fat diets emphasize eating foods higher in complex carbohydrates and fiber.

If You Decide to Design Your Own Diet Plan, Include the Three Strategies

As we noted earlier, a healthful and effective weight-loss plan involves making a modest reduction in your energy intake, incorporating physical activity into each day, and practicing changes in behavior that can help you reduce your energy intake and increase your energy expenditure. Following are some guidelines for designing your own personalized diet plan that incorporates these strategies.

Set Realistic Goals

The first key to safe and effective weight loss is setting realistic goals related to how much weight to lose and how quickly to lose it. Although making gradual changes in body weight is frustrating for most people, this slower change is much more effective in maintaining weight loss over the long term. Ask yourself the question "How long did it take me to gain this extra weight?" If you are like most people, your answer is that it took 1 or more years, not just a few months. A fair expectation for weight loss is similarly gradual: experts recommend a pace of about 0.5 to 2 pounds per week. A weight-loss plan should never provide less than 1,200 kcal/day unless you are under a physician's supervision. Your weight-loss goals should also take into consideration any health-related concerns you have. After checking with your physician, you may decide initially to set a goal of simply maintaining your current weight and preventing additional weight gain. After your weight has remained stable for several weeks, you might then write down realistic goals for weight loss.

Goals that are more likely to be realistic and achievable share the following characteristics:

- *They are specific.* Telling yourself "I will eat less this week" is not helpful because the goal is not specific. An example of a specific goal is "I will eat only half of my restaurant entrée tonight and take the rest home and eat it tomorrow for lunch."
- *They are reasonable.* If you are not presently physically active, it would be unreasonable to set a goal of exercising for 30 minutes every day. A more reasonable goal would be to exercise for 15 minutes per day, 3 days per week. Once you've achieved that goal, you can increase the frequency, intensity, and time of exercise according to the improvements in fitness that you have experienced.
- *They are measurable.* Effective goals are ones you can measure. An example is "I will lose at least half a pound by May 1st" or "I will substitute drinking water for my regular soft drink at lunch each day this week." Recording your specific, measurable goals will help you determine whether you are achieving them.

By monitoring your progress regularly, you can determine whether you are meeting your goals or whether you need to revise them based on accomplishments or challenges that arise.

Eat Smaller Portions of Lower-Fat Foods

The portion sizes of foods offered and sold in restaurants have expanded considerably over the past 40 years. One of the most challenging issues related to food is understanding what a healthful portion size is and how to reduce the portion sizes of foods that we eat.

Recent studies indicate that, when children and adults are presented with large portion sizes of foods and beverages, they eat more energy overall and do not respond

QUICK TIPS

Controlling Portion Sizes

✓ To help increase your understanding of the portion sizes of packaged foods, measure out the amount of food that is identified as 1 serving on the Nutrition Facts Panel, and eat it from a plate or bowl instead of straight out of the box or bag.

✓ Try using smaller dishes, bowls, and glasses. This will make your portion appear larger, and you'll be eating or drinking less.

✓ When cooking at home, put a serving of the entrée on your plate; then freeze any leftovers in single-serving containers. This way, you won't be tempted to eat the whole batch before the food goes bad, and you'll have ready-made servings for future meals.

✓ To help you fill up, take second helpings of plain vegetables. That way, dessert may not seem so tempting!

✓ When buying snacks, go for single-serving, prepackaged items. If you buy larger bags or boxes, divide the snack into single-serving bags.

✓ When you have a treat, such as ice cream, measure out 1/2 cup, eat it slowly, and enjoy it!

✓ To test your understanding of what exactly constitutes a serving size, take the "Portion Distortion" interactive quiz from the National Institutes of Health. See Web Resources at the end of this chapter for the link.

to cues of fullness.[25,26] Thus, it has been suggested that effective weight-loss strategies include reducing both the portion size and the energy density of foods consumed and replacing energy-dense beverages with low-Calorie or noncaloric beverages.[26]

What specific changes can you make to reduce your energy intake and stay healthy? Here are some helpful suggestions from the Weight-Control Information Network.[27]

Now that you have your portion sizes under control, what can you do to reduce the saturated fat and energy content of the portions you *do* eat? Remember that people trying to lose weight should aim for a total fat intake of 15–25% of total energy intake and a saturated fat intake of 10% or below. This goal can be achieved by eliminating extra fats, such as butter, cheese sauces, mayonnaise, and snack foods (such as ice cream, doughnuts, and cakes). Save these foods as occasional special treats. Select lower-fat versions of the foods listed in the USDA Food Patterns. This means selecting leaner cuts of meat (such as the white meat of poultry and extra-lean ground beef) and reduced-fat or skim dairy products and selecting lower-fat preparation methods (such as baking and broiling instead of frying). It also means switching from a sugar-filled beverage to a low-Calorie or noncaloric beverage during and between meals.

In addition, try to increase the number of times each day that you choose foods that are relatively low in energy density. These include salads (with low-Calorie or noncaloric dressings), fruits, vegetables, and broth-based soups. These foods are low in energy and high in fiber, water, and nutrients. Because they contain relatively more water and fiber than more energy-dense foods, they can help you feel satiated without having to consume large amounts of energy.

Figure 11.10 illustrates two sets of meals, one higher in energy and one lower in energy. You can see from this figure that simple changes to a meal, such as choosing lower-fat dairy products, smaller portion sizes, and foods that are relatively less dense in energy, can reduce energy intake without sacrificing taste, pleasure, or nutritional quality!

Participate in Regular Physical Activity

Why is being physically active so important for achieving changes in body weight and for maintaining a healthful body weight? Of course, we expend extra energy during physical activity, but there's more to it than that because exercise alone (without a reduction of energy intake) does not result in dramatic decreases in body weight. Instead, one of the most important reasons for being regularly active is that it helps us maintain or increase our lean body mass and our BMR. In contrast, energy restriction alone causes us to lose lean body mass. As you've learned, the more lean body mass we have, the more energy we expend over the long term.

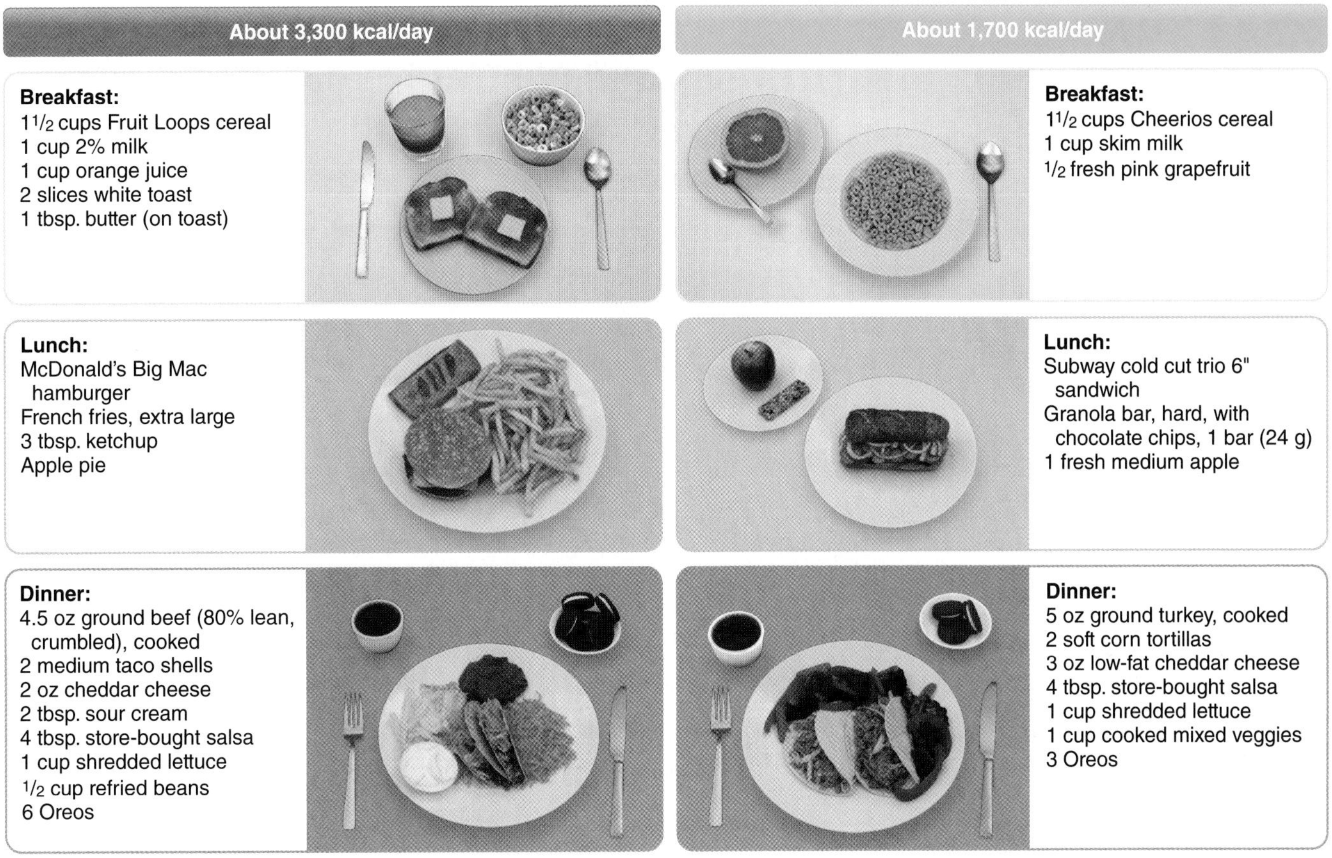
About 3,300 kcal/day
About 1,700 kcal/day
Breakfast:
1 1/2 cups Fruit Loops cereal
1 cup 2% milk
1 cup orange juice
2 slices white toast
1 tbsp. butter (on toast)
Breakfast:
1 1/2 cups Cheerios cereal
1 cup skim milk
1/2 fresh pink grapefruit
Lunch:
McDonald's Big Mac hamburger
French fries, extra large
3 tbsp. ketchup
Apple pie
Lunch:
Subway cold cut trio 6" sandwich
Granola bar, hard, with chocolate chips, 1 bar (24 g)
1 fresh medium apple
Dinner:
4.5 oz ground beef (80% lean, crumbled), cooked
2 medium taco shells
2 oz cheddar cheese
2 tbsp. sour cream
4 tbsp. store-bought salsa
1 cup shredded lettuce
1/2 cup refried beans
6 Oreos
Dinner:
5 oz ground turkey, cooked
2 soft corn tortillas
3 oz low-fat cheddar cheese
4 tbsp. store-bought salsa
1 cup shredded lettuce
1 cup cooked mixed veggies
3 Oreos

Figure 11.10 The energy density of two sets of meals. The set on the left is higher in energy density, while the set on the right is lower in energy density and the preferred choice for a person trying to lose weight.

The National Weight Control Registry is an ongoing project documenting the habits of people who have lost at least 30 pounds and kept their weight off for at least 1 year. Of the 784 people studied thus far, the average weight loss was 66 pounds, and the group maintained the minimum weight-loss criteria of 30 pounds for more than 5 years.[28] Almost all of the people (89%) reported changing both physical activity and dietary intake to lose weight and maintain weight loss. No one form of exercise seems to be most effective, but many people report doing some form of aerobic exercise (such as bicycling, walking, running, aerobic dance, step aerobics, or hiking) and weight lifting at least 45 minutes most days of the week. In fact, on average,

QUICK TIPS

Overcoming Barriers to Physical Activity

✓ *I don't have enough time!* An active lifestyle doesn't have to consume all your free time. Try to do a minimum of 30 minutes of moderate activity most—preferably all—days of the week. If you can, do 45 minutes. But remember, you don't have to get in all of your daily activity in one go! Be active for a few minutes at a time throughout your day. Walk from your dorm or apartment to classes, if possible. Instead of meeting friends for lunch, meet them for a lunchtime walk, jog, or workout. Break up study sessions with 3 minutes of jumping jacks. Skip the elevator and take the stairs. When you're talking on the phone, pace instead of sitting still.

✓ *I can't manage the details!* Bust this excuse by keeping clean clothes, shoes, water, and equipment for physical activity in a convenient place. If time management is an obstacle, enroll in a scheduled fitness class, yoga class, sports activity, walking group, or running club. Put it on your schedule of academic classes and make it part of your weekly routine.

✓ *I just don't like to work out!* You don't have to! Try dancing, roller blading, walking, hiking, swimming, tennis, or any other activity you enjoy.

✓ *I can't stay motivated.* Friends can help. Use the "buddy" system by exercising with a friend and calling each other when you need encouragement to stay motivated. Or keep a journal or log of your daily physical activity. Write your week's goal at the top of the page (such as "Walk to and from campus each day, and at least 10 minutes on campus at lunch"). Then track your progress. You can also use the form in **Figure 11.11**. If you achieve your goal for the week, reward yourself with a massage, a new song for your iPod, or some other nonfood treat.

My Weekly Activity Goals

Week 1 Goals

I commit to begin____________________(type of activity) for ____________________minutes on

❑ Monday ❑ Tuesday ❑ Wednesday
❑ Thursday ❑ Friday ❑ Saturday ❑ Sunday

Week 2 Goals

I commit to begin____________________(type of activity) for ____________________minutes on

❑ Monday ❑ Tuesday ❑ Wednesday
❑ Thursday ❑ Friday ❑ Saturday ❑ Sunday

Week 3 Goals

I commit to begin____________________(type of activity) for ____________________minutes on

❑ Monday ❑ Tuesday ❑ Wednesday
❑ Thursday ❑ Friday ❑ Saturday ❑ Sunday

Week 4 and Beyond

I commit to begin____________________(type of activity) for ____________________minutes on

❑ Monday ❑ Tuesday ❑ Wednesday
❑ Thursday ❑ Friday ❑ Saturday ❑ Sunday

Figure 11.11 Use this goal-setting card to help you set—and reach—weekly activity goals.
Data from Weight-Control Information Network. 2010. NIH Publication No. 10-4352. www.win.niddk.nih.gov/publications/active.htm

this group expended more than 2,800 kcal each week through physical activity! While very few weight-loss studies have documented long-term maintenance of weight loss, those that have find that only people who are regularly active are able to maintain most of their weight loss.

In addition to expending energy and maintaining lean body mass and BMR, regular physical activity improves our mood, results in a higher quality of sleep, increases self-esteem, and gives us a sense of accomplishment (see Chapter 12 for more benefits of regular physical activity). All of these changes enhance our ability to engage in long-term healthful lifestyle behaviors.

What specific changes can you make to increase your level of physical activity? We'll have plenty of practical suggestions in Chapter 12, but to get you warmed up, it might help to start identifying—and overcoming—your barriers to an active life. Here are some ideas.

Incorporate Appropriate Behavior Modifications into Daily Life

Successful weight loss and long-term maintenance of a healthful weight require people to modify their behaviors. Some of the behavior modifications related to food and physical activity have been discussed in the previous sections. Here are a few more practical changes you can make to help you lose weight and keep it off.

RECAP Achieving and maintaining a healthful body weight involves gradual reductions in energy intake, such as by eating smaller portion sizes and limiting dietary fat; engaging in regular physical activity; and applying appropriate behavior modification techniques. Fad diets do not use these strategies and do not result in long-term, healthful weight change. Diets based on macronutrient composition may promote long-term weight loss, but some have unhealthful side effects. Using dietary supplements to lose weight is controversial and can be dangerous.

QUICK TIPS

Modifying Your Behaviors Related to Food

- ✓ Shop for food only when you're not hungry.
- ✓ Avoid buying problem foods—that is, foods that you may have difficulty eating in moderate amounts.
- ✓ Avoid purchasing high-fat, high-sugar food from vending machines and convenience stores.
- ✓ Avoid feelings of deprivation by eating small, regular meals throughout the day.
- ✓ Eat only at set times in one location. Do not eat while studying, working, driving, watching television, and so forth.
- ✓ Slow down while eating.
- ✓ Keep a log of what you eat, when, and why. As discussed previously (Chapter 3), try to identify social or emotional cues that cause you to overeat, such as getting a poor grade on an exam or feeling lonely. Then strategize about nonfood-related ways to cope, such as phoning a sympathetic friend.
- ✓ Save high-fat, high-kilocalorie snack foods (such as ice cream, doughnuts, and cakes) for occasional special treats.
- ✓ Whether at home or dining out, share food with others.
- ✓ Prepare healthful snacks to take along with you, so that you won't be tempted by foods from vending machines, fast-food restaurants, and so forth.
- ✓ Chew food slowly, taking at least 20 minutes to eat a full meal, stopping at once if you begin to feel full.
- ✓ Always use appropriate utensils.
- ✓ Leave food on your plate or store it for the next meal.
- ✓ Don't punish yourself for deviating from your plan (and you will—everyone does). Ask others to avoid responding to any slips you make.

What About Underweight?

As defined earlier in this chapter, underweight occurs when a person has too little body fat to maintain health. People with a BMI of less than 18.5 kg/m^2 are typically considered underweight. Being underweight can be just as unhealthful as being obese, because it increases the risk for infections and illness and impairs the body's ability to recover. Some people are healthy but underweight because of their genetics and/or because they are very physically active and consume adequate energy to maintain their underweight status but not enough to gain weight. In others, underweight is due to heavy smoking; an underlying disease, such as cancer or HIV infection; or an eating disorder, such as anorexia nervosa (see the ***In Depth*** on eating disorders that follows Chapter 12).

With so much emphasis in the United States on obesity and weight loss, some find it surprising that many people are trying to gain weight. People looking to gain weight include those who are underweight to the extent that it is compromising their health and many athletes who are attempting to increase their strength and power for competition.

To gain weight, people must eat more energy than they expend. While overeating large amounts of foods high in saturated fats (such as bacon, sausage, and cheese) can cause weight gain, doing this without exercising is not considered healthful because most of the weight gained is fat, and high-fat diets increase our risks for cardiovascular and other diseases. Unless there are medical reasons to eat a high-fat

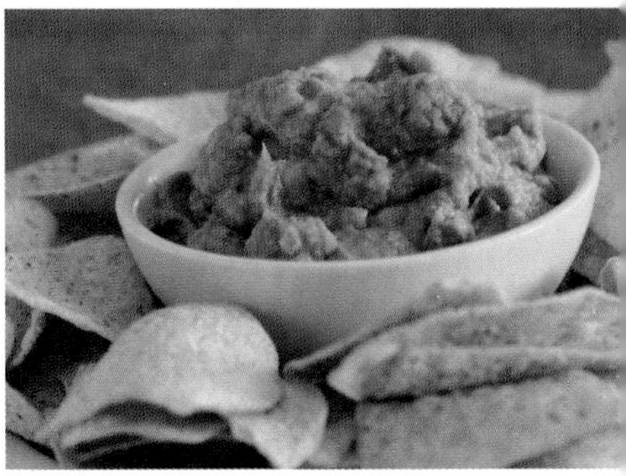

Eating frequent nutrient- and energy-dense snacks can help promote weight gain.

diet, it is recommended that people trying to gain weight eat a diet that is relatively low in dietary fat (less than 30% of total Calories) and relatively high in complex carbohydrates (55% of total Calories). Recommendations for weight gain include:

- Eat a diet that includes about 500–1,000 kcal/day more than is needed to maintain present body weight. Although we don't know exactly how much extra energy is needed to gain 1 pound, estimates range from 3,000 to 3,500 kcal. Thus, eating 500–1,000 kcal/day in excess should result in a gain of 1–2 pounds of weight each week.
- Eat frequently, including meals and numerous snacks throughout the day. Many underweight people do not take the time to eat often enough.
- Avoid the use of tobacco products, as they depress appetite and increase metabolic rate, and both of these effects oppose weight gain. Tobacco use also causes lung, mouth, and esophageal cancers.
- Exercise regularly and incorporate weight lifting or some other form of resistance training into your exercise routine. This form of exercise is most effective in increasing muscle mass. Performing aerobic exercise (such as walking, running, bicycling, or swimming) at least 30 minutes for 3 days per week will help you maintain a healthy cardiovascular system.

The key to gaining weight is to eat frequent meals throughout the day and to select energy-dense foods. When selecting foods that are higher in fat, make sure they are higher in polyunsaturated and monounsaturated fats (such as peanut butter, olive and canola oils, and avocados). For instance, smoothies and milkshakes made with low-fat milk or yogurt are a great way to take in a lot of energy. Eating peanut butter with fruit or celery and including salad dressings on your salad are other ways to increase the energy density of foods. The biggest challenge to weight gain is setting aside time to eat; by packing a lot of foods to take with you throughout the day, you can increase your opportunities to eat more.

RECAP Weight gain can be achieved by eating about 500–1,000 kcal/day more than is needed to maintain present weight and by performing weight lifting and aerobic exercise. Eating frequent meals throughout the day, selecting healthy foods that are energy dense, and avoiding the use of tobacco products are strategies that can assist with healthy weight gain.

HOT TOPIC

Using Dietary Supplements to Lose Weight—Should You Consider It?

As we explored ***In Depth*** following Chapter 10, dangerous or ineffective supplements can be marketed and sold without meeting the FDA's strict safety and quality standards. Moreover, the FDA can pull a dietary supplement from the shelves only if it can prove that the supplement is dangerous. So if you want to lose weight—should you consider an over-the-counter weight-loss supplement?

Consumers have a variety of weight-loss products to choose from. Some of the most common are the mineral chromium, spirulina (blue-green algae), ginseng (a root used in Chinese medicine), chitosan (derived from the exoskeleton of crustaceans), green tea, and psyllium (a source of fiber).[29,30] These products are popular despite the fact that studies find insufficient evidence to support their use. Some products marketed for weight loss do indeed increase metabolic rate and decrease appetite; however, they create these effects because they contain *stimulants*, substances that speed up physiologic processes. Use of these substances is controversial and may be dangerous, as excessive increases in heart rate and blood pressure can occur.

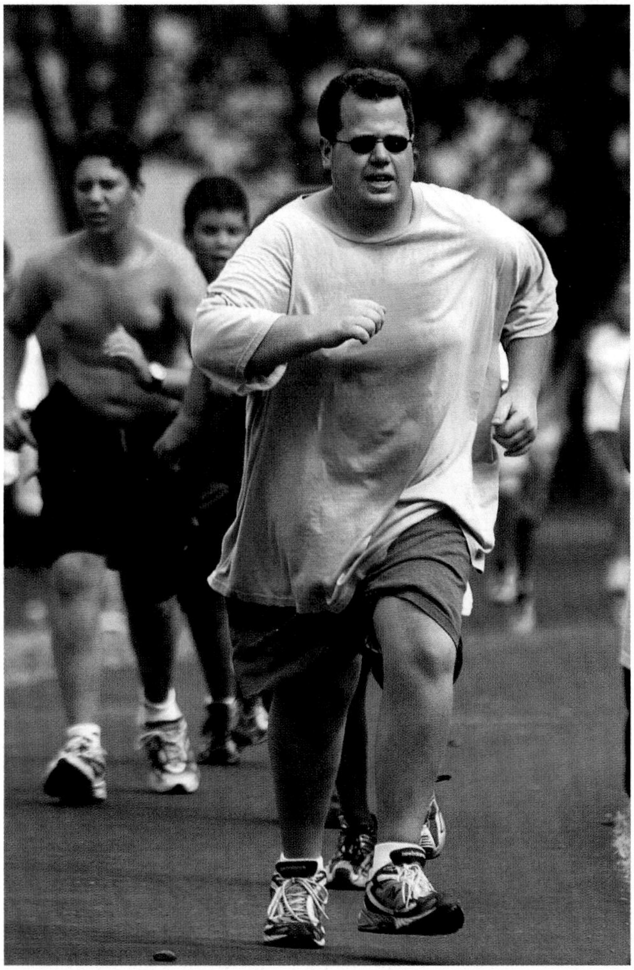

Increased physical activity can help many obese people succeed in losing weight and keeping it off.

goals. Other people have tried to follow healthful weight-loss suggestions for years and have not been successful. In response to these challenges, prescription drugs have been developed to assist people with weight loss. These drugs typically act as appetite suppressants and may increase satiety.

Weight-loss medications should be used only with proper supervision from a physician. Physician involvement is so critical because many drugs developed for weight loss have side effects. Some have even proven deadly. Fenfluramine (brand name Pondimin), dexfenfluramine (brand name Redux), and a combination of phentermine and fenfluramine (called phen-fen) are appetite-suppressing drugs that were banned from the market in 1996. These drugs, while resulting in more weight loss than diet alone, were found to cause two life-threatening conditions: primary pulmonary hypertension and valvular heart disease. Although these drugs were banned many years ago, they still illustrate that the treatment of obesity through pharmacologic means is neither simple nor risk-free.

Two Prescribed Medications Are Available

Two prescription weight-loss drugs are currently available: sibutramine and orlistat. Their long-term safety and efficacy are still being explored.

Sibutramine (brand name Meridia) is an appetite suppressant that can cause increased heart rate and blood pressure in some people. Because many people who are overweight or obese have high blood pressure and are at increased risk for heart disease, these side effects could limit the widespread use of this drug. However, in one study, combining sibutramine therapy with medically supervised aerobic exercise and a low-fat diet resulted in significant weight loss and a significant decrease in heart rate and blood pressure.[14] In addition to increased blood pressure, side effects of sibutramine include dry mouth, anorexia, constipation, insomnia, dizziness, and nausea.

Orlistat (brand name Xenical) is a drug that inhibits the absorption of dietary fat from the intestinal tract, which can result in weight loss in some people. Recent research shows that orlistat results in significant weight loss in obese adolescents, and adults experience significant weight loss and improved blood lipid profiles when orlistat is combined with an energy-restricted diet.[15,16] The side effects of orlistat include abdominal pain, fatty and loose stools, leaky stools, flatulence, and decreased absorption of fat-soluble nutrients, such as vitamins E and D.

Prescription Weight-Loss Medications Are Not for Everyone

Although the use of prescribed weight-loss medications is associated with side effects and a certain level of risk, they are justified for people who are obese. That's because the health risks of obesity override the risks of the medications. Specifically, prescription weight-loss medications are advised for people who have the following:

- A BMI greater than or equal to 30 kg/m^2
- A BMI greater than or equal to 27 kg/m^2 who also have other significant health risk factors, such as heart disease, high blood pressure, and type 2 diabetes

These medications should be used only while under a physician's supervision, so that progress and health risks can be closely monitored. They

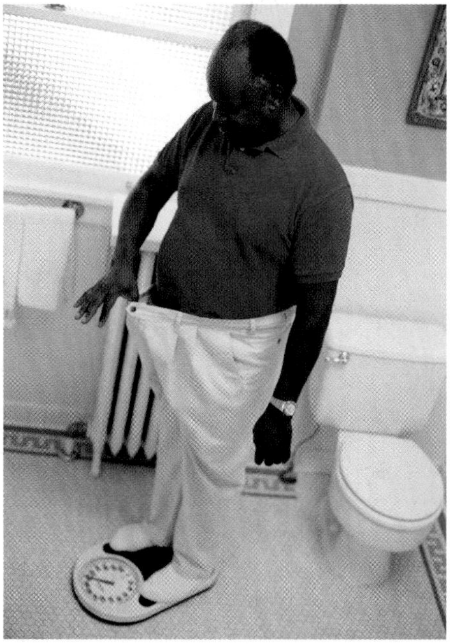

Some people find that combining lifestyle changes with prescription medications increases their success in losing weight.

are most effective when combined with a program that supports energy restriction, regular exercise, and increased physical activity throughout the day.

Surgery Can Be Used to Treat Morbid Obesity

For people who are morbidly obese, surgery may be recommended. Generally, surgery is advised in people with a BMI greater than or equal to 40 kg/m^2 or in people with a BMI greater than or equal to 35 kg/m^2 who have other life-threatening conditions, such as diabetes, hypertension, or elevated cholesterol levels.[12] The three most common types of weight-loss surgery performed are gastroplasty, gastric bypass, and gastric banding **(Figure 2)**.

- *Vertical banded gastroplasty* involves partitioning, or "stapling," a small section of the stomach to reduce total food intake.
- *Gastric bypass surgery* involves attaching the lower part of the small intestine to the stomach, so that food bypasses most of the stomach and the duodenum of the small intestine. This results in both a smaller stomach pouch, which restricts food intake, and significantly less absorption of food in the intestine.
- *Gastric banding* is a relatively new procedure in which stomach size is reduced using a constricting band, thus restricting food intake.

Surgery is considered the last resort for morbidly obese people who have not been able to lose weight with energy restriction, exercise, and medications. This is because the risks of surgery in people with morbid obesity are extremely high. They include increased incidence of infections, the formation of blood clots, and adverse reactions to anesthesia. After the surgery, these people may face a lifetime of problems with chronic diarrhea, vomiting, intolerance to dairy products and other foods, dehydration, and nutritional deficiencies resulting from alterations in nutrient digestion and absorption that occur with bypass procedures. Thus, the potential benefits of the procedure must outweigh the risks. It is critical that each surgery candidate be carefully screened by a trained physician. If the immediate threat of serious disease and death is more dangerous than the risks associated with surgery, then the procedure is justified.

Are these surgical procedures successful in reducing obesity? About one-third to one-half of people who received obesity surgery lose significant amounts of weight and keep this weight off for at least 5 years. The reasons that one-half to two-thirds do not experience long-term success are

- Inability to eat less over time, even with a smaller stomach
- Loosening of staples and gastric bands and enlargement of stomach pouch
- Failure to survive the surgery or the postoperative recovery period

Although these surgical procedures are extremely risky, many of those who survive the surgery lose weight, maintain much of this weight loss over time, reduce their risk for type 2 diabetes and cardiovascular disease, and may even improve their ability to stay physically active over a prolonged period of time.[17]

Liposuction is a cosmetic surgical procedure that removes fat cells from localized areas in the body. It is not recommended or typically used to treat obesity or morbid obesity. Instead, it is often used by normal-weight or mildly overweight people to "spot reduce" fat from various areas of the body. This procedure is not without risks; blood clots, skin and nerve damage, adverse drug reactions, and

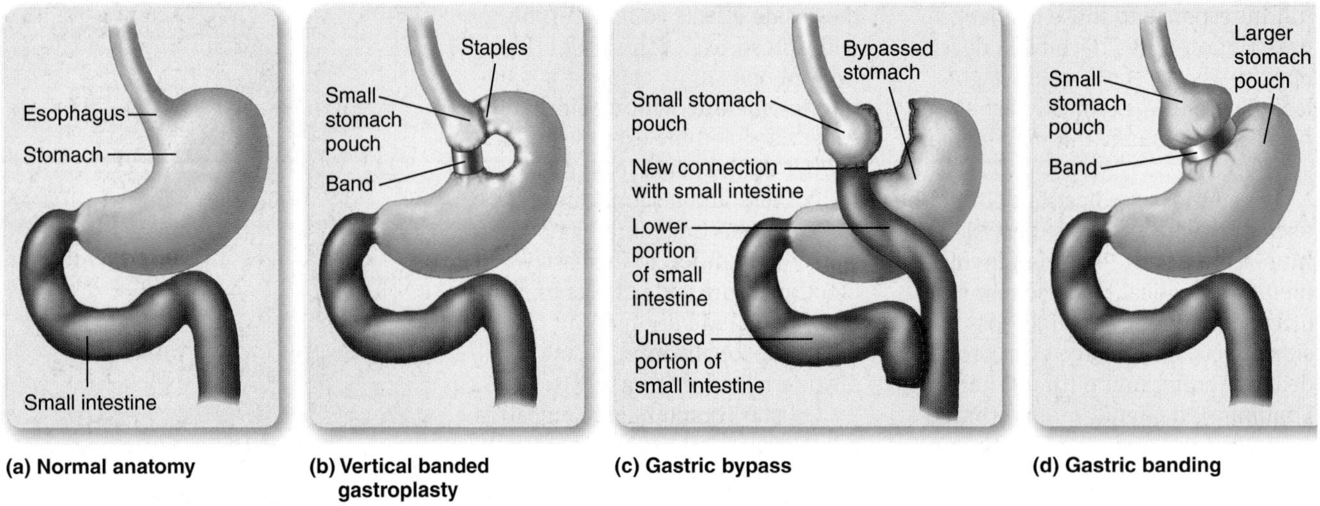

Figure 2 Various forms of surgery alter the normal anatomy **(a)** of the gastrointestinal tract to result in weight loss. Vertical banded gastroplasty **(b)**, gastric bypass **(c)**, and gastric banding **(d)** are three surgical procedures used to reduce morbid obesity.

NUTRI-CASE JUDY

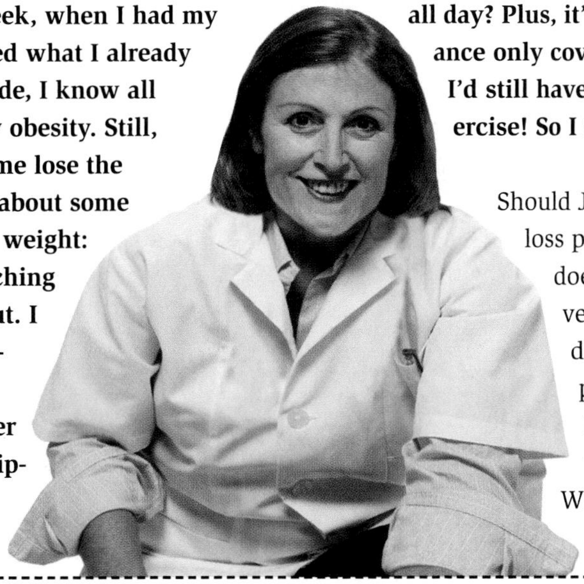

"All my life I've tried to lose weight. But nothing ever works, and when I go off a diet, I always end up fatter than when I started out! And last week, when I had my annual checkup, my doctor confirmed what I already knew—I'm obese! Being a nurse's aide, I know all about the health problems caused by obesity. Still, knowing how bad it is doesn't help me lose the weight and keep it off. So we talked about some slow and steady strategies for losing weight: I promised I'd do a better job of watching my diet and that I'd start working out. I asked my doctor about using weight-loss pills from the drugstore, but he said no way, they're mostly just water pills. Then he wrote me out a prescription for a *real* weight-loss drug. I haven't filled it yet, though, because he said it could give me stomach pain and diarrhea, and how can I manage that when I have to work all day? Plus, it's expensive and my insurance only covers part of it. Worst of all, I'd still have to stick to my diet and exercise! So I figure, why bother?"

Should Judy bother with the weight-loss prescription? Given that Judy does have a demanding job and very little discretionary income, do you feel that, for her, the potential benefits—including long-term benefits—outweigh the side effects and cost? Why or why not?

perforation injuries occur as a result of liposuction. It can also cause deformations in the area where the fat is removed. This procedure is not the solution to long-term weight loss, as the millions of fat cells that remain in the body after liposuction enlarge if the person continues to overeat. In addition, although liposuction may reduce the fat content of a localized area, it does not reduce a person's risk for the diseases that are more common among overweight or obese people. Only traditional weight loss with diet and exercise can reduce body fat and the risks for chronic diseases.

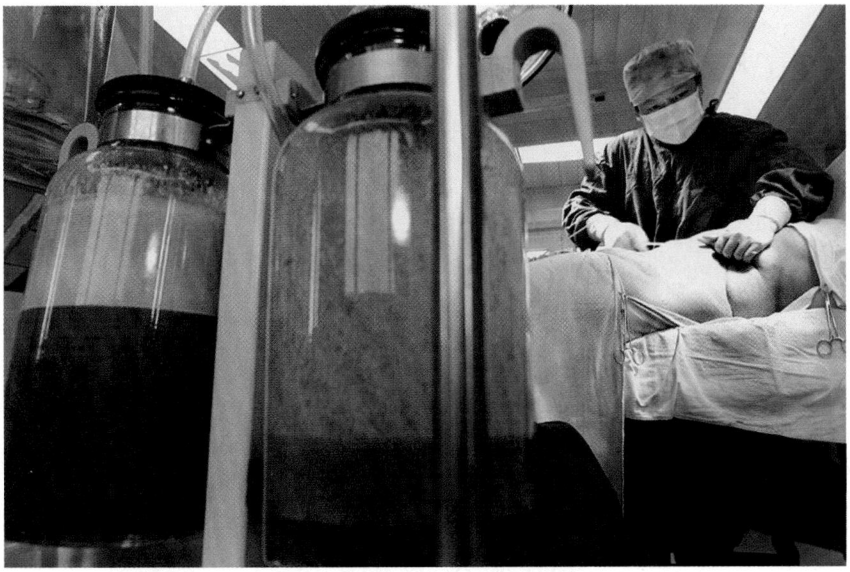

Liposuction removes fat cells from specific areas of the body.

Web Resources

www.oa.org
Overeaters Anonymous

Visit this site to learn about ways to reduce compulsive overeating.

www.nhlbi.nih.gov/health/dci/Diseases/obe/obe_treatments
National Heart, Lung, and Blood Institute Overweight and Obesity Site

Visit this site to find out more about various treatment options for overweight and obesity.

www.win.niddk.nih.gov
Weight Control Information Network

This site, from the National Institute of Diabetes and Digestive and Kidney Diseases (NIDDK), offers information, brochures, and other tools on obesity, weight control, physical activity, and related nutritional issues.

12 Nutrition and Physical Activity: Keys to Good Health

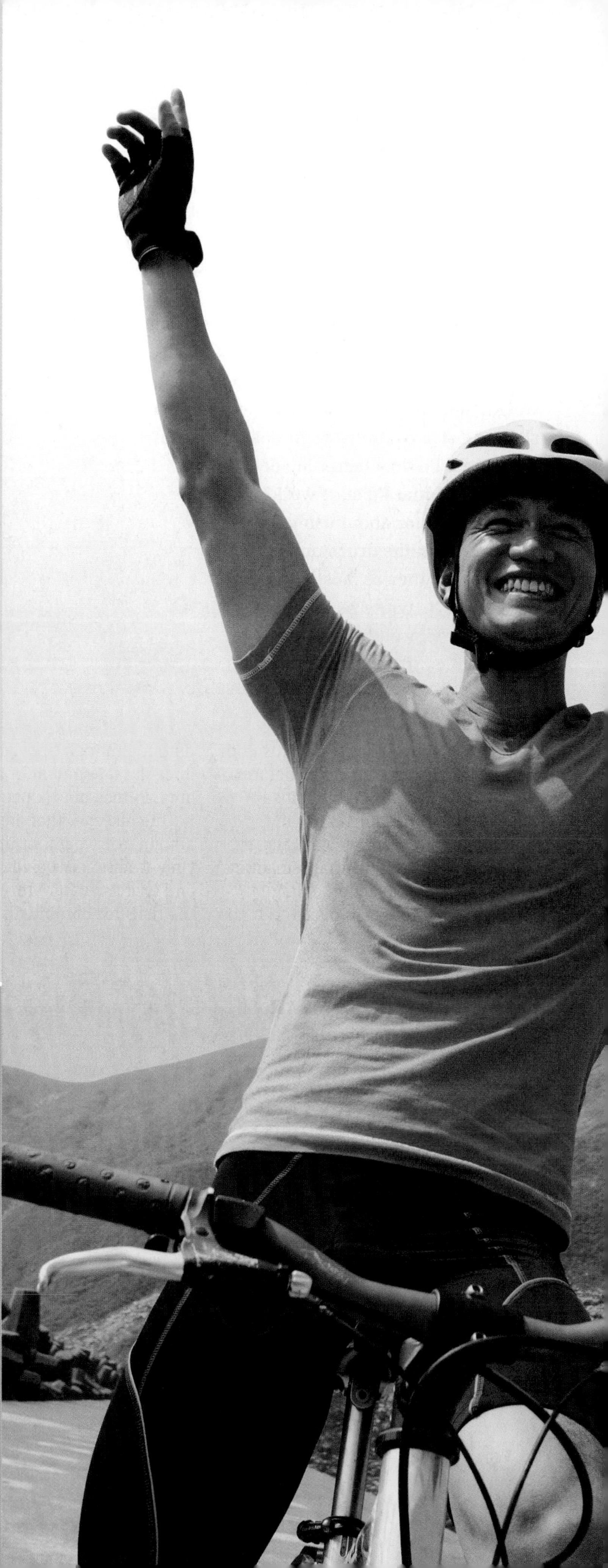

CHAPTER OBJECTIVES

After reading this chapter you will be able to:

1. **Explain the differences between physical activity and exercise, p. 412.**
2. **Define the four components of fitness, p. 412.**
3. **List at least four health benefits of being physically active on a regular basis, pp. 412–413.**
4. **Describe the FIT principle and calculate your maximal and training heart rate range, pp. 415–417.**
5. **List and describe at least three processes we use to break down fuels to support physical activity, pp. 419–423.**
6. **Discuss at least three changes in nutrient needs that can occur in response to an increase in physical activity or vigorous exercise training, pp. 425–430.**
7. **Define the term *ergogenic aids* and discuss the potential benefits and risks of at least four ergogenic aids that are currently on the market, pp. 434–436.**

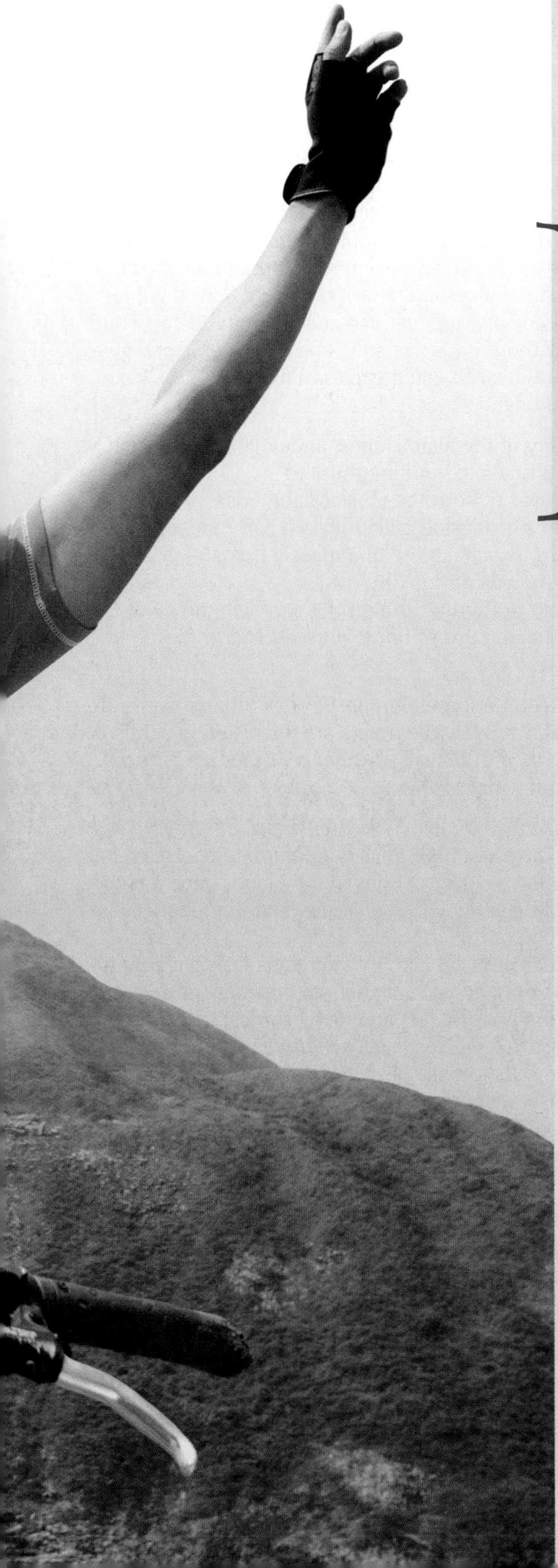

Test Yourself

1. **T F Despite the multitude of health benefits of participating in regular physical activity, more than half of all Americans are insufficiently active.**

2. **T F Eating extra protein helps us build muscle.**

3. **T F Most ergogenic aids are not effective, and many can be dangerous or cause serious health consequences.**

Test Yourself answers can be found at the end of the chapter.

In the summer of 2009, Millie Bolton of Ohio and Glenn Dody of Arizona each took the gold medal for the 400-meter dash in track and field at the National Senior Games. Bolton clocked 2 minutes, 31 seconds, and Dody's time was 1 minute, 42 seconds. If these performance times don't amaze you, perhaps they will when you consider these athletes' ages: both were competing in the class for 85- to 89-year-olds!

There's no doubt about it: regular physical activity dramatically improves strength, stamina, health, and quality of life—throughout the life span. But what qualifies as "regular physical activity"? In other words, how much do we need to do to reap the benefits? And if we do become more active, does our diet have to change, too?

Healthy eating practices and regular physical activity are like two sides of the same coin, interacting in a variety of ways to improve our strength and stamina and increase our resistance to many chronic diseases and acute illnesses. In fact, the nutrition and physical activity recommendations for reducing your risk for heart disease also reduce your risk for high blood pressure, type 2 diabetes, obesity, and some forms of cancer! In this chapter, we'll define physical activity, identify its many benefits, and discuss the nutrients needed to maintain an active life.

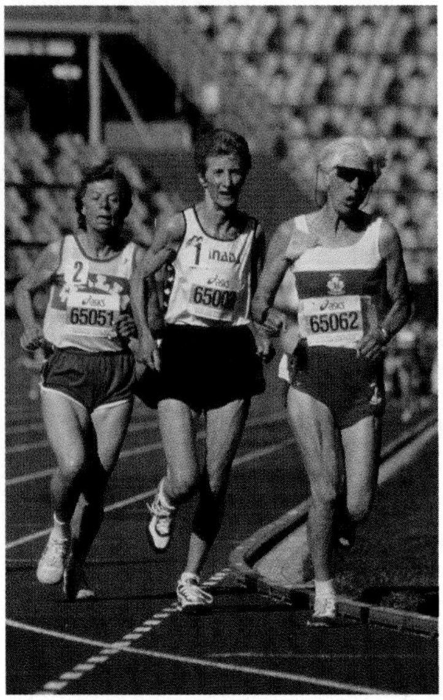

With the help of a nutritious diet, many people are able to remain physically active—and even competitive—throughout adult life.

Why Engage in Physical Activity?

A lot of people are looking for a "magic pill" that will help them maintain weight loss, reduce their risk for diseases, make them feel better, and improve their quality of sleep. Although many people are not aware of it, regular physical activity is this magic pill. **Physical activity** is any movement produced by muscles that increases energy expenditure. Different categories of physical activity include occupational, household, leisure-time, and transportation.[1] **Leisure-time physical activity** is any activity not related to a person's occupation and includes competitive sports, planned exercise training, and recreational activities such as hiking, walking, and bicycling. **Exercise** is therefore considered a subcategory of leisure-time physical activity and refers to activity that is purposeful, planned, and structured.[2]

The current recommendations for physical activity include accumulating at least 30 minutes of moderate physical activity on most, preferably all, days of the week. One of the most important benefits of regular physical activity is that it increases our physical fitness. **Physical fitness** is a state of being that arises largely from the interaction between nutrition and physical activity. It is defined as the ability to carry out daily tasks with vigor and alertness, without undue fatigue, and with ample energy to enjoy leisure-time pursuits and meet unforeseen emergencies.[1] Physical fitness has several components[3] **(Table 12.1)**, including:

- *Cardiorespiratory fitness* is the ability of the heart, lungs, and circulatory system to efficiently supply oxygen and nutrients to working muscles.
- *Musculoskeletal fitness* involves fitness of both the muscles and bones. It includes *muscular strength*, the maximal force or tension level that can be produced by a muscle group, and *muscular endurance,* the ability of a muscle to maintain submaximal force levels for extended periods of time.
- *Flexibility* is the ability to move a joint fluidly through the complete range of motion, and *body composition* is the amount of bone, muscle, and fat tissue in the body.

Although many people are interested in improving their physical fitness, some are more interested in maintaining general fitness, while others are interested in achieving higher levels of fitness to optimize their athletic performance. Other benefits of regular physical activity include the following:

- *It reduces our risks for, and complications of, heart disease, stroke, and high blood pressure.* Regular physical activity increases high-density lipoprotein cholesterol (HDL, the "good" cholesterol) and lowers triglycerides in the blood, improves the strength of the heart, helps maintain healthy blood pressure, and limits the progression of atherosclerosis (hardening of the arteries).
- *It reduces our risk for obesity.* Regular physical activity maintains lean body mass and promotes more healthful levels of body fat, may help in appetite control, and increases energy expenditure and the use of fat as an energy source.
- *It reduces our risk for type 2 diabetes.* Regular physical activity enhances the action of insulin, which improves the cells' uptake of glucose from the blood, and it can improve blood glucose control in people with diabetes, which in turn reduces the risk for, or delays the onset of, diabetes-related complications.

physical activity Any movement produced by muscles that increases energy expenditure; includes occupational, household, leisure-time, and transportation activities.

leisure-time physical activity Any activity not related to a person's occupation; includes competitive sports, recreational activities, and planned exercise training.

exercise A subcategory of leisure-time physical activity; any activity that is purposeful, planned, and structured.

physical fitness The ability to carry out daily tasks with vigor and alertness, without undue fatigue, and with ample energy to enjoy leisure-time pursuits and meet unforeseen emergencies.

TABLE 12.1 The Components of Fitness

Fitness Component	Examples of Activities One Can Do to Achieve Fitness in Each Component
Cardiorespiratory	Aerobic-type activities, such as walking, running, swimming, cross-country skiing
Musculoskeletal fitness:	Resistance training, weight lifting, calisthenics, sit-ups, push-ups
Muscular strength	Weight lifting or related activities using heavier weights with few repetitions
Muscular endurance	Weight lifting or related activities using lighter weights with more repetitions
Flexibility	Stretching exercises, yoga
Body composition	Aerobic exercise, resistance training

- *It reduces our risk for osteoporosis.* Regular physical activity strengthens bones and enhances muscular strength and flexibility, thereby reducing the likelihood of falls and the incidence of fractures and other injuries when falls occur.
- *It potentially reduces our risk for colon cancer.* Although the exact role that physical activity may play in reducing colon cancer risk is still unknown, we do know that regular physical activity enhances gastric motility, which reduces the transit time of potential cancer-causing agents through the gut.

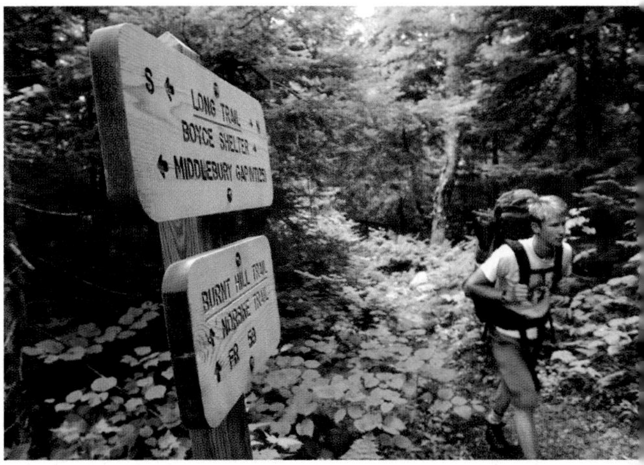

Hiking is a leisure-time physical activity that can contribute to your physical fitness.

Regular physical activity is also known to improve our sleep patterns, reduce our risk for upper respiratory infections by improving immune function, improve self-esteem, and reduce anxiety and mental stress. It also can be effective in treating mild and moderate depression. During pregnancy, regular physical activity helps maintain the mother's fitness and muscle tone and helps control weight gain. It is also associated with a reduced risk for pregnancy-related complications.[4]

Despite the plethora of benefits derived from regular physical activity, most people find that this magic pill is not easy to swallow. In fact, most people in the United States are physically inactive. The Centers for Disease Control and Prevention reports that over half of all U.S. adults do not do enough physical activity to meet national health recommendations, and almost 25% of adults in the United States admit to doing no leisure-time physical activity at all.[5,6] These statistics mirror the reported increases in obesity, heart disease, and type 2 diabetes in industrialized countries.

This trend toward inadequate physical activity levels is also occurring in young people. Only 37% of young people are meeting the recommended 60 minutes per day on 5 or more days per week.[7] Although physical education (PE) is part of the mandated curriculum in most states, only 28.4% of high school students attend PE classes daily, and only 6.4% of middle schools offer daily PE for the entire school year.[8] Since our habits related to eating and physical activity are formed early in life, it is imperative that we provide opportunities for children and adolescents to engage in regular, enjoyable physical activity. An active lifestyle during childhood increases the likelihood of a healthier life as an adult.

RECAP **Physical activity is any movement produced by muscles that increases energy expenditure. Physical fitness is the ability to carry out daily tasks with vigor and alertness, without undue fatigue, and with ample energy to enjoy leisure-time pursuits and meet unforeseen emergencies. Physical activity provides a multitude of health benefits, including reducing our risks for obesity and many chronic diseases and relieving anxiety and stress. Despite the many health benefits of physical activity, most people in the United States, including many children, are inactive.**

What Is a Sound Fitness Program?

There are several widely recognized qualities of a sound fitness program, as well as guidelines to help you design one that is right for you. These are explored here. Keep in mind that people with heart disease, high blood pressure, diabetes, obesity, osteoporosis, asthma, or arthritis should get approval to exercise from their healthcare practitioner prior to starting a fitness program. In addition, a medical evaluation should be conducted before starting an exercise program for an apparently healthy but currently inactive man 40 years or older or woman 50 years or older.

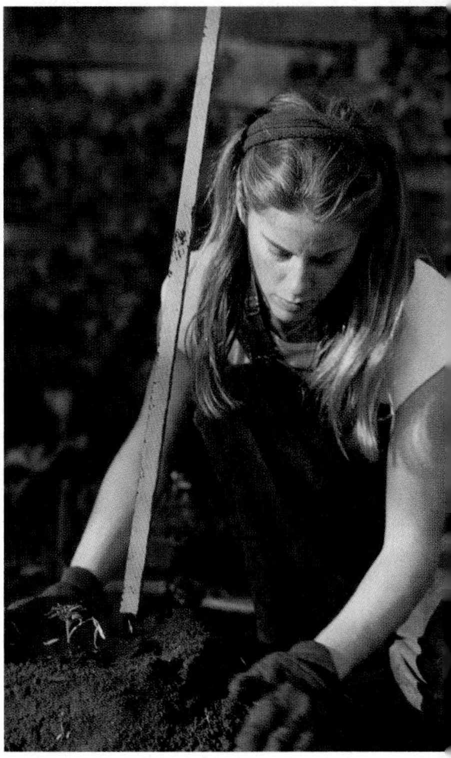

Moderate physical activity, such as gardening, helps maintain overall health.

A Sound Fitness Program Meets Your Personal Goals

A fitness program that may be ideal for you is not necessarily right for everyone. Before designing or evaluating any program, it is important to define your personal fitness goals. Do you want to prevent osteoporosis, diabetes, or another chronic disease that runs in your family? Do you simply want to increase your energy and stamina? Or do you intend to compete in athletic events? Each of these scenarios requires a unique fitness program.

For example, if you want to train for athletic competition, a traditional approach that includes planned, purposive exercise sessions under the guidance of a trainer or coach would probably be most beneficial. Or if you want to achieve cardiorespiratory fitness, participating in an aerobics class at least three times per week may be recommended.

In contrast, if your goal is to maintain your overall health, you might do better to follow the 1996 report of the Surgeon General on achieving health through regular physical activity.[1] This report emphasizes that significant health benefits, including reducing your risk for chronic diseases (such as heart disease, osteoporosis, and type 2 diabetes), can be achieved by participating in a moderate amount of physical activity (such as 45 minutes of gardening, 20 minutes of brisk walking, or 30 minutes of basketball) on most, if not all, days of the week. These health benefits occur even when the time spent performing the physical activities is cumulative (for example, brisk walking for 10 minutes three times per day). While these guidelines are appropriate for achieving health benefits, they are not necessarily of sufficient intensity and duration to improve physical fitness.

Recently, the Institute of Medicine published guidelines stating that the minimum amount of physical activity that should be done each day to maintain health and fitness is 60 minutes—not 30 minutes, as published in the Surgeon General's report.[1,9] This discrepancy in fitness guidelines has caused some confusion among consumers. Refer to the Nutrition Debate at the end of this chapter to learn more about this controversy.

A Sound Fitness Program Is Varied, Consistent, . . . and Fun!

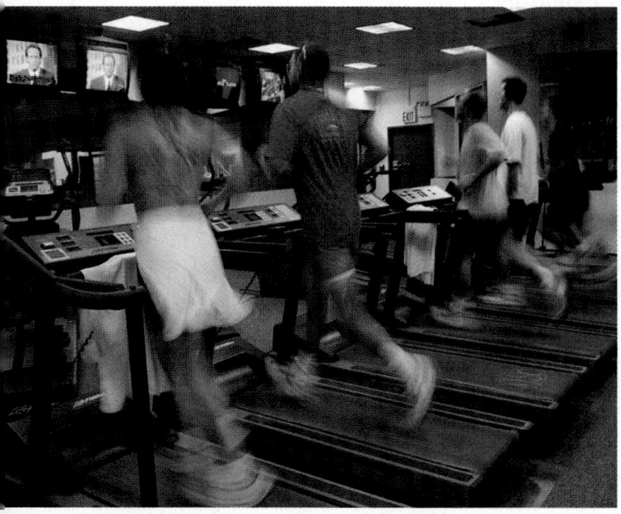

Watching television or reading can provide variety while running on a treadmill.

One of the most important goals for everyone is fun; unless you enjoy being active, you will find it very difficult to maintain your physical fitness. If you enjoy the outdoors, hiking, camping, fishing, and rock climbing are potential activities for you. If you would rather exercise with friends on your lunch break, walking, climbing stairs, and bicycle riding may be more appropriate. Or you may prefer to use the programs and equipment at your local fitness club or purchase your own treadmill and free weights.

Variety is critical to maintaining your fitness. While some people enjoy doing similar activities day after day, most of us get bored with the same fitness routine. Incorporating a variety of activities into your fitness program will help maintain your interest and increase your enjoyment while you are active. Variety can be achieved by engaging in different indoor and outdoor activities on different days of the week, taking a different route when you walk each day, or watching different TV programs or listening to music while you ride a stationary bicycle or work out on a rowing machine. This smorgasbord of activities can increase your activity level without leading to monotony and boredom.

A useful tool has been developed to help you increase the variety of your physical activity choices (Figure 12.1). The **Physical Activity Pyramid** makes recommendations for the type and amount of activity you should do weekly to increase your physical activity level. The bottom of the pyramid describes activities that should be done every day, including walking more, taking the stairs instead of the elevator, and working in your garden. Aerobic types of exercises (such as bicycling and brisk walking) and recreational activities (such as soccer, tennis, and basketball) should be done three to five times each week, for at least 20 or 30 minutes. Flexibility, strength, and leisure activities should be done two or three times each week. The

Physical Activity Pyramid A pyramid-shaped graphic that suggests types and amounts of activity that should be done weekly to increase physical activity levels.

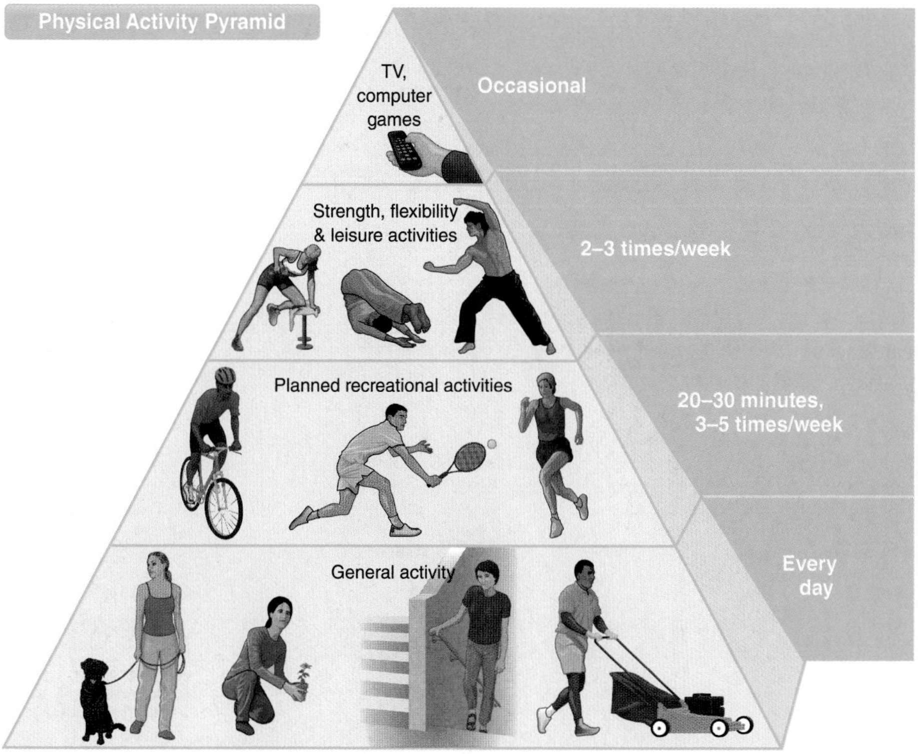

Figure 12.1 You can use this Physical Activity Pyramid as a guide to increase your level of physical activity.
Data from Corbin, C. B., and R. D. Pangrazi. 1998. Physical Activity Pyramid rebuffs peak experience. *ACSM's Health Fitness J.* 2(1). Copyright © 1998. Used with permission.

top of the pyramid emphasizes things we should do less of, including watching TV, playing computer games, and sitting for more than 30 minutes at one time.

It is important to understand that you cannot do just one activity to achieve overall fitness because every activity is specific to a certain fitness component. Refer back to Table 12.1, and notice the various activities listed as examples for the various components. For instance, participating in aerobic-type activities will improve cardiorespiratory fitness but will do little to improve muscular strength. To achieve that goal, we must participate in some form of **resistance training,** or exercises in which our muscles work against resistance. Flexibility is achieved by participating in stretching activities. By following the recommendations put forth in the Physical Activity Pyramid, you can achieve physical fitness in all components.

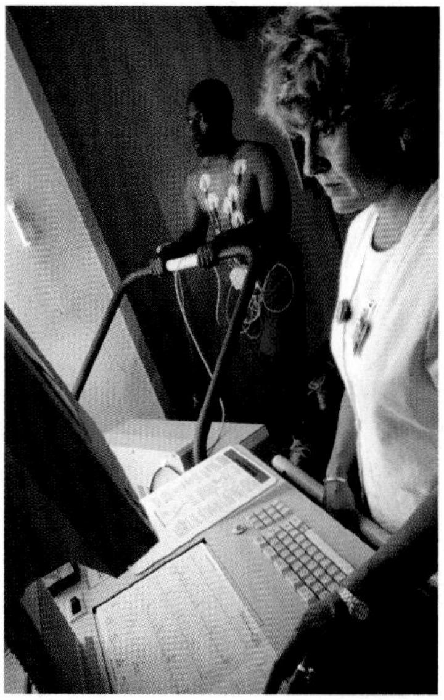

Testing in a fitness lab is the most accurate way to determine maximal heart rate.

A Sound Fitness Program Appropriately Overloads the Body

In order to improve your fitness, you must place an extra physical demand on your body. This is referred to as the **overload principle.** A word of caution is in order here: *the overload principle does not advocate subjecting your body to inappropriately high stress* because this can lead to exhaustion and injuries. In contrast, an appropriate overload on various body systems will result in healthy improvements in fitness.

To achieve an appropriate overload, you should consider three factors, collectively known as the **FIT principle:** *f*requency, *i*ntensity, and *t*ime of activity. You can use the FIT principle to design either a general physical fitness program or a performance-based exercise program. **Figure 12.2** shows how the FIT principle applies to a cardiorespiratory, musculoskeletal, and flexibility fitness program. Let's consider each of the FIT principle's three factors in more detail.

Frequency

Frequency refers to the number of activity sessions per week. Depending on your goals for fitness, the frequency of your activities will vary. To achieve cardiorespiratory fitness, you should train more than 2 days per week. On the other hand, training

resistance training Exercises in which our muscles act against resistance.

overload principle Placing an extra physical demand on your body in order to improve your fitness level.

FIT principle The principle used to achieve an appropriate overload for physical training; FIT stands for frequency, intensity, and time of activity.

frequency The number of activity sessions per week you perform.

	Frequency	Intensity	Time
Cardiorespiratory fitness 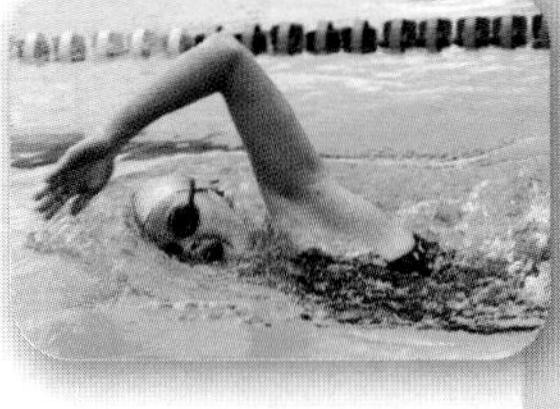	3–5 days per week	64–90% maximal heart rate	At least 20 consecutive minutes
Muscular fitness 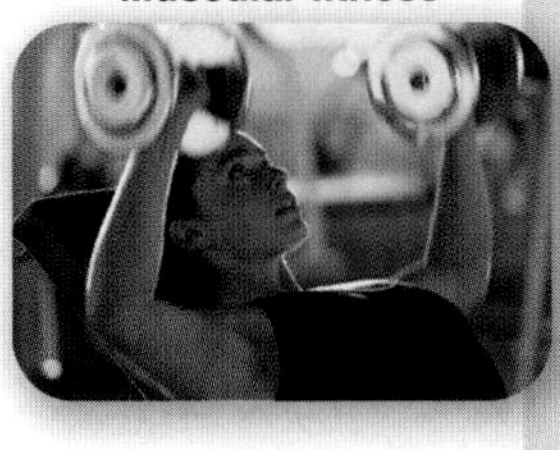	2–3 days per week	70–85% maximal weight you can lift	1–3 sets of 8–12 lifts* for each set *A minimum of 8–10 exercises involving the major muscle groups such as arms, shoulders, chest, abdomen, back, hips, and legs, is recommended.
Flexibility 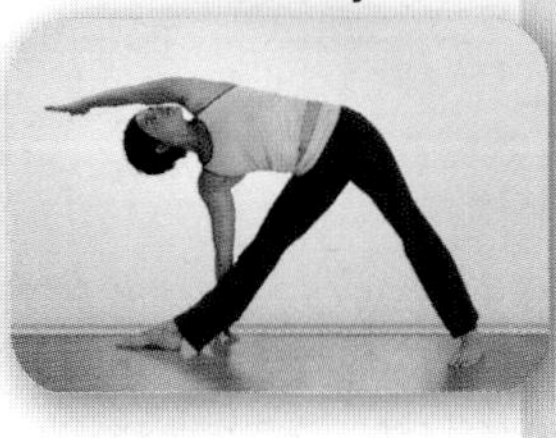	2–4 days per week	Stretching through full range of motion	2–4 repetitions per stretch* *Hold each stretch for 15–30 seconds.

Figure 12.2 Using the FIT principle to achieve cardiorespiratory and musculoskeletal fitness and flexibility.

more than 5 days per week does not cause significant gains in fitness but can substantially increase your risk for injury. Training 3 to 5 days per week appears optimal to achieve and maintain cardiorespiratory fitness. In contrast, only 2 to 3 days are needed to achieve musculoskeletal fitness.

Intensity

Intensity refers to the amount of effort expended or to how difficult the activity is to perform. In general, **low-intensity activities** are those that cause very mild increases in breathing, sweating, and heart rate, while **moderate-intensity activities** cause moderate increases in these responses. **Vigorous-intensity activities** produce significant increases in breathing, sweating, and heart rate, so that talking is difficult when exercising.

Traditionally, heart rate has been used to indicate level of intensity during aerobic activities. You can calculate the range of exercise intensity that is appropriate for you by estimating your **maximal heart rate,** which is the rate at which your heart beats during maximal intensity exercise (see the You Do the Math box on the next page). Maximal heart rate is estimated by subtracting your age from 220. The Centers for Disease Control and Prevention recommends that to achieve moderate-intensity physical activity, your target heart rate should be 50–70% of your estimated maximal heart rate; to achieve vigorous-intensity physical activity, your target heart rate should be 70–85% of your estimated maximal heart rate.[10] People who are older or who have been inactive for a long time may want to exercise at the lower end of the moderate-intensity range. Those who are more physically fit or are striving for a more rapid improvement in fitness may want to exercise at the higher end of the

intensity The amount of effort expended during the activity, or how difficult the activity is to perform.

low-intensity activities Activities that cause very mild increases in breathing, sweating, and heart rate.

moderate-intensity activities Activities that cause moderate increases in breathing, sweating, and heart rate.

vigorous-intensity activities Activities that produce significant increases in breathing, sweating, and heart rate; talking is difficult when exercising at a vigorous intensity.

maximal heart rate The rate at which your heart beats during maximal-intensity exercise.

YOU DO THE MATH

Calculating Your Maximal and Training Heart Rate Range

Judy was recently diagnosed with type 2 diabetes, and her healthcare provider has recommended she begin an exercise program. She is considered obese according to her body mass index, and she has not been regularly active since she was a teenager. Judy's goals are to improve her cardiorespiratory fitness and achieve and maintain a more healthful weight. Fortunately, Valley Hospital, where she works as a nurse's aide, recently opened a small fitness center for the use of its employees. Judy plans to begin by either walking on the treadmill or riding the stationary bicycle at the fitness center during her lunch break.

Judy needs to exercise at an intensity that will help her improve her cardiorespiratory fitness and lose weight. She is 38 years of age, is obese, has type 2 diabetes, and has been approved to do moderate-intensity activity by her healthcare provider. She does a lot of walking and lifting in her work as a nurse's aide, and her doctor has recommended that she start her program by setting her training heart rate range at 50%; once her fitness improves, she can work toward exercising at 75% of her maximal heart rate.

Let's calculate Judy's maximal heart rate values:

- Maximal heart rate: 220 – age = 220 – 38 = 182 beats per minute (bpm)
- Lower end of intensity range: 50% of 182 bpm = 0.50 × 182 bpm = 91 bpm
- Higher end of intensity range: 75% of 182 bpm = 0.75 × 182 bpm = 137 bpm

Because Judy is a trained nurse's aide, she is skilled at measuring a heart rate, or pulse. To measure your own pulse,

- Place your second (index) and third (middle) fingers on the inside of your wrist, just below the wrist crease and near the thumb. Press lightly to feel your pulse. Don't press too hard, or you will occlude the artery and be unable to feel its pulsation.
- If you can't feel your pulse at your wrist, try the carotid artery at your neck. This is located below your ear, on the side of your neck directly below your jaw. Press lightly against your neck under the jaw bone to find your pulse.
- Begin counting your pulse with the count of "zero;" then count each beat for 15 seconds.
- Multiply that value by 4 to estimate heart rate over 1 minute.
- Do not take your pulse with your thumb, as it has its own pulse, which would prevent you from getting an accurate estimate of your heart rate.

As you can see from these calculations, when Judy walks on the treadmill or rides the bicycle, her heart rate should be between 91 and 137 bpm; this will put her in her aerobic training zone and allow her to achieve cardiorespiratory fitness. It will also help her lose weight.

vigorous-intensity range. Competitive athletes generally train at a higher intensity, around 80–95% of their maximal heart rate.

Although the calculation *220 – age* has been used extensively for years to predict maximal heart rate, it was never intended to represent everyone's true maximal heart rate or to be used as the standard of aerobic training intensity. The most accurate way to determine your own maximal heart rate is to complete a maximal exercise test in a fitness laboratory; however, this test is not commonly conducted with the general public and can be very expensive. Although not completely accurate, the estimated maximal heart rate method can still be used to give you a general idea of your aerobic training range.

Time of Activity

Time of activity refers to how long each session lasts. To achieve general health, you can do multiple short bouts of activity that add up to 30 minutes each day. However, to achieve higher levels of fitness, it is important that the activities be done for at least 20 to 30 consecutive minutes.

For example, let's say you want to compete in triathlons. To be successful during the running segment of the triathlon, you will need to be able to run for at least 5 miles. Thus, it is appropriate for you to train so that you can complete 5 miles during one session and still have enough energy to swim and bicycle during the race. You will need to consistently train at a distance of 5 miles; you will also benefit from running longer distances.

time of activity The period of time that an exercise session lasts.

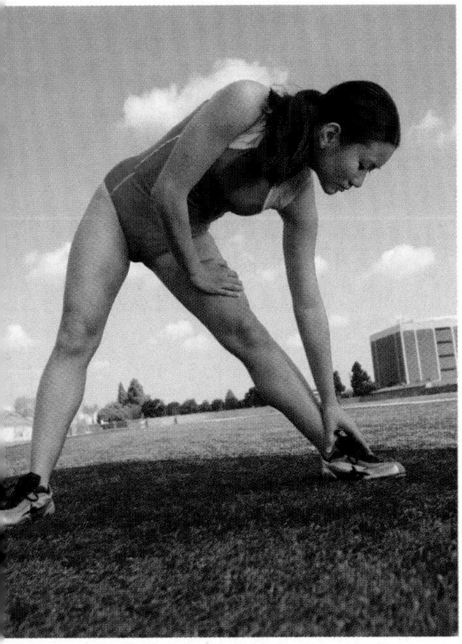

Stretching should be included in the warm-up before and the cool-down after exercise.

A Sound Fitness Plan Includes a Warm-Up and a Cool-Down Period

To properly prepare for and recover from an exercise session, warm-up and cool-down activities should be performed. **Warm-up,** which properly prepares muscles for exertion by increasing blood flow and temperature, includes general activities (such as stretching and calisthenics) and specific activities that prepare you for the actual activity (such as jogging or swinging a golf club). The warm-up should be brief (5 to 10 minutes), gradual, and sufficient to increase muscle and body temperature, but it should not cause fatigue or deplete energy stores.

Cool-down activities are done after the exercise session. The cool-down should be gradual, allowing your body to recover slowly, with ample stretching as well as a lower-intensity version of some of the same activities you performed during the exercise session. Cool-down after exercise assists in the prevention of injury and may help reduce muscle soreness.

Simple Changes Can Boost Your Physical Activity

There are 1,440 minutes in every day. Spend just 30 of those minutes in physical activity, and you'll be taking an important step toward improving your health. Here are some tips adapted from the Centers for Disease Control and Prevention and the United States Department of Health and Human Services for working daily activity into your life:[11,12]

QUICK TIPS

Increasing Your Physical Activity

- ✓ Walk as often and as far as possible: park your car farther away from your dorm, lecture hall, or shops; walk to school or work; go for a brisk walk between classes; get on or off the bus one stop away from your destination.
- ✓ Take the stairs instead of the elevator.
- ✓ Exercise while watching television—for example, by doing sit-ups, stretching, or using a treadmill or stationary bike.
- ✓ Put on a CD and dance!
- ✓ Get an exercise partner: join a friend for walks, hikes, cycling, skating, tennis, or a fitness class.
- ✓ Take up a group sport.
- ✓ Register for a class from the physical education department in an activity you've never tried before, maybe yoga or fencing.
- ✓ Register for a dance class, such as jazz, tap, or ballroom.
- ✓ Join a health club, gym, or YMCA/YWCA and use the swimming pool, weights, rock-climbing wall, and other facilities.
- ✓ Join an activity-based club, such as a skating or hiking club.

If you have been inactive for a while, use a sensible approach by starting out slowly. Gradually build up the time you spend doing the activity by adding a few minutes every few days until you reach 30 minutes a day. As this 30-minute minimum becomes easier, gradually increase either the length of time you spend in activity, the intensity of the activities you choose, or both.

RECAP **A sound fitness program must meet your personal fitness goals. It should be fun and include variety and consistency to help you maintain interest and achieve fitness in all components. It must also place an extra physical demand, or an overload, on your body. To achieve appropriate overload, follow the FIT principle: *frequency* refers to the number of activity sessions per week; *intensity* refers to how difficult the activity is to perform, and *time* refers to how long each activity session lasts. Warm-up and cool-down activities help the body prepare for and recover from exertion.**

warm-up Activities that prepare you for an exercise bout, including stretching, calisthenics, and movements specific to the exercise bout; also called preliminary exercise.

cool-down Activities done after an exercise session is completed; should be gradual and allow your body to slowly recover from exercise.

What Fuels Our Activities?

In order to perform exercise, or muscular work, we must be able to generate energy. The common currency of energy for virtually all cells in the body is **adenosine triphosphate,** or ATP. As you might guess from its name, a molecule of ATP includes an organic compound called adenosine and three phosphate groups **(Figure 12.3)**. When one of the phosphates is cleaved, or broken away, from ATP, energy is released. The products remaining after this reaction are adenosine diphosphate (ADP) and an independent inorganic phosphate group (P_i). In a mirror image of this reaction, the body regenerates ATP by adding a phosphate group back to ADP. In this way, we continually provide energy to our cells.

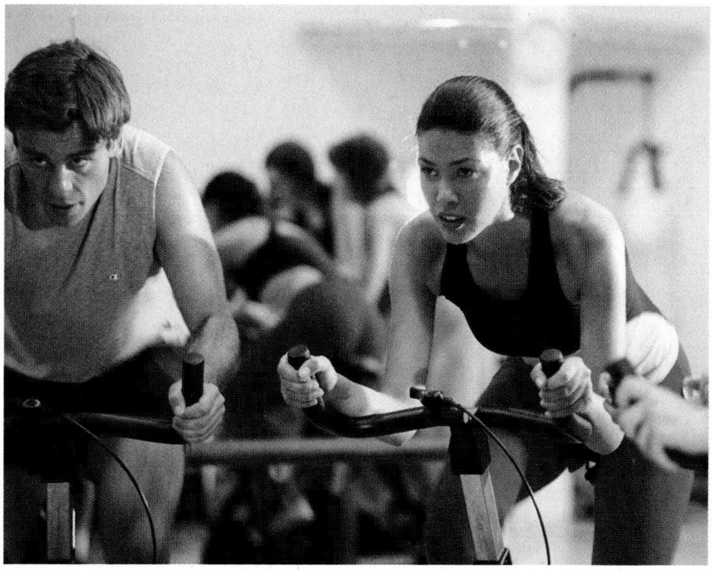

The amount of daily physical activity you should participate in is determined by your personal fitness goals.

The amount of ATP stored in a muscle cell is very limited; it can keep the muscle active for only about 1 to 3 seconds. Thus, we need to generate ATP from other sources to fuel activities for longer periods of time. Fortunately, we are able to generate ATP from the breakdown of carbohydrate, fat, and protein, providing our cells with a variety of sources from which to receive energy. The primary energy systems that provide energy for physical activities are the adenosine triphosphate–creatine phosphate (ATP-CP) energy system and the anaerobic and aerobic breakdown of carbohydrates. Our body also generates energy from the breakdown of fats. As you will see, the type, intensity, and duration of the activities performed determine the amount of ATP needed and therefore the energy system that is used.

The ATP-CP Energy System Uses Creatine Phosphate to Regenerate ATP

As previously mentioned, muscle cells store only enough ATP to maintain activity for 1 to 3 seconds. When more energy is needed, a high-energy compound called **creatine phosphate (CP)** (also called *phosphocreatine,* or *PCr*) can be broken down to support the regeneration of ATP **(Figure 12.4)**. Because this reaction can occur in the absence of oxygen, it is referred to as an **anaerobic** (meaning "without oxygen") reaction.

Muscle tissue contains about four to six times as much CP as ATP, but there is still not enough CP available to fuel long-term activity. CP is used the most during very

adenosine triphosphate (ATP) The common currency of energy for virtually all cells of the body.

creatine phosphate (CP) A high-energy compound that can be broken down for energy and used to regenerate ATP.

anaerobic Means "without oxygen;" the term used to refer to metabolic reactions that occur in the absence of oxygen.

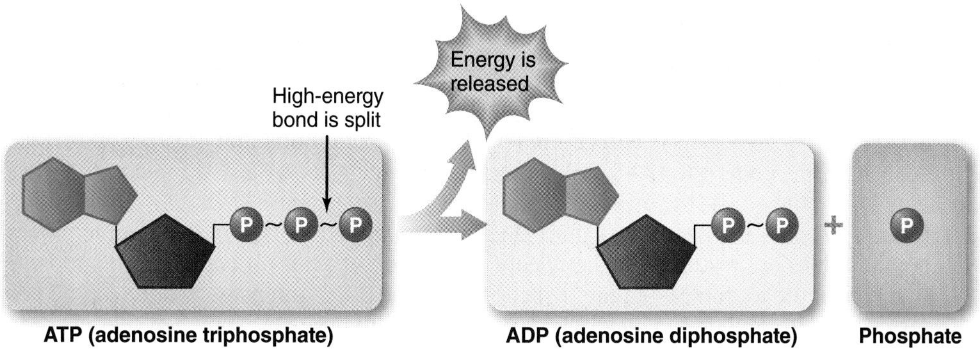

Figure 12.3 Structure of adenosine triphosphate (ATP). Energy is produced when ATP is split into adenosine diphosphate (ADP) and inorganic phosphate (P_i).

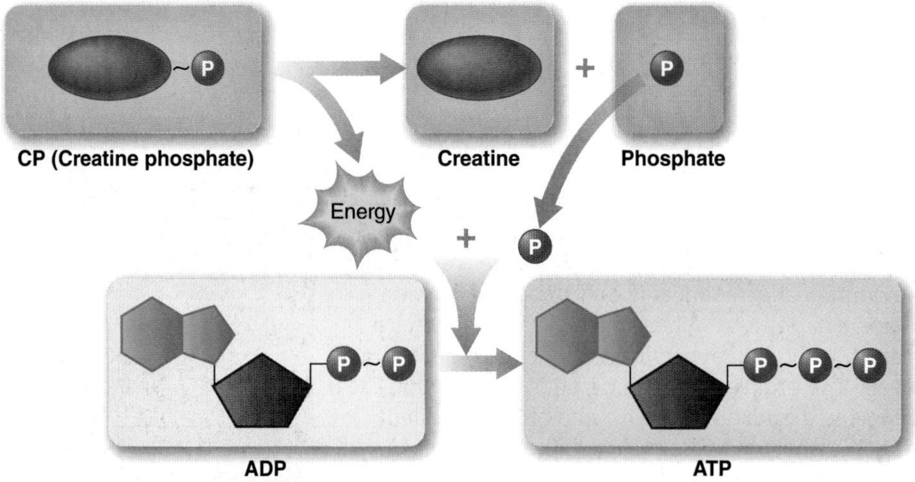

Figure 12.4 When the compound creatine phosphate (CP) is broken down into a molecule of creatine and an independent phosphate molecule, energy is released. This energy, along with the independent phosphate molecule, can then be used to regenerate ATP.

intense, short bouts of activity, such as lifting, jumping, and sprinting (**Figure 12.5**). Together, our stores of ATP and CP can support a *maximal* physical effort for only about 3 to 15 seconds. We must rely on other energy sources, such as carbohydrate and fat, to support activities of longer duration.

The Breakdown of Carbohydrates Provides Energy for Both Brief and Long-Term Exercise

During activities lasting about 30 seconds to 3 minutes, our body needs an energy source that can be used quickly to produce ATP. The breakdown of carbohydrates, specifically glucose, provides this quick energy in a process called **glycolysis.** The most common source of glucose during exercise comes from glycogen stored in the muscles and glucose found in the blood. As shown in **Figure 12.6**, for every glucose molecule that goes through glycolysis, two ATP molecules are produced. The primary end product of glycolysis is **pyruvic acid.**

When oxygen availability is limited in the cell, pyruvic acid is converted to **lactic acid.** For years it was assumed that lactic acid was a useless, even potentially toxic, by-product of high-intensity exercise. We now know that lactic acid is an important intermediate of glucose breakdown and that it plays a critical role in supplying fuel for working muscles, the heart, and resting tissues (see the Nutrition Myth or Fact box on page 422).

The major advantage of glycolysis is that it is the fastest way that we can regenerate ATP for exercise, other than the ATP-CP system. However, this high rate of ATP production can be sustained only briefly, generally less than 3 minutes. To perform exercise that lasts longer than 3 minutes, we must rely on the aerobic energy system to provide adequate ATP.

To generate even more ATP molecules, pyruvic acid can go through additional metabolic pathways in the presence of oxygen (see Figure 12.6). Although this process is slower than glycolysis occurring under anaerobic conditions, the breakdown of 1 glucose molecule going through aerobic metabolism yields 36 to 38 ATP molecules for energy, while the anaerobic process yields only 2 ATP molecules. Thus, this aerobic process supplies eighteen times more energy! Another advantage of the aerobic process is that it does not result in the significant production of acids and other compounds that contribute to muscle fatigue, which means that a low-intensity activity can be performed for hours. Aerobic metabolism of glucose is the primary source of fuel for our muscles during activities lasting from 3 minutes to 4 hours (see Figure 12.5).

As you learned in Chapter 4, we can store only a limited amount of glycogen in our body. An average, well-nourished man who weighs about 154 pounds (70 kg) can

glycolysis The breakdown of glucose; yields two ATP molecules and two pyruvic acid molecules for each molecule of glucose.

pyruvic acid The primary end product of glycolysis.

lactic acid A compound that results when pyruvic acid is metabolized in the presence of insufficient oxygen.

store about 200 to 500 g of muscle glycogen, which is equal to 800 to 2,000 kcal of energy. Although trained athletes can store more muscle glycogen than the average person, even their bodies do not have enough stored glycogen to provide an unlimited energy supply for long-term activities. Thus, we also need a fuel source that is very abundant and can be broken down under aerobic conditions, so that it can support activities of lower intensity and longer duration. This fuel source is fat.

Aerobic Breakdown of Fats Supports Exercise of Low Intensity and Long Duration

When we refer to fat as a fuel source, we mean stored triglycerides, which is the primary storage form of fat in our cells. As you learned in Chapter 5, a triglyceride molecule is composed of a glycerol backbone attached to three fatty acid molecules (see Figure 5.1 in Chapter 5). It is these fatty acid molecules that provide much of the energy we need to support long-term activity. Fatty acids are classified by their length—that is, by the number of carbons they contain. The longer the fatty acid, the more ATP that can be generated from its breakdown. For instance, palmitic acid is a fatty acid with 16 carbons. If palmitic acid is broken down completely, it yields 129 ATP molecules! Obviously, far more energy is produced from this one fatty acid molecule than from the aerobic breakdown of a glucose molecule.

There are two major advantages of using fat as a fuel. First, fat is an abundant energy source, even in lean people. For example, a man who weighs 154 pounds (70 kg) who has a body fat level of 10% has approximately 15 pounds of body fat, which is equivalent to more than 50,000 kcal of energy! This is significantly more energy than can be provided by his stored muscle glycogen (800 to 2,000 kcal). Second, fat provides 9 kcal of energy per gram, more than twice as much energy per gram as carbohydrate. The primary disadvantage of using fat as a fuel is that the breakdown process is relatively slow; thus, fat is used predominantly as a fuel source during activities of lower intensity and longer duration. Fat is also our primary energy source during rest, sitting, and standing in place.

What specific activities are primarily fueled by fat? Walking long distances uses fat stores, as does hiking, long-distance cycling, and other low- to moderate-intensity forms of exercise. Fat is also an important fuel source during endurance events, such as marathons (26.2 miles) and ultra-marathon races (49.9 miles). Endurance exercise training improves our ability to use fat for energy, which may be one reason that people who exercise regularly tend to have lower body fat levels than people who do not exercise.

It is important to remember that we are almost always using some combination of carbohydrate and fat for energy. At rest, we use very little carbohydrate, relying mostly on fat. However this does not mean that we can reduce our body fat by resting and doing very little activity! As discussed in Chapter 11, to lose weight and reduce body fat, a person needs to exercise regularly and reduce energy intake, so that negative energy balance results. During

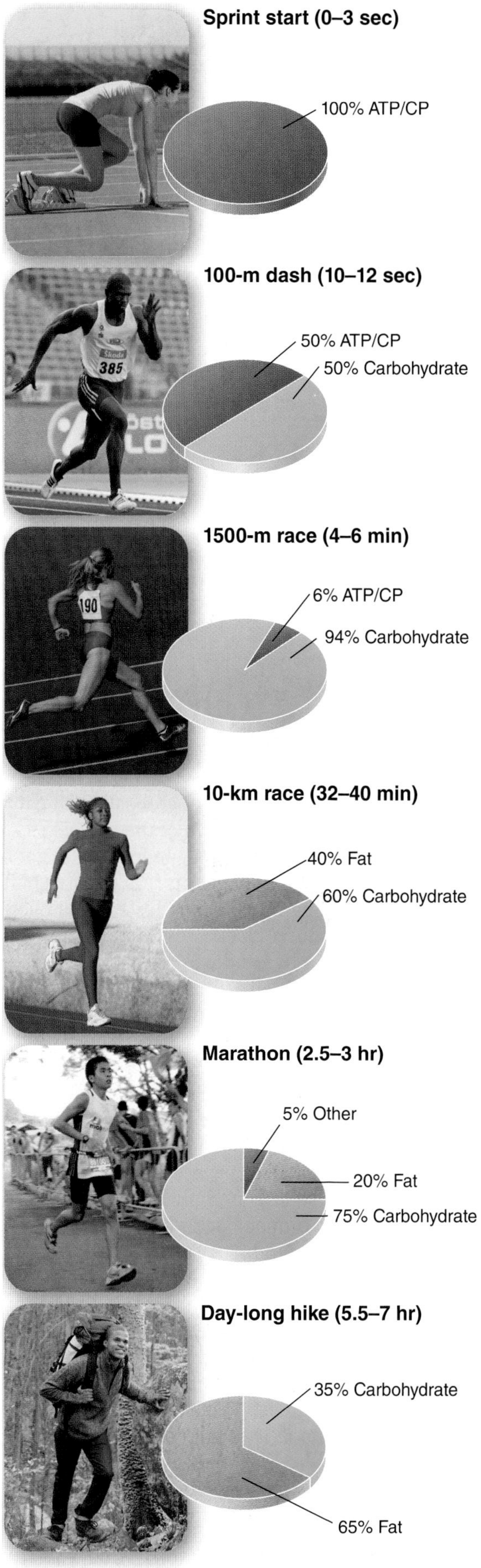

Figure 12.5 The relative contributions of ATP–CP, carbohydrate, and fat to activities of various durations and intensities.

Figure 12.6 The breakdown of one molecule of glucose, or the process of glycolysis, yields two molecules of pyruvic acid and two ATP molecules. The further metabolism of pyruvic acid in the presence of insufficient oxygen (anaerobic process) results in the production of lactic acid. The metabolism of pyruvic acid in the presence of adequate oxygen (aerobic process) yields 36 to 38 molecules of ATP.

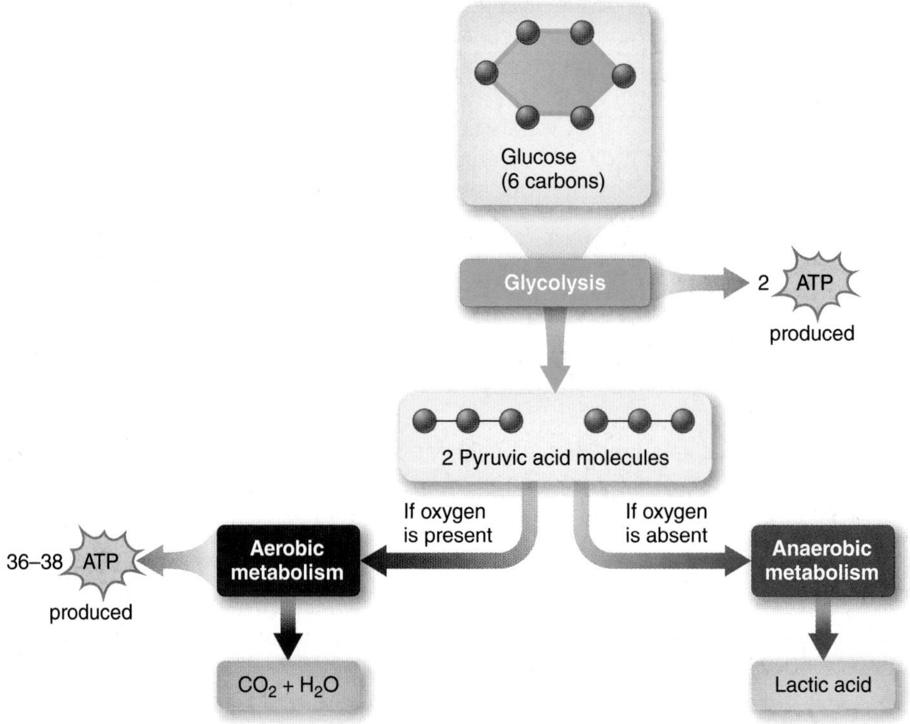

NUTRITION MYTH OR FACT?

Does Lactic Acid Cause Muscle Fatigue and Soreness?

Theo and his teammates won their basketball game last night, but just barely. With two of the players sick, Theo got more court time than usual, and when he got back to the dorm, he could hardly get his legs to carry him up the stairs. This morning, Theo's muscles ache all over, and he wonders if a buildup of lactic acid is to blame.

Lactic acid is a by-product of glycolysis. For many years, both scientists and athletes believed that lactic acid caused muscle fatigue and soreness. Does recent scientific evidence support this belief?

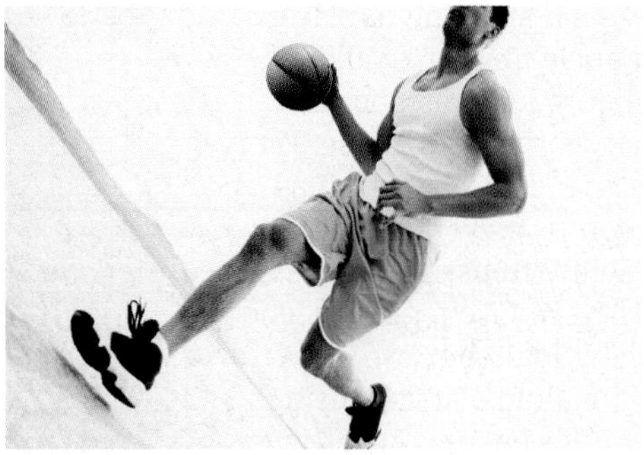

The exact causes of muscle fatigue are not known, and there appear to be many contributing factors. Recent evidence suggests that fatigue may be due not only to the accumulation of many acids and other metabolic by-products, such as inorganic phosphate,[13] but also to the depletion of creatine phosphate and changes in calcium in the cells that affect muscle contraction. Depletion of muscle glycogen, liver glycogen, and blood glucose, as well as psychological factors, can all contribute to fatigue.[14] Thus, it appears that lactic acid only contributes to fatigue but does not cause fatigue independently.

So what causes muscle soreness? As with fatigue, there are probably many factors. It is hypothesized that soreness usually results from microscopic tears in the muscle fibers as a result of strenuous exercise. This damage triggers an inflammatory reaction, which causes an influx of fluid and various chemicals to the damaged area. These substances work to remove damaged tissue and initiate tissue repair, but they may also stimulate pain. However, it appears highly unlikely that lactic acid is an independent cause of muscle soreness.

Recent studies indicate that lactic acid is produced even under aerobic conditions! This means it is produced at rest as well as during exercise at any intensity. The reasons for this constant production of lactic acid are still being studied. What we do know is that lactic acid is an important fuel for resting tissues, for working cardiac and skeletal muscles, and even for the brain both at rest and during exercise.[15,16] That's right—skeletal muscles not only *produce* lactic acid but also *use* it for energy, both directly and after it is converted into glucose and glycogen in the liver. We also know that endurance training improves the muscles' ability to use lactic acid for energy. Thus, contrary to being a waste product of glucose metabolism, lactic acid is actually an important energy source for muscle cells during rest and exercise.

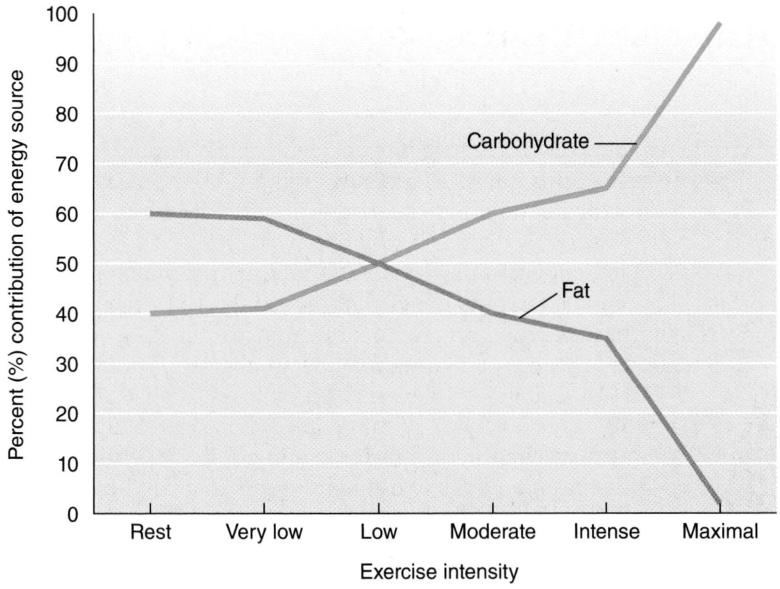

Figure 12.7 For most daily activities, including exercise, we use a mixture of carbohydrate and fat for energy. At lower exercise intensities, we rely more on fat as a fuel source. As exercise intensity increases, we rely more on carbohydrate for energy.
Data from Brooks, G. A., and J. Mercier. 1994. Balance of carbohydrate and lipid utilization during exercise: the "crossover" concept. *J. Appl. Physiol.* 76(6):2253–2261.

maximal exercise (at 90–100% effort), we are using virtually all carbohydrate. However, most activities we do each day involve some use of both fuels (**Figure 12.7**).

When it comes to eating properly to support regular physical activity or exercise training, the nutrient to focus on is carbohydrate. This is because most people store more than enough fat to support exercise, whereas our storage of carbohydrate is limited. It is especially important that we maintain adequate stores of glycogen for moderate to intense exercise. Dietary recommendations for fat, carbohydrate, and protein are reviewed later in this chapter.

Amino Acids Are Not Major Sources of Fuel during Exercise

Proteins, or more specifically amino acids, are not major energy sources during exercise. As discussed in Chapter 6, amino acids can be used directly for energy if necessary, but they are more often used to make glucose to maintain our blood glucose levels during exercise. Amino acids also help build and repair tissues after exercise. Depending on the intensity and duration of the activity, amino acids may contribute about 1–6% of the energy needed.[17]

Given this, why is it that so many people are concerned about their protein intakes? As you learned in Chapter 6, our muscles are not stimulated to grow when we eat extra dietary protein. Only appropriate physical training can stimulate our muscles to grow and strengthen. Thus, while we need enough dietary protein to support activity and recovery, consuming very high amounts does not provide an added benefit. The protein needs of athletes are only slightly higher than the needs of non-athletes, and most of us eat more than enough protein to support even the highest requirements for competitive athletes! Thus, there is generally no need for recreationally active people or even competitive athletes to consume protein or amino acid supplements.

RECAP The amount of ATP stored in a muscle cell is limited and can keep a muscle active for only about 1 to 3 seconds. For intense activities lasting about 3 to 15 seconds, creatine phosphate can be broken down to provide energy and support the regeneration of ATP. To support activities that last from 30 seconds to 2 minutes, energy is produced from glycolysis. Fatty acids can be broken down aerobically to support activities of low intensity and longer duration. The two major advantages of using fat as a fuel are that it is an abundant energy source and it provides more than twice the energy per gram as compared with carbohydrate. Amino acids may contribute from 3% to 6% of the energy needed during exercise, depending on the intensity and duration of the activity. Amino acids help build and repair tissues after exercise.

What Kind of Diet Supports Physical Activity?

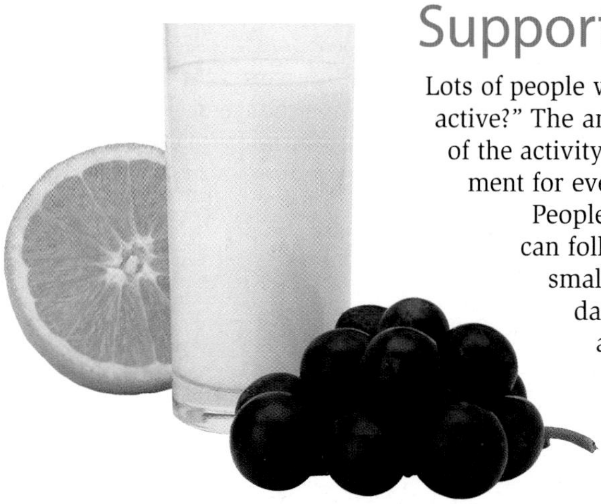

Small snacks can be helpful to meet daily energy demands.

Lots of people wonder, "Do my nutrient needs change if I become more physically active?" The answer to this question depends on the type, intensity, and duration of the activity in which you participate. It is not necessarily true that our requirement for every nutrient is greater if we are physically active.

People who are performing moderate-intensity daily activities for health can follow the dietary guidelines put forth in the USDA Food Guide. For smaller or less active people, the lower end of the range of recommendations for each food group may be appropriate. For larger or more active people, the higher end of the range is suggested. Modifications may be necessary for people who exercise vigorously every day, particularly for athletes training for competition. **Table 12.2** provides an overview of the nutrients that can be affected by regular, vigorous exercise training. Each of these nutrients is described in more detail in the following section.[18]

TABLE 12.2 Suggested Intakes of Nutrients to Support Vigorous Exercise

Nutrient	Functions	Suggested Intake
Energy	Supports exercise, activities of daily living, and basic body functions	Depends on body size and the type, intensity, and duration of activity. For many female athletes: 1,800 to 3,500 kcal/day For many male athletes: 2,500 to 7,500 kcal/day
Carbohydrate	Provides energy, maintains adequate muscle glycogen and blood glucose; high complex carbohydrate foods provide vitamins and minerals	45–65% of total energy intake Depending on sport and gender, should consume 6–10 g of carbohydrate per kg body weight per day
Fat	Provides energy, fat-soluble vitamins, and essential fatty acids; supports production of hormones and transport of nutrients	20–35% of total energy intake
Protein	Helps build and maintain muscle; provides building material for glucose; energy source during endurance exercise; aids recovery from exercise	10–35% of total energy intake Endurance athletes: 1.2–1.4 g per kg body weight Strength athletes: 1.2–1.7 g per kg body weight
Water	Maintains temperature regulation (adequate cooling); maintains blood volume and blood pressure; supports all cell functions	Consume fluid before, during, and after exercise Consume enough to maintain body weight Consume at least 8 cups (64 fl. oz) of water daily to maintain regular health and activity Athletes may need up to 10 liters (170 fl. oz) every day; more is required if exercising in a hot environment
B-vitamins	Critical for energy production from carbohydrate, fat, and protein	May need slightly more (one to two times the RDA) for thiamin, riboflavin, and vitamin B_6
Calcium	Builds and maintains bone mass; assists with nervous system function, muscle contraction, hormone function, and transport of nutrients across cell membrane	Meet the current AI: 14–18 years: 1,300 mg/day 19–70 years: 1,000 mg/day 71 and older: 1,200 mg/day
Iron	Primarily responsible for the transport of oxygen in blood to cells; assists with energy production	Consume at least the RDA: Males: 14–18 years: 11 mg/day 19 and older: 8 mg/day Females: 14–18 years: 15 mg/day 19–50 years: 18 mg/day 51 and older: 8 mg/day

Vigorous Exercise Increases Energy Needs

Athletes generally have higher energy needs than moderately physically active or sedentary people. The amount of extra energy needed to support regular training is determined by the type, intensity, and duration of the activity. In addition, the energy needs of male athletes are higher than those of female athletes because male athletes weigh more, have more muscle mass, and expend more energy during activity. This is relative, of course: a large woman who trains 3 to 5 hours each day will probably need more energy than a small man who trains 1 hour each day. The energy needs of athletes can range from only 1,500 to 1,800 kcal/day for a small female gymnast to more than 7,500 kcal/day for a male cyclist competing in the Tour de France cross-country cycling race!

Figure 12.8 shows a sample of meals that total 1,800 kcal per day and 4,000 kcal per day, with the carbohydrate content of these meals meeting more than 60% of total energy intake. As you can see, athletes who require more than 4,000 kcal per day need to consume very large quantities of food. However, the heavy demands of daily physical training, work, school, and family responsibilities often leave these athletes with little time to eat adequately. Thus, many athletes meet their energy demands by planning regular meals and snacks and **grazing** (eating small meals throughout the day) consistently. They may also take advantage of the energy-dense snack foods and meal replacements specifically designed for athletes participating in vigorous training. These steps help athletes maintain their blood glucose and energy stores.

grazing Consistently eating small meals throughout the day; done by many athletes to meet their high energy demands.

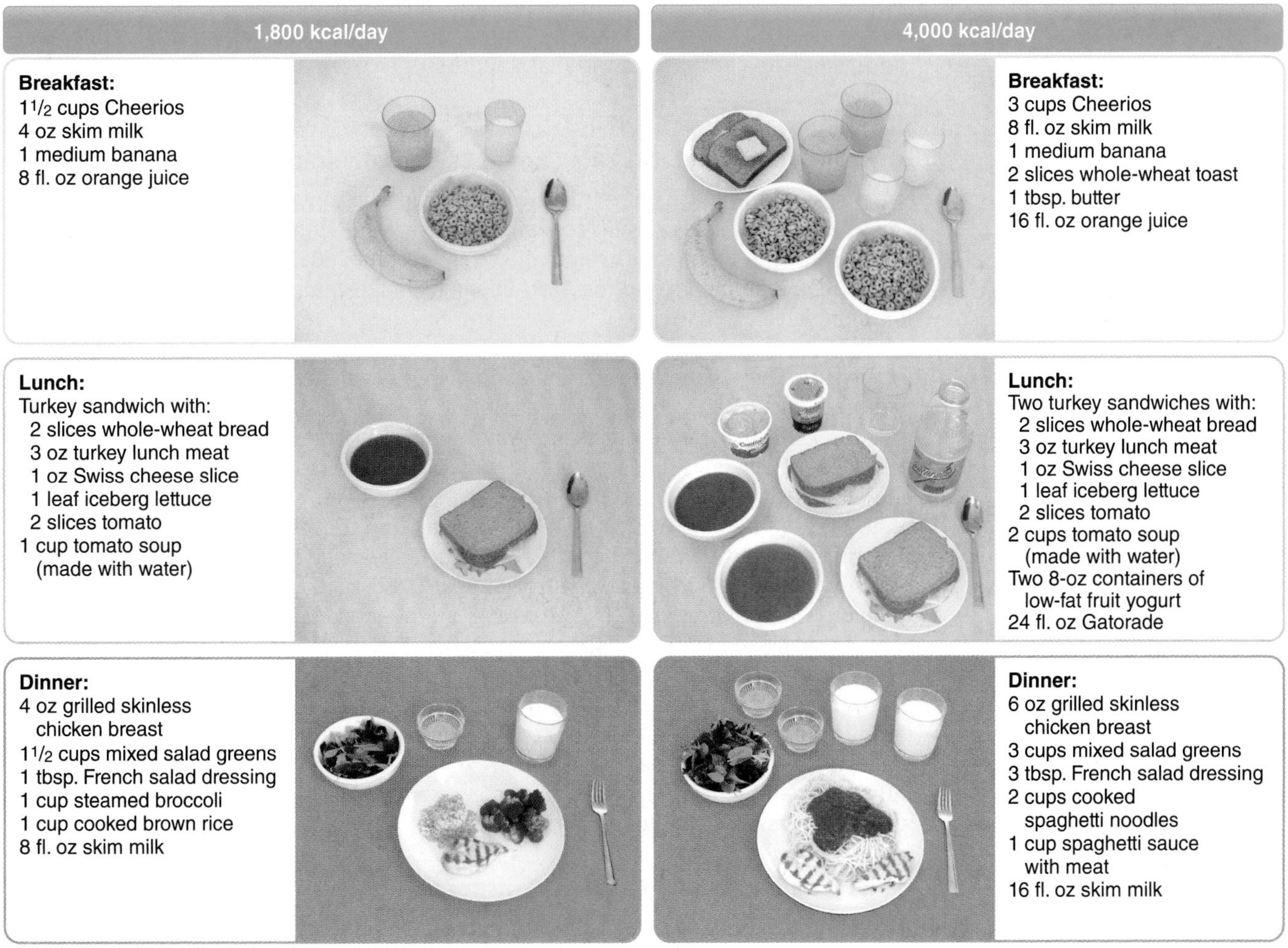
1,800 kcal/day
4,000 kcal/day
Breakfast:
1 1/2 cups Cheerios
4 oz skim milk
1 medium banana
8 fl. oz orange juice
Breakfast:
3 cups Cheerios
8 fl. oz skim milk
1 medium banana
2 slices whole-wheat toast
1 tbsp. butter
16 fl. oz orange juice
Lunch:
Turkey sandwich with:
2 slices whole-wheat bread
3 oz turkey lunch meat
1 oz Swiss cheese slice
1 leaf iceberg lettuce
2 slices tomato
1 cup tomato soup (made with water)
Lunch:
Two turkey sandwiches with:
2 slices whole-wheat bread
3 oz turkey lunch meat
1 oz Swiss cheese slice
1 leaf iceberg lettuce
2 slices tomato
2 cups tomato soup (made with water)
Two 8-oz containers of low-fat fruit yogurt
24 fl. oz Gatorade
Dinner:
4 oz grilled skinless chicken breast
1 1/2 cups mixed salad greens
1 tbsp. French salad dressing
1 cup steamed broccoli
1 cup cooked brown rice
8 fl. oz skim milk
Dinner:
6 oz grilled skinless chicken breast
3 cups mixed salad greens
3 tbsp. French salad dressing
2 cups cooked spaghetti noodles
1 cup spaghetti sauce with meat
16 fl. oz skim milk

Figure 12.8 High-carbohydrate (approximately 60% of total energy) meals that contain approximately 1,800 kcal/day (on left) and 4,000 kcal/day (on right). Athletes, particularly those with very high energy needs, must plan their meals carefully to meet energy demands.

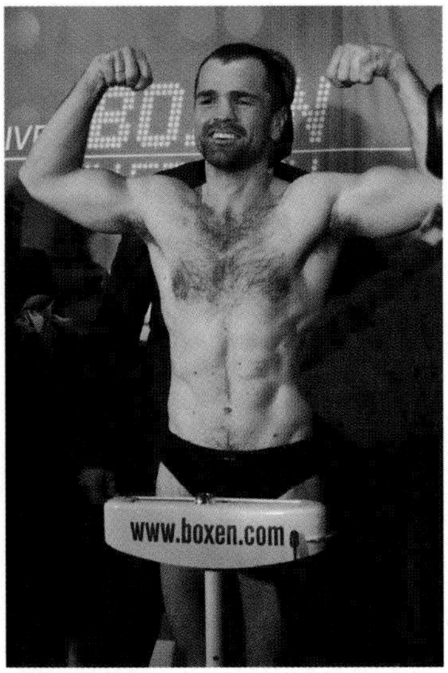

Some athletes diet to meet a predefined weight category.

If an athlete is losing body weight, then his or her energy intake is inadequate. Conversely, weight gain may indicate that energy intake is too high. Weight maintenance is generally recommended to maximize performance. If weight loss is warranted, food intake should be lowered no more than 200 to 500 kcal/day, and athletes should try to lose weight prior to the competitive season, if at all possible. Weight gain may be necessary for some athletes and can usually be accomplished by consuming 500 to 700 kcal/day more than needed for weight maintenance. The extra energy should come from a healthy balance of carbohydrate (45–60% of total energy intake), fat (20–35% of total energy intake), and protein (10–35% of total energy intake).

Many athletes are concerned about their weight. Jockeys, boxers, wrestlers, judo athletes, and others are required to "make weight"—to meet a predefined weight category. Others, such as distance runners, gymnasts, figure skaters, and dancers, are required to maintain a very lean figure for performance and aesthetic reasons. These athletes tend to eat less energy than they need to support vigorous training, which puts them at risk for inadequate intakes of all nutrients. These athletes are also at a higher risk of suffering from health consequences resulting from poor energy and nutrient intake, including eating disorders, osteoporosis, menstrual disturbances, dehydration, heat and physical injuries, and even death.

Carbohydrate Needs Increase for Many Active People

As you know, carbohydrate (in the form of glucose) is one of the primary sources of energy needed to support exercise. Both endurance athletes and strength athletes require adequate carbohydrate to maintain their glycogen stores and provide quick energy.

How Much of an Athlete's Diet Should Be Carbohydrate?

You may recall from Chapter 4 that the AMDR for carbohydrates is 45–65% of total energy intake. Athletes should consume carbohydrate within this recommended range. Although high-carbohydrate diets (greater than 60% of total energy intake) have been recommended in the past, this percentage value may not be appropriate for all athletes.

To illustrate the importance of carbohydrate intake for athletes, let's see what happens to Theo when he participates in a study designed to determine how carbohydrate intake affects glycogen stores during a period of heavy training. Theo was asked to go to the exercise laboratory at the university and ride a stationary bicycle for 2 hours a day for 3 consecutive days at 75% of his maximal heart rate. Before and after each ride, samples of muscle tissue were taken from his thighs to determine the amount of glycogen stored in the working muscles. Theo performed these rides under two different experimental conditions—once when he had eaten a high-carbohydrate diet (80% of total energy intake) and again when he had eaten a moderate-carbohydrate diet (40% of total energy intake). As you can see in **Figure 12.9**, Theo's muscle glycogen levels decreased dramatically after each training session. More important, his muscle glycogen levels did not recover to baseline levels over the 3 days when Theo ate the lower-carbohydrate diet. He was able to maintain his muscle glycogen levels only when he was eating the higher-carbohydrate diet. Theo also told the researchers that completing the 2-hour rides was much more difficult when he had eaten the moderate-carbohydrate diet as compared to when he ate the diet that was higher in carbohydrate.

When Should Carbohydrates Be Consumed?

It is important for athletes not only to consume enough carbohydrate to maintain glycogen stores but also to time their intake optimally. Our body stores glycogen very rapidly during the first 24 hours of recovery from exercise, with the highest storage rates occurring during the first few hours.[19] Higher carbohydrate intakes during the first 24 hours of recovery from exercise are associated with higher amounts of glucose being stored as muscle glycogen. A daily carbohydrate intake of approximately 6 to

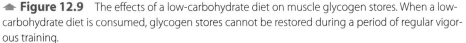

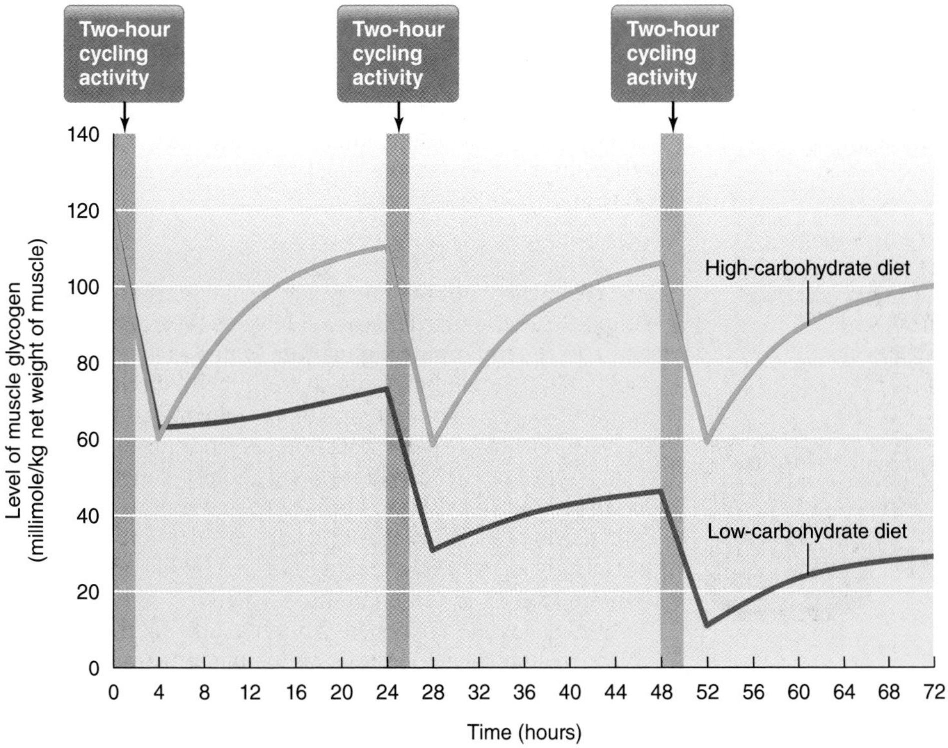

Figure 12.9 The effects of a low-carbohydrate diet on muscle glycogen stores. When a low-carbohydrate diet is consumed, glycogen stores cannot be restored during a period of regular vigorous training.

Data from Costill, D. L., and J. M. Miller. 1980. Nutrition for endurance sport: CHO and fluid balance. *Int. J. Sports Med.* 1:2–14. Copyright © 1980 Georg Thieme Verlag. Used with permission.

10 g of carbohydrate per kg body weight will optimize muscle glycogen stores in many athletes. However, this need might be much greater in athletes who are training heavily daily, as they have less time to recover and require more carbohydrate to support both training and storage needs.

If an athlete has to perform or participate in training bouts that are scheduled less than 8 hours apart, then he or she should try to consume enough carbohydrate in the few hours following training to allow for ample glycogen storage. However, with a longer recovery time (generally 12 hours or more), the athlete can eat when he or she chooses, and glycogen levels should be restored as long as the total carbohydrate eaten is sufficient.

Interestingly, studies have shown that muscle glycogen can be restored to adequate levels in the muscle whether the food is eaten in small, multiple snacks or in larger meals,[19] although some studies show enhanced muscle glycogen storage during the first 4 to 6 hours of recovery when athletes are fed large amounts of carbohydrate every 15 to 30 minutes.[20,21] There is also evidence that consuming high glycemic index foods during the immediate postrecovery period results in higher glycogen storage than is achieved as a result of eating low glycemic index foods. This may be due to a greater malabsorption of the carbohydrate in low glycemic index foods, as these foods contain more indigestible forms of carbohydrate.[19]

What Food Sources of Carbohydrates Are Good for Athletes?

What are good carbohydrate sources to support vigorous training? In general, complex, less processed carbohydrate foods, such as whole grains and cereals, fruits, vegetables, and juices, are excellent sources that also supply fiber, vitamins, and minerals. Guidelines recommend that intake of simple sugars be less than 10% of total energy intake, but some athletes who require very large energy intakes to support training may need to consume more. In addition, as previously mentioned, glycogen storage can be enhanced by consuming foods with a high glycemic index immediately postrecovery. Thus, there are advantages to consuming a wide variety of carbohydrate sources.

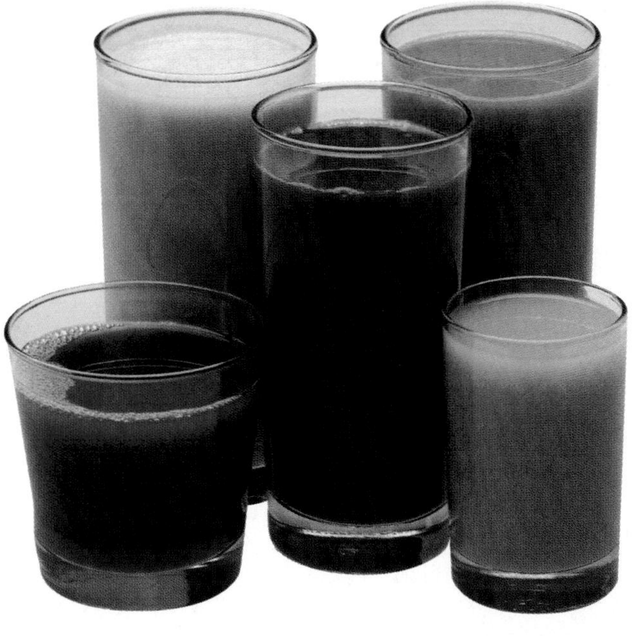

Fruit and vegetable juices can be a good source of carbohydrates.

As a result of time constraints, many athletes have difficulties consuming enough food to meet carbohydrate demands. Thus, many sports drinks and energy bars have been designed to help athletes increase their carbohydrate intake. **Table 12.3,** below, identifies some energy bars and other simple, inexpensive snacks and meals that contain 50 to 100 g of carbohydrate.

When Does Carbohydrate Loading Make Sense?

As you know, carbohydrate is a critical energy source to support exercise, particularly endurance-type activities. Because of the importance of carbohydrates as an exercise fuel and our limited capacity to store them, discovering ways to maximize our storage of carbohydrates has been at the forefront of sports nutrition research for many years. The practice of **carbohydrate loading,** also called *glycogen loading,* involves altering both exercise duration and carbohydrate intake such that it maximizes the amount of muscle glycogen. **Table 12.4** reviews a schedule for carbohydrate loading for an endurance athlete.

Athletes who may benefit from maximizing muscle glycogen stores include those competing in marathons, ultra-marathons, long-distance swimming, cross-country skiing, and triathlons. Athletes who compete in baseball, American football, 10-kilometer runs, walking, hiking, weight lifting, and most swimming events will not gain any performance benefits from this practice, nor will people who regularly participate in moderately intense physical activities to maintain fitness.

It is important to realize that carbohydrate loading does not always improve performance. There are many adverse side effects of this practice, including extreme gastrointestinal distress, particularly diarrhea. We store water along with the extra glycogen in our muscles, which leaves many athletes feeling heavy and sluggish. Athletes who want to try carbohydrate loading should experiment prior to competition to determine whether it is an acceptable and beneficial approach for them.

carbohydrate loading Also known as glycogen loading. A process that involves altering training and carbohydrate intake, so that muscle glycogen storage is maximized.

TABLE 12.3 Carbohydrate and Total Energy in Various Foods

Food	Amount	Carbohydrate (g)	Energy from Carbohydrate (%)	Total Energy (kcal)
Sweetened applesauce	1 cup	50	97	207
Large apple with	1 each	50	82	248
Saltine crackers	8 each			
Whole-wheat bread	1-oz slice	50	71	282
with jelly	4 tsp.			
and skim milk	12 fl. oz			
Spaghetti (cooked)	1 cup	50	75	268
with tomato sauce	1/4 cup			
Brown rice (cooked)	1 cup	100	88	450
with mixed vegetables	1/2 cup			
and apple juice	12 fl. oz			
Grape-Nuts cereal	1/2 cup	100	84	473
with raisins	3/8 cup			
and skim milk	8 fl. oz			
Clif Bar (chocolate chip)	2.4 oz	45	72	250
Meta-Rx (fudge brownie)	3.53 oz	48	60	320
Power Bar (chocolate)	2.25 oz	42	75	225
PR Bar Ironman	2 oz	24	42	230

Data from Manore, M. M., N. L. Meyer, and J. Thompson. 2009. *Sport Nutrition for Health and Performance,* 2nd ed. Champaign, IL: Human Kinetics.

TABLE 12.4 Recommended Carbohydrate Loading Guidelines for Endurance Athletes

Days Prior to Event	Exercise Duration (minutes) at 70% Maximal Effort	Carbohydrate Content of Diet (g/kg of body weight)
6	90	5
5	40	5
4	40	5
3	20	10
2	20	10
1	Rest	10
Day of race	Competition	Precompetition food and fluid

Data from Coleman, E. 2006. Carbohydrate and exercise. In: Dunford, M., ed. *Sports Nutrition,* 4th ed. Chicago, IL: The American Dietetic Association. Used with permission.

Moderate Fat Consumption Is Enough to Support Most Activities

As you have learned, fat is an important energy source for both moderate physical activity and vigorous endurance training. When athletes reach a physically trained state, they are able to use more fat for energy; in other words, they become better "fat burners." This can also occur in people who are not athletes but who regularly participate in aerobic-type fitness activities. This training effect occurs for a number of reasons, including an increase in the number and activity of various enzymes involved in fat metabolism, improved ability of the muscle to store fat, and improved ability to extract fat from the blood for use during exercise. By using fat as a fuel, athletes can spare carbohydrate, so that they can use it during prolonged, intense training or competition.

Many athletes concerned with body weight and physical appearance believe they should eat less than 15% of their total energy intake as fat, but this is inadequate for vigorous activity. Instead, a fat intake of 20–35% of total energy intake is generally recommended for most athletes, with less than 10% of total energy intake as saturated fat.

These recommendations are also put forth for non-athletes. Recall from Chapter 5 that fat provides not only energy but also fat-soluble vitamins and essential fatty acids that are critical to maintaining general health. If fat consumption is too low, inadequate levels of these nutrients can eventually prove detrimental to training and performance. Athletes who have chronic disease risk factors, such as high blood lipids, high blood pressure, or unhealthful blood glucose levels, should work with their physician to adjust their intake of fat and carbohydrate according to their health risks.

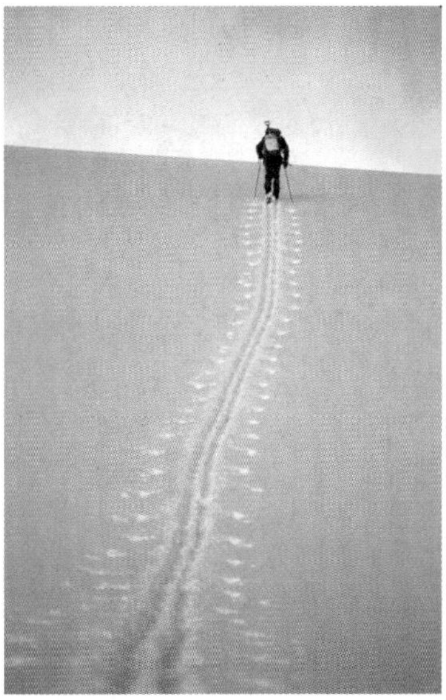

Carbohydrate loading may benefit endurance athletes, such as cross-country skiers.

Many Athletes Have Increased Protein Needs

The protein intakes suggested for competitive athletes and moderately active people are given in **Table 12.5**. Let's consider the terminology used in the table:

- Competitive male and female endurance athletes train 5 to 7 days per week for more than an hour each day; many of these individuals may train for 3 to 6 hours per day. These athletes need significantly more protein than the current RDA of 0.8 g of protein per kg body weight.
- Resistance athletes focus on building and maintaining muscle mass and strength. Those who are already trained need less protein than those who are initiating training. Studies do not support the claim that consuming more than 2 g of protein per kg body weight improves protein synthesis, muscle strength, or performance.[17]
- Moderate-intensity endurance athletes are people exercising four or five times per week for 45 to 60 minutes each time; these individuals may compete in community races and other activities. Their protein needs are only modestly increased above the RDA.

TABLE 12.5 Estimated Protein Requirements for Athletes

Group	Protein Requirements (g/kg of body weight)
Competitive male and female athletes	1.4–1.6
Moderate-intensity endurance athletes	1.2
Recreational endurance athletes	0.8–1.0
Football, power sports players	1.4–1.7
Resistance athletes, weight lifters (early training)	1.5–1.7
Resistance athletes, weight lifters (steady-state training)	1.0–1.2

Data from Tarnopolsky, M. 2006. Protein and amino acid needs for training and bulking up. In: Burke, L., and Deakin, V., eds. *Clinical Sports Nutrition*, 3rd ed. New York: McGraw-Hill.

- Recreational endurance athletes are people who exercise four or five times per week for 30 minutes at less than 60% of their maximal effort. These individuals have a protein need that is equal to or only slightly higher than the RDA.

As noted previously, most inactive people and many athletes in the United States consume more than enough protein to support their needs.[22] However, some athletes do not consume enough protein; these typically include individuals with very low energy intakes, vegetarians or vegans who do not consume high-protein food sources, and young athletes who are growing and are not aware of their higher protein needs.

In 1995, Dr. Barry Sears published *The Zone: A Dietary Road Map,* a book that claims numerous benefits of a high-protein, low-carbohydrate diet for athletes.[23] Since that time, Sears has published several additional books espousing the same principles, which are still being recommended to both athletes and non-athletes. As you learned in Chapter 11, low-carbohydrate, high-protein diets are quite popular, especially among people who want to lose weight (see Nutrition Debate box in Chapter 11). Unlike many of the current high-protein diets, the Zone Diet was developed and marketed specifically for competitive athletes. It recommends that athletes eat a 40–30–30 diet, or one composed of 40% carbohydrate, 30% fat, and 30% protein. Dr. Sears claims that high-carbohydrate diets impair athletic performance because of unhealthy effects of insulin. These claims have never been supported by research—in fact, many of Dr. Sears's claims are not consistent with human physiology. The primary problem with the Zone Diet for athletes is that it is too low in both energy and carbohydrate to support training and performance.

As described in Chapter 6, high-quality protein sources include lean meats, poultry, fish, eggs and egg whites, low-fat dairy products, legumes, and soy products. By following the USDA Food Guide and meeting energy needs, people of all fitness levels can consume more than enough protein without the use of supplements or specially formulated foods.

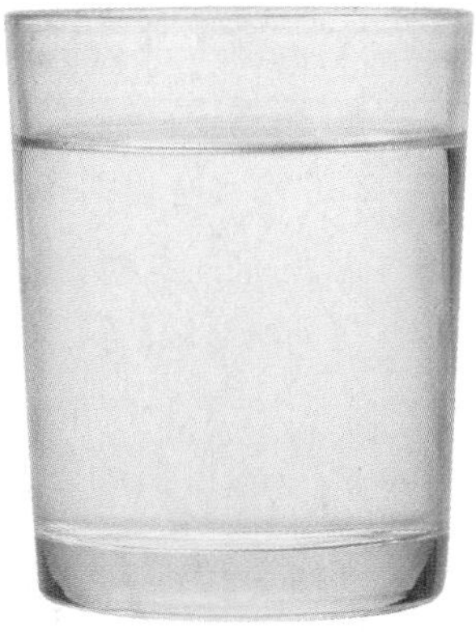

Water is essential for maintaining fluid balance and preventing dehydration.

RECAP **The type, intensity, and duration of activities a person participates in determine his or her nutrient needs. Carbohydrate needs may increase for some active people. In general, athletes should consume 45–65% of their total energy as carbohydrate. Carbohydrate loading involves altering physical training and the diet such that the storage of muscle glycogen is maximized. Active people use more fat than carbohydrates for energy because they experience an increase in the number and activity of the enzymes involved in fat metabolism, and they have an improved ability to store fat and extract it from the blood for use during exercise. A dietary fat intake of 20–35% is recommended for athletes, with less than 10% of total energy intake as saturated fat. Although protein needs can be higher for athletes, most people in the United States already consume more than twice their daily needs for protein.**

Regular Exercise Increases Our Need for Fluids

A detailed discussion of fluid and electrolyte balance is provided in Chapter 7. In this chapter, we will focus on the role of water during exercise.

Cooling Mechanisms

Heat production can increase fifteen to twenty times during heavy exercise! The primary way in which we dissipate this heat is through sweating, which is also called **evaporative cooling.** When body temperature rises, more blood (which contains water) flows to the surface of the skin. Heat is carried in this way from the core of our body to the surface of our skin. By sweating, the water (and body heat) leaves our body, and the air around us picks up the evaporating water from our skin, cooling our body.

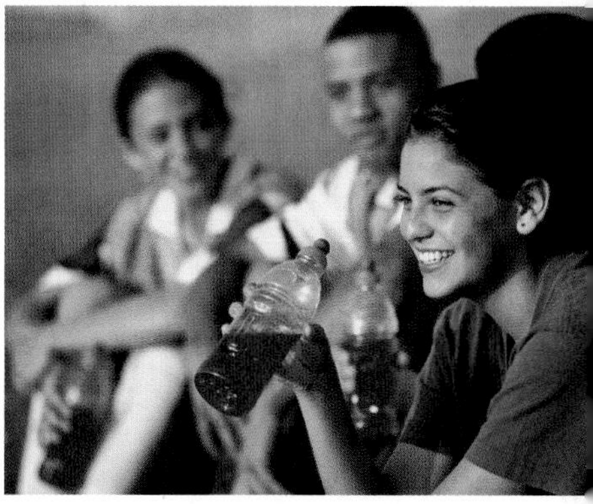

Drinking sports beverages during training and competition lasting more than 1 hour replaces fluid, carbohydrates, and electrolytes.

Dehydration and Heat-Related Illnesses

Heat illnesses occur because when we exercise in the heat, our muscles and skin constantly compete for blood flow. When there is no longer enough blood flow to provide adequate blood to both our muscles and our skin, muscle blood flow takes priority and evaporative cooling is inhibited. Exercising in heat plus humidity is especially dangerous because whereas the heat dramatically raises body temperature, the high humidity inhibits evaporative cooling; that is, the environmental air is already so saturated with water that it is unable to absorb the water in sweat. Body temperature becomes dangerously high, and heat illness is likely.

It is important to remember that dehydration significantly increases our risk for heat illnesses. In **Figure 12.10**, specific signs of dehydration during heavy exercise are listed. Review the ***In Depth*** following Chapter 7 for more information on specific heat-related illnesses in which fluid intake plays a role.

Guidelines for Proper Fluid Replacement

How can we prevent dehydration and heat illnesses? Obviously, adequate fluid intake is critical before, during, and after exercise. Unfortunately, our thirst mechanism cannot be relied upon to signal when we need to drink. If we rely only on our feelings of thirst, we will not consume enough fluid to support exercise.

General fluid replacement recommendations are based on maintaining body weight. As discussed in Chapter 7, athletes who are training and competing in hot environments should weigh themselves before and after the training session or event and should regain the weight lost over the subsequent 24-hour period. They should avoid losing more than 2–3% of body weight during exercise, as performance can be impaired with fluid losses as small as 1% of body weight.

Table 12.6 reviews the guidelines for proper fluid replacement. For activities lasting less than 1 hour, plain water is generally adequate to replace fluid losses. However, for training and competition lasting longer than 1 hour in any weather, sports

evaporative cooling Another term for sweating, which is the primary way in which we dissipate heat.

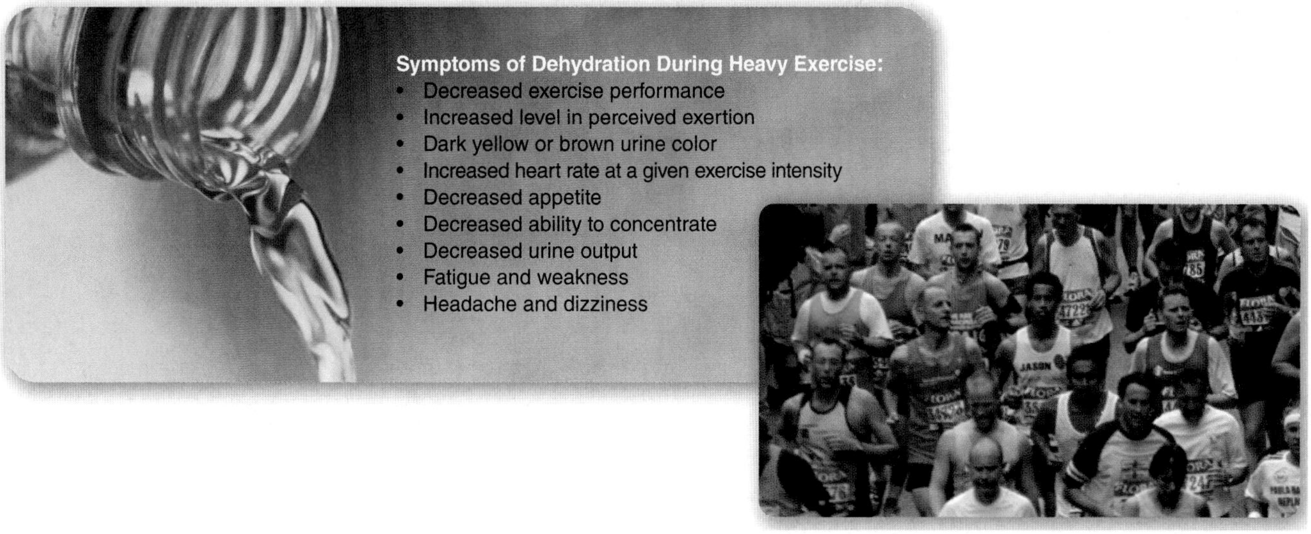
Symptoms of Dehydration During Heavy Exercise:
• Decreased exercise performance
• Increased level in perceived exertion
• Dark yellow or brown urine color
• Increased heart rate at a given exercise intensity
• Decreased appetite
• Decreased ability to concentrate
• Decreased urine output
• Fatigue and weakness
• Headache and dizziness

Figure 12.10 Symptoms of dehydration during heavy exercise.

TABLE 12.6 Guidelines for Fluid Replacement

Activity Level	Environment	Fluid Requirements (liters per day)
Sedentary	Cool	2–3
Active	Cool	3–6
Sedentary	Warm	3–5
Active	Warm	5–10

Before Exercise or Competition:

- Drink adequate fluids during the 24 hours before event; should be able to maintain body weight.
- Slowly drink about 0.17 to 0.24 fl. oz per kg body weight of water or a sports drink at least 4 hours prior to exercise or event to allow time for excretion of excess fluid prior to event.
- Slowly drink another 0.10 to 0.17 fl. oz per kg body weight about 2 hours before event.
- Consuming beverages with sodium and/or small amounts of salted snacks at a meal will help stimulate thirst and retain fluids consumed.

During Exercise or Competition:

- Drink early and regularly throughout event to sufficiently replace all water lost through sweating.
- Amount and rate of fluid replacement depend on individual sweating rate, exercise duration, weather conditions, and opportunities to drink.
- Fluids should be cooler than the environmental temperature and flavored to enhance taste and promote fluid replacement.

During Exercise or Competition That Lasts More Than 1 Hour:

- Fluid replacement beverage should contain 5–10% carbohydrate to maintain blood glucose levels; sodium and other electrolytes should be included in the beverage in amounts of 0.5–0.7 g of sodium per liter of water to replace the sodium lost by sweating.

Following Exercise or Competition:

- Consume about 3 cups of fluid for each pound of body weight lost.
- Fluids after exercise should contain water to restore hydration status, carbohydrates to replenish glycogen stores, and electrolytes (for example, sodium and potassium) to speed rehydration.
- Consume enough fluid to permit regular urination and to ensure the urine color is very light or light yellow in color; drinking about 125–150% of fluid loss is usually sufficient to ensure complete rehydration.

In General:

- Products that contain fructose should be limited, as these may cause gastrointestinal distress.
- Caffeine and alcohol should be avoided, as these products increase urine output and reduce fluid retention.
- Carbonated beverages should be avoided, as they reduce the desire for fluid intake due to stomach fullness.

Data from Murray, R. 1997. Drink more! Advice from a world class expert. *ACSM's Health and Fitness Journal* 1:19–23; American College of Sports Medicine Position Stand. 2007. Exercise and fluid replacement. *Med. Sci. Sports Exerc.* 39(2):377–390; and Casa, D. J., L. E. Armstrong, S. K. Hillman, S. J. Montain, R. V. Reiff, B. S. E. Rich, W. O. Roberts, and J. A. Stone. 2000. National Athletic Trainers' Association position statement: fluid replacement for athletes. *J. Athlet. Train.* 35:212–224.

beverages containing carbohydrates and electrolytes are recommended. These beverages are also recommended for people who will not drink enough water because they don't like the taste. If drinking these beverages will guarantee adequate hydration, they are appropriate to use. For more specific information about sports beverages, refer to Chapter 7, page 247.

Inadequate Intakes of Some Vitamins and Minerals Can Diminish Health and Performance

When individuals train vigorously for athletic events, their requirements for certain vitamins and minerals may be altered. Many highly active people do not eat enough food or a variety of foods that allows them to consume enough of these nutrients, yet it is imperative that active people do their very best to eat an adequate, varied, and balanced diet to try to meet the increased needs associated with vigorous training.

B-Vitamins

The B-vitamins are directly involved in energy metabolism (see pages 328–341). There is reliable evidence that the requirements of active people for thiamin, riboflavin, and vitamin B_6 may be slightly higher than the current RDA due to increased production of energy in active people and inadequate dietary intake in some individuals.[22] However, these increased needs are easily met by consuming adequate energy and a lot of complex carbohydrates, fruits, and vegetables. Athletes and physically active people at risk for poor B-vitamin status are those who consume inadequate energy or who consume mostly refined carbohydrate foods, such as soda pop and sugary snacks. Vegan athletes and active individuals may be at risk for inadequate intake of vitamin B_{12}. Food sources enriched with this nutrient include soy and cereal products.

Calcium and the Female Athlete Triad

Calcium supports proper muscle contraction and ensures bone health (see pages 296–301). Calcium intakes are inadequate for most women in the United States, including both sedentary and active women. This is most likely due to a failure to consume foods that are high in calcium, particularly dairy products. While vigorous training does not appear to increase our need for calcium, we need to consume enough calcium to support bone health. If we do not, stress fractures and severe loss of bone can result.

Some female athletes suffer from a syndrome known as the *female athlete triad.* This condition is discussed in the ***In Depth*** following this chapter. In the female athlete triad, nutritional inadequacies cause irregularities in the menstrual cycle and hormonal disturbances that lead to a significant loss of bone mass. Thus, for female athletes, consuming the recommended amounts of calcium is critical. For female athletes who are physically small and have lower energy intakes, calcium supplementation may be needed to meet current recommendations.

Iron

Iron is a part of the hemoglobin molecule and is critical for the transport of oxygen in our blood to our cells and working muscles. Iron also is involved in energy production. Research has shown that active individuals lose more iron in the sweat, feces, and urine than do inactive individuals and that endurance runners lose iron when their red blood cells break down in their feet due to the high impact of running.[24] Female athletes and non-athletes lose more iron than male athletes because of menstrual blood losses, and females in general tend to eat less iron in their diet. Vegetarian athletes and active people may also consume less iron. Thus, many athletes and active people are at higher risk for iron deficiency. Depending on its severity, poor iron status can impair athletic performance and our ability to maintain regular physical activity.

Not all athletes suffer from iron deficiency. A phenomenon known as *sports anemia* was identified in the 1960s. Sports anemia is not true anemia, but a transient decrease in iron stores that occurs at the start of an exercise program for some people, and it is seen in athletes who increase their training intensity. Exercise training increases the amount of water in our blood (called *plasma volume*); however, the amount of hemoglobin does not increase until later in the training period. Thus, the iron content in the blood appears to be low but instead is falsely depressed due to increases in plasma volume. Sports anemia, since it is not true anemia, does not affect performance.

The stages of iron deficiency are described on pages 352–354. In general, it appears that physically active females are at relatively high risk of suffering from the first stage of iron depletion, in which iron stores are low.[25,26] Because of this, it is suggested that blood tests of iron stores and monitoring of dietary iron intake be done routinely for active females.[22] In some cases, iron needs cannot be met through the diet, and supplementation is necessary. Iron supplementation should be done with a physician's approval and proper medical supervision.

NUTRI-CASE THEO

"Ever since I did that cycling test in the fitness lab, I've been watching my carbohydrates. Lately, I've been topping 500 grams of carbs a day. But now I'm beginning to wonder, am I getting enough protein? I'm starting to feel really wiped out, especially after games. We've won four out of the last five games, and I'm giving it everything I've got, but today I was really dragging myself through practice. I'm eating about 150 grams of protein a day, but I think I'm going to try one of those protein powders they sell at my gym. I guess I just feel like, when I'm competing, I need some added insurance."

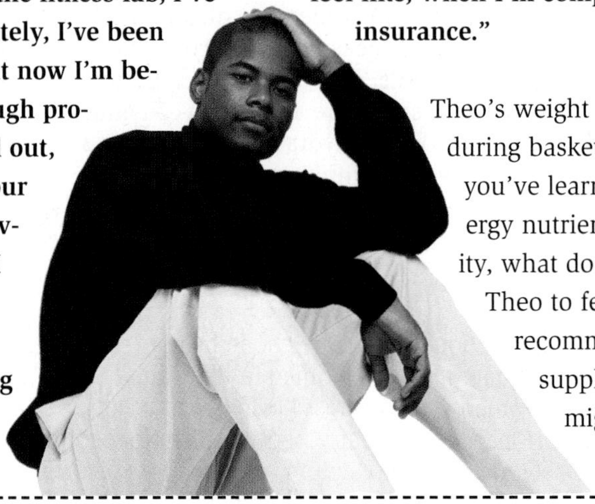

Theo's weight averages about 190 pounds during basketball season. Given what you've learned about the role of the energy nutrients in vigorous physical activity, what do you think might be causing Theo to feel "wiped out"? Would you recommend that Theo try the protein supplement? What other strategies might be helpful for him to consider?

RECAP **Regular exercise increases fluid needs. Fluid is critical to cool our internal body temperature and prevent heat illnesses. Dehydration is a serious threat during exercise in extreme heat and high humidity. Active people may need more thiamin, riboflavin, and vitamin B_6 than inactive people. Exercise itself does not increase our calcium needs, but most women, including active women, do not consume enough calcium. Some female athletes suffer from the female athlete triad, a condition that involves the interaction of low energy availability, osteoporosis, and amenorrhea. Many active individuals require more iron, particularly female athletes and vegetarian athletes.**

Are Ergogenic Aids Necessary for Active People?

Many competitive athletes and even some recreationally active people search continually for that something extra that will enhance their performance. **Ergogenic aids** are substances used to improve exercise and athletic performance. For example, nutrition supplements can be classified as ergogenic aids, as can anabolic steroids and other pharmaceuticals. Interestingly, people report using ergogenic aids not only to enhance athletic performance but also to improve their physical appearance, prevent or treat injuries, treat diseases, and help them cope with stress. Some people even report using them because of peer pressure!

As you have learned in this chapter, adequate nutrition is critical to athletic performance and to regular physical activity, and products such as sports bars and beverages can help athletes maintain their competitive edge. However, as we will explore shortly, many of these products are not effective, some are dangerous, and most are very expensive. For the average consumer, it is virtually impossible to track the latest research findings for these products. In addition, many have not been adequately studied, and unsubstantiated false claims surrounding them are rampant. How can you become a more educated consumer about ergogenic aids?

ergogenic aids Substances used to improve exercise and athletic performance.

New ergogenic aids are available virtually every month, and keeping track of these substances is a daunting task. It is therefore not possible to discuss every available product in this chapter. However, a brief review of a number of currently popular ergogenic aids is provided.

Anabolic Products Are Touted as Muscle and Strength Enhancers

Many ergogenic aids are said to be **anabolic,** meaning that they build muscle and increase strength. Most anabolic substances promise to increase testosterone, which is the hormone that is associated with male sex characteristics and that increases muscle size and strength. Although some anabolic substances are effective, they are generally associated with harmful side effects.

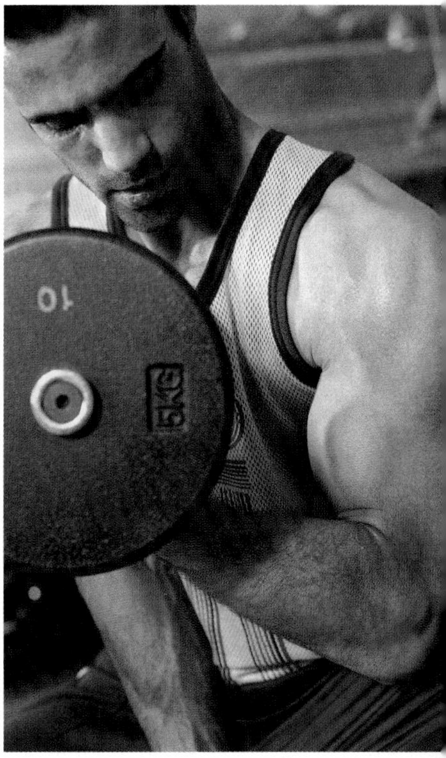

Anabolic substances are often marketed to people wishing to increase muscle size, but carry risks for harmful side effects.

Anabolic Steroids

Anabolic steroids are testosterone-based drugs that have been used extensively by strength and power athletes. Anabolic steroids are known to be effective in increasing muscle size, strength, power, and speed. However, these products are illegal in the United States, and their use is banned by all major collegiate and professional sports organizations, in addition to both the U.S. and the International Olympic Committees. The following are proven long-term and irreversible effects of steroid use:

- infertility
- early closure of the plates of the long bones, resulting in permanent shortened stature
- shriveled testicles, enlarged breast tissue (that can be removed only surgically), and other signs of "feminization" in men
- enlarged clitoris, facial hair growth, and other signs of "masculinization" in women
- increased risk for certain forms of cancer
- liver damage
- unhealthful changes in blood lipids
- hypertension
- severe acne
- hair thinning or baldness
- disorders such as depression, delusions, sleep disturbances, and extreme anger (so-called roid rage)

Androstenedione and Dehydroepiandrosterone

Androstenedione ("andro") and dehydroepiandrosterone (DHEA) are precursors of testosterone. Manufacturers of these products claim that taking them will increase testosterone levels and muscle strength. Androstenedione became very popular after baseball player Mark McGwire claimed he used it during the time he was breaking home run records. A national survey found that, in 2002, about one of every forty high-school seniors had used it in the past year.[27] Contrary to popular claims, recent

HOT TOPIC

Ergogenic Aids: Let the Buyer Beware?

The sale of ergogenic aids is a multibillion-dollar industry, and some companies resort to misleading claims to boost their share of the market. Beware of the following deceptive tactics used to market ergogenic aids:

1. Taking published research out of context, applying the findings in an unproven manner, or having inappropriate control over study results. Some companies claim that research has been done or is currently being done, but fail to provide specific information.
2. Paying celebrities to endorse products—remember that testimonials can be faked, bought, and exaggerated.
3. Stating that the product is patented and that this proves its effectiveness. Patents are granted to indicate differences among products.
4. Advertizing through infomercials and mass-media marketing videos. Although the Federal Trade Commission (FTC) regulates false claims in advertising, products are generally investigated only if they pose significant public danger.
5. Offering mail-order fitness evaluations or anabolic measurements. Most of these evaluations are inappropriate and inaccurate.

anabolic The term applied to a substance that builds muscle and increases strength.

studies have found that neither androstenedione nor DHEA increases testosterone levels, and androstenedione has been shown to increase the risk for heart disease in men aged 35 to 65.[28] There are no studies that support claims that these products improve strength or increase muscle mass.

Gamma-Hydroxybutyric Acid

Gamma-hydroxybutyric acid, or GHB, has been promoted as an alternative to anabolic steroids for building muscle. The production and sale of GHB have never been approved in the United States; however, it was illegally produced and sold on the black market. For many users, GHB caused only dizziness, tremors, or vomiting, but others experienced severe side effects, including seizures. Many people were hospitalized and some died.

After GHB was banned, a similar product (gamma-butyrolactone, or GBL) was marketed in its place. This product was also found to be dangerous and was removed from the market. Recently, another replacement product called BD, or 1,4-butanediol, was banned because it has caused at least seventy-one deaths, with forty more under investigation. BD is an industrial solvent and is listed on ingredient labels as tetramethylene glycol, butylene glycol, or sucol-B. Side effects include wild, aggressive behavior; nausea; incontinence; and sudden loss of consciousness.

Creatine

Creatine is a supplement that has become wildly popular with strength and power athletes. Creatine, or creatine phosphate, is found in meat and fish and stored in our muscles. As described earlier in this chapter, we use creatine phosphate (CP) to regenerate ATP. It is hypothesized that, by taking creatine supplements, individuals have more CP available to replenish ATP, which will prolong their ability to train and perform in short-term, explosive activities, such as weight lifting and sprinting. Between 1994 and 2010, more than 1,700 research articles related to creatine and exercise in humans were published. These studies indicate that creatine does not enhance performance in aerobic-type events, but it does enhance sprint performance in swimming, running, and cycling.[28–32] Other studies have shown that creatine increases the work performed and the amount of strength gained during resistance exercise.[31,33,34] Currently, creatine is not banned by any sports governing bodies, and many collegiate sports programs readily provide creatine supplements for their athletes.

In January 2001, the *New York Times* reported that the French government had claimed that creatine use could lead to cancer.[35] The news spread quickly across national and international news organizations and over the Internet. These claims were subsequently found to be false, as there are no studies in humans that suggest an increased risk for cancer with creatine use. In fact, numerous studies show an anticancer effect for creatine.[36,37] Although side effects such as dehydration, muscle cramps, and gastrointestinal disturbances have been reported with creatine use, there is very little information on how the long-term use of creatine impacts health. Further research is needed to determine the effectiveness and safety of creatine use over prolonged periods of time.

Some Products Are Said to Optimize Fuel Use during Exercise

Certain ergogenic aids are touted as increasing energy levels and improving athletic performance by optimizing our use of fat, carbohydrate, and protein. The products reviewed here are caffeine, ephedrine, carnitine, chromium, and ribose.

Caffeine

Caffeine is a stimulant that makes us feel more alert and energetic, decreasing feelings of fatigue during exercise. Caffeine has been shown to increase the use of fat as a fuel during endurance exercise, which spares muscle glycogen and improves performance.[38,39] Energy drinks that contain high amounts of caffeine, such as Red Bull, have become popular with athletes and many college students. These drinks should be avoided during exercise, as severe dehydration can result due to the combination of fluid loss from exercise and caffeine consumption. It should be recognized that caffeine is a controlled or restricted drug in the athletic world, and athletes can be banned from Olympic competition if urine caffeine levels are too high. However, the amount of caffeine that is banned is quite high, and athletes would need to consume caffeine in pill form to reach this level. Side effects of caffeine use include increased blood pressure, increased heart rate, dizziness, insomnia, headache, and gastrointestinal distress.

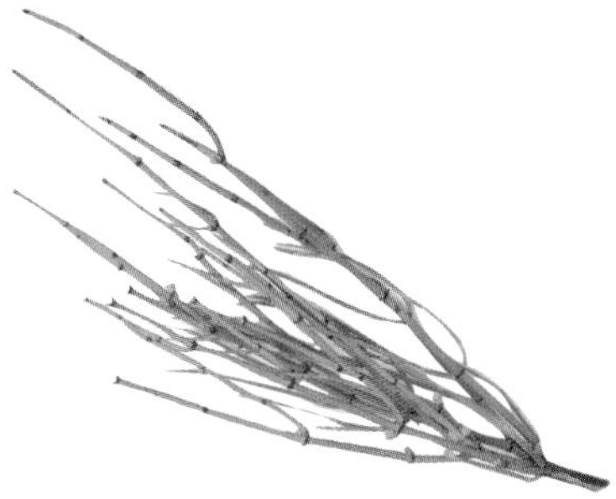

Ephedrine is made from the herb *Ephedra sinica* (Chinese ephedra).

Ephedrine

Ephedrine, also known as ephedra, Chinese ephedra, or *ma huang*, is a strong stimulant marketed as a weight-loss supplement and energy enhancer. In reality, many products sold as Chinese ephedra (or herbal ephedra) contain ephedrine from the laboratory and other stimulants, such as caffeine. The use of ephedra supplements does not appear to enhance performance, but supplements containing both caffeine and ephedra have been shown to prolong the amount of exercise that can be done until exhaustion is reached.[40] Ephedra is known to reduce body weight and body fat in sedentary women, but its impact on weight loss and body fat levels in athletes is unknown. Side effects of ephedra use include headaches, nausea, nervousness, anxiety, irregular heart rate, and high blood pressure, and at least seventeen deaths have been attributed to its use.[41] It is currently illegal to sell ephedra-containing supplements in the United States.

Carnitine

Carnitine is a compound made from amino acids that is found in the mitochondrial membrane of our cells. Carnitine helps shuttle fatty acids into the mitochondria, so that they can be used for energy. In theory, it has been proposed that exercise training depletes our cells of carnitine and that supplementation should increase the amount of carnitine in our cell membranes. By increasing cellular levels of carnitine, we should be able to improve our use of fat as a fuel source. Thus, carnitine is marketed not only as a performance-enhancing substance but also as a "fat burner." Research studies of carnitine supplementation do not support these claims, as neither the transport of fatty acids nor their oxidation appears to be enhanced with supplementation.[42,43] Use of carnitine supplements has not been associated with significant side effects.

Chromium

Chromium is a trace mineral that enhances insulin's action of increasing the transport of amino acids into the cell (see Chapter 10). It is found in whole-grain foods, cheese, nuts, mushrooms, and asparagus. It is theorized that many people are chromium deficient and that supplementation will enhance the uptake of amino acids into muscle cells, which will increase muscle growth and strength. Like carnitine, chromium is marketed as a fat burner, as it is speculated that its effect on insulin stimulates the brain to decrease food intake.[41] Chromium supplements are available as chromium picolinate and chromium nicotinate. Early studies of chromium supplementation showed promise, but more recent, better-designed studies do not support any benefit of chromium supplementation to muscle mass, muscle strength, body fat, or exercise performance.[44]

Ribose

Ribose is a five-carbon sugar that is critical to the production of ATP. Ribose supplementation is claimed to improve athletic performance by increasing work output and promoting a faster recovery time from vigorous training. While ribose has been shown to improve exercise tolerance in patients with heart disease,[45] several studies have reported that ribose supplementation has no impact on athletic performance.[46–48]

From this review of ergogenic aids, you can see that most of these products are not effective in enhancing athletic performance or optimizing muscle strength or body composition. It is important to be a savvy consumer when examining these products to make sure you are not wasting your money or putting your health at risk by using them.

RECAP **Ergogenic aids are substances used to improve exercise and athletic performance. Anabolic steroids are effective in increasing muscle size, power, and strength, but they are illegal and can cause serious health problems. Androstenedione and dehydroepiandrosterone are precursors of testosterone; neither of these products has been shown to effectively increase testosterone levels or to increase strength or muscle mass. Creatine supplements are popular and can enhance sprint performance in swimming, running, and cycling. Caffeine is a stimulant that increases the use of fat during exercise; its use in the athletic world is controlled. Ephedrine is a stimulant that has potentially fatal side effects. Carnitine, chromium, and ribose are marketed as ergogenic aids but studies do not support their effectiveness.**

Nutrition DEBATE
How Much Physical Activity Is Enough?

Your aerobics instructor tells you to work out at your target heart rate for 20 minutes a day, whereas your doctor tells you to walk for half an hour three or four times a week. A magazine article exhorts you to work out to the point of exhaustion, while a new weight-loss book claims that you can be perfectly healthy without ever breaking a sweat. As if these mixed messages about what constitutes "regular physical activity" weren't enough, a report from the Institute of Medicine (IOM), which contributed to the (previous release) 2005 Dietary Guidelines for Americans, inadvertently added to the confusion. This report recommended that Americans be active 60 minutes per day to optimize health.[9] This message appears contradictory to the Surgeon General's report published in 1996, which recommended that Americans accumulate 30 minutes of physical activity on most, if not all, days of the week to optimize health.[1]

So how much activity is really enough? To try to answer this question, let's take a closer look at how the two reports differ. The Surgeon General's report considers a combination of what we have learned from two types of studies not used by the IOM: exercise training studies and population-based epidemiological studies. *Exercise training studies* involve putting individuals through a clearly defined training program and assessing fitness and health outcomes. These studies consistently show that less fit and older individuals can significantly improve their cardiorespiratory fitness and reduce their risk for chronic diseases by participating in moderate levels of physical activity.[49,50] In contrast, *population-based epidemiological studies* compare self-reports of physical activity and/or fitness to rates of illness and mortality.[51,52] In other words, these studies do not assess the direct effect of exercise training; instead, they assess only the relationship between level of physical activity/fitness and rates of disease and premature death. These studies show that unfit, sedentary people suffer from the highest rates of disease and premature mortality and that increased physical activity significantly correlates to decreased risks for chronic diseases and premature mortality.

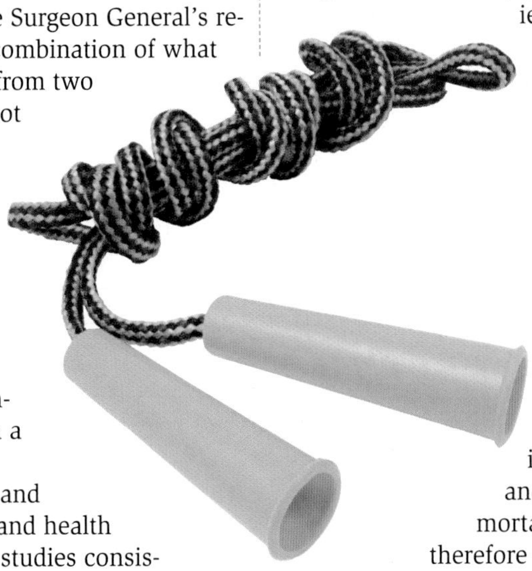

One challenge highlighted in the Surgeon General's report was how to determine the exact dose of exercise needed to improve physical fitness and health. Although the authors of this report acknowledged that using epidemiological studies to determine this dose was problematic, they pointed to studies indicating that expending an average of 150 kcal/day, which is equivalent to about 30 minutes of moderate physical activity per day, is associated with significant reductions in disease risk and premature mortality.[53–56] They therefore used this information to shape the recommendations put forth in the Surgeon General's report. It is important to emphasize that these recommendations were intended for individuals who are currently inactive. They were not intended to apply to individuals who are already doing more than 30 minutes of activity a day. In fact, the Surgeon General's report emphasizes that additional health and fitness benefits will result by doing more moderate-intensity physical activity or by substituting vigorous physical activities for those that are moderate in intensity.

In contrast, the IOM based its physical activity recommendations on metabolic studies determining the energy expenditure associated with maintaining a healthful body weight (defined as a BMI of 18.5 to 25 kg/m^2). After reviewing a large number of studies that assessed energy expenditure and BMI, the Institute of Medicine concluded that participating in about 60 minutes of moderately intense physical activity per day will move people from a very sedentary to an active lifestyle and will allow them to maintain a healthful body weight.

Although this recommendation appears to be very different from that of the Surgeon General's report, and may seem unrealistic, the IOM emphasizes that it includes all activities a person does above resting levels, including gardening, dog walking, housekeeping, and shopping.

So are these two recommendations really that different? Probably not. Nutrition experts, exercise physiologists, and other healthcare professionals all recognize that weight loss and healthful weight maintenance are easier to achieve by people who do more, not less, physical activity each day.

Chapter Review

Test Yourself ANSWERS

1. True. About 54% of Americans are insufficiently active, and almost 16% report doing no leisure activity at all.

2. False. Our muscles are not stimulated to grow when we eat extra protein, whether as food or supplements. Weight-bearing exercise appropriately stresses the body and produces increased muscle mass and strength.

3. True. Most ergogenic aids do not produce the results that are advertised. Many ergogenic aids, such as anabolic steroids and ephedrine, can actually cause serious health consequences, even death.

Find the Quack

When Brian joined the track team his first year in high school, he found his passion. Now in his third year of college, he's built a reputation as a winning distance runner, and he has several medals to prove it. One day his friend Jim, who is the track team's top sprinter, tells him about creatine supplements. Jim says that since he started using them several weeks ago, his performance times have improved. With an intercollegiate marathon event approaching, Brian is looking to improve his performance, so he goes online to check out the creatine supplements website Jim recommends. Here's what he learns:

- "Creatine is an amino acid synthesized by the body that plays a vital role in anaerobic energy production by regenerating ATP in skeletal muscle."
- "Creatine supplementation has been shown in several controlled studies to increase muscle stores of creatine and to improve performance in athletes whose sports rely heavily on the creatine phosphate anaerobic energy pathway." (The article cites six recent studies published in academic journals.)
- "Creatine supplementation is most effective for the performance of intense bursts of activity."
- "The manufacturer has on file more than 1,000 testimonials from satisfied customers whose athletic performance improved after taking creatine supplements."
- "The recommended dosage for an athlete's 'loading phase' varies according to gender, weight, and other factors, but a general recommendation is to consume four or five doses of 5 g each per day, for 5 to 7 days. This will fill the muscles' creatine phosphate stores to capacity. After this, a reduced maintenance dose of approximately 2–5 g/day is recommended. Taken as recommended, the supplements cost as little as $1 a day!"

1. Explain what the website article means by "the creatine phosphate anaerobic energy pathway."
2. Brian is a distance runner. Would you recommend he purchase creatine supplements? Why or why not?
3. Brian's track teammate Jim is a sprinter. Do you think it's possible that he has experienced physiologic benefits from creatine supplementation, or do you think his increased performance times are due to the placebo effect? Explain.
4. Recall the Hot Topic on deceptive practices used to market ergogenic aids. How many of these were employed by the creatine supplements website? Is this website an example of quackery? Why or why not?

Answers can be found on the companion website, at www.pearsonhighered.com/thompsonmanore.

Review Questions

1. For moderate-intensity exercise, the intensity range typically recommended is
   a. 25–50% of your estimated maximal heart rate.
   b. 35–75% of your estimated maximal heart rate.
   c. 50–70% of your estimated maximal heart rate.
   d. 75–95% of your estimated maximal heart rate.
2. The amount of ATP stored in a muscle cell can keep a muscle active for about
   a. 1 to 3 seconds.
   b. 10 to 30 seconds.
   c. 1 to 3 minutes.
   d. 1 to 3 hours.
3. To support a long afternoon of gardening, the body predominantly uses which nutrient for energy?
   a. carbohydrate
   b. fat
   c. amino acids
   d. lactic acid
4. Creatine
   a. seems to enhance performance in aerobic-type events.
   b. appears to increase an individual's risk for bladder cancer.
   c. seems to increase strength gained in resistance exercise.
   d. is stored in the liver.
5. Athletes participating in an intense athletic competition lasting more than 1 hour should
   a. drink caffeinated beverages to improve their performance while maintaining their hydration.
   b. drink plain warm water copiously both before and during the event in response to fluid losses from sweating and desire to drink.
   c. drink plain ice water both before and during the event in response to thirst.
   d. drink a beverage containing carbohydrate and electrolytes both before and during the event in amounts that balance hydration with energy, carbohydrate, and electrolyte needs.
6. True or false? A sound fitness program overloads the body.
7. True or false? A dietary fat intake of 20–35% is generally recommended for athletes.
8. True or false? Carbohydrate loading involves altering the duration and intensity of exercise and intake of carbohydrate such that the storage of fat is minimized.
9. True or false? Sports anemia is a chronic decrease in iron stores that occurs in some athletes who have been training intensely for several months to years.
10. True or false? FIT stands for frequency, intensity, and time.

Answers to Review Questions can be found at the back of this text, and additional essay questions and answers are located on the companion website at www.pearsonhighered.com/thompsonmanore.

Web Resources

www.americanheart.org
American Heart Association

The Healthy Lifestyle section of this site has sections on health tools, exercise and fitness, healthy diet, lifestyle management, and more.

www.acsm.org
American College of Sports Medicine

Click on "General Public" for guidelines on healthful aerobic activity and calculating your exercise heart rate range. You can also click on the "Fit Society Page" section to access ACSM's Fit Society Page newsletter.

www.cdc.gov/physicalactivity/everyone/guidelines
Centers for Disease Control and Prevention Physical Activity for Everyone

Visit on this site to learn more about how much physical activity is enough for children, adults, and older adults and how to set physical activity and fitness goals.

www.win.niddk.nih.gov/publications/physical
Weight Control Information Network

Find out more about healthy fitness programs from this website produced by the National Institute of Diabetes and Digestive and Kidney Diseases.

www.dietary-supplements.info.nih.gov
NIH Office of Dietary Supplements

Look on this National Institutes of Health site to learn more about the health effects of specific nutritional supplements.

www.nal.usda.gov/fnic
Food and Nutrition Information Center

Visit this site for links to detailed information about ergogenic aids and sports nutrition.

www.nutrition.arizona.edu/new
Nutrition Exercise Wellness

Check this University of Arizona site for information for athletes on nutrition, fluid intake, and ergogenic aids.

Disordered Eating

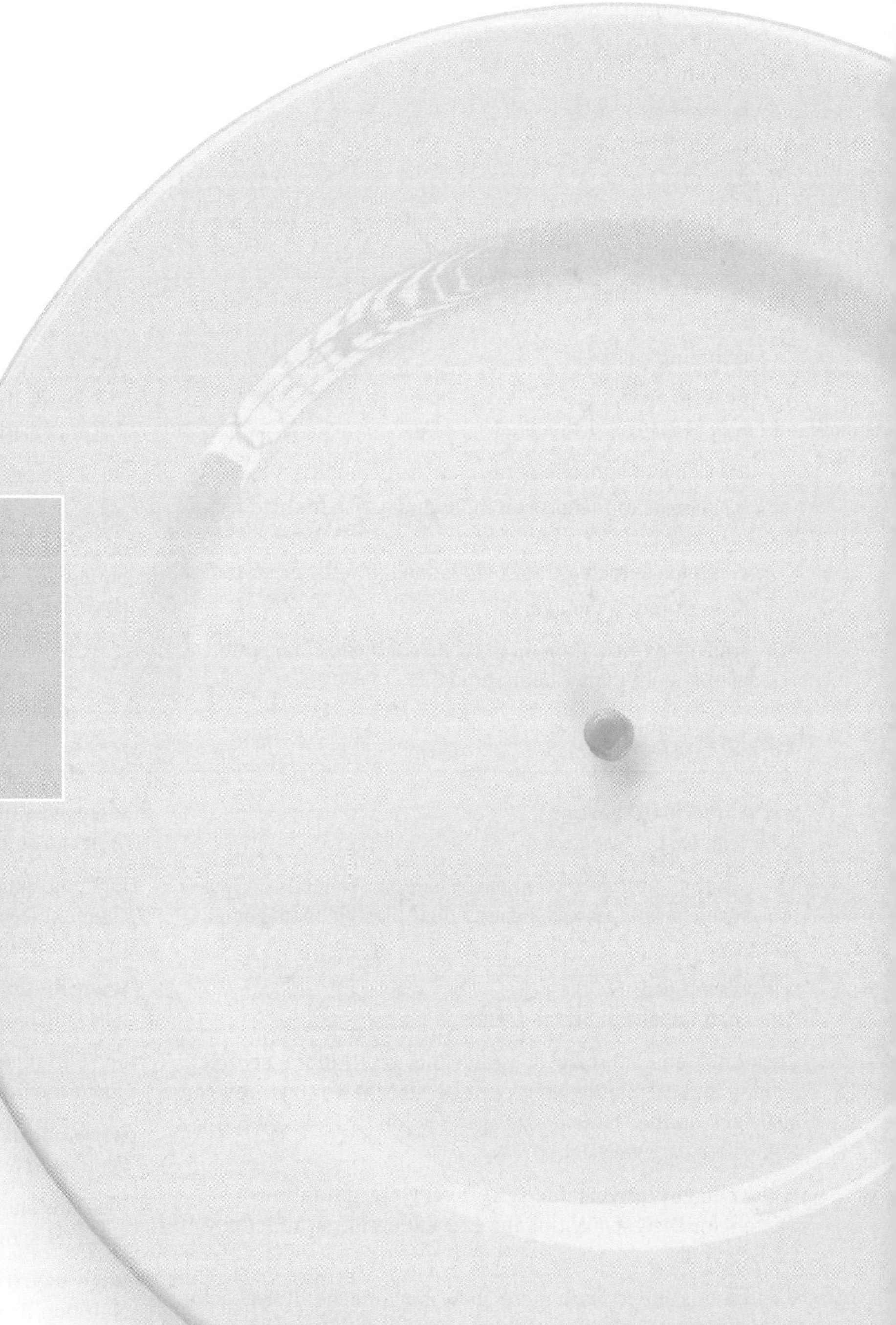

WANT TO FIND OUT. . .

- **what is the leading cause of death in females age 15 through 24?**
- **whether men experience disordered eating?**
- **what's keeping some overweight people up all night?**

READ ON.

On August 2, 2006, Uruguayan fashion model Luisel Ramos collapsed during a fashion show. Just 22 years old, she was pronounced dead of heart failure brought on by *anorexia nervosa,* a condition of self-imposed starvation. Family members said that, in the months prior to her death, she had adopted a diet of lettuce leaves and Diet Coke, and at 5′9″ tall, her weight had dropped to just 98 pounds. The following month, Madrid's "Fashion Week" responded to Ramos's death by banning from its runway fashion models who could not meet a minimum weight–height standard. A similar ruling was quickly adopted by the Milan fashion show, and several modeling agencies began to require prospective models to present medical records certifying that they are healthy. Although promising, such measures alone are clearly inadequate, and at least three more fashion models had died from self-starvation by the summer of 2008.

Do only models develop eating disorders, or can they occur in people like you? When does normal dieting cross the line into disordered eating? What early warning signs might tip you off that a friend was crossing that line? If you noticed the signs in a friend or family member, would you confront him or her? If so, what would you say? In the following pages, we explore ***In Depth*** some answers to these important questions.

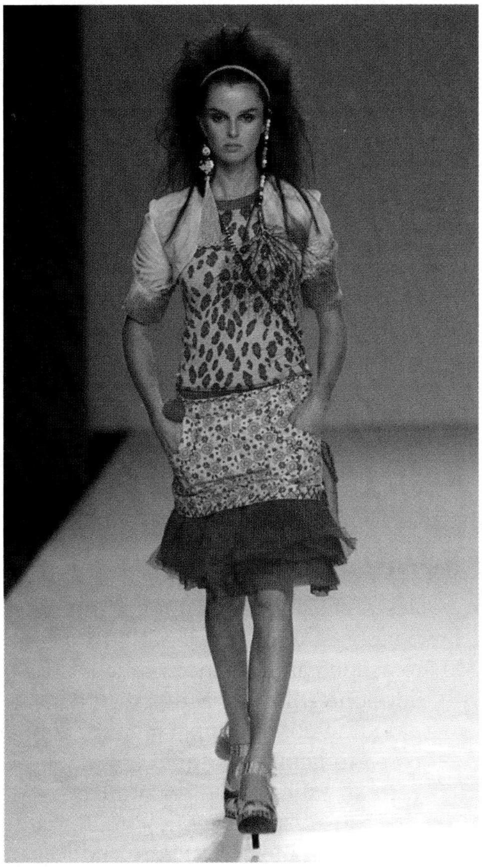

A string of models have died because of eating disorders.

Eating Behaviors Occur on a Continuum

Disordered eating is a general term used to describe a variety of atypical eating behaviors that people use to achieve or maintain a lower body weight. These behaviors may be as simple as going on and off diets or as extreme as refusing to eat any fat. Such behaviors don't usually continue for long enough to make the person seriously ill, nor do they significantly disrupt the person's normal routine.

In contrast, some people restrict their eating so much or for so long that they become dangerously underweight. These people have an **eating disorder,** a psychiatric condition that involves extreme body dissatisfaction and long-term eating patterns that negatively affect body functioning. The two more commonly diagnosed eating disorders are anorexia nervosa and bulimia nervosa. **Anorexia nervosa** is a potentially life-threatening eating disorder characterized by self-starvation, which eventually leads to a severe nutrient deficiency. In contrast, **bulimia nervosa** is characterized by recurrent episodes of extreme overeating and compensatory behaviors to prevent weight gain, such as self-induced vomiting, misuse of laxatives, fasting, excessive exercise, or several of these in combination. Both disorders will be discussed in more detail shortly.

When does normal dieting cross the line into disordered eating? Eating behaviors occur on a *continuum,* a spectrum that can't be divided neatly into parts. One example of a continuum is a rainbow—where exactly does the red end and the orange begin? Thinking about eating behaviors as a continuum makes it easier to understand how a person can progress from relatively normal eating behaviors to a pattern that is disordered.

Suppose that for several years you've skipped breakfast in favor of a mid-morning snack, but now you find yourself avoiding the cafeteria until early afternoon. Is this normal? To answer that question, you'd need to consider your feelings about food and your **body image**—the way you perceive your body.

Take a moment to take the self-test in the accompanying What About You? box. It will help you clarify how you feel about your body and about food and whether you're at risk for disordered eating.

Many Factors Contribute to Disordered Eating Behaviors

The factors that result in the development of disordered eating are very complex, but research indicates that a number of psychological, interpersonal, social, and biological factors may contribute in any particular individual.

disordered eating A variety of abnormal or atypical eating behaviors that are used to keep or maintain a lower body weight.

eating disorder A clinically diagnosed psychiatric disorder characterized by severe disturbances in body image and eating behaviors.

anorexia nervosa A serious, potentially life-threatening eating disorder characterized by self-starvation, which eventually leads to a deficiency in energy and the essential nutrients the body requires to function normally.

bulimia nervosa A serious eating disorder characterized by recurrent episodes of binge eating and recurrent inappropriate compensatory behaviors in order to prevent weight gain, such as self-induced vomiting, fasting, excessive exercise, or misuse of laxatives, diuretics, enemas, or other medications.

body image A person's perception of his or her body's appearance and functioning.

What About You?

Are You at Risk for Disordered Eating?

Take a look at the Eating Issues and Body Image Continuum figure **(Figure 1)** near this box. Which of the five columns best describes your feelings about food and your body? If you find yourself identifying with the statements on the left side of the continuum, you probably have few issues with food or body image. Most likely, you accept your body size and view food as a normal part of maintaining your health and fueling your daily physical activity.

As you progress to the right side of the continuum, food and body image become bigger issues, with food restriction becoming the norm. If you identify with the statements on the far right, you may be afraid of eating and dislike your body. If so, you should consult a healthcare professional as soon as possible. The earlier you seek treatment, the more likely it is you'll succeed in taking ownership of your body and developing a more healthful approach to food.

Influence of Genetic Factors

Overall, the diagnosis of anorexia nervosa and bulimia nervosa is several times more common in females, and in siblings and other blood relatives who also have the diagnosis, than in the general population.[1] This observation might imply the existence of an "eating disorder gene"; however, it is difficult to separate the contribution of genetic from other biological and social factors.[2]

Influence of Family

Research suggests that family conditioning, structure, and patterns of interaction can influence the development of an eating disorder. Based on observational studies, compared to families without a member with an eating disorder, families with an anorexic member show more rigidity in their family structure and less clear interpersonal boundaries, and they tend to avoid open discussions on topics of disagreement. Conversely, families with a member diagnosed with bulimia nervosa tend to have a less stable family organization and to be less nurturing, more angry, and more disruptive.[3] In addition, childhood physical or sexual abuse can increase the risk for an eating disorder.[4]

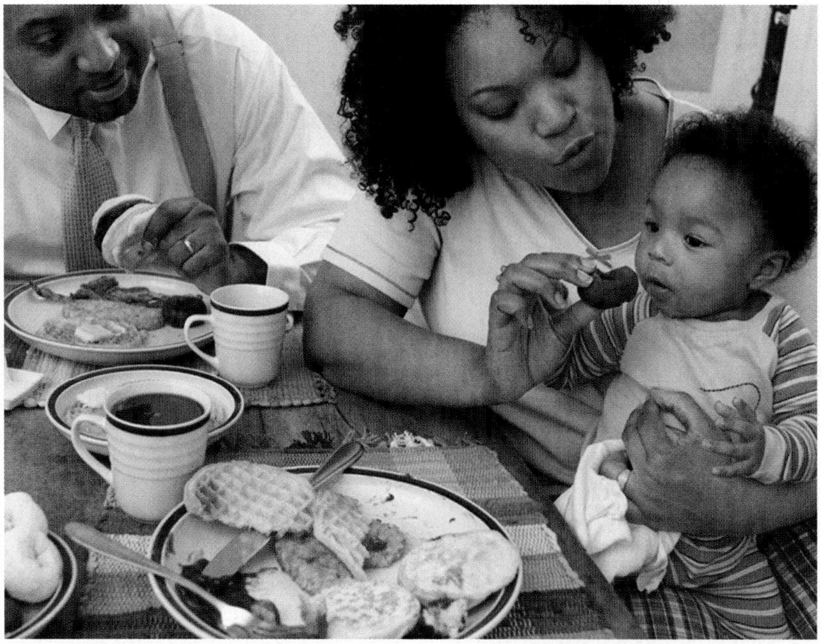

Family environment often influences when, what, and how much we eat.

Influence of Media

As media saturation has increased over the last century, so has the incidence of eating disorders among white women.[5] Every day, we are confronted with advertisements in which computer-enhanced images of lean, beautiful women promote everything from beer to cars **(Figure 2)**. Most adult men and women understand that these images are unrealistic, but adolescents, who are still developing a sense of their identity and body image, lack the same ability to distance themselves from what they see.[6] Because body image influences eating behaviors, it is not unlikely that the barrage of media models may be contributing to the increase in eating disorders. However, scientific evidence demonstrating that the media are *causing* increased eating disorders is difficult to obtain.

Influence of Social and Cultural Values

Eating disorders are significantly more common in white females in developed Western societies than in other women worldwide.[2] This may be due in part to the white Western culture's association of slenderness with health, wealth, and high fashion **(Figure 3)**. In contrast, until recently,

FOOD IS NOT AN ISSUE	CONCERNED/WELL	FOOD PREOCCUPIED/ OBSESSED	DISRUPTIVE EATING PATTERNS	EATING DISORDERED
• I am not concerned about what others think regarding what and how much I eat. • When I am upset or depressed I eat whatever I am hungry for without any guilt or shame. • I feel no guilt or shame no matter how much I eat or what I eat. • Food is an important part of my life but only occupies a small part of my time. • I trust my body to tell me what and how much to eat.	• I pay attention to what I eat in order to maintain a healthy body. • I may weigh more than what I like, but I enjoy eating and balance my pleasure with eating with my concern for a healthy body. • I am moderate and flexible in goals for eating well. • I try to follow Dietary Guidelines for healthy eating.	• I think about food a lot. • I feel I don't eat well most of the time. • It's hard for me to enjoy eating with others. • I feel ashamed when I eat more than others or more than what I feel I should be eating. • I am afraid of getting fat. • I wish I could change how much I want to eat and what I am hungry for.	• I have tried diet pills, laxatives, vomiting, or extra time exercising in order to lose or maintain my weight. • I have fasted or avoided eating for long periods of time in order to lose or maintain my weight. • I feel strong when I can restrict how much I eat. • Eating more than I wanted to makes me feel out of control.	• I regularly stuff myself and then exercise, vomit, or use diet pills or laxatives to get rid of the food or Calories. • My friends/family tell me I am too thin. • I am terrified of eating fat. • When I let myself eat, I have a hard time controlling the amount of food I eat. • I am afraid to eat in front of others.

BODY OWNERSHIP	BODY ACCEPTANCE	BODY PREOCCUPIED/ OBSESSED	DISTORTED BODY IMAGE	BODY HATE/ DISASSOCIATION
• Body image is not an issue for me. • My body is beautiful to me. • My feelings about my body are not influenced by society's concept of an ideal body shape. • I know that the significant others in my life will always find me attractive. • I trust my body to find the weight it needs to be at so I can move and feel confident about my physical body.	• I base my body image equally on social norms and my own self-concept. • I pay attention to my body and my appearance because it is important to me, but it only occupies a small part of my day. • I nourish my body so it has the strength and energy to achieve my physical goals. • I am able to assert myself and maintain a healthy body without losing my self-esteem.	• I spend a significant amount time viewing my body in the mirror. • I spend a significant amount time comparing my body to others. • I have days when I feel fat. • I am preoccupied with my body. • I accept society's ideal body shape and size as the best body shape and size. • I believe that I'd be more attractive if I were thinner, more muscular, etc.	• I spend a significant amount of time exercising and dieting to change my body. • My body shape and size keep me from dating or finding someone who will treat me the way I want to be treated. • I have considered changing or have changed my body shape and size through surgical means so I can accept myself. • I wish I could change the way I look in the mirror.	• I often feel separated and distant from my body—as if it belongs to someone else. • I hate my body and I often isolate myself from others. • I don't see anything positive or even neutral about my body shape and size. • I don't believe others when they tell me I look OK. • I hate the way I look in the mirror.

Figure 1 The Eating Issues and Body Image Continuum. The progression from normal eating (far left) to eating disorders (far right) occurs on a continuum.

Data from Smiley, L., L. King, and H. Avery. University of Arizona Campus Health Service. Original Continuum, C. Shlaalak. Preventive Medicine and Public Health.

the prevailing view in developing societies has been that excess body fat is desirable as a sign of health and material abundance.

The members of society with whom we most often interact—our family members, friends, classmates, and co-workers—also influence the way we see ourselves. Their comments related to our body weight or shape can be particularly hurtful—enough so to cause some people to start down the path of disordered eating. For example, individuals with bulimia nervosa report that they perceived greater pressure from their peers to be thin than controls, while research shows that peer teasing about weight increases body dissatisfaction and eating disturbances.[7] Thus, our comments to others regarding their weight do count.

Influence of Personality

A number of studies suggest that people with anorexia nervosa exhibit increased rates of obsessive-compulsive behaviors and perfectionism. They also tend to be socially inhibited, compliant, and emotionally restrained.[8] Unfortunately, many studies observe these behaviors only in individuals who are very ill and in a state of starvation, which may affect personality. Thus, it is difficult to determine if personality is a contributing factor or an effect of the disorder.

In contrast to people with anorexia nervosa, people with bulimia nervosa tend to be more impulsive, have low self-esteem, and demonstrate an extroverted, erratic personality style that

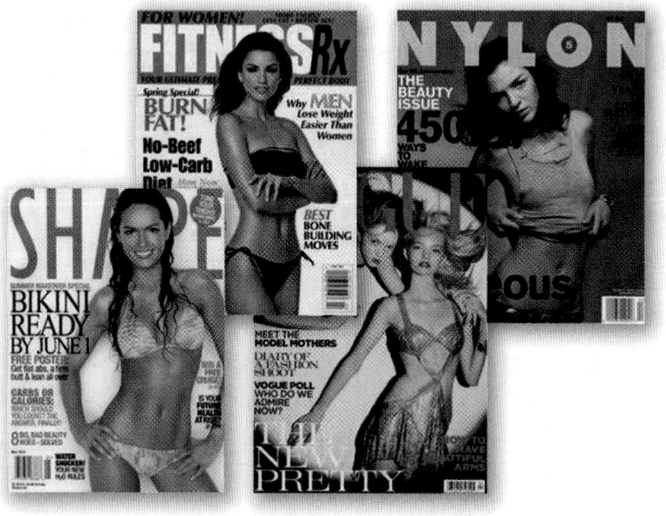

Figure 2 Photos of celebrities and models are often airbrushed or otherwise altered to "enhance" physical appearance. Unfortunately, many people regard these as accurate portrayals and strive to reach an unrealistic level of physical beauty.

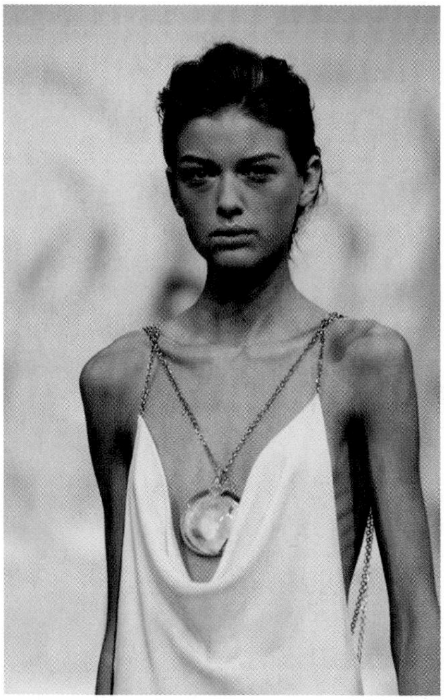

Figure 3 The preferred look among runway models can require extreme emaciation, often achieved by self-starvation and/or drug abuse.

seeks attention and admiration. In these people, negative moods are more likely to cause overeating than food restriction.[8]

Anorexia Nervosa Is a Potentially Deadly Eating Disorder

According to the American Psychiatric Association, 90–95% of individuals with anorexia nervosa are young girls or women.[1] Approximately 0.5–1% of American women develop anorexia, and between 5% and 20% will die from complications of the disorder within 10 years of the initial diagnosis.[4] These statistics make anorexia nervosa the most common and deadly psychiatric disorder diagnosed in women and the leading cause of death in females between the ages of 15 and 24 years.[4] As the statistics indicate, anorexia nervosa also occurs in males, but the prevalence is much lower than in females.[2,9]

Signs and Symptoms of Anorexia Nervosa

The classic sign of anorexia nervosa is an extremely restrictive eating pattern that leads to self-starvation (**Figure 4**). These individuals may fast completely, restrict energy intake to only a few kilocalories per day, or eliminate all but one or two food groups from their diet. They also have an intense fear of weight gain, and even small amounts (such as 1–2 lb) trigger high stress and anxiety.

In females, **amenorrhea** (no menstrual periods for at least 3 months) is a common feature of anorexia nervosa. It occurs when a young woman consumes insufficient energy to maintain normal body functions.

The American Psychiatric Association identifies the following conditions of anorexia nervosa:[10]

- Refusal to maintain body weight at or above a minimally normal weight for age and height
- Intense fear of gaining weight or becoming fat, even though considered underweight by all medical criteria

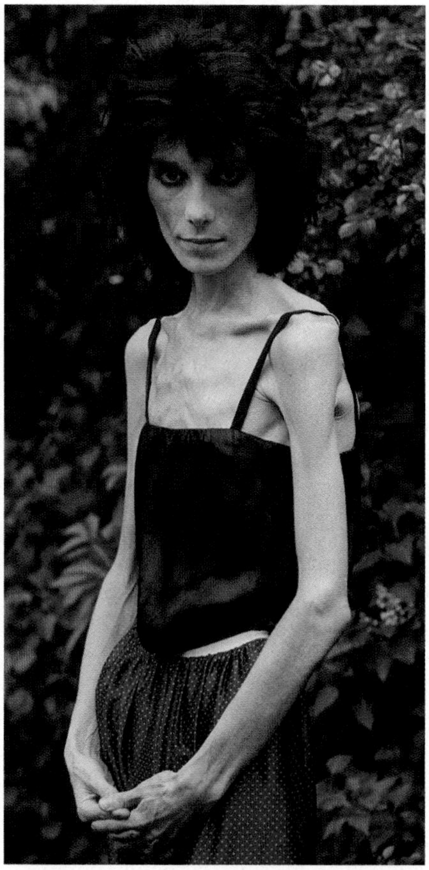

Figure 4 People with *anorexia nervosa* experience an extreme drive for thinness, resulting in potentially fatal weight loss.

---

amenorrhea The absence of menstruation. In females who had previously been menstruating, it is defined as the absence of menstrual periods for 3 or more months.

HOT TOPIC

Muscle Dysmorphia: The Male Eating Disorder?

Is there an eating disorder unique to men? Recently, experts have defined a disorder called muscle dysmorphia. Men with muscle dysmorphia perceive themselves as small and frail, even though they may actually be large and muscular. They spend long hours lifting weights, but no matter how "chiseled" they become, their biology cannot match their idealized body size and shape.[12]

A common behavior of men with muscle dysmorphia is abuse of performance-enhancing drugs. Additionally, men with muscle dysmorphia tend to consume excessive amounts of high-protein foods and dietary supplements, such as protein powders.

Men with muscle dysmorphia share some characteristics with men and women with other eating disorders. For instance, they report "feeling fat" and express significant discomfort with the idea of exposing their bodies to others. They also have increased rates of mental illness.[13]

Outward indications that someone is struggling with muscle dysmorphia include:

- Rigid and excessive weight training
- Strict adherence to a high-protein, muscle-enhancing diet
- Use of muscle-enhancing drugs or supplements
- Avoiding social engagements that might interfere with following a strict diet or training schedule
- Frequent and critical body self-evaluation

Muscle dysmorphia can cause distress and despair. Therapy can help.

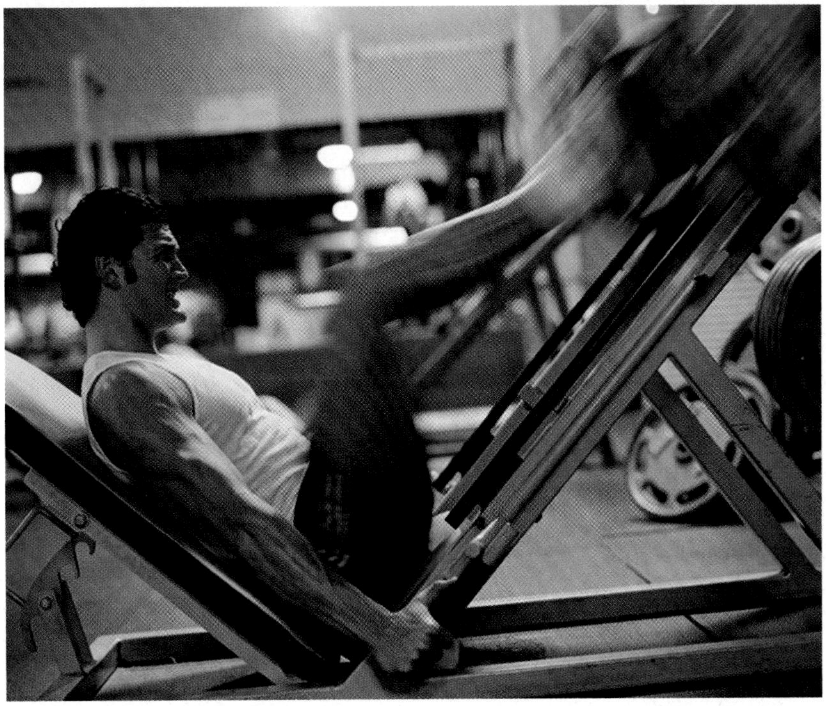

Men are more likely than women to exercise excessively in an effort to control their weight.

- Disturbance in the way in which one's body weight or shape is experienced, undue influence of body weight or shape on self-evaluation, or denial of the seriousness of the current low body weight
- Amenorrhea in females who are past puberty; a woman is considered to have amenorrhea if her periods occur only when given hormones, such as estrogen or oral contraceptives

The signs of an eating disorder, such as anorexia nervosa, may be somewhat different in males. Females with eating disorders say they *feel* fat even though they typically are normal weight or even underweight before they develop the disorder. In contrast, males who develop eating disorders are more likely to have actually *been* overweight or even obese.[9,11] Thus, the male's fear of "getting fat again" is based on reality. In addition, males with disordered eating are less concerned with actual body weight (scale weight) than females but are more concerned with body composition (percentage of muscle mass compared to fat mass).

The methods that men and women use to achieve weight loss also appear to differ. Males are more likely to use excessive exercise as a means of weight control, whereas females tend to use severe energy restriction, vomiting, and laxative abuse. These weight-control differences may stem from sociocultural biases; that is, dieting is considered to be more acceptable for women, whereas the overwhelming sociocultural belief is that "real men don't diet."[11]

Health Risks of Anorexia Nervosa

Left untreated, anorexia nervosa eventually leads to a deficiency in energy and other nutrients that are required by the body to function normally. The body will then use stored fat and lean tissue (such as organ and muscle tissue) as an energy source to maintain brain tissue and vital body functions. The body will also shut down or reduce nonvital body functions to conserve energy. Electrolyte imbalances can lead to heart failure and death. **Figure 5** highlights many of the health problems that occur in people with anorexia nervosa. The best chance of recovery is when an individual receives intensive treatment early.

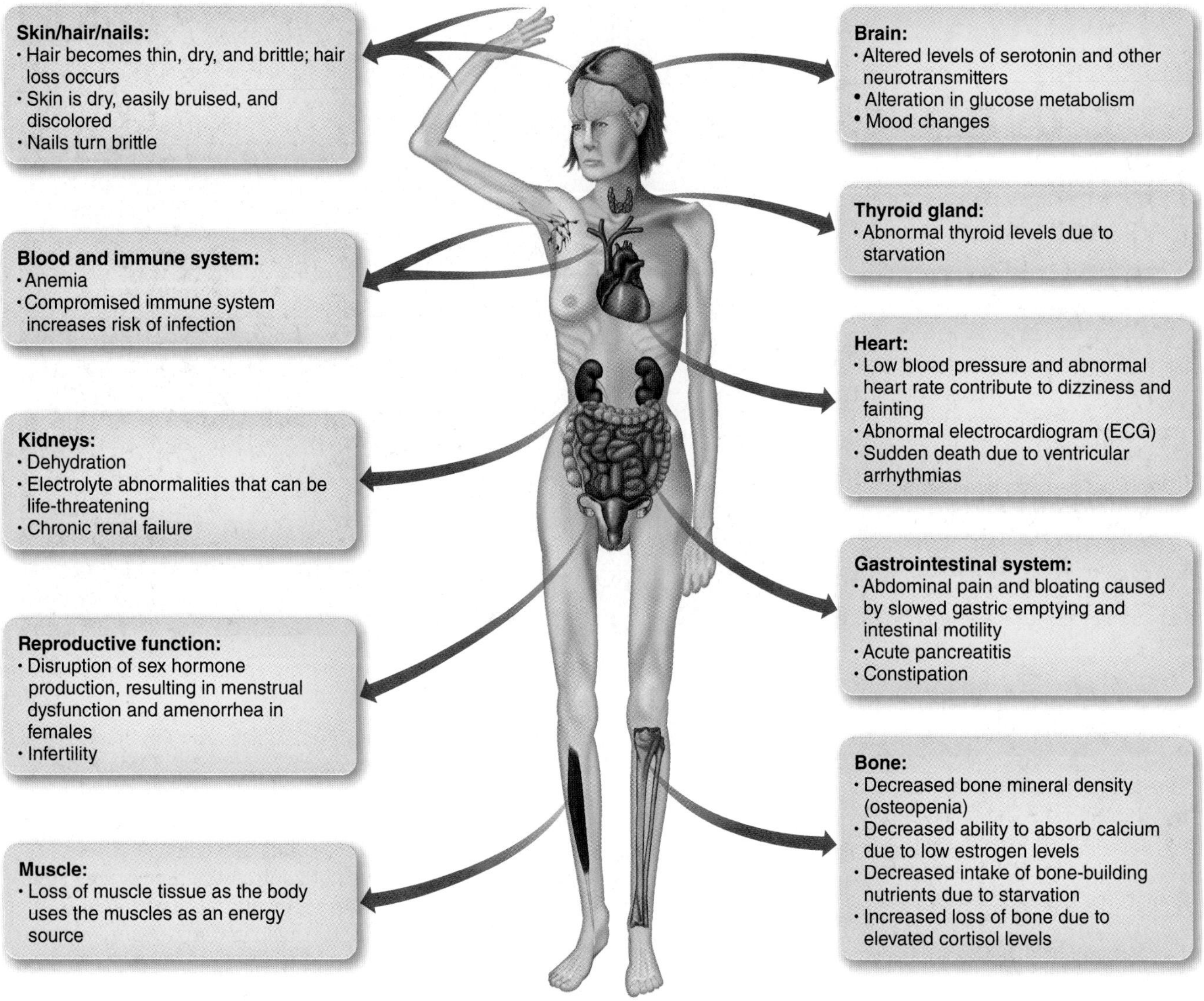
Skin/hair/nails:
• Hair becomes thin, dry, and brittle; hair loss occurs
• Skin is dry, easily bruised, and discolored
• Nails turn brittle
Blood and immune system:
• Anemia
• Compromised immune system increases risk of infection
Kidneys:
• Dehydration
• Electrolyte abnormalities that can be life-threatening
• Chronic renal failure
Reproductive function:
• Disruption of sex hormone production, resulting in menstrual dysfunction and amenorrhea in females
• Infertility
Muscle:
• Loss of muscle tissue as the body uses the muscles as an energy source
Brain:
• Altered levels of serotonin and other neurotransmitters
• Alteration in glucose metabolism
• Mood changes
Thyroid gland:
• Abnormal thyroid levels due to starvation
Heart:
• Low blood pressure and abnormal heart rate contribute to dizziness and fainting
• Abnormal electrocardiogram (ECG)
• Sudden death due to ventricular arrhythmias
Gastrointestinal system:
• Abdominal pain and bloating caused by slowed gastric emptying and intestinal motility
• Acute pancreatitis
• Constipation
Bone:
• Decreased bone mineral density (osteopenia)
• Decreased ability to absorb calcium due to low estrogen levels
• Decreased intake of bone-building nutrients due to starvation
• Increased loss of bone due to elevated cortisol levels

Figure 5 The impact of *anorexia nervosa* on the body.

Bulimia Nervosa Is Characterized by Bingeing and Purging

Bulimia nervosa is an eating disorder characterized by repeated episodes of **binge eating** followed by some form of **purging.** While binge eating, the person feels a loss of self-control, including an inability to end the binge once it has started.[14] At the same time, the person feels a sense of euphoria not unlike a drug-induced high. A "binge" is usually defined as a quantity of food that is large for the person and for the amount of time in which it is eaten **(Figure 6)**. For example, a person may eat a dozen brownies with 2 quarts of ice cream in 30 minutes.

The prevalence of bulimia nervosa is higher than that of anorexia nervosa and is estimated to affect 1–4% of women. Like anorexia nervosa, bulimia nervosa is found predominately in women: six to ten females are diagnosed for every one male. The mortality rate is lower than for anorexia nervosa, with 1% of patients dying within 10 years of diagnosis.[4]

Although the prevalence of bulimia nervosa is much higher in women, rates for men are significant in some predominantly "thin-build" sports in which participants are encouraged to maintain a low body weight (for instance, horse racing, wrestling, crew, and gymnastics). Individuals in these sports typically do not have all the characteristics of bulimia nervosa, however, and the purging behaviors they practice usually stop once the sport is discontinued.

An individual with bulimia nervosa typically purges after most episodes, but not necessarily on every occasion, and weight gain as a

---

binge eating Consumption of a large amount of food in a short period of time, usually accompanied by a feeling of loss of self-control.

purging An attempt to rid the body of unwanted food by vomiting or other compensatory means, such as excessive exercise, fasting, or laxative abuse.

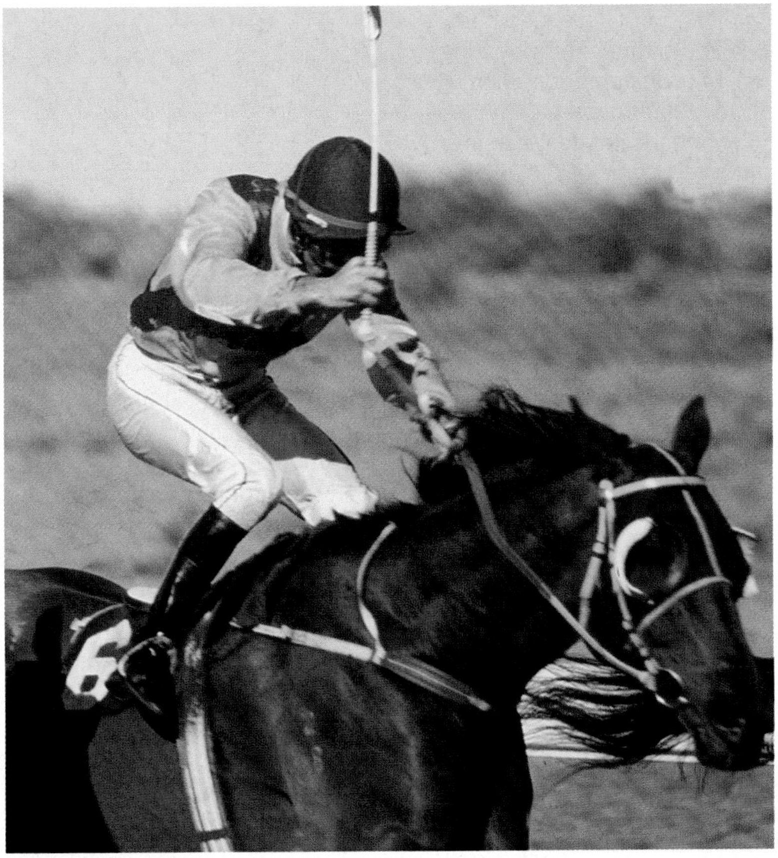

Men who participate in "thin-build" sports, such as jockeys, have a higher risk for *bulimia nervosa* than men who do not.

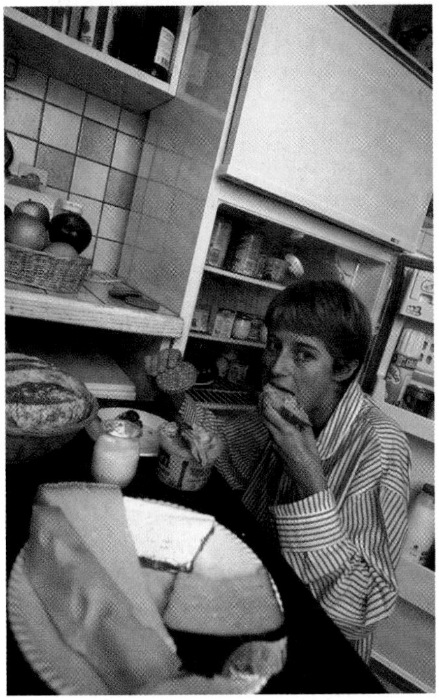

Figure 6 People with *bulimia nervosa* can consume relatively large amounts of food in brief periods of time.

result of binge eating can be significant. Methods of purging include vomiting, laxative or diuretic abuse, enemas, fasting, or excessive exercise. For example, after a binge, a runner may increase her daily mileage to equal the "calculated" energy content of the binge.

Symptoms of Bulimia Nervosa

As with anorexia nervosa, the American Psychiatric Association has identified conditions of bulimia nervosa:[10]

- Recurrent episodes of binge eating, such as eating a large amount of food within a short period of time (about 2 hours).
- Recurrent inappropriate compensatory behavior in order to prevent weight gain, such as self-induced vomiting; misuse of laxatives, diuretics, enemas, or other medications; fasting; or excessive exercise.
- Binge eating occuring on average at least twice a week for 3 months.
- Body shape and weight unduly influencing self-evaluation.
- The disturbance not necessarily occuring exclusively during episodes of anorexia nervosa. Some individuals will have periods of binge eating and then periods of starvation, which makes classification of their disorder difficult.

How can you tell if someone has bulimia nervosa? In addition to the recurrent and frequent binge eating and purging episodes, the National Institutes of Health have identified the following symptoms of bulimia nervosa:

- chronically inflamed and sore throat
- swollen glands in the neck and below the jaw
- worn tooth enamel and increasingly sensitive and decaying teeth as a result of exposure to stomach acids
- gastroesophageal reflux disorder
- intestinal distress and irritation from laxative abuse
- kidney problems from diuretic abuse
- severe dehydration from purging of fluids

Health Risks of Bulimia Nervosa

The destructive behaviors of bulimia nervosa can lead to illness and even death. The most common health consequences associated with bulimia nervosa are the following:

- Electrolyte imbalance typically caused by dehydration and the loss of potassium and sodium from the body from frequent vomiting. This can lead to irregular heartbeat and even heart failure and death.
- Gastrointestinal problems: inflammation, ulceration, and possible rupture of the esophagus and stomach from frequent bingeing and vomiting. Chronic irregular bowel movements and

constipation may result in people with bulimia who chronically abuse laxatives.
- Dental problems: tooth decay and staining from stomach acids released during frequent vomiting

As with anorexia nervosa, the chance of recovery from bulimia nervosa increases, and the negative effects on health decrease, if the disorder is detected and treated at an early stage. Familiarity with the warning signs of bulimia nervosa can help you identify friends and family members who might be at risk.

Binge-Eating Disorder Can Cause Significant Weight Gain

When was the last time a friend or relative confessed to you about "going on an eating binge"? Most likely, the person explained that the behavior followed some sort of stressful event, such as a problem at work, the breakup of a relationship, or a poor grade on an exam. Many people have one or two binge episodes every year or so, in response to stress. But in people with **binge-eating disorder,** the behavior occurs an average of twice a week or more and is not usually followed by purging. This lack of compensation for the binge distinguishes binge-eating disorder from bulimia nervosa and explains why the person tends to gain a lot of weight.

The prevalence of binge-eating disorder is estimated to be 2–3% of the adult population and 8% of the obese population.[15] In contrast to anorexia and bulimia, binge-eating disorder is also common in men. Our current food environment, which offers an abundance of good-tasting, cheap food any time of the day, makes it difficult for people with binge-eating disorder to avoid food triggers.

As you would expect, the increased energy intake associated with binge eating significantly increases a person's risk of being overweight or obese. In addition, the types of foods individuals typically consume during a binge episode are high in fat and sugar, which can increase blood lipids. Finally, the stress associated with binge eating can have psychological consequences, such as low self-esteem, avoidance of social contact, depression, and negative thoughts related to body size.

Night-Eating Syndrome Can Lead to Obesity

Night-eating syndrome was first described in a group of patients who were not hungry in the morning but spent the evening and night eating and reported insomnia. Like binge-eating disorder, it is associated with obesity because, although night eaters don't binge, they do consume significant energy in their frequent snacks, and they don't compensate for the excess energy intake.

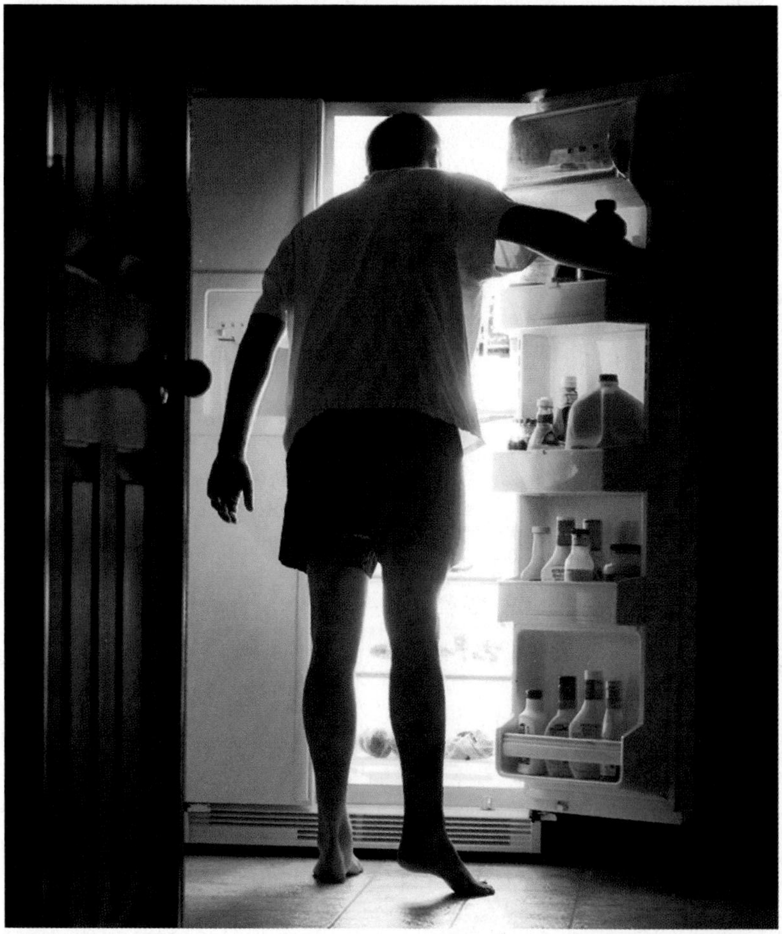

People with night-eating syndrome consume most of their daily energy between 8 PM and 6 AM.

binge-eating disorder A disorder characterized by binge eating an average of twice a week or more, typically without compensatory purging.

night-eating syndrome A disorder characterized by intake of the majority of the day's energy between 8:00 PM and 6:00 AM. Individuals with this disorder also experience mood and sleep disorders.

Symptoms of Night-Eating Syndrome

The distinguishing characteristic of night-eating syndrome is the time during which most of the day's energy intake occurs. Night eaters eat relatively little during the day, consuming the majority of their energy between 8:00 PM and 6:00 AM. They even get up in the night to eat. Night eating is also characterized by a depressed mood and insomnia. In short, night eaters appear to have a unique combination of three disorders: an eating disorder, a sleep disorder, and a mood disorder.[16]

Health Risks of Night-Eating Syndrome

Night-eating syndrome is important clinically because of its association with obesity, which increases the risk for several chronic diseases, including heart disease, high blood pressure, stroke, type 2 diabetes, and arthritis. Obesity also increases the risk for sleep apnea, which can further disrupt the night eater's already abnormal sleeping pattern.

The Female Athlete Triad Consists of Three Disorders

The **female athlete triad** is a serious syndrome that consists of three clinical conditions in some physically active females: (1) low energy availability (such as inadequate energy intake to maintain menstrual function or to cover energy expended in exercise) (with or without eating disorders), (2) amenorrhea (the absence of menstruation), and (3) osteoporosis[17] **(Figure 7)**.Certain sports that strongly emphasize leanness or a thin body build may place a young girl or a woman at risk for the female athlete triad. These sports typically include figure skating, gymnastics, and diving; classical ballet dancers are also at increased risk for the disorder.

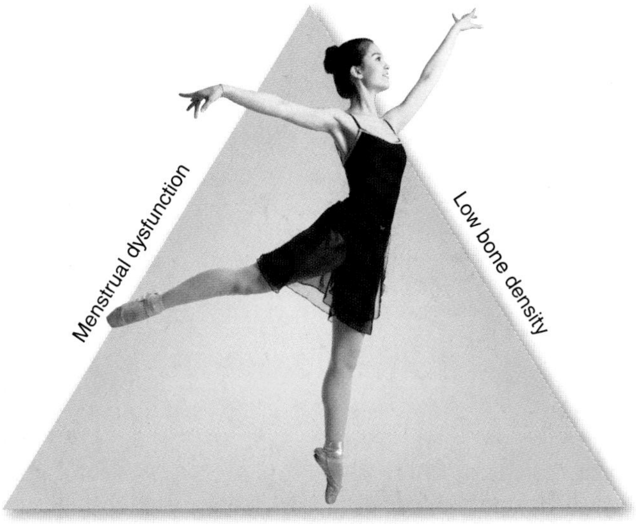
Menstrual dysfunction
Low bone density
Low energy availability

Figure 7 The female athlete triad is a syndrome composed of three coexisting disorders: low energy availability (with or without eating disorders), menstrual dysfunction (such as amenorrhea), and osteoporosis. Energy availability is defined as dietary energy intake minus exercise energy expenditure.

Components of the Female Athlete Triad

Active women experience the general social and cultural demands placed on women to be thin, as well as pressure from their coach, teammates, judges, and/or spectators to meet weight standards or body-size expectations for their sport. Failure to meet these standards can result in severe consequences, such as being cut from the team, losing an athletic scholarship, or decreased participation with the team.

As the pressure to be thin mounts, active women may restrict their energy intake, typically by engaging in disordered eating behaviors. Energy restriction combined with high levels of physical activity can disrupt the menstrual cycle and result in amenorrhea. Menstrual dysfunction can also occur in active women who are not dieting and don't have an eating disorder. These women are simply not eating enough to cover the energy costs of their exercise training and all the other energy demands of the body and daily living. Female athletes with menstrual dysfunction, regardless of the cause, typically have reduced levels of the reproductive hormones, such as estrogen and progesterone. When estrogen levels in the body are low, it is difficult for bone to retain calcium, and gradual loss of bone mass occurs. Thus, many female athletes develop premature bone loss (osteoporosis) and are at increased risk for fractures.

female athlete triad A serious syndrome that consists of three clinical conditions in some physically active females: low energy availability (with or without eating disorders), amenorrhea, and osteoporosis.

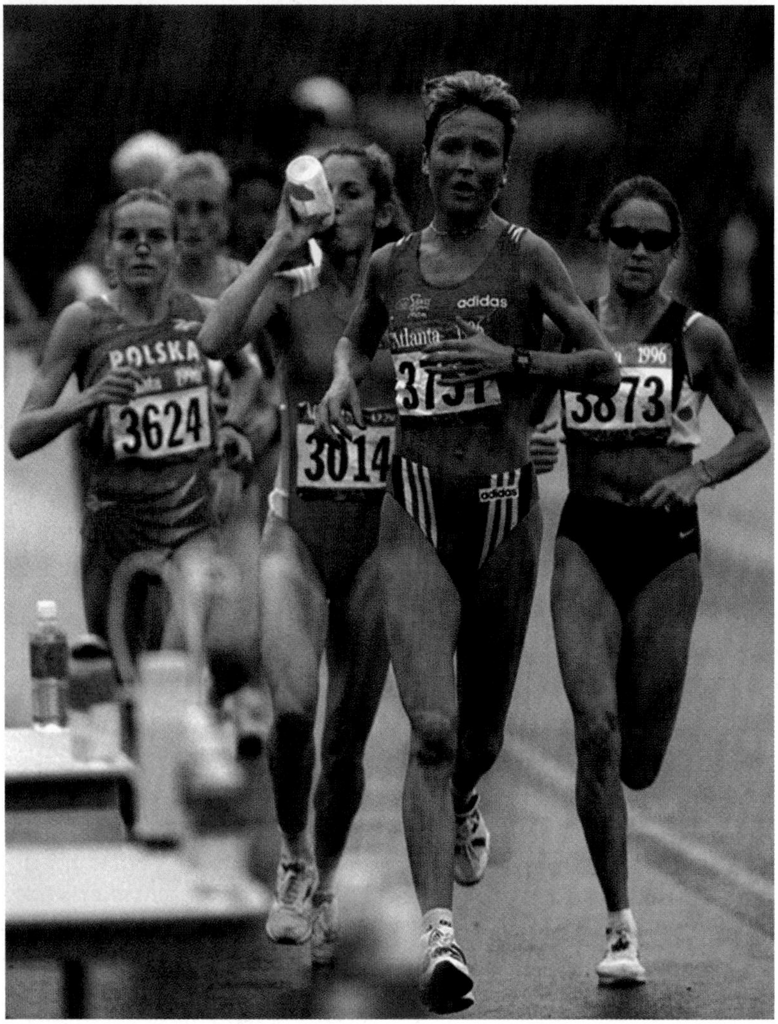

Sports that emphasize leanness, or that require athletes to wear body-contouring clothing, increase the risk for female athlete triad.

Recognizing and Treating the Female Athlete Triad

Recognition of an athlete with one or more of the components of the female athlete triad can be difficult, especially if the athlete is reluctant to be honest when questioned about the symptoms. For this reason, familiarity with the early warning signs is critical. These include excessive dieting and/or weight loss, excessive exercise, stress fractures, and self-esteem that appears to be dictated by body weight and shape.

Treating an athlete requires a multidisciplinary approach. This means that the sports medicine team, sports dietitian, exercise physiologist, psychologist, coach, trainer, parents, friends of the athlete, and athlete all must work together.

Treatment for Disordered Eating Requires a Multidisciplinary Approach

As with any health problem, prevention is the best treatment for disordered eating. People having trouble with eating and body image issues need help to deal with these issues before they develop into something more serious.

Treating anyone with disordered eating requires a multidisciplinary approach, which typically includes the physician and psychologist, a nutritionist, and family members. The severity of the eating disorder will dictate the treatment. Patients who are severely underweight, display signs of malnutrition, are medically unstable, or are suicidal may require immediate hospitalization. Conversely, patients who are underweight but are still medically stable may enter an outpatient program designed to meet their specific needs.

Do you have a friend you suspect has an eating disorder? Discussing a friend's eating behaviors can be difficult. It is important to choose an appropriate time and place to raise your concerns and to listen closely and with great sensitivity to your friend's feelings. It is also important to locate a health professional specializing in eating disorders whom you can recommend. If you are at a university or college, check with the student health center to see what resources it has. Finally, the National Eating Disorders Association provides a list of steps to consider before talking to your friend about his or her eating disorder.[18] You can find it under Information and Resources at its website listed in Web Resources.

NUTRI-CASE LIZ

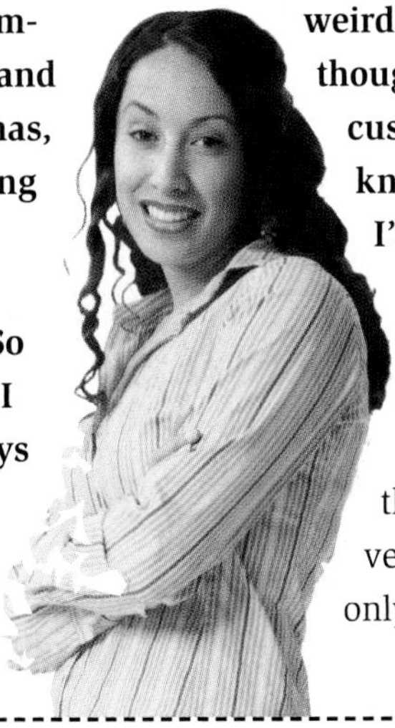

"I used to dance with a really cool modern company, where everybody looked sort of healthy and 'real.' No waifs! When they folded after Christmas, I was disappointed, but this spring, I'm planning to audition for the City Ballet. My best friend dances with them, and she told me that they won't even look at anybody over 100 pounds. So I've just put myself on a strict diet. Most days, I come in under 1,200 Calories, though some days I cheat and then I feel so out of control. Last week, my dance teacher stopped me after class and asked me whether or not I was menstruating. I thought that was a pretty weird question, so I just said sure, but when I thought about it, I realized that I've been so focused and stressed out lately that I really don't know! The audition is only a week away, so I'm going on a juice fast this weekend. I've just got to make it into the City Ballet!"

What factors increase Liz's risk for the female athlete triad? What, if anything, do you think Liz's dance teacher should do? Is intervention even necessary, since the audition is only a week away?

Web Resources

www.harriscentermgh.org
Harris Center, Massachusetts General Hospital

This site provides information about current eating disorder research, as well as sections on understanding eating disorders and resources for those with eating disorders.

www.nimh.nih.gov
National Institute of Mental Health (NIMH) Office of Communications and Public Liaison

Search this site for "disordered eating" or "eating disorders" to find numerous articles on the subject.

www.anad.org
National Association of Anorexia Nervosa and Associated Disorders

Visit this site for information and resources about eating disorders.

www.nationaleatingdisorders.org
National Eating Disorders Association

This site is dedicated to expanding public understanding of eating disorders and promoting access to treatment for those affected and support for their families.

13 Food Safety and Technology: Impact on Consumers

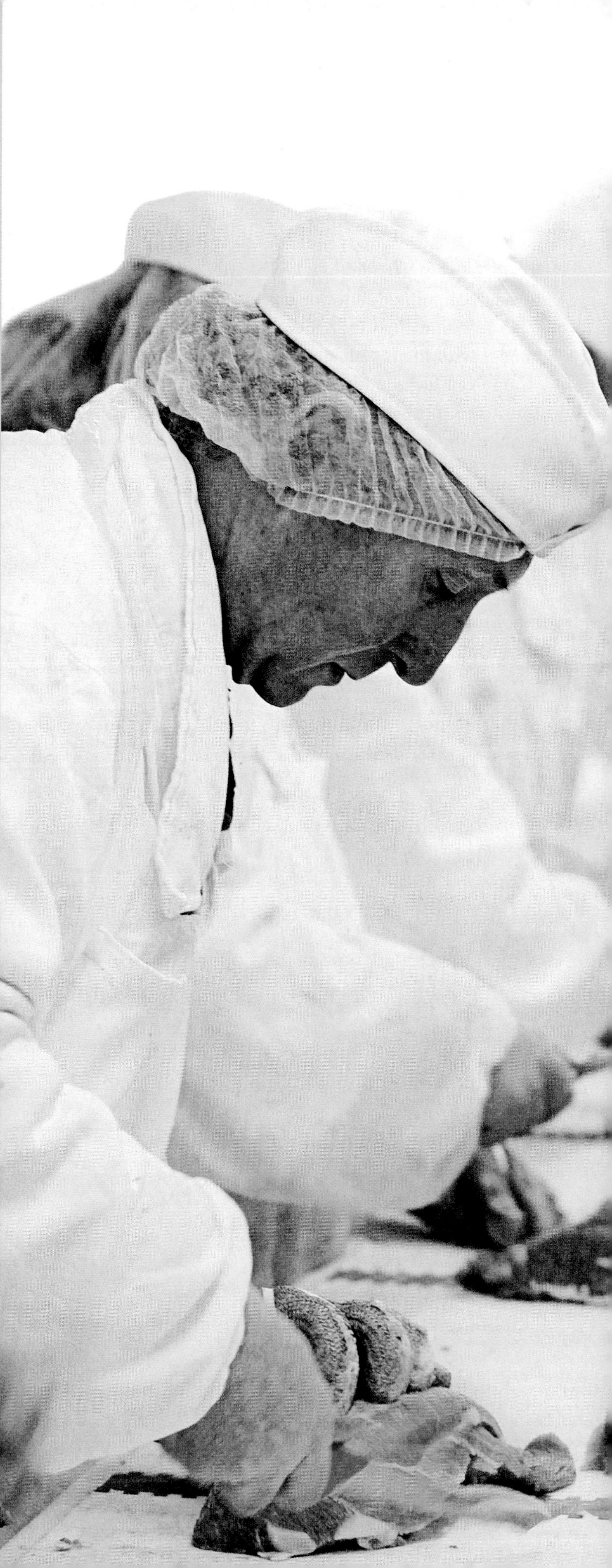

CHAPTER OBJECTIVES

After reading this chapter you will be able to:

1. **Identify the types of contaminants involved in food-borne illness, pp. 457–461.**
2. **Describe strategies for preventing food-borne illness at home, while eating out, and when traveling to other countries, pp. 465–472.**
3. **Discuss the advantages of newer food-preservation methods, such as innovative packaging techniques and irradiation, over traditional methods used to preserve foods, pp. 473–476.**
4. **Debate the safety of food additives, including the role of the GRAS list, pp. 476–478.**
5. **Describe the process of genetic modification and discuss its potential risks and benefits pp. 479–480.**
6. **Describe the process by which persistent organic pollutants accumulate in foods, pp. 480–482.**
7. **Discuss the benefits and safety concerns related to pesticides, pp. 482–484.**
8. **Explain the current system of labeling for organic foods, p. 485.**

nightmares or hallucinations, but the illness is rarely fatal and typically resolves within a few weeks.[20]

Potatoes that have turned green contain the toxin solanine, which forms during the greening process. The green color is actually due to chlorophyll, a harmless pigment that forms when the potatoes are exposed to light. Although the production of solanine occurs simultaneously with the production of chlorophyll, the two processes are separate and unrelated.[21] Although there is a potential for toxicity from consuming potatoes with a very high solanine content, because solanine formation occurs near the potato's skin, the green areas can be cut away to remove any toxins. A good guide is to taste a small piece of the potato after the green areas have been removed. If the potato tastes bitter, then throw it away. If you're in doubt, or if you're serving the potato to someone with allergies or compromised immunity, you should discard the potato. You can avoid the greening of potatoes by storing them for only short periods in a dark cupboard or brown paper bag in a cool area. Wash the potato to expose its color, and cut away and discard any green areas. Cooked potatoes cannot turn green or produce solanine, but cooking green potatoes does not remove the chlorophyll or solanine that is formed prior to cooking.

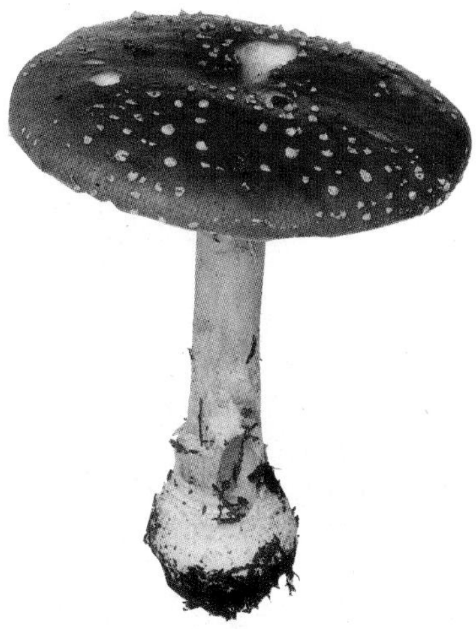

Figure 13.5 Some mushrooms, such as this fly agaric, contain toxins that can cause illness or even death.

The Body Responds to Contaminated Foods with Acute Illness

Many food-borne microbes are killed in the mouth by antimicrobial enzymes in saliva or in the stomach by hydrochloric acid. Any microbe that survives these chemical assaults will usually trigger vomiting and/or diarrhea as the gastrointestinal tract attempts to expel the offender. Simultaneously, the white blood cells of the immune system will be activated, and a generalized inflammatory response will cause the person to experience nausea, fatigue, fever, and muscle cramps. Depending on the state of one's health, the precise microbe involved, and the number of microbes ingested, the symptoms can range from mild to severe, including double vision, loss of muscle control, and excessive or bloody diarrhea. As noted earlier, some cases, if left untreated, can result in death.

To diagnose a food-borne illness, a specimen must be obtained and cultured. This means the specimen is analyzed in a laboratory setting in which the offending microorganisms are grown in a specific chemical medium. Stool (fecal) cultures are usually analyzed, especially if diarrhea is a symptom. Blood is cultured if the patient has a high fever. Treatment usually involves keeping the person hydrated and comfortable, as most food-borne illness tends to be self-limiting; the person's vomiting and/or diarrhea, although unpleasant, rid the body of the offending agent. In treating botulism, the patient's intestinal tract is flushed repeatedly to remove the microorganisms, and antibodies are injected to neutralize its deadly toxin.

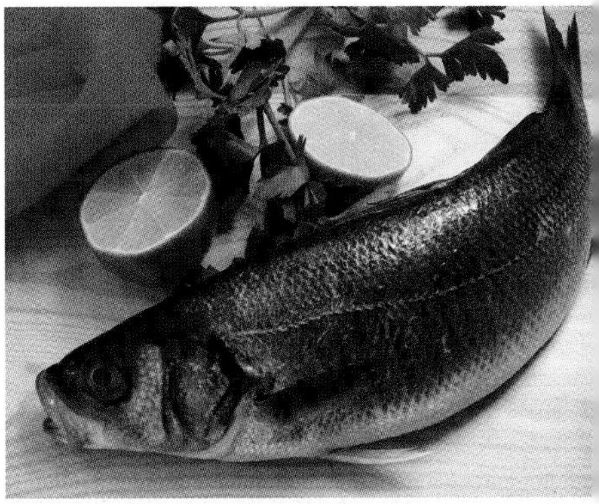

Sea bass may look appealing, but like several other large, predatory tropical fish, can be contaminated with a high concentration of marine toxins.

In the United States, all confirmed cases of food-borne illness must be reported to the state health department, which in turn reports these illnesses to the CDC in Atlanta, Georgia. The CDC monitors its reports for indications of epidemics of food-borne illness and assists local and state agencies in controlling such outbreaks.

Certain Conditions Help Microorganisms Multiply in Foods

Given the correct environmental conditions, microorganisms can thrive in many types of food. Four factors affect the survival and reproduction of food microorganisms:

- *Temperature.* Many microorganisms capable of causing human illness thrive at warm temperatures, from about 40°F to 140°F (4°C to 60°C). You can think of this range of temperatures as the **danger zone.** These microorganisms can be destroyed by thoroughly heating or cooking foods, and their reproduction can be slowed by refrigeration and freezing. We'll identify safe cooking and food-storage temperatures later in this chapter.

danger zone The range of temperature at which many microorganisms capable of causing human illness thrive; about 40°F to 140°F (4°C to 60°C).

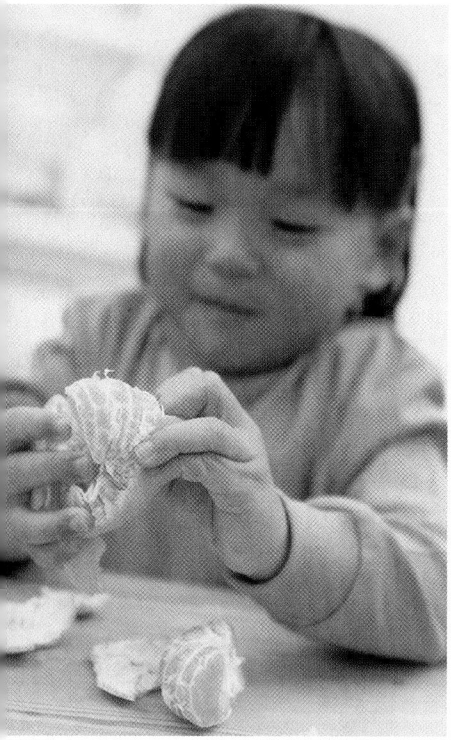

Peels protect foods against contamination; however, you should still wash fruit before peeling.

- *Humidity.* Many microorganisms require a high level of moisture; thus, foods such as boxed dried pasta do not make suitable microbial homes, although cooked pasta left at room temperature would prove hospitable.
- *Acidity.* Most microorganisms have a preferred range of acidity, or pH, in which they thrive. For instance, *Clostridium botulinum* thrives in alkaline environments. It cannot grow or produce its toxin in acidic environments, so the risk for botulism is decreased in citrus fruits, pickles, and tomato-based foods. In contrast, alkaline foods, such as fish and low-acid vegetables, are a magnet for *C. botulinum.*
- *Oxygen content.* Many microorganisms require oxygen to function; thus, food-preservation techniques that remove oxygen, such as industrial canning and bottling, keep foods safe for consumption. Because *C. botulinum* thrives in an oxygen-free environment, the canning process heats foods to an extremely high temperature to destroy this organism.

In addition, microorganisms need an entryway into a food. Just as our skin protects our body from microbial invasion, the peels, rinds, and shells of many foods seal off access to the nutrients within. Eggshells are a good example of a natural food barrier. Once such a barrier is removed, however, the food loses its primary defense against contamination.

RECAP **Food infections result from the consumption of food containing living microorganisms, such as bacteria, whereas food intoxications result from consuming food in which microbes have secreted toxins. Some foods develop toxins independently of microbes. The body has several defense mechanisms, such as saliva, stomach acid, vomiting, diarrhea, and the inflammatory response, which help rid us of offending microorganisms or their toxins. In order to reproduce in foods, microbes require a precise range of temperature, humidity, acidity, and oxygen content.**

How Can Food-Borne Illness Be Prevented?

Foods of animal origin are most commonly associated with food-borne illness. These include not only raw meat, poultry, and fish but also eggs, shellfish, and unpasteurized milk. Fruits and vegetables can also cause problems when they are consumed unwashed and raw. For example, in 2006, more than 200 people became ill and 3 died after eating raw spinach contaminated with *E. coli,* and this was quickly followed by an outbreak of salmonellosis traced to fresh tomatoes.[22] So how can you

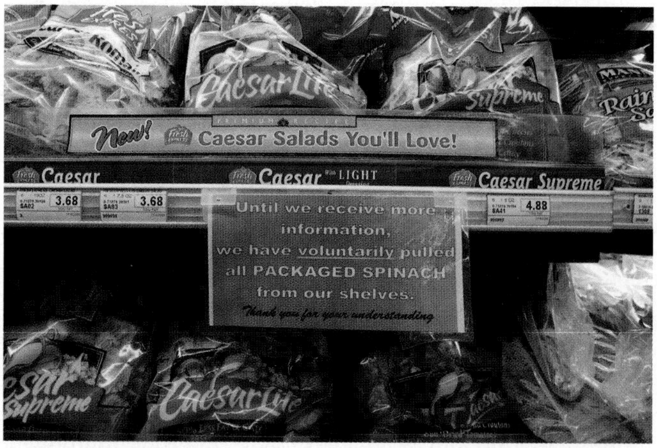

Spinach was pulled from supermarket shelves during an *E. coli* outbreak in 2006.

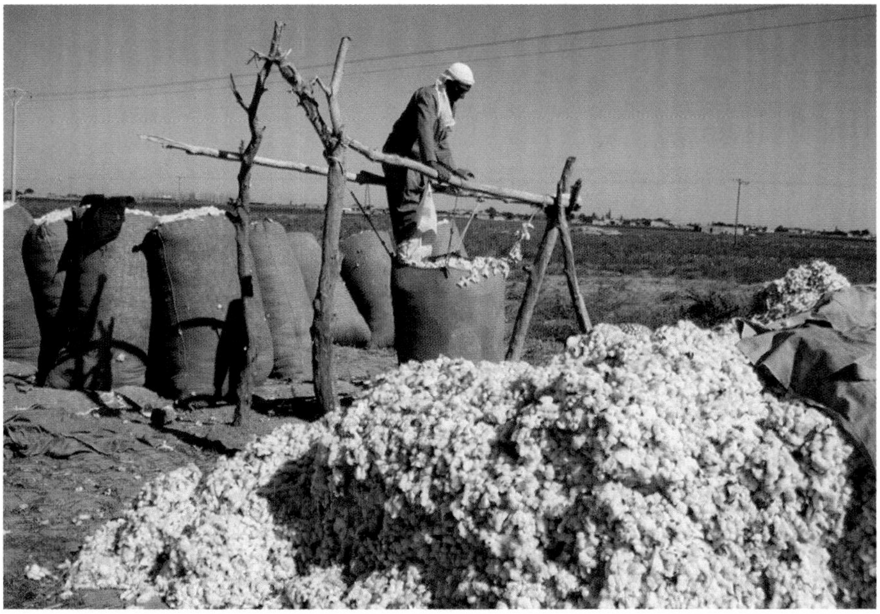

Cotton is a cash crop that farmers often grow instead of local food crops.

plete the soil of nutrients and reduce crop yield. The use of agricultural land for **cash crops,** such as cotton, coffee, and tobacco, may replace land use for local food crops, such as sorghum and corn. The end result may be less food available for local consumption.

Lack of Infrastructure

Many developing countries lack roads and transportation into rural areas. This limits available food to whatever can be produced locally. Lack of electricity and refrigeration can limit storage and allow the spoilage of even local foods before they can be used. Other crucial aspects of infrastructure are irrigation systems, sanitation services, communication systems, an adequate healthcare delivery system, and adequate public education.

Impact of Disease

Disease reduces the work capacity of individuals, and this in turn reduces their ability to ward off poverty and malnutrition. This vicious cycle is demonstrated by the AIDS epidemic. In sub-Saharan Africa, more than 5% of adults are infected with HIV, and 2 million died from AIDS in 2008.[8] Because AIDS most commonly strikes young adults who are the primary wage earners in their families, their illness or death orphans their children, impoverishes their elderly parents, and devastates their communities. By creating populations in which children and the elderly predominate, the AIDS epidemic has exacerbated the risk for undernutrition in many developing countries.

Unequal Distribution

The world produces a surplus of food. In 2009, the number of hungry people worldwide increased to unprecedented levels, despite the fact that the world food harvests in 2008 and 2009 were the largest on record.[9] The major cause of unequal distribution of food within a community is, of course, poverty. At greatest risk are people who do not own enough land to grow their own food and must work to buy food in areas where employment opportunities are scarce.

Unequal distribution also occurs because of cultural biases. In some communities, limited food is distributed first to men and boys and only secondarily to women and girls. Food distribution to the elderly is also sometimes limited. Access to food also can differ by ethnicity and religion. For example, higher mortality was documented in some ethnic and religious groups during the drought-induced famine in northern Ethiopia in the 1980s.[10]

What Health Problems Result from Undernutrition?

Undernutrition can cause a wide variety of health problems. The most common are discussed here.

Increased Infant and Child Mortality

Undernutrition increases by close to 50% the likelihood that a child will die between birth and age 5.[11] In 2009, in industrialized countries, the infant mortality rate was only 5 per 1,000, and the childhood mortality rate (the rate of deaths for all children under 5) was 6 per 1,000. In contrast, in the least developed countries of the world, the infant mortality rate was 84 per 1,000 and the child mortality rate was 103 per 1,000.[12]

Increased Vulnerability to Infection

We noted earlier that the most common way that undernutrition kills infants and children is by making them more vulnerable to infectious diseases, such as pneumonia and infectious diarrhea. By decreasing a child's general health, malnutrition increases the likelihood that the child will not survive infection. Moreover, infection exacerbates malnutrition by decreasing appetite, causing vomiting and diarrhea, and generally weakening the immune system. A vicious cycle of malnutrition, infection, worsening malnutrition, and increased vulnerability to infection develops.

Macronutrient Deficiencies

Marasmus is a disease of children that results from grossly inadequate intakes of energy. As we explained in Chapter 6, it commonly occurs when chronic food shortages reduce children's total energy intake. As a result,

cash crops Crops grown to be sold rather than eaten, such as cotton, tobacco, jute, and sugarcane.

the children slowly starve to death. Typically, their weakened immune system makes them highly vulnerable to infection; thus, they often die from pneumonia or from dehydration caused by diarrhea. Alternatively, they suffer heart failure from a weakened heart muscle.

Kwashiorkor is a disease of toddlers who have recently been weaned from breast milk, which is replaced with a watery porridge that has inadequate and poor-quality protein. The lack of dietary protein causes edema, because the level of protein in the blood is inadequate to keep fluids from seeping into the tissue spaces. Edema swells the child's belly and makes the face and limbs appear adequately nourished. The child experiences severe wasting of muscle tissue and easily succumbs to infection.

Micronutrient Deficiencies

Undernourished people are at risk for a variety of micronutrient deficiencies. Iron deficiency is the world's most common nutrient deficiency. It increases the risk for infection, premature birth, low birth weight, and maternal death during or immediately following childbirth. It also impairs children's ability to learn and adults' ability to work. Iodine deficiency is responsible for mental impairment in children and goiter in adults. Zinc deficiency reduces growth and immune function. Deficiency of vitamin B_{12} can result in severe cognitive impairment. Lack of sufficient vitamin A in the diet is a preventable cause of night blindness in children. Adding iron, iodine, zinc, B-vitamins, and vitamin A to common foods, such as salt and flour, costs only about 30 cents per person reached per year and is a major initiative of several international aid organizations.[13]

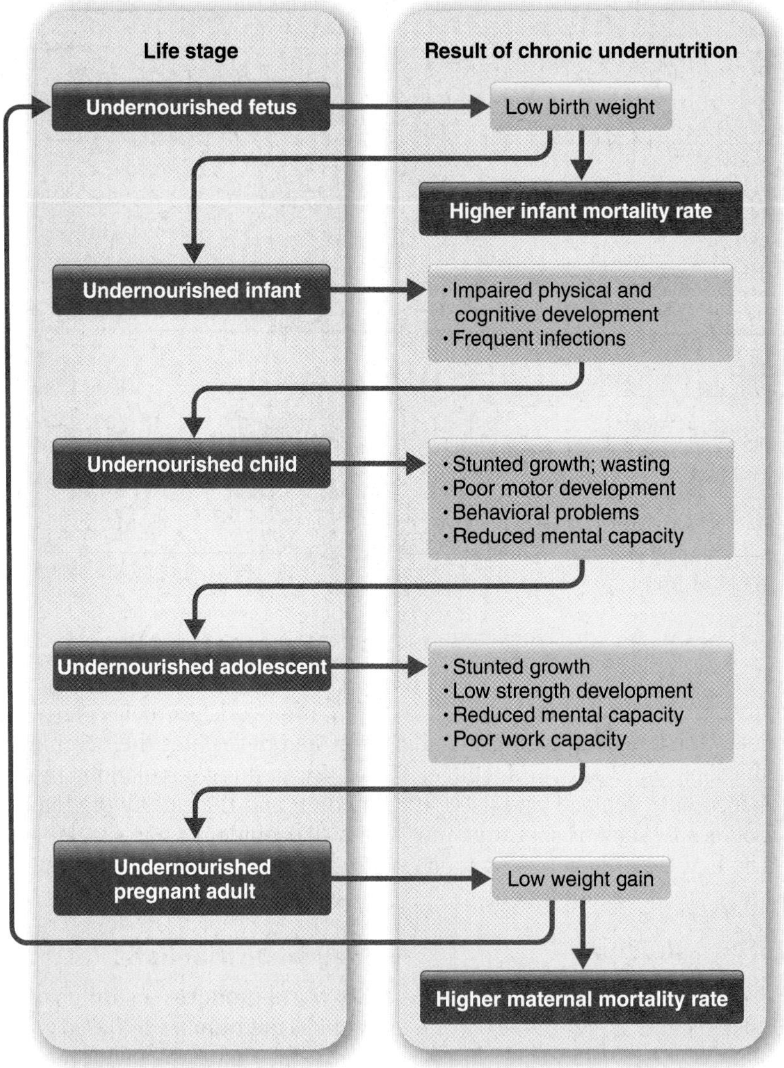

Figure 2 Acute and long-term effects of malnutrition throughout the life cycle.

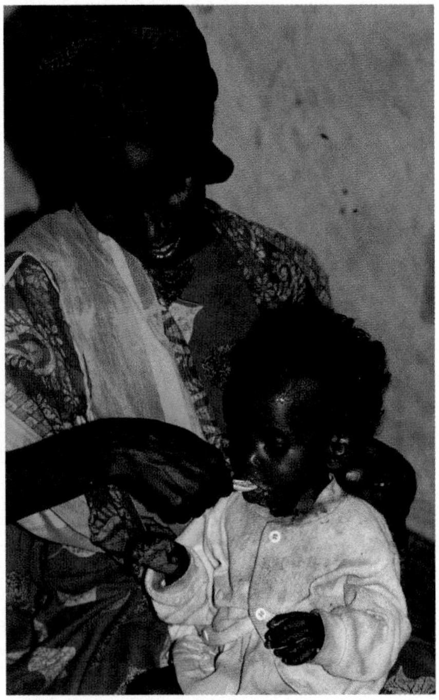

In developing nations, providing vitamin A supplements to children under age 5 has significantly reduced mortality.

Poor Work Capacity in Adults

The debilitating weakness caused by undernutrition affects the productivity of adults in many developing nations. It is especially detrimental when manual labor involved in subsistence farming is the main source of food and income. Nutrient deficiency also contributes to poor work capacity. Iron-deficiency anemia is particularly debilitating because of iron's role in oxygen transport.

Figure 2 illustrates the varied and cruel effects of chronic undernutrition throughout the life span. As you can see, the cycle is perpetuated across generations when undernourished women give birth to undernourished infants.

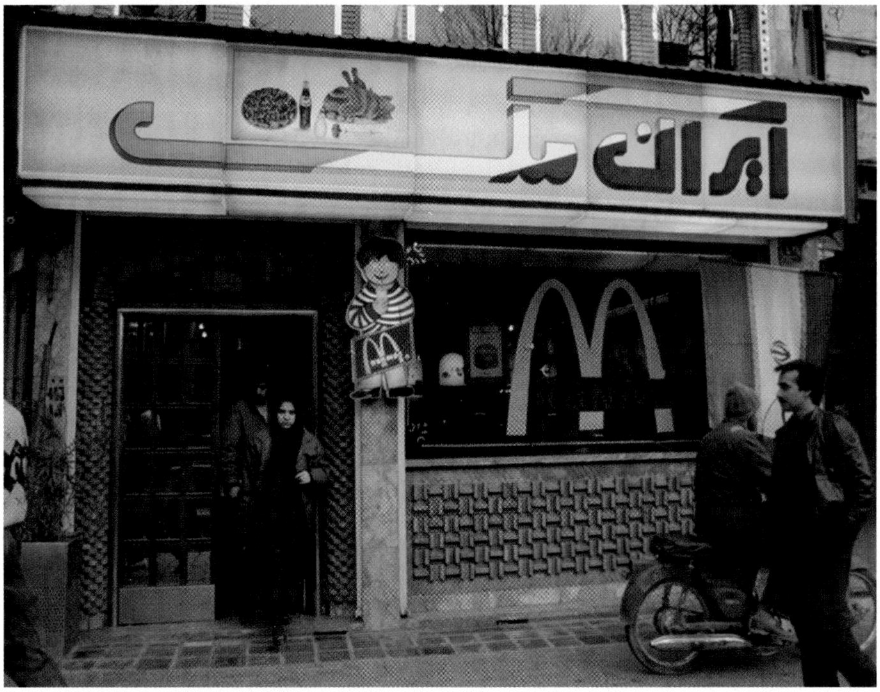

Overnutrition is becoming a global concern now that low-cost, energy-dense foods are becoming widely available.

Why Is Obesity a Growing Problem in Developing Nations?

People living in countries with growing economies, such as Egypt, Brazil, and China, enjoy increased food availability and variety. Unfortunately, their new diet usually includes more processed foods with high energy density due to added fat and sugar, including snack foods and fast foods. These foods are usually less expensive than traditional foods, such as fish, milk, and fresh fruits and vegetables.[14] This shift in dietary pattern as poverty is relieved is called the **nutrition transition.** And while the population is consuming more energy, greater access to motorized transportation and a decrease in manual labor are reducing their energy expenditure. The result of this equation is overnutrition.

In addition, there is now significant evidence linking undernutrition during fetal life to overnutrition in adulthood. The hypothesis known as "fetal origins of adult disease" states that fetal adaptations to poor maternal nutrition help the child during times of food shortages but make the child susceptible to obesity and chronic disease when food is plentiful.[15] For example, when a mother is malnourished during pregnancy, her newborn will tend to have a low birth weight but be relatively fat. This may occur because the fetal body has favored growth of the brain, which is more than 50% fat, at the expense of muscle tissue. Researchers theorize that this adaptation may prompt a permanent physiologic tendency to gain fat tissue when food is plentiful.[16]

Given these factors, it is not surprising that countries throughout the world have been experiencing an alarming increase in the prevalence of obesity. The World Health Organization (WHO) estimates that, since 1980, obesity rates have increased threefold or more. In 2010, 300 million adults worldwide were clinically obese, and the WHO predicts that, by 2015, more than 700 million will be obese.[17] As we have pointed out throughout this text, overweight and obesity increase the risk for cardiovascular disease, type 2 diabetes, and some cancers. Of these, type 2 diabetes is fast becoming an especially significant burden in the developing world. The WHO predicts that, by 2020, deaths due to diabetes will increase worldwide by more than 50%.[17]

Malnutrition in the United States

As we discussed in Chapter 11, overnutrition is becoming a national health crisis. A majority of Americans are now overweight or obese, and the prevalence of type 2 diabetes and other chronic diseases associated with obesity is increasing. Paradoxically, obesity is increasingly a problem of the poor. That's in part because, for many poor families, the priority is to maximize caloric intake for each dollar spent. This can lead to an overconsumption of Calories and a less healthful diet. Energy-dense foods with longer shelf lives, such as cookies, chips, and soft drinks, are less expensive than perishable foods, such as fresh produce. They also tend to have a higher satiety value, keeping hunger at bay for longer. For example, $1.50 will buy about half of one sweet red pepper, or an entire package of store-brand cookies. If you were hungry and had just a few dollars to spend for groceries, which would you purchase? Moreover, research suggests that, during periods of insufficient income, poor mothers restrict their food intake in favor of their children. Such chronic ups and downs of food intake can contribute to obesity.[18]

How many people in the United States are affected by this inability to reliably purchase healthful food? As shown in **Figure 3**, the U.S. Department of Agriculture (USDA) estimates that 14.6% of U.S. households, comprising 49.1 million Americans, including 16.7 million children, suffer

---

nutrition transition A shift in dietary pattern toward greater food security, greater variety of foods, and more foods with high energy density; associated with increased incidence of obesity and chronic disease.

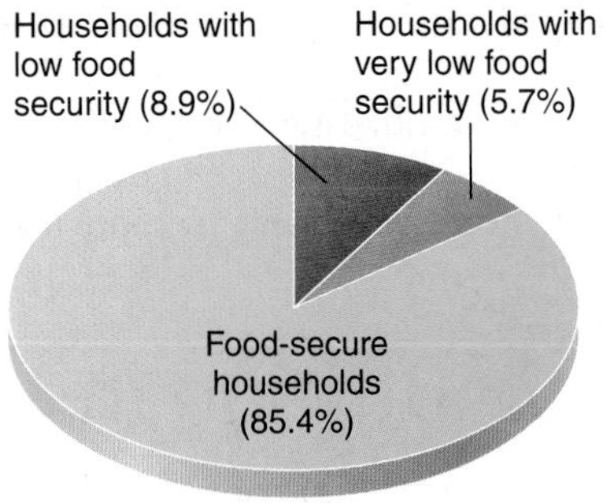

Figure 3 Food security status of U.S. households in 2008. Note: Food-insecure households include those with low food security and with very low food security.
Data from the Economic Research Service (ERS) using data from the December 2008 Current Population Survey Food Security Supplement. www.ers.usda.gov/Briefing/FoodSecurity/Stats_Graphics.htm.

food insecurity.[19] This means that they are unable to obtain enough food to meet their physical needs every day.

Most at risk are families with an income below the official U.S. poverty level ($21,834 for a family of four in 2008). Of these, 42% experience food insecurity.[19] Also at great risk are families consisting of single mothers and their children: in 2008, 37.2% of households with children headed by a single woman experienced food insecurity.[19] In addition, black and Hispanic households have higher rates of food insecurity (25–27%) than average.[19] Other vulnerable groups are the homeless, the unemployed, migrant laborers, and other workers in minimum-wage jobs.

In 2008, more than 5 million American children lived in homes with *very low food security,* meaning that the normal eating patterns of one or more household members were disrupted and food intake was reduced at times during the year. Typically in these homes, children are protected from substantial reduction in food intake; however, in 2008, more than 1 million of these children lived in homes where they, too, were forced to skip meals, cut portions, or otherwise forgo food.[19]

What Can Be Done to Relieve Malnutrition?

To combat malnutrition and achieve global food security, long-term solutions are critical. We discuss some of the most effective here.

Global Solutions

Among the most important long-term solutions for improving the health and nutrition of children worldwide are programs that encourage breastfeeding. This is because breast milk provides optimal nutrition for the healthy growth of the newborn and contains antibodies that protect against infections. In contrast, feeding infants with formula increases the infant's risk for diarrhea if the powder is mixed with unsanitary water. The WHO sponsors programs to encourage breastfeeding throughout the developing world.

Strategies to increase the immunization of children are helping reduce the rate of infectious disease in children worldwide. At the same time, supplying local health agencies with oral rehydration therapy, a simple solution of fluids and electrolytes that can be administered to children with diarrhea, is helping reduce deaths from dehydration.

Many international organizations help improve the nutrient status of the poor by encouraging national programs to enrich or fortify common foods, such as flour and salt, with micronutrients. Other programs provide micronutrients, such as vitamin A, as supplements. Many aid organizations foster the ability of poor communities to produce their own foods. For example, both USAID and the Peace Corps have agricultural education programs, the World Bank provides loans to fund small business ventures, and many non-profit and non-governmental organizations support community and family farms and gardens.

Another method for increasing local food production is **sustainable agriculture.** The goal of the sustainable agriculture movement is to develop local, site-specific farming methods that improve soil conservation, crop yields, and food security in a sustainable manner, minimizing the adverse environmental impact. For example, soil erosion can be controlled by the terracing of sloped land for the cultivation of crops **(Figure 4)**, by tillage that minimizes disturbance to the topsoil, and by the use of herbicides to remove weeds rather than hoeing. Another practice associated with sustainable agriculture is the use of **transgenic crops,** plant varieties that have had one or more genes altered to reduce the need for insecticides or to permit the cultivation of marginally fertile land.

Local Solutions

In the United States, several government programs help low-income citizens acquire food over extended periods of time. Among these programs are the Supplemental Nutrition Assistance Program (commonly referred to as "food stamps"), which helps low-income individuals of all ages; the Special Supplemental Nutrition Program for Women, Infants, and Children (WIC), which helps pregnant women and children to age 5; the National School Lunch and National School Breakfast Programs, which help low-income schoolchildren; and the Summer Food Service Program, which helps low-income children in the summer. The U.S. Department of Agriculture also sponsors programs to distribute emergency foods and surplus commodity foods to qualifying families. Foods may be distributed through charitable organizations or local or county agencies.

Many other local initiatives are underway in different communities. These include food banks, where qualifying clients can choose a variety of foods for their families; free meals, often distributed by churches or community centers; and gleaning, a prac-

---

food insecurity Circumstances in which households are uncertain of having, or unable to acquire, enough food to meet the needs of all their members because they have insufficient money or other resources for food.

sustainable agriculture Techniques of food production that preserve the environment indefinitely.

transgenic crops Plant varieties that have had one or more genes altered through the use of genetic technologies; also called genetically modified organisms, or GMOs.

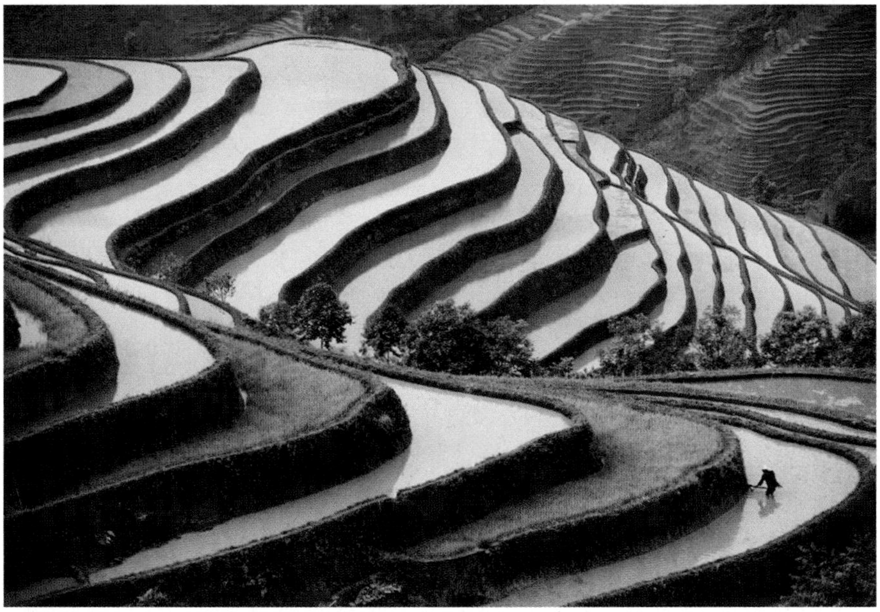

Figure 4 Terracing sloped land to avoid soil erosion is one practice of sustainable agriculture.

tice in which volunteers comb fields and orchards after harvesting and gather any remaining edible produce, then clean it and distribute it to the poor. Some community groups are fostering home gardens for poor inner-city residents, including raised beds, seeds, a drip irrigation system, and gardening classes, to give the residents immediate access to organic produce in neighborhoods with only fast-food outlets and liquor stores.

Get Involved!

Several times each year, college students from hundreds of campuses all over the United States gather to fight hunger. Members of the National Student Campaign Against Hunger and Homelessness, they hold Hunger Clean-Ups, staff relief agencies, solicit donations of food and money, and promote community activism. Their organization is just one of dozens in which you can get involved. For more information, see Web Resources at the end of this ***In Depth***. Also, the What About You? box (page 498) identifies more steps you can take to fight hunger in your role as consumer, student, and world citizen.

If you still wonder whether your acts can make a difference, consider the advice of the late historian and social activist Howard Zinn. He urged people to "just do something, to join with millions of others who will just do something, because all of those somethings, at certain points in history, come together and make the world better."[20]

NUTRI-CASE JUDY

"I never seem to be able to make ends meet. I keep hoping next month will be different, but rent and utilities eat up most of my paycheck, so when something unexpected happens, I'm short. Last week, my car broke down and I'm way behind on my credit card payments. Today, a collections guy called and said that, if I didn't pay at least $100 right away, they'd take me to court. When I got off the phone, I started to cry, and Hannah asked me what was wrong. When I told her how bad the money situation is, she thought we might qualify for food stamps. I have a full-time job, so I don't think we'll qualify, but even if we do, I wonder if it'll help much."

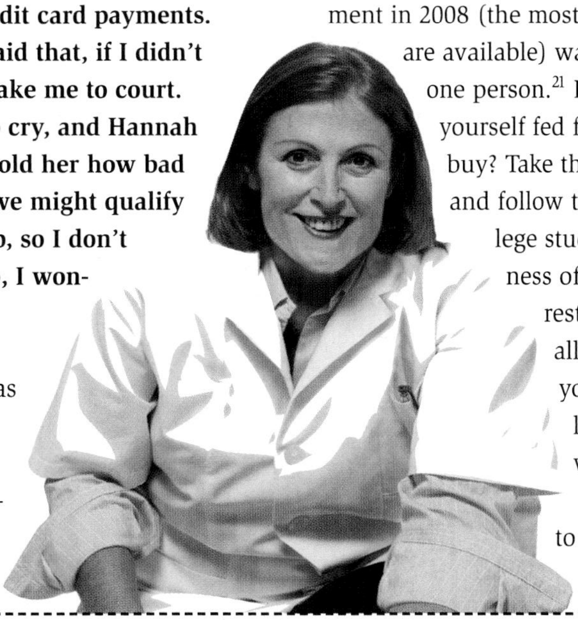

In 2009, the federal minimum wage was $7.25 an hour. As a nurse's aide, Judy earns $10 an hour, or $1,733 a month, making her eligible for the Supplemental Nutrition Assistance Program (food stamps). Are you surprised that someone making almost 40% more than the minimum wage, and working full-time, qualifies for food assistance? Before you're too certain that Judy's eligibility will solve her problems, consider that the average food stamp allotment in 2008 (the most recent year for which data are available) was about $101 per month for one person.[21] If you had just $25 to keep yourself fed for a week, what would you buy? Take this challenge one step further and follow the example of some U.S. college students to raise local awareness of food insecurity: for 1 week, restrict yourself to just $25 for all your food purchases. Let your campus newspaper and local media outlets know what you're doing, and ask readers to make donations to local food banks.

IN DEPTH

What About You?

Do Your Actions Contribute to Global Food Security?

Have you ever wondered whether your actions inadvertently contribute to the problem of world hunger? Or whether any efforts you make in your home or community can help feed people thousands of miles away? If so, you might want to reflect on your behaviors in each of three roles you play every day: consumer, student, and citizen of the world.

In your role as a Consumer, ask yourself:

☐ **What kinds of food products do I buy?**
Your purchases influence the types of foods that are manufactured and sold, and buying fewer processed foods saves energy.

1. Choose fresh, locally grown, organic foods more often to support local sustainability.
2. Choose whole or less processed versions of packaged foods (such as peanut butter made solely from ground peanuts or plain yogurt from a local dairy), rather than versions of foods made with high-fructose corn syrup, dyes, and other additives. This encourages increased production of the less processed foods.
3. Limit purchases of nutrient-poor foods and beverages to discourage their profitability. Also limit high-Calorie fast-food meals.

☐ **How often do I eat vegetarian?**
Vegetarian foods can be produced with less energy than animal-based foods; plus, livestock production contributes much higher levels of greenhouse gases to the environment. So every time you eat vegetarian, you save global energy and contribute to reductions in global warming.

1. Experiment with some recipes in a vegetarian cookbook. Try making at least one new vegetarian meal each week.
2. Introduce friends and family members to your new vegetarian dishes.
3. When eating out, choose restaurants that provide vegetarian menu choices. If the campus cafeteria or a favorite restaurant has no vegetarian choices, request that one or more be added to the menu.

☐ **How much do I eat?**
Eating just the Calories you need to maintain a healthy weight provides more of the global harvest for others and will likely reduce your use of limited medical resources.

1. To raise your consciousness about the physical experience of hunger, consider fasting for 1 day. If health or other reasons prevent you from fasting safely, try keeping silent during each meal throughout 1 day, so that you can more fully appreciate the food you're eating and reflect on those who do not enjoy food security.
2. For 1 week, keep track of how much food you throw away, and why. Do you put more food on your plate than you can eat? Do you allow foods stored in your refrigerator to spoil?

In your role as a Student, ask yourself:

☐ **How can I use what I have learned about nutrition to help feed my neighbors and the world?**

1. Join the National Student Campaign Against Hunger and Homelessness. If your campus doesn't have a branch, start one!
2. Research what local produce is available in each season. Write an article for your school newspaper, listing what is in season each month of the year and include two healthy, low-cost recipes using vegetables and fruits that are in season during the month your article will be published.
3. Create an entertaining skit or puppet show that encourages young children to eat healthful foods. Offer to entertain on the weekends at your local library, day-care center, or after-school community program.
4. Begin or join a food cooperative, community garden, or shared farming program. Donate a portion of your produce each week to a local food pantry.

☐ **What careers could I consider to promote global food security?**

1. If you are interested in teaching, you could become a member of the Peace Corps and teach nutrition in developing countries. If you want to teach in the United States, see the Feeding Minds Fighting Hunger website listed in the Web Resources for information on teaching young people about global nutrition.
2. If you are interested in science, you could help develop higher-yielding crops, better irrigation methods, or projects to improve food or water safety.
3. If you plan a career in business, you could enter the food industry and help market healthful, affordable foods.
4. If you pursue a career in healthcare, you could join an international medical corps working among the poor.

In your role as a World Citizen, ask yourself:

☐ **How can I improve the nutrition of people in my own community?**

1. You can volunteer at a local soup kitchen, homeless shelter, food bank, or community garden.
2. To combat obesity in your community, you can help increase opportunities for physical activity. Start a walking group, or volunteer to coach children in your favorite sport.

☐ **How can I improve the nutrition of people in developing nations?**

1. Donate time or money to one of the international agencies that work to provide relief from famine or chronic hunger. Check out options for charitable contributions and volunteer efforts at www.charitynavigator.org.
2. Research the global effects of protectionist agricultural subsidies in the United States and Europe; then write letters to your school or community newspaper, your elected officials, and political action groups, expressing your concerns.
3. Research the human rights records of international food companies whose products you buy. If you don't like what you find out, switch brands and write to the company and tell them why you did.
4. Vote for elected officials who support policies that help impoverished Americans and promote agricultural equity around the world.

Web Resources

www.actionagainsthunger.org
Action Against Hunger

This site explains the mission of an international organization that aids in food crises and promotes long-term food security. The site also explains how you can help.

www.secondharvest.org
America's Second Harvest

Check out this site for information on programs for fighting hunger in the United States.

www.bread.org
Bread for the World

Visit this site to learn about a faith-based effort to advocate local and global policies that help the poor obtain food.

www.care.org
CARE

This site links to CARE organizations working in many countries to improve economic conditions in over seventy developing nations.

www.doctorswithoutborders-usa.org
Doctors Without Borders, Starved for Attention Multimedia Campaign

See this site for a multimedia introduction to some of the key issues involved in battling global hunger.

www.feedingminds.org
Feeding Minds, Fighting Hunger

Visit this international electronic classroom to explore the problems of hunger, malnutrition, and food insecurity.

www.studentsagainsthunger.org
National Student Campaign Against Hunger and Homelessness

Visit this site to learn what students are doing to fight hunger, and how you can get involved.

www.hungerbanquet.org
Hunger Banquet

At this site, sponsored by Oxfam America, you can play a "hunger game" that confronts you with some of the same choices facing people in developing nations every day, or take a "hunger quiz" to find out how much you know about global hunger.

www.unicef.org
The United Nations Children's Fund

Visit this site to learn about international concerns affecting the world's children, including nutrient deficiencies and hunger.

www.who.int/nutrition/en
The World Health Organization Nutrition Site

Visit this site to learn about global malnutrition, micronutrient deficiencies, nutrition transition, and other issues of world hunger.

14 Nutrition Through the Life Cycle: Pregnancy and the First Year of Life

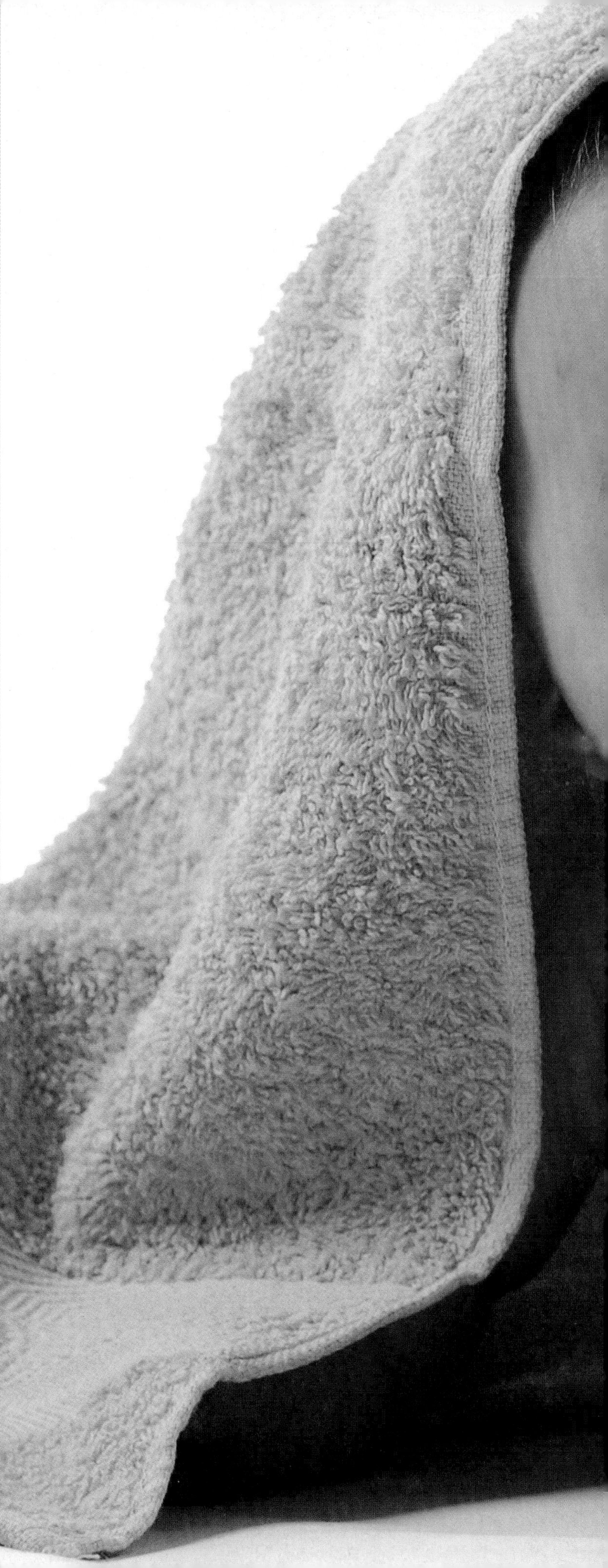

CHAPTER OBJECTIVES

After reading this chapter you will be able to:

1. **Explain why maintaining a nutritious diet is important for prospective parents even before conception, p. 502.**
2. **Describe the relationship between fetal development, physiologic changes in the mother, and increasing nutrient requirements during the course of a pregnancy, pp. 502–505.**
3. **Identify the range of optimal weight gain for a pregnant woman in the first, second, and third trimesters, pp. 505–507.**
4. **Describe the physiologic events that lead to lactation, pp. 517–518.**
5. **Compare and contrast the nutrient requirements of pregnant and lactating women, pp. 508–512 and 519–520.**
6. **Identify the primary advantages and most common challenges of breastfeeding, pp. 521–524.**
7. **Relate the growth and activity patterns of infants to their nutrient needs, pp. 525–530.**
8. **Discuss some common nutrition-related concerns for infants, pp. 530–532.**

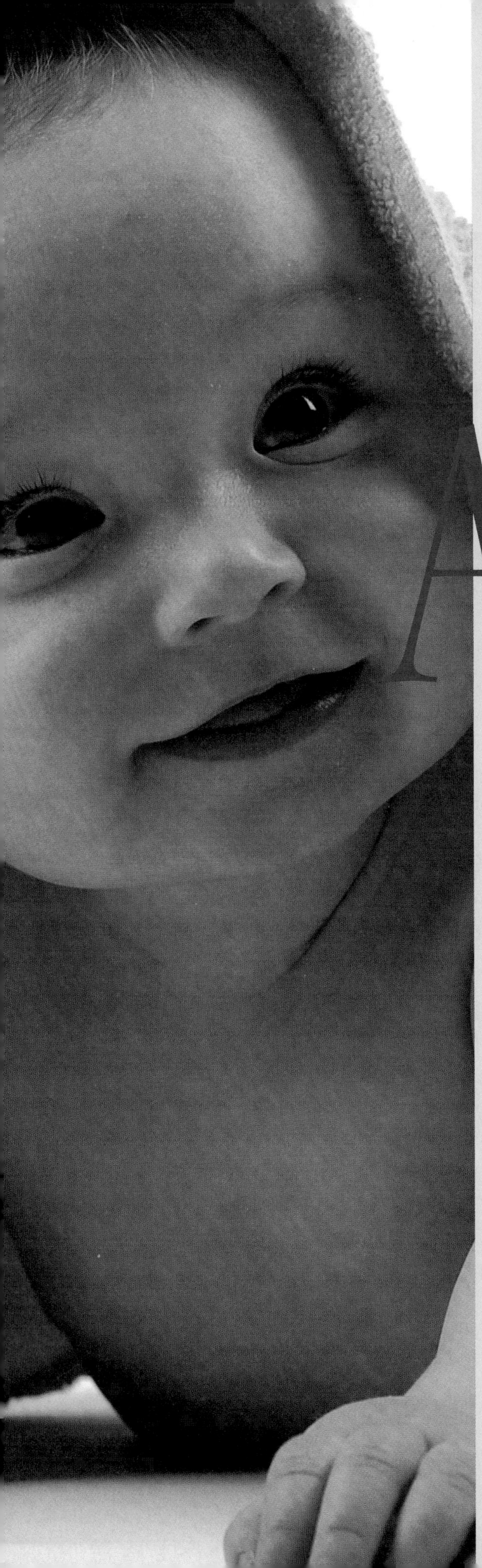

Test Yourself

1. **T F A pregnant woman needs to consume twice as many Calories as she did prior to the pregnancy.**
2. **T F Breastfed infants tend to have fewer infections and allergies than formula-fed infants.**
3. **T F Most infants begin to require solid foods by about 3 months (12 weeks) of age.**

Test Yourself answers can be found at the end of the chapter.

An active, curious 2-year-old, Tomas brings joy and laughter to his parents and family. That wasn't always the case, however. Tomas weighed just over 3 lb 5 oz at birth—about half of what an average full-term newborn weighs. Even today, Tomas is still small for his age and continues to struggle with his coordination and speech. Although the United States has an extensive and expensive healthcare system, the numbers of low-, very-low-, and extremely low-birth-weight infants, such as Tomas, continue to increase, to more than 8% in 2006.[1] Moreover, our infant mortality rate—the number of deaths of infants before their first birthday—is higher than the rate in 44 other countries: in 2009, the United States recorded 6.22 infant deaths for every 1,000 live births, as compared to just 2.75 for Sweden and 2.31 for Singapore, the best-ranked.[2]

What contributes to these troubling statistics? What are the short- and long-term effects of low and extremely low birth weights on children? On a broader scale, what role does prenatal diet play in determining the future health and well-being of the child? Why is inadequate iron or folate intake especially dangerous to a pregnant woman and her fetus? What roles do other nutrients play in maternal, fetal, and infant health? In this chapter, we'll discuss how adequate nutrition supports fetal development, maintains the pregnant woman's health, and contributes to lactation. We'll then explore the nutrient needs of breastfeeding and formula-feeding infants.

Starting Out Right: Healthful Nutrition in Pregnancy

At no stage of life is nutrition more crucial than during fetal development and infancy. From conception through the end of the first year of life, adequate nutrition is essential for tissue formation, neurologic development, and bone growth, modeling, and remodeling. The ability to reach peak physical and intellectual potential in adult life is in part determined by the nutrition received during the earliest years of development.

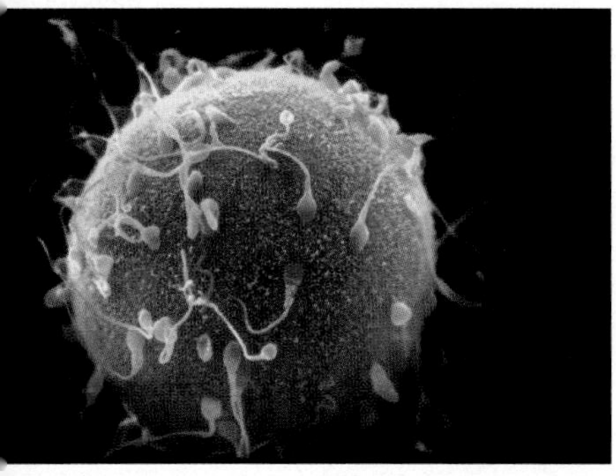

During conception, a sperm fertilizes an egg, creating a zygote.

Is Nutrition Important Before Conception?

Several factors make adequate nutrition important even before **conception,** the point at which a woman's ovum (egg) is fertilized with a man's sperm. First, some deficiency-related problems develop extremely early in the pregnancy, typically before the mother even realizes she is pregnant. An adequate and varied preconception diet reduces the risk for such problems during those first few weeks of life. For example, inadequate levels of folate during the first few weeks following conception can result in brain and spinal cord defects. This problem is discussed in more detail shortly. To reduce the incidence of such defects, federal guidelines advise all women capable of becoming pregnant to consume 400 μg of folic acid daily, whether or not they plan to become pregnant.

Second, adopting a healthful diet prior to conception includes the avoidance of alcohol, illegal drugs, and other known **teratogens** (substances that cause birth defects). Women should also consult their healthcare provider about their consumption of caffeine, medications, herbs, and supplements, and if they smoke they should attempt to quit.

Third, a healthful diet and an appropriate level of physical activity can help women achieve and maintain an optimal body weight prior to pregnancy. Women with a pre-pregnancy body mass index (BMI) between 19.8 and 26.0 kg/m^2 have the best chance of a successful pregnancy.[1] As we will discuss shortly, women with a BMI above or below this range are at greater risk for pregnancy-related complications.

Finally, maintaining a balanced and nourishing diet before conception reduces a woman's risk of developing a nutrition-related disorder during her pregnancy. These disorders, which we discuss later in the chapter, include gestational diabetes and hypertensive disorders. Although genetic and metabolic abnormalities are beyond the woman's control, following a healthful diet prior to conception is something a woman can do to help her fetus develop into a healthy baby.

The man's nutrition prior to pregnancy is important as well, since malnutrition contributes to abnormalities in sperm.[2] Both sperm number and motility (ability to move) are reduced by alcohol consumption, as well as by the use of certain prescription and illegal drugs. Finally, infections accompanied by a high fever can destroy sperm, so to the extent that adequate nutrition keeps the immune system strong, it also promotes a man's fertility.

Are you ready to have a child? The decision to become pregnant is often complex and it is best to plan ahead. It's important to understand the realities of becoming a parent before making the decision to start a family. Several online self-assessments are available that can help you decide if you are personally ready to take on the role of parenthood. See Web Resources at the end of this chapter for details.

Why Is Nutrition Important During Pregnancy?

A balanced, nourishing diet is important throughout pregnancy to provide the nutrients needed to support fetal development without depriving the mother of the nutrients she needs to maintain her own health. It also minimizes the risk of excess energy intake. A full-term pregnancy lasts 38 to 42 weeks and is divided into three **trimesters,** with each trimester lasting about 13 to 14 weeks.

conception (also called *fertilization*) The uniting of an ovum (egg) and sperm to create a fertilized egg, or zygote.

teratogen Any substance that can cause a birth defect.

trimester Any one of three stages of pregnancy, each lasting 13 to 14 weeks.

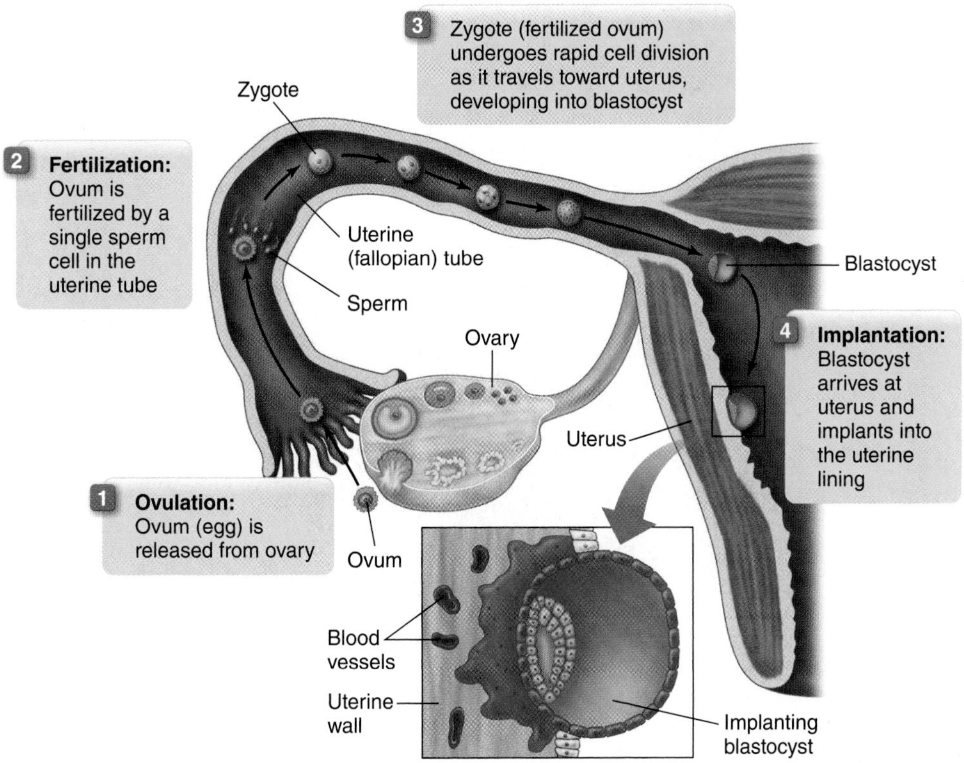
3 Zygote (fertilized ovum) undergoes rapid cell division as it travels toward uterus, developing into blastocyst
Zygote
2 Fertilization: Ovum is fertilized by a single sperm cell in the uterine tube
Uterine (fallopian) tube
Sperm
Blastocyst
Ovary
4 Implantation: Blastocyst arrives at uterus and implants into the uterine lining
Uterus
1 Ovulation: Ovum (egg) is released from ovary
Ovum
Blood vessels
Uterine wall
Implanting blastocyst

Figure 14.1 Ovulation, conception, and implantation.

The First Trimester

About once each month, a non-pregnant woman of childbearing age experiences **ovulation,** the release of an ovum (egg cell) from an ovary. The ovum is then drawn into the uterine tube. The first trimester of pregnancy begins when the ovum and sperm unite to form a single, fertilized cell called a **zygote.** As the zygote travels through the uterine tube, it divides into a ball of 12 to 16 cells, which, at about day 4, arrives in the uterus **(Figure 14.1)**. By day 10, the inner portion of the zygote, called the *blastocyst,* has implanted into the uterine lining. The outer portion becomes part of the placenta, which is discussed shortly.

Further cell growth, multiplication, and differentiation occur, resulting in the formation of an **embryo.** Over the next 6 weeks, embryonic tissues continue to differentiate and fold into a primitive, tubelike structure with limb buds, organs, and facial features recognizable as human **(Figure 14.2)**. It isn't surprising, then, that the embryo is most vulnerable to teratogens during this time. Not only alcohol and illegal drugs, but also some prescription and over-the-counter medications, megadoses of certain

ovulation The release of an ovum (egg) from a woman's ovary.

zygote A fertilized egg (ovum) consisting of a single cell.

embryo The human growth and developmental stage lasting from the third week to the end of the eighth week after fertilization.

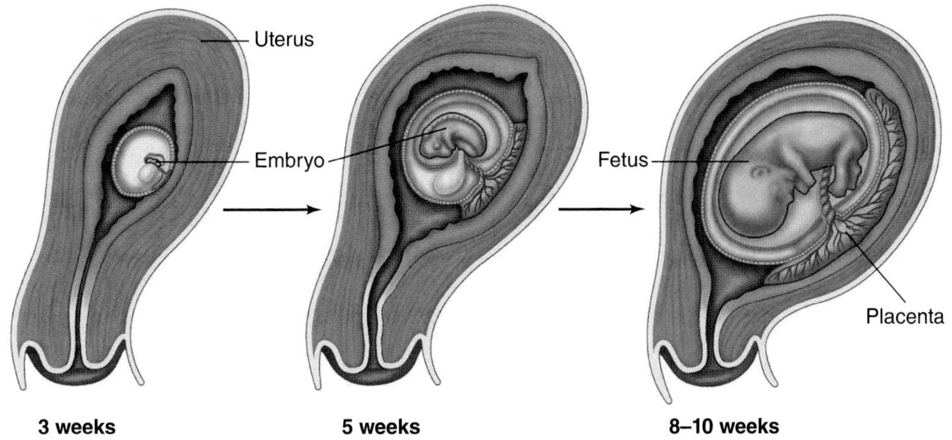
Uterus
Embryo
Fetus
Placenta
3 weeks
5 weeks
8–10 weeks

Figure 14.2 Human embryonic development during the first 10 weeks. Organ systems are most vulnerable to teratogens during this time, when cells are dividing and differentiating.

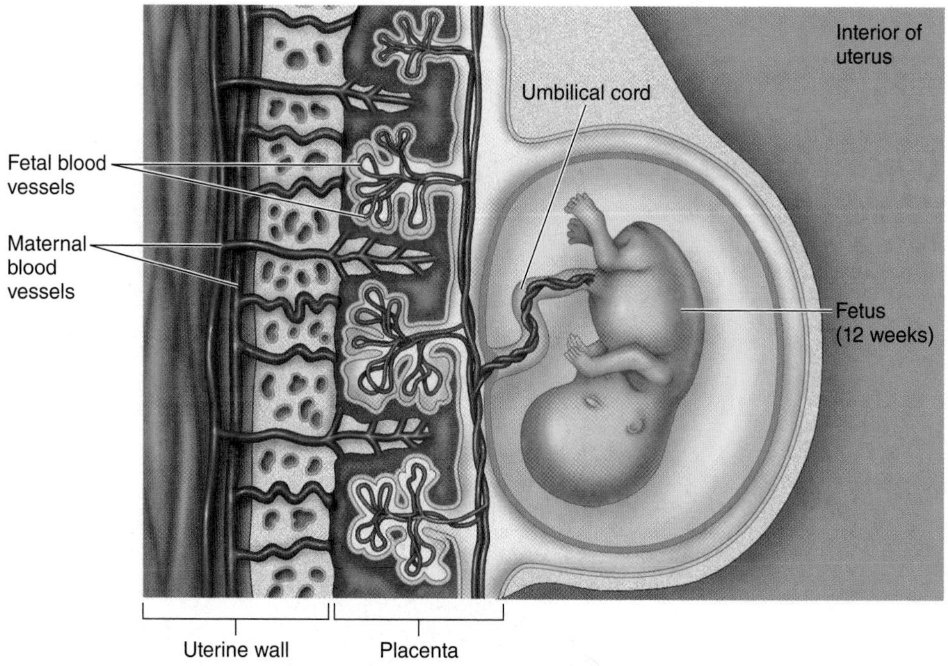

Figure 14.3 Placental development. The placenta is formed from both embryonic and maternal tissues. When the placenta is fully functional, fetal blood vessels and maternal blood vessels are intimately intertwined, allowing the exchange of nutrients and wastes between the two. The mother transfers nutrients and oxygen to the fetus, and the fetus transfers wastes to the mother for disposal.

supplements, several herbs, some viruses, cigarette smoking, and radiation can interfere with embryonic development and cause birth defects. In some cases, the damage is so severe that the pregnancy is naturally terminated in a **spontaneous abortion** (*miscarriage*), most of which occur in the first trimester.

During the first weeks of pregnancy, the embryo obtains its nutrients from cells lining the uterus. But by the fourth week, a primitive **placenta** has formed in the uterus from both embryonic and maternal tissue. Within a few more weeks, the placenta will be a fully functioning organ, through which the mother will provide nutrients and remove fetal wastes **(Figure 14.3)**.

By the end of the embryonic stage, about 8 weeks postconception, the embryo's tissues and organs have differentiated dramatically. A primitive skeleton, including fingers and toes, has formed. Muscles have begun to develop in the trunk and limbs, and some movement is possible. A primitive heart has begun to beat, and the digestive organs are becoming distinct. The brain has differentiated, and the head has a mouth, eyespots with eyelids, and primitive ears.

The third month of pregnancy marks the transition from embryo to **fetus.** To support its dramatic growth, the fetus requires abundant nutrients from the placenta. It is connected to the fetal circulatory system via the **umbilical cord,** an extension of fetal blood vessels emerging from the fetus's navel (called the *umbilicus*). Blood rich in oxygen and nutrients flows through the placenta and into the umbilical vein (Figure 14.3). Wastes are excreted in blood returning from the fetus to the placenta via the umbilical arteries. Although many people think there is a mixing of blood from the fetus and the mother, the two blood supplies remain separate. Nutrients move from the maternal blood into the fetal blood and waste products are transferred out of the fetal blood into the maternal blood.

spontaneous abortion (also called *miscarriage*) The natural termination of a pregnancy and expulsion of pregnancy tissues because of a genetic, developmental, or physiologic abnormality that is so severe that the pregnancy cannot be maintained.

placenta A pregnancy-specific organ formed from both maternal and embryonic tissues. It is responsible for oxygen, nutrient, and waste exchange between mother and fetus.

fetus The human growth and developmental stage lasting from the beginning of the ninth week after conception to birth.

umbilical cord The cord containing the arteries and veins that connect the baby (from the navel) to the mother via the placenta.

The Second Trimester

During the second trimester (weeks 14 to 27 of pregnancy), the fetus continues to grow and mature. It develops the ability to suck its thumb, to hear, and to open and close its eyes in response to light. At the beginning of the second trimester, the fetus is about 3 inches long and weighs about 1.5 pounds. By the end of this trimester, it is generally over a foot long and weighs more than 2 pounds. Some babies born prematurely in the last weeks of the second trimester survive with intensive care.

The Third Trimester

During the third trimester (weeks 28 to birth), the fetus gains nearly half its body length and three-quarters of its body weight! At birth, an average baby will be approximately 18 to 22 inches long and weigh about 7.5 pounds **(Figure 14.4)**. Brain growth (which continues to be rapid for the first 2 years of life) is also quite remarkable and the lungs become fully mature. The fetus acquires eyebrows, eyelashes, and hair on the head. Because of the intense growth and maturation of the fetus during the third trimester, it continues to be critical that the mother eat an adequate and balanced diet.

Impact of Nutrition on Maturity and Birth Weight

An adequate, nourishing diet is one of the most important variables under a woman's control for increasing the chances for birth of a mature newborn (at 38 to 42 weeks of **gestation**). Proper nutrition also increases the likelihood that the newborn's weight will be appropriate for his or her gestational age. Generally, a birth weight of at least 5.5 pounds is considered a marker of a successful pregnancy.

An undernourished mother who gains too little weight during her pregnancy is more likely to give birth to a **low birth weight** baby than a woman with appropriate nutritional intake.[3] An infant weighing less than 2,500 g (about 5.5 pounds) at birth is considered to be of low birth weight and an infant weighing less than 1,500 g (about 3.3 pounds) is termed very low birth weight. Both groups are at increased risk for infection, learning disabilities, impaired physical development, and death in the first year of life **(Figure 14.5)**. Many low- and very low birth weight babies are born **preterm**—that is, before 38 weeks' gestation. Others are born at term but are small for gestational age; in other words, they weigh less than would be expected. Although nutrition is not the only factor contributing to maturity and birth weight, its role cannot be overstated.

RECAP **A full-term pregnancy lasts from 38 to 42 weeks and is traditionally divided into trimesters lasting 13 to 14 weeks. During the first trimester, cells differentiate and divide rapidly to form the various tissues of the human body. Vulnerability to nutrient deficiencies, toxicities, and teratogens is highest during this trimester. The second and third trimesters are characterized by continued growth and maturation of organ systems. Nutrition is important before and throughout pregnancy to maintain the mother's health, support fetal development, and increase the likelihood that the baby will be born after 37 weeks and will weigh at least 5.5 pounds.**

How Much Weight Should a Pregnant Woman Gain?

Recommendations for weight gain vary according to a woman's weight *before* she became pregnant and whether she is expecting a single or multiple birth **(Table 14.1)**. The average recommended weight gain for women of normal pre-pregnancy weight is 25 to 35 pounds; underweight women should gain a little more than this amount,

TABLE 14.1 Recommended Weight Gain for Women During Pregnancy

Pre-Pregnancy Weight Status	Body Mass Index (kg/m^2)	Recommended Weight Gain (lb)
Normal	18.5–24.9	25–35
Underweight	<18.5	28–40
Overweight	25.0–29.9	15–25

gestation The period of intrauterine development from conception to birth.

low birth weight Having a weight of less than 5.5 pounds at birth.

preterm The birth of a baby prior to 38 weeks' gestation.

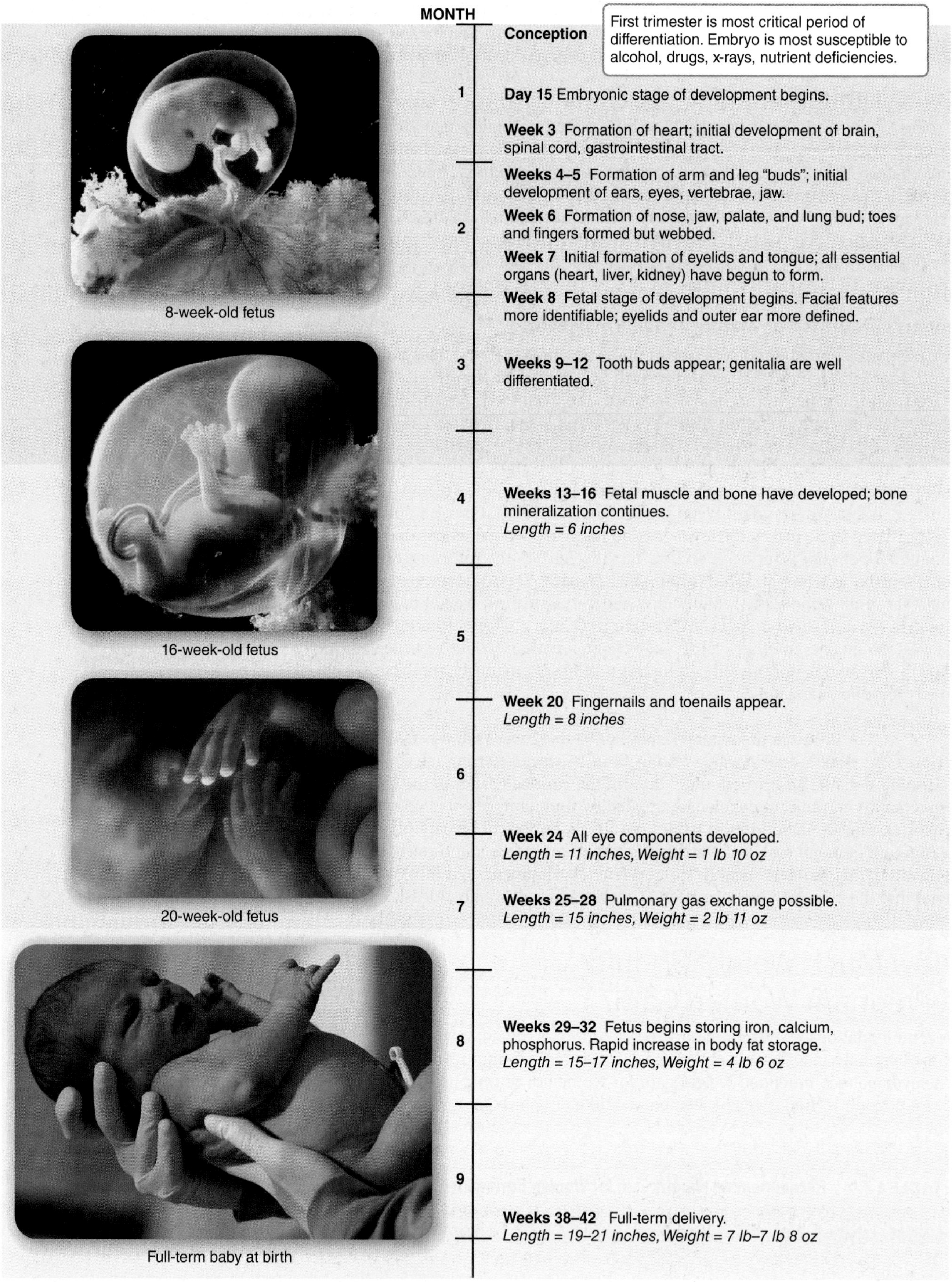

MONTH
Conception
First trimester is most critical period of differentiation. Embryo is most susceptible to alcohol, drugs, x-rays, nutrient deficiencies.
1
Day 15 Embryonic stage of development begins.
Week 3 Formation of heart; initial development of brain, spinal cord, gastrointestinal tract.
Weeks 4–5 Formation of arm and leg "buds"; initial development of ears, eyes, vertebrae, jaw.
2
Week 6 Formation of nose, jaw, palate, and lung bud; toes and fingers formed but webbed.
Week 7 Initial formation of eyelids and tongue; all essential organs (heart, liver, kidney) have begun to form.
Week 8 Fetal stage of development begins. Facial features more identifiable; eyelids and outer ear more defined.
8-week-old fetus
3
Weeks 9–12 Tooth buds appear; genitalia are well differentiated.
4
Weeks 13–16 Fetal muscle and bone have developed; bone mineralization continues.
Length = 6 inches
16-week-old fetus
5
Week 20 Fingernails and toenails appear.
Length = 8 inches
6
Week 24 All eye components developed.
Length = 11 inches, Weight = 1 lb 10 oz
7
Weeks 25–28 Pulmonary gas exchange possible.
Length = 15 inches, Weight = 2 lb 11 oz
20-week-old fetus
8
Weeks 29–32 Fetus begins storing iron, calcium, phosphorus. Rapid increase in body fat storage.
Length = 15–17 inches, Weight = 4 lb 6 oz
9
Weeks 38–42 Full-term delivery.
Length = 19–21 inches, Weight = 7 lb–7 lb 8 oz
Full-term baby at birth

Figure 14.4 A timeline of embryonic and fetal development.

activity among pregnant women, is an excellent low-impact choice. Women who were avid runners before pregnancy can often continue to run, although they may need to limit the distance and intensity of their runs.

RECAP About half of all pregnant women experience morning sickness. Heartburn and constipation in pregnancy are related to hormonal relaxation of smooth muscle. Gestational diabetes and hypertensive disorders can seriously affect maternal and fetal well-being. The nutrient needs of pregnant adolescents are so high that adequate nourishment becomes difficult. Women who follow a vegan diet usually need to consume supplements during pregnancy. Caffeine intake should be limited and the use of alcohol, cigarettes, and illegal drugs should be completely avoided during pregnancy. Safe food choices and handling practices are especially important during pregnancy. Exercise (provided the mother has no contraindications) can enhance the health of a pregnant woman.

NUTRI-CASE JUDY

"Back when I was pregnant with Hannah, the doctor told me I had gestational diabetes but said I shouldn't worry about it. He said I didn't need any medication, and I don't remember changing my diet. In fact, I just kept eating whatever I wanted, and by the time Hannah was born, I had gained almost 60 pounds. I never did lose all that extra weight."

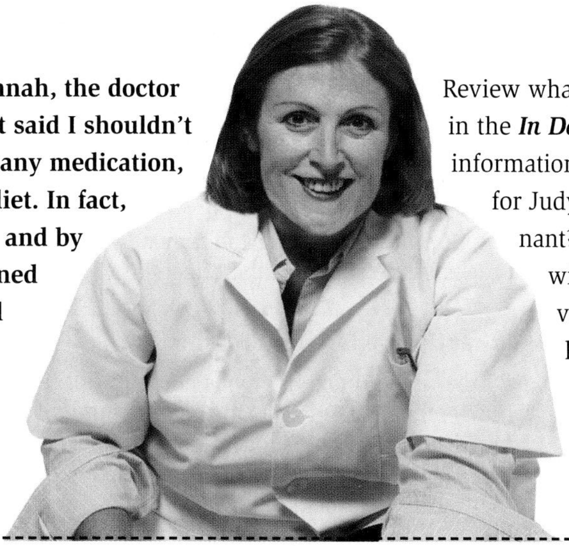

Review what you learned about diabetes in the ***In Depth*** on pages 137–141. What information would have been important for Judy to learn while she was pregnant? Is it common for women with gestational diabetes to develop type 2 diabetes years later? What are some things Judy could have done to lower her risk for type 2 diabetes?

Lactation: Nutrition for Breastfeeding Mothers

Throughout most of human history, infants have thrived on only one food: breast milk. But during the first half of the 20th century, commercially prepared infant formulas slowly began to replace breast milk as the mother's preferred feeding method. Aggressive marketing campaigns convinced many families, even in developing nations, to switch. Soon formula-feeding had become a status symbol, proof of the family's wealth and modern thinking. In the 1970s, this trend began to reverse with a renewed appreciation for the natural simplicity of breastfeeding. At the same time, several international organizations, including the World Health Organization, UNICEF, and La Leche League, began to promote the nutritional, immunologic, financial, and emotional advantages of breastfeeding and developed programs to encourage and support breastfeeding worldwide. These efforts have paid off: in 2005, almost 75% of new mothers initiated breastfeeding in the hospital and over 43% of mothers were still breastfeeding their babies at 6 months of age.[27] Worldwide, more than half of all women breastfeed exclusively for at least 6 months, but rates of initiation and continuation of breastfeeding vary greatly between countries. For example, rates of initiation of breastfeeding are extremely low in Eastern Europe and Central Asia, whereas the highest rates are in Latin America, the Caribbean, and Eastern and Northern Africa.[28]

How, exactly, does breastfeeding occur? What nutrients are important for breastfeeding mothers? And what exactly are the advantages that everyone is talking about? The answers to these questions are presented in the following sections.

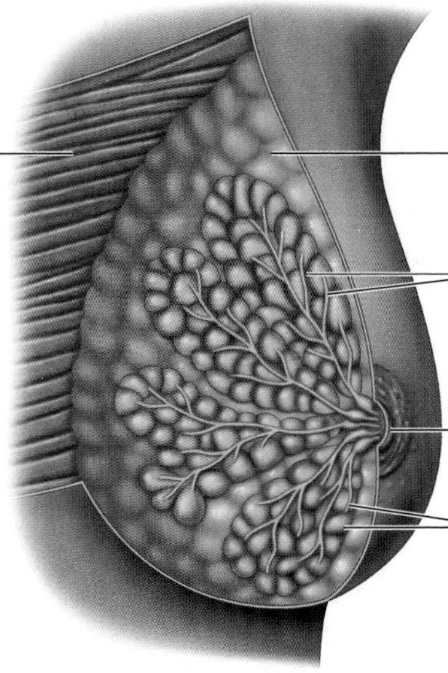

Figure 14.8 Anatomy of the breast. During pregnancy, estrogen and progesterone secreted by the placenta foster the preparation of breast tissue for lactation. This process includes breast enlargement and development of the milk-producing glands, or alveoli.

How Does Lactation Occur?

Lactation, the production of breast milk, is a process that is set in motion during pregnancy in response to several hormones. Once established, lactation can be sustained as long as the mammary glands continue to receive the proper stimuli.

The Body Prepares During Pregnancy

Throughout pregnancy, the placenta produces estrogen and progesterone. In addition to performing various functions to maintain the pregnancy, these hormones prepare the breasts physically for lactation. The breasts increase in size, and milk-producing glands (alveoli) and milk ducts are formed (**Figure 14.8**). Toward the end of pregnancy, the hormone *prolactin* increases. Prolactin is released by the anterior pituitary gland and is responsible for milk synthesis. However, estrogen and progesterone suppress the effects of prolactin during pregnancy.

What Happens After Childbirth

By the time a pregnancy has come to full term, the level of prolactin is about ten times higher than it was at the beginning of pregnancy. At birth, the suppressive effect of estrogen and progesterone ends, and prolactin is free to stimulate milk production. The first substance to be released is **colostrum,** sometimes called pre-milk or first milk. It is thick, yellowish in color, and rich in protein and micronutrients, and it includes antibodies that help protect the newborn from infection. Colostrum also contains a factor that fosters the growth of a particular species of "friendly" bacteria in the infant gastrointestinal tract. These bacteria in turn prevent the growth of other, potentially harmful bacteria. Finally, colostrum has a laxative effect in infants, helping the infant expel *meconium,* the sticky "first stool."

Within 2 to 4 days in most women, colostrum is fully replaced by mature milk. Mature breast milk contains protein, fat, and carbohydrate (in the form of the sugar lactose). Much of the protein and fat is synthesized in the breast, while the rest enters the milk from the mother's bloodstream.

Mother–Infant Interaction Maintains Milk Production

Continued, sustained breast milk production depends entirely on infant suckling (or a similar stimulus, such as a mechanical breast pump). Infant suckling stimulates the continued production of prolactin, which in turn stimulates more milk production. The longer and more vigorous the feeding, the more milk will be produced. Thus, even multiples (twins, triplets) can be successfully breastfed.

Prolactin allows for milk to be produced, but that milk has to move through the milk ducts to the nipple in order to reach the baby's mouth. The hormone responsible for this "let down" of milk is *oxytocin.* Like prolactin, oxytocin is produced by the pituitary gland, and its production is dependent on the suckling stimulus at the beginning of a feeding (**Figure 14.9**). This response usually occurs within 10 to 30 seconds but can be significantly inhibited by stress. Finding a relaxed environment in which to breastfeed is therefore important.

lactation The production of breast milk.

colostrum The first fluid made and secreted by the breasts from late in pregnancy to about a week after birth. It is rich in immune factors and protein.

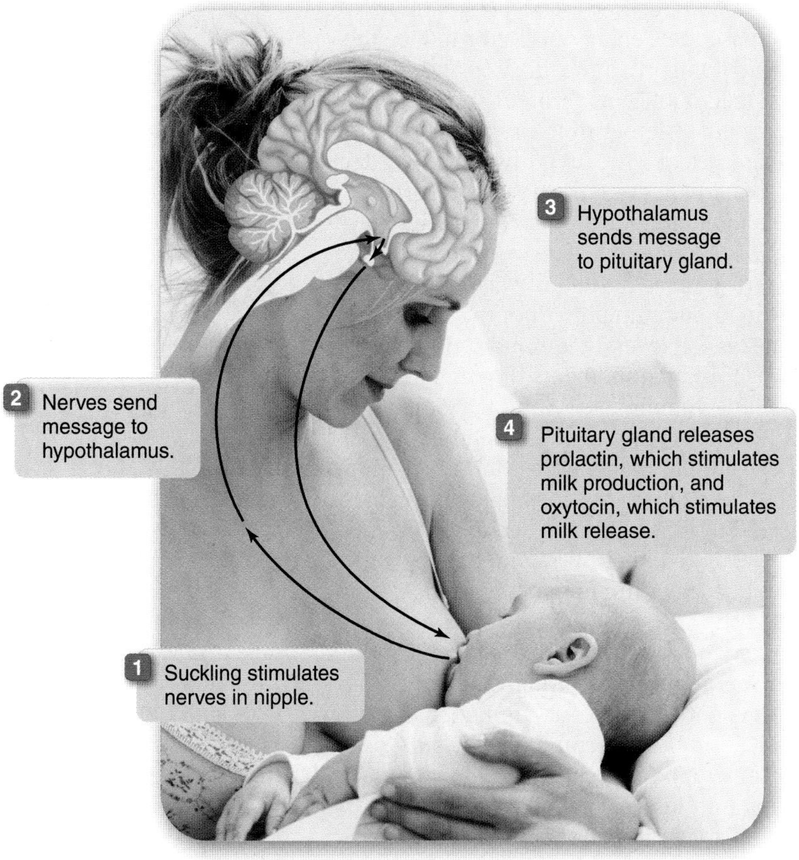

1 Suckling stimulates nerves in nipple.
2 Nerves send message to hypothalamus.
3 Hypothalamus sends message to pituitary gland.
4 Pituitary gland releases prolactin, which stimulates milk production, and oxytocin, which stimulates milk release.

Figure 14.9 Sustained milk production depends on the mother–child interaction during breastfeeding, specifically the suckling of the infant. Suckling stimulates the continued production of prolactin, which is responsible for milk production, and oxytocin, which is responsible for the letdown response.

What Are a Breastfeeding Woman's Nutrient Needs?

You might be surprised to learn that breastfeeding requires even more energy than pregnancy! This is because breast milk has to supply an adequate amount of all the nutrients an infant needs to grow and develop.

Nutrient Recommendations for Breastfeeding Women

It is estimated that milk production requires about 700 to 800 kcal/day. It is generally recommended that lactating women 19 and older consume 330 kcal/day above their pre-pregnancy energy needs during the first 6 months of lactation and 400 additional kcal/day during the second 6 months. This additional energy is sufficient to support adequate milk production. The remaining energy deficit will assist in the gradual loss of excess fat and body weight gained during pregnancy. It is critical that lactating women avoid severe energy restriction, as this practice can result in decreased milk production.

The weight loss that occurs during breastfeeding should be gradual, approximately 1 to 4 pounds per month. Both breastfeeding and participation in regular physical activity can assist with weight loss. The 2010 Dietary Guidelines for Americans confirm that neither occasional nor regular exercise negatively affects a woman's ability to breastfeed successfully. Some active women, however, may lose too much weight during breastfeeding and must either increase their energy intake or reduce their activity level to maintain health.

Of the macronutrients, protein and carbohydrate needs are different from pregnancy requirements. Increases of 15 to 20 g of protein per day and 80 g of carbohydrate per day above pre-pregnancy requirements are recommended during lactation. Women who breastfeed also need good dietary sources of the fatty acid DHA to support the rapid brain growth of the newborn.

The needs for several vitamins and minerals increase over the requirements of pregnancy. These include vitamins A, C, and E; riboflavin; vitamin B_{12}; biotin; and choline and the minerals copper, chromium, manganese, iodine, selenium, and zinc. The requirement for folate during lactation is 500 µg/day, which is decreased from the 600 µg/day required during pregnancy, but it is still higher than pre-pregnancy needs (400 µg/day).

Requirements for iron decrease significantly during lactation, to a mere 9 mg/day. This is because iron is not a significant component of breast milk, and breastfeeding usually suppresses menstruation for at least a few months, minimizing iron losses.

Calcium is a significant component of breast milk; however, as in pregnancy, calcium absorption is enhanced during lactation, and urinary loss of calcium is decreased. In addition, some calcium appears to come from the demineralization of the mother's bones, and increased dietary calcium does not prevent this. Thus, the recommended intake for calcium for a lactating woman is unchanged from pregnancy and non-pregnant guidelines—that is, 1,000 mg/day (for mothers over age 18). Because of their own continuing growth, however, teen mothers who are breastfeeding should continue to consume 1,300 mg/day. Typically, if calcium intake is adequate, a woman's bone density returns to normal shortly after lactation ends.

HOT TOPIC

Can a Mother Breastfeed Her Adopted Baby?

It might sound impossible, but it's not! Some women who wish to breastfeed their adopted baby have induced lactation by stimulating production of the hormones that naturally cause milk production and letdown. How? The most common method is to pump both breasts using a hospital-grade breast pump three times a day, beginning about 2 months before the expected adoption date. The woman's physician can also prescribe pharmaceutical estrogen, progesterone, or other medications that mimic the effects of pregnancy. If used, these are discontinued before breastfeeding begins, at which point the infant's suckling should stimulate and maintain milk production.[29]

MyPyramid For Moms
MyPyramid.gov

MyPyramid for Moms has specific dietary advice for women who are exclusively or partially breastfeeding their infants.

Do Breastfeeding Women Need Supplements?

If a breastfeeding woman appropriately increases her energy intake, and does so with nutrient-dense foods, her nutrient needs can usually be met without supplements. However, there is nothing wrong with taking a basic multivitamin for insurance, as long as it is not considered a substitute for proper nutrition. Lactating women should consume omega-3 fatty acids in either fish or supplements to increase the levels of DHA in their breast milk in order to support the infant's developing nervous system. Women who don't consume dairy products should monitor their calcium intake carefully.

Fluid Recommendations for Breastfeeding Women

Because extra fluid is expended with every feeding, lactating women need to consume about an extra quart (about 1 liter) of fluid per day. This extra fluid facilitates milk production and reduces risk for dehydration. Many women report that, within a minute or two of beginning to nurse their baby, they become intensely thirsty. To prevent this thirst and achieve the recommended fluid intake, women are encouraged to drink a nutritious beverage, such as water, juice, or milk, each time they nurse their baby. However, it is not good practice to drink hot beverages while nursing because accidental spills could burn the infant.

RECAP **Lactation is the result of the coordinated effort of several hormones, including estrogen, progesterone, prolactin, and oxytocin. Breasts are prepared for lactation during pregnancy, and infant suckling provides the stimulus that sustains the production of the prolactin and oxytocin needed to maintain the milk supply. It is recommended that lactating women consume an extra 300–400 kcal/day above pre-pregnancy energy intake, including increased protein, DHA, certain vitamins and minerals, and fluids. The requirements for folate and iron decrease from pregnancy levels, while the requirement for calcium remains the same.**

Getting Real About Breastfeeding: Advantages and Challenges

Breastfeeding is the perfect way to nourish a baby for its first 6 months of life. However, the technique does require patience and practice, and teaching by an experienced mother or a certified lactation consultant is important. La Leche League International (see Web Resources at the end of this chapter) and "Baby Friendly" hospitals can provide ongoing support and advice. For some women, illness, medication use, or other factors may make breastfeeding a difficult choice. The decision to breastfeed or use formula must be made by each family after careful consideration of all the factors that apply to their situation.

Advantages of Breastfeeding

As adept as formula manufacturers have been at simulating the components of breast milk, an exact replica has never been produced. In addition, there are benefits that mother and baby can access only through breastfeeding.[30]

Nutritional Quality of Breast Milk The amount and types of protein in breast milk are ideally suited to the human infant. The main protein in breast milk, lactalbumin, is easily digested in infants' immature gastrointestinal tracts, reducing the risk for gastric distress. Other proteins in breast milk bind iron and prevent the growth of harmful bacteria that require iron. Antibodies from the mother are additional proteins that help prevent infection while the infant's immune system is still immature. Certain proteins in human milk improve the absorption of iron; this is important, since breast milk is low in iron. Cow's milk contains too much protein for infants, and the types of protein in cow's milk are harder for the infant to digest.

The primary carbohydrate in milk is lactose, a disaccharide composed of glucose and galactose. The galactose component is important in nervous system development. Lactose provides energy and prevents ketosis in the infant, promotes the growth of beneficial bacteria, and increases the absorption of calcium. Breast milk has more lactose than cow's milk does, reinforcing the advantages of the breastfeeding process.

The amounts and types of fats in breast milk are ideally suited to the human infant. DHA and arachidonic acid (ARA) have been shown to be essential for growth and development of the infant's nervous system and for development of the retina of the eyes. Until 2002, these fatty acids were omitted from commercial infant formulas in the United States, although they have been available in formulas in other parts of the world for the better part of a decade. Interestingly, the concentration of DHA in breast milk varies considerably, reflecting the amount of DHA in the mother's diet, and is highest in women who regularly consume fish.

The fat content of breast milk, which is higher than that of whole cow's milk, changes according to the gestational age of the infant and during the course of every feeding: The milk that is initially released (called *foremilk*) is watery and low in fat,

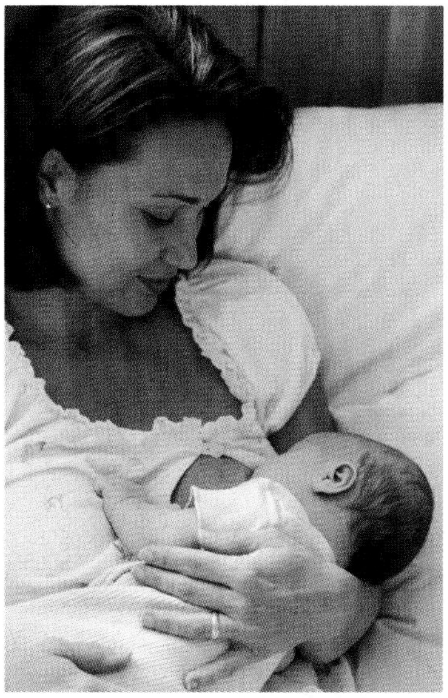

Breastfeeding has benefits for both the mother and her infant.

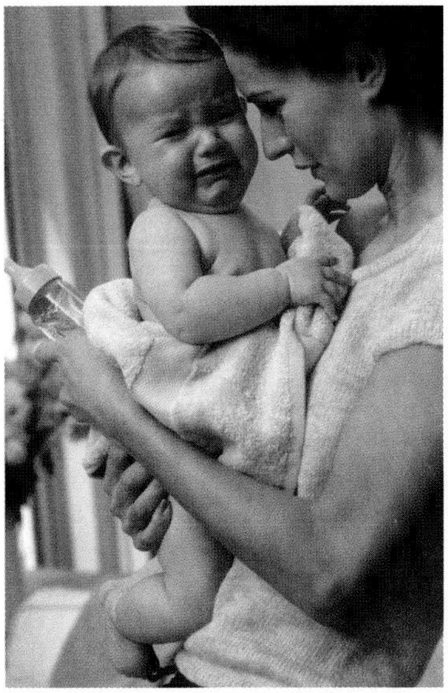

Some breastfed babies refuse to take a bottle.

somewhat like skim milk. This milk is thought to satisfy the infant's initial thirst. As the feeding progresses, the milk acquires more fat and becomes more like whole milk. Finally, the very last 5% or so of the milk produced during a feeding (called the *hindmilk*) is very high in fat, similar to cream. This milk is thought to satiate the infant. It is important to let infants suckle for at least 20 minutes at each feeding, so that they get this hindmilk. Breast milk is also relatively high in cholesterol, which supports the rapid growth and development of the brain.

Another important aspect of breastfeeding (or any type of feeding) is the fluid it provides the infant. Because of their small size, infants are at risk for dehydration, which is one reason feedings must be consistent and frequent. This topic will be discussed at greater length in the section on infant nutrition.

In terms of micronutrients, breast milk is a good source of readily absorbed calcium and magnesium. It is low in iron, but the iron it does contain is easily absorbed. Since healthy full-term infants store iron in preparation for the first few months of life, most experts agree that their iron needs can be met by breast milk alone for the first 6 months, after which iron-rich foods are needed. Although breast milk has some vitamin D, the American Academy of Pediatrics recommends that all breast-fed infants be provided a vitamin D supplement, particularly those infants with highly pigmented skin.[1]

Breast milk composition continues to change as the infant grows and develops. Because of this ability to change as the baby changes, breast milk alone is entirely sufficient to sustain infant growth for the first 6 months of life. In addition, exclusively breast-fed infants maintain total control over their food intake, allowing them to self-regulate energy intake during a critical period of growth and development. Some researchers believe this self-regulation accounts for the finding that breast-fed babies grow in length and weight at a slower rate than formula-fed infants. The relationship between breastfeeding and lifelong patterns of weight gain are explored in more detail in the Nutrition Debate at the end of this chapter.

Throughout the next 6 months of infancy, as solid foods are gradually introduced, breast milk remains the baby's primary source of superior-quality nutrition. The American Academy of Pediatrics recommends exclusive breastfeeding for the first 6 months of life, continuing breastfeeding for at least the first year of life, and, if acceptable within the family, into the second year of life.[31]

Protection from Infections, Allergies, and Residues Immune factors from the mother, including antibodies and immune cells, are passed directly from the mother to the newborn through breast milk. These factors provide important disease protection for the infant while its immune system is still immature. It has been shown that breast-fed infants have a lower incidence of respiratory tract, gastrointestinal tract, and urinary tract infections than formula-fed infants. Even a few weeks of breastfeeding is beneficial, but the longer a child is breastfed, the greater the level of passive immunity from the mother. In the United States, infant mortality rates are reduced by 21% in breast-fed infants.[31]

In addition, breast milk is nonallergenic, and breastfeeding is associated with a reduced risk for allergies during childhood and adulthood. Breast-fed babies also have fewer ear infections, die less frequently from **sudden infant death syndrome (SIDS)**, and have a decreased chance of developing diabetes, overweight and obesity, and chronic digestive disorders.

Exclusively breast-fed infants are also protected from exposure to known and unknown contaminants and residues that may be found in baby bottles and cans of infant formulas. Recent concerns have centered on bisphenol A (BPA), a toxic chemical that has been found in some brands of reusable bottles and formula cans. See the Hot Topic in Chapter 13, page 475.

sudden infant death syndrome (SIDS) The sudden death of a previously healthy infant; the most common cause of death in infants over 1 month of age.

Physiologic Benefits for Mother Breastfeeding causes uterine contractions, which quicken the return of the uterus to pre-pregnancy size and reduce bleeding. Many women also find that breastfeeding helps them lose the weight they gained during pregnancy, particularly if it continues for more than 6 months. In addition, breastfeeding appears to be associated with a decreased risk for breast cancer.[32] The relationship between breastfeeding and osteoporosis is still unclear, and more research on this topic is needed.[33]

Breastfeeding also suppresses ovulation, lengthening the time between pregnancies and giving a mother's body the chance to recover before she conceives again. This benefit can be life-saving for malnourished women living in countries that discourage or outlaw the use of contraceptives. Ovulation may not cease completely, however, so it is still possible to become pregnant while breastfeeding. Healthcare providers typically recommend the use of additional birth control methods while breastfeeding to avoid another conception occurring too soon to allow a mother's body to recover from the earlier pregnancy.

Mother–Infant Bonding Breastfeeding is among the most intimate of human interactions. Ideally, it is a quiet time away from distractions when mother and baby begin to develop an enduring bond of affection known as *attachment*. Breastfeeding enhances attachment by providing the opportunity for frequent, direct skin-to-skin contact, which stimulates the baby's sense of touch and is a primary means of communication. Most hospitals now permit round-the-clock rooming-in of breast-fed infants in order to optimize the initiation and continuation of breastfeeding. The cuddling and intense watching that occur during breastfeeding begin to teach the mother and baby about the other's behavioral cues. Breastfeeding also reassures the mother that she is providing the best possible nutrition for her baby.

Undoubtedly, bottle-feeding does not preclude parent–infant attachment! As long as attention is paid to closeness, cuddling, and skin and eye contact, bottle-feeding can foster bonding as well.

Convenience and Cost Breast milk is always ready, clean, at the right temperature, and available on demand, whenever and wherever it's needed. In the middle of the night, when the baby wakes up hungry, a breastfeeding mother can respond almost instantaneously, and both are soon back to sleep. In contrast, formula-feeding is a time-consuming process: parents have to continually wash and sterilize bottles, and each batch of formula must be mixed and heated to the proper temperature.

In addition, breastfeeding costs nothing other than the price of a modest amount of additional food for the mother. In contrast, formula can be relatively expensive, and there are the additional costs of bottles and other supplies, as well as the cost of energy used for washing and sterilization. A hidden cost of formula-feeding is its effect on the environment: the energy used and waste produced during formula manufacturing, marketing, shipping and distribution, preparation, and disposal of used packaging. In contrast, breastfeeding is environmentally responsible, using no external energy and producing no external wastes.

Challenges Associated with Breastfeeding

For some women and infants, breastfeeding is easy from the very first day. Others experience some initial difficulty, but with support from an experienced nurse, lactation consultant, or volunteer mother from La Leche League, the experience becomes successful and pleasurable. In contrast, some families encounter difficulties that make formula-feeding their best choice. This section discusses some challenges that may impede the success of breastfeeding.

Effects of Drugs and Other Substances on Breast Milk Many substances, including illegal, prescription, and over-the-counter drugs, pass into breast milk. Breastfeeding mothers should inform their physician that they are breastfeeding. If a safe and effective form of a necessary medication cannot be found, the mother will have to avoid breastfeeding while she is taking the drug. During this time, she can pump and discard her breast milk, so that her milk supply will be adequate when she resumes breastfeeding.

Caffeine, alcohol, and nicotine also enter breast milk. Caffeine can make the baby agitated and fussy, whereas alcohol can make the baby sleepy, depress the central nervous system, and slow motor development, in addition to inhibiting the mother's milk supply. Women who are breastfeeding should abstain from alcohol, since it easily passes into the breast milk at levels equal to blood alcohol concentrations. Nicotine also passes into breast milk; therefore, it is best for the woman to quit smoking altogether.

Environmental contaminants, including pesticides, industrial solvents, dioxins, and heavy metals (such as lead and mercury), can pass into breast milk when breastfeeding mothers are exposed to these chemicals. Mothers can limit their infants' exposure to these harmful substances by controlling their own environments. Fresh fruits and vegetables should be thoroughly washed and peeled to minimize exposure to pesticides and fertilizer residues. Exposure to paint fumes, gasoline, solvents, and similar products should be greatly limited. Even with some exposure to these environmental contaminants, U.S. and international health agencies all agree that the benefits of breastfeeding almost always outweigh potential concerns.[34]

Food components that pass into the breast milk may seem innocuous; however, some substances, such as those found in garlic, onions, peppers, broccoli, and cabbage, are distasteful enough to the infant to prevent proper feeding. Some babies have allergic reactions to foods the mother has eaten, such as wheat, cow's milk, eggs, or citrus, and suffer gastrointestinal upset, diaper rash, or another reaction. The offending foods must then be identified and avoided.

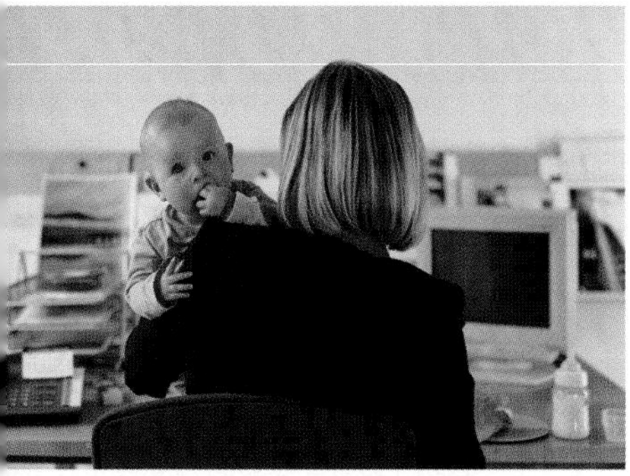

Working moms can be discouraged from—or supported in—breastfeeding in a variety of ways.

Maternal HIV Infection HIV, which causes AIDS, can be transmitted from mother to baby through breast milk. Thus, HIV-positive women in the United States and Canada are encouraged to feed their infants formula. This recommendation does not apply to all women worldwide, however, since the low cost and sanitary nature of breast milk, as compared to the potential for waterborne diseases with formula-feeding, often make breastfeeding the best choice for women in developing countries, even among populations with high rates of HIV infection and exposure.[35]

Conflict Between Breastfeeding and the Mother's Employment Breast milk is absorbed more readily than formula, making more frequent feedings necessary. Newborns commonly require breastfeedings every 1 to 3 hours versus every 2 to 4 hours for formula-feedings. Mothers who are exclusively breastfeeding and return to work within the first 6 months after the baby's birth must leave several bottles of pumped breast milk for others to feed the baby in their absence each day. This means that working women have to pump their breasts to express the breast milk during the workday. This can be a challenge in companies that do not provide the time, space, and privacy required.

Work-related travel is also a concern: if the mother needs to be away from home for longer than 24 to 48 hours, she can typically pump and freeze enough breast milk for others to give the baby in her absence. When longer business trips are required, some mothers take the baby with them and arrange for childcare at their destination. Others resort to pumping, freezing, and shipping breast milk home via overnight mail. Understandably, many women cite returning to work as the reason they switch to formula-feeding.[36]

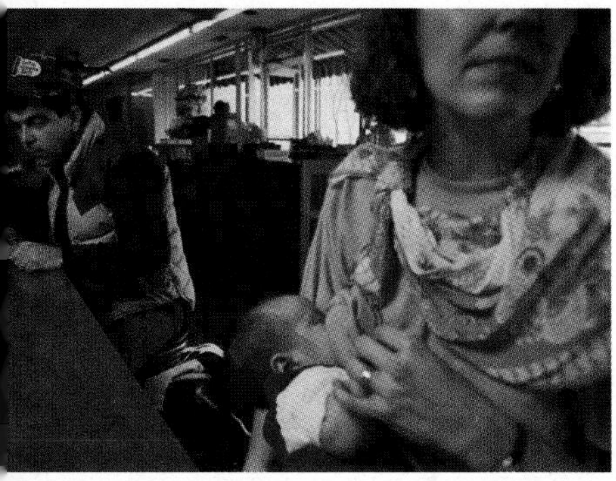

Although a much more common practice today than in the past, breastfeeding in public can still meet with disapproval.

Some working women successfully combine breastfeeding with commercial formula-feeding. For example, a woman might breastfeed in the morning before she leaves for work, as soon as she returns home, and once again before retiring at night. The remainder of the feedings are formula given by the infant's father or a childcare provider. Women who choose supplemental formula-feedings usually find that their bodies adapt quickly to the change and produce ample milk for the remaining breastfeedings.

Social Concerns In North America, women have been conditioned to keep their breasts covered in public, even when feeding an infant. However, public places are beginning to be more accommodating for nursing mothers. For example, separate nursing rooms can often be found adjacent to, but not within, public restrooms. Some states have passed legislation preserving a woman's right to breastfeed in public. Special nursing clothing or judicious placement of a scarf or shawl allows women to breastfeed discreetly. When women feel free to breastfeed in public, the baby's feeding schedule becomes much less confining.

What About Bonding for Fathers and Siblings?

With all the attention given to attachment between a breastfeeding mother and her infant, it is easy for fathers and siblings to feel left out. One option that allows other family members to participate in infant feeding is to supplement breastfeedings with bottle-feedings of stored breast milk or formula. If a family decides to share infant feeding in this manner, bottle-feedings can begin as soon as breastfeeding has become well established. That way, the infant will not become confused by the artificial nipple. Fathers and other family members can also bond with the infant when bathing and/or clothing the infant, as well as through everyday cuddling and play.

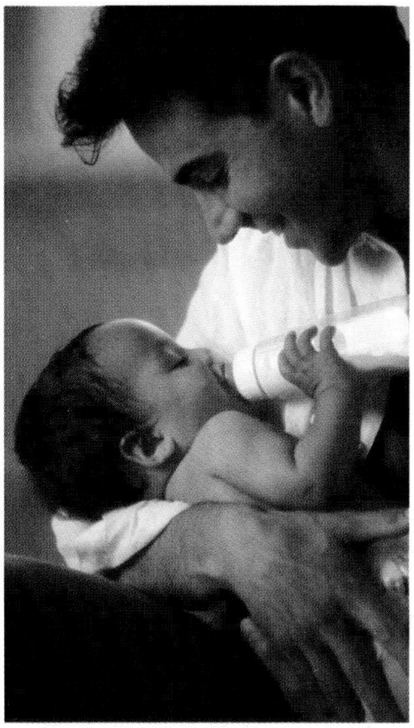

Fathers and siblings can bond with infants through bottle-feeding and other forms of close contact.

RECAP **Breastfeeding provides many benefits to both mother and newborn, including superior nutrition, heightened immunity, mother–infant bonding, convenience, and cost. However, breastfeeding may not be the best option for every family. The mother may need to use a medication that enters the breast milk and makes it unsafe for consumption. A mother's job may interfere with the baby's requirement for frequent feedings. The infant's father and siblings can participate in feedings using a bottle filled with either pumped breast milk or formula.**

Infant Nutrition: From Birth to 1 Year

Most first-time parents are amazed at how rapidly their infant grows. Optimal nutrition is extremely important during the first year, as the baby's organs and nervous system continue to develop and the baby grows physically. In fact, physicians use length and weight measurements as the main tools for assessing an infant's nutritional status. These measurements are plotted on growth charts (there are separate charts for boys and girls), which track an infant's growth over time (**Figure 14.10**). Although every infant is unique, in general, physicians look for a correlation between length and weight. In other words, an infant who is in the 60th percentile for length is usually in about the 50th to 70th percentile for weight. An infant who is in the 90th percentile for weight but is in the 20th percentile for length might be overfed. Consistency over time is also a consideration: for example, an infant who suddenly drops well below her established profile for weight might be underfed or ill.

Typical Infant Growth and Activity Patterns

Babies' basal metabolic rates are high, in part because their body surface area is large compared to their body size. Still, their limited physical activity keeps total energy expenditure relatively low. For the first few months of life, an infant's activities consist mainly of eating and sleeping. As the first year progresses, the repertoire of activity gradually expands to include rolling over, sitting up, crawling, standing, and finally taking the first few wobbly steps. Nevertheless, relatively few Calories are expended in movement, and the primary use of energy is to support growth.

In the first year of life, an infant generally grows about 10 inches in length and triples in weight—a growth rate more rapid than will ever occur again. Not surprisingly, energy needs per unit body weight are also the highest they will ever be in order to support this phenomenal growth and metabolism.

Part of the rapid growth of an infant involves the brain, the growth of which is more rapid during the first year than at any other time. To accommodate such a large increase in brain size, infants' heads are typically quite large in proportion to the rest of their body. Pediatricians use head circumference as an additional tool for the assessment of growth and nutritional status. After around 18 months of age, the rate of brain growth slows, and gradually the body "catches up" to head size.

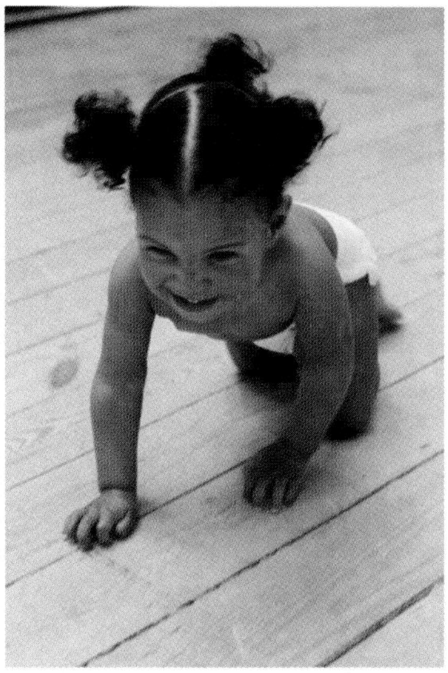

An infant's physical activity will progress beyond crawling before the first year of life is over.

Nutrient Needs for Infants

Three characteristics of infants combine to make their nutritional needs unique: (1) their high energy needs per unit body weight to support rapid growth, (2) their immature digestive tract and kidneys, and (3) their small size.

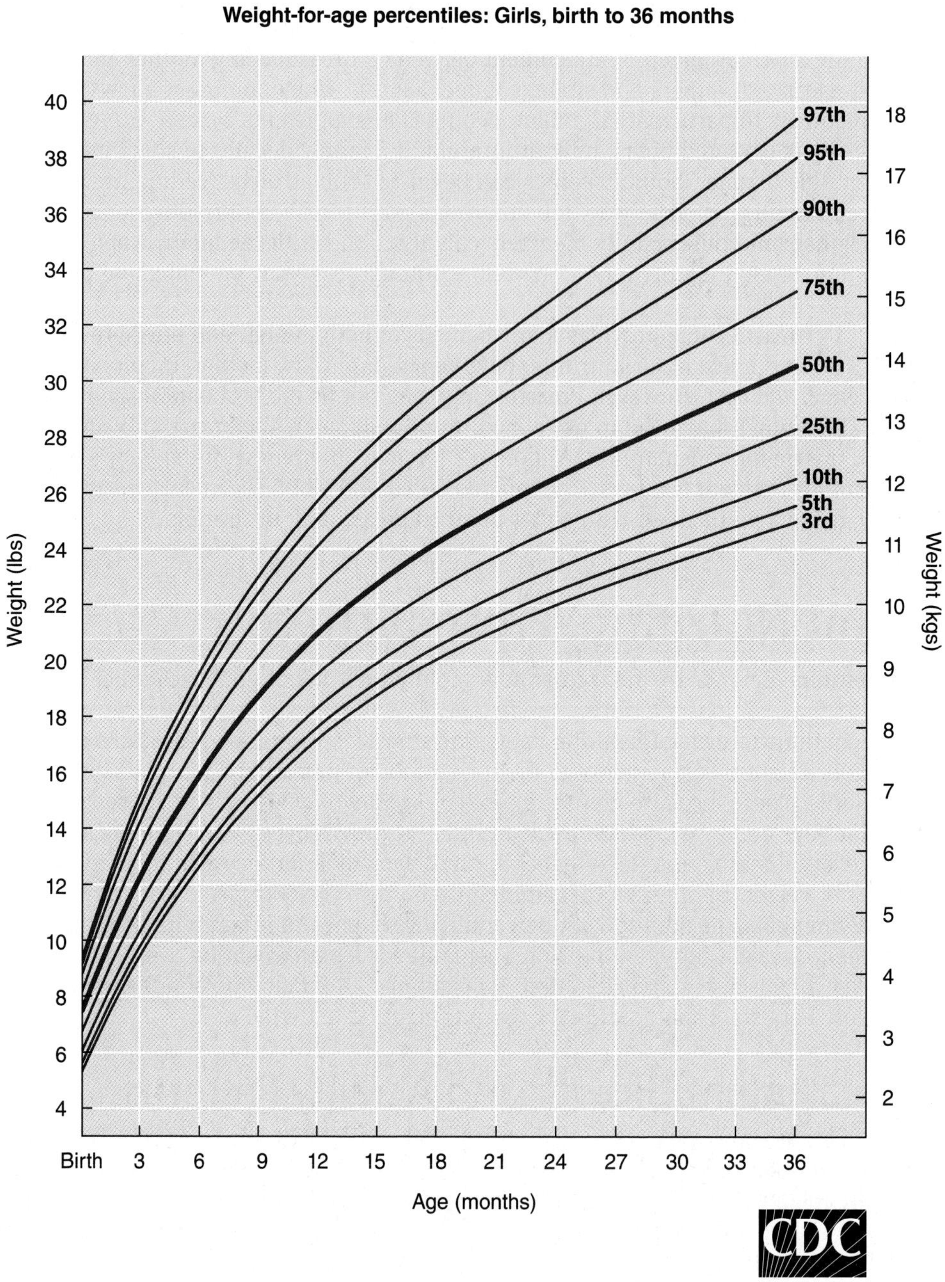

Figure 14.10 This weight-for-age growth chart is a much smaller version of charts used by healthcare practitioners to monitor and assess the growth of an infant/toddler from birth to 36 months. This example shows the growth curves of girls over time, each at different percentiles.

Data from the National Center for Health Statistics in collaboration with the National Center for Chronic Disease Prevention and Health Promotion, 2000, www.cdc.gov/growthcharts/data/set1clinical/cj411018.pdf.

Macronutrient Needs of Infants

An infant needs to consume about 40–50 kcal/lb of body weight per day. This amounts to about 600–650 kcal/day at around 6 months of age. Given the immature digestive tract and kidneys of infants, as well as their high fluid needs, providing this much energy may seem difficult. Fortunately, breast milk and commercial formulas are energy dense, contributing about 650 kcal/quart of fluid. When solid foods are introduced after about 4 to 6 months of age, they provide even more energy in addition to the breast milk or formula.

Infants are not merely small versions of adults. The proportions of macronutrients they require differ from adult proportions, as do the types of food they can tolerate. It is generally agreed that about 40–50% of an infant's energy should come from fat during the first year of life and that fat intake below this level can be harmful before the age of 2. Given the high energy needs of infants, it makes sense to take advantage of the energy density of fat (9 kcal/g) to help meet these requirements. Breast milk and commercial formulas are both high in fat (about 50% of total energy). In addition, specific fatty acids are essential for the rapid brain growth and nervous system development that happens in the first 1 to 2 years of life. Breast milk is an excellent source of the fatty acids arachidonic acid (AA) and docosahexaenoic acid (DHA), although DHA levels vary considerably with the mother's diet. Many formula manufacturers now add AA and DHA to their products.

Infants 0 to 6 months of age need approximately 9 g of protein/day, while infants 7 to 12 months need almost 10 g/day. These amounts accommodate an infant's rapid growth. Infants have immature kidneys, which are not able to process and excrete the excess nitrogen groups from higher-protein diets; thus, no more than 20% of an infant's daily energy requirement should come from protein. Breast milk and commercial formulas both provide adequate total protein and appropriate essential amino acids to support growth and development.

The recommended intake for carbohydrate is set at 60 g/day for infants 0 to 6 months of age and 95 g/day for infants 7 to 12 months old. These levels reflect the lactose content of human milk, which is used as the reference point for most infant nutrient guidelines.

Micronutrient Needs of Infants

Infants need micronutrients to accommodate their rapid growth and development. The micronutrients of particular concern are iron, vitamin D, zinc, fluoride, and iodide. Fortunately, breast milk and commercial formulas provide most of the micronutrients needed for infant growth and development, with some special considerations, discussed shortly.

In addition, all infants are routinely given an injection of vitamin K shortly after birth. This provides vitamin K until the infant's intestine can develop its own healthful bacteria, which then contribute to the infant's supply of vitamin K.

Do Infants Need Supplements?

Breast milk and commercial formulas provide most of the vitamins and minerals infants need. However, several micronutrients may warrant supplementation. For breast-fed infants, a supplement containing vitamin D is commonly prescribed from birth to around 6 months of age, even in sunny climates, because exposure of a young infant's skin to adequate direct sunlight for vitamin D synthesis is not advised.[37] Vitamin D deficiency is actually quite common among U.S. infants with dark skin and those with limited sunlight exposure.[1] Breast-fed infants also require additional iron beginning no later than 6 months of age because the infant's iron stores become depleted and breast milk is a poor source of iron. Iron is extremely important for cognitive development and prevention of iron-deficiency anemia. Starting solid foods (infant rice cereal) fortified with iron at 4 to 6 months of age can serve as an additional iron source. In addition, if the mother is a vegan, her breast milk may be low in vitamin B_{12}, and a supplement of this vitamin should be given to the baby. Fluoride is important for strong tooth development, but fluoride supplementation is not recommended during the first 6 months of life.

For formula-fed infants, supplementation depends on the formula composition and the water supply used to make the formula. Many formulas are already fortified with iron, for example, and some municipal water supplies contain fluoride. If this is the case, and the baby is getting adequate vitamin D, then an extra supplement may not be necessary.

If a supplement is given, the dose should be considered carefully. The supplement should be formulated specifically for infants, and the daily dose should not be exceeded. High doses of micronutrients can be dangerous. Too much iron can be

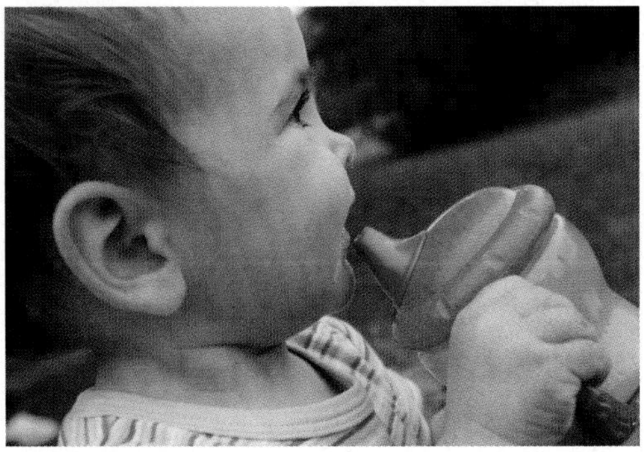

Infants are at high risk for dehydration, but breast milk and formula are almost always adequate to meet their fluid needs.

fatal, too much fluoride can cause discoloration and pitting of the teeth, and too much vitamin D can lead to calcification of soft tissue, such as the kidneys.

Fluid Recommendations for Infants

Fluid is critical for everyone, but for infants the balance is more delicate for two reasons. First, because infants are so small, they proportionally lose more water through evaporation than adults. Second, their kidneys are immature and unable to concentrate urine. Hence, they are at even greater risk for dehydration. An infant needs about 2 oz of fluid per pound of body weight, and either breast milk or formula is almost always enough to provide this amount. Experts recently confirmed that "infants exclusively fed human milk do not require supplemental water."[12] However, certain conditions, such as diarrhea, vomiting, fever, or hot weather, can greatly increase fluid loss. In these instances, supplemental fluid, ideally as water, may be necessary. Since too much fluid can be particularly dangerous for an infant, supplemental fluids (whether water or an infant electrolyte formula) should be given only under the advice of a physician. Generally, it is advised that supplemental fluids not exceed 4 oz per day, and parents should avoid giving sugar water, fruit juices, or any sweetened beverage in a bottle. Parents can be sure that their infant's fluid intake is appropriate if the infant produces six to eight wet diapers per day.

What Types of Formula Are Available?

We discussed the advantages of breastfeeding earlier in this chapter, and indeed both national and international healthcare organizations consider breastfeeding the best choice for infant nutrition, when possible. However, if breastfeeding is not feasible, several types of commercial formulas provide nutritious alternatives. By law, formula manufacturers must meet minimum and maximum standards for 29 different nutrients.

Most formulas are based on cow's milk proteins, casein and whey, that have been modified to make them more appropriate for human infants. The sugars lactose and sucrose, alone or in combination, provide carbohydrates, and vegetable oils and/or microbiologically produced fatty acids provide the fat component. Recently, some manufacturers have added other nutrients, such as the fatty acids AA and DHA, to more closely mimic the nutrient profile of human milk. This chapter's Nutrition Label Activity gives you the opportunity to review some of these ingredients.

Soy-based formulas are a viable alternative for infants who are lactose intolerant (although this is rare in infants) or cannot tolerate the proteins in cow's milk–based formulas. Soy formulas may also satisfy the requirements of families who are strict vegans. However, soy-based formulas are not without controversy. Because soy contains isoflavones, or plant forms of estrogens, there is some concern over the effects these compounds have on growing infants. Babies can also have allergic reactions to soy-based formulas.[38] Soy-based formulas are not the same as soy milk, which is not suitable for infant feeding.

There are specialized formula preparations for specific medical conditions. Some contain proteins that have been predigested, for example, or have compositions designed to accommodate certain diseases. Some have been specially formulated for preterm infants, older infants, and toddlers. The final choice of formula should depend on infant tolerance, stage of infant development, cost, and the advice of the infant's pediatrician. It is important to note that the use of cow's milk (fresh, dried, evaporated, or condensed) is inappropriate for infants under the age of 1 year, as is the use of goat's milk.

When Do Infants Begin to Need Solid Foods?

Infants begin to need solid, or complementary, foods at around 6 months of age. Before this age, several factors make most infants unable to consume solid food.

NUTRITION LABEL ACTIVITY

Reading Infant Food Labels

Imagine that you are a new parent shopping for infant formula. **Figure 14.11** shows the label from a typical can of formula. As you can see, the ingredients list is long and has many technical terms. Even well-informed parents would probably be stumped by many of them. Fortunately, with the information you learned in previous chapters, you can probably answer the following questions.

Figure 14.11 An infant formula label. Notice that there is a long list of ingredients and no % Daily Value.

- The first ingredient listed is a modified form of *whey protein*. What common food is the source of whey?
- The fourth ingredient listed is *lactose*. Is lactose a form of protein, fat, or carbohydrate? Why is it important for infants?
- The front label states that the formula has a blend of *docosahexaenoic acid (DHA)* and *arachidonic acid (ARA)*. Are DHA and ARA forms of protein, fat, or carbohydrate? Why are these two nutrients thought to be important for infants?

The label also claims that this formula is "Our Closest Formula to Breast Milk." Can you think of some differences between breast milk and this formula that still exist?

Look at the list of nutrients on the label. You'll notice that there is no "% Daily Value" column, which you see on most food labels. The next time you are at the grocery store, look at other baby food items, such as baby cereal or pureed fruits. Do their labels simply list the nutrient content or is the "% Daily Value" column used? Why do you think infant formula has a different label format?

Let's say you are feeding a 6-month-old infant who needs about 500 kcal/day. Using the information from the nutrition section of the label, you can calculate the number of fluid ounces of formula the baby needs (this assumes that no cereal or other foods are eaten):

There are 100 kcal (Calories) per 5 fl. oz.

$$100 \text{ kcal} \div 5 \text{ fl. oz} = 20 \text{ kcal/fl. oz}$$

$$500 \text{ kcal} \div 20 \text{ kcal/fl. oz} = 25 \text{ fl. oz of formula}$$

per day to meet the baby's energy needs

A 6-month-old infant needs about 210 mg calcium per day. Based on an intake of 25 fl. oz of formula per day, as just calculated, you can use the label nutrition information to calculate the amount of calcium that is provided:

There are 78 mg calcium per 5 fl. oz serving of formula.

$$78 \text{ mg} \div 5 \text{ fl. oz} = 15.6 \text{ mg calcium per fl. oz}$$

$$15.6 \text{ mg calcium per fl. oz} \times 25 \text{ fl. oz} = 390 \text{ mg of calcium per day}$$

You can see that the infant's need for calcium is easily met by the formula alone.

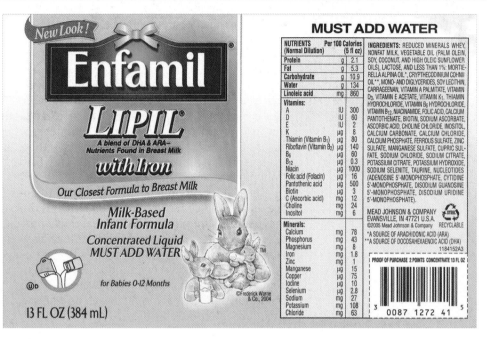

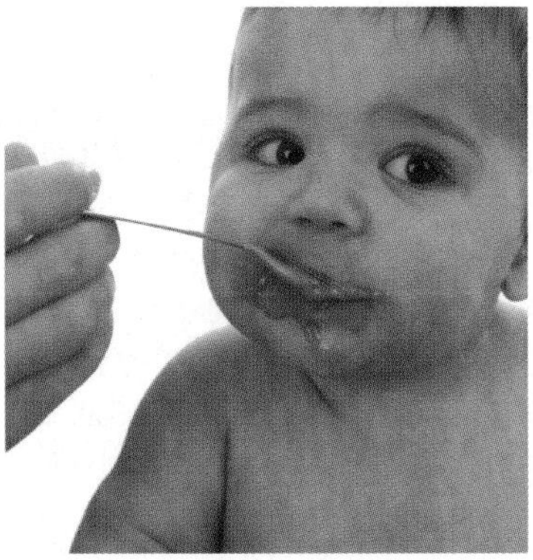

The extrusion reflex will push solid food out of an infant's mouth.

One factor is the *extrusion reflex*. During infant feeding, the suckling response depends on a particular movement of the tongue that draws liquid out of the breast or bottle. But when solid foods are introduced with a spoon, this tongue movement (the extrusion reflex) causes the baby to push most of the food back out of the mouth. The extrusion reflex begins to lessen around 4 to 5 months of age.

Another factor is muscle development. To minimize the risk for choking, the infant must have gained muscular control of the head and neck and be able to sit up (with or without support).

Still another part of being ready for solid foods is sufficient maturity of the digestive and kidney systems. While infants can digest and absorb lactose from birth, the ability to digest starch does not fully develop until the age of 3 to 4 months. If an infant is fed cereal, for example, before he can digest the starch, diarrhea and discomfort may develop. In addition, early introduction of solid foods can lead to improper absorption of intact, undigested proteins, setting the stage for allergies. Finally, the kidneys must have matured so that they are better able to process nitrogen wastes from proteins and concentrate urine.

The need for solid foods is also related to nutrient needs. At about 6 months of age, infant iron stores become depleted; thus, iron-fortified infant cereals are often the first foods introduced. Rice cereal rarely provokes an allergic response and is easy to digest. Once a child reaches 6 months of age, other single-grain cereals, strained vegetables, fruits, and protein sources can gradually be incorporated into the diet.

Infant foods should be introduced one at a time, with no other new foods for about 1 week, so that parents can watch for signs of allergies, such as a rash, gastrointestinal problems, a runny nose, or wheezing. Gradually, a variety of foods should be introduced by the end of the first year. Commercial baby foods are convenient, nutritious, and typically made without added salt or sugar; however, home-prepared baby foods are usually cheaper and reflect the cultural food patterns of the family. Throughout the first year, solid foods should only be a supplement to, not a substitute for, breast milk or iron-fortified formula. Infants still need the nutrient density and energy that breast milk and formula provide.

What *Not* to Feed an Infant

The following foods should never be offered to an infant:

- *Foods that can cause choking.* Infants cannot adequately chew foods such as grapes, hot dogs, nuts, popcorn, raw carrots, raisins, and hard candies. These can cause choking.
- *Corn syrup and honey.* These may contain spores of the bacterium *Clostridium botulinum*. These spores can germinate and grow into viable bacteria in the immature digestive tract of infants, whereupon they produce a potent toxin, which can be fatal. Children older than 1 year can safely consume these substances because their digestive tract is mature enough to kill any *C. botulinum* bacteria.
- *Goat's milk.* Goat's milk is notoriously low in many nutrients that infants need, such as folate, vitamin C, vitamin D, and iron.
- *Cow's milk.* For children under 1 year, cow's milk is too concentrated in minerals and protein and contains too few carbohydrates to meet infant energy needs. Infants can begin to consume whole cow's milk after the age of 1 year. Infants and toddlers should not be given reduced-fat cow's milk before the age of 2, as it does not contain enough fat and is too high in mineral content for the kidneys to handle effectively. Infants should not be given evaporated milk or sweetened condensed milk.
- *Too much salt and sugar.* Infant foods should not be seasoned with salt or other seasonings. Naturally occurring sugars, such as those found in fruits, can provide needed energy. Cookies, cakes, and other excessively sweet, processed foods should be avoided.
- *Too much breast milk or formula.* As nutritious as breast milk and formula are, once infants reach the age of 6 months, solid foods should be introduced gradually. Six months of age is a critical time; it is when a baby's iron stores begin to be

depleted. Over-reliance on breast milk or formula can limit the infant's intake of iron-rich foods, resulting in a condition known as *milk anemia*. In addition, infants are physically and psychologically ready to eat solid foods at this time, and solid foods can help appease their increasing appetites. Between 6 months and the time of weaning (from breast or bottle), solid foods should gradually make up an increasing proportion of the infant's diet.

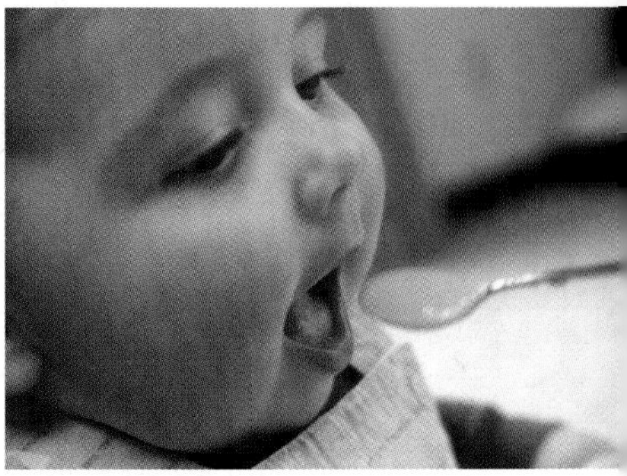

Early introduction of solid foods may play a role in the development of food allergies, especially if infants are introduced to highly allergenic foods early on.

Nutrition-Related Concerns for Infants

Nutrition is one of the biggest concerns of new parents. Infants cannot speak, and their cries are sometimes indecipherable. Feeding time can be very frustrating for parents, especially if the child is not eating, is not growing appropriately, or has problems such as diarrhea, vomiting, or persistent skin rashes. The following are some nutrition-related concerns for infants.

Allergies

Many foods have the potential to stimulate an allergic reaction (see pages 101–103). Breastfeeding helps deter allergy development, as does delaying the introduction of solid foods until the age of 6 months. One of the most common allergies in infants is to the proteins in cow's milk–based formulas. Egg whites, peanuts, and wheat are other common triggers of food allergies. Symptoms vary but may include gastrointestinal distress, such as diarrhea, constipation, bloating, blood in the stool, and vomiting. As stated earlier, every food should be introduced in isolation, so that any allergic reaction can be identified and the offending food avoided.

Dehydration

Whether the cause is diarrhea, vomiting, or inadequate fluid intake, dehydration is extremely dangerous to infants and, if left untreated, can quickly result in death. The factors behind infants' increased risk for dehydration were discussed on pages 528–529. Treatment includes providing fluids, a task that is difficult if vomiting is occurring. In some cases, the physician may recommend that a pediatric electrolyte solution be administered on a temporary basis. In more severe cases, hospitalization may be necessary. If possible, breastfeeding should continue throughout an illness. A physician should be consulted concerning formula-feeding and solid foods.

Colic

Perhaps nothing is more frustrating to new parents than the relentless crying spells of some infants, typically referred to as **colic.** In this condition, newborns and young infants who appear happy, healthy, and well nourished suddenly begin to cry or even shriek, continuing for several minutes to 3 hours or more, no matter what their caregiver does to console them. The spells tend to occur at the same time of day, typically late in the afternoon or early in the evening, and often occur daily for a period of several weeks. Overstimulation of the nervous system, feeding too rapidly, swallowing of air, and intestinal gas pain are considered possible culprits, but the precise cause is unknown.

As with allergies, if a colicky infant is breastfed, breastfeeding should be continued, but the mother should try to determine whether eating certain foods seems to prompt crying and, if so, eliminate the offending food(s) from her diet. Formula-fed infants may benefit from a change in type of formula. In the worst cases of colic, a physician may prescribe medication. Fortunately, most cases disappear spontaneously, possibly because of the maturity of the gastrointestinal tract, around 3 months of age.

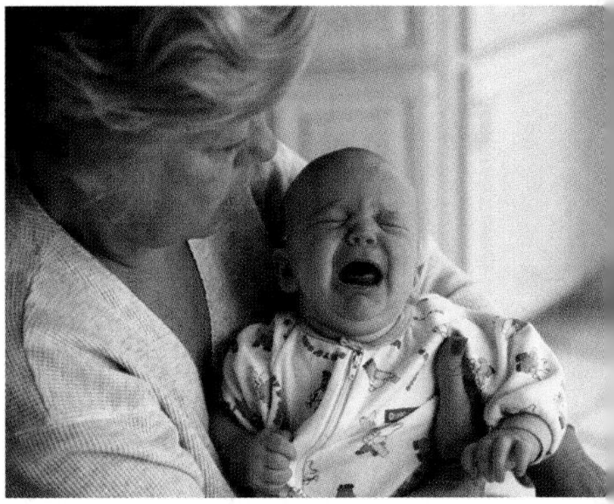

Colicky babies will begin crying for no apparent reason, even if they otherwise appear well nourished and happy.

Anemia

As stated earlier, full-term infants are born with sufficient iron stores to last for approximately the first 6 months of life. In older infants and toddlers, however, iron is

colic A condition of inconsolable infant crying that lasts for hours at a time.

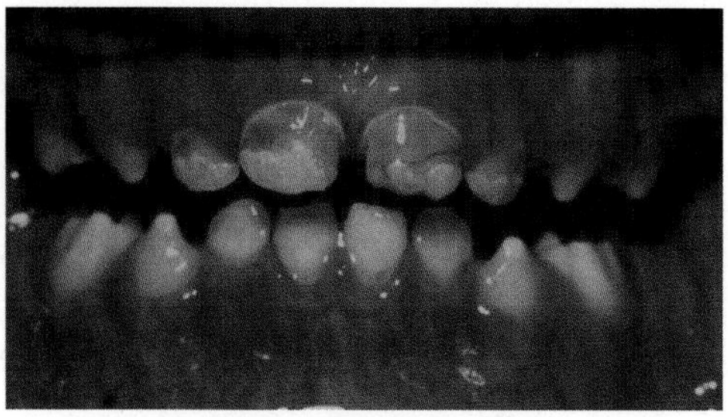

Figure 14.12 Leaving a baby alone with a bottle can result in the tooth decay of nursing bottle syndrome.

the mineral most likely to be deficient. Iron-deficiency anemia causes pallor, lethargy, and impaired growth. Iron-fortified formula is a good source for formula-fed infants. Some pediatricians prescribe a supplement containing iron especially formulated for infants. Iron for older infants is typically supplied by iron-fortified rice cereal.

Nursing Bottle Syndrome

Infants should not be left alone with a bottle, whether lying down or sitting up. As infants manipulate the nipple of the bottle in their mouth, the high-carbohydrate fluid (whether breast milk, formula, or fruit juice) drips out, coming into prolonged contact with the developing teeth. This high-carbohydrate fluid provides an optimal food source for the bacteria that are the underlying cause of **dental caries** (cavities). Severe tooth decay can result (**Figure 14.12**). Encouraging the use of a cup around the age of 8 months helps prevent nursing bottle syndrome, along with weaning the baby from a bottle entirely by the age of 15 to 18 months.

Lead Poisoning

Lead is especially toxic to infants and children because their brain and central nervous system are still developing. Lead poisoning can result in decreased mental capacity, behavioral problems, impaired growth, impaired hearing, and other problems. Unfortunately, leaded pipes and lead paint can still be found in older homes and buildings. The following measures can reduce lead exposure:

- Allowing tap water to run for a minute or so before use, to clear the pipes of any lead-contaminated water
- Using only cold tap water for drinking and cooking, as hot tap water is more likely to leach lead
- Professionally removing lead-based paint or painting over it with latex paint

RECAP **Infancy is characterized by the most rapid growth a human being will ever experience, and appropriate growth is the most reliable long-term indicator of adequate infant nutrition. Infants need large amounts of energy per unit body weight to keep up with growth. Breast milk or iron-fortified formula provides all necessary nutrients for the first 6 months of life. After that, solid foods can gradually be introduced into an infant's diet. Micronutrient supplements should be given only if prescribed. Infants must be monitored for allergies, dehydration, and other signs of distress.**

dental caries Dental erosion and decay caused by acid-secreting bacteria in the mouth and on the teeth. The acid produced is a by-product of bacterial metabolism of carbohydrates deposited on the teeth.

Nutrition DEBATE
Should Breastfeeding Throughout Infancy Be Mandatory?

The year is 2021. Obesity rates have remained unacceptably high, especially among children, many of whom are experiencing high blood glucose, high blood pressure, and other signs of metabolic syndrome. In this climate, Marcy goes shopping for infant formula. Although her daughter Sidney has been exclusively breastfed since her birth 4 months ago, Marcy needs to go back to work full-time and has decided to switch to formula. At the check-out, Marcy is horrified at the price of the can of powdered formula she has selected. "It's not our fault," the clerk replies. "There's a new state surcharge to discourage families from using formula!"

If this scenario sounds preposterous, you might be interested to learn that some healthcare providers are actually proposing that states implement a system of rewards for breastfeeding and penalties for formula-feeding—and a surcharge like the one just described is among the various proposals. Why? What's behind these recommendations, and could they ever become law? Let's have a look.

As obesity rates have climbed, more researchers have posed the question "Do adults and children who were breastfed as infants have lower rates of obesity than adults and children who were formula-fed?"[39–44] These researchers point to the theory of *metabolic programming,* which states that infant-feeding practices and other factors in early postnatal life greatly influence an infant's physiology and subsequent risk for obesity and chronic diseases. Supporting this theory is the established fact that breast-fed infants grow in length and weight at a slower rate than formula-fed infants. But does this lower weight persist into childhood and adulthood?

While some studies show no protective effect, most have concluded that breastfeeding for longer than 3 to 6 months does, in fact, lower rates of child and adult overweight and obesity.[39–42] Some researchers have found that exclusive breastfeeding provides greater protection than partial breastfeeding and that, the longer breastfeeding persists, the greater the protection against obesity.[39, 43]

The obesity risk reduction may stem from the lower protein and energy intakes of breast-fed infants, alterations in insulin secretion, and/or differences in metabolism.[43] In contrast, rapid weight gain during infancy, which is more common among formula-fed infants, is associated with a higher risk for obesity later in life.[39]

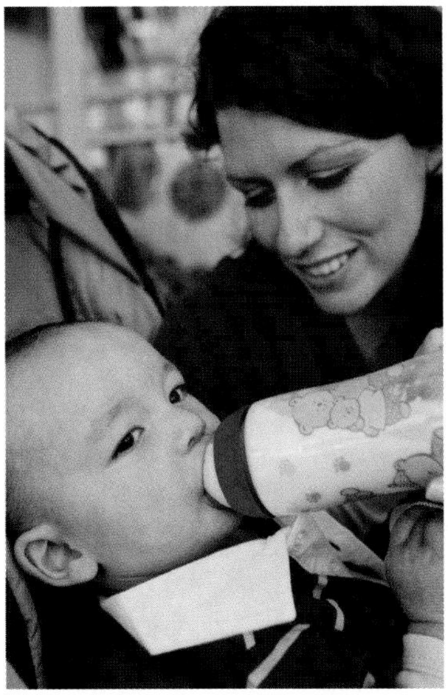

Formula-feeding has been associated with an increased risk for obesity in childhood and adulthood.

Some scientists have suggested that differences in feeding patterns influence the risk for obesity: formula-fed infants suck at a faster and more powerful rate, consume a larger volume at each feeding, and have fewer feedings per day with longer intervals between feedings compared to breasted infants.[44] It is possible that these differences translate into different eating habits as the infant transitions to child and adult diets.

The data from these studies prompt a complex question: does this difference in weight gain suggest that our society should do more to encourage or even require prolonged breastfeeding? Before you answer, consider the costs of obesity: as you have learned in previous chapters of this book, obesity is a well-established risk factor for heart disease, stroke, type 2 diabetes, and some forms of cancer. What's more, obesity-related costs account for 5–7% of annual U.S. healthcare expenditures, an estimated $100 billion annually, with additional costs related to lost productivity, reduced longevity, and impaired quality of life.[45]

Given this staggering financial burden of obesity, and the fact that much of it is borne by the public in the form of higher healthcare costs and insurance premiums, not to mention reduced tax revenues (from lost productivity) and increased disability payments, should we legislate actions that could reduce obesity rates? After all, we have laws restricting sales of alcohol and tobacco to adults, and most states tax these products heavily. These laws were enacted not only to improve the public health but also to reduce the financial burden of disease on the American public. Although some would argue that such laws take away our "personal freedoms," others point out that they protect primarily children and adolescents, either from the poor choices of their parents or from the harmful consequences of their own choices, which they are too young to fully understand.

If breastfeeding were conclusively shown to lower obesity rates, should it be encouraged via incentives and surcharges, or even required by law? Or do you believe the decision to breast- or formula-feed an infant should rest only with the family? At what point does "the public good" override personal freedoms, especially in an area as individualized as infant-feeding?

Chapter Review

Test Yourself ANSWERS

1. False. Pregnant women need only 350–450 additional Calories per day, and only during the second and third trimesters of pregnancy. This is an increase of only 20% or less, not a doubling of Calories.

2. True. Breast milk contains various immune factors (antibodies and immune system cells) from the mother that protect the infant against infection. The nutrients in breast milk are structured to be easily digested by an infant, resulting in fewer symptoms of gastrointestinal distress and fewer allergies.

3. False. Most infants do not have a physiologic need for solid food until about 6 months of age.

Find the Quack

Three weeks ago, Kaitlyn gave birth to her first child, Sean, whom she has been breastfeeding successfully. Or at least she thinks so. But sometimes she finds herself wondering whether her breast milk is providing everything her son needs to grow up healthy and strong. This afternoon, while Sean naps, she leafs through a magazine and notices an ad for infant formula; it looks so thick and creamy in comparison to her breast milk, which looks thin and watery. On the next page, she sees another ad. "Are you breastfeeding?" it asks. "If so, congratulations on making this healthy choice. But how can you be sure you're meeting all of your infant's nutrient needs?" Attracted by the healthy-looking newborn in the photo, Kaitlyn reads the full-page ad, which promotes an infant vitamin supplement called First Days "ID" Drops. She reads:

- "Mother's milk provides almost all the nutrition a growing baby needs. But two vital nutrients are low in breast milk. These are iron and vitamin D."
- "Both iron and vitamin D are low in breast milk. Both are critical to your baby's growth and health."
- "Available without a prescription, First Days "ID" Drops will provide your baby with the level of iron and vitamin D he or she needs."
- "For pennies a day, First Days "ID" Drops will safeguard your baby's growth and health."

1. Kaitlyn is consuming a diet rich in iron and vitamin D. Nevertheless, might her breast milk be low in these two nutrients? Why or why not?
2. Kaitlyn's newborn, Sean, is 3 weeks old. Does Sean need to consume iron in either breast milk or a supplement? Why or why not? Does Sean need supplemental vitamin D? Why or why not?
3. The ad states that First Days "ID" Drops are "available without a prescription." Should Kaitlyn consult her health-care provider before giving her baby these drops? Why or why not?
4. Does the ad for First Days "ID" Drops suggest that this is a legitimate product, or would you characterize it as an example of quackery? Defend your position.

Answers can be found on the companion website, at www.pearsonhighered.com/thompsonmanore.

Review Questions

1. Folate deficiency in the first weeks after conception has been linked with which of the following problems in the newborn?
   a. anemia
   b. neural tube defects
   c. low birth weight
   d. preterm delivery
2. Which of the following hormones is responsible for the letdown response?
   a. progesterone
   b. estrogen
   c. oxytocin
   d. prolactin
3. Which of the following nutrients should be added to the diet of breast-fed infants when they are around 6 months of age?
   a. fiber
   b. fat
   c. iron
   d. vitamin A
4. A pregnancy weight gain of 28 to 40 pounds is recommended for
   a. all women.
   b. women who begin their pregnancy underweight.
   c. women who begin their pregnancy overweight.
   d. women who begin their pregnancy at a normal weight.
5. The best solid food to introduce first to infants is
   a. Cream of Wheat cereal.
   b. applesauce.
   c. teething biscuits.
   d. iron-fortified rice cereal.
6. True or false? Major developmental errors and birth defects are most likely to occur in the third trimester of pregnancy.
7. True or false? Women who are breastfeeding require a higher energy intake than they needed when they were pregnant.
8. True or false? Growth is a key indicator of adequate infant nutrition.
9. True or false? Caffeine crosses the placenta and reaches the fetus, but it does not enter breast milk.
10. True or false? If gestational diabetes is uncontrolled, the fetus may not receive enough glucose and may be born small for gestational age.

Answers to Review Questions can be found at the back of this text, and additional essay questions and answers are located on the companion website at www.pearsonhighered.com/thompsonmanore.

Web Resources

www.drspock.com/toolsforyou/quiz
Dr. Spock.com

Check out this website for a quiz testing your readiness for parenthood. You can also use links within the quiz to find out how much it'll cost you!

www.aappolicy.aappublications.org
American Academy of Pediatrics

Visit this website for information on infants' and children's health. Searches can be performed for topics such as "neural tube defects" and "infant formulas."

www.fnic.nal.usda.gov
Food and Nutrition Information Center

Click on See Topics A–Z and then Child Nutrition and Health for a list of infant nutrition topics and a listing of child nutrition programs, links, and resources.

www.emedicine.com/ped
eMedicine: Pediatrics

Select Toxicology and then Toxicity, Iron to learn about accidental iron poisoning and its signs in children and infants.

www.marchofdimes.com
March of Dimes

Click on During Your Pregnancy to find links on nutrition during pregnancy, exercise, and things to avoid.

www.diabetes.org
American Diabetes Association

Search for "gestational diabetes" to find information about diabetes that develops during pregnancy.

www.lalecheleague.org
La Leche League

Search this site to find multiple articles on the health effects of breastfeeding for mother and infant.

www.obgyn.net
OBGYN.net

Visit this site to learn about pregnancy health and nutrition, as well as breastfeeding and infant nutrition.

www.nofas.org
National Organization on Fetal Alcohol Syndrome

This site provides news and information relating to fetal alcohol syndrome.

www.helppregnantsmokersquit.org
The National Partnership for Smoke-Free Families

This site was created for healthcare providers and smokers with the purpose of educating about the dangers of smoking while pregnant and providing tools to help pregnant smokers quit.

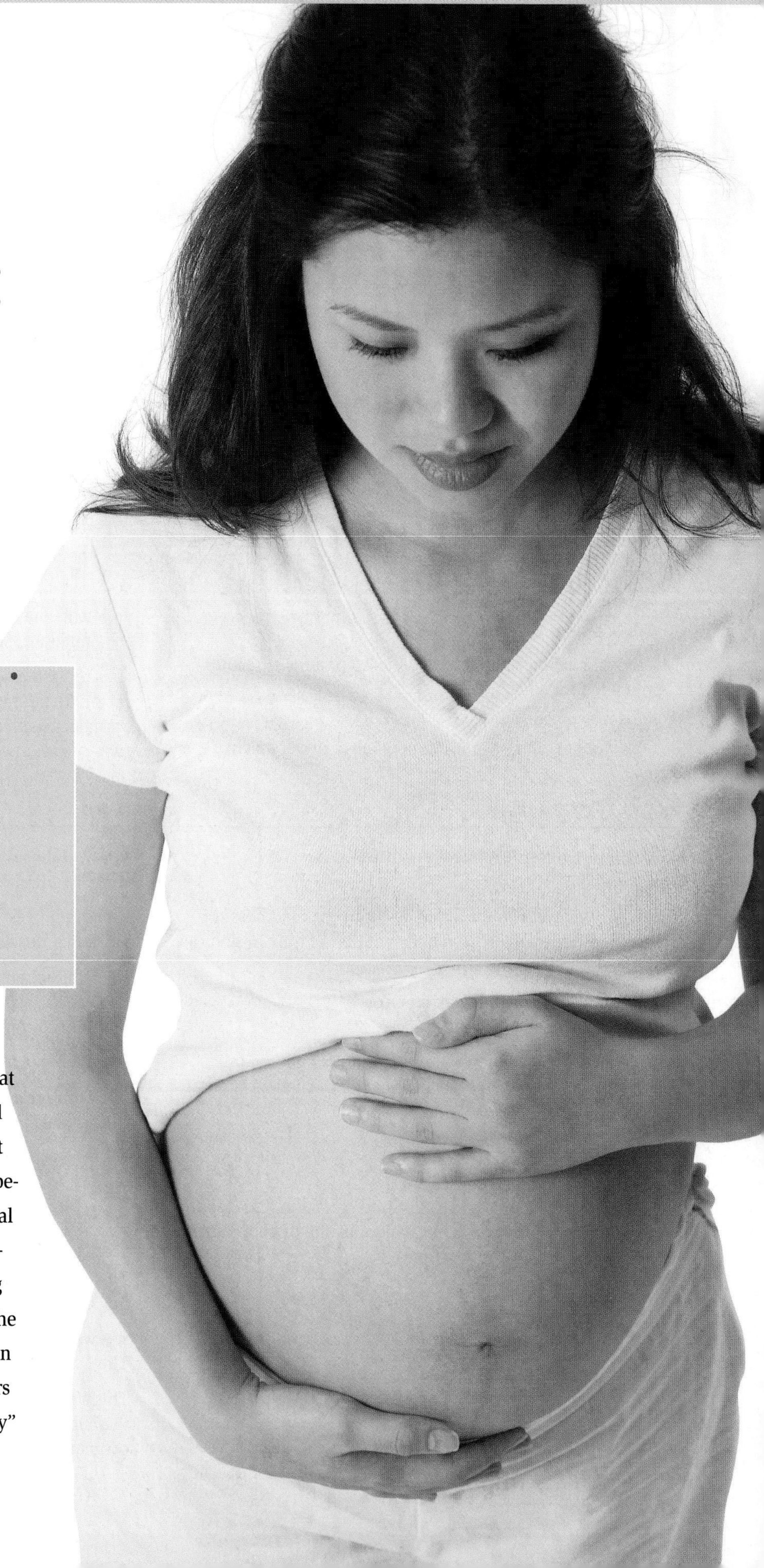

The Fetal Environment: A Lasting Impression

WANT TO FIND OUT. . .

- why an undernourished fetus is more likely to become an obese adult?
- about the consequences of excessive nutrient availability during fetal development?
- what the link is between maternal smoking and adult-onset diabetes?

READ ON.

Would you be surprised to learn that your risk of developing obesity and certain chronic diseases as an adult can be influenced by what happened even before your birth? It's true. Over the last several decades, a growing body of evidence has revealed that the fetal environment, including the mother's nutritional status, influences the risks for obesity and chronic diseases later in life. To describe this relationship, researchers have coined the phrases "fetal origins theory" and "developmental origins of adult health and disease." This *In Depth* explores this relationship and describes the lifelong effects of a variety of factors in the fetal environment.

Exposure to Famine

Some of the earliest research into the fetal origins theory investigated the health of adults born during or shortly after a famine in the Netherlands in 1944 and 1945, that resulted from an extended German embargo during World War II. Because the Dutch maintained an excellent system of healthcare records, scientists were able to learn important information about not only pregnancy outcomes but also the health of the offspring of the Dutch famine victims over the next 60 years. Not surprisingly, maternal weight gain and infant birth weight were much lower than normal. What was surprising, however, was the long-term impact of the famine on babies born there during this period as they progressed through adulthood.[1,2]

In any circumstances, exposure to famine during the first trimester of pregnancy results in a much higher risk among the offspring for obesity, abdominal obesity, coronary heart disease, abnormal serum lipid profile, and metabolic syndrome during adulthood. If a pregnancy progresses to the third trimester by the time a famine begins, there is a higher rate of glucose intolerance and type 2 diabetes in adulthood (**Figure 1**).[1]

Why, you might wonder, would low pregnancy weight gain and low birth weight lead to an increased risk for overweight, obesity, heart disease, high blood pressure, abnormal blood lipids, stroke, diabetes, premature death, and even schizophrenia, some 50 years later? While there are many theories, most relate to a process known as **fetal adaptation.**[3,4] In this process, a fetus exposed to a harmful environment, such as maternal starvation or malnutrition, goes into survival mode. The body's production of various hormones may shift in favor of those that promote energy storage, the activity of certain enzymes may increase or decrease, and the size and functioning of body organs such as the liver, kidneys, and pancreas may change. There may even be changes in the activation—and thus the expression—of certain genes. Although these adaptations are beneficial to the fetus, allowing it to survive the harmful prenatal environment, the same hormonal, enzymatic, organ, and genetic changes may contribute to the development of chronic diseases over the life span (see Figure 1).

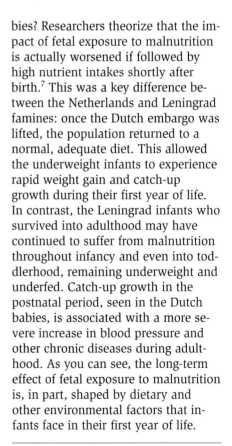

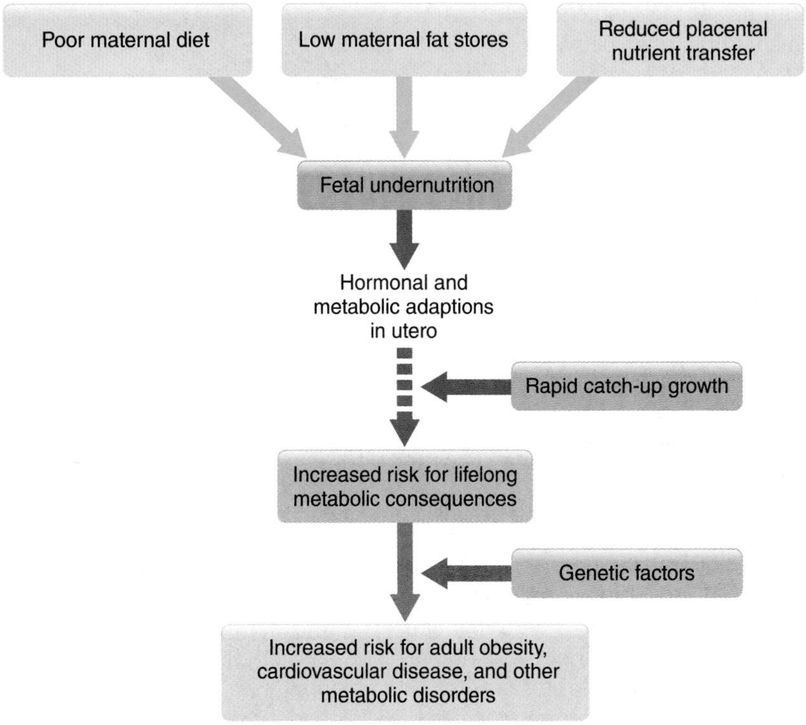

Figure 1 Fetal origins of adult diseases are complex and interrelated.[5]

The Dutch Famine Study provided some of the earliest evidence supporting the fetal origins theory, but the results of many other "natural experiments" suggest that the effects of the prenatal environment on adult health depend quite heavily on the precise circumstances in each situation. For example, the Russian city of Leningrad was under siege during World War II for over 2 1/2 years; as a result, the population experienced starvation—over a million people died. However, adults who were born during this period did not have the same increased disease risks as those found in the adults exposed, *in utero,* to the Dutch famine.[5,6] How can this be, since the Leningrad babies were exposed to conditions far worse than those experienced by the Dutch babies? Researchers theorize that the impact of fetal exposure to malnutrition is actually worsened if followed by high nutrient intakes shortly after birth.[7] This was a key difference between the Netherlands and Leningrad famines: once the Dutch embargo was lifted, the population returned to a normal, adequate diet. This allowed the underweight infants to experience rapid weight gain and catch-up growth during their first year of life. In contrast, the Leningrad infants who survived into adulthood may have continued to suffer from malnutrition throughout infancy and even into toddlerhood, remaining underweight and underfed. Catch-up growth in the postnatal period, seen in the Dutch babies, is associated with a more severe increase in blood pressure and other chronic diseases during adulthood. As you can see, the long-term effect of fetal exposure to malnutrition is, in part, shaped by dietary and other environmental factors that infants face in their first year of life.

fetal adaptation The process by which a fetus's metabolism, hormone production, and other physiologic processes shift in response to factors, such as inadequate energy intake, in the maternal environment.

Studies of the medical records of Finnish adults born between 1934 and 1944, periods of great economic stress for that country, have also confirmed the link between fetal malnutrition, early childhood weight gain, and risk for chronic disease as an adult. The higher the childhood BMI, the greater the risk of developing insulin resistance and heart disease in adulthood.[8]

More recently, people born during weather- and war-related famines in Africa and other parts of the world have provided researchers with additional information on the impact of the fetal environment on adult health/disease outcomes. These more recent studies, including ones from South Africa and the Democratic Republic of Congo, confirm that low birth weight is associated with higher blood pressure in childhood and adolescence.[9] Cardiovascular disease is now the second most common cause of adult death in sub-Saharan Africa, in stark contrast to previous decades, when infectious diseases accounted for the majority of deaths. In addition, half of the cardiovascular deaths in the sub-Saharan population were among adults 30 to 69 years of age, a far younger age than is seen in the United States and other developed nations[8] **(Figure 2)**.

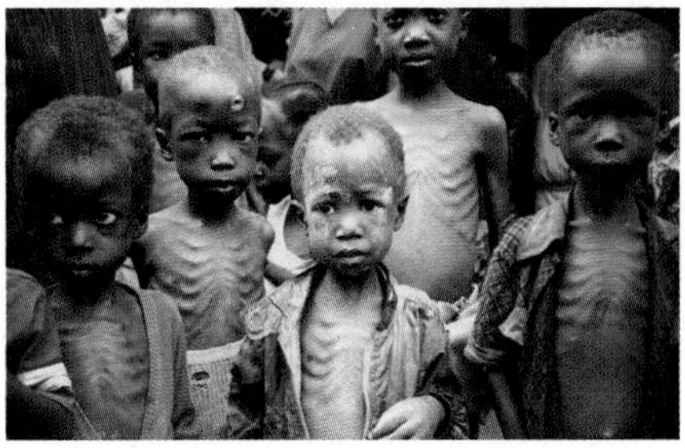

Figure 2 The consequences of childhood starvation are often lifelong.

Exposure to Specific Nutrient Deficiencies

By definition, a famine is a widespread lack or severe reduction in all food. Thus, research on the long-term health effects of famines cannot identify or describe the impact of *in utero* deficiencies of specific nutrients. Other studies, however, have been able to look at specific food patterns and nutrient intakes to determine the possible effects on the future health of the offspring. For example, evidence suggests long-term consequences of the following maternal deficiencies:[4,10]

- Low maternal intake of calcium increases the risk for hypertension in the offspring.
- Poor maternal folate status has been linked not only to neural tube defects in the newborn but also to early signs of atherosclerosis in adult offspring.
- Low maternal intake of fish, possibly a marker for DHA or omega-3 fatty acid intake, has been associated with developmental delays in childhood.
- Maternal zinc deficiency may account for some of the metabolic abnormalities and disease risks seen in adult offspring.

Thus, fetal stressors that influence adult health include not only starvation and inadequate energy but also specific nutrient deficiencies.

Exposure to Dietary Excesses

While our discussion so far has focused on maternal deficiencies, very strong evidence also links maternal dietary excesses to poor health outcomes in adult offspring. Maternal obesity has been linked not only to an increased risk for childhood and adult[11,12] obesity but also to changes in the "programming" of the fetal brain, resulting in altered feeding behaviors.[13] Maternal obesity is also linked to a higher risk for birth defects, many of which have lifelong implications for health.[14] Infants born to overweight or obese women have higher rates of spina bifida and other neural tube defects, heart defects, cleft lip and palate, and abnormalities of their arms and/or legs. These birth defects are more likely to occur in women who are obese prior to their pregnancies or who gain an excessive amount of weight during their pregnancies. Population studies have also reported an association between high birth weight, common in infants born to obese women, and in increased risk for breast cancer in adulthood.

Maternal diabetes and its high-glucose environment has been shown to greatly increase the risk for type 2 diabetes,[15] overweight, and metabolic syndrome[16] in adult offspring. The children of these diabetic women are up to eight times more likely to develop type 2 diabetes or pre-diabetes as adults compared to the general population. High blood levels of triglycerides, an increased waist circumference, and increased blood pressure are other measures of adult-onset diseases associated with maternal diabetes.

While research on prenatal exposure to excessive levels of individual nutrients typically is done with animal models, some human research results are available. It is known, for example, that a high maternal intake of vitamin A as retinol (but not as its precursor, beta-carotene) is associated with an increased risk for congenital heart defects,[17] skull abnormalities, and other defects.[18] Scientists continue to investigate the possible lifelong effects of other nutrient excesses, including the impact of high maternal intake of sodium on the risk for hypertension in adult offspring and the effect of high maternal saturated fat intake on the risk for congenital defects.

In short, research suggests that there are lifelong consequences to any type of nutrient imbalance during pregnancy, whether the imbalance is a total energy deficit, a single nutrient deficiency, or an energy or nutrient excess.

Exposure to Alcohol, Tobacco, and Other Toxic Agents

You've already learned of the lifelong impact of fetal alcohol syndrome, resulting from exposure to high maternal blood alcohol levels in

NUTRI-CASE HANNAH

"In my nutrition class, I learned that having a mother with diabetes increases the risk that you'll develop diabetes in childhood or adulthood. That helps me understand why my blood sugar test showed I have pre-diabetes, but it doesn't help me understand what to do about it."

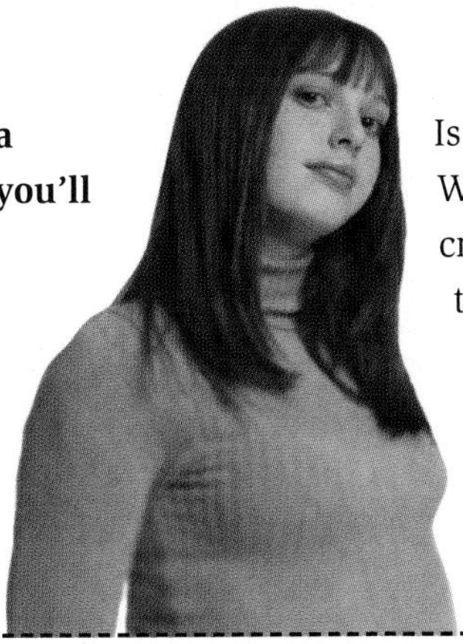

Is Hannah destined to develop type 2 diabetes? Why or why not? Identify the factors that increase her risk, as well as the steps she can take to reduce her blood glucose levels and avoid the disease. If necessary, review the ***In Depth*** essay on diabetes on pages 137–141.

the ***In Depth*** following chapter 1 (pages 35–36). In addition, maternal smoking has been shown to negatively impact the long-term health of the offspring. Not only are the offspring of women who smoked during pregnancy at high risk for preterm delivery and low birth weight, but they are also at higher risk for childhood allergies and respiratory diseases, adult-onset high blood pressure, childhood behavioral problems,[4] and cleft lip and palate.[19] New evidence also confirms a link between maternal smoking and increased risk for adult-onset diabetes among offspring, as well as a lifelong higher risk for obesity.[20]

Not surprisingly, maternal exposure to lead and other environmental pollutants also has lifelong implications for offspring.[21] Maternal lead exposure increases the offspring's risk for developmental delays, behavioral and learning problems, and hearing loss, whereas exposure to mercury can result in irreversible damage to the nervous system and subsequent learning disabilities. In each of these examples, the mother's dietary intake and her immediate environment can lead to harmful effects that persist into and throughout adulthood.

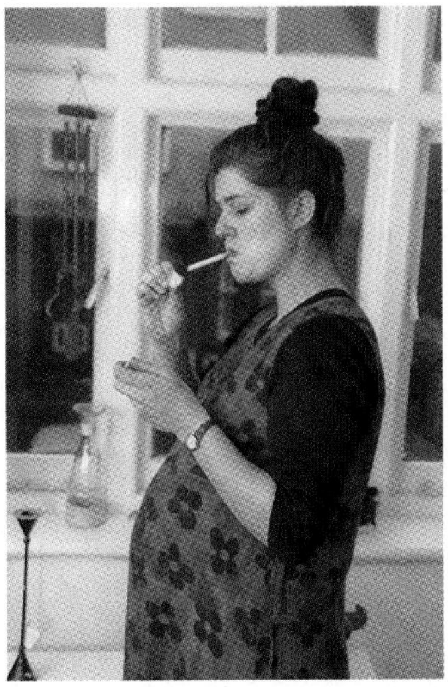

Maternal smoking is extremely harmful to the fetus, and increases the risk for a variety of health problems in childhood and adulthood.

Implications for Your Health

What does this research on fetal origins of adult disease mean to you? If your mother experienced some type of nutritional, metabolic, or environmental stress during pregnancy, are you doomed to suffer from one or more of the health problems mentioned earlier? Although there is not yet a definitive answer, it is important to remember that this research is looking at "risk" and "susceptibility" in terms of populations. In other words, all of this research reported on large groups of people, not individuals. Moreover, it calculated increases in risk for—or susceptibility to—certain conditions, but it did not and cannot condemn anyone to any particular disease.

Any type of fetal programming or genetic influence that develops as a result of the fetal environment is just one factor in your wellness. A much more significant influence is your own lifestyle, especially your personal food choices, dietary patterns, activity habits, alcohol intake, and smoking. In fact, the Centers for Disease Control and Prevention cite these as the primary factors influencing your risk of actually experiencing any of the most common chronic diseases.[22] In short, you have the power to optimize your health by making smart lifestyle choices every day.

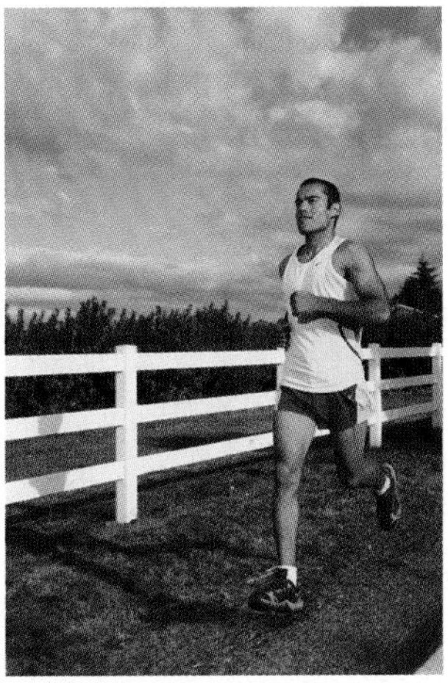

Regular physical activity is one of the most significant factors in maintaining wellness.

Web Resources

www.marchofdimes.com
March of Dimes

This website provides information on the potential risks of maternal dietary imbalances and exposure to environmental pollutants.

www.epa.gov/mercury/exposure
Environmental Protection Agency

The latest information on health effects of mercury can be found in this resource.

15 Nutrition Through the Life Cycle: Childhood to Late Adulthood

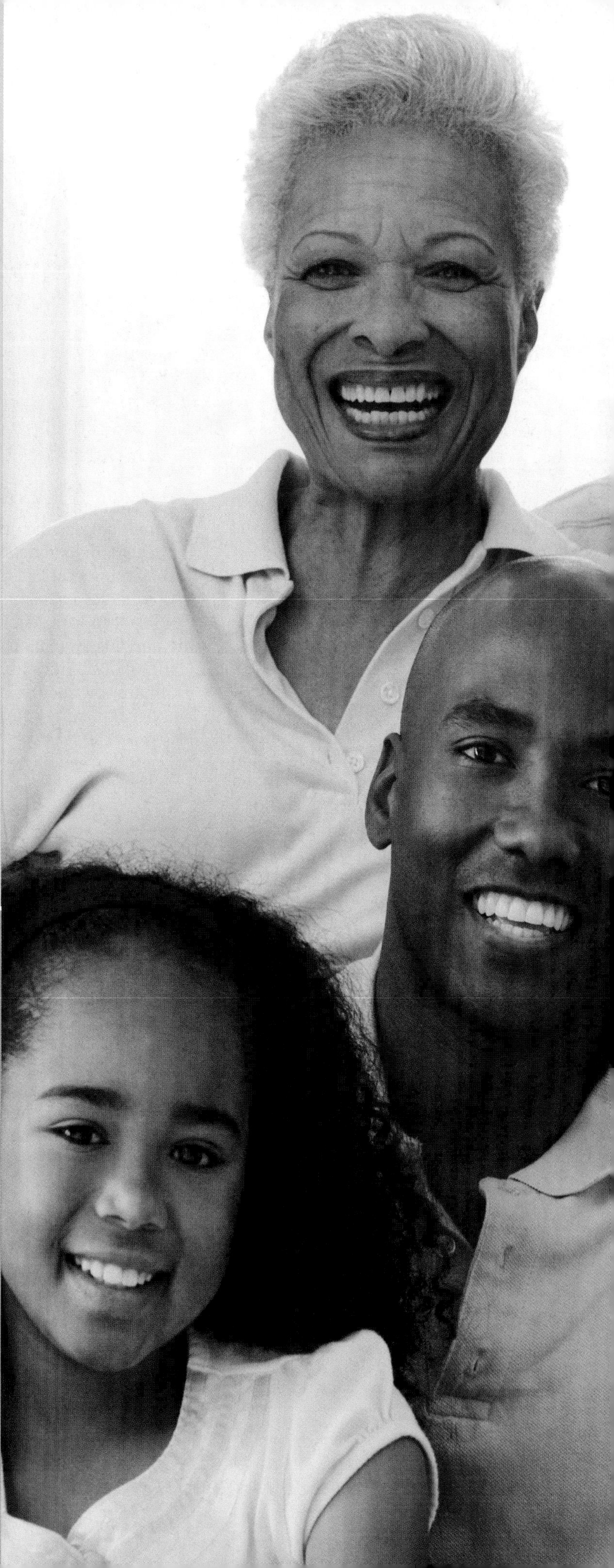

CHAPTER OBJECTIVES

After reading this chapter you will be able to:

1. **Compare and contrast the nutrient needs of toddlers and children, pp. 542–545, and 547–550.**
2. **List at least three nutrients of concern when feeding a vegan diet to young children, pp. 546–548.**
3. **Define puberty and describe how it influences changes in body composition, pp. 554–555.**
4. **Explain why adequate intakes of calcium and vitamin D are particularly important during the adolescent years, p. 556.**
5. **List at least two factors that can increase the risk for obesity during childhood and adolescence, pp. 560–561.**
6. **Identify at least three physiologic changes that occur with aging and describe how they affect the nutrient needs of older adults, pp. 562–564.**
7. **Describe two reasons why older adults may not be able to drink adequate amounts of fluid, p. 567.**
8. **Discuss several changes in health that can contribute to inadequate nutrient intake in older adults, pp. 567–570.**

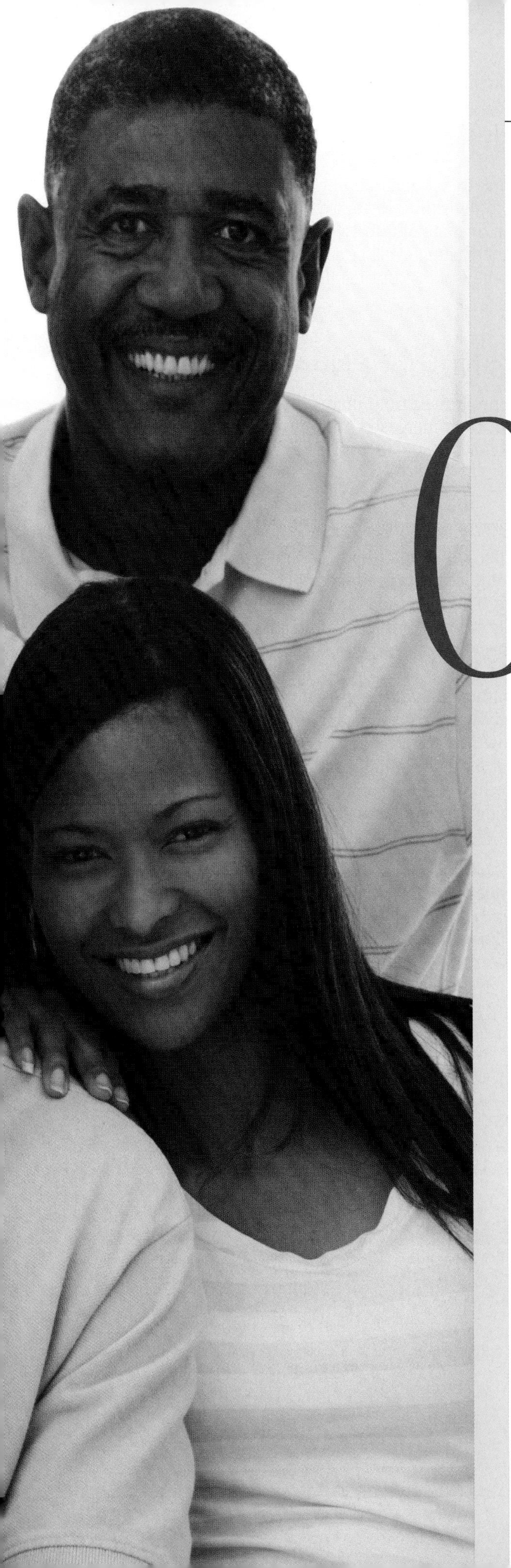

Test Yourself

1. **T F** **It is now believed that diet has virtually no role in the development of acne.**
2. **T F** **Participating in regular physical activity can delay or reduce some of the loss of muscle mass that occurs with aging.**
3. **T F** **Experts agree that, within the next 20–30 years, the human life span will exceed 150 years.**

Test Yourself answers can be found at the end of the chapter.

On Sunday afternoons, the Sophat family gathers for dinner at the Long Beach apartment of their 88-year-old matriarch, Leng. Only 5 feet tall, Leng is as thin as a rail, as is her 70-year-old daughter and 67-year-old son. But when her granddaughters, who are cooking the family meal, send everyone to the table, a change becomes evident. Almost all of Leng's grandchildren and their spouses are overweight, as are most of her great-grandchildren. Even her "darling," 9-year-old Teddy, is chubby. Leng worries about everyone's weight. Back home in Cambodia, overweight was rare and a sign of health, but here in America, it seems to bring illness. One of her grandsons has had a heart attack, and many in her family have been diagnosed with type 2 diabetes. Leng's family isn't alone in their weight problems: in the United States, more than 10% of toddlers and preschoolers (2 to 5 years), nearly 20% of children (6 to 11 years) and 18% of youth (12 to 19 years) are classified as obese, leading to both short- and long-term health problems.[1]

Why are the rates of obesity and its associated chronic diseases so high, and what can be done to promote weight management across the life span? How do our nutrient needs change as we grow and age, and what other nutrition-related concerns develop in each life stage? This chapter will help you answer these questions.

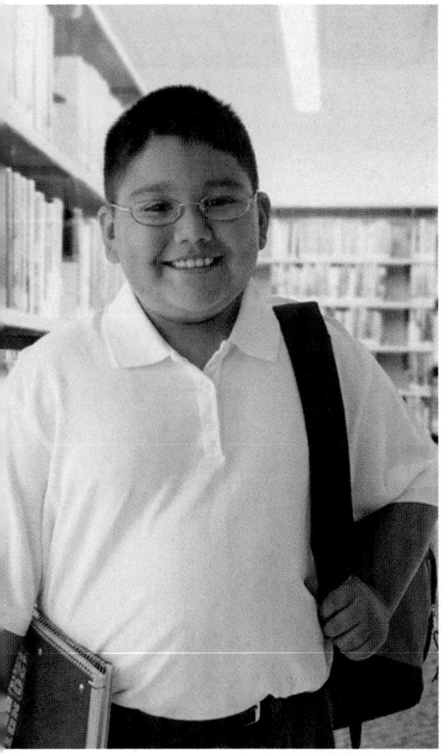

American children of all ethnicities experience overweight and obesity.

Nutrition for Toddlers

As babies begin to walk and explore, they transition out of infancy and into the active world of toddlers. From their first to their third birthday, a toddler will grow a total of about 5.5 to 7.5 inches and gain an average of 9 to 11 pounds. Toddlers need to consume a lot of energy to fuel their increasing levels of activity as they explore their ever-expanding world and develop new skills. But feeding a toddler raises new challenges for parents and caregivers.

What Are a Toddler's Nutrient Needs?

Nutrient needs increase as a child progresses from infancy to toddlerhood. Although toddlers' rate of growth has slowed, their increased nutrient needs reflect their larger body size and increased activity. Refer to **Table 15.1** for a review of specific nutrient recommendations.

Energy and Macronutrient Recommendations for Toddlers

Although the energy requirement per kilogram of body weight for toddlers is slightly less than for infants, *total* energy requirements are higher because toddlers are larger and much more active than infants. The estimated energy requirements (EERs) vary according to the toddler's age, body weight, and level of activity.[2] In general, toddlers should consume a diet that provides enough energy to sustain a healthy and appropriate rate of growth.

Although there is currently insufficient evidence to set a DRI for fat for toddlers, healthy toddlers of appropriate body weight should consume 30–40% of their total daily energy intake as fat.[2] We know that fat provides a concentrated source of energy in a relatively small amount of food, and this is important for toddlers, especially those who are fussy eaters or have little appetite. Fat is also necessary to support the toddler's continuously developing nervous system.

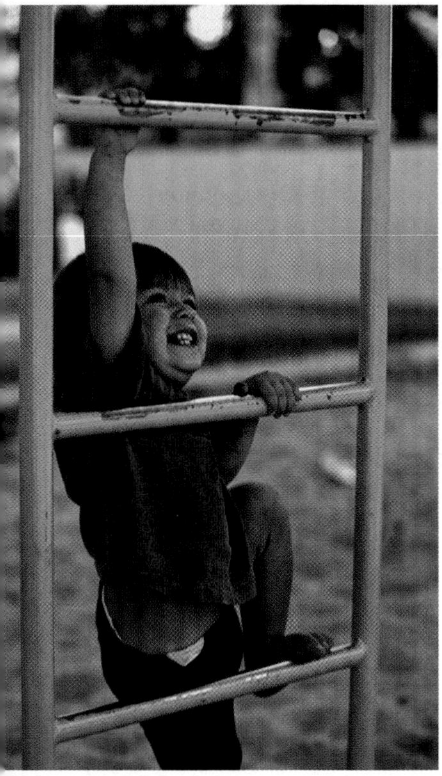

Toddlers expend significant amounts of energy actively exploring their world.

TABLE 15.1 Nutrient Recommendations for Children and Adolescents

Nutrient	Toddlers (1–3 years)	Children (4–8 years)	Children (9–13 years)	Adolescents (14–18 years)
Fat	No DRI	No DRI	No DRI	No DRI
Protein	1.10 g/kg body weight per day	0.95 g/kg body weight per day	0.95 g/kg body weight per day	0.85 g/kg body weight per day
Carbohydrate	130 g/day	130 g/day	130 g/day	130 g/day
Vitamin A	300 µg/day	400 µg/day	600 µg/day	Boys = 900 µg/day Girls = 700 µg/day
Vitamin C	15 mg/day	25 mg/day	45 mg/day	Boys = 75 mg/day Girls = 65 mg/day
Vitamin E	6 mg/day	7 mg/day	11 mg/day	15 mg/day
Calcium	700 mg/day	1,000 mg/day	1,300 mg/day	1,300 mg/day
Iron	7 mg/day	10 mg/day	8 mg/day	Boys = 11 mg/day Girls = 15 mg/day
Zinc	3 mg/day	5 mg/day	8 mg/day	Boys = 11 mg/day Girls = 9 mg/day
Fluid	1.3 liters/day	1.7 liters/day	Boys = 2.4 liters/day Girls = 2.1 liters/day	Boys = 3.3 liters/day Girls = 2.3 liters/day

Toddlers' protein needs increase modestly because they weigh more than infants and are still growing rapidly. The RDA for protein for toddlers is 1.10 g/kg body weight per day, or approximately 13 g of protein daily.[2] Remember that 2 cups of milk alone provide 16 g of protein; thus, most toddlers have little trouble meeting their protein needs.

The RDA for carbohydrate for toddlers is 130 g/day, and carbohydrate intake should be about 45–65% of total energy intake.[2] As is the case for older children and adults, most of the carbohydrates eaten should be complex, and refined carbohydrates from high-fat/high-sugar items, such as desserts and snack foods, should be kept to a minimum. Fruits and fruit juices are nutritious sources of simple carbohydrates; however, too much fruit juice can displace other foods and can cause diarrhea. The American Academy of Pediatrics recommends that the intake of fruit juice be limited to 4–6 fl. oz/day for children 1 to 6 years of age.[3]

Adequate fiber is important for toddlers to maintain regularity. The AI is 14 g of fiber per 1,000 kcal of energy, or, on average, 19 g/day.[2] Whole-grain breads and cereals and fresh fruits and vegetables are healthful choices for toddlers. Too much fiber, however, can inhibit the absorption of iron, zinc, and other essential nutrients, harm the toddler's small digestive tract, and cause satiation before the toddler has consumed adequate nutrients.

Determining the macronutrient requirements of toddlers can be challenging. See the You Do the Math box on page 544 for an analysis of the macronutrient levels in one toddler's daily diet.

Micronutrient Recommendations for Toddlers

As toddlers grow, their micronutrient needs increase (Table 15.1). Of particular concern with toddlers is an adequate intake of the minerals calcium and iron.

Calcium is necessary for children to promote optimal bone mass, which continues to accumulate until early adulthood. For toddlers, the AI for calcium is 700 mg/day.[4] Dairy products are excellent sources of calcium. When a child reaches the age of 1 year, whole cow's milk can be given; however, reduced-fat milk (2% or less) should *not* be given until age 2 due to the relatively high need for total energy. If dairy products are not feasible, calcium-fortified orange juice or soy milk can supply calcium, or children's calcium supplements can be given. Toddlers generally cannot consume enough food to depend on alternate calcium sources, such as dark-green vegetables.

Iron-deficiency anemia is the most common nutrient deficiency in young children in the United States and around the world. Iron-deficiency anemia can affect a child's energy level, attention span, and mood. The RDA for iron for toddlers is 7 mg/day.[5] Good sources of well-absorbed heme iron include lean meats, fish, and poultry; non-heme iron is provided by eggs, legumes, greens, and fortified foods, such as breakfast cereals. When toddlers consume non-heme sources of iron, eating vitamin C at the same meal will enhance the absorption of iron from these sources.

Given toddlers' typically erratic eating habits, pediatricians often recommend a multivitamin and mineral supplement as a precaution against deficiencies. The toddler's physician or dentist may also prescribe a fluoride supplement, if the community water supply is not fluoridated. Any supplement given should be formulated especially for toddlers, and the recommended dose should not be exceeded. A supplement should not contain more than 100% of the Daily Value of any nutrient per dose. Toddlers are at particularly high risk of overdosing on iron supplements, so parents must be careful to keep such products out of reach of their children.

Fluid Recommendations for Toddlers

Toddlers lose less fluid from evaporation than infants, and their more mature kidneys are able to concentrate urine, thereby sparing fluid. However, as toddlers become active, they start to lose significant fluid through sweat, especially in hot weather. Parents need to make sure an active toddler is drinking adequately. The recommended fluid intake for toddlers—about 4 cups as beverages, including drinking water—is listed in Table 15.1.[6] Suggested beverages are plain water, milk and soy milk, diluted fruit juice, and foods high in water content, such as vegetables and fruits.

YOU DO THE MATH

Is This Menu Good for a Toddler?

A dedicated mother and father want to provide the best nutrition for their son, Ethan, who is now 1 1/2 years old and has just been completely weaned from breast milk. Ethan weighs about 26 pounds (11.8 kg). In the accompanying table is a typical day's menu for Ethan. Grams of protein, fat, and carbohydrate are given for each food. The day's total energy intake is 1,168 kcal. Calculate the percentage of Ethan's Calories that come from protein, fat, and carbohydrate (the numbers may not add up to exactly 100% because of rounding). In what areas are Ethan's parents doing well, and where can they improve?

Note: This activity focuses on the macronutrients. It does not ask you to consider Ethan's intake of micronutrients or fluids.

Meal	Foods	Protein (g)	Fat (g)	Carbohydrate (g)
Breakfast	Oatmeal (1/2 cup, cooked)	2.5	1.5	13.5
	Brown sugar (1 tsp.)	0	0	4
	Milk (1%, 4 fl. oz)	4	1.25	5.5
	Grape juice (4 fl. oz)	0	0	20
Mid-morning snack	Banana slices (1 small banana)	0	0	16
	Yogurt (nonfat, fruit-flavored l, 3 fl. oz)	5.5	0	15.5
	Orange juice (4 fl. oz)	1	0	13
Lunch	Whole-wheat bread (1 slice)	1.5	0.5	10
	Peanut butter (1 tbsp.)	4	8	3.5
	Strawberry jam (1 tbsp.)	0	0	13
	Carrots (cooked, 1/8 cup)	0	0	2
	Applesauce (sweetened, 1/4 cup)	0	0	12
	Milk (1%, 4 fl. oz)	4	1.25	5.5
Afternoon snack	Bagel (1/2)	3	1	20
	American cheese product (1 slice)	3	5	1
	Water	0	0	0
Dinner	Scrambled egg (1)	11	5	1
	Baby food spinach (3 oz)	2	0.5	5.5
	Whole-wheat toast (1 slice)	1.5	0.5	10
	Mandarin orange slices (1/4 cup)	0.5	0	10
	Milk (1%, 4 fl. oz)	4	1.25	5.5

Calculations:

There is a total of 47.5 g protein in Ethan's menu.

$$47.5 \text{ g} \times 4 \text{ kcal/g} = 190 \text{ kcal}$$
$$190 \text{ kcal protein}/1{,}168 \text{ total kcal} \times 100 = 16\% \text{ protein}$$

There is a total of 25.75 g fat in Ethan's menu.

$$25.75 \text{ g} \times 9 \text{ kcal/g} = 232 \text{ kcal}$$
$$232 \text{ kcal fat}/1{,}168 \text{ total kcal} \times 100 = 20\% \text{ fat}$$

There is a total of 186.5 g carbohydrate in Ethan's menu.

$$186.5 \text{ g} \times 4 \text{ kcal/g} = 746 \text{ kcal}$$
$$746 \text{ kcal carbohydrate}/1{,}168 \text{ total kcal} \times 100 = 64\% \text{ carbohydrate}$$

Analysis:

Ethan's parents are doing very well at offering a wide variety of foods from various food groups; they are especially doing well with fruits and vegetables. Also, according to his estimated energy requirement, Ethan requires about 970 kcal/day, and he is consuming 1,168 kcal/day, thus meeting his energy needs.

Ethan's total carbohydrate intake for the day is 186.5 g, which is higher than the RDA of 130 g/day; however, this value falls within the recommended 45–65% of total energy intake that should come from carbohydrates. Thus, high carbohydrate intake is adequate to meet his energy needs.

However, Ethan is being offered far more than enough protein. The DRI for protein for toddlers is about 13 g/day, and Ethan is eating more than three times that much!

It is also readily apparent that Ethan is being offered too little fat for his age. Toddlers need at least 30–40% of their total energy intake from fat, and Ethan is consuming only about 20% of his Calories from fat. He should be drinking whole milk, not 1% milk. He should occasionally be offered higher-fat foods, such as cheese for his snacks or macaroni and cheese for a meal. Yogurt is fine, but it shouldn't be nonfat at Ethan's age. In conclusion, Ethan's parents should continue to offer a variety of nutritious foods but should shift some of the energy Ethan currently consumes as protein and carbohydrate to fat.

RECAP Growth during toddlerhood is slower than during infancy; however, toddlers are highly active, and total energy, fat, and protein requirements are higher for toddlers than for infants. While all forms of milk can be used to meet calcium requirements, until age 2, toddlers should drink energy-rich whole milk rather than reduced-fat milk. Iron deficiency can be avoided by feeding toddlers lean meats/fish/poultry, eggs, and iron-fortified foods. Toddlers need to drink about 4 cups of water or other beverages per day.

Encouraging Nutritious Food Choices with Toddlers

Parents and pediatricians have long known that toddlers tend to be choosy about what they eat. Some avoid entire food groups, such as all meats or vegetables. Others will refuse all but one or two favorite foods (such as peanut butter on crackers) for several days or longer. Still others eat extremely small amounts, seemingly satisfied by a single slice of apple or two bites of toast. These behaviors frustrate and worry many parents, but in fact, as long as a variety of healthful food is available, most toddlers have the ability to match their intake with their needs. A toddler will most likely make up for one day's deficiency later on in the week. Parents who offer only nutritious foods can feel confident that their children are being well fed, even if a child's choices seem odd or erratic on any particular day. Food should never be "forced" on a child, as doing so sets the stage for eating and control issues later in life.

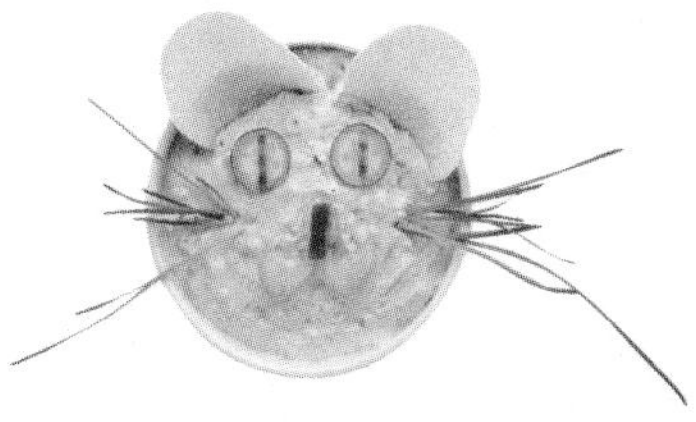

Figure 15.1 Most toddlers are delighted by food prepared in a fun way.

It is also important to recognize that toddlers' stomachs are still very small, and they cannot consume all of the Calories they need in three meals. Toddlers need small meals, alternated with nutritious snacks, every 2 to 3 hours. A successful technique is to create a snack tray filled with small portions of nutritious food choices, such as one-third of a banana, two pieces of cheese, and two whole-grain crackers, and leave it within reach of the child's play area. The child can then "graze" on these healthful foods while he or she plays. A snack tray plus a spill-proof cup of milk or water is particularly useful on car trips.

Foods prepared for toddlers should be developmentally appropriate. Nuts, carrots, grapes, raisins, and cherry tomatoes are difficult for a toddler to chew and pose a choking hazard. Foods should be soft and sliced into strips or wedges that are easy for children to grasp. As the child develops more teeth and becomes more coordinated, the range of food can expand.

Foods prepared for toddlers can also be fun **(Figure 15.1)**. Parents can use cookie cutters to turn a peanut butter sandwich into a pumpkin face, or arrange cooked peas or carrot slices to look like a smiling face on top of mashed potatoes. Juice and yogurt can be frozen into "popsicles" or blended into "milkshakes."

Even at mealtime, portion sizes should be small. One tablespoon of a food for each year of age constitutes a serving throughout the toddler and preschool years **(Figure 15.2)**. Realistic portion sizes can give toddlers a sense of accomplishment when they "eat it all up" and minimize parents' fears that their child is not eating enough.

New foods should be introduced gradually. Most toddlers are leery of new foods, spicy foods, hot (temperature) foods, mixed foods (such as casseroles), and foods with strange textures. A helpful rule is to encourage the child to eat at least one bite of a new food: if the child does not want the rest, nothing negative should be said and the child should be praised just for the willingness to try. The food should be reintroduced a few weeks later. Eventually, after several tries, the child might accept it. Parents should

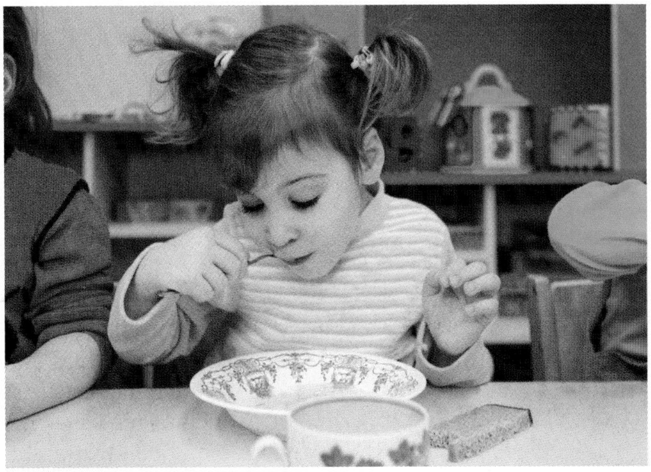

Figure 15.2 Portion sizes for preschoolers are much smaller than those for older children. Use the following guideline: 1 tbsp. of the food for each year of age equals 1 serving. For example, 2 tbsp. of rice, 2 tbsp. of black beans, and 2 tbsp. of chopped tomatoes is appropriate for a 2-year-old.

never bribe with food—for example, promising dessert if the child finishes her squash. Bribing teaches children that food can be used to reward and manipulate. Instead, parents can try to positively reinforce good behaviors—for example, "Wow! You ate every bite of your squash! That's going to help you grow big and strong!"

Role modeling is important, since toddlers mimic older children and adults: if they see their parents eating a variety of healthful foods, they are likely to do so as well. Providing limited healthful alternatives will also help toddlers make nutritious food choices. For example, parents might say, "It's snack time! Would you like apples and cheese or bananas and yogurt?" Finally, toddlers are more likely to eat food they help prepare: encourage them to assist in the preparation of simple foods, such as helping pour a bowl of cereal or helping arrange the raw vegetables on a plate.

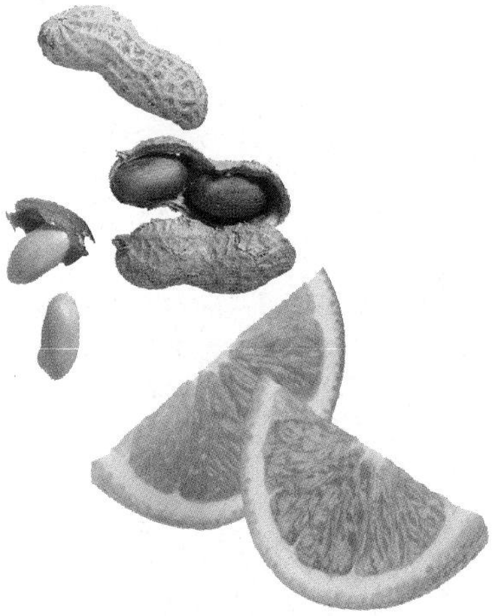

Foods that may cause allergies, such as peanuts and citrus fruits, should be introduced to toddlers one at a time.

Nutrition-Related Concerns for Toddlers

Just as toddlers have their own specific nutrient needs, they also have toddler-specific nutrition concerns, while others continue from infancy.

Continued Allergy Watch

As during infancy, new foods should be presented one at a time, and the toddler should be monitored for allergic reactions for a week before additional new foods are introduced. To prevent the development of food allergies, even foods that are established in the diet should be rotated, rather than served every day.

Overweight: A Concern Now?

Believe it or not, the signs of a tendency toward overweight can occur as early as the toddler years. Toddlers should *not* be denied nutritious food; however, they should not be forced or encouraged to eat when they are full. In the toddler years, a child who is above the 80th percentile for weight (one who weighs more than 80% of children of the same age and height) should be monitored. These children should be encouraged and supported in increasing their physical activity, and, as for all children, their intake of foods with low nutritional value should be limited. See the discussion on pages 560–561 for more information on obesity in children.

Vegetarian Families

For toddlers, a lacto-ovo-vegetarian diet, in which dairy foods and eggs are included, can be as wholesome as a diet including meats and fish. However, because red meat is an important source of zinc and heme iron, families who do not serve red meat must be careful to include enough zinc and iron from other sources in their child's diet. And a fast-growing young child needs specific nutrients in their early years for normal functioning and healthy development.

In contrast, a vegan diet, in which no foods of animal origin are consumed, poses several potential nutritional risks for toddlers:

- Protein—Vegan diets can be too low in total protein or protein quality for toddlers, who need adequate amounts of high-quality protein for growth and increasing activity. Few toddlers can consume enough legumes and whole grains to provide sufficient protein. The high fiber content of legumes and whole grains results in a rapid sense of fullness for toddlers, decreasing their total food intake. Soy-based products are excellent sources of dietary protein.
- Calcium—Children who consume no milk, yogurt, or cheese are at risk for calcium deficiency. As with protein, few children can consume enough calcium from plant sources to meet their daily requirement. Although some brands of soy milk and rice milk, and certain fruit juices and cereals, are now fortified with calcium, supplementation is advised.
- Zinc and iron—These minerals are also commonly low in vegan diets due to the absence of meat, poultry, and seafood. While both of these minerals are found in legumes, young children simply cannot eat enough legumes to meet their iron and zinc needs.

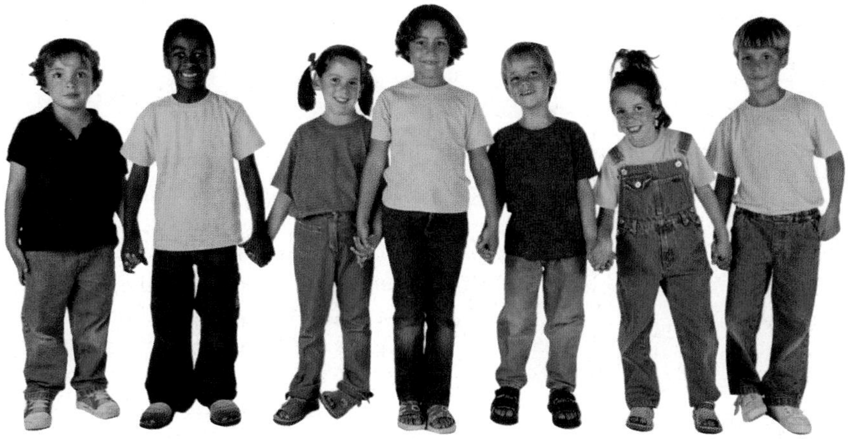

Children grow an average of 2 to 4 inches per year.

- Vitamins D and B_{12}—Children consuming strict vegan diets are at risk for deficiencies of both of these vitamins. Some cereals and soy milks are fortified with vitamin D; however, many toddlers may still need a vitamin D–containing supplement. Vitamin B_{12} is not available in any amount from plant foods and must be supplemented.
- Fiber—Vegan diets often contain a higher amount of fiber than is recommended for toddlers, resulting in lowered absorption of iron and zinc, as well as the early onset of fullness or satiety.

Although adults following a vegan diet have the ability to choose alternative foods and/or supplements to meet the demands for these nutrients, toddlers depend on their parents to make appropriate food choices for them. If parents are determined to maintain a vegan diet for their toddler, choosing to include fortified juices, soy milk, and other soy products, along with an appropriate pediatric supplement and ongoing consultation with a pediatrician, can ensure adequate nutrition in the toddler's diet.

The practice of feeding a vegan diet to infants and young children is highly controversial. See the Nutrition Myth or Fact? box (page 548) for more information about this controversy.

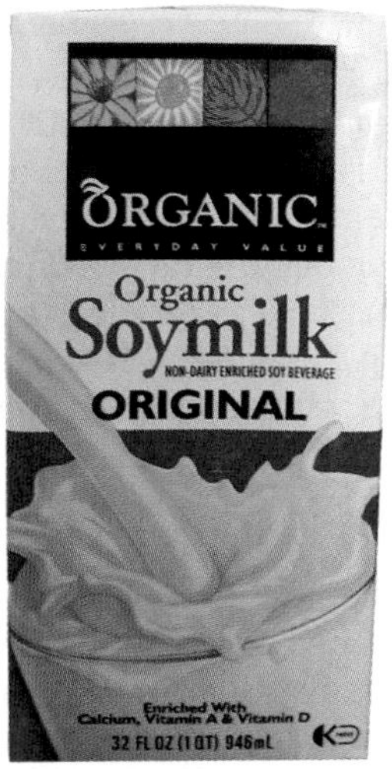

Enriched foods, such as fortified soy milk, should be given to toddlers consuming vegan diets.

RECAP **Toddlers require small, frequent, nutritious meals and snacks, and food should be cut in small pieces, so that it is easy to handle, mash, and swallow. Because toddlers are becoming more independent and can self-feed, parents need to be alert for choking and should watch for allergies and monitor weight gain. Role modeling by parents and access to ample healthful foods can help toddlers make nutritious choices. Feeding vegan diets to toddlers poses the potential for deficiencies in protein, calcium, zinc, iron, vitamin D, and vitamin B_{12}.**

Nutrition for Preschool and School-Age Children

During the preschool and school-age years, children become even more active, but their growth rate slows. Children grow an average of 2 to 4 inches per year at a slow and steady pace, the "calm before the storm" of adolescence, when growth rates again become very rapid. For children age 6–11 years, the USDA has produced a MyPyramid for Kids poster **(Figure 15.3)** advising children to "Eat Right. Exercise. Have Fun." The nutrient requirements and nutrition issues of importance to preschool and school-age children are discussed in this section.

What Are a Child's Nutrient Needs?

Until the age of 8 or 9 years, the nutrient needs of young boys and girls do not differ; because of this, the DRI values for the macronutrients, fiber, and micronutrients are

NUTRITION MYTH OR FACT?

Are Vegan Diets Appropriate for Young Children?

A glance at the headlines reveals that feeding a vegan diet to young children is a controversial issue. Supporters of veganism state that any consumption of animal products is wrong and that feeding animal products to children is forcing them into a life of obesity and chronic diet-related diseases. Some feel that the consumption of animal products wastes natural resources and contributes to environmental damage and is therefore morally wrong. Those who oppose veganism for young children assert that feeding a vegan diet to toddlers and developing children deprives them of the essential nutrients for both body and brain functioning that can be found only in animal products. Some people even suggest that veganism for young children is, in essence, a form of child abuse.

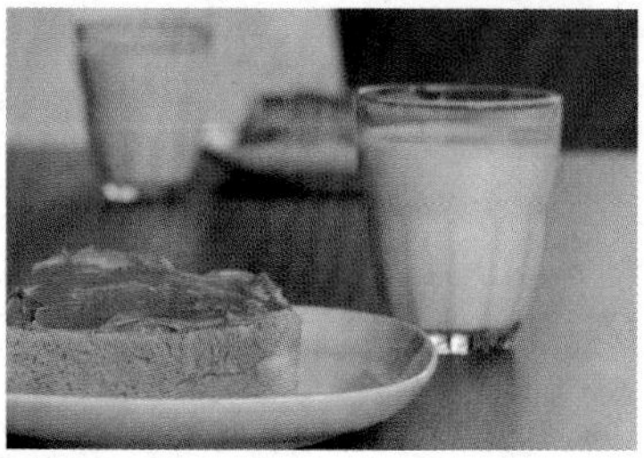

Most nutrition experts recommend a more moderate diet—one that includes fish, dairy products, and eggs—rather than a vegan diet for young children. This snack of a peanut butter sandwich and milk is a healthful choice.

As with many controversies, there is some truth on both sides. For example, there have been documented cases of children failing to thrive, and even dying, on extreme vegan diets.[7,8] Cases of protein deficiency as well as vitamin B_{12} and other micronutrient deficiencies have been cited in vegan children. The nutrients of concern are found primarily or almost exclusively in animal products, and deficiencies can have serious and lifelong consequences. For example, not all of the neurologic impairments caused by vitamin B_{12} deficiency can be reversed by timely B_{12} supplement intervention. In addition, inadequate zinc, calcium, vitamin D, and omega-3 fatty acids can result in impaired bone growth and strength, failure to reach peak bone mass, and impaired development.

However, a close inspection of the cases of nutrition-related illness in children due to veganism reveals that lack of education, fanaticism, and/or extremism is usually at the root of the problem. Informed parents following a responsible vegan diet, in conjunction with pediatric monitoring, are rarely involved. Such cases point to the vital importance of education in the challenges of administering this diet to young children. Specifically, parents need to know *which nutrients are not available in plant products and therefore must be supplemented*. They also need to understand that typical vegan diets are high in fiber and low in fat, a combination that can be dangerous for very young children.[9] Moreover, certain staples of the vegan diet, such as wheat, soy, and nuts, commonly provoke allergic reactions in children; when this happens, finding a plant-based substitute that contains adequate nutrients can be very challenging.

Both the American Dietetic Association[10] and the American Academy of Pediatrics have stated that a vegan diet can promote normal growth and development in childhood. Well-planned vegan diets in infancy and childhood do not impair childhood growth, although vegetarian children tend to be slightly smaller and leaner.[10,11] It has also been shown that well-planned vegan diets can have no negative effect on final adult height or weight. Parents should ensure that adequate supplements and/or fortified foods are consumed to account for the nutrients that are normally found in animal products. Many health organizations, however, continue to advocate a more moderate approach during the early childhood years. There are several reasons for this level of caution:

- Some vegan parents are not adequately educated on the planning of meals, the balancing of foods, and the inclusion of supplements to ensure adequate intake of all nutrients.
- Most young children are picky eaters and are hesitant to eat certain food groups, particularly vegetables, a staple in the vegan diet.
- The high fiber content of vegan diets may not be appropriate for very young children.
- Children on vegan diets may require slightly higher amounts of dietary protein due to the lower digestibility and quality of plant proteins.
- Young children have small stomachs, and they are not able to consume enough plant-based foods to ensure adequate intakes of all nutrients and energy.

Because of these concerns, most nutrition experts advise parents to take a more moderate dietary approach, one that emphasizes plant foods but also includes some animal-based foods, such as fish, dairy, and/or eggs.

Once children reach school age, the low fat, abundant fiber, antioxidants, and many micronutrients in a vegan diet will promote their health as they progress into adulthood. However, those who consume animal products can also live a healthful life and reduce their risk for chronic diseases by choosing low-fat, nutrient-dense foods, such as lean meats, nonfat dairy products, whole grains, and fruits and vegetables. When a varied diet is consumed, there are fewer worries about consuming adequate amounts of all nutrients.

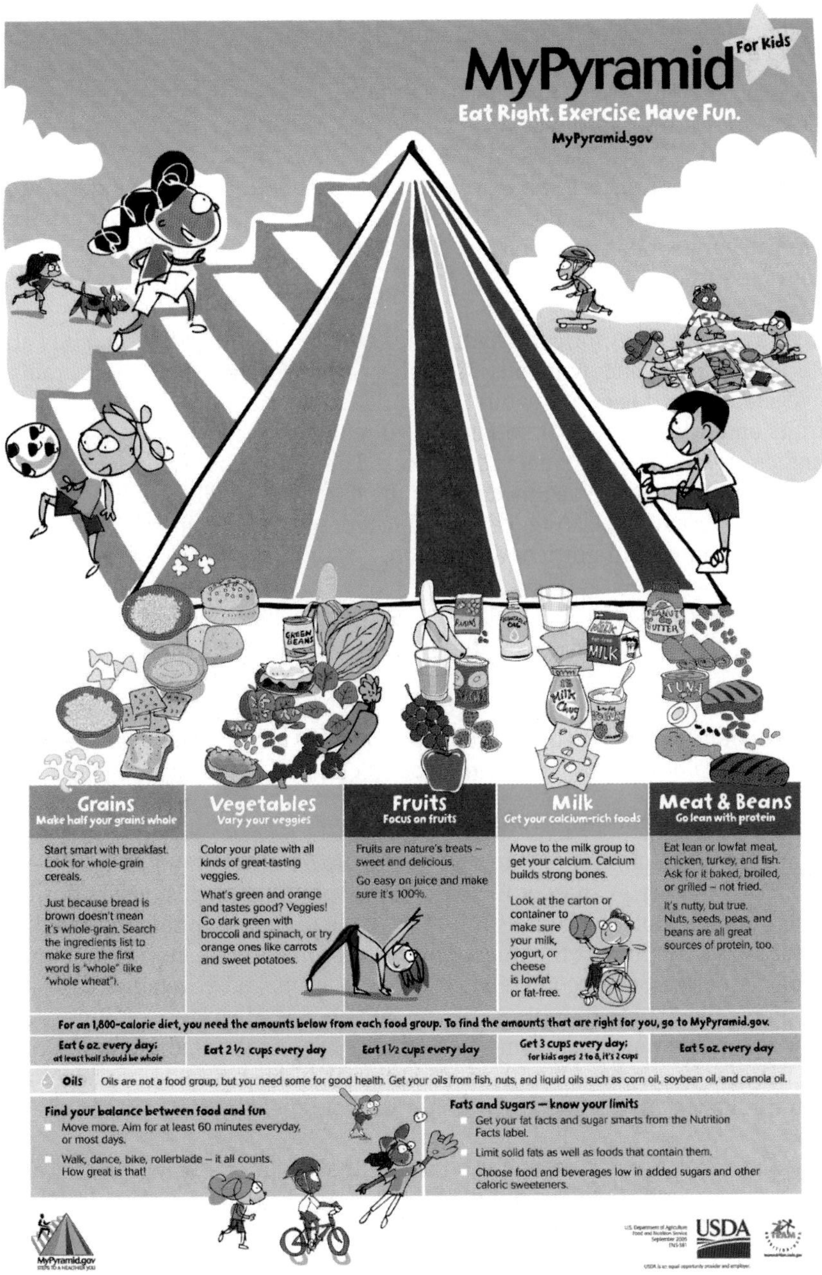

Figure 15.3 MyPyramid for Kids. This graphic illustrates the nutritional needs of children and encourages them to "Eat Right. Exercise. Have Fun."

grouped together for children age 4 to 8 years. The beginning of sexual maturation, however, has a dramatic impact on the nutrient needs of children. Boys' and girls' bodies develop differently in response to gender-specific hormones. These changes in sexual maturation can begin subtly between the ages of 8 and 9 years; thus, the DRI values are separately defined for boys and girls age 9 to 13 years.[2] Table 15.1 (page 542) identifies the nutrient needs of children and adolescents.

Energy and Macronutrient Recommendations for Children

Total energy requirements continue to increase throughout childhood because of increasing body size and, for some children, higher levels of physical activity. The estimated energy requirement (EER) varies according to the child's age, body weight, and level of activity. Parents should provide diets that allow for normal growth and support physical activity while minimizing the risk for excess weight gain.

Fat Although dietary fat remains a key macronutrient in the preschool years, total fat intake should gradually be reduced to a level closer to that of an adult, 25–35% of total energy.[2] One easy way to start reducing dietary fat is to gradually introduce lower-fat dairy products, such as 2% or 1% milk, and to minimize the intake of fried foods. A diet providing fewer than 25% of Calories from fat is not recommended for children, as they are still growing, developing, and maturing. Foods such as meats and dairy products should not be withheld solely because of their fat content, since they have important nutrient value. In fact, parents should avoid putting too much emphasis on fat at this age. Impressionable and peer-influenced children can easily be led to categorize foods as "good" or "bad," leading to skewed views of food and inappropriate eating habits.

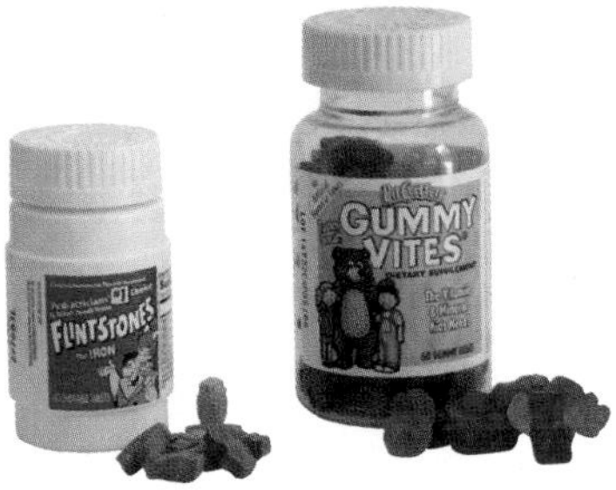

Children's multivitamins often appear in shapes or bright colors.

Carbohydrate The RDA for carbohydrate for children is 130 g/day, which is about 45–65% of total daily energy intake.[2] Complex carbohydrates from whole grains, fruits, vegetables, and legumes should be emphasized. Simple sugars should come from fruits and fruit juices, with foods high in refined sugars, such as cakes, cookies, and candies, saved for occasional indulgences. The AI for fiber for children is 14 g/1,000 kcal of energy consumed.[2] As is the case with toddlers, too much fiber can be harmful because it can make a child feel prematurely full and interfere with adequate food intake and nutrient absorption.

Protein As you can see in Table 15.1, the protein recommendation for boys and girls is 0.95 g/kg body weight per day.[2] Although the recommended protein intake per kg body weight for children age 4 to 13 years is lower than that of toddlers, the total protein intake of school-age children is higher due to their higher body weight. Lean meats/fish/poultry, lower-fat dairy products, soy-based foods, and legumes are nutritious sources of protein that can be provided to children of all ages.

Micronutrient Recommendations for Children

The need for most micronutrients increases slightly for children up to age 8 because of their increasing size. A sharper increase in micronutrient needs occurs during the transition into full adolescence; this increase is due to the beginning of sexual maturation and in preparation for the impending adolescent growth spurt. Children who fail to consume the USDA-recommended 4 cups of fruits and vegetables each day may become deficient in vitamins A, C, and E. Minerals of concern continue to be calcium, iron, and zinc, which come primarily from animal-based foods.[4,5] Notice that the RDA for iron is based on the assumption that most girls do not begin menstruation until after age 13.[5] Refer to Table 15.1 for a review of the nutrient needs of children.

If there is any concern that a child's nutrient needs are not being met for any reason (for instance, breakfasts are skipped, lunches are traded, or parents lack money for nourishing food), a pediatric vitamin/mineral supplement that provides no more than 100% of the daily value for the micronutrients may help correct any existing deficit.

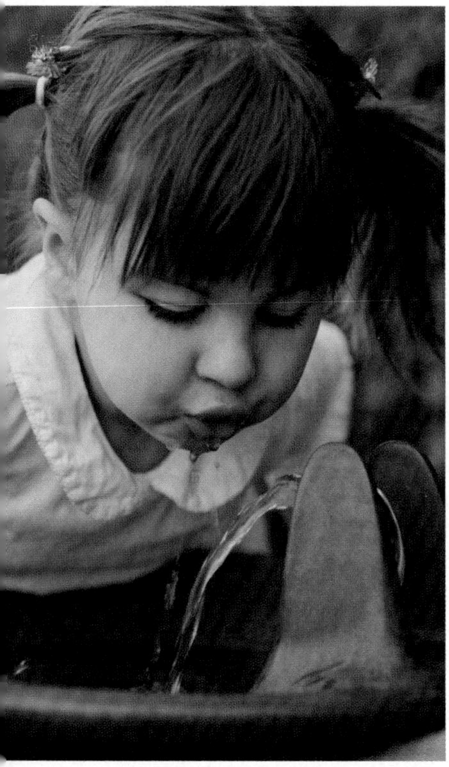

Fluid intake is important for children, who may become so involved in their play that they ignore the sensation of thirst.

Fluid Recommendations for Children

The fluid recommendations for children are about 5–8 cups as beverages, including drinking water (Table 15.1). The exact amount of fluid needed varies according to a child's level of physical activity and the weather conditions. At this point in life, children are mostly in control of their own fluid intake. However, as they engage in physical activity at school and in sports and play, young children in particular may need reminders to drink in order to stay properly hydrated, especially if the weather is hot.

RECAP **Total protein and energy needs are higher for children due to their larger size and higher activity levels. Dietary fat should be gradually reduced to the level of 25–35% of total energy. Calcium, iron, and zinc requirements are higher for children than toddlers. Children need to drink from 5 to 8 cups of water and other beverages throughout the day.**

Encouraging Nutritious Food Choices with Children

Peer pressure can be extremely difficult for both parents and their children to deal with during this life stage. Most children want to feel as if they "belong," and they admire and like to emulate children they believe to be popular. If the popular children at school are eating chips and drinking sugared soft drinks, it may be hard for a child to eat a peanut butter on whole-wheat sandwich, apple, and low-fat milk without embarrassment.

One strategy for combating peer pressure is to introduce kids to "cool" role models, such as star athletes and popular entertainers who follow nutritious diets. Involving children in growing their own food, shopping, and preparing meals is also a good idea. If they have input into what is going into their bodies, children may be more likely to take an active role in their health. In addition, adults should consistently model healthful eating and physical activity patterns.

What Is the Effect of School Attendance on Nutrition?

Children's school attendance can affect their nutrition in several ways. First, in the hectic time between waking and getting out the door, many children minimize or skip breakfast completely. Many nutrition and education experts believe that children who skip breakfast are at increased risk for behavioral and learning problems associated with hunger in the classroom. Public schools offer low- or no-cost school breakfasts to help children optimize their nutrient intake and avoid these problems, but not all children take advantage of them. You've probably heard people say that breakfast is the most important meal of the day. Is that so? Read the Nutrition Myth or Fact? box on page 552 to find out.

Another consequence of attending school is that, with little or no supervision of what they eat, children do not always consume appropriate types or amounts of food. They may spend their lunchtime talking or playing with friends rather than eating. If they purchase a school lunch, they might not like all the foods being served, or their friends might influence them to skip certain foods with comments such as "This broccoli's nasty!" Even homemade lunches that contain nutritious foods may be left uneaten or traded for less nutritious fare.

Finally, some schools continue to sell soft drinks, chips, and sweets at bake sales and other fund-raisers. Also, despite recent legislation and industry-sponsored initiatives, some schools still have vending machines offering snacks that are high in energy, sugar, and fat. Eating too many of these foods, either in place of or in addition to lunch, can lead to overweight and potential nutrient deficiencies.

Are School Lunches Nutritious?

On the surface, the answer to this question is "yes." Although the National School Lunch Program (NSLP) guidelines are based on old (1989) nutrient standards, all school lunches must meet updated total fat, saturated fat, and sodium requirements set by federal guidelines. Every lunch must provide one-third of the 1989 RDAs for protein, vitamin A, vitamin C, iron, calcium, and energy.[12] School meals must also comply with the Healthy Meals for Healthy Americans Act.

However, when this question is examined in more detail, the answer is not so clear. First, despite the recent implementation of new dietary guidelines, very few school lunch programs actually meet them: virtually none meet the sodium guideline, about 60% meet the total fat guideline (no more than 30% of total energy); and less than one-third meet the saturated fat guideline (no more than 10% of total energy).[13] Second, the nutrients a student *gets* depends on what the student actually *eats*. School lunch programs do not have to meet the federal guidelines every day, but only over the course of a week's meals. As a result, the school lunches that students actually eat tend to be higher in fat than the guideline because students tend to favor pizza, hamburgers, hot dogs, and french fries over the more nutritious, lower-fat entrées and side dishes offered. Third, some schools actually have fast-food restaurants

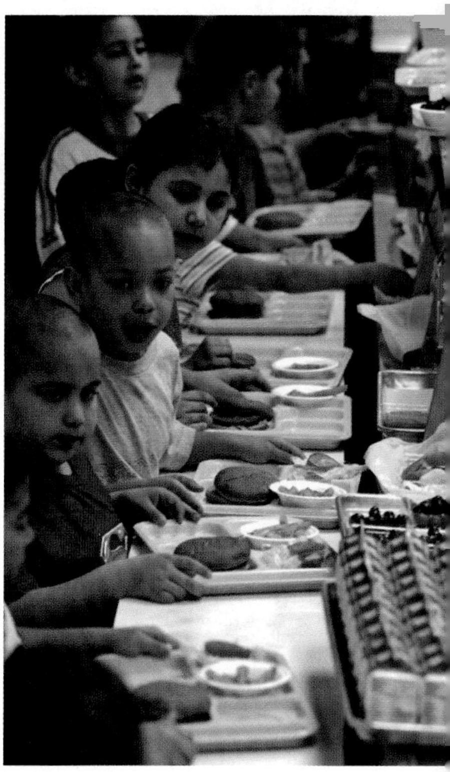

School-age children may receive a standard school lunch, but many choose less healthful foods when given the opportunity.

NUTRITION MYTH OR FACT?

Is Breakfast the Most Important Meal of the Day?

What did you eat for breakfast this morning? Whole-grain cereal with low-fat milk? A strawberry Pop-Tart? Or nothing at all? What does it matter, anyway? Sure, you've heard the saying that breakfast is the most important meal of the day, but that's just a myth—isn't it? As long as you eat a nutritious lunch and dinner, why should breakfast matter?

Over the past 20 years, dozens of published research studies have confirmed the importance of a healthful breakfast. Many of these studies highlight the ability of breakfast to support our physical and mental functioning. Let's examine the evidence for this claim.

The word *breakfast* was first used as a verb meaning "to break the fast"—that is, to end the hours of fasting that naturally occur while we sleep. When we fast, our body breaks down stored nutrients to provide fuel for the resting body. First, cells break down glycogen stores in the liver and muscle tissues, using the newly released glucose for energy. These stores last about 12 hours. But people who skip breakfast typically go without food for much longer than that: if they finish dinner about 7:00 PM and don't eat again until noon the next day, they are fasting (going without fuel) for 17 hours! Long before that point, essentially all stored glycogen is used up, and the body has turned to fatty acids and amino acids as fuel sources.

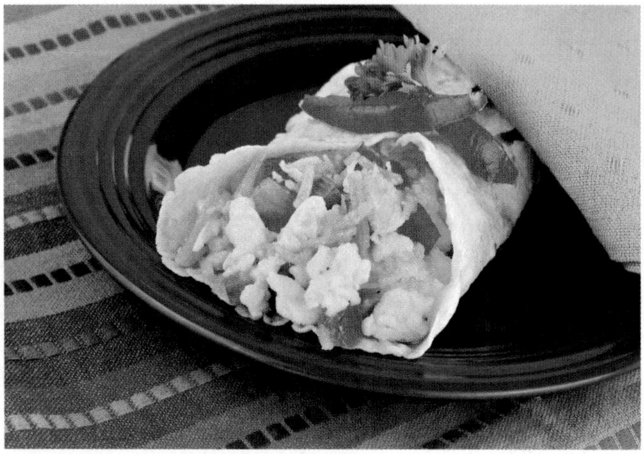

Breakfast doesn't have to be boring! A breakfast burrito with scrambled eggs, low-fat cheese, and vegetables wrapped in a whole-grain tortilla provides energy and nutrients to start your day off right.

If you're like most people, when your blood glucose is low, you are not only hungry but also weak, shaky, and irritable, and you have poor concentration. So it's not surprising that children and teens who skip breakfast don't function as well as their breakfast-eating peers: their physical, academic, and behavioral performances are all negatively affected.[14,15] Recent research confirms the following conclusions:

- Missing breakfast and experiencing hunger impair students' ability to learn. Exam scores are lower, their attention span is reduced, and they have more behavioral problems than students who arrive at school in a well-nourished state.
- Eating breakfast at school helps students perform better on demanding mental tasks and improves attention and memory. Children who eat a complete breakfast make fewer mistakes and work faster in math and vocabulary.
- Breakfast improves students' behavior, decreases their tardiness, and improves their school attendance.

What do you think? Is breakfast the most important meal of the day? And what—if anything—will you be having for breakfast tomorrow?

selling their food in competition with the school lunch program! Thus, even though school lunches as *planned* are considered a healthful choice, children may not be getting the benefit of these meals.

The good news is that most states have adopted policies that limit the types of competitive foods that can be sold on school campuses to ensure a more healthful food environment. The Institute of Medicine has also developed a set of nutrition standards for foods and beverages sold in schools.[16] At the local level, attention to nutrition is resulting in the offering of healthful alternatives, such as salad bars, and is changing how foods are bought and prepared by food service staff. The School Nutrition Association promotes "nutrition integrity" for all schools, emphasizing healthy diets, appropriate physical activity, and school-based nutrition education. These nutrition professionals also promote the goal of increasing the consumption of whole grains, fruits, and vegetables to adequately nourish all students while minimizing the risk for obesity.[17]

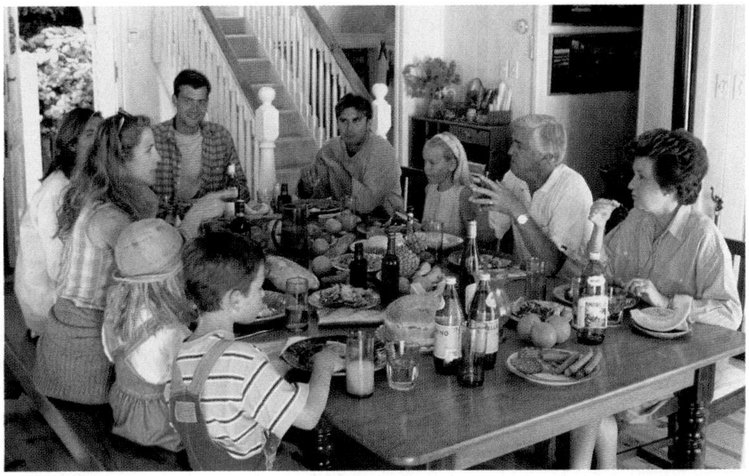

Families should try to have shared meals with their children whenever possible.

and pastries. Schools can set aside land or construct raised beds for vegetable gardens, and food service providers can use the produce in lunch menus. Consistent and repeated school-based messages on good nutrition can reinforce the efforts of parents and healthcare providers.

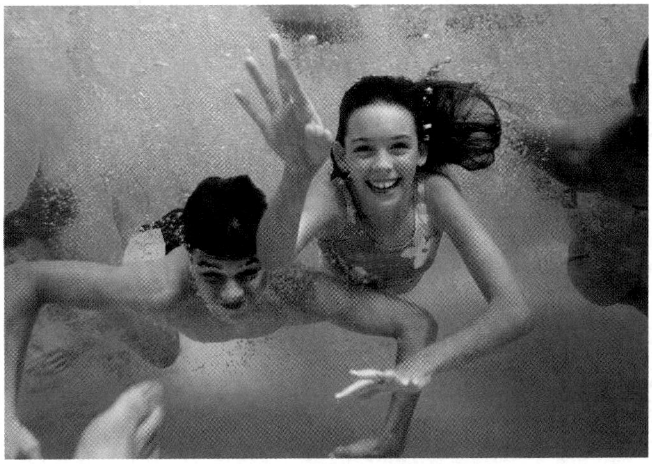

Regular physical activity is important for adolescents.

Prevention Through an Active Lifestyle

Increased energy expenditure through increased physical activity is essential for successful weight management among children. The Institute of Medicine recommends that children participate in daily physical activity and exercise for at least an hour each day.[2] For younger children, this can be divided into two or three shorter sessions, allowing them to regroup, recoup, and refocus between activity sessions. The 2008 Physical Activity Guidelines for Americans also advise bone- and muscle-strengthening activities at least 3 days each week.[30] Overweight children are more likely to engage in physical activities that are noncompetitive, fun, and structured in a way that allows them to proceed at their own pace. Children should be exposed to a variety of activities, so that they move different muscles, play at various intensities, avoid boredom, and find out what they like and don't like to do. The American Dietetic Association has a specific Fitness Pyramid for Kids to help guide children toward a physically active lifestyle **(Figure 15.6)**.

RECAP **Obesity is an important concern for children of all ages, their families, and their communities. Parents should model healthy eating and activity behaviors. Schools play an important role in providing nutritious breakfasts and lunches and varied opportunities for daily physical activity.**

Nutrition for Older Adults

The U.S. population is getting older each year. Consider the following statistics:

- In 2007, average life expectancy at birth reached 77.9 years.[31]
- It is estimated that, by the year 2030, the elderly (those 65 years and above) will account for about 20% of Americans.[31,32]

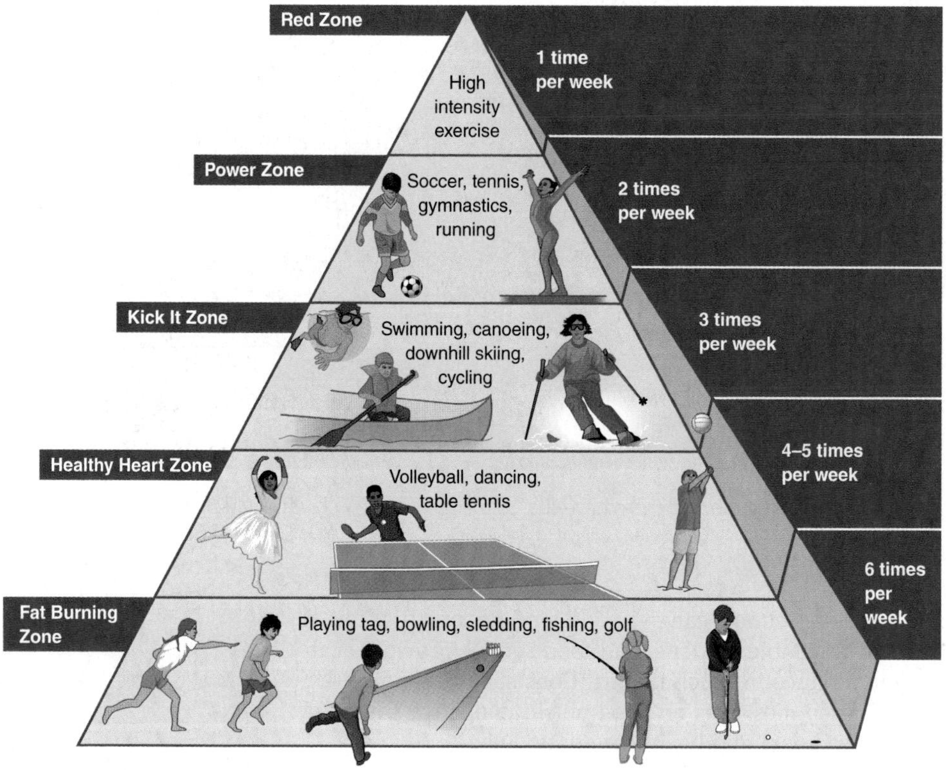

Figure 15.6 The American Dietetic Association's Fitness Pyramid for Kids[33] gives guidelines for the duration, intensity, and frequency of various types of activities that are appropriate for children age 2 to 11 years.

Data from the American Dietetic Association National Center for Nutrition and Dietetics, Kids Activity Pyramid, www.fitness.gov/10tips.htm.

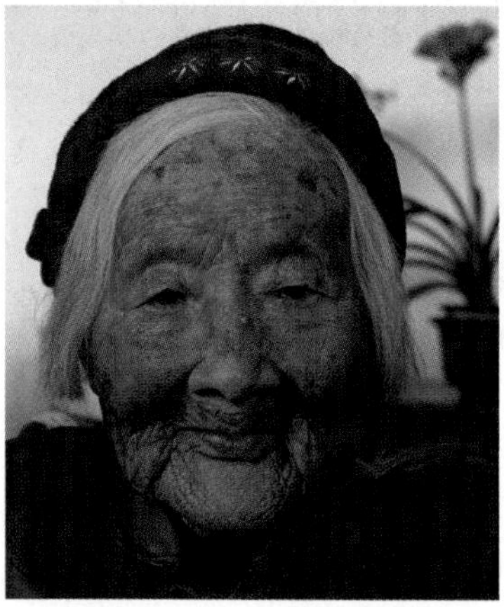

Centenarians represent the future of U.S. elderly.

- People 85 years of age and older currently represent the fastest-growing U.S. population subgroup, projected to increase from 4.2 million in 2000 to over 20 million by the year 2050.
- The number of *centenarians,* persons over the age of 100 years, and *super centenarians,* over 110 years, continues to grow as well. These so-called very elderly or oldest old account for the majority of healthcare expenditures and nursing home admissions in the United States.

These statistics have important nutrition-related implications even for younger adults, since a nutritious diet and regular physical activity throughout life can help prevent or delay the onset of chronic diseases and keep adults happy and productive in their later years. Throughout this book, our exploration of nutrition and physical activity has focused mainly on young and middle-age adults. In the following section, we discuss the unique nutritional needs and concerns of older adults, and we identify ways in which diet and lifestyle affect the aging process.

What Physiologic Changes Accompany Aging?

Older adulthood is a time in which body systems begin to slow and degenerate. If the following discussion of this degeneration seems disturbing or depressing, remember that the changes described are at least partly within an individual's control. For instance, some of the decrease in muscle mass, bone mass, and muscle strength is due to low physical activity levels. In addition, there are intriguing lines of research actively searching for a modern-day "Fountain of Youth," some of which are discussed ***In Depth*** following this chapter.

Age-Related Changes in Sensory Perception

For most individuals, eating is a social and pleasurable process; the sights, sounds, odors, and textures associated with food stimulate and enhance one's appetite. However, odor, taste, touch, and vision all decline with age and negatively affect the food intake and nutritional status of older adults.

It has been estimated that over half of older adults experience a significant impairment in their sense of smell. The nerve receptors for taste and smell are complementary; thus, enjoyment of food relies heavily on the sense of smell. Older adults who cannot adequately appreciate the appealing aromas of food may be unable to fully enjoy the foods offered in a meal. While often a simple consequence of aging, loss of odor perception can also be caused by a zinc deficiency or a medication. If this is the case, a zinc supplement or change of medication may be a simple solution. Taste perception dims as well, especially the ability to detect salt and bitter tastes. The ability to perceive sweetness and sourness also declines, but to a lesser extent.

Loss of visual acuity has unexpected consequences for the nutritional health of older adults. Many have difficulty reading food labels, including nutrient information and "pull dates" for perishable foods. Driving skills decline, limiting the ability of some older Americans to get to a market offering healthful, affordable foods. Older adults with vision loss may not be able to see the temperature knobs on stoves or the controls on microwave ovens and may therefore choose cold meals, such as sandwiches, rather than meals that require heating. Also, the visual appeal of a colorful, attractively arranged plate of food is lost to visually impaired elderly people, further reducing their desire to eat healthful meals.

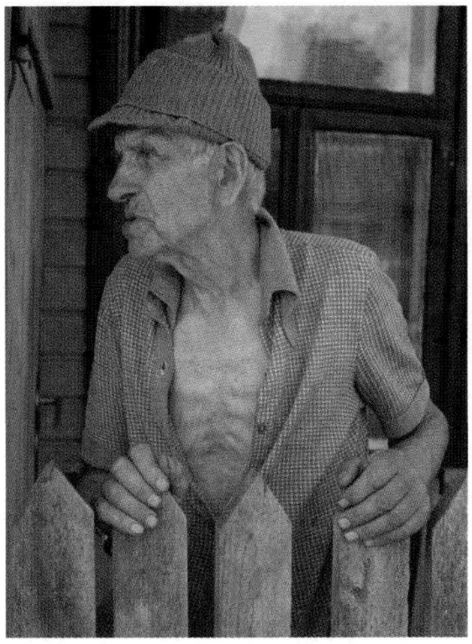

A variety of gastrointestinal and other physiologic changes can lead to weight loss in older adults.

Age-Related Changes in Gastrointestinal Function

Significant changes in the mouth, stomach, intestinal tract, and related organs occur with aging. Some of these changes can increase the risk for nutrient deficiency.

With increasing age, salivary production declines. A dry mouth reduces taste perception, increases tooth decay, and makes chewing and swallowing more difficult. Thus, a diet rich in moist foods, including fruits and vegetables; sauces or gravies on meats; and high-fluid desserts, such as puddings, is advised. Difficulty swallowing foods can also result from a stroke or a condition such as Parkinsonism. Smooth, thick foods, such as cream soups, applesauce, milkshakes, fruit nectars, and puddings, are usually well tolerated. Older adults are also at risk for a reduced secretion of gastric acid, which limits the absorption of minerals such as calcium, iron, and zinc and food sources of folic acid and vitamin B_{12}. A lack of intrinsic factor greatly reduces the absorption of vitamin B_{12} (see Chapter 10). These elderly, therefore, benefit from vitamin B_{12} supplements and/or B_{12} shots.

Age-Related Changes in Body Composition

With aging, body fat increases and muscle mass declines.[34] It has been estimated that women and men lose 20–25% of their lean body mass, respectively, as they age from 35 to 70 years. The decreased production of certain hormones, including testosterone and growth hormone, and chronic diseases contribute to this loss of muscle, as do poor diet and an inactive lifestyle. Along with adequate dietary intake, regular physical activity, including strength or resistance training, can help older adults maintain their muscle mass and strength, delaying or preventing the need for institutionalization.

Body fat increases from young adulthood through middle age, peaking at approximately 55–65 years of age, then declining in persons over the age of 70. With aging, body fat shifts from subcutaneous stores, just below the skin, to internal, or visceral, fat stores. Older men and women tend to deposit more fat in their abdominal region compared to younger adults. Among women, this shift in body fat stores is most dramatic after the onset of menopause and coincides with an increased risk for heart disease, diabetes, and metabolic syndrome.

Bone mineral density declines with age and may eventually drop to the critical fracture zone. Among older women, the onset of menopause leads to a sudden and dramatic loss of bone due to the lack of estrogen. Although it is less dramatic, elderly men also experience this loss of bone, due in part to decreasing levels of testosterone. In addition to the well-known benefits of calcium and vitamin D, intakes of vitamins A, C, and K, phosphorus, magnesium, fluoride, and protein are now recognized as influencing bone density. As noted in the Nutrition Debate on page 571, bone health can be promoted through regular weight-bearing activity in adults well into their nineties and beyond.

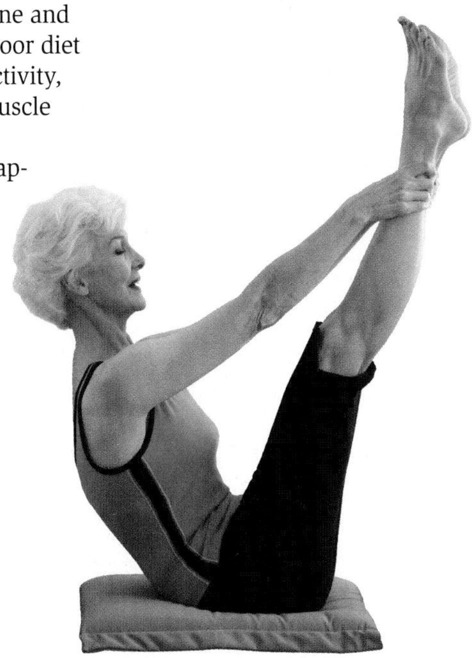

Regular physical activity slows age-related loss of muscle mass.

RECAP The physiologic changes that can occur with aging include sensory declines; an impaired ability to chew, swallow, and absorb and metabolize various nutrients; a loss of muscle mass and lean tissue; increased fat mass; and decreased bone density. These age-related changes influence the nutritional needs of older adults and their ability to consume a healthful diet.

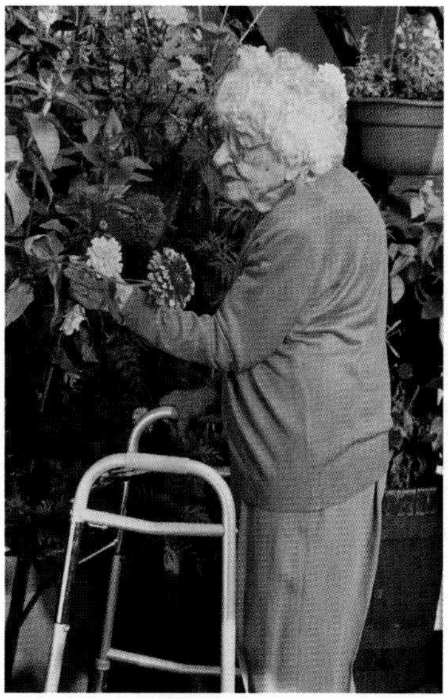

A less physically active lifestyle will lead to lower total energy requirements in older adults.

What Are an Older Adult's Nutrient Needs?

The requirements for many nutrients are the same for older adults as for young and middle-aged adults. A few nutrient requirements increase, and a few are actually lower. **Table 15.2** identifies the nutrient recommendations that change, as well as the physiologic reasons behind these changes.

Energy and Macronutrient Recommendations for Older Adults

The energy needs of older adults are lower than those of younger adults. This decrease is due to a loss of muscle mass and lean tissue, a reduction in thyroid hormones, and a less physically active lifestyle. It is estimated that total daily energy expenditure decreases approximately 10 kcal each year for men and 7 kcal each year for women ages 19 and older.[2] This means that a woman who needs 2,000 kcal at age 20 needs just 1,650 at age 70. Some of this decrease in energy expenditure is an inevitable response to aging, but some of the decrease can be delayed or minimized by staying physically active. To avoid weight gain, older adults need to consume a diet high in nutrient-dense foods but not too high in energy. Refer to the ***In Depth*** following this chapter to learn more about the theory of caloric restriction, which proposes that low-energy diets may significantly prolong lives.

Fat As with other age groups, there is no DRI for total fat intake for older adults.[2] However, to reduce their risk for heart disease and other chronic diseases, it is recommended that their total fat intake remain within 20–35% of total daily energy intake, with no more than 10% of total energy intake coming from saturated fat.

Carbohydrate The RDA for carbohydrate for older adults is 130 g/day.[2] As with all other age groups, this level of carbohydrate is sufficient to support brain glucose utilization. Complex carbohydrates should be emphasized over simple sugars: it is recommended that older individuals consume a diet that contains no more than 30% of total energy intake as sugars.[2] The fiber recommendations are slightly lower for older

TABLE 15.2 Nutrient Recommendations That Change with Increased Age

Changes in Nutrient Recommendations	Rationale for Changes
Vitamin D Increased need for vitamin D from 600 IU/day for adults age 18 to 70 years and to 800 IU/day for adults over age 70 years	Decreased bone density Decreased ability to synthesize vitamin D in the skin
Calcium Increased need for calcium from 1,000 mg/day for adults to 1,000 to 1,200 mg/day for adults 50 years of age and older	Decreased bone density Decreased absorption of dietary calcium
Fiber Decreased need for fiber from 38 g/day for young men to 30 g/day for men 51 years and older; decreases for women from 25 g/day for young women to 21 g/day for women 51 years and older	Decreased energy intake
B-Vitamins Increased need for vitamin B_6 and need for vitamin B_{12} as a supplement or from fortified foods	Lower levels of stomach acid Decreased absorption of food B_{12} from gastrointestinal tract Increased need to reduce homocysteine levels and to optimize immune function

adults than for younger adults because older adults eat less energy. After age 50, 30 g of fiber per day for men and 21 g for women is assumed sufficient to reduce the risks for constipation and diverticular disease, maintain healthful blood levels of glucose and lipids, and provide good sources of nutrient-dense, low-energy foods.

Protein The DRI for protein is the same for adults of all ages: 0.80 g protein/kg body weight per day.[2] Some researchers have argued for a protein allowance of 1.0 to 1.2 g protein/kg body weight for older adults in order to optimize their protein status; however, the issue remains unresolved.[35,36] Protein is important to help minimize the loss of muscle and lean tissue, optimize healing after injury or disease, maintain immunity, and help prevent excessive bone loss. Many protein-rich foods are also important sources of the vitamins and minerals that are typically low in the diets of older adults; thus, protein is an important nutrient for this age group.

Micronutrient Recommendations for Older Adults

The vitamins and minerals of particular concern for older adults are identified in Table 15.2.

Calcium and Vitamin D Preventing or minimizing the consequences of osteoporosis is a top priority for older adults. The requirements for both calcium and vitamin D are higher because of a reduced absorption of calcium from the gut, along with reduced production of vitamin D in the skin. Many older adults are at risk for vitamin D deficiency because they are institutionalized and are not exposed to adequate amounts of sunlight. The widespread use of sunscreen has lowered the risk for skin cancer among older adults; however, these products also block the sunlight needed for vitamin D synthesis in the skin. It is critical that older adults consume foods that are high in calcium and vitamin D and, when needed, use supplements. The Tufts Modified MyPyramid for Older Adults **(Figure 15.7)** recommends calcium and vitamin D supplements, along with the routine use of vitamin B_{12} supplements.

Iron Iron needs decrease with aging. This decrease is primarily due to reduced muscle and lean tissue in both men and women and the cessation of menstruation in women. The decreased need for iron in older men is not significant enough to change the recommendations for iron intake in this group; thus, the RDA for iron is the same for older and younger men, 8 mg/day. However, the RDA for iron for older women is 8 mg/day, which is 10 mg/day lower than the RDA for younger women.[5] Heme iron from meat, fish, and poultry represents the most available source of dietary iron; however, some older adults reduce their intake of these foods due to cost and possibly to difficulties in chewing and swallowing. Fortified grains and cereals, as well as legumes, greens, and dried fruits, can provide additional iron in the diet.

Zinc Although zinc recommendations are the same for all adults, it is a critical nutrient for optimizing immune function and wound healing in older adults. Zinc intake can be inadequate in older adults for the same reasons that heme iron intake may be deficient: red meats, poultry, and fish are relatively expensive, and older adults may have a difficult time chewing meats due to loss of teeth and/or the use of dentures.

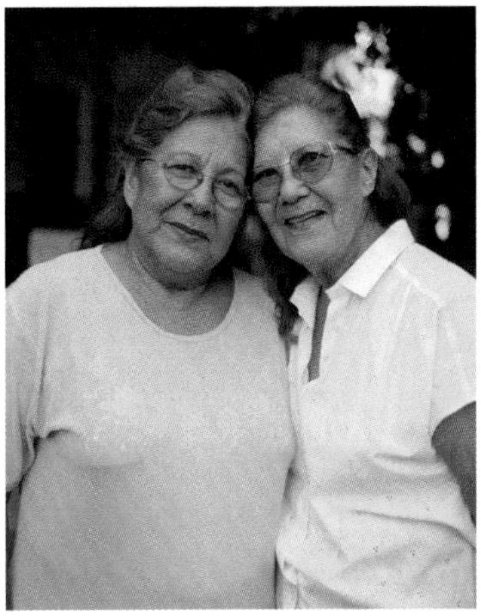

Older adults have unique nutritional needs.

Vitamins C and E Although it is speculated that older adults have increased oxidative stress, the recommendations for the antioxidant vitamins C and E are the same as for younger adults. While some research suggests that taking supplements containing vitamins C and E can lower the risk for age-related vision impairment, it is not possible to reach a conclusion regarding the benefits of supplementation.

B-vitamins Older adults need to pay close attention to their intake of the B-vitamins—specifically, vitamin B_{12}, vitamin B_6, and folate.[37] As discussed in detail in Chapter 10, inadequate intakes of these nutrients increase the levels of the amino acid homocysteine in the blood, and elevated homocysteine levels have been associated with an increased risk for cardiovascular, cerebrovascular, and peripheral vascular diseases.[38] These diseases are common among older adults.

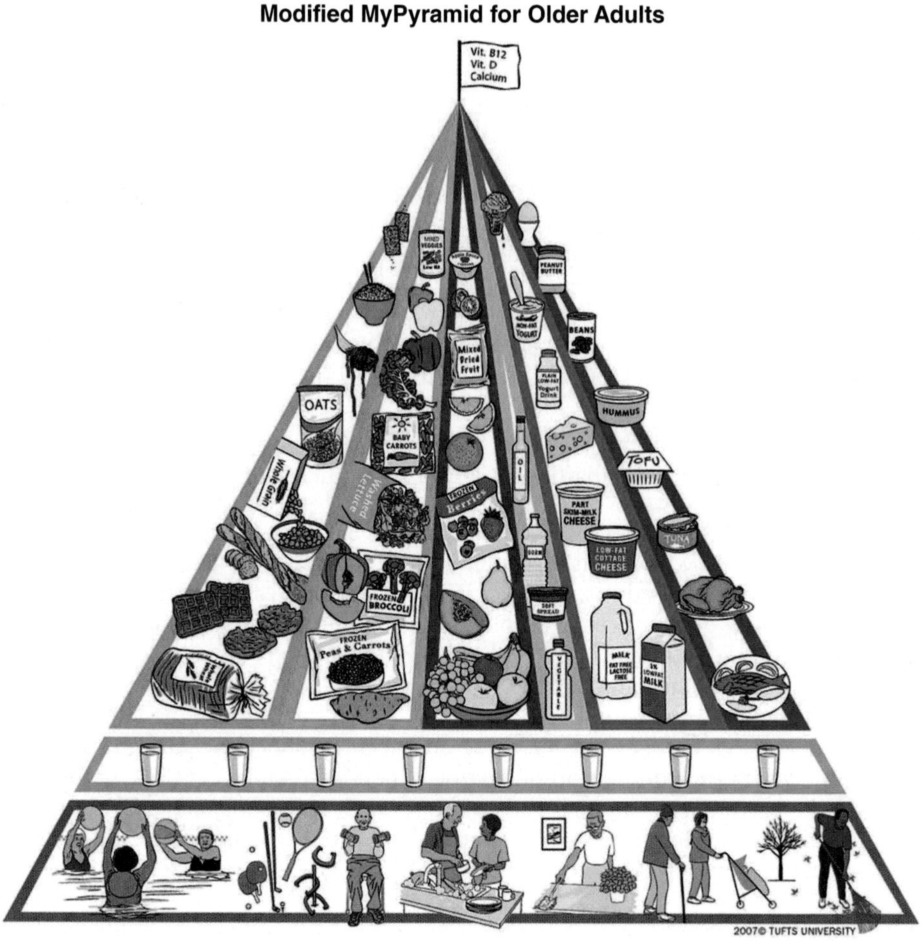

Figure 15.7 The Tufts Modified MyPyramid for Older Adults highlights the need for fluids, physical activity, and supplemental calcium and vitamins B_{12} and D.
Data from © Tufts University, www.nutrition.tufts.edu/docs/pdf/releases/ModifiedMyPyramid.pdf.

The RDA for both folate and vitamin B_{12} is the same for younger and older adults, but up to 30% of older adults cannot absorb enough vitamin B_{12} from foods due to low stomach acid production. It is recommended that older adults consume supplements or foods that are fortified with vitamin B_{12} because the vitamin B_{12} in these sources is absorbed more readily. Vitamin B_{12} is also available via injection. Vitamin B_6 recommendations are slightly higher for older adults, as these higher levels appear necessary to reduce homocysteine levels and optimize immune function in this population.[37]

Vitamin A Vitamin A requirements are the same for adults of all ages; however, older adults should be careful not to consume more than the RDA, as the absorption of vitamin A is actually greater in older adults. Thus, this group is at greater risk for vitamin A toxicity, which can cause liver damage and neurologic problems. In addition, high intakes of vitamin A by older adults have been linked to increased risk for hip fractures.[5] While older adults should avoid high dietary vitamin A and high-potency vitamin A supplements, consuming fruits and vegetables high in beta-carotene or other carotenoids is safe and does not lead to vitamin A toxicity.

A variety of factors may limit an older adult's ability to eat healthfully. These include limited financial resources that prevent some older people from buying nutrient-dense foods on a regular basis, reduced appetite, social isolation, an inability to prepare foods, and illnesses and physiologic changes that limit the absorption and metabolism of many nutrients. Thus, some older adults may benefit from taking a multivitamin and mineral supplement that contains no more than the RDA for all the nutrients contained in the supplement. Additional supplementation may be necessary for nutrients such as calcium, vitamin D, and vitamin B_{12}. However, supplementation with individual nutrients should be done only under the supervision of the individual's

HOT TOPIC

Senior Supplements: A Marketing Ploy?

Are the so-called "silver" supplements really better for seniors than ordinary formulations? Only minor differences exist between most standard and silver products. Let's take a look.

Iron and tin are omitted from the silver supplement, and vitamin K is reduced. Why? Eliminating iron lowers a senior's increased risk for iron overload. Since tin has no Daily Value or DRI, there is no justification for including it. Also, many seniors take prescription anti-clotting medications, so less vitamin K reduces the risk for a negative drug–nutrient interaction.

Silver supplements provide 40 mg more calcium, which helps supply the additional 200 mg of calcium that older adults need. Vitamins E and B_6 are also increased. The DRI for vitamin E does not change with age; however, increased oxidative stress and age-associated eye disorders explain the modest increase in the silver version. The increase in vitamin B_6 may help lower serum homocysteine, and the silver supplement provides four times more vitamin B_{12}. Why? Many adults over age 50 malabsorb vitamin B_{12} from foods so it is better absorbed in a supplement. Seniors should evaluate the potential benefits of silver supplements; their differences can be small but appropriate.

primary healthcare provider, as the risk of nutrient toxicity is high in this population.

Fluid Recommendations for Older Adults

The AI for fluid is the same for older and younger adults.[6] Men should consume 3.7 liters of total water per day, which includes 3.0 liters (about 13 cups) as beverages, including drinking water. Women should consume 2.7 liters of total water per day, which includes 2.2 liters (about 9 cups) as beverages. Kidney function changes with age, and the thirst mechanism of older people can be impaired. These changes can result in chronic dehydration and hypernatremia (elevated blood sodium levels) in this population. Some older adults intentionally limit their beverage intake because they have urinary incontinence or don't want to be awakened for nighttime urination. This practice can endanger their health, so it is important for them to seek treatment for the incontinence and continue to drink plenty of fluids.

RECAP **Older adults have lower energy needs due to their loss of lean tissue and lower physical activity levels. Older adults should consume 20–35% of total energy as fat and 45–65% of their energy as carbohydrate. Protein recommendations are the same as for younger adults. The micronutrients of concern are calcium, vitamin D, iron, zinc, vitamin B_{12}, vitamin B_6, and folate. Older adults need to carefully select nutrient-dense foods to meet their micronutrient needs, and supplementation may be necessary. Older adults are at risk for chronic dehydration. Men need to drink about 13 cups of water and other beverages per day, and women need about 9 cups.**

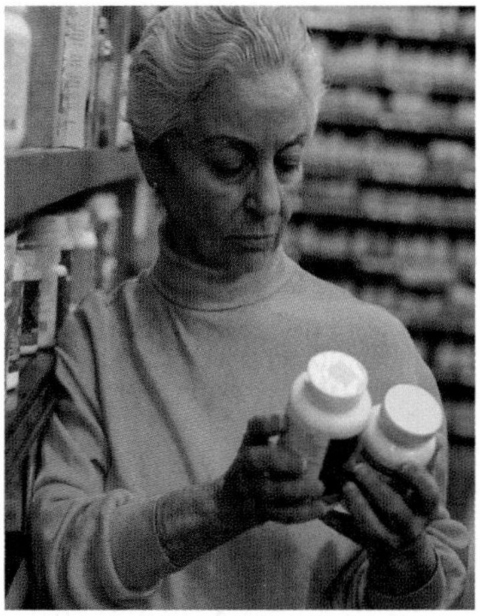

Many supplements are targeted at the elderly.

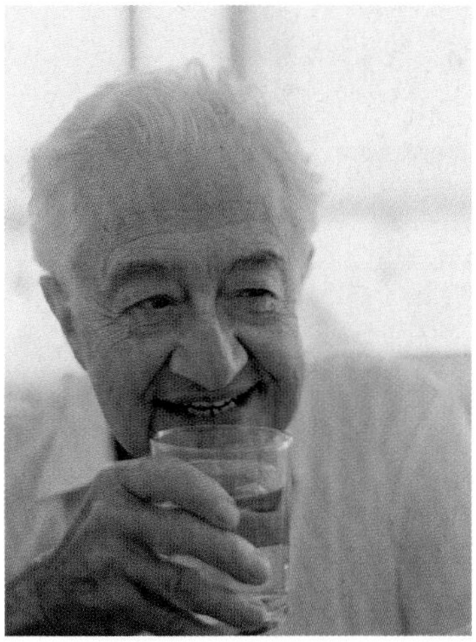

Older adults need the same amount of fluids as other adults.

Nutrition-Related Concerns for Older Adults

Older adults have a number of unique nutritional concerns. In addition to overweight and underweight, they commonly face dental problems, eye disorders, and potential interactions between nutrients and medications. Also, some older adults face financial difficulties that affect their nutritional choices. Each of these concerns is discussed briefly in the following sections.

Overweight and Underweight: A Delicate Balancing Act

Not surprisingly, overweight and obesity are of concern to older adults. Over the past decade, U.S. rates of obesity among the elderly have more than doubled. It is estimated that 78% of men and 71% of women between the ages of 65 and 74 are overweight or obese, while the incidence drops to 66% (men) and 63% (women) for those 75 years and older.[38] The elderly population as a whole has a high risk for heart disease, hypertension, type 2 diabetes, and cancer, and these diseases are more prevalent in older adults who are overweight or obese. Obesity increases the severity and consequences of osteoarthritis, limits mobility, and is associated with functional declines in daily activities.[39] In contrast, overweight can be protective against osteoporosis and fall-related fractures in older adults.

Underweight is also risky for older adults; mortality rates are actually higher in the underweight elderly than in the overweight elderly.[40] Significantly underweight older adults have fewer protein reserves to call upon during periods of catabolic stress, such as post-surgery or trauma, and are more susceptible to infection. Inappropriate weight loss suggests inadequate energy intake, which also implies inadequate nutrient intake. Chronic deficiencies of protein, vitamins, and minerals leave older adults at risk for poor wound healing and a depressed immune response.

Gerontologists have identified "nine Ds" that account for most cases of geriatric weight loss (**Figure 15.8**). Several of these factors promote weight loss by reducing energy intake, others by increasing energy expenditure or loss of nutrients.

Dental Health Issues

Diet plays an important role in the maintenance of dental health in the elderly. Vitamin B-complex deficiencies contribute to irritation, inflammation, and cracking of the lips and tongue, whereas vitamin C deficiency increases the risk for periodontal (gum) disease. A lack of adequate calcium, vitamin D, and protein contributes to bone loss in the oral cavity, which increases risk for tooth loss. Saliva helps neutralize the decay-promoting acids produced by oral bacteria; however, with aging, saliva production decreases.

Despite great advances in dental health, older adults remain at high risk of losing some or all of their teeth, suffering from gum disease, or having poorly fitting dentures. These conditions cause considerable mouth pain and make chewing difficult and sometimes embarrassing. Thus, older adults may avoid eating foods such as meats and firm fruits and vegetables, leading to nutrient deficiencies. Older adults can compensate for a loss of chewing ability by selecting soft, protein-rich foods, such as eggs, peanut butter, cheese, yogurt, ground meat, fish, and well-cooked legumes. Red meats and poultry can be stewed or cooked in liquid for a long period of time. Oatmeal and other whole-

Figure 15.8 The nine Ds of geriatric weight loss. Many factors contribute to inappropriate weight loss in the elderly.

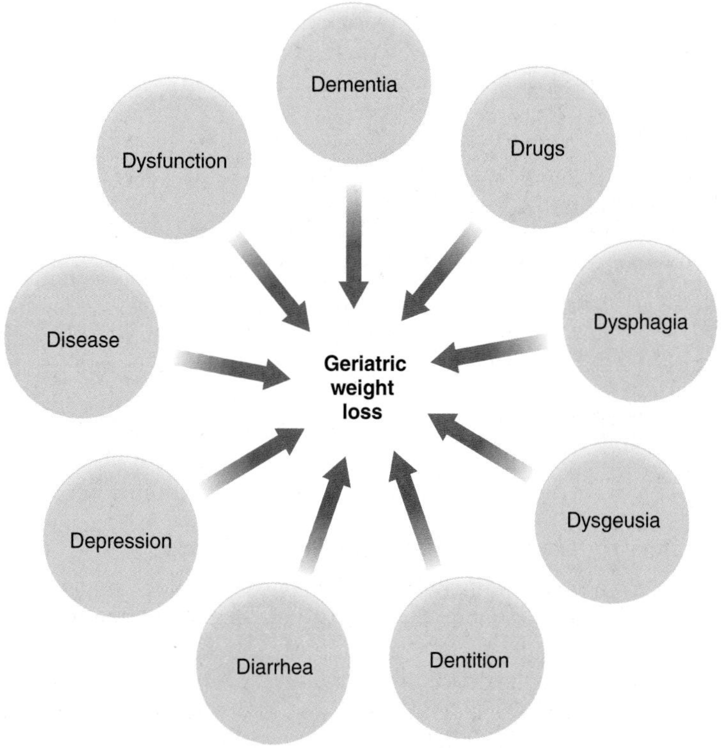

grain cooked cereals can provide needed fiber, as do mashed berries and bananas, ripened melons, and canned vegetables. Shredded and minced raw vegetables can be added to dishes. With planning, older adults with oral health problems can maintain a varied, healthful diet.

Age-Related Eye Diseases

Two age-related eye disorders are responsible for vision impairment and blindness in older adults. *Macular degeneration* is damage to the macula, a portion of the retina of the eye (**Figure 15.9a**). It is the most common cause of blindness in the U.S. elderly. A *cataract* is a cloudiness in the lens of the eye (Figure 15.9b). This condition affects 20% of adults in their sixties and almost 70% of those in their eighties. Although these are different conditions, sunlight exposure and smoking are lifestyle practices that increase the risk for both.

Recent research suggests, but does not prove, that dietary choices may slow the progress of these two degenerative eye diseases, saving millions of dollars and preventing or delaying the functional losses associated with impaired vision. Several studies have shown the beneficial effects of antioxidants, including vitamins C and E, on cataract formation, whereas others have reported no significant benefit. Two phytochemicals, lutein and zeaxanthin, have also been identified as protective by some, but not all, studies. These four antioxidants, as well as zinc, may also provide protection against macular degeneration. Although the research is not yet conclusive, older adults can benefit by consuming foods rich in these nutrients, primarily colorful fruits and vegetables, nuts, and whole grains. Vision-enhancing nutrient supplements remain an unproved therapy.

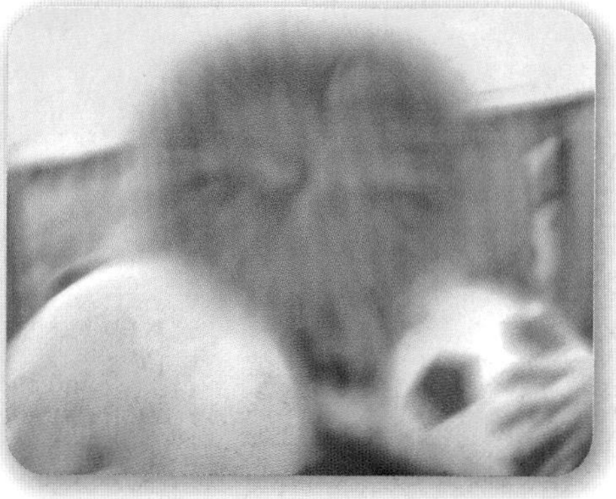

(a)

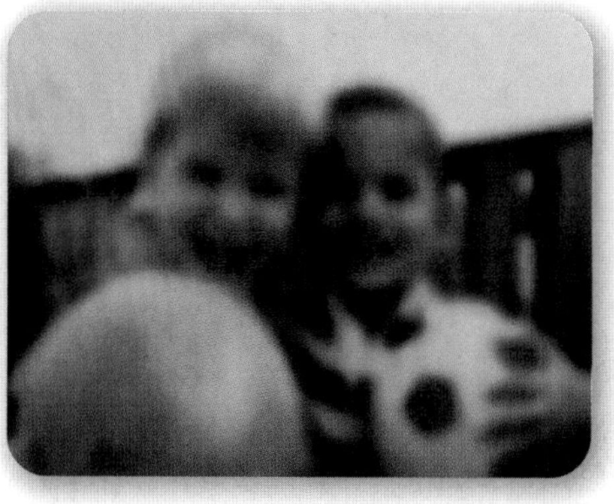

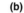

(b)

Figure 15.9 These photos simulate two forms of vision loss common in older adults. **(a)** Macular degeneration results in a loss of central vision. **(b)** Cataracts impair vision across the visual field.[42]

Interactions Between Medications and Nutrition

Although persons 65 years of age and above account for only 13% of the U.S. population, they are prescribed about 35% of all medications, and they experience almost 40% of all adverse drug effects, in part because of *polypharmacy*, or the use of multiple drugs.[41] Almost one-third of older U.S. adults use five or more prescription medications at any given time, while 15% use five or more dietary supplements on a regular basis. The use of over-the-counter drugs adds to the potential for harmful interactions: more than half of all older adults use five or more products (prescription medications, over-the-counter drugs, and/or dietary supplements) at the same time. It should come as no surprise, then, that older adults make more than 175,000 emergency room visits annually for medication-related problems.

Medications interact not only with each other but also with nutrients and other food components. Some medications increase or decrease food intake, while others alter nutrient digestion, absorption, or excretion. Several drugs negatively affect the metabolism of nutrients such as vitamin D, folate, and vitamin B_6. **Table 15.3** summarizes some of the more common drug–nutrient interactions.

Financial Problems

Approximately 9% of elderly men and women in the United States experience some form of food insecurity at least once a year.[43] In response to this problem, the federal government has developed a network of food and nutrition services for older Americans. These services are typically coordinated with state and local governments, as well as non-profit or community organizations. They include the following:

- *Supplemental Nutrition Assessment Program (SNAP):* Previously known as the Food Stamp program, this USDA program is the primary food assistance program for low-income households. It is designed to meet the basic nutritional needs of eligible people of all ages. Participants are provided with a monthly allotment, typically in the form of a pre-paid debit card or food coupons. There are very few restrictions on the foods that can be purchased under this plan.
- *Child and Adult Care Program:* This program provides healthy meals and snacks to older and functionally impaired adults in qualified adult day-care settings. While only

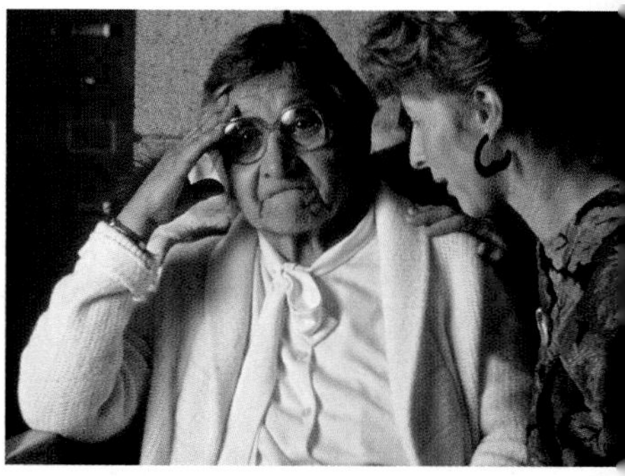

Financial problems can affect an older adult's nutritional status.

TABLE 15.3 Examples of Common Drug–Nutrient Interactions

Category of Drug	Interactions
Antacids	May decrease the absorption of iron, calcium, folate, vitamin B_{12}
Antibiotics	May reduce the absorption of calcium, fat-soluble vitamins; reduces the production of vitamin K by gut bacteria
Anticonvulsants	Interfere with activation of vitamin D
Anticoagulants ("blood thinners")	Reduce the activity of vitamin K
Antidepressants	May cause weight gain as a result of increased appetite
Antiretroviral agents (used in treatment of HIV/AIDS)	Reduce absorption of most nutrients
Aspirin	Lowers blood folate levels; increases iron loss due to gastrointestinal bleeding
Diuretics	May increase urinary excretion of potassium, sodium, calcium, magnesium; may cause retention of potassium, other electrolytes
Laxatives	Increase fecal excretion of dietary fat, fat-soluble vitamins, calcium and other minerals

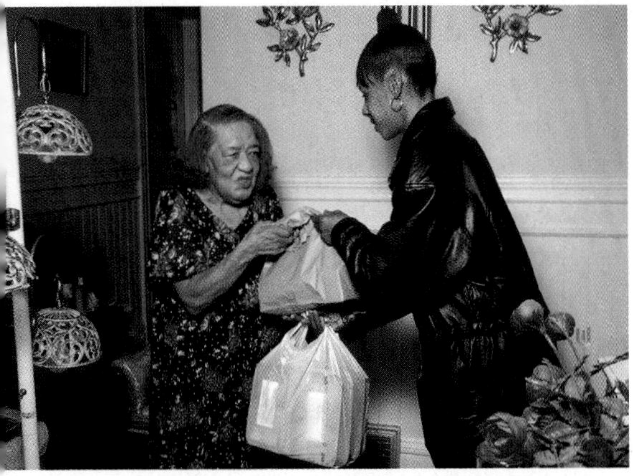

For homebound, disabled, and older adults, community programs such as Meals on Wheels provide nourishing, balanced meals as well as vital social contact.

2% of program funds are in support of adult care programs, they are a valuable source of revenue for the religious and community agencies that run the programs.

- *Commodity Supplemental Food Program:* This program targets low-income pregnant women, infants and young children, and older adults. Income guidelines must be met. Specific commodity foods are distributed, including cereals, peanut butter, dry beans, rice or pasta, and canned juice, fruits, vegetables, meat, poultry, and tuna. Unlike food stamps, this program is not intended to provide a complete array of foods.
- *Senior Farmers' Market Nutrition Program:* This program, sponsored by the USDA, provides coupons to low-income seniors, so that they can buy eligible foods at farmers' markets and roadside stands. Seniors enjoy the nutritional benefits of fresh produce and the opportunity to increase the variety of their meals.
- *Nutrition Services Incentive Program:* The Department of Health and Human Services provides cash and USDA commodity foods to state agencies for meals for senior citizens. There are no income criteria; any person 60 years or older (plus his or her spouse, even if younger) can take part in this program. Meals, designed to provide one-third of the RDA for key nutrients, are served at senior centers located in community complexes, public housing units, religious centers, schools, and similar locations. Some centers provide "bag dinners" for evening meals, and others send home meals on Fridays for consumption over the weekend. For qualified elders, meals can be delivered to their homes through the Meals on Wheels program. Although the meals are free, participants are encouraged to contribute what they can to cover the cost of each meal.

Participation in the Nutrition Services Incentive Program improves the dietary quality and nutrient intakes of older adults; however, the program may have a long waiting list and be unable to meet the current demand in the community.

RECAP **Overweight and obesity are important concerns for older adults, as they increase the risk for chronic diseases. Underweight is also a concern, as it can lead to increased illness and injury. Older adults may lose their sense of smell and taste, and dental and vision problems can limit their intake of meats, fruits, and vegetables, leading to nutrient deficiencies. Medications and certain nutrients can have adverse interactions. Several government and community programs are available for older adults in need of food assistance.**

Nutrition DEBATE

Physical Activity in Older Adulthood: Should Seniors "Go for the Gold"?

Recent information from the Centers for Disease Control and Prevention (CDC) confirms that participation in vigorous activity is uncommon among older adults: fewer than 14% of the "young elderly" (65–74 years) and only 7% of the "older elderly" (75 years and above) report participating in a regular program of vigorous exercise.[44]

We know that physically active elders live longer and enjoy better health. A regular program of physical activity lowers the risk for heart disease, hypertension, type 2 diabetes, obesity, depression, and cognitive decline or dementia. The complications of arthritis can also be reduced with appropriate exercise, as can the risk for falls and bone fractures. The need for healthcare visits, diagnostic tests, medication, and other treatments to control blood glucose, serum cholesterol, blood pressure, and other factors in chronic illness can be reduced or eliminated with regular exercise.

How much physical activity do older adults need in order to achieve these health benefits—and does moderate activity count, or should seniors "go for the gold"? Here are the most recent CDC guidelines:

- Aerobic activity: Seniors should engage in a minimum of 150 minutes of moderate-intensity aerobic activity (brisk walking, bicycling, swimming) or 75 minutes of vigorous aerobic activity (running or jogging) every week.
- Muscle strengthening: Seniors should engage in muscle-strengthening activities, such as resistance or strength training, on 2 or more days a week.[45] Muscle-strengthening activities should work all the major muscle groups, including the legs, arms, hips, back, abdomen, chest, and shoulders. Free weights, weight machines, resistance bands, push-ups, and heavy physical work (digging, shoveling) all contribute to muscle strengthening. Older adults can gain even greater health benefits by increasing their aerobic exercise to either 300 minutes of moderate-intensity or 150 minutes of vigorous activity each week.
- Flexibility and balance: Seniors should do a few minutes of flexibility exercises, such as stretches and yoga, most days of the week. Daily balance exercises are also important to reduce the risk for falls as we age. Toe raises, side leg raises, and rear leg swings are examples of balance activities; tai chi is another popular way to improve balance.

Are older adults more susceptible to injury or harm from vigorous exercise? A review of exercise-related sudden cardiac death in adults concluded that vigorous activity can, in fact, increase the risk for heart attack and/or sudden cardiac death in susceptible persons.[46] But who qualifies as susceptible? At greatest risk are people who perform activities at an intensity or a duration they are not used to. Think of the "weekend warrior": a person who is very sedentary most days of the week but goes "all out" on a Saturday afternoon. This person is at high risk for a heart attack or sudden cardiac death during or shortly after vigorous activity. A second vulnerable group includes older adults with diagnosed or undiagnosed heart disease. Seniors may also be more vulnerable to dehydration, heat stress, fractures, falls, knee pain, and muscle soreness or stiffness with intense exercise.[46]

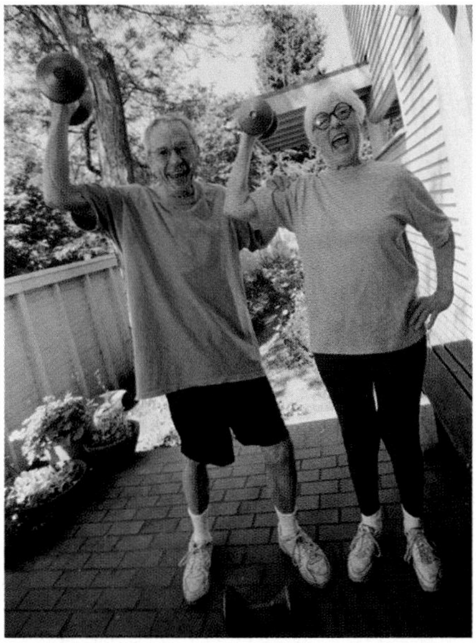

To minimize the risk for exercise-related cardiac events and other complications of vigorous exercise, older adults should follow these guidelines:

- All older adults should be carefully evaluated by their healthcare provider to determine the optimal types, intensities, and duration of physical activities appropriate for them.
- Older adults should be familiar with the signs of cardiac impairment: shortness of breath, chest pain, neck pain, dizziness or palpitations, and unusual fatigue. They should seek immediate medical care if any of these symptoms develop during or shortly after activity. Older adults should recognize the need to modify their activity patterns under conditions of stress, such as very cold temperatures, high heat or humidity, or a period of illness, such as the flu.
- Older adults should exercise in rooms with appropriate temperature, ventilation, and lighting; wear appropriate clothing and comfortable shoes; and have water readily available.
- Older adults should engage in supervised warm-up and cool-down activities.

The benefits of regular physical activity by older adults almost always far outweigh the potential risks, even at relatively high levels of intensity—the payoff is better health, more independence, less disability, and a longer, happier life!

Chapter Review

Test Yourself ANSWERS

1. True. Experts agree that food choices, including the consumption of fried foods, chocolate, and sodas, have virtually no impact on the development of acne.

2. True. Although a reduction in muscle mass and lean tissue is inevitable with aging, some of this loss can be attenuated with regular physical activity.

3. False. It is unlikely that the human life span will exceed 125 years.

Find the Quack

Sal is having lunch at the golf club with his friend Donald. Normally, they spend most of their time discussing their game, which Sal usually wins and Donald often complains that he's lost because of his painful joints. But today is different. Donald shows Sal something he's just received free in the mail: *Longevity Today* magazine. He says there are articles in it that prove that most of the problems of aging can be cured by a remedy containing a substance called procaine. Sal shakes his head. "Sounds like a scam to me!"

"But these articles are written by doctors," his friend insists. "And scientists. And one is even written by a former nutrition consultant for the Olympics! For instance," he continues, stabbing his finger at a particular page, "here's an article written by an M.D. that says that this procaine stuff 'reverses the physical and cognitive effects of aging, including hypertension, enlarged prostate, joint pain, constipation, and even depression!' That's a quote!"

Sal laughs. "One pill is supposed to do all that?"

"They cite studies!" Donald exclaims. "Listen: 'Clinical trials in Europe, Asia, and the United States have consistently demonstrated the benefits of procaine as an anti-aging wonder drug.' It's only 20 bucks for a month's supply. I say it's worth a try."

Sal shrugs. "Listen, Donald, if you want to throw away your money, go ahead. But I'd rather save my 20 bucks and take Doris out for a walk on the beach at sunset. That's my anti-aging remedy!"

1. Look up procaine in a reputable online encyclopedia or another source. What is it, and what is behind the claims for its anti-aging properties?
2. Donald is impressed by the authorship of the articles he read in *Longevity Today* magazine—physicians, scientists, and a nutrition consultant—and by the fact that the articles "cite studies." Are you? Why or why not?
3. Comment on the fact that Donald received *Longevity Today* magazine free in the mail.
4. What do you think of Sal's "anti-aging remedy"?

Answers can be found on the companion website, at www.pearsonhighered.com/thompsonmanore.

Review Questions

1. Which of the following nutrients is needed in increased amounts in older adulthood?
   a. fiber
   b. vitamin D
   c. iron
   d. vitamin A
2. Carbohydrate should make up what percentage of total energy for children?
   a. 25–40%
   b. 35–50%
   c. 45–65%
   d. 65–85%
3. Which of the following is a major nutrition-related concern for toddlers?
   a. lacto-ovo-vegetarianism
   b. skipping breakfast
   c. botulism
   d. allergies
4. Which of the following breakfasts would be most appropriate to serve a 20-month-old child?
   a. 1/2 cup of iron-fortified cooked oat cereal, 2 tbsp. of mashed pineapple, and 1 cup of whole milk
   b. 2 tbsp. of nonfat yogurt, 2 tbsp. of applesauce, one slice of melba toast spread with strawberry preserves, and 1 cup of calcium-fortified orange juice
   c. 1/2 cup of iron-fortified cooked oat cereal, 1/4 cup of cubed pineapple, and 1 cup of low-fat milk
   d. two small link sausages cut in 1-inch pieces, 2 tbsp. of scrambled egg, one slice of whole-wheat toast, four cherry tomatoes, 2 tbsp. of applesauce, and 1 cup of whole milk
5. Which of the following statements about cigarette smoking is true?
   a. Cigarette smoking can interfere with the metabolism of nutrients.
   b. Cigarette smoking commonly causes food cravings, known as "the munchies."
   c. Cigarette smoking is the number one cause of death in adolescents.
   d. All of the above statements are true.
6. True or false? Preschool children are too young to understand and be influenced by their parents' examples.
7. True or false? The food choice patterns of children are heavily influenced by circumstances at school.
8. True or false? High-potency vitamin A supplements are an effective treatment for acne.
9. True or false? Mortality rates are higher in the underweight elderly than in the overweight elderly.
10. True or false? Regular participation in strengthening and aerobic exercises slows age-related loss of muscle mass.

Answers to Review Questions can be found at the back of this text, and additional essay questions and answers are located on the companion website at www.pearsonhighered.com/thompsonmanore.

Web Resources

www.kidsnutrition.org
USDA/ARS Children's Nutrition Research Center

This site provides information about current research projects, nutrition web links, and consumer and nutrition news.

www.keepkidshealthy.com
Keep Kids Healthy.com

Find information about nutrition and health for toddlers, children, and adolescents on this website.

www.cdc.gov
The Centers for Disease Control and Prevention

Click on Life Stages & Populations; then you can select topics such as Adolescents & Teens or Older Adults & Seniors.

www.vrg.org
The Vegetarian Resource Group

Learn more about vegetarianism for all ages. Included on the site are sections for teens and kids, as well as recipes and eating guides.

www.nichd.nih.gov/milk
Milk Matters

This website provides practical tips and menus for children and adolescents.

www.nutrition.wsu.edu/ebet/toolkit
Eat Better, Eat Together

This website offers educational materials for strengthening family meal time. Suggestions for community events, media interviews, and educational materials are available.

www.fns.usda.gov
USDA Food & Nutrition Service

Read about government programs to provide food to people of all ages, including school meals programs, the Child and Adult Care Food program, and the WIC program.

Searching for the Fountain of Youth

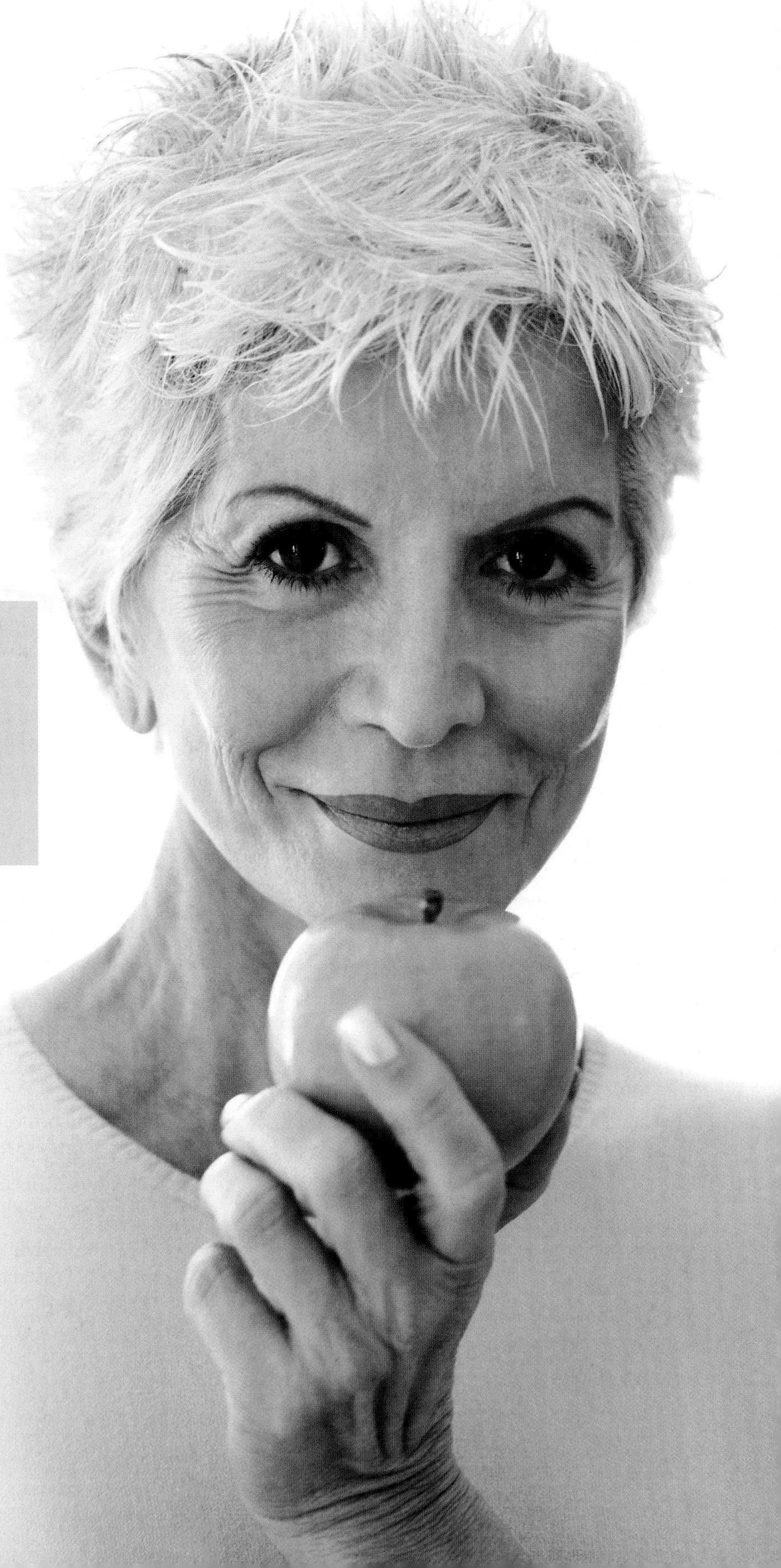

WANT TO FIND OUT...

- **whether Calorie restriction can extend your life span?**
- **how dietary supplements affect longevity?**
- **if you're on track toward a long and healthy life?**

READ ON.

How old do you want to live to be—80 years, 90, 100? Worldwide, throughout human history, legends have told of a "fountain of youth," which reverses decades of aging in anyone who drinks its waters. Of course, no one believes such tales any longer, but pick up a fashion or fitness magazine and you're likely to find modern equivalents: anti-aging diets, supplements, cosmetics, spa treatments, and other therapies. For instance, if you were to read that you could live to celebrate your 100th birthday in good health by eating about a quarter less than your current energy intake, would you do

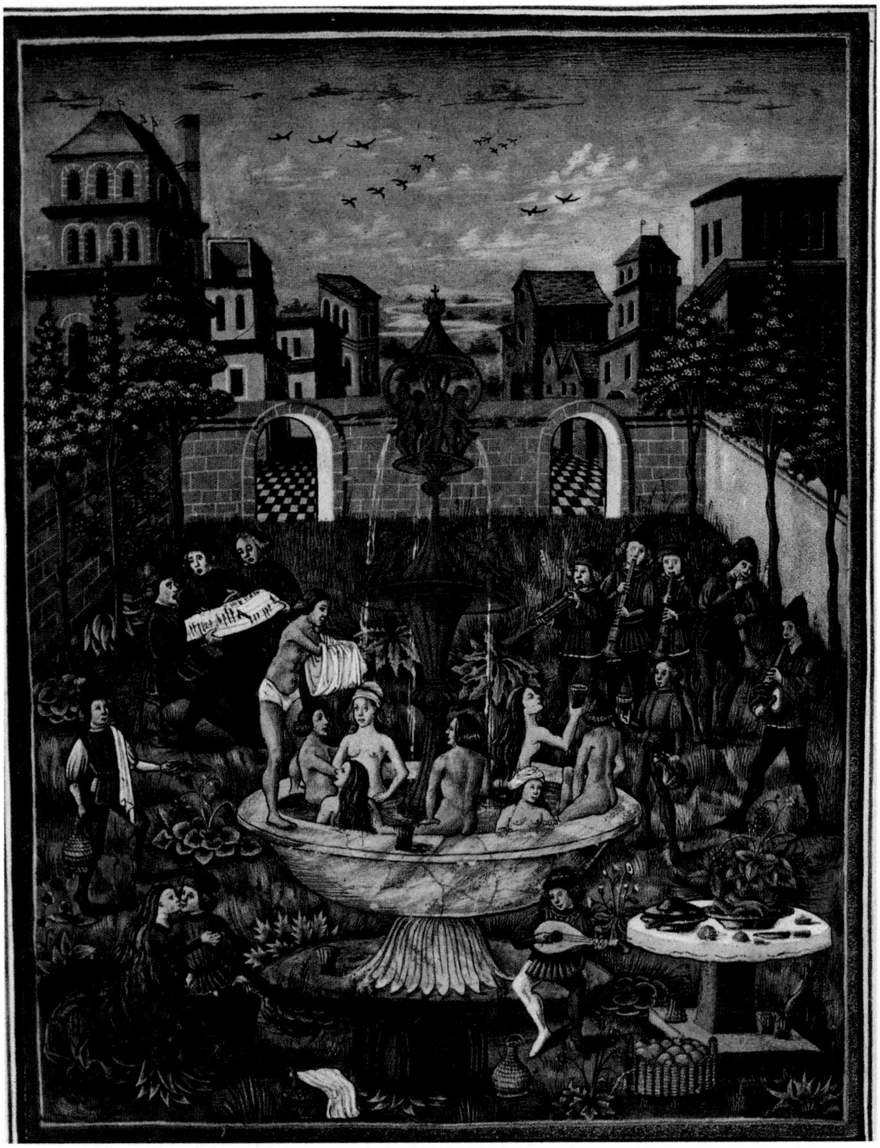

We may no longer believe in an actual "fountain of youth," but our search for health and longevity continues today.

it? If there were a supplement ad that claimed the product could give you an extra decade of healthful living, would you buy it? Or would you assume that these are just fairy tales, too?

Believe it or not, a growing number of people are trying such approaches in an effort to extend both their youthfulness and their longevity. Are these measures effective? What other actions can you take right now to live longer in good health? Let's find out.

Does Calorie Restriction Increase Life Span?

The practice known as *Calorie restriction (CR)* has been getting a lot of media attention lately. Although researchers haven't defined a precise number of Calories, or level of nutrients, that qualifies as a Calorie-restricted diet, the practice typically involves eating fewer Calories than your body needs to maintain your normal weight—while getting enough vitamins and other nutrients to keep your body functioning in good health. In general—allowing for differences in how many Calories people are consuming prior to CR, as well as their gender, age, body composition, level of activity, and so forth—CR may call for a person to consume 20–30% fewer Calories than usual.[1]

Effects of Calorie Restriction

Research over many years has consistently shown that CR can significantly extend the life span of small animals, such as rats, mice, fish, flies, and yeast cells.[2] Research with monkeys has followed more recently, with similar results. But only in the past few years have researchers begun to design and conduct studies of CR in humans. The results of these preliminary studies suggest that CR can also improve the metabolic measures of health in humans and thus may be able to extend the human life span.[3]

How might CR prolong life span? The answer to this question is not fully understood, but it is thought that the reduction in metabolic rate that occurs with restricting energy intake results in a much lower production of free radicals, which in turn reduces oxidative damage to DNA, cell membranes, and other cell structures, possibly lowering chronic disease risk and prolonging life. Calorie restriction also causes marked improvements in insulin sensitivity and other hormonal changes that can lower the risk for chronic diseases, such as heart disease, stroke, and diabetes. There is also evidence that CR can alter gene expression in ways that reduce the effects of aging and lower the risk for cancer and other diseases. The following are some of the metabolic effects of CR reported in several, but not all, human studies:[2-4]

- Decreased fat mass and lean body mass
- Decreased insulin levels and improved insulin sensitivity, decreased fasting blood glucose levels

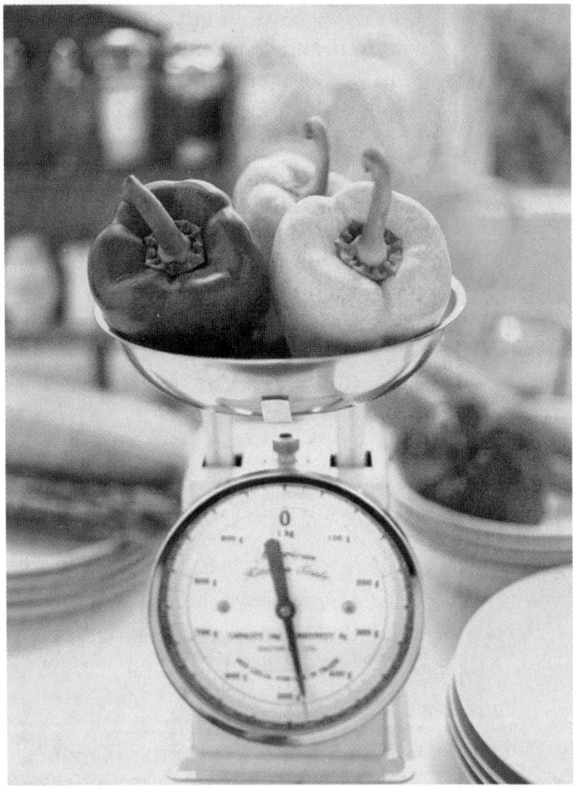

On a Calorie-restricted diet, all food must be highly nutritious, and both nutrients and energy must be calculated precisely.

- Decreased core body temperature and blood pressure
- Decreased serum LDL- and total cholesterol, increased serum HDL-cholesterol
- Decreased energy expenditure, beyond that expected for the weight loss that occurred, which suggests a generalized slowing of metabolic rate
- Decreased oxidative stress (i.e., reduced cell degeneration from free radicals)
- Reduced levels of DNA damage
- Lower levels of chronic inflammation
- Protective changes in various hormone levels

It's important to emphasize that the species known to live longer with CR are fed highly nutritious diets. Conditions such as starvation, anorexia nervosa, and wasting diseases, such as cancer, in which energy and nutrient intakes are severely restricted, do *not* result in prolonged life. In fact, these conditions are associated with increased risks for illness and premature death.

It's also essential to understand that the benefits of CR are seen as correlating to the age at which a person begins the program. In other words, the later in life the CR protocol is started, the less the expected benefit. For example, if a person did not start CR until the age of 55 years, he or she would be expected to gain only about 4 months of extended life![3]

Challenges of Calorie Restriction

Although the benefits of CR appear promising, the research data supporting them in humans is still preliminary. Research that could precisely study and measure the results of CR in humans may never be conducted because of logistical and ethical concerns. For instance, finding enough people to participate in any research study over the course of their lifetime would be extremely difficult. In addition, most people find it very challenging to follow a Calorie-restricted diet for even a few months; compliance with this type of diet for 80 years or more may be almost impossible. There are also ethical concerns about potential malnutrition in study participants.

In the absence of high-quality human studies, several CR groups, including the Caloric Restriction Society[5–7] and the "CRONies" (people in the group Caloric Restriction with Optimal Nutrition), have provided researchers with some data. Most of the members of the Caloric Restriction Society are men with an average age of 50 years, and 75% of CRONies are men in their late thirties or mid-fifties. One report indicated that most CRONies had followed the CR diet for about 10 years, although some had restricted their caloric intake for longer.[3] CRONies also reportedly reduce their caloric intake by about 30%. Overall, the members of CR groups report improved blood lipids and the other health benefits listed earlier. Still, researchers lack specific data on how well free-living adults actually follow the rigid and extensive demands of CR protocols.[1]

You may be wondering how much less energy *you* would have to consume to meet the definition of Calorie restriction—and when you'd have to begin. It has been estimated that humans would need to restrict their typical caloric intake by at least 20% for 40 years or more in order to gain an additional 4–5 years of healthy living. If you normally eat about 2,000 kcal/day, a 20% reduction would require an energy intake of about 1,600 kcal/day. Although this amount of energy reduction does not seem excessive, it would be very difficult to achieve every day for a lifetime—particularly if you lived to be over 100 years of age!

Also keep in mind that this diet must be of very high nutritional quality. This requirement presents a huge number of challenges, including the meticulous planning of meals; the preparation of most, if not all, of your own foods; limited options for eating meals outside of your home; and the challenge of working the demands of your special diet around the eating behaviors of family members and friends.

Also, those who follow the CR program report several side effects. The top three complaints are constant hunger, frequently feeling cold, and a loss of libido (sex drive).[3] Finally, the long-term effects of the diet are not known. There is concern that, if initiated in early adulthood, CR would reduce bone density, increasing the risk for osteoporosis. It could also lead to inappropriate loss of muscle mass. And because the production of female reproductive hormones is linked to a certain level of body fat, CR could impair a woman's fertility. Interestingly, as noted earlier, most of the members of the Caloric Restriction Society and the CRONies are men.

Alternatives to Calorie Restriction

An interesting alternative to Calorie restriction is the practice of *intermittent fasting (IF)*, also known as every-other-day-feeding (EODF) or alternate-day fasting (ADF).[8] This approach, which does *not* reduce average caloric intake but simply alters the pattern of food consumption, has also been shown in animals to prolong life span and improve a range of metabolic measures of health. Although not as well studied as Calorie restriction, IF has produced beneficial changes in insulin and glucose status, blood lipid levels, and blood pressure in humans in at least some studies.

Additionally, some researchers have proposed that limiting total protein intake, which is much easier to implement than extreme Calorie restriction, may limit the onset of cancer and aging. As noted in Chapter 6, surveys indicate that Americans eat 15–17% of their total daily energy intake as protein, so limiting total protein might mean consuming a diet with 10% of energy intake from protein, which is still within the AMDR. While this reduction may be challenging for those who follow a "meat and potatoes" diet, others would find this dietary modification very easy to follow over the long term.

Finally, research suggests that exercise-induced leanness may slow the aging process without the need for Calorie restriction.[2] That is, it may not be the energy intake per se that extends life span but the overall energy balance a person maintains. For example, a person would not have to strictly limit energy or Calorie intake as long as his or her activity (energy expenditure) were high enough to maintain a lean body profile (low percent body fat, high muscle mass).

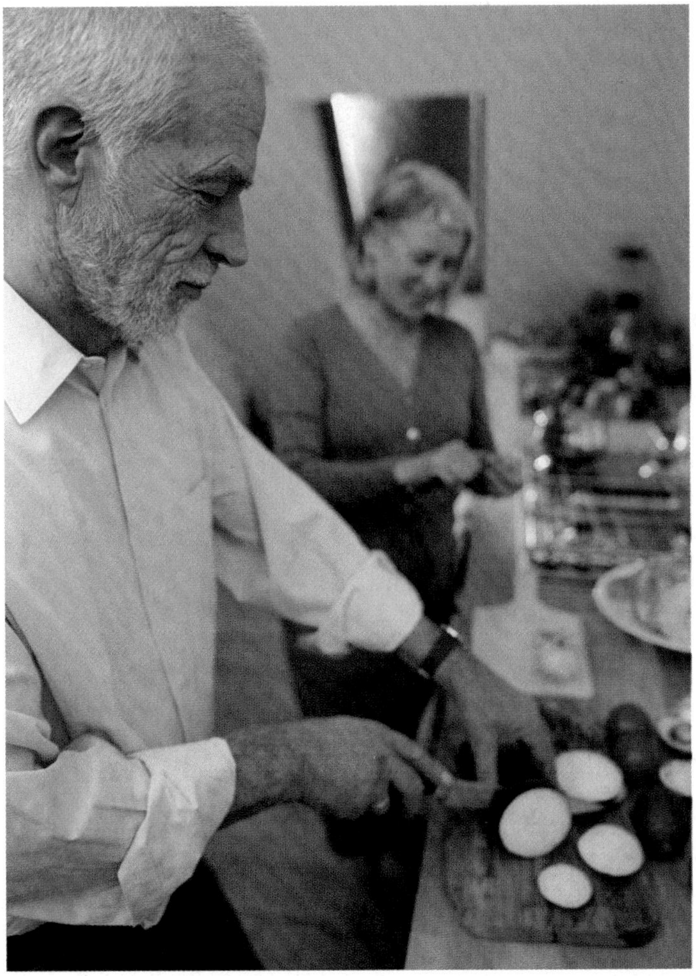

Maintaining an energy-restricted diet that is also highly nutritious requires significant planning and preparation of most of your own meals.

Can Supplements Slow Aging?

Recently, some researchers have speculated that consuming the optimum level of nutrients can maximize a person's healthy life span.[9] Can supplements take the place of whole foods in providing this "optimum level of nutrients"? And can other ingredients, besides vitamins and minerals, also slow aging?

The anti-aging market is said to generate about $50 billion in total revenues, with individual patients spending as much as $4,000 to $20,000 annually on a variety of treatments. Primary among these are "anti-aging" or "age-management" supplements. Some of these supplements provide specific vitamins and minerals, while others provide exotic "metabolites," "glandular extracts," or "food concentrates." Many of these products are heavily marketed and, as just noted, can be very expensive. Are they worth the investment? Let's take a look at some of the research into supplements promoted for longevity.

Many well-designed, carefully conducted research studies have looked at the effect of vitamin and/or mineral supplements on chronic disease risk and rates of death, or mortality. Antioxidants such as vitamins A, E, and C and beta-carotene have gotten the most attention.[10] Unfortunately, not even one trial of these nutrients (alone or in combination) has shown them to lower rates of death from heart disease or other causes. In fact, several of the studies actually reported a *higher* rate of death with high doses of vitamins A or E and of beta-carotene supplements.[11] However, a

NUTRI-CASE GUSTAVO

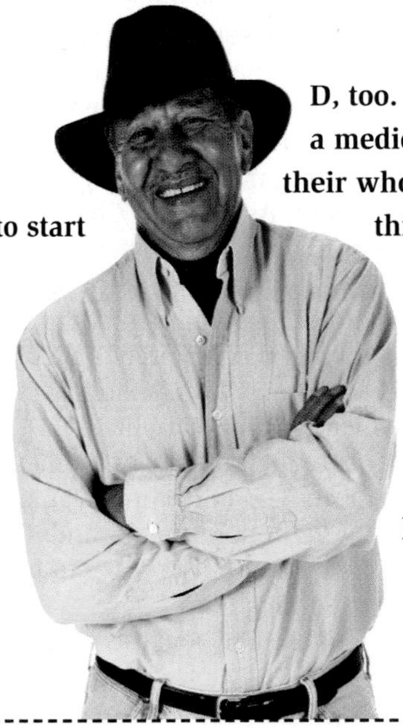

"I don't believe in taking pills. If you eat good food, you get everything you need and it's the way nature intended it. My daughter kept nagging my wife and me to start taking B vitamins and some kind of Chinese herb with a name I can't pronounce. She said we need this stuff because when people get to be our age they have problems with their nerves and circulation. I didn't fall for it, but my wife did, and then her doctor told her she needs calcium pills and vitamin D, too. The kitchen counter is starting to look like a medicine cabinet! Our ancestors never took pills their whole lives! So how come we need them? I think the whole thing is a hoax to get you to empty your wallet."

Would you support Gustavo's decision to avoid taking supplements? Given what you have learned in previous Nutri-Cases about Gustavo's wife, would you support or oppose her taking ginkgo biloba, B vitamins, calcium, or vitamin D? Explain your choices.

quick search on your computer will open up a world of promises, all guaranteeing better health and longer life spans, if you use these supplements!

Other supplements that claim to enhance longevity include products based on

- food extracts, such as resveratrol from red wines, and other foods
- herbals, including Siberian ginseng, ginkgo biloba, and various combinations of Eastern botanicals
- animal extracts, such as royal jelly and dried glandulars
- hormone-based preparations, such as DHEA (dehydroepiandrosterone), human growth hormone, and melatonin
- metabolites, such as alpha lipoic acid

Manufacturers promote these products with claims such as "used since prehistoric times," "revered in Eastern cultures," and "nature's own therapeutic powers." However, no well-designed research studies support the claims of life-extending effectiveness for any of these products in humans.

Moreover, researchers have been unable to identify any plausible scientific explanations for why or how these supplements might increase longevity in humans.

More disturbingly, like antioxidant supplements, many of these non-nutrient supplements have serious side effects. For example, ginkgo can cause gastrointestinal upset, nausea, diarrhea, headache, dizziness, or an allergic reaction.[12] Human growth hormone can contribute to heart disease and diabetes and cause joint pain, muscle pain, and other symptoms.[13] DHEA may decrease HDL-cholesterol and increase the risk for certain types of cancer. However, despite these concerns, the sales of such supplements continue to grow.[14]

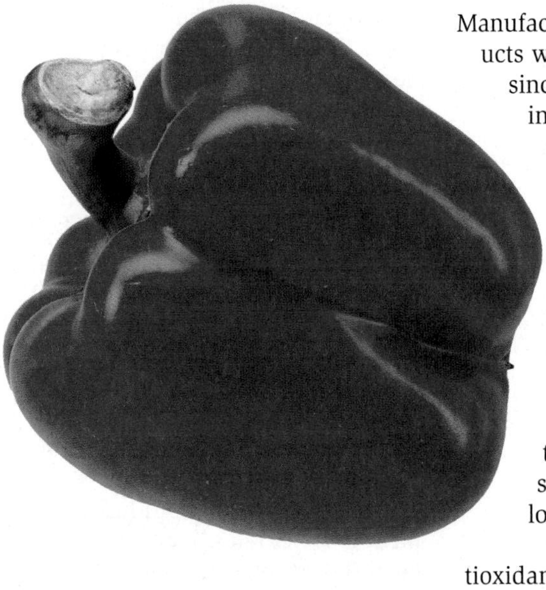

Anyone can benefit from the antioxidant nutrients in fresh fruits and vegetables. Antioxidant supplements are not necessary, and they may be harmful.

Are Your Actions Today Promoting a Longer, Healthier Life?

The debate over the effectiveness and safety of CR, IF, and the variety of anti-aging supplements will continue as more research is conducted. In the meantime, what can you do to increase your chances of living a long and healthful life? The U.S. Centers for Disease Control and Prevention (CDC) reminds us that chronic disease is responsible for seven out of every ten American deaths. Moreover, just four behaviors, all within our control, are responsible for much of the illness, suffering, and early death

What About You?

How Long Are You Likely to Live?

First, let's get one thing straight: no "longevity calculator," game, or quiz, no matter how complex or high-tech, can predict how long you'll live. That's not only because death from traumatic injury is unpredictable, but also because chronic diseases, as we've discussed throughout this text, are multifactorial, and we have a long way to go before we understand fully how all the factors interact to produce or prevent disease. That said, studies of large populations have demonstrably linked certain behaviors with an increased life span. These include regular physical activity, a nourishing diet, no tobacco use, and no excessive alcohol consumption. These factors are included in *all* longevity tools. In addition, most tools ask about other factors, such as drug abuse, stress, sleep quality and duration, seat belt use, and social support. Want to learn more? If so, you'll find longevity games and quizzes on many websites. Here are two popular options:

The Longevity Game

www.northwesternmutual.com/learning-center/the-longevity-game
This game, from the Northwestern Mutual Life Insurance Company, was developed using the company's actuarial statistics tracking longevity for more than 150 years.

Living to 100

www.livingto100.com
This quiz, developed by Dr. Thomas Perls, has forty questions related to your family and health. It provides some brief feedback and a list of suggested lifestyle changes to improve your health.

associated with chronic disease:[15,16] They are:

- Lack of physical activity
- Poor nutrition
- Tobacco use
- Excessive alcohol consumption

So if you want to live a longer, healthier life, the CDC advises that you adopt the health habits highlighted in the Quick Tips box.

Maybe you're already engaging in these healthful behaviors but still wonder how long you're likely to live. If so, check out the What About You? feature box for some fun longevity quizzes: your results might make you laugh, or put you on track to more healthful choices starting today!

QUICK TIPS

Promoting Your Longevity

✓ Engage in at least 30 minutes of moderate physical activity most days of the week.

✓ Eat a diet based on the USDA Food Guide.

✓ Use only the nutrient supplements that have been recommended to you by your healthcare provider and within the recommended amounts.

✓ Maintain a healthful weight and body composition. Both underweight and overweight are associated with increased mortality. (See Chapter 11.)

✓ If you smoke or use any other form of tobacco, stop. If you don't smoke, don't start. On average, smokers die 13 to 14 years earlier than non-smokers.[13]

✓ If you drink alcohol, do so only in moderation, meaning no more than two drinks per day for men and one drink per day for women. The health risks of alcohol were discussed ***In Depth*** following Chapter 1 on pages 28–37.

Web Resources

www.nia.nih.gov
The National Institute on Aging

The National Institute on Aging provides information about how older adults can benefit from physical activity and a good diet.

www.nihseniorhealth.gov

National Institutes of Health, Senior Health

This website, written in large print, offers up-to-date information on popular health topics for older Americans.

www.agingblueprint.org/partnership

American College of Sports Medicine, Active Aging Partnership

Get information for health professionals and the general public on The National Blueprint: Increasing Physical Activity Among Adults Age 50 and Older.

www.aarp.org/health/fitness

The American Association of Retired Persons

Visit this gateway site for a wide range of articles on promoting physical activity in older adults.

APPENDIX A

DIETARY GUIDELINES, UPPER INTAKE LEVELS, AND DIETARY REFERENCE INTAKES

DIETARY GUIDELINES FOR AMERICANS, 2010

Key Recommendations for Each Area of the Guidelines:

Adequate Nutrients Within Calorie Needs

a. Consume a variety of nutrient-dense foods and beverages within and among the basic food groups while choosing foods that limit the intake of saturated and *trans* fats, cholesterol, added sugars, salt, and alcohol.

b. Meet recommended intakes by adopting a balanced eating pattern, such as the USDA Food Patterns or the DASH Eating Plan.

Weight Management

a. To maintain body weight in a healthy range, balance Calories from foods and beverages with Calories expended.

b. To prevent gradual weight gain over time, make small decreases in food and beverage Calories and increase physical activity.

Physical Activity

a. Engage in regular physical activity and reduce sedentary activities to promote health, psychological well-being, and a healthy body weight.

b. Achieve physical fitness by including cardiovascular conditioning, stretching exercises for flexibility, and resistance exercises or calisthenics for muscle strength and endurance.

Food Groups to Encourage

a. Consume a sufficient amount of fruits and vegetables while staying within energy needs. Two cups of fruit and 2 1/2 cups of vegetables per day are recommended for a reference 2,000-Calorie intake, with higher or lower amounts depending on the Calorie level.

b. Choose a variety of fruits and vegetables each day. In particular, select from all five vegetable subgroups (dark green, orange, legumes, starchy vegetables, and other vegetables) several times a week.

c. Consume 3 or more ounce-equivalents of whole-grain products per day, with the rest of the recommended grains coming from enriched or whole-grain products.

d. Consume 3 cups per day of fat-free or low-fat milk or equivalent milk products.

Fats

a. Consume less than 10% of Calories from saturated fatty acids and less than 300 mg/day of cholesterol, and keep *trans* fatty acid consumption as low as possible.

b. Keep total fat intake between 20 and 35% of Calories, with most fats coming from sources of polyunsaturated and monounsaturated fatty acids, such as fish, nuts, and vegetable oils.

c. Choose foods that are lean, low-fat, or fat-free, and limit intake of fats and oils high in saturated and/or *trans* fatty acids.

Carbohydrates

a. Choose fiber-rich fruits, vegetables, and whole grains often.

b. Choose and prepare foods and beverages with little added sugars or caloric sweeteners, such as amounts suggested by the USDA Food Patterns and the DASH Eating Plan.

c. Reduce the incidence of dental caries by practicing good oral hygiene and consuming sugar- and starch-containing foods and beverages less frequently.

Sodium and Potassium

a. Consume less than 2,300 mg (approximately 1 tsp of salt) of sodium per day.

b. Consume potassium-rich foods, such as fruits and vegetables.

Alcoholic Beverages

a. Those who choose to drink alcoholic beverages should do so sensibly and in moderation—defined as the consumption of up to one drink per day for women and up to two drinks per day for men.

b. Alcoholic beverages should not be consumed by some individuals, including those who cannot restrict their alcohol intake, women of childbearing age who may become pregnant, pregnant and lactating women, children and adolescents, individuals taking medications that can interact with alcohol, and those with specific medical conditions.

c. Alcoholic beverages should be avoided by individuals engaging in activities that require attention, skill, or coordination, such as driving or operating machinery.

Food Safety

a. To avoid microbial food-borne illness, clean hands, food contact surfaces, and fruits and vegetables; separate raw, cooked, and ready-to-eat foods; cook foods to a safe temperature; and refrigerate perishable food promptly and defrost foods properly. Meat and poultry should not be washed or rinsed.

b. Avoid unpasteurized milk or products made from unpasteurized milk or juices, or raw or partially cooked eggs, meat, or poultry.

There are additional key recommendations for specific population groups. You can access all the Guidelines on the web at www.healthierus.gov/dietaryguidelines.

Data from U.S. Department of Agriculture, and U.S. Department of Health and Human Services. 2010. Dietary Guidelines for Americans, 2010. 7th ed. Available at www.healthierus.gov/dietaryguidelines.

TOLERABLE UPPER INTAKE LEVELS(UL[a])

Vitamins

Life-Stage Group	Vitamin A (µg/d)[b]	Vitamin C (mg/d)	Vitamin D (IU/d)	Vitamin E (mg/d)[c,d]	Niacin (mg/d)[d]	Vitamin B_6 (mg/d)	Folate (µg/d)[d]	Choline (g/d)
Infants								
0–6 mo	600	ND[e]	1,000	ND	ND	ND	ND	ND
7–12 mo	600	ND	1,500	ND	ND	ND	ND	ND
Children								
1–3 y	600	400	2,500	200	10	30	300	1.0
4–8 y	900	650	3,000	300	15	40	400	1.0
Males, Females								
9–13 y	1,700	1,200	4,000	600	20	60	600	2.0
14–18 y	2,800	1,800	4,000	800	30	80	800	3.0
19–70 y	3,000	2,000	4,000	1,000	35	100	1,000	3.5
>70 y	3,000	2,000	4,000	1,000	35	100	1,000	3.5
Pregnancy								
≤18 y	2,800	1,800	4,000	800	30	80	800	3.0
19–50 y	3,000	2,000	4,000	1,000	35	100	1,000	3.5
Lactation								
≤18 y	2,800	1,800	4,000	800	30	80	800	3.0
19–50 y	3,000	2,000	4,000	1,000	35	100	1,000	3.5

Elements

Life-Stage Group	Boron (mg/d)	Calcium (mg/d)	Copper (µg/d)	Fluoride (mg/d)	Iodine (µg/d)	Iron (mg/d)	Magnesium (mg/d)[f]	Manganese (mg/d)	Molybdenum (µg/d)	Nickel (mg/d)	Phosphorus (g/d)	Selenium (µg/d)	Vanadium (mg/d)[g]	Zinc (mg/d)
Infants														
0–6 mo	ND	1,000	ND	0.7	ND	40	ND	ND	ND	ND	ND	45	ND	4
7–12 mo	ND	1,500	ND	0.9	ND	40	ND	ND	ND	ND	ND	60	ND	5
Children														
1–3 y	3	2,500	1,000	1.3	200	40	65	2	300	0.2	3	90	ND	7
4–8 y	6	2,500	3,000	2.2	300	40	110	3	600	0.3	3	150	ND	12
Males, Females														
9–13 y	11	3,000	5,000	10	600	40	350	6	1,100	0.6	4	280	ND	23
14–18 y	17	3,000	8,000	10	900	45	350	9	1,700	1.0	4	400	ND	34
19–50 y	20	2,500	10,000	10	1,100	45	350	11	2,000	1.0	4	400	1.8	40
51–70 y	20	2,000	10,000	10	1,100	45	350	11	2,000	1.0	4	400	1.8	40
>70 y	20	2,000	10,000	10	1,100	45	350	11	2,000	1.0	3	400	1.8	40
Pregnancy														
≤18y	17	3,000	8,000	10	900	45	350	9	1,700	1.0	3.5	400	ND	34
19–50 y	20	2,500	10,000	10	1,100	45	350	11	2,000	1.0	3.5	400	ND	40
Lactation														
≤18y	17	3,000	8,000	10	900	45	350	9	1,700	1.0	4	400	ND	34
19–50 y	20	2,500	10,000	10	1,100	45	350	11	2,000	1.0	4	400	ND	40

Data from the Dietary Reference Intakes series, National Academies Press. Copyright 1997, 1998, 2000, 2001, and 2010, by the National Academy of Sciences. These reports may be accessed via www.nap.edu. Courtesy of the National Academies Press, Washington, DC. Reprinted with permission.

[a] UL = The maximum level of daily nutrient intake that is likely to pose no risk of adverse effects. Unless otherwise specified, the UL represents total intake from food, water, and supplements. Due to lack of suitable data, ULs could not be established for vitamin K, thiamin, riboflavin, vitamin B_{12}, pantothenic acid, biotin, or carotenoids. In the absence of ULs, extra caution may be warranted in consuming levels above recommended intakes.

[b] As preformed vitamin A only.

[c] As α-tocopherol; applies to any form of supplemental α-tocopherol.

[d] The ULs for vitamin E, niacin, and folate apply to synthetic forms obtained from supplements, fortified foods, or a combination of the two.

[e] ND = Not determinable due to lack of data of adverse effects in this age group and concern with regard to lack of ability to handle excess amounts. Source of intake should be from food only to prevent high levels of intake.

[f] The ULs for magnesium represent intake from a pharmacological agent only and do not include intake from food and water.

[g] Although vanadium in food has not been shown to cause adverse effects in humans, there is no justification for adding vanadium to food, and vanadium supplements should be used with caution. The UL is based on adverse effects in laboratory animals, and this data could be used to set a UL for adults but not children and adolescents.

DIETARY REFERENCE INTAKES: RDA, AI*, (AMDR)

Macronutrients

Life-Stage Group	Carbohydrate—Total Digestible (g/d)	Total Fiber (g/d)	Total Fat (g/d)	n-6 polyunsaturated fatty acids (linoleic acid) (g/d)	n-3 polyunsaturated fatty acids (?-linoleic acid) (g/d)	Protein and Amino Acids (g/d)[a]
Infants						
0–6 mo	60* (ND[b])[c]	ND	31*	4.4* (ND)	0.5* (ND)	9.1* (ND)
7–12 mo	95* (ND)	ND	30*	4.6* (ND)	0.5* (ND)	13.5 (ND)
Children						
1–3 y	130 (45–65)	19*	(30–40)	7* (5–10)	0.7* (0.6–1.2)	13 (5–20)
4–8 y	130 (45–65)	25*	(25–35)	10* (5–10)	0.9* (0.6–1.2)	19 (10–30)
Males						
9–13 y	130 (45–65)	31*	(25–35)	12* (5–10)	1.2* (0.6–1.2)	34 (10–30)
14–18 y	130 (45–65)	38*	(25–35)	16* (5–10)	1.6* (0.6–1.2)	52 (10–30)
19–30 y	130 (45–65)	38*	(20–35)	17* (5–10)	1.6* (0.6–1.2)	56 (10–35)
31–50 y	130 (45–65)	38*	(20–35)	17* (5–10)	1.6* (0.6–1.2)	56 (10–35)
51–70 y	130 (45–65)	30*	(20–35)	14* (5–10)	1.6* (0.6–1.2)	56 (10–35)
>70 y	130 (45–65)	30*	(20–35)	14* (5–10)	1.6* (0.6–1.2)	56 (10–35)
Females						
9–13 y	130 (45–65)	26*	(25–35)	10* (5–10)	1.0* (0.6–1.2)	34 (10–30)
14–18 y	130 (45–65)	26*	(25–35)	11* (5–10)	1.1* (0.6–1.2)	46 (10–30)
19–30 y	130 (45–65)	25*	(20–35)	12* (5–10)	1.1* (0.6–1.2)	46 (10–35)
31–50 y	130 (45–65)	25*	(20–35)	12* (5–10)	1.1* (0.6–1.2)	46 (10–35)
51–70 y	130 (45–65)	21*	(20–35)	11* (5–10)	1.1* (0.6–1.2)	46 (10–35)
>70 y	130 (45–65)	21*	(20–35)	11* (5–10)	1.1* (0.6–1.2)	46 (10–35)
Pregnancy						
≤18 y	175 (45–65)	28*	(20–35)	13* (5–10)	1.4* (0.6–1.2)	71 (10–35)
19–30 y	175 (45–65)	28*	(20–35)	13* (5–10)	1.4* (0.6–1.2)	71 (10–35)
31–50 y	(45–65)	28*	(20–35)	13* (5–10)	1.4* (0.6–1.2)	71 (10–35)
Lactation						
≤18 y	210 (45–65)	29*	(20–35)	13* (5–10)	1.3* (0.6–1.2)	71 (10–35)
19–30 y	210 (45–65)	29*	(20–35)	13* (5–10)	1.3* (0.6–1.2)	71 (10–35)
31–50 y	210 (45–65)	29*	(20–35)	13* (5–10)	1.3* (0.6–1.2)	71 (10–35)

Data from "Dietary Reference Intakes for Energy, Carbohydrates, Fiber, Fat, Fatty Acids, Cholesterol, Protein, and Amino Acids (Macronutrients)," © 2002 by the National Academy of Sciences, courtesy of the National Academies Press, Washington, DC. Reprinted with permission.

Note: This table is adapted from the DRI reports, see www.nap.edu. It lists Recommended Dietary Allowances (RDAs), with Adequate Intakes (AIs) indicated by an asterisk (*), and Acceptable Macronutrient Distribution Range (AMDR) data provided in parentheses. RDAs and AIs may both be used as goals for individual intake. RDAs are set to meet the needs of almost all (97% to 98%) individuals in a group. For healthy breastfed infants, the AI is the mean intake. The AI for other life stage and gender groups is believed to cover the needs of all individuals in the group, but lack of data prevent being able to specify with confidence the percentage of individuals covered by this intake.

[a] Based on 1.5 g/kg/day for infants, 1.1 g/kg/day for 1–3 y, 0.95 g/kg/day for 4–13 y, 0.85 g/kg/day for 14–18 y, 0.8 g/kg/day for adults, and 1.1 g/kg/day for pregnant (using pre-pregnancy weight) and lactating women.

[b] ND = Not determinable due to lack of data of adverse effects in this age group and concern with regard to lack of ability to handle excess amounts. Source of intake should be from food only to prevent high levels of intake.

[c] Data in parentheses are Acceptable Macronutrient Distribution Range (AMDR). This is the range of intake for a particular energy source that is associated with reduced risk of chronic disease while providing intakes of essential nutrients. If an individual consumes in excess of the AMDR, there is a potential of increasing the risk of chronic diseases and/or insufficient intakes of essential nutrients.

DIETARY REFERENCE INTAKES: RDA, AI*

Vitamins

Life-Stage Group	Vitamin A (μg/d)[a]	Vitamin D (IU/d)[b]	Vitamin E (mg/d)[c]	Vitamin K (μg/d)	Thiamin (mg/d)	Riboflavin (mg/d)	Niacin (mg/d)[d]	Pantothenic Acid (mg/d)	Biotin (μg/d)	Vitamin B_6 (mg/d)	Folate (μg/d)[e]	Vitamin B_{12} (μg/d)	Vitamin C (mg/d)	Choline (mg/d)
Infants														
0–6 mo	400*	400*	4*	2.0*	0.2*	0.3*	2*	1.7*	5*	0.1*	65*	0.4*	40*	125*
7–12 mo	500*	400*	5*	2.5*	0.3*	0.4*	4*	1.8*	6*	0.3*	80*	0.5*	50*	150*
Children														
1–3 y	300	600	6	30*	0.5	0.5	6	2*	8*	0.5	150	0.9	15	200*
4–8 y	400	600	7	55*	0.6	0.6	8	3*	12*	0.6	200	1.2	25	250*
Males														
9–13 y	600	600	11	60*	0.9	0.9	12	4*	20*	1.0	300	1.8	45	375*
14–18 y	900	600	15	75*	1.2	1.3	16	5*	25*	1.3	400	2.4	75	550*
19–30 y	900	600	15	120*	1.2	1.3	16	5*	30*	1.3	400	2.4	90	550*
31–50 y	900	600	15	120*	1.2	1.3	16	5*	30*	1.3	400	2.4	90	550*
51–70 y	900	600	15	120*	1.2	1.3	16	5*	30*	1.7	400	2.4	90	550*
>70 y	900	800	15	120*	1.2	1.3	16	5*	30*	1.7	400	2.4	90	550*
Females														
9–13 y	600	600	11	60*	0.9	0.9	12	4*	20*	1.0	300	1.8	45	375*
14–18 y	700	600	15	75*	1.0	1.0	14	5*	25*	1.2	400	2.4	65	400*
19–30 y	700	600	15	90*	1.1	1.1	14	5*	30*	1.3	400	2.4	75	425*
31–50 y	700	600	15	90*	1.1	1.1	14	5*	30*	1.3	400	2.4	75	425*
51–70 y	700	600	15	90*	1.1	1.1	14	5*	30*	1.5	400	2.4	75	425*
>70 y	700	800	15	90*	1.1	1.1	14	5*	30*	1.5	400	2.4	75	425*
Pregnancy														
≤18 y	750	600	15	75*	1.4	1.4	18	6*	30*	1.9	600	2.6	80	450*
19–30 y	770	600	15	90*	1.4	1.4	18	6*	30*	1.9	600	2.6	85	450*
31–50 y	770	600	15	90*	1.4	1.4	18	6*	30*	1.9	600	2.6	85	450*
Lactation														
≤18 y	1,200	600	19	75*	1.4	1.4	17	7*	35*	2.0	500	2.8	115	550*
19–30 y	1,300	600	19	90*	1.4	1.4	17	7*	35*	2.0	500	2.8	120	550*
31–50 y	1,300	600	19	90*	1.4	1.4	17	7*	35*	2.0	500	2.8	120	550*

Data from the Dietary Reference Intakes series, National Academies Press. Copyright 1997, 1998, 2000, 2001, and 2010, by the National Academy of Sciences. These reports may be accessed via www.nap.edu. Courtesy of the National Academies Press, Washington, DC. Reprinted with permission.

Note: This table is adapted from the DRI reports; see www.nap.edu. It lists Recommended Dietary Allowances (RDAs), with Adequate Intakes (AIs) indicated by an asterisk (*). RDAs and AIs may both be used as goals for individual intake. RDAs are set to meet the needs of almost all (97 percent to 98 percent) individuals in a group. For healthy breastfed infants, the AI is the mean intake. The AI for other life stage and gender groups is believed to cover the needs of all individuals in the group, but lack of data prevent being able to specify with confidence the percentage of individuals covered by this intake.

[a] Given as retinal activity equivalents (RAE).

[b] Also known as calciferol. The DRI values are based on the absence of adequate exposure to sunlight.

[c] Also known as α-tocopherol.

[d] Given as niacin equivalents (NE), except for infants 0–6 months, which are expressed as preformed niacin.

[e] Given as dietary folate equivalents (DFE).

APPENDIX D

U.S. EXCHANGE LISTS FOR MEAL PLANNING

Starch List

1 starch choice = 15 g carbohydrate, 0–3 g protein, 0–1 g fat, and 80 cal

Icon Key

☺ = More than 3 g of dietary fiber per serving.

! = Extra fat, or prepared with added fat. (Count as 1 starch + 1 fat.)

🧂 = 480 mg or more of sodium per serving.

Food	Serving Size
Bread	
Bagel, 4 oz	¼ (1 oz)
! Biscuit, 2½" across	1
Bread	
☺ reduced-Calorie	2 slices (1½ oz)
white, whole-grain, pumpernickel, rye, unfrosted raisin	1 slice (1 oz)
Chapatti, small, 6" across	1
! Cornbread, 1¾" cube	1 (1½ oz)
English muffin	½
Hot dog bun or hamburger bun	½ (1 oz)
Naan, 8" by 2"	¼
Pancake, 4" across, ¼" thick	1
Pita, 6" across	½
Roll, plain small	1 (1 oz)
! Stuffing, bread	⅓ cup
! Taco shell, 5" across	2
Tortilla	
Corn, 6" across	1
Flour, 6" across	1
Flour, 10" across	⅓ tortilla
! Waffle, 4"-square or 4" across	1
Cereals and Grains	
Barley, cooked	⅓ cup
Bran, dry	
☺ oat	¼ c
☺ wheat	½ c
☺ Bulgur (cooked)	½ c
Cereals	½ c
☺ bran	½ c
cooked (oats, oatmeal)	½ c
puffed	1½ c
shredded wheat, plain	½ c
sugar-coated	½ c
unsweetened, ready-to-eat	¾ c
Couscous	⅓ c
Granola	
low-fat	¼ c
! regular	¼ c
Grits, cooked	½ c
Kasha	½ c
Millet, cooked	⅓ c
Muesli	¼ c
Pasta, cooked	⅓ c
Polenta, cooked	⅓ c
Quinoa, cooked	⅓ c
Rice, white or brown, cooked	⅓ c
Tabbouleh (tabouli), prepared	½ c
Wheat germ, dry	3 tbs
Wild rice, cooked	½ c
Starchy Vegetables	
Cassava	⅓ c
Corn	½ c
on cob, large	½ cob (5 oz)
☺ Hominy, canned	¾ c
☺ Mixed vegetables with corn, peas, or pasta	1 c
☺ Parsnips	½ c
☺ Peas, green	½ c
Plantain, ripe	⅓ c
Potato	
baked with skin	¼ large (3 oz)
boiled, all kinds	½ c or ½ medium (3 oz)
! mashed, with milk and fat	½ c
French fried (oven-baked)	1 cup (2 oz)
☺ Pumpkin, canned, no sugar added	1 c
Spaghetti/pasta sauce	½ c
☺ Squash, winter (acorn, butternut)	1 c
☺ Succotash	½ c
Yam, sweet potato, plain	½ c
Crackers and Snacks	
Animal crackers	8
Crackers	
! round-butter type	6
saltine-type	6
! sandwich-style, cheese or peanut butter filling	3
! whole-wheat regular	2–5 (¾ oz)
☺ whole-wheat lower fat or crispbreads	2–5 (¾ oz)
Graham crackers, 2½" square	3

Food	Serving Size
Matzoh	¾ oz
Melba toast, about 2" by 4" piece	4 pieces
Oyster crackers	20
Crackers and Snacks	
Popcorn	3 c
! ☻ with butter	3 c
☻ no fat added	3 c
☻ lower fat	3 c
Pretzels	¾ oz
Rice cakes, 4" across	2
Snack chips	
fat-free or baked (tortilla, potato), baked pita chips	15–20 (¾ oz)
! regular (tortilla, potato)	9–13 (¾ oz)

Food	Serving Size
Beans, Peas, and Lentils	
(Count as 1 starch + 1 lean meat)	
☻ Baked beans	⅓ c
☻ Beans, cooked (black, garbanzo, kidney, lima, navy, pinto, white)	½ c
☻ Lentils, cooked (brown, green, yellow)	½ c
☻ Peas, cooked (black-eyed, split)	½ c
🧂 ☻ Refried beans, canned	½ c

Fruit List

1 fruit choice = 15 g carbohydrate, 0 g protein, 0 g fat, and 60 cal

Weight includes skin, core, seeds, and rind.

Icon Key

☻ = More than 3 g of dietary fiber per serving.

! = Extra fat, or prepared with added fat.

🧂 = 480 mg or more of sodium per serving.

Food	Serving Size
Apples	
unpeeled, small	1 (4 oz)
dried	4 rings
Applesauce, unsweetened	½ c
Apricots	
canned	½ c
dried	8 halves
☻ fresh	4 whole (5½ oz)
Banana, extra small	1 (4 oz)
☻ Blackberries	¾ c
Blueberries	¾ c
Cantaloupe, small	⅓ melon or 1 c cubed (11 oz)
Cherries	
sweet, canned	½ c
sweet, fresh	12 (3 oz)
Dates	3
Dried fruits (blueberries, cherries, cranberries, mixed fruit, raisins)	2 tbs
Figs	
dried	1½
☻ fresh	1½ large or 2 medium (3½ oz)
Fruit cocktail	½ c
Grapefruit	
large	½ (11 oz)
sections, canned	¾ c

Food	Serving Size
Grapes, small	17 (3 oz)
Honeydew melon	1 slice or 1 c cubed (10 oz)
☻ Kiwi	1 (3½ oz)
Mandarin oranges, canned	¾ c
Mango, small	½ fruit (5½ oz) or ½ c
Nectarine, small	1 (5 oz)
☻ Orange, small	1 (6½ oz)
Papaya	½ fruit or 1 c cubed (8 oz)
Peaches	
canned	½ c
fresh, medium	1 (6 oz)
Pears	
canned	½ c
fresh, large	½ (4 oz)
Pineapple	
canned	½ c
fresh	¾ c
Plums	
canned	½ c
dried (prunes)	3
small	2 (5 oz)
☻ Raspberries	1 c
☻ Strawberries	1¼ c whole berries

Food	Serving Size	Food	Serving Size
Tangerines, small	2 (8 oz)	Grape juice	⅓ c
Watermelon	1 slice or 1¼ c cubes (13½ oz)	Grapefruit juice	½ c
Fruit Juice		Orange juice	½ c
Apple juice/cider	½ c	Pineapple juice	½ c
Fruit juice blends, 100% juice	⅓ c	Prune juice	⅓ c

Milk and Yogurts

1 milk choice = 12 g carbohydrate and 8 g protein

Food	Serving Size	Count as
Fat-free or Low-Fat (1%)		
(0–3 g fat per serving, 100 Calories per serving)		
Milk, buttermilk, acidophilus milk, Lactaid	1 c	1 fat-free milk
Evaporated milk	½ c	1 fat-free milk
Yogurt, plain or flavored with an artificial sweetener	⅔ c (6 oz)	1 fat-free milk
Reduced-fat (2%)		
(5 g fat per serving, 120 Calories per serving)		
Milk, acidophilus milk, kefir, Lactaid	1 c	1 reduced-fat milk
Yogurt, plain	⅔ c (6 oz)	1 reduced-fat milk
Whole		
(8 g fat per serving, 160 Calories per serving)		
Milk, buttermilk, goat's milk	1 c	1 whole milk
Evaporated milk	½ c	1 whole milk
Yogurt, plain	8 oz	1 whole milk
Dairy-Like Foods		
Chocolate milk		
fat-free	1 c	1 fat-free milk + 1 carbohydrate
whole	1 c	1 whole milk + 1 carbohydrate
Eggnog, whole milk	½ c	1 carbohydrate + 2 fats
Rice drink		
flavored, low-fat	1 c	2 carbohydrates
plain, fat-free	1 c	1 carbohydrate
Smoothies, flavored, regular	10 oz	1 fat-free milk + 2½ carbohydrates
Soy milk		
light	1 c	1 carbohydrate + ½ fat
regular, plain	1 c	1 carbohydrate + 1 fat
Yogurt		
and juice blends	1 c	1 fat-free milk + 1 carbohydrate
low carbohydrate (less than 6 g carbohydrate per choice)	⅔ c (6 oz)	½ fat-free milk
with fruit, low-fat	⅔ c (6 oz)	1 fat-free milk + 1 carbohydrate

Sweets, Desserts, and Other Carbohydrates List

1 other carbohydrate choice = 15 g carbohydrate and variable protein, fat, and Calories.

Icon Key

🧂 = 480 mg or more of sodium per serving.

Food	Serving Size	Count as
Beverages, Soda, and Energy/Sports Drinks		
Cranberry juice cocktail	½ c	1 carbohydrate
Energy drink	1 can (8.3 oz)	2 carbohydrates
Fruit drink or lemonade	1 c (8 oz)	2 carbohydrates
Hot chocolate		
regular	1 envelope added to 8 oz water	1 carbohydrate + 1 fat
sugar-free or light	1 envelope added to 8 oz water	1 carbohydrate
Soft drink (soda), regular	1 can (12 oz)	2½ carbohydrates
Sports drink	1 cup (8 oz)	1 carbohydrate
Brownies, Cake, Cookies, Gelatin, Pie, and Pudding		
Brownie, small, unfrosted	1¼" square, ⅞" high (about 1 oz)	1 carbohydrate + 1 fat
Cake		
angel food, unfrosted	1/12 of cake (about 2 oz)	2 carbohydrates
frosted	2" square (about 2 oz)	2 carbohydrates + 1 fat
unfrosted	2" square (about 2 oz)	1 carbohydrate + 1 fat
Cookies		
chocolate chip	2 cookies (2¼" across)	1 carbohydrate + 2 fats
gingersnap	3 cookies	1 carbohydrate
sandwich, with creme filling	2 small (about ⅔ oz)	1 carbohydrate + 1 fat
sugar-free	3 small or 1 large (¾ oz–1oz)	1 carbohydrate + 1–2 fats
vanilla wafer	5 cookies	1 carbohydrate + 1 fat
Cupcake, frosted	1 small (about 1¾ oz)	2 carbohydrates + 1–1½ fats
Fruit cobbler	½ c (3½ oz)	3 carbohydrates + 1 fat
Gelatin, regular	½ c	1 carbohydrate
Pie		
commercially prepared fruit, 2 crusts	⅙ of 8" pie	3 carbohydrates + 2 fats
pumpkin or custard	⅛ of 8" pie	1½ carbohydrates + 1½ fats
Pudding		
regular (made with reduced-fat milk)	½ c	2 carbohydrates
sugar-free, or sugar-free and fat-free (made with fat-free milk)	½ c	1 carbohydrate
Candy, Spreads, Sweets, Sweeteners, Syrups, and Toppings		
Candy bar, chocolate/peanut	2 "fun size" bars (1 oz)	1½ carbohydrates + 1½ fats
Candy, hard	3 pieces	1 carbohydrate
Chocolate "kisses"	5 pieces	1 carbohydrate + 1 fat
Coffee creamer		
dry, flavored	4 tsp	½ carbohydrate + ½ fat
liquid, flavored	2 tbsp	1 carbohydrate
Fruit snacks, chewy (pureed fruit concentrate)	1 roll (¾ oz)	1 carbohydrate
Fruit spreads, 100% fruit	1½ tbs	1 carbohydrate
Honey	1 tbsp	1 carbohydrate

Food	Serving Size	Count as
Jam or jelly, regular	1 tbs	1 carbohydrate
Sugar	1 tbs	1 carbohydrate
Syrup		
chocolate	2 tbs	2 carbohydrates
light (pancake type)	2 tbs	1 carbohydrate
regular (pancake type)	1 tbs	1 carbohydrate
Condiments and Sauces		
Barbeque sauce	3 tbs	1 carbohydrate
Cranberry sauce, jellied	¼ c	1½ carbohydrates
Gravy, canned or bottled	½ c	½ carbohydrate + ½ fat
Salad dressing, fat-free, low-fat, cream-based	3 tbs	1 carbohydrate
Sweet and sour sauce	3 tbs	1 carbohydrate
Doughnuts, Muffins, Pastries, and Sweet Breads		
Banana nut bread	1" slice (1 oz)	2 carbohydrates + 1 fat
Doughnut		
cake, plain	1 medium, (1½ oz)	1½ carbohydrates + 2 fats
yeast type, glazed	3¾" across (2 oz)	2 carbohydrates + 2 fats
Muffin (4 oz)	¼ muffin (1 oz)	1 carbohydrate + ½ fat
Sweet roll or Danish	1 (2½ oz)	2½ carbohydrates + 2 fats
Frozen Bars, Frozen Dessert, Frozen Yogurt, and Ice Cream		
Frozen pops	1	½ carbohydrate
Fruit juice bars, frozen, 100% juice	1 bar (3 oz)	1 carbohydrate
Ice cream		
fat-free	½ c	1-½ carbohydrates
light	½ c	1 carbohydrate + 1 fat
no sugar added	½ c	1 carbohydrate + 1 fat
regular	½ c	1 carbohydrate + 2 fats
Sherbet, sorbet	½ c	2 carbohydrates
Yogurt, frozen		
fat-free	⅓ c	1 carbohydrate
regular	½ c	1 carbohydrate + 0–1 fat
Granola Bars, Meal Replacement Bars/Shakes, and Trail Mix		
Granola or snack bar, regular or low-fat	1 bar (1 oz)	1½ carbohydrates
Meal replacement bar	1 bar (1⅓ oz)	1½ carbohydrates + 0–1 fat
Meal replacement bar	1 bar (2 oz)	2 carbohydrates + 1 fat
Meal replacement shake, reduced-Calorie	1 can (10–11 oz)	1½ carbohydrates + 0–1 fat
Trail mix		
candy/nut-based	1 oz	1 carbohydrates + 2 fats
dried-fruit-based	1 oz	1 carbohydrate + 1 fat

Nonstarchy Vegetable List

1 vegetable choice = 5 g carbohydrate, 2 g protein, 0 g fat, 25 cal

Icon Key

☻ = More than 3 g of dietary fiber per serving.

🧂 = 480 mg or more of sodium per serving.

Amaranth or Chinese spinach
Artichoke
Artichoke hearts
Asparagus
Baby corn
Bamboo shoots
Beans (green, wax, Italian)
Bean sprouts
Beets
🧂 Borscht
Broccoli
☻ Brussels sprouts
Cabbage (green, bok choy, Chinese)
☻ Carrots
Cauliflower
Celery
☻ Chayote
Coleslaw, packaged, no dressing
Cucumber
Eggplant
Gourds (bitter, bottle, luffa, bitter melon)
Green onions or scallions
Greens (collard, kale, mustard, turnip)
Hearts of palm
Jicama
Kohlrabi
Leeks
Mixed vegetables (without corn, peas, or pasta)
Mung bean sprouts
Mushrooms, all kinds, fresh
Okra
Onions
Oriental radish or daikon
Pea pods
☻ Peppers (all varieties)
Radishes
Rutabaga
🧂 Sauerkraut
Soybean sprouts
Spinach
Squash (summer, crookneck, zucchini)
Sugar pea snaps
☻ Swiss chard
Tomato
Tomatoes, canned
🧂 Tomato sauce
🧂 Tomato/vegetable juice
Turnips
Water chestnuts
Yard-long beans

Meat and Meat Substitutes List

Icon Key

! = Extra fat, or prepared with added fat. (Add an additional fat choice to this food.)

🧂 = 480 mg or more of sodium per serving (based on the sodium content of a typical 3-oz serving of meat, unless 1 or 2 is the normal serving size).

Food	Amount
Lean Meats and Meat Substitutes *(1 lean meat choice = 7 g protein, 0–3 g fat, 100 Calories)*	
Beef: Select or Choice grades trimmed of fat: ground round, roast (chuck, rib, rump), round, sirloin, steak (cubed, flank, porterhouse, T-bone), tenderloin	1 oz
🧂 Beef jerky	1 oz
Cheeses with 3 g of fat or less per oz	1 oz
Cottage cheese	¼ cup
Egg substitutes, plain	¼ cup
Egg whites	2
Fish, fresh or frozen, plain: catfish, cod, flounder, haddock, halibut, orange roughy, salmon, tilapia, trout, tuna	1 oz
🧂 *Fish, smoked:* herring or salmon (lox)	1 oz
Game: buffalo, ostrich, rabbit, venison	1 oz
🧂 Hot dog with 3 g of fat or less per oz (8 dogs per 14 oz package) (*Note: May be high in carbohydrate.*)	1
Lamb: chop, leg, or roast	1 oz
Organ meats: heart, kidney, liver (*Note: May be high in cholesterol*)	1 oz

Food	Amount
Oysters, fresh or frozen	6 medium
Pork, lean	
🧂 Canadian bacon	1 oz
rib or loin chop/roast, ham, tenderloin	1 oz
Poultry without skin: Cornish hen, chicken, domestic duck or goose (well drained of fat), turkey	1 oz
Processed sandwich meats with 3 g of fat or less per oz: chipped beef, deli thin-sliced meats, turkey ham, turkey kielbasa, turkey pastrami	1 oz
Salmon, canned	1 oz
Sardines, canned	2 medium
🧂 Sausage with 3 g or less fat per oz	1 oz
Shellfish: clams, crab, imitation shellfish, lobster, scallops, shrimp	1 oz
Tuna, canned in water or oil, drained	1 oz
Veal: Lean chop, roast	1 oz
Medium-Fat Meat and Meat Substitutes	
(1 medium-fat meat choice = 7 g protein, 4–7 g fat, and 130 Calories)	
Beef: corned beef, ground beef, meatloaf, Prime grades trimmed of fat (prime rib), short ribs, tongue	1 oz
Cheeses with 4–7 g of fat per oz: feta, mozzarella, pasteurized processed cheese spread, reduced-fat cheeses, string	1 oz
Egg (*Note: High in cholesterol, limit to 3 per week.*)	1
Fish, any fried product	1 oz
Lamb: ground, rib roast	1 oz
Pork: cutlet, shoulder roast	1 oz
Poultry: chicken with skin; dove, pheasant, wild duck, or goose; fried chicken; ground turkey	1 oz
Ricotta cheese	2 oz or ¼ c
🧂 Sausage with 4–7 g fat per oz	1 oz
Veal: Cutlet (no breading)	1 oz
High-Fat Meat and Substitutes[a]	
(1 high-fat meat choice = 7 g protein, 8+ g fat, 150 Calories)	
Bacon	
🧂 pork	2 slices (16 slices per lb or 1 oz each, before cooking)
🧂 turkey	3 slices (½ oz each before cooking)
Cheese, regular: American, bleu, brie, cheddar, hard goat, Monterey Jack, queso, Swiss	1 oz
🧂 ! *Hot dog:* beef, pork, or combination (10 per lb-sized package)	1
🧂 *Hot dog:* turkey or chicken (10 per lb-sized package)	1
Pork: ground, sausage, spareribs	1 oz
Processed sandwich meats with 8 g of fat or more per oz: bologna, pastrami, hard salami	1 oz
🧂 *Sausage with 8 g of fat or more per oz:* bratwurst, chorizo, Italian, knockwurst, Polish, smoked, summer	1 oz

[a]These foods are high in saturated fat, cholesterol, and Calories and may raise blood cholesterol levels if eaten on a regular basis. Try to eat 3 or fewer servings from this group per week.

Plant-Based Proteins

Because carbohydrate content varies among plant-based proteins, you should read the food label.

Icon Key

☻ = More than 3 g of dietary fiber per serving.

🧂 = 480 mg or more of sodium per serving (based on the sodium content of a typical 3-oz serving of meat, unless 1 or 2 oz is the normal serving size).

Food	Amount	Count as
"Bacon" strips, soy-based	3 strips	1 medium-fat meat
☻ Baked beans	⅓ c	1 starch + 1 lean meat
☻ *Beans, cooked:* black, garbanzo, kidney, lima, navy, pinto, white	½ c	1 starch + 1 lean meat
☻ "Beef" or "sausage" crumbles, soy-based	2 oz	½ carbohydrate + 1 lean meat
"Chicken" nuggets, soy-based	2 nuggets (1½ oz)	½ carbohydrate + 1 medium-fat meat
☻ Edamame	½ c	½ carbohydrate + 1 lean meat
Falafel (spiced chickpea and wheat patties)	3 patties (about 2 inches across)	1 carbohydrate + 1 high-fat meat
Hot dog, soy-based	1 (1½ oz)	½ carbohydrate + 1 lean meat
☻ Hummus	⅓ c	1 carbohydrate + 1 high-fat meat

Food	Amount	Count as
Lentils, brown, green, or yellow	½ c	1 carbohydrate + 1 lean meat
Meatless burger, soy-based	3 oz	½ carbohydrate + 2 lean meats
Meatless burger, vegetable- and starch-based	1 patty (about 2½ oz)	1 carbohydrate + 2 lean meats
Nut spreads: almond butter, cashew butter, peanut butter, soy nut butter	1 tbs	1 high-fat meat
Peas, cooked: black-eyed and split peas	½ c	1 starch + 1 lean meat
Refried beans, canned	½ c	1 starch + 1 lean meat
"Sausage" patties, soy-based	1 (1½ oz)	1 medium-fat meat
Soy nuts, unsalted	¾ oz	½ carbohydrate + 1 medium-fat meat
Tempeh	¼ cup	1 medium-fat meat
Tofu	4 oz (½ cup)	1 medium-fat meat
Tofu, light	4 oz (½ cup)	1 lean meat

Fat List

Icon Key

1 fat choice = 5 g fat, 45 cal

= 480 mg or more of sodium per serving.

Food	Serving Size
Unsaturated Fats—Monounsaturated Fats	
Avocado, medium	2 tbs (1 oz)
Nut butters (trans fat-free): almond butter, cashew butter, peanut butter (smooth or crunchy)	1½ tsp
Nuts	
almonds	6 nuts
Brazil	2 nuts
cashews	6 nuts
filberts (hazelnuts)	5 nuts
macadamia	3 nuts
mixed (50% peanuts)	6 nuts
peanuts	10 nuts
pecans	4 halves
pistachios	16 nuts
Oil: canola, olive, peanut	1 tsp
Olives	
black (ripe)	8 large
green, stuffed	10 large
Polyunsaturated Fats	
Margarine: lower-fat spread (30% to 50% vegetable oil, *trans* fat-free)	1 tbs
Margarine: stick, tub (*trans* fat-free), or squeeze (*trans* fat-free)	1 tsp
Mayonnaise	
reduced-fat	1 tbs
regular	1 tsp
Mayonnaise-style salad dressing	
reduced-fat	1 tbs
regular	2 tsp
Nuts	
Pignolia (pine nuts)	1 tbs
walnuts, English	4 halves
Oil: corn, cottonseed, flaxseed, grape seed, safflower, soybean, sunflower	1 tsp
Oil: made from soybean and canola oil—Enova	1 tsp
Plant stanol esters	
light	1 tbs
regular	2 tsp
Salad dressing	
reduced-fat (*Note: May be high in carbohydrate.)*	2 tbs
regular	1 tbs
Seeds	1 tbs
flaxseed, whole	1 tbs
pumpkin, sunflower	1 tbs
sesame seeds	1 tbs
Tahini or sesame paste	2 tsp
Saturated Fats	
Bacon, cooked, regular or turkey	1 slice
Butter	
reduced-fat	1 tbs
stick	1 tsp
whipped	2 tsp
Butter blends made with oil	
reduced-fat or light	1 tbs
regular	1½ tsp
Chitterlings, boiled	2 tbs (½ oz)
Coconut, sweetened, shredded	2 tbs

Food	Serving Size
Coconut milk	
light	⅓ c
regular	1½ tbs
Cream	
half and half	2 tbs
heavy	1 tbs
light	1½ tbs
whipped	2 tbs
whipped, pressurized	¼ c
Cream cheese	
reduced-fat	1½ tbs (¾ oz)
regular	1 tbs (½ oz)
Lard	1 tsp
Oil: coconut, palm, palm kernel	1 tsp
Salt pork	¼ oz
Shortening, solid	1 tsp
Sour cream	
reduced-fat or light	3 tbs
regular	2 tbs

Free Foods List

A *free food* is any food or drink that has less than 20 Calories and 5 g or less of carbohydrate per serving. Foods with a serving size listed should be limited to three servings per day. Foods listed without a serving size can be eaten as often as you like.

Icon Key

🧂 = 480 mg or more of sodium per serving.

Food	Serving Size
Low Carbohydrate Foods	
Cabbage, raw	½ c
Candy, hard (regular or sugar-free)	1 piece
Carrots, cauliflower, or green beans, cooked	¼ c
Cranberries, sweetened with sugar substitute	½ c
Cucumber, sliced	½ c
Gelatin	
dessert, sugar-free	
unflavored	
Gum	
Jam or jelly, light or no sugar added	2 tsp
Rhubarb, sweetened with sugar substitute	½ c
Salad greens	
Sugar substitutes (artificial sweeteners)	
Syrup, sugar-free	2 tbs
Modified Fat Foods with Carbohydrate	
Cream cheese, fat-free	1 tbs (½ oz)
Creamers	
nondairy, liquid	1 tbs
nondairy, powdered	2 tsp
Margarine spread	
fat-free	1 tbs
reduced-fat	1 tsp
Mayonnaise	
fat-free	1 tbs
reduced-fat	1 tsp
Mayonnaise-style salad dressing	
fat-free	1 tbs
reduced-fat	1 tsp
Salad dressing	
fat-free or low-fat	1 tbs
fat-free, Italian	2 tbs
Sour cream, fat-free, reduced-fat	1 tbs
Whipped topping	
light or fat-free	2 tbs
regular	1 tbs
Condiments	
Barbecue sauce	2 tsp
Catsup (ketchup)	1 tbs
Honey mustard	1 tbs
Horseradish	
Lemon juice	
Miso	1½ tsp
Mustard	
Parmesan cheese, freshly grated	1 tbs
Pickle relish	1 tbs
Pickles	
🧂 dill	1½ medium
sweet, bread and butter	2 slices
sweet, gherkin	¾ oz
Salsa	¼ c
🧂 Soy sauce, regular or light	1 tbs
Sweet and sour sauce	2 tsp
Sweet chili sauce	2 tsp
Taco sauce	1 tbs
Vinegar	
Yogurt, any type	2 tbs

Drinks/Mixes

Any food on this list—without serving size listed—can be consumed in any moderate amount.

Icon Key

🧂 = 480 mg or more of sodium per serving.

🧂 Bouillon, broth, consommé	Diet soft drinks, sugar-free
Bouillon or broth, low sodium	Drink mixes, sugar-free
Carbonated or mineral water	Tea, unsweetened or with sugar substitute
Club soda	Tonic water, diet
Cocoa powder, unsweetened (1 tbs)	Water
Coffee, unsweetened or with sugar substitute	Water, flavored, carbohydrate free

Seasonings

Any food on this list can be consumed in any moderate amount.

Flavoring extracts (for example, vanilla, almond, peppermint)	Spices
Garlic	Hot pepper sauce
Herbs, fresh or dried	Wine, used in cooking
Nonstick cooking spray	Worcestershire sauce
Pimento	

Combination Foods List

Icon Key

☻ = More than 3 g of dietary fiber per serving.

🧂 = 600 mg or more of sodium per serving (for combination food main dishes/meals).

Food	Serving Size	Count as
Entrées		
🧂 Casserole type (tuna noodle, lasagna, spaghetti with meatballs, chili with beans, macaroni and cheese)	1 c (8 oz)	2 carbohydrates + 2 medium-fat meats
🧂 Stews (beef/other meats and vegetables)	1 c (8 oz)	1 carbohydrate + 1 medium-fat meat + 0–3 fats
Tuna salad or chicken salad	½ c (3½ oz)	½ carbohydrate + 2 lean meats + 1 fat
Frozen Meals/Entrées		
🧂☻ Burrito (beef and bean)	1 (5 oz)	3 carbohydrates + 1 lean meat + 2 fats
🧂 Dinner-type meal	generally 14–17 oz	3 carbohydrates + 3 medium-fat meats + 3 fats
🧂 Entrée or meal with less than 340 Calories	about 8–11 oz	2–3 carbohydrates + 1–2 lean meats
Pizza		
🧂 cheese/vegetarian thin crust	¼ of 12" (4½ to 5 oz)	2 carbohydrates + 2 medium-fat meats
🧂 meat topping, thin crust	¼ of 12" (5 oz)	2 carbohydrates + 2 medium-fat meats, + 1½ fats
🧂 Pocket sandwich	1 (4½ oz)	3 carbohydrates + 1 lean meat + 1–2 fats
🧂 Pot pie	1 (7 oz)	2½ carbohydrates + 1 medium-fat meat + 3 fats
Salads (Deli-Style)		
Coleslaw	½ c	1 carbohydrate + 1½ fats
Macaroni/pasta salad	½ c	2 carbohydrates + 3 fats
🧂 Potato salad	½ c	1½ carbohydrates + 1–2 fats
Soups		
🧂 Bean, lentil, or split pea	1 cup	1 carbohydrate + 1 lean meat

Food	Serving Size	Count as
🧂 Chowder (made with milk)	1 c (8 oz)	1 carbohydrate + 1 lean meat + 1½ fats
🧂 Cream (made with water)	1 c (8 oz)	1 carbohydrate + 1 fat
🧂 Instant	6 oz prepared	1 carbohydrate
🧂 with beans or lentils	8 oz prepared	2½ carbohydrates + 1 lean meat
🧂 Miso soup	1 c	½ carbohydrate + 1 fat
🧂 Oriental noodle	1 c	2 carbohydrates + 2 fats
Rice (congee)	1 c	1 carbohydrate
🧂 Tomato (made with water)	1 c (8 oz)	1 carbohydrate
🧂 Vegetable beef, chicken noodle, or other broth-type	1 c (8 oz)	1 carbohydrate

Fast Foods List[a]

Icon Key

☻ = More than 3 g of dietary fiber per serving.

! = Extra fat, or prepared with added fat.

🧂 = 600 mg or more sodium per serving (for fast food main dishes/meals).

Food	Serving Size	Exchanges per Serving
Breakfast Sandwiches		
🧂 Egg, cheese, meat, English muffin	1 sandwich	2 carbohydrates + 2 medium-fat meats
🧂 Sausage biscuit sandwich	1 sandwich	2 carbohydrates + 2 high-fat meats + 3½ fats
Main Dishes/Entrees		
🧂☻ Burrito (beef and beans)	1 (about 8 oz)	3 carbohydrates + 3 medium-fat meats + 3 fats
🧂 Chicken breast, breaded and fried	1 (about 5 oz)	1 carbohydrate + 4 medium-fat meats
Chicken drumstick, breaded and fried	1 (about 2 oz)	2 medium-fat meats
🧂 Chicken nuggets	6 (about 3½ oz)	1 carbohydrate + 2 medium-fat meats + 1 fat
🧂 Chicken thigh, breaded and fried	1 (about 4 oz)	½ carbohydrate + 3 medium-fat meats + 1½ fats
🧂 Chicken wings, hot	6 (5 oz)	5 medium-fat meats + 1½ fats
Oriental		
🧂 Beef/chicken/shrimp with vegetables in sauce	1 c (about 5 oz)	1 carbohydrate + 1 lean meat + 1 fat
🧂 Egg roll, meat	1 (about 3 oz)	1 carbohydrate + 1 lean meat + 1 fat
Fried rice, meatless	½ c	1½ carbohydrates + 1½ fats
🧂 Meat and sweet sauce (orange chicken)	1 c	3 carbohydrates + 3 medium-fat meats + 2 fats
🧂☻ Noodles and vegetables in sauce (chow mein, lo mein)	1 c	2 carbohydrates + 1 fat
Pizza		
🧂 Cheese, pepperoni, regular crust	⅛ of 14" (about 4 oz)	2½ carbohydrates + 1 medium-fat meat + 1½ fats
🧂 Cheese/vegetarian, thin crust	¼ of 12" (about 6 oz)	2½ carbohydrates + 2 medium-fat meats + 1½ fats
Sandwiches		
🧂 Chicken sandwich, grilled	1	3 carbohydrates + 4 lean meats
🧂 Chicken sandwich, crispy	1	3½ carbohydrates + 3 medium-fat meats + 1 fat
Fish sandwich with tartar sauce	1	2½ carbohydrates + 2 medium-fat meats + 2 fats
Hamburger		
🧂 large with cheese	1	2½ carbohydrates + 4 medium-fat meats + 1 fat
regular	1	2 carbohydrates + 1 medium-fat meat + 1 fat
🧂 Hot dog with bun	1	1 carbohydrate + 1 high-fat meat + 1 fat
Submarine sandwich		
🧂 less than 6 grams fat	6" sub	3 carbohydrates + 2 lean meats
🧂 regular	6" sub	3½ carbohydrates + 2 medium-fat meats + 1 fat

[a] The choices in the Fast Foods list are not specific fast food meals or items, but are estimates based on popular foods. You can get specific nutrition information for almost every fast food or restaurant chain. Ask the restaurant or check its website for nutrition information about your favorite fast foods.

Food	Serving Size	Exchanges per Serving
Taco, hard or soft shell (meat and cheese)	1 small	1 carbohydrate + 1 medium-fat meat + 1½ fats
Salads		
Salad, main dish (grilled chcken type, no dressing or croutons)	salad	1 carbohydrate + 4 lean meats
Salad, side, no dressing or cheese	Small (about 5 oz)	1 vegetable
Sides/Appetizers		
! French fries, restaurant style	Small	3 carbohydrates + 3 fats
Medium		4 carbohydrates + 4 fats
Large		5 carbohydrates + 6 fats
Nachos with cheese	Small (about 4½ oz)	2½ carbohydrates + 4 fats
Onion rings	1 serving (about 3 oz)	2½ carbohydrates + 3 fats
Desserts		
Milkshake, any flavor	12 oz	6 carbohydrates + 2 fats
Soft-serve ice cream cone	1 small	2½ carbohydrates + 1 fat

Alcohol List

In general, 1 alcohol choice (½ oz absolute alcohol) has about 100 Calories.

Alcoholic Beverage	Serving Size	Count as
Beer		
light (4.2%)	12 fl. oz	1 alcohol equivalent + ½ carbohydrate
regular (4.9%)	12 fl. oz	1 alcohol equivalent + 1 carbohydrate
Distilled spirits: vodka, rum, gin, whiskey, 80 or 86 proof	1½ fl. oz	1 alcohol equivalent
Liqueur, coffee (53 proof)	1 fl. oz	1 alcohol equivalent + 1 carbohydrate
Sake	1 fl. oz	½ alcohol equivalent
Wine		
dessert (sherry)	3½ fl. oz	1 alcohol equivalent + 1 carbohydrate
dry, red or white (10%)	5 fl. oz	1 alcohol equivalent

STATURE-FOR-AGE CHARTS

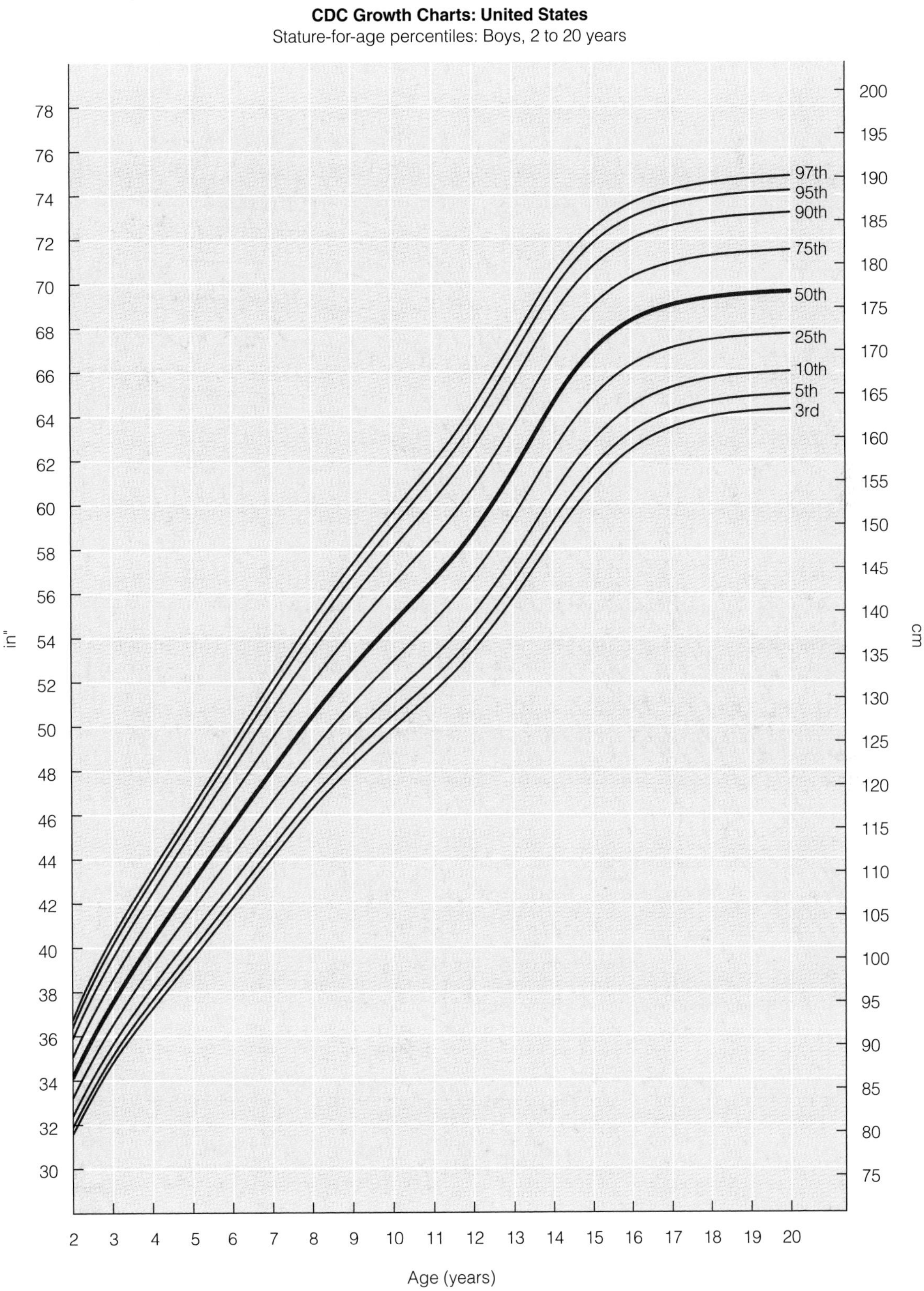

Published May 30, 2000.
Data from: The National Center for Health Statistics in collaboration with the National Center for Chronic Disease Prevention and Health Promotion (2000).

CDC
SAFER • HEALTHIER • PEOPLE™

CDC Growth Charts: United States

Stature-for-age percentiles: Girls, 2 to 20 years

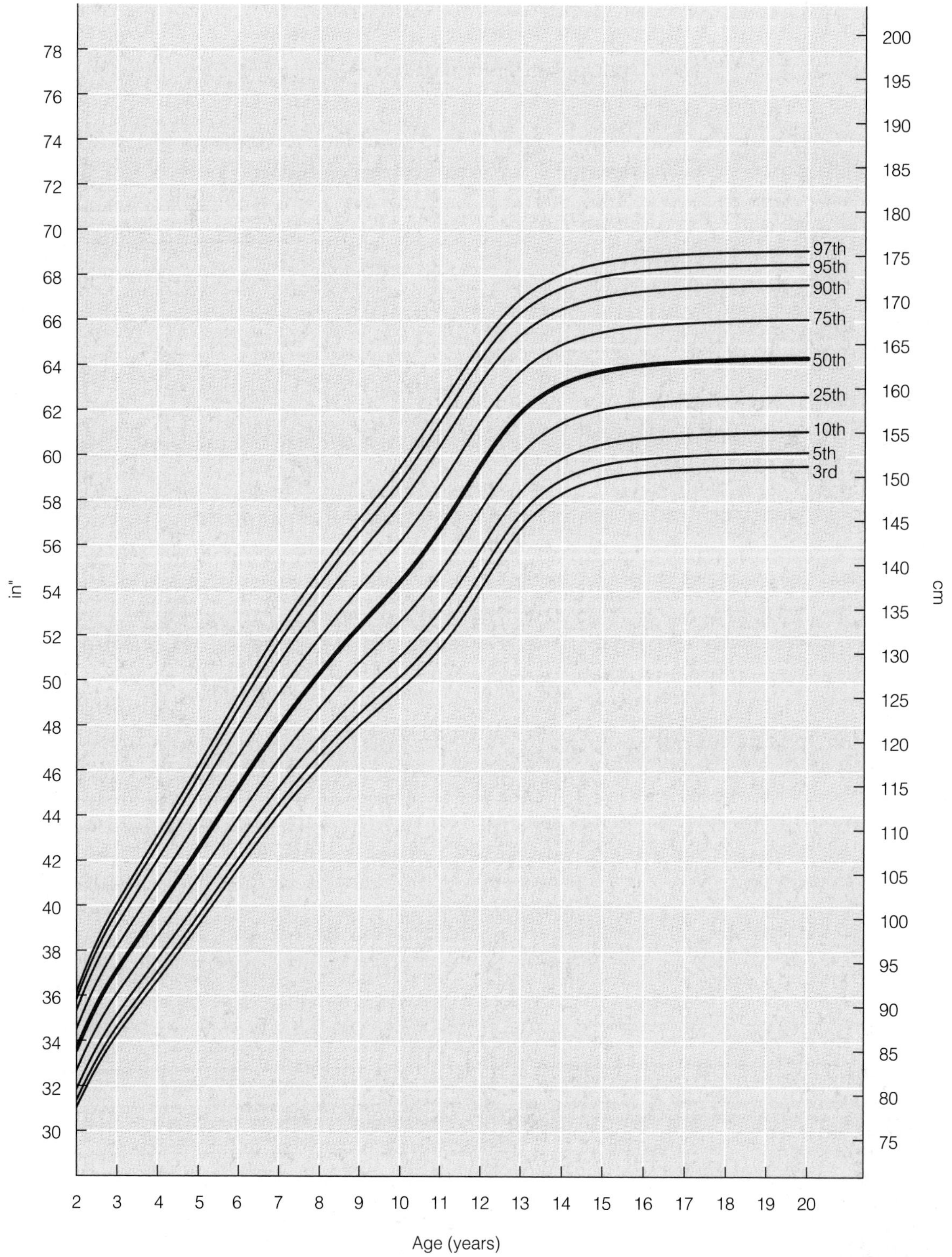

Published May 30, 2000.

Data from: The National Center for Health Statistics in collaboration with the National Center for Chronic Disease Prevention and Health Promotion (2000).

SAFER • HEALTHIER • PEOPLE™

APPENDIX F ORGANIZATIONS AND RESOURCES

ACADEMIC JOURNALS

International Journal of Sport Nutrition and Exercise Metabolism
Human Kinetics
P.O. Box 5076
Champaign, IL 61825-5076
(800) 747-4457
www.humankinetics.com/IJSNEM

Journal of Nutrition
Department of Nutrition
Pennsylvania State University
126-S Henderson Building
University Park, PA 16802-6504
(814) 865-4721
www.nutrition.org

Nutrition Research
Elsevier: Journals Customer Service
6277 Sea Harbor Drive
Orlando, FL 32887
(877) 839-7126
www.journals.elsevierhealth.com/periodicals/NTR

Nutrition
Elsevier: Journals Customer Service
6277 Sea Harbor Drive
Orlando, FL 32887
(877) 839-7126
www.journals.elsevierhealth.com/periodicals/NUT

Nutrition Reviews
International Life Sciences Institute
Subscription Office
P.O. Box 830430
Birmingham, AL 35283
(800) 633-4931
www.ingentaconnect.com/content/ilsi/nure

Obesity Research
North American Association for the Study of Obesity (NAASO)
8630 Fenton Street, Suite 918
Silver Spring, MD 20910
(301) 563-6526
www.obesityresearch.org

International Journal of Obesity
Journal of the International Association for the Study of ObesityNature Publishing Group
The Macmillan Building
4 Crinan Street
London N1 9XW
United Kingdom
www.nature.com/ijo

Journal of the American Medical Association
American Medical Association
P.O. Box 10946
Chicago, IL 60610-0946
(800) 262-2350
www.jama.ama-assn.org

New England Journal of Medicine
10 Shattuck Street
Boston, MA 02115-6094
(617) 734-9800
www.content.nejm.org

American Journal of Clinical Nutrition
The American Journal of Clinical Nutrition
9650 Rockville Pike
Bethesda, MD 20814-3998
(301) 634-7038
www.ajcn.org

Journal of the American Dietetic Association
Elsevier, Health Sciences Division
Subscription Customer Service
6277 Sea Harbor Drive
Orlando, FL 32887
(800) 654-2452
www.adajournal.org

AGING

Administration on Aging
U.S. Health & Human Services
200 Independence Avenue, SW
Washington, DC 20201
(877) 696-6775
www.aoa.gov

American Association of Retired Persons (AARP)
601 E. Street, NW
Washington, DC 20049
(888) 687-2277
www.aarp.org

Health and Age
Sponsored by the Novartis Foundation for Gerontology & The Web-Based Health Education Foundation
Robert Griffith, MD
Executive Director
573 Vista de la Ciudad
Santa Fe, NM 87501
www.healthandage.com

National Council on the Aging
300 D Street, SW, Suite 801
Washington, DC 20024
(202) 479-1200
www.ncoa.org

International Osteoporosis Foundation
5 Rue Perdtemps
1260 Nyon
Switzerland
41 22 994 01 00
www.osteofound.org

National Institute on Aging
Building 31, Room 5C27
31 Center Drive, MSC 2292
Bethesda, MD 20892
(301) 496-1752
www.nia.nih.gov

Osteoporosis and Related Bone Diseases National Resource Center
2 AMS Circle
Bethesda, MD 20892-3676
(800) 624-BONE
www.osteo.org

American Geriatrics Society
The Empire State Building
350 Fifth Avenue, Suite 801
New York, NY 10118
(212) 308-1414
www.americangeriatrics.org

National Osteoporosis Foundation
1232 22nd Street, NW
Washington, DC 20037-1292
(202) 223-2226
www.nof.org

ALCOHOL AND DRUG ABUSE

National Institute on Drug Abuse
6001 Executive Boulevard, Room 5213
Bethesda, MD 20892-9561
(301) 443-1124
www.nida.nih.gov

National Institute on Alcohol Abuse and Alcoholism
5635 Fishers Lane, MSC 9304
Bethesda, MD 20892-9304
www.niaaa.nih.gov

Alcoholics Anonymous
Grand Central Station
P.O. Box 459
New York, NY 10163
www.alcoholics-anonymous.org

Narcotics Anonymous
P.O. Box 9999
Van Nuys, California 91409
(818) 773-9999
www.na.org

National Council on Alcoholism and Drug Dependence
20 Exchange Place, Suite 2902
New York, NY 10005
(212) 269-7797
www.ncadd.org

National Clearinghouse for Alcohol and Drug Information
11420 Rockville Pike
Rockville, MD 20852
(800) 729-6686
www.health.org

CANADIAN GOVERNMENT

Health Canada
A.L. 0900C2
Ottawa, ON
K1A 0K9
(613) 957-2991
www.hc-sc.gc.ca/english

National Institute of Nutrition
408 Queen Street, 3rd Floor
Ottawa, ON K1R 5A7
(613) 235-3355
www.nin.ca/public_html

Agricultural and Agri-Food Canada
Public Information Request Service
Sir John Carling Building
930 Carling Avenue
Ottawa, ON K1A 0C5
(613) 759-1000
www.arg.gc.ca

Bureau of Nutritional Sciences
Sir Frederick G. Banting Research Centre
Tunney's Pasture (2203A)
Ottawa, ON K1A 0L2
(613) 957-0352
www.hc-sc.gc.ca/food-aliment/ns-sc/e_nutrition.html

Canadian Food Inspection Agency
59 Camelot Drive
Ottawa, ON K1A 0Y9
(613) 225-2342
www.inspection.gc.ca/english/toce.shtml

Canadian Institute for Health Information
CIHI Ottawa
377 Dalhousie Street, Suite 200
Ottawa, ON K1N 9N8
(613) 241-7860
www.cihi.ca

Canadian Public Health Association
1565 Carling Avenue, Suite 400
Ottawa, ON K1Z 8R1
(613) 725-3769
www.cpha.ca

CANADIAN NUTRITION AND PROFESSIONAL ORGANIZATIONS

Dietitians of Canada
480 University Avenue, Suite 604
Toronto, ON M5G 1V2
(416) 596-0857
www.dietitians.ca

Canadian Diabetes Association
National Life Building
1400-522 University Avenue
Toronto, ON M5G 2R5
(800) 226-8464
www.diabetes.ca

National Eating Disorder Information Centre
CW 1-211, 200 Elizabeth Street
Toronto, ON M5G 2C4
(866) NEDIC-20
www.nedic.ca

Canadian Pediatric Society
100-2204 Walkley Road
Ottawa, ON K1G 4G8
(613) 526-9397
www.cps.ca

Canadian Dietetic Association
480 University Avenue, Suite 604
Toronto, ON M5G 1V2
(416) 596-0857
www.dietitians.ca

DISORDERED EATING

American Psychiatric Association
1000 Wilson Boulevard, Suite 1825
Arlington, VA 22209
(703) 907-7300
www.psych.org

Harvard Eating Disorders Center
WACC 725
15 Parkman Street
Boston, MA 02114
(617) 236-7766
www.hedc.org

National Institute of Mental Health
Office of Communications
6001 Executive Boulevard, Room 8184, MSC 9663
Bethesda, MD 20892
(866) 615-6464
www.nimh.nih.gov

National Association of Anorexia Nervosa and Associated Disorders (ANAD)
Box 7
Highland Park, IL 60035
(847) 831-3438
www.anad.org

National Eating Disorders Association
603 Stewart Street, Suite 803
Seattle, WA 98101
(206) 382-3587
www.nationaleatingdisorders.org

Eating Disorder Referral and Information Center
2923 Sandy Pointe, Suite 6
Del Mar, CA 92014
(858) 792-7463
www.edreferral.com

Anorexia Nervosa and Related Eating Disorders, Inc. (ANRED)
E-mail: jarinor@rio.com
www.anred.com

Overeaters Anonymous
P.O. Box 44020
Rio Rancho, NM 87174
(505) 891-2664
www.oa.org

EXERCISE, PHYSICAL ACTIVITY, AND SPORTS

American College of Sports Medicine (ACSM)
P.O. Box 1440
Indianapolis, IN 46206-1440
(317) 637-9200
www.acsm.org

American Physical Therapy Association (ASNA)
1111 North Fairfax Street
Alexandria, VA 22314
(800) 999-APTA
www.apta.org

Gatorade Sports Science Institute (GSSI)
617 West Main Street
Barrington, IL 60010
(800) 616-GSSI
www.gssiweb.com

National Coalition for Promoting Physical Activity (NCPPA)
1010 Massachusetts Avenue, Suite 350
Washington, DC 20001
(202) 454-7518
www.ncppa.org

Sports, Wellness, Eating Disorder and Cardiovascular Nutritionists (SCAN)
P.O. Box 60820
Colorado Springs, CO 80960
(719) 635-6005
www.scandpg.org

President's Council on Physical Fitness and Sports
Department W
200 Independence Avenue, SW
Room 738-H
Washington, DC 20201-0004
(202) 690-9000
www.fitness.gov

American Council on Exercise
4851 Paramount Drive
San Diego, CA 92123
(858) 279-8227
www.acefitness.org

The International Association for Fitness Professionals (IDEA)
10455 Pacific Center Court
San Diego, CA 92121
(800) 999-4332, ext. 7
www.ideafit.com

FOOD SAFETY

Food Marketing Institute
655 15th Street, NW
Washington, DC 20005
(202) 452-8444
www.fmi.org

Agency for Toxic Substances and Disease Registry (ATSDR)
ORO Washington Office
Ariel Rios Building
1200 Pennsylvania Avenue, NW
M/C 5204G
Washington, DC 20460
(888) 422-8737
www.atsdr.cdc.gov

Food Allergy and Anaphylaxis Network
11781 Lee Jackson Highway, Suite 160
Fairfax, VA 22033-3309
(800) 929-4040
www.foodallergy.org

Foodsafety.gov
www.foodsafety.gov

The USDA Food Safety and Inspection Service
Food Safety and Inspection Service
United States Department of Agriculture
Washington, DC 20250
www.fsis.usda.gov

Consumer Reports
Web Site Customer Relations Department
101 Truman Avenue
Yonkers, NY 10703
www.consumerreports.org

Center for Science in the Public Interest: Food Safety
1875 Connecticut Avenue, NW
Washington, DC 20009
(202) 332-9110
www.cspinet.org/foodsafety

Center for Food Safety and Applied Nutrition
5100 Paint Branch Parkway
College Park, MD 20740
(888) SAFEFOOD
www.cfsan.fda.gov

Food Safety Project
Dan Henroid, MS, RD, CFSP
HRIM Extension Specialist and Website Coordinator
Hotel, Restaurant and Institution Management
9e MacKay Hall
Iowa State University
Ames, IA 50011
(515) 294-3527
www.extension.iastate.edu/foodsafety

Organic Consumers Association
6101 Cliff Estate Road
Little Marais, MN 55614
(218) 226-4164
www.organicconsumers.org

INFANCY AND CHILDHOOD

Administration for Children and Families
370 L'Enfant Promenade, SW
Washington, DC 20447
www.acf.dhhs.gov

The American Academy of Pediatrics
141 Northwest Point Boulevard
Elk Grove Village, IL 60007
(847) 434-4000
www.aap.org

Kidnetic.com
E-mail: contactus@kidnetic.com
www.kidnetic.com

Kidshealth: The Nemours Foundation
12735 West Gran Bay Parkway
Jacksonville, FL 32258
(866) 390-3610
www.kidshealth.org

National Center for Education in Maternal and Child Health
Georgetown University
Box 571272
Washington, DC 20057
(202) 784-9770
www.ncemch.org

Birth Defects Research for Children, Inc.
930 Woodcock Road, Suite 225
Orlando, FL 32803
(407) 895-0802
www.birthdefects.org

USDA/ARS Children's Nutrition Research Center at Baylor College of Medicine
1100 Bates Street
Houston, TX 77030
www.kidsnutrition.org

Keep Kids Healthy.com
www.keepkidshealthy.com

INTERNATIONAL AGENCIES

UNICEF
3 United Nations Plaza
New York, NY 10017
(212) 326-7000
www.unicef.org

World Health Organization
Avenue Appia 20
1211 Geneva 27
Switzerland
41 22 791 21 11
www.who.int/en

The Stockholm Convention on Persistent Organic Pollutants
11–13 Chemin des Anémones
1219 Châtelaine
Geneva, Switzerland
41 22 917 8191
www.pops.int

Food and Agricultural Organization of the United Nations
Viale delle Terme di Caracalla
00100 Rome, Italy
39 06 57051
www.fao.org

International Food Information Council Foundation
1100 Connecticut Avenue, NW
Suite 430
Washington, DC 20036
(202) 296-6540

PREGNANCY AND LACTATION

San Diego County Breastfeeding Coalition
c/o Children's Hospital and Health Center
3020 Children's Way, MC 5073
San Diego, CA 92123
(800) 371-MILK
www.breastfeeding.org

National Alliance for Breastfeeding Advocacy
Barbara Heiser, Executive Director
9684 Oak Hill Drive
Ellicott City, MD 21042-6321
OR
Marsha Walker, Executive Director
254 Conant Road
Weston, MA 02493-1756
www.naba-breastfeeding.org

American College of Obstetricians and Gynecologists
409 12th Street, SW, P.O. Box 96920
Washington, DC 20090
www.acog.org

La Leche League
1400 N. Meacham Road
Schaumburg, IL 60173
(847) 519-7730
www.lalecheleague.org

National Organization on Fetal Alcohol Syndrome
900 17th Street, NW
Suite 910
Washington, DC 20006
(800) 66 NOFAS
www.nofas.org

March of Dimes Birth Defects Foundation
1275 Mamaroneck Avenue
White Plains, NY 10605
(888) 663-4637
www.modimes.org

PROFESSIONAL NUTRITION ORGANIZATIONS

Association of Departments and Programs of Nutrition (ANDP)
Dr. Marilynn Schnepf, ANDP Chair
316 Ruth Leverton Hall
Nutrition and Health Sciences
University of Nebraska-Lincoln
Lincoln, NE 68583-0806
www.andpnet.org

North American Association for the Study of Obesity (NAASO)
8630 Fenton Street, Suite 918
Silver Spring, MD 20910
(301) 563-6526
www.naaso.org

American Dental Association
211 East Chicago Avenue
Chicago, IL 60611-2678
(312) 440-2500
www.ada.org

American Heart Association
National Center
7272 Greenville Avenue
Dallas, TX 75231
(800) 242-8721
www.americanheart.org

American Dietetic Association (ADA)
120 South Riverside Plaza, Suite 2000
Chicago, IL 60606-6995
(800) 877-1600
www.eatright.org

The American Society for Nutrition (ASN)
9650 Rockville Pike, Suite L-4500
Bethesda, MD 20814-3998
(301) 634-7050
www.nutrition.org

The Society for Nutrition Education
7150 Winton Drive, Suite 300
Indianapolis, IN 46268
(800) 235-6690
www.sne.org

American College of Nutrition
300 S. Duncan Avenue, Suite 225
Clearwater, FL 33755
(727) 446-6086
www.amcollnutr.org

American Obesity Association
1250 24th Street, NW, Suite 300
Washington, DC 20037
(800) 98-OBESE

American Council on Health and Science
1995 Broadway
Second Floor
New York, NY 10023
(212) 362-7044
www.acsh.org

American Diabetes Association
ATTN: National Call Center
1701 North Beauregard Street
Alexandria, VA 22311
(800) 342-2383
www.diabetes.org

Institute of Food Technologies
525 W. Van Buren, Suite 1000
Chicago, IL 60607
(312) 782-8424
www.ift.org

ILSI Human Nutrition Institute
One Thomas Circle, Ninth Floor
Washington, DC 20005
(202) 659-0524
www.hni.ilsi.org

TRADE ORGANIZATIONS

American Meat Institute
1700 North Moore Street
Suite 1600
Arlington, VA 22209
(703) 841-2400
www.meatami.com

National Dairy Council
10255 W. Higgins Road, Suite 900
Rosemont, IL 60018
(312) 240-2880
www.nationaldairycouncil.org

United Fresh Fruit and Vegetable Association
1901 Pennsylvania Ave. NW, Suite 1100
Washington, DC 20006
(202) 303-3400
www.uffva.org

U.S.A. Rice Federation
Washington, DC
4301 North Fairfax Drive, Suite 425
Arlington, VA 22203
(703) 236-2300
www.usarice.com

U.S. GOVERNMENT

The USDA National Organic Program
Agricultural Marketing Service
USDA-AMS-TMP-NOP
Room 4008-South Building
1400 Independence Avenue, SW
Washington, DC 20250-0020
(202) 720-3252
www.ams.usda.gov

U.S. Department of Health and Human Services
200 Independence Avenue, SW
Washington, DC 20201
(877) 696-6775
www.os.dhhs.gov

Food and Drug Administration (FDA)
5600 Fishers Lane
Rockville, MD 20857
(888) 463-6332
www.fda.gov

Environmental Protection Agency
Ariel Rios Building
1200 Pennsylvania Avenue, NW
Washington, DC 20460
(202) 272-0167
www.epa.gov

Federal Trade Commission
600 Pennsylvania Avenue, NW
Washington, DC 20580
(202) 326-2222
www.ftc.gov

Partnership for Healthy Weight Management
www.consumer.gov/weightloss

Office of Dietary Supplements
National Institutes of Health
6100 Executive Boulevard, Room 3B01, MSC 7517
Bethesda, MD 20892
(301) 435-2920
www.dietary-supplements.info.nih.gov

Nutrient Data Laboratory Homepage
Beltsville Human Nutrition Center
10300 Baltimore Avenue
Building 307-C, Room 117
BARC-East
Beltsville, MD 20705
(301) 504-8157
www.nal.usda.gov/fnic/foodcomp

National Digestive Disease Clearinghouse
2 Information Way
Bethesda, MD 20892-3570
(800) 891-5389
www.digestive.niddk.nih.gov

The National Cancer Institute
NCI Public Inquiries Office
Suite 3036A
6116 Executive Boulevard, MSC 8322
Bethesda, MD 20892-8322
(800) 4-CANCER
www.cancer.gov

The National Eye Institute
31 Center Drive, MSC 2510
Bethesda, MD 20892-2510
(301) 496-5248
www.nei.nih.gov

The National Heart, Lung, and Blood Institute
Building 31, Room 5A52
31 Center Drive, MSC 2486
Bethesda, MD 20892
(301) 592-8573
www.nhlbi.nih.gov

Institute of Diabetes and Digestive and Kidney Diseases
Office of Communications and Public Liaison
NIDDK, NIH, Building 31, Room 9A04
Center Drive, MSC 2560
Bethesda, MD 20892
(301) 496-4000
www.niddk.nih.gov

National Center for Complementary and Alternative Medicine
NCCAM Clearinghouse
P.O. Box 7923
Gaithersburg, MD 20898
(888) 644-6226
www.nccam.nih.gov

U.S. Department of Agriculture (USDA)
14th Street, SW
Washington, DC 20250
(202) 720-2791
www.usda.gov

Centers for Disease Control and Prevention (CDC)
1600 Clifton Rd
Atlanta, GA 30333
(404) 639-3311 / Public Inquiries: (800) 311-3435
www.cdc.gov

National Institutes of Health (NIH)
9000 Rockville Pike
Bethesda, MD 20892
(301) 496-4000
www.nih.gov

Food and Nutrition Information Center
Agricultural Research Service, USDA
National Agricultural Library, Room 105
10301 Baltimore Avenue
Beltsville, MD 20705-2351
(301) 504-5719
www.nal.usda.gov/fnic

National Institute of Allergy and Infectious Diseases
NIAID Office of Communications and Public Liaison
6610 Rockledge Drive, MSC 6612
Bethesda, MD 20892
(301) 496-5717
www.niaid.nih.gov

WEIGHT AND HEALTH MANAGEMENT

The Vegetarian Resource Group
P.O. Box 1463, Dept. IN
Baltimore, MD 21203
(410) 366-VEGE
www.vrg.org

American Obesity Association
1250 24th Street, NW
Suite 300
Washington, DC 20037
(202) 776-7711
www.obesity.org

Anemia Lifeline
(888) 722-4407
www.anemia.com

The Arc
(301) 565-3842
E-mail: info@thearc.org
www.thearc.org

Bottled Water Web
P.O. Box 5658
Santa Barbara, CA 93150
(805) 879-1564
www.bottledwaterweb.com

The Food and Nutrition Board
Institute of Medicine
500 Fifth Street, NW
Washington, DC 20001
(202) 334-2352
www.iom.edu/board.asp?id-3788

The Calorie Control Council
www.caloriecontrol.org

TOPS (Take Off Pounds Sensibly)
4575 South Fifth Street
P.O. Box 07360
Milwaukee, WI 53207
(800) 932-8677
www.tops.org

Shape Up America!
15009 Native Dancer Road
N. Potomac, MD 20878
(240) 631-6533
www.shapeup.org

WORLD HUNGER

Center on Hunger, Poverty, and Nutrition Policy
Tufts University
Medford, MA 02155
(617) 627-3020
www.tufts.edu/nutrition

Freedom from Hunger
1644 DaVinci Court
Davis, CA 95616
(800) 708-2555
www.freefromhunger.org

Oxfam International
1112 16th Street, NW, Suite 600
Washington, DC 20036
(202) 496-1170
www.oxfam.org

WorldWatch Institute
1776 Massachusetts Avenue, NW
Washington, DC 20036
(202) 452-1999
www.worldwatch.org

Food First
398 60th Street
Oakland, CA 94618
(510) 654-4400
www.foodfirst.org

The Hunger Project
15 East 26th Street
New York, NY 10010
(212) 251-9100
www.thp.org

U.S. Agency for International Development
Information Center
Ronald Reagan Building
Washington, DC 20523
(202) 712-0000
www.usaid.gov

APPENDIX G THE USDA FOOD GUIDE EVOLUTION

EARLY HISTORY OF FOOD GUIDES

Did you know that in the United States food guides in one form or another have been around for over 125 years?

That's right. Back in 1885 a college chemistry professor named Wilber Olin Atwater helped bring the fledgling science of nutrition to a broader audience by introducing dietary standards that became the basis for the first U.S. food guide. Those early standards focused on defining the daily needs of an "average man" for proteins and Calories. They soon expanded into food composition tables with three sweeping categories: protein, fat, and carbohydrate; mineral matter; and "fuel values." As early as 1902, Atwater advocated for three foundational nutritional principles that we still support today: variety, proportionality, and moderation in food choices and eating.

These ideas were adapted a few years later by a nutritionist named Caroline Hunt, who developed a food "buying" guide divided into five categories: meats and proteins; cereals and starches; vegetables and fruits; fatty foods; and sugar.

From the 1930s to the early 1970s, these guidelines kept changing—from twelve food groups to seven to four, and from there to a "Hassle-Free" guide that briefly increased the number of groups back up to five. Although critics identified many drawbacks of these approaches, they were necessary attempts to provide Americans with reliable guidelines based on the best scientific data and practices available at the time.

CONTEMPORARY FOOD GUIDES: FROM PYRAMID TO PLATE

By the early 1980s, public health experts began to recognize that, to be effective, a national food guide had to reflect key philosophical values. These core values included the following:

- it must encompass a broad focus on *overall health*;
- it should emphasize the use of *current research*;
- it should be an approach that includes the *total diet*, rather than parts or pieces;
- it should be *useful*;
- it should be *realistic*;
- it should be *flexible*;
- it should be *practical*;
- and it must be *evolutionary*, able to adapt as new information comes to light.

These values guided the development of the USDA Food Guide Pyramid, released in 1992, which also was the first guide to include a graphic representation of the Dietary Guidelines for Americans—in the shape of a pyramid. The 1992 Guide included the following components:

- Nutritional Goals
- Food Groups
- Serving Sizes
- Nutrient Profiles
- Numbers of Servings

The 1992 Guide did not have an enthusiastic reception. Instead, critics quickly began pointing out flaws in the design, recommendations, and ease of use. Many nutritionists trying to use the Guide to teach different population groups basic nutrition messages found that it was out of touch with people's day-to-day lives. Back to the drawing board!

The USDA addressed these complaints by revising—and then radically reinventing—the 1992 Guide. Let's take a look at this evolution of the USDA Food Guide over the past two decades by examining the following graphics.

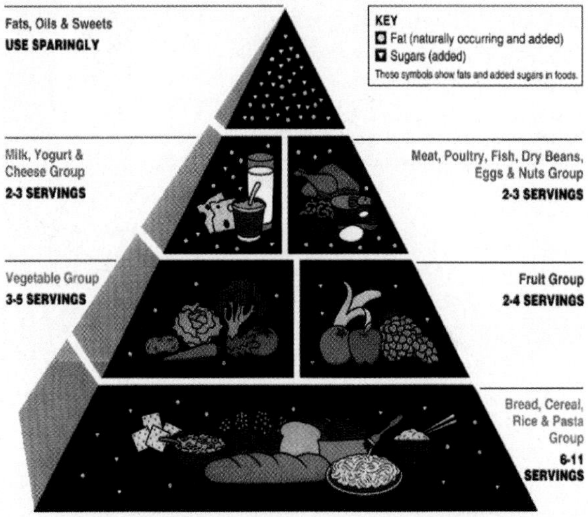

The 1992 Food Guide Pyramid. This representation of the USDA guidelines took several years to develop and attempted to convey in a single image all the key aspects of a nutritional guide.

The USDA revised the Guide in 2005 to address concerns regarding the recommendations and ease of use for a general audience. The result was the MyPyramid Food Guidance System, which retained the "pyramid" graphic, but in a simpler presentation that included an emphasis on daily physical activity, and introduced an interactive MyPyramid website where consumers could enter personal data and print out a personalized guide.

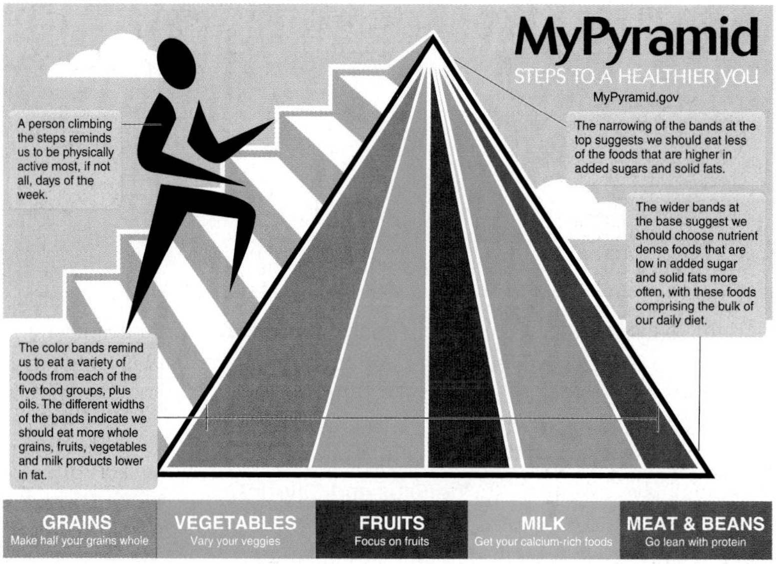

In May 2011 the USDA again changed the food guide—this time dramatically. Dropping the pyramid concept, as well as the previous attempts to teach detailed lessons about foods and physical activity, the new MyPlate guide uses simple icons to directly convey a few key pointers for maintaining a healthy diet. The accompanying website, www.choosemyplate.gov, includes more detailed information as well as interactive tools and multimedia for professionals and consumers.

Data adapted from: www.nal.usda.gov/fnic/history/hist.htm and http://www.choosemyplate.gov/downloads/MyPlate/ABriefHistoryOfUSDAFoodGuides.pdf.

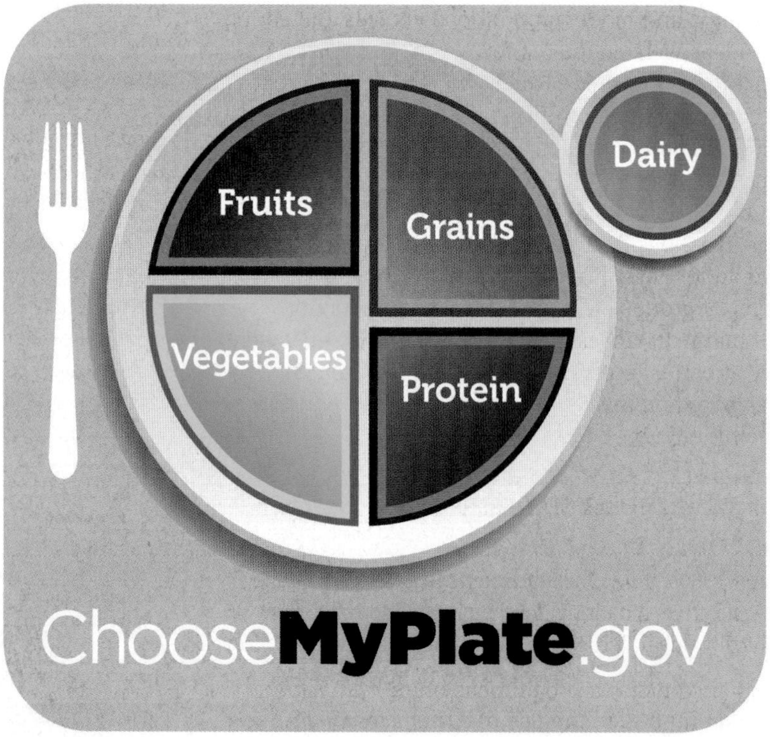

REFERENCES

Chapter 1

1. Kraut, A. Dr. Joseph Goldberger & the War on Pellagra. National Institutes of Health, Office of NIH History. Available at http://www.history.nih.gov/exhibits/goldberger and H. Markel. 2003. The New Yorker who changed the diet of the South. *New York Times* 12 August, 2003:D5.
2. Institute of Medicine, Food and Nutrition Board. 2003. *Dietary Reference Intakes: Applications in Dietary Planning.* Washington, DC: National Academies Press.
3. Institute of Medicine, Food and Nutrition Board. 2002. *Dietary Reference Intakes for Energy, Carbohydrates, Fiber, Fat, Protein and Amino Acids (Macronutrients).* Washington, DC: National Academies Press.
4. Fogel, J., and SBS Shlivko. 2010. Weight Problems and Spam E-mail for Weight Loss Products. *Southern Medical Journal.* January 2010. Vol. 103. Issue 1. pp. 31–36.
5. U.S. Department of Health and Human Services. Centers for Disease Control and Prevention. 2009. Health Risks in the United States. Behavioral Risk Factor Surveillance System: At a Glance, 2009. Available at http://www.cdc.gov/chronicdisease/resources/publications/AAG/brfss.htm.
6. Watters, E. 2006. DNA is not destiny. *Discover* 27(11):32–75.
7. The NCMHD Center of Excellence for Nutritional Genomics. Retrieved April 2007, from http://nutrigenomics.ucdavis.edu.
8. Johnson, N., and J. Kaput. 2003. Nutrigenomics: an emerging scientific discipline. *Food Technology* 57(4):60–67.
9. Grierson, B. 2003. What your genes want you to eat. *New York Times*, May 4.
10. Wallace, K. 2007. Diet, exercise may lower colon cancer risk [television broadcast]. CBS News, March 15.
11. Kaput, J., and R. Rodriguez. 2004. Nutritional genomics: the next frontier in the postgenomic era. *Physiological Genomics* 16:166–177.

In Depth: Alcohol

1. Dufour, M. C., L. Archer, and E. Gordis. 1992. Alcohol and the elderly. *Clin. Geriatr. Med.* 8:127–141.
2. Gunzerath, L., V. Faden, S. Zakhari, and K. Warren. 2004. National Institute on Alcohol Abuse and Alcoholism Report on moderate drinking. *Alcohol. Clin. Exp. Res.* 28L:829–847.
3. Stranges, S., T. Wu, J. M. Born., et al. 2004. Relationship of alcohol drinking pattern to risk of hypertension. *Hypertension* 44:813–819.
4. Meister, K. A., E. M. Whelan, and R. Kava. 2000. The health effects of moderate alcohol intake in humans: an epidemiologic review. *Crit. Rev. Clin. Lab. Sci.* 37:261–296.
5. Caton, S. J., M. Ball, A. Ahern, et al. 2004. Dose-dependent effects of alcohol on appetite and food intake. *Physiol. Behav.* 81:51–58.
6. National Institute of Alcohol Abuser and Alcoholism. NIAA Council approves definition of binge drinking. http://pubs.niaaa.nih.gov/publications/Newsletter/winter2004/Newsletter_Number3.pdf. NIAA Newsletter 2004: 3:3.
7. Nelson, D. E., T. S. Naimi, R. D. Brewer, J. Bolen, and H. E. Wells. 2004. Metropolitan-area estimates of binge drinking in the United States. *Am. J. Pub. Health* 94:663–671.
8. Naimi, T. S., R. D. Brewer, A. Mokdad, C. Denny, and M. K. Serdula. 2003. Binge drinking among US adults. 289:70–79.
9. National Institute on Alcohol Abuse and Alcoholism (NIAAA). 2007. A Snapshot of High-Risk College Drinking Consequences. www.collegedrinkingprevention.gov/facts/snapshot.aspx.
10. Oscar-Berman, M., and K. Marinkovic. 2003. Alcoholism and the brain: an overview. *Alc. Res. Health* 27:161–173.
11. Brown, S. A., S. F. Tapert, E. Granholm, and D. C. Delis. 2000. Neurocognitive functioning of adolescents: effects of protracted alcohol use. *Alc. Clin. Exp. Res.* 24:164–171.
12. National Institute on Alcohol Abuse and Alcoholism (NIAAA). 2006. Young Adult Drinking. *Alcohol Alert*, No. 68, April 2006.
13. Bagnardi, V., M. Blangiardo, C. La Vecchia, and G. Corrao. 2001. Alcohol consumption and the risk of cancer: a meta-analysis. *Alc. Res. Health* 25:263–270.
14. Inoue, M., and S. Tsugane for the JPHC Study Group. 2004. Impact of alcohol drinking on total cancer risk: data from a large-scale population-based cohort study in Japan. *Brit. J. Cancer* 92:182–187.
15. National Institute on Alcohol Abuse and Alcoholism (NIAAA). 2007. A Snapshot of High-Risk College Drinking Consequences. www.collegedrinkingprevention.gov/facts/snapshot.aspx.
16. Sokol, R. J., et al. 2003. Fetal alcohol spectrum disorder. *JAMA* 290:2996–2999.
17. National Institute on Alcohol Abuse and Alcoholism (NIAAA). 2005. Alcohol: How to Cut Down on Your Drinking. www.collegedrinkingprevention.gov/facts/cutdrinking.aspx.

Chapter 2

1. Ogden, C. L., M. D. Carroll, and K. M. Flegal. 2008. High body mass index for age among US children and adolescents, 2003–2006. *JAMA* 299(20): 2401–2405.
2. U.S. Department of Health and Human Services (USDHHS) and U.S. Department of Agriculture (USDA). 2010. Dietary Guidelines for Americans, 2010, 7th edn. Washington, DC: U.S. Government Printing Office. www.healthierus.gov/dietaryguidelines.
3. Nielsen, S. J., and B. M. Popkin. 2003. Patterns and trends in food portion sizes, 1977–1998. *JAMA* 289(4):450–453.
4. Food and Nutrition Information Center. 2006. Dietary Guidance. Ethnic/Cultural Food Pyramid. http://fnic.nal.usda.gov/nal_display/index.php?info_center=4&tax_level=3&tax_subject=256&topic_id=1348&level3_id=5732.
5. Taylor, P., C. Funk, and P. Craighill. 2006. Eating More; Enjoying Less. Pew Research Center. A Social Trends Report. http://pewresearch.org/assets/social/pdf/Eating.pdf. (Accessed March 2007.)
6. Ogden, C. L., M. D. Carroll, M. A. McDowell, and K. M. Flegal. 2007. Obesity Among Adults in the United States—No Change Since 2003-2004. NCHS data brief no 1. Hyattsville, MD: National Center for Health Statistics. Available at http://www.cdc.gov/nchs/data/databriefs/db01.pdf.
7. Institute of Food Technologists. Functional foods: Opportunities and challenges. IFT Expert Report.Available at http://members.ift.org/NR/rdonlyres/4D40132D-B06B-4F2B-9753-CE18B73E187E/0/OnePagerIntro.pdf.
8. Federal Register, October 25, 2006 (Volume 71, Number 206). From the Federal Register Online via GPO Access [wais.access.gpo.gov] [DOCID:fr25oc06-12] Food and Drug Administration, HHS; 21 CFR Parts 101 and 170 [Docket No. 2002P-0122] (formerly 02P-0122). Conventional Foods Being Marketed as "Functional Foods"; Public Hearing; Request for Comments.
9. U.S. Food and Drug Administration (FDA). 2006. Docket No. 2006D-0480. Draft Guidance for Industry on Complementary and

Alternative Medicine Products and Their Regulation by the Food and Drug Administration.
10. Saier, M. H., Jr., and N. M. Mansour. 2005. Probiotics and prebiotics in human health. *J. Mol. Microbiol. Biotechnol.* 10(1):22–25.
11. Doron, S., and S. L. Gorbach. 2006. Probiotics: Their role in the treatment and prevention of diseases. *Expert Rev. Anti-Infect. Ther.* 4(2):261–275.
12. Ezendam, J., and H. van Loveren. 2006. Probiotics: Immunomodulation and evaluation of safety and efficacy. *Nutr. Rev.* 64(1):1–14.
13. Sanders, M. E., D. C.Walker, K. M. Walker, K. Aoyama, and T. R. Klaenhammer. 1996. Performance of commercial cultures in fluid milk applications. *J. Dairy Sci.* 79:943–955.

In Depth: Phytochemicals

1. Liu, R. H. 2003. Health benefits of fruit and vegetables are from additive and synergistic combinations of phytochemicals. *Am. J. Clin. Nutr.* 78(suppl.):517S–520S.
2. Panel on Dietary Antioxidants and Related Compounds. Subcommittee on Upper Reference Levels of Nutrients and Interpretation and Uses of Dietary Reference Intakes. Standing Committee on the Scientific Evaluation of Dietary Reference Intakes. Food and Nutrition Board. Institute of Medicine. 2000. Dietary Reference Intakes for Vitamin C, Vitamin E, Selenium, and Carotenoids.Washington, DC: National Academies Press.
3. Chun, O. K., et al. 2007. Estimated dietary flavonoid intake and major food sources of US adults. *J. Nutr.* 137:1244–1252.
4. Melton, L. 2006. The antioxidant myth: A medical fairy tale. *New Sci.* 2563:40–43.
5. Linus Pauling Institute, Oregon State University. 2005. Micronutrient information center: Flavonoids. Available at http://lpi.oregonstate.edu/infocenter/phytochemicals/flavonoids.
6. Beauchamp, G. K., R. S. Keast, D. Morel, J. Lin, J. Pika, Q. Han, C. H. Lee, A. B. Smith, and P. A. Breslin. 2005. Ibuprofen-like activity in extra virgin olive oil. *Nature* 437:45–46.
7. Liu, R. H. 2004. Potential synergy of phytochemicals in cancer prevention:Mechanism of action. *J. Nutr.* 134:3479S–3485S.
8. Boileau, T. W.-M., et al. 2003. Prostate carcinogenesis in N-methyl-N-nitrosurea (NMU)-testosterone-treated rats fed tomato powder, lycopene, and energy-restricted diets. *J. Natl. Cancer Inst.* 95:1578–1586.
9. Milner, J. A. 2001. A historical perspective on garlic and cancer. *J. Nutr.* 131:1027S–1031S.
10. Rice S., and S. A.Whitehead. 2006. Phytoestrogens and breast cancer—promoters or protectors? *Endocr. Relat. Cancer* 13(4):995–1015.
11. Meyskens, F. L., and E. Szabo. 2005. Diet and cancer: The disconnect between epidemiology and randomized clinical trials. *Cancer Epidemiol. Biomarkers Prev.* 14(6):1366–1369.
12. The Alpha-Tocopherol, Beta-Carotene Cancer Prevention Study Group. 1994. The effect of vitamin E and beta carotene on the incidence of lung cancer and other cancers in male smokers. *N. Engl. J. Med.* 330(15):1029–1035.
13. Omenn, G. S., et al. 1996. Risk factors for lung cancer and for intervention effects in CARET, the Beta-Carotene and Retinol Efficacy Trial. *J. Natl. Cancer Inst.* 88(21):1550–1559.
14. U.S. Preventive Services Task Force. 2003. Routine vitamin supplementation to prevent cancer and cardiovascular disease: Recommendations and rationale. *Ann. Intern. Med.* 139(1):51–55.
15. Baur, J. A., et al. 2006. Resveratrol improves health and survival of mice on a high calorie diet. *Nature* 444:337–342.
16. Lagouge, M., et al. 2006. Resveratrol improves mitochondrial function and protects against metabolic disease by activating SIRT1 and PGC-1alpha. *Cell* 27(6):1109–1122.

Chapter 3

1. Orr, J., and B. Davy. 2005. Dietary influences on peripheral hormones regulating energy intake: potential applications for weight management. *J. Am. Diet. Assoc.* 105:1115–1124; Astrup, A. 2005. The satiating power of protein—a key to obesity prevention? *Am. J. Cl. Nutr.* Vol. 82 No. 1, 1–2, July 2005. Available at www.ajcn.org/cgi/content/full/82/1/1.
2. Pollack, A. 2009. Medicine's Elusive Goal: A Safe Weight-Loss Drug. *The New York Times*, October 17, 2009. www.nytimes.com/2009/10/17/business/17obesity.html?_r=1&scp=1&sq=appetite%20suppressants&st=cse.
3. Davidson, N. O. 2003. Intestinal lipid absorption. In: Yamada, T., D. H. Alpers, N. Kaplowitz, L. Laine, C. Owyang, and D. W. Powell, eds. *Textbook of Gastroenterology*, Vol. 1, 4th edn. Philadelphia: Lippincott Williams & Wilkins.
4. National Institute of Diabetes and Digestive and Kidney Diseases (NIDDK). 2007. Heartburn, Gastroesophageal Reflux (GER), and Gastroesophageal Reflux Disease (GERD). NIH Publication No. 07-0882. http://digestive.niddk.nih.gov/ddiseases/pubs/gerd/index.htm.
5. Bauman, R. 2011. *Microbiology*, 3rd edn. San Francisco: Benjamin Cummings.
6. National Institute of Diabetes and Digestive and Kidney Diseases (NIDDK). 2004. H. pylori and Peptic Ulcer. NIH Publication No. 05-4225. http://digestive.niddk.nih.gov/ddiseases/pubs/hpylori/.
7. National Institute of Diabetes and Digestive and Kidney Diseases (NIDDK). 2004. NSAIDs and Peptic Ulcers. NIH Publication No. 04-4644. Available at http://digestive.niddk.nih.gov/ddiseases/pubs/nsaids/index.htm.
8. National Institute of Diabetes and Digestive and Kidney Diseases (NIDDK). 2007. Diarrhea. NIH Publication No. 07–2749. http://digestive.niddk.nih.gov/ddiseases/pubs/diarrhea/index.htm.
9. DuPont, H. L. 2006. New insights and directions in traveler's diarrhea. Gastroenterol. *Clin. N. Am.* 35(2):337–353, viii–ix.
10. National Institute of Diabetes and Digestive and Kidney Diseases (NIDDK). 2007. Diarrhea. NIH Publication No. 07-2749. http://digestive.niddk.nih.gov/ddiseases/pubs/diarrhea/index.htm.
11. Lewis, C. July–August 2001. Irritable Bowel Syndrome: A Poorly Understood Disorder. *FDA Consumer Magazine*. www.fda.gov/fdac/features/2001/401_ibs.html.
12. National Institute of Diabetes and Digestive and Kidney Diseases (NIDDK). 2007. Irritable Bowel Syndrome. NIH Publication No. 07-693. http://digestive.niddk.nih.gov/ddiseases/pubs/ibs/.
13. Mayo Clinic. 2009. Colon cleansing: Is it helpful or harmful? Mayo Foundation for Medical Education and Research. Available at: www.mayoclinic.com/health/colon-cleansing/AN00065; WebMD. 2009. Natural Colon Cleansing: Is It Necessary? WebMD Medical Reference. Available at www.webmd.com/balance/natural-colon-cleansing-is-it-necessary.
14. Picco, M. 2008. Detox diets: Do they offer any health benefits? Mayo Foundation for Medical Education and Research. Available at: www.mayoclinic.com/health/detox-diets/AN015334.
15. Mayo Clinic, op. cit.; Picco, op. cit.; Ellin, A. 2009. Flush Those Toxins! Eh, Not So Fast. *The New York Times*. January 22, 2009. Available at www.nytimes.com/2009/01/22/fashion/22skin.html.

In Depth: Disorders Related to Specific Foods

1. National Institute of Diabetes and Digestive and Kidney Diseases (NIDDK). 2009. Lactose Intolerance. NIH Publication No. 09-2751. http://digestive.niddk.nih.gov/ddiseases/pubs/lactoseintolerance/.
2. U.S. Food and Drug Administration (FDA). December 20, 2005. FDA to Require Food Manufacturers to List Food Allergens. FDA News. www.fda.gov/bbs/topics/NEWS/2005/NEW01281.html.
3. U.S. Food and Drug Administration (FDA). July 18, 2006. Information for Consumers: Food Allergen Labeling and Consumer

Protection Act of 2004 Questions and Answers. www.cfsan.fda.gov/∼dms/alrgqa.html.

4. National Institutes of Health (NIH). 2009. Allergy Testing. Medline Plus. Available at www.nlm.nih.gov/medlineplus/ency/article/003519.htm.
5. National Institute of Diabetes and Digestive and Kidney Diseases (NIDDK). September 2008. Celiac Disease. NIH Publication No. 08-4269. http://digestive.niddk.nih.gov/ddiseases/pubs/celiac/.
6. National Institutes of Health. June 2004. NIH Consensus Development Conference on Celiac Disease. http://consensus.nih.gov/2004/2004CeliacDisease118html.htm.

Chapter 4

1. Sears, B. 1995. The Zone. A Dietary Road Map. New York: HarperCollins Publishers.
2. Steward, H. L., M. C. Bethea, S. S. Andrews, and L. A. Balart. 1995. Sugar Busters! Cut Sugar to Trim Fat. New York: Ballantine Books.
3. Atkins, R. C. 1992. Dr. Atkins' New Diet Revolution. New York: M. Evans & Company, Inc.
4. Topping, D. L., and P. M. Clifton. 2001. Short-chain fatty acids and human colonic function: roles of resistant starch and nonstarch polysaccharides. *Physiol. Rev.* 81:1031–1064.
5. Pan, J. W., D. L. Rothman, K. L. Behar, D. T. Stein, and H. P. Hetherington. 2000. Human brain α-hydroxybutyrate and lactate increase in fasting-induced ketosis. *J. Cerebral Blood Flow Metabol.* 20:1502–1507.
6. Institute of Medicine, Food and Nutrition Board. 2002. Dietary Reference Intakes for Energy, Carbohydrates, Fiber, Fat, Protein and Amino Acids (Macronutrients). Washington, DC: The National Academy of Sciences.
7. Romijn, J. A., E. F. Coyle, L. S. Sidossis, A. Gastaldelli, J. F. Horowitz, E. Endert, and R. R. Wolfe. 1993. Regulation of endogenous fat and carbohydrate metabolism in relation to exercise intensity and duration. *Am. J. Physiol.* 265 [Endocrinol. Metab. 28]: E380–E391.
8. Foster-Powell, K., S. H. A. Holt, and J. C. Brand-Miller. 2002. International table of glycemic index and glycemic load values: 2002. *Am. J. Clin. Nutr.* 76:5–56.
9. Liu, S., J. E. Manson, M. J. Stampfer, M. D. Holmes, F. B. Hu, S. E. Hankinson, and W. C. Willett. 2001. Dietary glycemic load assessed by food-frequency questionnaire in relation to plasma high-density-lipoprotein cholesterol and fasting plasma triacylglycerols in postmenopausal women. *Am. J. Clin. Nutr.* 73:560–566.
10. Sloth, B., I. Krog-Mikkelsen, A. Flint, I. Tetens, I. Björck, S. Vinoy, H. Elmståhl, A. Astrup, V. Lang, and A. Raben. 2004. No difference in body weight decrease between a low-glycemic-index and a high-glycemic-index diet but reduced LDL cholesterol after 10-wk ad libitum intake of the low-glycemic-index diet. *Am. J. Clin. Nutr.* 80:337–347.
11. Buyken, A. E., M. Toeller, G. Heitkamp, G. Karamanos, B. Rottiers, R. Muggeo, and M. Fuller. 2001. Glycemic index in the diet of European outpatients with type 1 diabetes: relations to glycated hemoglobin and serum lipids. *Am. J. Clin. Nutr.* 73:574–581.
12. Augustin, L. S. A., C. Galeone, L. Dal Maso, C. Pelucchi, V. Ramazzotti, D. J. A. Jenkins, M. Montella, R. Talamini, E. Negri, S. Franceschi, and C. La Vecchia. 2004. Glycemic index, glycemic load and risk of prostate cancer. Int. *J. Cancer* 112: 446–450.
13. U.S. Department of Health and Human Services (USDHHS) and U.S. Department of Agriculture (USDA). 2010. Dietary Guidelines for Americans, 2010, 7th edn. Washington, DC: U.S. Government Printing Office. www.healthierus.gov/dietaryguidelines.
14. U.S. Department of Health and Human Services (USDHHS) and U.S. Department of Agriculture (USDA). 2006. Eating healthier and feeling better using the Nutrition Facts Label. www.cfsan.fda.gov/∼acrobat/nutfacts.pdf.
15. Howard, B. V., and J. Wylie-Rosett. 2002. Sugar and cardiovascular disease. A statement for healthcare professionals from the Committee on Nutrition of the Council on Nutrition, Physical Activity, and Metabolism of the American Heart Association. *Circulation* 106:523–527.
16. Meyer, K. A., L. H. Kushi, D. R. Jacobs, J. Slavin, T. A. Sellers, and A. R. Folsom. 2000. Carbohydrates, dietary fiber, and incident type 2 diabetes in older women. *Am. J. Clin. Nutr.* 71:921–930.
17. Schultze, M. B., J. E. Manson, D. S. Ludwig, G. A. Colditz, M. J. Stampfer, W. C. Willett, and F. B. Hu. 2004. Sugar-sweetened beverages, weight gain, and incidence of type 2 diabetes in young and middle-aged women. *JAMA*. 292:927–934.
18. Colditz, G. A., J. E. Manson, M. J. Stampfer, B. Rosner, W. C. Willett, and F. E. Speizer. 1992. Diet and risk of clinical diabetes in women. *Am. J. Clin. Nutr.* 55:1018–1023.
19. International Food Information Council Foundation. 2009. Facts About Low-Calorie Sweeteners. http://www.foodinsight.org/Content/6/LCS%20Fact%20Sheet_11-09.pdf.
20. Bray, G. A., S. J. Nielsen, and B. M. Popkin. 2004. Consumption of high-fructose corn syrup in beverages may play a role in the epidemic of obesity. *Am. J. Clin. Nutr.* 79:537–543.
21. Wilkinson Enns, C., S. J. Mickle, and J. D. Goldman. 2002. Trends in food and nutrient intakes by children in the United States. Family Econ. *Nutr. Rev.* 14:56–68.
22. Harnack, L., J. Stang, and M. Story. 1999. Soft drink consumption among U.S. children and adolescents: nutritional consequences. *J. Am. Diet. Assoc.* 99:436–441.
23. Ebbeling, C. B., H. A. Feldman, S. K. Osganian, V. R. Chomitz, S. H. Ellenbogen, and D. S. Ludwig. 2006. Effects of decreasing sugar-sweetened beverage consumption on body weight in adolescents: a randomized, controlled pilot study. *Pediatrics* 117:673–680.
24. Jacobson, M. F. 2004. Letter to the editor. High-fructose corn syrup and the obesity epidemic. *Am. J. Clin. Nutr.* 80:1081–1090.
25. Lê, K.-A., D. Faeh, R. Stettler, M. Ith, R. Kreis, P. Vermathen, C. Boesch, E. Ravussin, and L. Tappy. 2006. A 4-wk high-fructose diet alters lipid metabolism without affecting insulin sensitivity or ectopic lipids in healthy humans. *Am. J. Clin. Nutr.* 84:1374–1379.26.
26. Elliott, S. S., N. L. Keim, J. S. Stern, K. Teff, and P. J. Havel. 2002. Fructose, weight gain, and the insulin resistance syndrome. *Am. J. Clin. Nutr.* 76:911–922.

In Depth: Diabetes

1. Kleinfield, N. R. 2006. Diabetes and its awful toll quietly emerge as a crisis. The New York Times. January 9, 2006. http://www.nytimes.com/2006/01/09/nyregion/nyregionspecial5/09diabetes.html.
2. National Diabetes Information Clearinghouse (NDIC). 2008. National Diabetes Statistics, 2007. National Institutes of Health Publication No. 08–3892. http://diabetes.niddk.nih.gov/dm/pubs/statistics/index.htm#y_people.
3. American Diabetes Association. 2010. Genetics of diabetes. Available online at http://www.diabetes.org/diabetes-basics/genetics-of-diabetes.html.
4. Grundy, S. M., J. I. Cleeman, S. R. Daniels, K. A. Donato, R. H. Exkel, B. A. Franklin, D. J. Gordon, R. M. Krauss, P. J. Savage, S. C. Smith, J. A. Spertus, and F. Costa. 2005. Diagnosis and management of the metabolic syndrome: An American Heart Association/National Heart, Lung, and Blood Institute scientific statement. *Circulation* 112(17):2735–2752.
5. Huang, T. T.-K., Kempf, A. M., Strother, M. L., Li, C., Lee, R. E., Harris, K. J., and Kaur, H. 2004. Overweight and components of the metabolic syndrome in college students. *Diab. Care* 27(12): 3000–3001.

6. American College Health Association (ACHA) National College Health Assessment (NCHA). 2008. ACHA NCHA II. Reference Group Executive Summary. http://www.achancha.org/reports_ACHA-NCHAII.html.
7. Pan, X. P., G. W. Li, Y. H. Hu, J. X. Wang, W. Y. Yang, Z. X. An, Z. X. Hu, J. Lin, J. Z. Xiao, H. B. Cao, P. A. Liu, X. G. Jiang, Y. Y. Jiang, J. P. Wang., H. Zheng, H. Zhang, P. H. Bennett, and B. V. Howard. 1997. Effects of diet and exercise in preventing NIDDM in people with impaired glucose tolerance. *Diabetes Care* 20:537–544.
8. American College of Sports Medicine (ACSM). 2000. Position stand: Exercise and type 2 diabetes. *Med. Sci. Sports Exerc.* 32:1345–1360.

Chapter 5

1. Champe, P. C., R. A. Harvey, and D. R. Ferrier. 2008. Lippincott's Illustrated Reviews: Biochemistry. 4th ed. Philadelphia: Lippincott Williams & Wilkins.
2. Lichtenstein A. H., L. J. Appel, M. Brands, M. Carnethon, S. Daniels, H. A. Franch, B. Franklin, P. Kris-Ethergon, W. S. Harris, B. Howard, N. Karanja, M. Lefevre, L. Rudel, F. Sancks, L. Van Horn, M. Winston, and J. Wylie-Rosett. 2006. Diet and lifestyle recommendations revision 2006: A scientific statement from the American Heart Association Nutrition Committee. *Circulation* 114:82–96.
3. Smith, C., A. D. Marks, and M. Lieberman. 2005. Mark's Basic Medical Biochemistry: A Clinical Approach. 2nd ed. Philadelphia: Lippincott Williams & Wilkins.
4. Wijendran, V., and K. C. Hayes. 2004. Dietary n-6 and n-3 fatty acid balance and cardiovascular health. *Annu. Rev. Nutr.* 24:597–615.
5. Din, J. N., D. E. Newby, and A. D. Flapan. 2004. Omega 3 fatty acids and cardiovascular disease—fishing for a natural treatment. *British Med. J.* 328(3):30–35.
6. Jebb, S. A., A. M. Prentice, G. R. Goldberg, P. R. Murgatroyd, A. E. Black, and W. A. Coward. 1996. Changes in macronutrient balance during over- and underfeeding assessed by 12-d continuous whole-body calorimetry. *Am. J. Clin. Nutr.* 64:259–266.
7. Institute of Medicine, Food and Nutrition Board. 2002. Dietary Reference Intakes for Energy, Carbohydrate, Fiber, Fat, Fatty Acids, Cholesterol, Protein, and Amino Acids (Macronutrients). Washington, DC: National Academies Press.
8. USDA, What we eat in America. Agricultural Research Service (ARS), 2009. http://www.ars.usdagov/research/projects/projects.htm?ACCN_NO=415257.
9. Jonnalagadda S. S. Jones J. M. 2005. Position of the American Dietetic Association: Fat Replacers. *J Am Diet Assoc.* 205:266–275.
10. Briefel, R. R., and C. L. Johnson. 2004. Secular trends in dietary intake in the United States. *Annu. Rev. Nutr.* 24:401–431.
11. Cialdella-Kam L. C., Manore M. M. 2009. Macronutrient requirements of active individuals: An Update. *Nutrition Today.* 44(3):104–111.
12. Rodriguez N. R., DiMarco N. M., Langley S. 2009. Postiion of the American Dietetic Association, Dietitians of Canada, and the American College of Sports Medicine: Nutrition and Athletic Performance. *J. Am. Diet. Assoc.* 109:509–527.
13. Lichtenstein, A. H., and L. Van Horn. 1998. Very low fat diets. *Circulation* 98:935–939.
14. Calloway, C. W. 1998. The role of fat-modified foods in the American diet. *Nutr. Today* 33:156–163.
15. Sigman-Grant, M. 1997. Can you have your low-fat cake and eat it too? The role of fat-modified products. *J. Am. Diet. Assoc.* 97(suppl.):S76–S81.
16. Expert Panel on Detection, Evaluation, and Treatment of High Blood Cholesterol in Adults, National Institutes of Health. 2001. Executive summary of the Third Report of the National Cholesterol Education Program (NCEP) Expert Panel on Detection, Evaluation, and Treatment of High Blood Cholesterol in Adults (Adult Treatment Panel III). *JAMA* 285(19):2486–2509.
17. USDA, Weighing in on Fats. Agricultural Research Service (ARS), 2008. http://www.ars.usda.gov/is/AR/archive/mar08/fats0308.htm.
18. Ratnayake W. M. N., M. R. L. L'Abee, S. Farnworth, L. Dumais, C. Gagnon, B. Lampi, V. Casey, D. Mohottalage, I. Rondeau, and L. Underhill. Trans fatty acids: Current contents in Canadian food and estimated intake levels for the Canadian population. *J AOAC International.* 92(5):1258–1276.
19. Teegala S. M., W. C. Willett, and D. Mazaffarian. 2009. Consumption and health effects of Trans fatty acids: a review. *J. AOAC International.* 92(5):1250–1257.
20. Mozaffarian, D., M. B. Katan, A. Ascherio, M. J. Stampher, and W. C. Willet. 2006. Trans fatty acids and cardiovascular disease. *N. Engl. J. Med.* 354(15):1601–1613.
21. New York Department of Health and Mental Hygiene, Board of Health. 2006. Notice of Adoption of an Amendment (81.08) to Article 81 of the New York City Health Code to Restrict the Service of Products Containing Artificial Trans Fats at All Food Service Establishments. December 5, 2006. www.nyc.gov/html/doh/downloads/pdf/public/notice-adoption-hc-art81-08.pdf.
22. Sabastian R., C. Enns, J. Goldman, and A. Moshfegh. 2008. Effect of fast food consumption on dietary intake and likelood of meeting MyPyramid recommendations in adults: Results from What We Eat in America, NHANES 2003–04. *FASEB Journal* 22:868.7.
23. Kim, Y. I. 2001. Nutrition and cancer. In: Bowman, B. A., and R. M. Russell, eds. Present Knowledge in Nutrition, 8th edn. Washington, DC: International Life Sciences Institute Press.
24. Kris-Etherton, P. M., and S. Innis. 2007. Position of the American Dietetic Association and Dietitians of Canada: Dietary fatty acid. *J. Am. Diet. Assoc.* 107:1599–1611.
25. Willett, W. C. 1999. Diet, nutrition and the prevention of cancer. In: Shils, M. E., J. A. Olsen, M. Shike, and A. C. Ross, eds. Modern Nutrition in Health and Disease, 9th edn. Baltimore: Williams & Wilkins.
26. Prentice, R. L., C. Bette, R. Chlebowski, et al. 2006. Low-fat dietary patterns and risk of invasive breast cancer. The Women's Health Initiative Randomized Controlled Dietary Modification Trial. *JAMA* 295:629–642.
27. Ormrod D. J., C. C. Holmes, and T. E. Miller. 1998. Dietary chitosan inhibits hypercholesterolaemia and atherogenesis in the apolipoprotein E-deficient mouse model of atherosclerosis. *Atherosclerosis.* 138(2):329–334.
28. Mhurchu C. N., C. Dunshea-Mooij, D. Bennet, and A. Rodgers. 2005a. Effect of chitosan on weight loss in overweight and obese individuals: a systemic review of randomized control trials. *Obesity Rev* 6:35–42.
29. Mhurchu C. N., C. A. Dunshea-Mooij, D. Bennett, and A. Rodgers. 2005b. Chitosan for overweight or obesity. Cochrane database of systematic reviews (Online) (Cochrane Database Syst Rev) 2005(3): CD003892. 2005b.
30. Pittler M. H., and E. Ernst. 2004 Dietary supplements for body-weight reduction: a systematic review. *Am. J. Clin. Nutr.* 79(4):529–536.
31. Kaats G. R., J. E. Michalek, and H. G. Preuss. 2006. Evaluating efficacy of a chitosan product using a double-blinded, placebo-controlled protocol. *J. Am. Coll. Nutr.* 25(5):389–394.
32. Gades M. D., and J. S. Stern. 2005. Chitosan supplementation and fat absorption in men and women. *J. Am. Diet. Assoc.* 105:72–77.

In Depth: Cardiovascular Disease

1. Wilson, P. W. F. 2004. CDC/AHA workshop on markers of inflammation and cardiovascular disease. Application to clinical and public health practice. Ability of inflammatory markers to predict disease in asymptomatic patients. A background paper. Circulation 110:e568–e571.
2. Ostchega Y., S. S. Yoon, J. Hughes, and T. Louise. 2008. Hypertension awareness, treatment and control—continued

disparities in adults: United States, 2005–2006. National Center for Health Statistics (NCHS) data brief no. Hyattsville, MD: NCHS.

3. Lloyd-Jones D., R. J. Adams, T. M. Brown, M. Carnethon, S. Dai, G. DeSimone, et al. 2010. Heart Disease and Stroke Statistics 2010 Update. A Report from the American Heart Association. *Circulation* 121:e1–e170.
4. National Center for Chronic Disease Prevention and Health Promotion (NCCDPHP). 2008. Division for Heart Disease and Stroke Prevention addressing the nation's leading killers. At a glance 2008. Available online at http://www.cdc.gov/print.do?url=http://www.cdc.gov/nccdphp/publications/AAG/dhdsp.htm.
5. Hahn, R. A., and G. W. Heath. 1998. Cardiovascular disease risk factors and preventive practices among adults—United States, 1994: a behavioral risk factor atlas. *Morbid. Mortal. Wkly. Rep.* 47(SS-5):35–69.
6. Rippe, J. M., T. J. Angelopoulos, and L. Zukley. 2007. The rationale for intervention to reduce the risk of coronary heart disease. *Am. J. Lifestyle Med.* 1(1):10–19.
7. Marwick T. H., M. D. Hordern, T. Miller, D. A. Chyun, A. G. Bertoni, R. S. Blumenthal, G. Philippides, and A. Rocchini. 2009. Exercise training for type 2 diabetes Mellitus: Impact on cardiovascular risk: A Scientific Statement from the American Heart Association. *Circulation.* 119:3244–3262.
8. Department of Health and Human Services (DHHS). 2008. Physical Activity Guidelines Advisory Committee, Phyiscal Activity Guidelines Advisory Committee Report, 2008. Washington DC.
9. Dept of Health and Human Services (DHHS), Centers for Disease Control and Prevention (CDC), Smoking and Tobacco Use, Frequently Asked questions. Accessed, Feb. 2010. http://apps.nccd.cdc.gov/osh_faq/topic.aspx?TopicID=8#11.
10. Libby P., P. M. Ridker, and A. Maseri. 2002. Inflammation and atherosclerosis. *Circulation* 105:1135–1143.
11. Kris-Etherton, P. M., W. S. Harris, L. J. Appel, and the Nutrition Committee of the American Heart Association. 2002. Fish consumption, fish oil, omega-3 fatty acids and cardiovascular disease. *Circulation* 106:2747–2757.
12. Harris, W. S. 1997. n-3 Fatty acids and serum lipoproteins: human studies. *Am. J. Clin. Nutr.* 65(suppl.):1645S–1654S.
13. Zoeller, R. F. 2007. Physical activity and fitness in the prevention of coronary heart disease and associated risk factors. *Am. J. Lifestyle Med.* 1(1):29–33.
14. Cotton P. A., A. F. Subar, J. E. Friday, and A. Cook. 2004. Dietary sources of nutrients among US adults, 1994–1996. *J. Am. Diet. Assoc.* 104:921–931.
15. Expert Panel on Detection, Evaluation, and Treatment of High Blood Cholesterol in Adults, National Institutes of Health. 2001. Executive summary of the Third Report of the National Cholesterol Education Program (NCEP) Expert Panel on Detection, Evaluation, and Treatment of High Blood Cholesterol in Adults (Adult Treatment Panel III). *JAMA* 285(19):2486–2509.
16. Lichtenstein A. H., L. J. Appel, M. Brands, M. Carnethon, S. Daniels, H. A. Franch, B. Franklin, P. Kris-Ethergon, W. S. Harris, B. Howard, N. Karanja, M. Lefevre, L. Rudel, F. Sancks, L. Van Horn, M. Winston, and J. Wylie-Rosett. 2006. Diet and lifestyle recommendations revision 2006: A scientific statement from the American Heart Association Nutrition Committee. *Circulation* 114:82–96.
17. Gidding S. S., A. H. Lichtenstein, M. S. Faith, A. Karpyn, J. A. Mennella, B. Popkin, J. Rowe, L. Van Horn, and L. Whitsel. 2009. Implementing American Heart Association Pediatric and Adult Nutrition Guidelines. *Circulation.* 119:1161–1175.
18. Institute of Medicine, Food and Nutrition Board. 2002. Dietary Reference Intakes for Energy, Carbohydrate, Fiber, Fat, Fatty Acids, Cholesterol, Protein, and Amino Acids (Macronutrients). Washington, DC: National Academies Press.
19. Blumenthal, J. A., A. Sherwood, E. C. D. Gullette, M. Babyak, R. Waugh, A. Georgiades, L. W. Craighead, D. Tweedy, M. Feinglos, M. Applebaum, J. Hayano, and A. Hinderliter. 2000. Exercise and weight loss reduce blood pressure in men and women with mild hypertension. *Arch. Intern Med.* 160:1947–1958.
20. Appel, L. J., T. J. Moare, E. Obarzanek, W. M. Vollmer, L. P. Svetkey, F. M. Sacks, G. A. Bray, T. M. Vogt, J. A. Cutler, M. M. Windhauser, P. H. Lin, and N. Karanja. 1997. A clinical trial of the effecs of dietary patterns on blood pressure. *New Engl. J. Medicine.* 336:1117–1124.
21. Sacks, F. M., L. P. Svetkey, W. M. Vollmer, L. J. Appel, G. A. Bray, D. Harsha, E. Obarzanek, P. R. Conlin, E. R. Miller III, D. G. Simons-Morton, N. Karanja, and P. H. Lin. 2001. Effects of blood pressure on reduced dietary sodium and the Dietary Approaches to Stop Hypertension (DASH) diet. *New Engl. J. Medicine.* 244:3–10.

Chapter 6

1. Bennett, J., and C. Lewis. 2001. Very Vegetarian. Nashville: Rutledge Hill Press.
2. Vegetarian Resource Group. 2009. Vegetarian Journal Available online at www.vrg.org/press/2009poll.htm.
3. McDowell, M. A., R. R. Briefel, K. Alaimo, A. M. Bischof, C. R. Caughman, M. D. Carroll, C. M. Lona, and C. L. Johnson. 1994. Energy and macronutrient intakes of persons ages 2 months and over in the United States: Third National Health and Nutrition Examination Survey, Phase I 1988–1991. *Adv. Data* 255:1–24.
4. Tillotson, J. L., G. E. Bartsch, D. Gorder, G. A. Grandits, and J. Stamler. 1997. Food group and nutrient intakes at baseline in the Multiple Risk Factor Intervention Trial. *Am. J. Clin. Nutr.* 65(suppl.):228S–257S.
5. Smit, E., J. Nieto, C. J. Crespo, and P. Mitchell. 1999. Estimates of animal and plant protein intake in US adults: results from the Third National Health and Nutrition Examination Survey, 1988–1991. *J. Am. Diet. Assoc.* 99:813–820.
6. Manore, M. M, N. L. Meyer, and J. Thompson. 2009. Sport Nutrition for Health and Performance. 2nd Edition. Champaign, IL: Human Kinetics.
7. Fraser, G. E., J. Sabaté, W. L. Beeson, and M. Strahan. 1992. A possible protective effect of nut consumption on risk of coronary heart disease. *Arch. Intern. Med.* 152:1416–1424.
8. Hu, F. B., M. J. Stampfer, J. E. Manson, E. B. Rimm, G. A. Colditz, B. A. Rosner, F. E. Speizer, C. H. Hennekens, and W. C.Willett. 1998. Frequent nut consumption and risk of coronary heart disease in women: Prospective cohort study. *BMJ* 317:1341–1345.
9. Albert, C. M., J. M. Gaziano,W. C.Willett, J. E. Mason, and C. H. Hennekens. 2002. Nut consumption and decreased risk of sudden cardiac death in the Physicians' Health Study. *Arch. Intern. Med.* 162:1382–1387.
10. American Dietetic Association and Dietitians of Canada. 2003. Position of the American Dietetic Association and Dietitians of Canada: Vegetarian diets. *J. Am. Diet. Assoc.* 103(6):748–765.
11. Klopp, S. A., C. J. Heiss, and H. S. Smith. 2003. Self-reported vegetarianism may be a marker for college women at risk for disordered eating. *J. Am. Diet. Assoc.* 103(6):745–747.
12. Institute of Medicine, Food and Nutrition Board. 2002. Dietary Reference Intakes for Energy, Carbohydrate, Fiber, Fat, Fatty Acids, Cholesterol, Protein, and Amino Acids (Macronutrients). Washington, DC: National Academies Press.
13. Fleming, R. M. 2000. The effect of high-protein diets on coronary blood flow. *Angiology* 51:817–826.
14. Leitzmann, C. 2005.Vegetarian diets: what are the advantages? *Forum Nutr.* 57:147–156.
15. Szeto, Y. T., T. C. Y. Kwok, and I. F. F. Benzie. 2004. Effects of a long-term vegetarian diet on biomarkers of antioxidant status and cardiovascular disease risk. *Nutrition* 20:863–866.
16. Munger, R. G., J. R. Cerhan, and B. C.-H. Chiu. 1999. Prospective study of dietary protein intake and risk of hip fracture in postmenopausal women. *Am. J. Clin. Nutr.* 69:147–152.

17. Alekel, D. L., A. St. Germain, C. T. Peterson, K. B. Hanson, J. W. Stewart, and T. Toda. 2000. Isoflavone-rich soy protein isolate attenuates bone loss in the lumbar spine of perimenopausal women. *Am. J. Clin. Nutr.* 72:844–852.
18. Kontessis, P., I. Bossinakou, L. Sarika, E. Iliopoulou, A. Papantoniou, R. Trevisan, D. Roussi, K. Stipsanelli, S. Grigorakis, and A. Souvatzoglou. 1995. Renal, metabolic, and hormonal responses to proteins of different origin in normotensive, non-proteinuric type 1 diabetic patients. *Diabetes Care* 18:1233–1240.
19. American Diabetes Association (ADA). 2003. Evidence-based nutrition principles and recommendations for the treatment and prevention of diabetes and related complications. *Diabet. Care* 26:S51–S61.
20. Poortmans, J. R., and O. Dellalieux. 2000. Do regular high protein diets have potential health risks on kidney function in athletes? *Int. J. Sport Nutr.* 10:2.
21. Food and Agriculture Organization. 2006. Livestock a major threat to environment: Remedies urgently needed. FAO Newsroom. 29 November. www.fao.org/newsroom/en/news/2006/1000448/index.html.
22. Eshel, G., and P. Martin. 2006. Diet, energy and global warming. Earth Interactions (March)10:1–17. http://geosci.uchicago.edu/~gidon/papers/nutri/nutri.html.
23. Jowit, J. 2008. UN says eat less meat to curb global warming. The Observer (September 7). www.guardian.co.uk/environment/2008/sep/07/food.foodanddrink.
24. National Cattlemen's Beef Association. 2010. Beef Industry Myths and Facts. http://www.beefusa.org/beefFactoidFighter.aspx.

In Depth: Vitamins and Minerals: Micronutrients with Macro Powers

1. Institute of Medicine, Food and Nutrition Board. 2001. Dietary Reference Intakes for Vitamin A, Vitamin K, Arsenic, Boron, Chromium, Copper, Iodine, Iron, Manganese, Molybdenum, Nickel, Silicon, Vanadium, and Zinc. Washington, DC: National Academy Press.
2. Bjelakovic, G., D. Nikolova, L. L. Gluud, R. G. Simonetti, and C. Gluud. 2007. Mortality in randomized trials of antioxidant supplements for primary and secondary prevention. *J. Am. Med. Assoc.* 297:842–857.
3. Penniston, K. L., and S. A. Tanumihardjo. 2006. The acute and chronic toxic effects of vitamin A. *Am. J. Clin. Nutr.* 83:191–201.
4. Pollan, M. 2007. The age of nutritionism. *The New York Times Magazine*, January 28.
5. Stover, P. J. 2006. Influence of human genetic variation on nutritional requirements. *Am. J. Clin. Nutr.* 83:436S–443S.

Chapter 7

1. Almond, C. S. D., A. Y. Shin, E. B. Fortescue, R. C. Mannix, D. Wypij, B. A. Binstadt, C. N. Duncan, D. P. Olson, A. E. Salerno, J. W. Newburger, and D. S. Greenes. 2005. Hyponatremia among runners in the Boston Marathon. *N. Engl. J. Med.* 352:1150–1156.
2. Institute of Medicine. 2004. Dietary Reference Intakes for Water, Potassium, Sodium, Chloride, and Sulfate. Washington, DC: National Academies Press.
3. Godek, S. F., A. R. Bartolozzi, R. Burkholder, E. Sugarman, and C. Peduzzi. 2008. Sweat rates and fluid turnover in professional football players: a comparison of national football league linemen and backs. *J. Athletic Training* 43:184–189.
4. Smith, T. 2008. Bottled water consumption continues to rise worldwide. TimesDaily.com. Available at http://www.timesdaily.com/article/20081020/ARTICLES/810200321?Title=Bottled-water-consumption-continues-to-rise-worldwide.
5. Brody, J. 2007. You are also what you drink. *New York Times*, Personal Health; March 27, 2007, Section F.
6. U.S. Department of Health and Human Services (USDHHS) and U.S. Department of Agriculture (USDA). 2010. Dietary Guidelines for Americans, 2010. 7th ed. Washington, DC: U.S. Government Printing Office. Available at www.healthierus.gov/dietaryguidelines.
7. The University of Maine Cooperative Extension. 2007. Sodium content of your food. http://www.umext.maine.edu/onlinepubs/htmpubs/4059.htm.
8. Frassetto, L. A., R. C. Morris, D. E. Sellmeyer, and A. Sebastian. 2008. Adverse effects of sodium chloride on bone in the aging human population resulting from habitual consumption of typical American diets. *J. Nutr.* 138:419S–422S.
9. McGill, C. R., V. L. Fulgoni, D. DiRienzo, P. J. Huth, A. C. Kurilich, and G. D. Miller. 2008. Contributions of dairy products to dietary potassium intake in the United States population. *J. Am. College Nutr.* 27:44–50.
10. Hew-Butler, T., J. C. Ayus, C. Kipps, R. J. Maughan, S. Mettler, W. H. Meeuwisse, A. J. Page, S. A. Reid, N. J. Rehrer, W. O. Roberts, I. R. Rogers, M. H. Rosner, A. J. Siegel, D. B. Speedy, K. J. Stuempfle, J. G. Verbalis, L. B. Weschler, and P. Wharam. 2008. Statement of the second international exercise-associated hyponatremia consensus development conference, New Zealand, 2007. *Clin. J. Sport Med.* 18:111–121.
11. Speedy, D. B., T. D. Noakes, I. R. Rogers, J. M. Thompson, R. G. Campbell, J. A. Kuttner, D. R. Boswell, S. Wright, and M. Hamlin. 1999. Hyponatremia in ultradistance triathletes. *Med. Sci. Sports Exerc.* 31:809–815.
12. Manore, M., N. L. Meyer, and J. Thompson. 2009. Sport Nutrition for Health and Performance, 2nd ed. Champaign, IL: Human Kinetics (117).
13. Sawka, M. N., L. M. Burke, E. R. Eichner, R. J. Maughan, S. J. Montain, and N. S. Stachenfeld. 2007. American College of Sports Medicine Position Stand: Exercise and fluid replacement. *Med. Sci. Sports Exer.* 39:377–390.

Chapter 8

1. Institute of Medicine. Food and Nutrition Board. 2000. Dietary Reference Intakes for Vitamin C, Vitamin E, Selenium and Carotenoids. Washington, DC: National Academy Press.
2. The HOPE and HOPE-TOO Trial Investigators. 2005. Effects of long-term vitamin E supplementation on cardiovascular events and cancer. A randomized controlled trial. *JAMA* 293:1338–1347.
3. Sesso, H. D., J. E. Buring, W. G. Christen, T. Kurth, C. Belanger, J. MacFadyn, V. Bubes, J. E. Manson, R. J. Glynn, and J. M. Gaziano. 2008. Vitamins E and C in the prevention of cardiovascular disease in men: The Physicians' Health Study II randomized controlled trial. *JAMA* 300(18):2123–2133.
4. Ford, E. S., and A. Sowell. 1999. Serum alpha-tocopherol status in the United States population: findings from the Third National Health and Nutrition Examination Survey. *Am. J. Epidemiol.* 150(3):290–300.
5. Yeomans, V. C., J. Linseisen, and G. Wolfram. 2005. Interactive effects of polyphenols, tocopherol, and ascorbic acid on the Cu2+-mediated oxidative modification of human low density lipoproteins. *Eur. J. Nutr.* 44(7): 422–428.
6. Hemilä, H., E. Chalker, B. Treacy, and B. Douglas. 2007. Vitamin C for preventing and treating the common cold. Cochrane Database of Systematic Reviews. Issue 3. Art. No. CD000980. DOI: 10.1002/14651858.CD000980.pub3.
7. Burri, B. J. 1997. Beta-carotene and human health: a review of current research. *Nutr. Res.* 17:547–580.
8. U.S. Department of Agriculture (USDA), Agricultural Research Service. 2009. USDA National Nutrient Database for Standard Reference, Release 22. Available at http://www.ars.usda.gov/ba/bhnrc/ndl.
9. Larsson, S., L. Bergkvist, I. Näslund, J. Rutegård, and A. Wolk. 2007. Vitamin A, retinol, and carotenoids and the risk of gastric cancer: a prospective cohort study. *Am. J. Clin. Nutr.* 85:497–503.
10. Livrea, M. A., L. Tesoriere, A. Bongiorno, A. M. Pintaudi, M. Ciaccio, and A. Riccio. 1995. Contribution of vitamin A to the

oxidation resistance of human low density lipoproteins. *Free Radic. Biol. Med.* 18:401–409.

11. Gutteridge, J. M. C., and B. Halliwell. 1994. Antioxidants in Nutrition, Health, and Disease. Oxford, UK: Oxford University Press.
12. Institute of Medicine. Food and Nutrition Board. 2001. Dietary Reference Intakes for Vitamin A, Vitamin K, Arsenic, Boron, Chromium, Copper, Iodine, Iron, Manganese, Molybdenum, Nickel, Silicon, Vanadium, and Zinc. Washington, DC: National Academy Press.
13. El-akawi, Z., N. Abdel-Latif, and K. Abdul-Razzak. 2006. Does the plasma level of vitamins A and E affect acne condition? *Clin. Experimen. Dermatol.* 31:430–434.
14. World Health Organization (WHO). 2009. Micronutrient deficiencies. Vitamin A deficiency. Available at http://www.who.int/nutrition/topics/vad/en/.
15. Albanes, D., O. P. Heinonen, J. K. Huttunen, P. R. Taylor, J. Virtamo, B. K. Edwards, J. Haapakoski, M. Rautalahti, A. M. Hartman, J. Palmgren, and P. Greenwald. 1995. Effects of alpha-tocopherol and beta-carotene supplements on cancer incidence in the Alpha-Tocopherol Beta-Carotene Cancer Prevention Study. *Am. J. Clin. Nutr.* 62(suppl.):1427S–1430S.
16. Omenn, G. S., G. E. Goodman, M. D. Thornquist, J. Balmes, M. R. Cullen, A. Glass, J. P. Keogh, F. L. Meyskens, B. Valanis, J. H. Williams, S. Barnhart, and S. Hammar. 1996. Effects of a combination of beta carotene and vitamin A on lung cancer and cardiovascular disease. *New Engl. J. Med.* 334:1150–1155.
17. Joshipura, K. J., F. B. Hu, J. E. Manson, M. J. Stampfer, E. B. Rimm, F. E. Speizer, G. Colditz, A. Ascherio, B. Rosner, D. Spiegelman, and W. C. Willett. 2001. The effect of fruit and vegetable intake on risk for coronary heart disease. *Ann. Intern. Med.* 134:1106–1114.
18. Liu, S., I.-M. Lee, U. Ajani, S. R. Cole, J. E. Buring, and J. E. Manson. 2001. Intake of vegetables rich in carotenoids and risk of coronary heart disease in men: The Physicians' Health Study. *Intl. J. Epidemiol.* 30:130–135.
19. The Alpha-Tocopherol, Beta-Carotene Cancer Prevention Study Group (The ATBC Study Group). 1994. The effect of vitamin E and beta carotene on the incidence of lung cancer and other cancers in male smokers. *N. Engl. J. Med.* 330:1029–1035.
20. Lee, I. M., N. R. Cook, J. M. Gaziano, D. Gordon, P. M. Ridker, J. E. Manson, C. H. Hennekens, and J. E. Buring. 2005. Vitamin E in the primary prevention of cardiovascular disease and cancer: The Women's Health Study: A randomized controlled trial. *JAMA* 294(1):56–65.
21. Geleijnse, J. M., L. J. Launer, D. A. M. van der Kuip, A. Hofman, and J. C. M. Witteman. 2002. Inverse association of tea and flavonoid intakes with incident myocardial infarction: The Rotterdam Study. *Am. J. Clin. Nutr.* 75:880–886.

In Depth: Cancer

1. American Cancer Society. 2009. Cancer Facts & Figures 2009. Available at www.cancer.org/downloads/STT/500809web.pdf.
2. McConnell, T. H. 2007. The Nature of Disease: Pathology for the Health Professions. Baltimore: Lippincott Williams & Wilkins. p. 96.
3. National Cancer Institute. 2009. Common Cancer Types. Available at www.cancer.gov/cancertopics/commoncancers.
4. American Cancer Society. 2007. Cancer atlas. Available at http://www.cancer.org/downloads/AA/CancerAtlas02.pdf.
5. American Cancer Society. 2009. ACS guide to quitting smoking. Available at http://www.cancer.org/docroot/PED/content/PED_10_13X_Guide_for_Quitting_Smoking.asp?sitearea=PED.
6. U.S. Department of Health and Human Services (USDHHS). 2004. The Health Consequences of Smoking: A Report of the Surgeon General. Washington, DC: U.S. Department of Health and Human Services, Centers for Disease Control and Prevention, National Center for Chronic Disease Prevention and Health Promotion, Office on Smoking and Health.
7. Thune, I., and A. S. Furberg. 2001. Physical activity and cancer risk: Dose-response and cancer, all sites and site-specific. *Med. Sci. Sports Exerc.* 33(suppl.):S530–S550.
8. Pfahlberg, A., K. F. Kolmel, and O. Gefeller. 2002. Adult vs. childhood susceptibility to melanoma. Is there a difference? *Arch. Dermatol.* 138:1234–1235.
9. Heinonen, O. P., D. Albanes, J. Virtamo, P. R. Taylor, J. K. Huttunen, A. M. Hartman, J. Haapakoski, N. Malila, M. Rautalahti, S. Ripatti, H. Maepaa, and International Agency for Research on Cancer (IARC). 2007. The association of use of sunbeds with cutaneous malignant melanoma and other skin cancers: A systematic review. *Int. J. Cancer* 120:1116–1122.
10. American Cancer Society. 2010. Signs and Symptoms of Cancer. January 6. Available at www.cancer.org/docroot/CRI/content/CRI_2_4_3X_What_are_the_signs_and_symptoms_of_cancer.asp?
11. American Cancer Society. 2009. Learning About New Ways to Prevent Cancer. March 6. Available at www.cancer.org/docroot/PED/PED_14_Learning_About_New_Cancer_Prevention_Methods.asp?
12. American Cancer Society. 2008. The Great American Health Challenge: Fitting in Fitness. September 28. Available at www.cancer.org/docroot/subsite/greatamericans/content/Fitting_in_Fitness.asp.
13. Greenwald P., C. K. Clifford, and J. A. Milner. 2001. Diet and cancer prevention. *Eur. J. Cancer* 37:948–965.

Chapter 9

1. United States Department of Agriculture, Economic Research Service. 2008. Dietary assessment of major trends in U.S. food consumption, 1970-2005. Economic Information Bulletin No. EIB-33, 1-27. www.ers.usda/Publications/EIB33/.EIB33_ReportSummary.html.
2. Ho, A. Y. Y., and A. W. C. Kung. 2005. Determinants of peak bone mineral density and bone area in young women. *J. Bone Miner. Metab.* 23:470–475.
3. Chevalley, T., R. Rizzoli, D. Hans, S. Ferrari, and J. P. Bonjour. 2005. Interaction between calcium intake and menarcheal age on bone mass gain: an eight-year follow-up study from prepuberty to postmenarche. *J. Clin. Endocrinol. Metab.* 90:44–51.
4. Kindblom, J. M., M. Lorentzon, E. Norjavaara, A. Hellqvist, S. Nilsson, D. Mellström, and C. Ohlsson. 2006. Pubertal timing predicts previous fractures and BMD in young adult men: the GOOD study. *J. Bone Min. Res.* 21:790–795.
5. Institute of Medicine, Food and Nutrition Board. 1997. Dietary Reference Intakes for Calcium, Phosphorus, Magnesium, Vitamin D, and Fluoride. Washington, DC: National Academies Press.
6. Keller, J. L., A. J. Lanou, and N. D. Barnard. 2002. The consumer cost of calcium from food and supplements. *J. Am. Diet. Assoc.* 102:1669–1671.
7. Nusser, S. M., A. L. Carriquiry, K. W. Dodd, and W. A. Fuller. 1996. A semiparametric transformation approach to estimating usual daily intake distributions. *J. Am. Stat. Assoc.* 91:1440–1449.
8. Ross, E. A., N. J. Szabo, and I. R. Tebbett. 2000. Lead content of calcium supplements. *JAMA* 284:1425–1433.
9. Massey, L. K., H. Roman-Smith, and R. A. Sutton. 1993. Effect of dietary oxalate and calcium on urinary oxalate and risk of formation of calcium oxalate kidney stones. *J. Am. Diet. Assoc.* 93:901–906.
10. Zemel, M. B., W. Thompson, A. Milstead, K. Morris, and P. Campbell. 2004. Calcium and dairy acceleration of weight and fat loss during energy restriction in obese adults. *Obes. Res.* 12:582–590.
11. Bowen, J., M. Noakes, and P. M. Clifton. 2005. Effect of calcium and dairy foods in high protein, energy-restricted diets on weight loss and metabolic parameters in overweight adults. *Int. J. Obes.* 29:957–965.
12. United States Department of Agriculture (USDA), Agricultural Research Service. 2007. News and Events. Weight loss study focuses on dairy foods. www.ars.usda.gov/IS/pr/2007/070427.htm.

13. Holick, M. F., L. Y. Matsuoka, and J. Wortsman. 1989. Age, vitamin D, and solar ultraviolet. *Lancet* 2:1104–1105.

14. Need, A. G., H. A. Morris, M. Horowitz, and C. Nordin. 1993. Effects of skin thickness, age, body fat, and sunlight on serum 25-hydroxyvitamin D. *Am. J. Clin. Nutr.* 58:882–885.

15. Florez, H., R. Martinez, W. Chacra, N. Strickman-Stein, and S. Levis. 2007. Outdoor exercise reduces the risk of hypovitaminosis D in the obese. *J. Steroid Biochem. Mol. Biol.* 103:679–681.

16. Holick, M. F. 2005. The vitamin D epidemic and its health consequences. *J. Nutr.* 135:2739S–2748S.

17. Holick, M. F. 1994. McCollum Award Lecture, 1994: Vitamin D: new horizons for the 21st century. *Am. J. Clin. Nutr.* 60:619–630.

18. Lim, H. W., B. A. Gilchrist, K. D. Cooper, H. A. Bischoff-Ferrari, D. S. Rigel, W. H. Cyr, S. Miller, V. A. DeLeo, T. K. Lee, C. A. Demko, M. A. Weinstock, A. Young, L. S. Edwards, T. M. Johnson, and S. P. Stone. 2005. Sunlight, tanning booths, and vitamin D. *J. Am. Acad. Dermatol.* 52:868–876.

19. Heaney, R. P. 2005. The vitamin D requirement in health and disease. *J. Steroid Biochem. Molec. Biol.* 97:13–19.

20. Heaney, R. P. 2007. The case for improving vitamin D status. *J. Steroid Biochem. Molec. Biol.* 103:635–641.

21. Holick, M. F. 2006. Resurrection of vitamin D deficiency and rickets. *J. Clin. Invest.* 116:2062–2072.

22. Weisberg, P., K. S. Scanlon, R. Li, and M. E. Cogswell. 2004. Nutritional rickets among children in the United States: review of cases reported between 1986 and 2003. *Am. J. Clin. Nutr.* 80(suppl.):1697S–1705S.

23. Institute of Medicine, Food and Nutrition Board. 2002. Dietary Reference Intakes for Vitamin A, Vitamin K, Arsenic, Boron, Chromium, Copper, Iodine, Iron, Manganese, Molybdenum, Nickel, Silicon, Vanadium, and Zinc. Washington, DC: National Academies Press.

24. Wyshak, G., R. E. Frisch, T. E. Albright, N. L. Albright, I. Schiff, and J. Witschi. 1989. Nonalcoholic carbonated beverage consumption and bone fractures among women former college athletes. *J. Orthop.* Res. 7:91–99.

25. Wyshak, G., and R. E. Frisch. 1994. Carbonated beverages, dietary calcium, the dietary calcium/phosphorus ratio, and bone fractures in girls and boys. *J. Adolesc. Health* 15:210–215.

26. Wyshak, G. 2000. Teenaged girls, carbonated beverage consumption, and bone fractures. *Arch. Pediatr. Adolesc. Med.* 154:610–613.

27. Heaney, R. P., and K. Rafferty. 2001. Carbonated beverages and urinary calcium excretion. *Am. J. Clin. Nutr.* 74:343–347.

28. Paolisso G., S. Sgambato, A. Gambardella, G. Pizza, P. Tesauro, M. Varricchio, and F. D'Onofrio. 1992. Daily magnesium supplements improve glucose handling in elderly subjects. *Am. J. Clin. Nutr.* 55:1161–1167.

29. Larsson, S. C., L. Bergkvist, and A. Wolk. 2005. Magnesium intake in relation to risk of colorectal cancer in women. *JAMA* 293:86–89.

30. Pak, C. Y., K. Sakhaee, B. Adams-Huet, V. Piziak, R. D. Peterson, and J. R. Poindexter. 1995. Treatment of postmenopausal osteoporosis with slow-release sodium fluoride. Final report of a randomized controlled trial. *Ann. Int. Med.* 123:401–408.

31. Reginster, J. Y., D. Felsenberg, I. Pavo, J. Stepan, J. Payer, H. Resch, C. C. Glüer, D. Mühlenbacher, D. Quail, H. Schmitt, and T. Nickelsen. 2003. Effect of raloxifene combined with monofluorophosphate as compared with monofluorophosphate alone in postmenopausal women with low bone mass: a randomized, controlled trial. *Osteoporosis Int.* 14:741–749.

32. Ringe, J. D., A. Dorst, H. Faber, C. Kipshoven, L. C. Rovati, and I. Setnikar. 2005. Efficacy of etidronate and sequential monofluorophosphate in severe postmenopausal osteoporosis: a pilot study. *Rheumatol. Int.* 25:296–300.

33. American Dietetic Association. 2005. Position of the American Dietetic Association: the impact of fluoride on health. *J. Am. Diet. Assoc.* 105:1620–1628.

34. U.S. Department of Health and Human Services. Public Health Service. 1991. Review of Fluoride: Benefits and Risks. Report of the Ad Hoc Subcommittee on Fluoride of the Committee to Coordinate Environmental Health and Related Programs. www.health.gov/environment/ReviewofFluoride/default.htm. (Accessed April 2007.)

35. Ginde, A. A., M. C. Liu, and C. A. Camargo, Jr. 2009. Demographic differences and trends of vitamin D insufficiency in the U.S. population, 1988-2004. *Arch. Intern. Med.* 169:626–632.

36. Weaver, C. M., and J. C. Fleet. 2004. Vitamin D requirements: Current and future. *Am. J. Clin. Nutr.* 80(suppl):1735S–1739S.

37. Adams, J. S. and M. Hewison. 2010. Update on vitamin *D. J. Clin. Endocrinol. Metab.* 95:471–478.

38. Yetley, E. A., B. Brulé, M. C. Cheney, C. D. Davis, K. A. Esslinger, P. W. F. Fischer, K. E. Friedl, L. S. Greene-Finestone, P. M. Guenther, D. M. Klurfeld, M. R. L'Abbe, and K. Y. McMurry. 2009. Dietary reference intakes for vitamin D: Justification for a review of the 1997 values. *Am. J. Clin. Nutr.* 89:719–727.

39. Looker, A. C., C. M. Pfeiffer, D. A. Lacher, R. L. Schleicher, M. F. Picciano, and E. A. Yetley. 2008. Serum 25-hydroxyvitamin D status of the U.S. population: 1988-1994 compared with 2000-2004. *Am. J. Clin. Nutr.* 88:1519–1527.

40. Wolpowitz, D., and B. A. Gilchrest. 2006. The vitamin D questions: how much do we need and how should we get it? *J. Am. Acad. Dermatol.* 54(2):301–317.

41. Lucas, R. M., and A. L. Ponsonby. 2006. Considering the potential benefits as well as adverse effects of sun exposure: Can all the potential benefits be provided by oral vitamin D supplementation? *Prog. Biophys. Molec. Biol.* 92:140–149.

42. Reichrath, J. 2006. The challenge resulting from positive and negative effects of sunlight: How much solar UV exposure is appropriate to balance between risks of vitamin D deficiency and skin cancer? *Prog. Biophys. Molec. Biol.* 92:9–16.

In Depth: Osteoporosis

1. National Osteoporosis Foundation. 2008. Osteoporosis Fast Facts. www.nof.org/osteoporosis/diseasefacts.htm.

2. International Osteoporosis Foundation. 2007. Facts and statistics about osteoporosis and its impact. Available at www.iofbonehealth.org/facts-and-statistics.html.

3. Feskanich, D., S. A. Korrick, S. L. Greenspan, H. N. Rosen, and G. A. Colditz. 1999. Moderate alcohol consumption and bone density among post-menopausal women. *J. Women's Health* 8:65–73.

4. Laitinen, K., M. Valimaki, and P. Keto. 1991. Bone mineral density measured by dual-energy x-ray absorptiometry in healthy Finnish women. *Calcif. Tissue Int.* 48:224–231.

5. Holbrook, T. L., and E. Barrett-Connor. 1993. A prospective study of alcohol consumption and bone mineral density. *BMJ* 306:1506–1509.

6. Felson, D. T., Y. Zhang, M. T. Hannan, W. B. Kannel, and D. P. Kiel. 1995. Alcohol intake and bone mineral density in elderly men and women. The Framingham Study. *Am. J. Epidemiol.* 142:485–492.

7. Rapuri, P. B., J. C. Gallagher, K. E. Balhorn, and K. L. Ryschon. 2000. Alcohol intake and bone metabolism in elderly women. *Am. J. Clin. Nutr.* 72:1206–1213.

8. Massey, L. K. 2001. Is caffeine a risk factor for bone loss in the elderly? *Am. J. Clin. Nutr.* 74:569–570.

9. Rapuri, P. B., J. C. Gallagher, H. K. Kinyamu, and K. L. Ryschon. 2001. Caffeine intake increases the rate of bone loss in elderly women and interacts with vitamin D receptor genotypes. *Am. J. Clin. Nutr.* 74:694–700.

10. Tucker, K. L., M. T. Hannan, H. Chen, L. A. Cupples, P. W. F. Wilson, and D. P. Kiel. 1999. Potassium, magnesium, and fruit and vegetable intakes are associated with greater bone mineral density in elderly men and women. *Am. J. Clin. Nutr.* 69:727–736.

11. Tucker, K. L., H. Chen, M. T. Hannan, L. A. Cupples, P. W. F. Wilson, D. Felson, and D. P. Kiel. 2002. Bone mineral density and dietary patterns in older adults: The Framingham Osteoporosis Study. *Am. J. Clin. Nutr.* 76:245–252.
12. Dawson-Hughes, B., and S. S. Harris. 2002. Calcium intake influences the association of protein intake with rates of bone loss in elderly men and women. *Am. J. Clin. Nutr.* 75:773–779.
13. Devine A., R. A. Criddle, I. M. Dick, D. A. Kerr, and R. L. Prince. 1995. A longitudinal study of the effect of sodium and calcium intakes on regional bone density in post-menopausal women. *Am. J. Clin. Nutr.* 62:740–745.
14. Institute of Medicine, Food and Nutrition Board. 1997. Dietary Reference Intakes for Calcium, Phosphorus, Magnesium, Vitamin D, and Fluoride. Washington, DC: National Academies Press.
15. South-Pal, J. E. 2001. Osteoporosis: Part II. Nonpharmacologic and pharmacologic treatment. *Am. Fam. Physician* 63:1121–1128.
16. Writing Group for the Women's Health Initiative Investigators. 2002. Risks and benefits of estrogen plus progestin in healthy postmenopausal women. Principal results from the Women's Health Initiative randomized control trial. *JAMA* 288:321–332.
17. Ross, E. A., N. J. Szabo, and I. R. Tebbett. 2000. Lead content of calcium supplements. *JAMA* 284:1425–1433.
18. Bischoff-Ferrari, H. A., W. C. Willett, J. B. Wong, A. E. Stuck, H. B. Staehelin, E. J. Orav, A. Thoma, D. P. Kiel, and J. Henschkowski. 2009. Prevention of nonvertabral fractures with oral vitamin D and dose dependency: a meta-analysis of randomized controlled trials. 169:551–561.
19. National Institutes of Health, Office of Dietary Supplements. 2009. Dietary supplement fact sheet: vitamin D. ods.od.nih.gov/factsheets/vitamind.asp.

Chapter 10

1. Bernstein, L. 2000. Dementia without a cause: Lack of vitamin B12 can cause dementia. *Discover Magazine,* February 2000.
2. Bates, C. J. 2006. Thiamin. In: Bowman, B. A., and R. M. Russel, eds. Present Knowledge in Nutrition, 9th edn., pp. 242–249. Washington, DC: ILSI Press.
3. McCollum, E. V. 1957. A History of Nutrition. Boston: Houghton Mifflin Co.
4. Day, E., P. Bentham, R. Callaghan, T. Kuruvilla, and S. George. 2004. Thiamine for Wernicke-Korsakoff Syndrome in people at risk from alcohol abuse (review). *Cochrane Database Syst. Rev.* 1:CD0040033.
5. McCormick, D. B. 2005. Riboflavin. In: Shils, M. E., M. Shike, A. C. Ross, B. Caballero, and R. Cousins, eds. Modern Nutrition in Health and Disease, 10th edn., pp. 434–441. Philadelphia: Lippincott Williams & Wilkins.
6. Rivlin, R. S. 2006. Riboflavin. In: Bowman, B. A., and R. M. Russel, eds. Present Knowledge in Nutrition, 9th edn., pp. 250–259. Washington, DC: ILSI Press.
7. Jacques, P. F., A. Taylor, S. Moeller, et al. 2005. Long-term nutrient intake and 5-year change in nuclear lens opacities. *Arch. Ophthalmol.* 123:571–526.
8. Jacob, R. A. 2006. Niacin. In: Bowman, B. A., and R. M. Russel, eds. Present Knowledge in Nutrition, 9th edn., pp. 260–268. Washington, DC: ILSI Press.
9. Jukes, T. H. 1990. Nutrition science from vitamins to molecular biology. *Annual Reviews of Nutrition*, 10:1–10.
10. Mackey, A. D., S. R. Davis, and J. F. Gregory III. 2006. Vitamin B6. In: Shils, M. E., M. Shike, A. C. Ross, B. Caballero, and R. Cousins, eds. *Modern Nutrition in Health and Disease,* 10th edn., pp. 452–261. Philadelphia: Lippincott Williams & Wilkins.
11. Boushey, C. J., S. A. Beresford, G. S. Omenn, and A. G. Motulsky. 1995. A quantitative assessment of plasma homocysteine as a risk factor for vascular disease. Probable benefits of increasing folic acid intakes. *JAMA* 274:1049–1057.
12. Joubert, L. M., and M. M. Manore. 2006. Exercise, nutrition and homocysteine. Int. *J. Sport Nutr. Exer. Metab.* 16:341–361.
13. Carmel, R. 2006. Folic acid. In: Shils, M. E., M. Shike, A. C. Ross, B. Caballero, and R. Cousins, eds. Modern Nutrition in Health and Disease, 10th edn., pp. 470–481. Philadelphia: Lippincott Williams & Wilkins.
14. Wyatt, K. M., P. W. Dimmock, P. W. Jones, and P. M. Shaughn O'Brien. 1999. Efficacy of vitamin B-6 in the treatment of premenstrual syndrome: Systemic review. *Br. J. Med.* 318:1375–1381.
15. Rapkin, A. 2003. The review of treatment of premenstrual syndrome & premenstrual dysphoric disorder. *Psychoneuroendocrinology* 28:39–53.
16. Schaumburg, H., J. Kaplan, A. Winderbank, N. Vick, S. Rasmus, D. Pleasure, and M. J. Brown. 1983. Sensory neuropathy from pyridoxine abuse: A new megavitamin syndrome. *N. Engl. J. Med.* 309:445–448.
17. Connolly, M., 2001. Premenstrual syndrome: An update on definitions, diagnosis and management. *Advances in Psychiatric Treatment* 7:469–477.
18. Kim, Y. 2006. Does a high folate intake increase the risk of breast cancer? *Nutr. Rev.* 64(10):468–475.
19. Institute of Medicine, Food and Nutrition Board. 1998. Dietary Reference Intakes for Thiamin, Riboflavin, Niacin, Vitamin B6, Folate, Vitamin B12, Pantothenic Acid, Biotin, and Choline. Washington, DC: National Academies Press.
20. Beresford, S. A., and C. J. Boushey. 1997. Homocysteine, folic acid, and cardiovascular disease risk. In: Bendich, A., and R. J. Deckelbaum, eds. Preventive Nutrition: The Comprehensive Guide for Health Professionals. Totowa, NJ: Humana Press.
21. Mayer, E. L., D. W. Jacobsen, and K. Robinson. 1996. Homocysteine and coronary atherosclerosis. *J. Am. Coll. Cardiol.* 27:517–527.
22. Sabler, S. P. 2006. Vitamin B12. In: Bowman, B. A., and R. M. Russel, eds. *Present Knowledge in Nutrition,* 9th edn., pp. 302–313. Washington, DC: ILSI Press.
23. Carmel, R. 2006. Cobalamin (vitamin B12). In: Shils, M. E., M. Shike, A. C. Ross, B. Caballero, and R. Cousins, eds. *Modern Nutrition in Health and Disease,* 10th edn., pp. 482–497. Philadelphia, PA: Lippincott Williams & Wilkins.
24. Miller, W. J., L. M. Rogers, and R. B. Rubker, 2006. Pantothenic acid. In: Bowman, B. A., and R. M. Russel, eds. *Present Knowledge in Nutrition,* 9th edn., pp. 327–339.Washington, DC: ILSI Press.
25. Combs G. F. The vitamins. 2008. Fundamental Aspects in Nutrition and Health. 3rd ed. Elsevier: San Francisco, p. 62.
26. Freake, H. C. 2006. Iodine. In: Stipanuk, M. H., ed. Biochemical and Physiological Aspects of Human Nutrition, 2nd Ed pp. 1068–1090. Philadelphia, PA: W. B. Saunders Co.
27. Evans, G. W. 1989. The effect of chromium picolinate on insulin controlled parameters in humans. Int. *J. Biosoc. Med. Res.* 11:163–180.
28. Hasten, D. L., E. P. Rome, D. B. Franks, and M. Hegsted. 1992. Effects of chromium picolinate on beginning weight training students. *Int. J. Sports Nutr.* 2:343–350.
29. Lukaski, H. C., W. W. Bolonchuk, W. A. Siders, and D. B. Milne. 1996. Chromium supplementation and resistance training: effects on body composition, strength, and trace element status of men. *Am. J. Clin. Nutr.* 63:954–965.
30. Hallmark, M. A., T. H. Reynolds, C. A. DeSouza, C. O. Dotson, R. A. Anderson, and M. A. Rogers. 1996. Effects of chromium and resistive training on muscle strength and body composition. *Med. Sci. Sports Exerc.* 28:139–144.
31. Pasman, W. J., M. S. Westerterp-Plantenga, and W. H. Saris. 1997. The effectiveness of long-term supplementation of carbohydrate, chromium, fibre and caffeine on weight maintenance. *Int. J. Obes. Relat. Metab. Disord.* 21:1143–1151.
32. Walker, L. S., M. G. Bemben, D. A. Bemben, and A. W. Knehans. 1998. Chromium picolinate effects on body composition and muscular performance in wrestlers. *Med. Sci. Sports Exerc.* 30:1730–1737.

33. Campbell, W. W., L. J. Joseph, S. L. Davey, D. Cyr-Campbell, R. A. Anderson, and W. J. Evans. 1999. Effects of resistance training and chromium picolinate on body composition and skeletal muscle in older men. *J. Appl. Physiol.* 86:29–39.

34. Volpe, S. L., H. W. Huang, K. Larpadisorn, and I. I. Lesser. 2001. Effect of chromium supplementation and exercise on body composition, resting metabolic rate and selected biochemical parameters in moderately obese women following an exercise program. *J. Am. Coll. Nutr.* 20:293–306.

35. Campbell, W. W., L. J. O. Joseph, R. A. Anderson, S. L. Davey, J. Hinton, and W. J. Evans. 2002. Effects of resistive training and chromium picolinate on body composition and skeletal muscle size in older women. *Int. J. Sports Nutr. Exerc. Metab.* 12:125–135.

36. Lukaski H. C., Siders W. A., Penland J. G. 2007. Chromium picolinate supplementation in women: effects on body weight, composition and iron status. *Nutr* 23:187–185.

37. Diaz M. L., B. A. Watkins, Y. Li, R. A. Anderson, and W. W. Campbell. 2008. Chromium picolinate and conjugated linoleic acid do not synergistically influence diet- and exercise-inudced changes in body composition and health indexes in overweight women. *J. Nutr Biochem* 19:61–68.

38. Booth, S. L., and J. W. Suttie. 1998. Dietary intake and adequacy of vitamin K. *J. Nutr.* 128:785–788.

39. Institute of Medicine, Food and Nutrition Board. 2001. Dietary Reference Intakes for Vitamin A, Vitamin K, Arsenic, Boron, Chromium, Copper, Iodine, Iron, Manganese, Molybdenum, Nickel, Silicon, Vanadium, and Zinc. Washington, DC: National Academies Press.

40. Feskanich, D., S. A. Korrick, S. L. Greenspan, H. N. Rosen, and G. A. Colditz. 1999. Moderate alcohol consumption and bone density among post-menopausal women. *J. Women's Health* 8:65–73.

41. Beard, J. 2006. Iron. In: Bowman, B. A., and R. M. Russel, eds. Present Knowledge in Nutrition, 9th edn., pp. 430–444. Washington, DC: ILSI Press.

42. U.S. Food and Drug Administration. 1997. Preventing Iron Poisoning in Children. FDA Backgrounder. www.cfsan.fda.gov/~dms/bgiron.html. (Accessed April 2007.)

43. Bacon, B. R., J. K. Olynyk, E. M. Brunt, R. S. Britton, and R. K. Wolff. 1999. HFE genotype in patients with hemochromatosis and other liver diseases. *Ann. Intern. Med.* 130:953–962.

44. National Institute of Allergy and Infectious Diseases, National Institutes of Health. 2007. The Common Cold. www3.niaid.nih.gov/topics/commonCold.

45. Prasad, A. 1996. Zinc: the biology and therapeutics of an ion. *Ann. Intern. Med.* 125:142–143.

46. Jackson, J. L., E. Lesho, and C. Peterson. 2000. Zinc and the common cold: A meta-analysis revisited. *J. Nutr.* 130:1512S–1515S.

47. Caruso, T. J., C. G. Prober, and J. M Gwaltney. 2007. Treatment of naturally acquired common colds with zinc: a structured review. *Clin. Infect Dis.* 45(5):569–574.

48. Chandra, R. K. 1984. Excessive intake of zinc impairs immune responses. *JAMA.* 252:1443–1446.

In Depth: Dietary Supplements: Necessity or Waste?

1. Nutrition Business Journal. 2009. 2009 U.S. Nutrition Industry Overview. Vol XIV, No 6/7, June/July. ©Penton Media, Inc.

2. Blendon, R. J., C. M. DesRoches, J. M. Benson, M. Brodie, and D. E. Altman. 2001. Americans' views on the use and regulation of dietary supplements. *Arch. Intern. Med.* 26:805–810.

3. U.S. Food and Drug Administration (FDA). Center for Food Safety and Applied Nutrition. 2008. Overview of dietary supplements. Available at http://www.cfsan.fda.gov/~dms/supplmnt.html.

4. U.S. Food and Drug Administration (FDA). Center for Food Safety and Applied Nutrition. May 07, 2009. Dietary supplements. Tips for the savvy supplement user: Making informed decisions and evaluating information. Available at http://www.cfsan.fda.gov/~dms/ds-savvy.html.

5. Dancho C., and M. M. Manore. 2001. Dietary supplement information on the World Wide Web. Sorting fact from fiction. *ACSM's Health and Fitness Journal* 5:7–12.

6. National Center for Complementary and Alternative Medicine. 2004. Herbal Supplements: Consider Safety, Too. Available at http://nccam.nih.gov/health/supplement-safety.

7. U.S. Government Accountability Office. (2010). Herbal Dietary Supplements: Examples of Deceptive or Questionable Marketing Practices and Potentially Dangerous Advice. May 26, 2010. GAO-10-662T. Available at: www.gao.gov/.

8. National Institutes of Health. 2005. Important information to know when you are taking Coumadin and Vitamin K. Available at: http://dietary-supplements.info.nih.gov/factsheets/cc/coumadin1.pdf.

9. American Dietetic Association. 2005. Dietary supplements. *J. Am. Diet. Assoc.* 102:460–470.

Chapter 11

1. Emme. 2009. Bio profile; books. http://emmestyle.com/about.

2. Stoynoff, N. 2008. Emme's cancer battle. People, January 21, pp. 99-101.

3. Manore, M. M, N. L. Meyer, and J. Thompson. 2009. Sport Nutrition for Health and Performance. 2nd Edition. Champaign, IL: Human Kinetics.

4. Wang, Y. 2004. Epidemiology of childhood obesity—methodological aspects and guidelines: what is new? *Int. J. Obes.* 23:S21–S28.

5. Deurenberg, P., M. Yap, and W. A. van Staveren. 1998. Body mass index and percent body fat: a meta analysis among different ethnic groups. *Int. J. Obes.* 22:1164–1171.

6. Shai, I., R. Jiang, J. E. Manson, M. J. Stampfer, W. C. Willett, G. A. Colditz, and F. B. Hu. 2006. Ethnicity, obesity, and risk of type 2 diabetes in women. *Diabet. Care* 29:1585–1590.

7. Zernike, K. 2004. U.S. body survey, head to toe, finds signs of expansion. *New York Times,* March 1, section 1.

8. Stunkard, A. J., T. I. A. Sorensen, C. Hanis, T. W. Teasdale, R. Chakraborty, W. J. Schull, and F. Schulsinger. 1986. An adoption study of human obesity. *N. Engl. J. Med.* 314:193–198.

9. Bouchard, C., A. Tremblay, J. P. Després, A. Nadeau, P. J. Lupien, G. Thériault, J. Dussault, S. Moorjani, S. Pinault, and G. Fournier. 1990. The response to long-term overfeeding in identical twins. *N. Engl. J. Med.* 322:1477–1482.

10. Hellerstein, M. 2001. No common energy currency: de novo lipogenesis as the road less traveled. *Am. J. Clin. Nutr.* 74:707–708.

11. Cummings, D. E., D. S. Weigle, R. S. Frayo, P. A. Breen, M. K. Ma, E. P. Dellinger, and J. Q. Purnell. 2002. Plasma ghrelin levels after diet-induced weight loss or gastric bypass surgery. *N. Engl. J. Med.* 346:1623–1630.

12. Druce, M. R., A. M. Wren, A. J. Park, J. E. Milton, M. Patterson, G. Frost, M. A. Ghatei, C. Small, and S. R. Bloom. 2005. Ghrelin increases food intake in obese as well as lean subjects. *Int. J. Obes.* 29:1130–1136.

13. Batterham, R. L., M. A. Cowley, C. J. Small, H. Herzog, M. A. Cohen, C. L. Dakin, A. M. Wren, A. E. Brynes, M. J. Low, M. A. Ghatel, R. D. Cone, and S. R. Bloom. 2002. Gut hormone PYY3-36 physiologically inhibits food intake. *Nature* 418:650–664.

14. Batterham, R. L., M. A. Cohen, S. M. Ellis, C. W. Le Roux, D. J. Withers, G. S. Frost, M. A. Ghatei, and S. R. Bloom. 2003. Inhibition of food intake in obese subjects by peptide YY3-36. *N. Engl. J. Med.* 349:941–948.

15. Virtanen, K. A., M. E. Lidell, J. Orava, M. Heglind, R. Westergren, T. Niemi, M. Taittonen, J. Laine, N-J. Savito, S. Enerbäck, and P. Nuutila. 2009. Functional brown adipose tissue in healthy adults. *N. Engl. J. Med.* 360(15):1518–1525.

16. Cypess, A. M., S. Lehman, G. Williams, I. Tal, D. Rodman, A. B. Goldfine, F. C. Kuo, E. L. Palmer, Y-H. Tseng, A. Doria, G. M. Kolodny, and C. R. Kahn. 2009. Identification and importance of brown adipose tissue in adult humans. *N. Engl. J. Med.* 360(15):1509–1517.

17. Eyler, A. E., D. Matson-Koffman, D. Rohm-Young, S. Wilcox, J. Wilbur, J. L. Thompson, B. Sanderson, and K. R. Evenson. 2003. Quantitative study of correlates of physical activity in women from diverse racial/ethnic groups: The Women's Cardiovascular Health Network Project. *Am. J. Prev. Med.* 25(3Si):93–103.

18. Eyler, A. E., D. Matson-Koffman, J. R. Vest, K. R. Evenson, B. Sanderson, J. L. Thompson, J. Wilbur, S. Wilcox, and D. Rohm-Young. 2002. Environmental, policy, and cultural factors related to physical activity in a diverse sample of women: The Women's Cardiovascular Health Network Project—Summary and Discussion. Women and Health. 36:123–134.

19. Pickett, K. E., S. Kelly, E. Brunner, T. Lobstein, and R. G. Wilkinson. 2005. Wider income gaps, wider waistbands? An ecological study of obesity and income inequality. *J. Epidemiol. Community Health* 59:670–674.

20. Elliott, S. 2005. Calories? Hah! Munch some mega M&M's. *New York Times,* August 5, section C5.

21. Koh-Banerjee, P., N. F. Chu, D. Spiegelman, B. Rosner, G. Colditz, W. Willett, and E. Rimm. 2003. Prospective study of the association of changes in dietary intake, physical activity, alcohol consumption, and smoking with 9-y gain in waist circumference among 16,587 U.S. men. *Am. J. Clin. Nutr.* 78:719–727.

22. Lumeng J. C., Forrest P., Appugliese D. P., Kaciroti N., Corwyn R. F., and Bradley R. H. 2010. Weight status as a predictor of being bullied in third through sixth grades. Pediatrics. e-publication ahead of print, doi:10.1542/peds.2009-0774. Published online May 3, 2010.

23. American Dietetic Association. 2002. Position of the American Dietetic Association: food and nutrition misinformation. *J. Am. Diet. Assoc.* 102(2):260–266.

24. Freedman, M. R., J. King, and E. Kennedy. 2001. Popular diets: a scientific review. *Obes. Res.* 9(suppl. 1):1S–40S.

25. Ello-Martin, J. A., J. H. Ledikwe, and B. J. Rolls. 2005. The influence of food portion size and energy density on energy intake: implications for weight management. *Am. J. Clin. Nutr.* 82(suppl.):236S–241S.

26. Flood, J. E., L. S. Roe, and B. J. Rolls. 2006. The effect of increased beverage portion size on energy intake at a meal. *J. Am. Diet. Assoc.* 106:1984–1990.

27. National Institute of Diabetes and Digestive and Kidney Diseases. Weight-control Information Network. 2009. Just Enough For You. About Food Portions. http://www.win.niddk.nih.gov/publications/just_enough.htm#home.

28. Klem, M. L., R. R. Wing, M. T. McGuire, H. M. Seagle, and J. O. Hill. 1997. A descriptive study of individuals successful at long-term maintenance of substantial weight loss. *Am. J. Clin. Nutr.* 66:239–246.

29. Saper, R. B., D. M. Eisenberg, and R. S. Phillips. 2004. Common dietary supplements for weight loss. *Am. Fam. Phys.* 70(9):1731–1738.

30. Allison, D. B., K. R. Fontaine, S. Heshka, J. L. Mentore, and S. B. Heymsfield. 2001. Alternative treatments for weight loss: a critical review. *Crit. Rev. Food Sci. Nutr.* 41(1):1–28.

31. Stern, L., N. Iqbal, P. Seshadri, K. L. Chicano, D. A. Daily, J. McGrory, M. Williams, E. J. Gracely, and F. F. Samaha. 2004. The effects of low-carbohydrate versus conventional weight loss diets in severely obese adults: One-year follow-up of a randomized trial. *Ann. Intern. Med.* 140:778–785.

32. Samaha, F. F., N. Iqbal, P. Seshadri, K. L. Chicano, D. A. Daily, J. McGrory, T. Williams, M. Williams, E. J. Gracely, and L. Stern. 2003. A low-carbohydrate as compared with a low-fat diet in severe obesity. *N. Engl. J. Med.* 348:2074–2081.

33. Foster, G. D., H. R. Wyatt, J. O. Hill, B. G. McGuckin, C. Brill, B. S. Mohammed, P. O. Szapary, D. J. Rader, J. S. Edman, and S. Klein. 2003. A randomized trial of a low-carbohydrate diet for obesity. *N. Engl. J. Med.* 348:2082–2090.

34. Bravata, D. M., L. Sanders, J. Huang, H. M. Krumholz, I. Olkin, C. D. Gardner, and D. M. Bravata. 2003. Efficacy and safety of low-carbohydrate diets. A systematic review. *JAMA* 289:1837–1850.

In Depth: Obesity

1. Dillon, S. 2007. Sorority evictions raise issue of looks and bias. The New York Times, February 25. Retrieved from www.nytimes.com/2007/02/25/education/25sorority.html?_r=1&scp=1&sq=sorority%20evictions&st=cse.

2. American Obesity Association. 2002. Discrimination. http://obesity1.tempdomainname.com/discrimination/employment.shtml.

3. Huizinga M. M., Cooper L. A., Bleich S. N., Clark J. M., Beach M. C. 2009. Physician respect for patients with obesity. *J. Gen. Intern.* Med. 24(11):1236–1239.

4. Flegal, K. M, M. D. Carroll, C. L. Ogden, and L. R. Curtin. 2010. Prevalence and trends in obesity among U.S. adults, 1999–2008. *JAMA* 303(3):235–241.

5. Grundy, S. M., B. Hansen, S. C. Smith, J. I. Cleeman, and R. A. Kahn. 2004. Clinical management of metabolic syndrome: Report of the American Heart Association/National Heart, Lung, and Blood Institute/American Diabetes Association Conference on Scientific Issues Related to Management. *Circulation* 109:551–556.

6. Department of Health and Human Services. National Institutes of Health. National Heart, Lung and Blood Institute. 2010. Diseases and conditions index. Metabolic syndrome. What is metabolic syndrome? Available at www.nhlbi.nih.gov/health/dci/Diseases/ms/ms_whatis.html.

7. Torgan, C. 2002. Childhood obesity on the rise. The NIH Word on Health. Available at http://www.nih.gov/news/WordonHealth/jun2002/childhoodobesity.htm.

8. Dietz, W. H. 1994. Critical periods in childhood for the development of obesity. *Am. J. Clin. Nutr.* 59:955–959.

9. Christakis, N. A. and J. H. Fowler. 2007. The spread of obesity in a large social network over 32 years. *N. Engl. J. Med.* 357(4):370–379.

10. National Institute of Diabetes and Digestive and Kidney Diseases. Weight-control Information Network. 2008. Understanding Adult Obesity. NIH Publication No. 06-3680 http://www.win.niddk.nih.gov/publications/understanding.htm#environmental.

11. Wing, R. R., and S. Phelan. 2005. Long-term weight loss maintenance. *Am. J. Clin. Nutr.* 82(1):222S–225S.

12. National Institutes of Health. National Heart, Lung, and Blood Institute. 1998. Clinical guidelines on the identification, evaluation, and treatment of overweight and obesity in adults. The Evidence Report. Available at www.nhlbi.nih.gov/guidelines/obesity/ob_gdlns.htm.

13. Institute of Medicine. Food and Nutrition Board. 2002. Dietary Reference Intakes for Energy, Carbohydrate, Fiber, Fat, Fatty Acids, Cholesterol, Protein, and Amino Acids (Macronutrients). Washington, DC: The National Academies Press.

14. Bérubé-Parent, S., D. Prud'homme, S. St-Pierre, E. Doucet, and A. Tremblay. 2001. Obesity treatment with a progressive clinical tri-therapy combining sibutramine and a supervised diet-exercise intervention. *Int. J. Obes.* 25:1144–1153.

15. Chanoine, J.-P., S. Hampl, C. Jensen, M. Boldrin, and J. Hauptman. 2005. Effect of orlistat on weight and body composition in obese adolescents. A randomized controlled trial. *JAMA* 293(23):2873–2883.

16. Hutton, B., and D. Fergusson. 2004. Changes in body weight and serum lipid profile in obese patients treated with orlistat in addition to a hypocaloric diet: A systemic review of randomized clinical trials. *Am. J. Clin. Nutr.* 80:1461–1468.

17. Sjöström, L., A-K. Lindroos, M. Peltonen, J. Torgerson, C. Bouchard, B. Carlsson, S. Dahlgren, B. Larsson, K. Narbro, C. D. Sjöström, M. Sullivan, and H. Wedel. 2004. Lifestyle, diabetes, and cardiovascular risk factors 10 years after bariatric surgery. *N. Engl. J. Med.* 351(26):2683–2693.

Chapter 12

1. U.S. Department of Health and Human Services. 1996. Physical Activity and Health: A Report of the Surgeon General. Atlanta, GA: U.S. Department of Health and Human Services, Centers for Disease Control and Prevention, National Centers for Chronic Disease Prevention and Health Promotion.
2. Caspersen, C. J., K. E. Powell, and G. M. Christensen. 1985. Physical activity, exercise, and physical fitness: definitions and distinctions for health-related research. *Publ. Health Rep.* 100:126–131.
3. Heyward, V. H. 2006. Advanced Fitness Assessment and Exercise Prescription, 5th ed. Champaign, IL: Human Kinetics.
4. Davidson, M. R., M. L. London, and P. W. Ladewig. 2008. Olds' Maternal-Newborn Nursing and Women's Health Across the Lifespan, 8th edn. Upper Saddle River, NJ: Prentice Hall Health.
5. Centers for Disease Control and Prevention (CDC). 2005. Adult participation in recommended levels of physical activity—United States, 2001 and 2003. *Morbid. Mortal. Wkly. Rep.* 54(47):1208–1212.
6. Department of Health and Human Services. Centers for Disease Control and Prevention (CDC). 2010. Physical Activity Statistics. 1988-2008 No Leisure Time Physical Activity Trend Chart. http://www.cdc.gov/nccdphp/dnpa/physical/stats/leisure_time.htm.
7. Department of Health and Human Services. Centers for Disease Control and Prevention (CDC). 2007. YRBSS. 2007 National Youth Risk Behavior Survey Overview. http://www.cdc.gov/HealthyYouth/yrbs/pdf/yrbs07_us_overview.pdf.
8. Pate, R. R., M. G. Davis, T. N. Robinson, E. J. Stone, T. L. McKenzie, and J. C. Young. 2006. Promoting physical activity in children and youth. A leadership role for schools: A scientific statement from the American Heart Association Council on Nutrition, Physical Activity and Metabolism (Physical Activity Committee) in collaboration with the Councils on Cardiovascular Disease in the Young and Cardiovascular Nursing. *Circulation* 114:1214–1224.
9. Institute of Medicine, Food and Nutrition Board. 2002. Dietary Reference Intakes for Energy, Carbohydrates, Fiber, Fat, Protein and Amino Acids (Macronutrients). Washington, DC: National Academies Press.
10. Centers for Disease Control and Prevention. 2010. Physical Activity for Everyone. Target Heart Rate and Estimated Maximum Heart Rate. http://www.cdc.gov/physicalactivity/everyone/measuring/heartrate.html.
11. Centers for Disease Control and Prevention. 2005. Physical activity for everyone: Making physical activity part of your life: Tips for being more active. Available at http://www.cdc.gov/nccdphp/dnpa/physical/life/tips.htm.
12. United States Department of Health and Human Services. 2005. Get active: Goals. Available at http://www.smallstep.gov/step_3/step_3_goals.html.
13. Westerblad, H., D. G. Allen, and J. Lännergren. 2002. Muscle fatigue: lactic acid or inorganic phosphate the major cause? *News Physiol. Sci.* 17(1):17–21.
14. Brooks, G. A. 2000. Intra- and extra-cellular lactate shuttles. *Med. Sci. Sports Exerc.* 32:790–799.
15. Brooks, G. A. 2009. Cell-cell and intracellular lactate shuttles. *J. Physiol.* 587(23):5591–5600.
16. van Hall G., M. Stromstad, P. Rasmussen, O. Jans, M. Zaar, C. Gam, B. Quistorff, N.H. Secher, and H.B. Nielsen. 2009. Blood lactate is an important energy source for the human brain. *J. Cerebral Blood Flow & Metab.* 29(6):1121–1129.
17. Tarnopolsky, M. 2010. Protein and amino acid needs for training and bulking up. In: Burke, L., and Deakin, V., eds. Clinical Sports Nutrition, 3rd edn. Sydney, Australia: McGraw-Hill, pp. 61–95.
18. American College of Sports Medicine, American Dietetic Association, and Dietitians of Canada. 2009. Nutrition and athletic performance. Joint position statement. *Med. Sci. Sports Exerc.* 41:709–731.
19. Burke, L. 2010. Nutrition for recovery after training and competition. In: Burke, L., and Deakin, V., eds. Clinical Sports Nutrition, 4th ed. Sydney, Australia: McGraw-Hill, pp. 358–392.
20. van Loon, L. J. C., W. H. M. Saris, M. Kruijshoop, and A. J. M. Wagenmakers. 2000. Maximizing postexercise muscle glycogen synthesis: carbohydrate supplementation and the application of amino acid or protein hydrolysate mixtures. *Am. J. Clin. Nutr.* 72:106–111.
21. Jentjens, R. L., L. J. C. van Loon, C. H. Mann, A. J. M. Wagenmakers, and A. E. Jeukendrup. 2001. Addition of protein and amino acids to carbohydrates does not enhance postexercise muscle glycogen synthesis. *J. Appl. Physiol.* 91:839–846.
22. Manore, M., N. L. Meyer, and J. Thompson. 2009. Sports Nutrition for Health and Performance. 2nd Edition. Champaign, IL: Human Kinetics (117).
23. Sears, B. 1995. The Zone: A Dietary Road Map. New York: HarperCollins Publishers.
24. Weaver, C. M., and S. Rajaram. 1992. Exercise and iron status. *J. Nutr.* 122:782–787.
25. Haymes, E. M. 1998. Trace minerals and exercise. In: Wolinsky, I., ed. Nutrition and Exercise and Sport. Boca Raton, FL: CRC Press, pp. 1997–2218.
26. Haymes, E. M., and P. M. Clarkson. 1998. Minerals and trace minerals. In: Berning, J. R., and Steen, S. N., eds. Nutrition and Sport and Exercise. Gaithersburg, MD: Aspen Publishers, pp. 77–107.
27. Food and Drug Administration (FDA). 2004. HHS Launches Crackdown on Products Containing Andro. http://www.fda.gov/NewsEvents/Newsroom/PressAnnouncements/2004/ucm108262.htm.
28. Broeder, C. E., J. Quindry, K. Brittingham, L. Panton, J. Thomson, S. Appakondu, K. Breuel, R. Byrd, J. Douglas, C. Earnest, C. Mitchell, M. Olson, T. Roy, and C. Yarlagadda. 2000. The Andro Project: physiological and hormonal influences of androstenedione supplementation in men 35 to 65 years old participating in a high-intensity resistance training program. *Arch. Intern. Med.* 160:3093–3104.
29. Balsom, P. D., K. Söderlund, B. Sjödin, and B. Ekblom. 1995. Skeletal muscle metabolism during short duration high-intensity exercise: influence of creatine supplementation. *Acta Physiol. Scand.* 1154:303–310.
30. Grindstaff, P. D., R. Kreider, R. Bishop, M. Wilson, L. Wood, C. Alexander, and A. Almada. 1997. Effects of creatine supplementation on repetitive sprint performance and body composition in competitive swimmers. *Int. J. Sport Nutr.* 7:330–346.
31. Kreider, R. B., M. Ferreira, M. Wilson, P. Grindstaff, S. Plisk, J. Reinardy, E. Cantler, and A. L. Almada. 1998. Effects of creatine supplementation on body composition, strength, and sprint performance. *Med. Sci. Sports Exerc.* 30:73–82.
32. Tarnopolsky, M. A., and D. P. MacLennan. 2000. Creatine monohydrate supplementation enhances high-intensity exercise performance in males and females. *Int. J. Sport Nutr. Exerc.* Metab. 10:452–463.
33. Kreider, R., M. Ferreira, M. Wilson, and A. L. Almada. 1999. Effects of calcium beta-hydroxy-beta-methylbutyrate (HMB) supplementation during resistance-training on markers of catabolism, body composition and strength. *Int. J. Sports Med.* 20(8):503–509.
34. Volek, J. S., N. D. Duncan, S. A. Mazzetti, R. S. Staron, M. Putukian, A. L. Gomez, D. R. Pearson, W. J. Fink, and W. J. Kraemer. 1999. Performance and muscle fiber adaptations to creatine supplementation and heavy resistance training. *Med. Sci. Sports Exerc.* 31:1147–1156.
35. Reuters. 2001. Creatine use could lead to cancer, French government reports. *New York Times*, January 25.
36. Jeong, K. S., S. J. Park, C. S. Lee, T. W. Kim, S. H. Kim, S. Y. Ryu, B. H. Williams, R. L. Veech, and Y. S. Lee. 2000. Effects of

cyclocreatine in rat hepatocarcinogenesis model. *Anticancer Res.* 20(3A):1627–1633.

37. Ara, G., L. M. Gravelin, R. Kaddurah-Daouk, and B. A. Teicher. 1998. Antitumor activity of creatine analogs produced by alterations in pancreatic hormones and glucose metabolism. *In Vivo* 12:223–231.
38. Anderson, M. E., C. R. Bruce, S. F. Fraser, N. K. Stepto, R. Klein, W. G. Hopkins, and J. A. Hawley. 2000. Improved 2000-meter rowing performance in competitive oarswomen after caffeine ingestion. *Int. J. Sport Nutr. Exerc. Metab.* 10:464–475.
39. Spriet, L. L., and R. A. Howlett. 2000. Caffeine. In: Maughan, R. J., ed. Nutrition in Sport. Oxford: Blackwell Science.
40. Bucci, L. 2000. Selected herbals and human exercise performance. *Am. J. Clin. Nutr.* 72:624S–636S.
41. Williams, M. H. 1998. The Ergogenics Edge. Champaign, IL: Human Kinetics.
42. Hawley, J. A. 2002. Effect of increased fat availability on metabolism and exercise capacity. *Med. Sci. Sports Exerc.* 34(9):1485–1491.
43. Heinonen, O. J. 1996. Carnitine and physical exercise. *Sports Med.* 22:109–132.
44. Vincent, J. B. 2003. The potential value and toxicity of chromium picolinate as a nutritional supplement, weight loss agent and muscle development agent. *Sports Med.* 33(3):213–230.
45. Pliml, W., T. von Arnim, A. Stablein, H. Hofmann, H. G. Zimmer, and E. Erdmann. 1992. Effects of ribose on exercise-induced ischaemia in stable coronary artery disease. *Lancet* 340(8818):507–510.
46. Earnest, C. P., G. M. Morss, F. Wyatt, A. N. Jordan, S. Colson, T. S. Church, Y. Fitzgerald, L. Autrey, R. Jurca, and A. Lucia. 2004. Effects of a commercial herbal-based formula on exercise performance in cyclists. *Med. Sci. Sports Exerc.* 36(3):504–509.
47. Hellsten, Y., L. Skadhauge, and J. Bangsbo. 2004. Effect of ribose supplementation on resynthesis of adenine nucleotides after intense intermittent training in humans. *Am. J. Physiol. Regul. Integr. Comp. Physiol.* 286:R182–R188.
48. Kreider, R. B., C. Melton, M. Greenwood, C. Rasmussen, J. Lundberg, C. Earnest, and A. Almada. 2003. Effects of oral D-ribose supplementation on anaerobic capacity and selected metabolic markers in healthy males. *Int. J. Sport Nutr. Exerc. Metab.* 13(1):76–86.
49. King, A. C., W. L. Haskell, C. B. Taylor, H. C. Kraemer, and R. F. DeBusk. 1991. Group- vs. home-based exercise training in healthy older men and women: a community-based clinical trial. *JAMA* 266:1535–1542.
50. Kohrt, W. M., M. T. Malley, A. R. Coggan, R. J. Spina, T. Ogawa, A. A. Ehsani, R. E. Bourey, W. H. Martin, 3rd, and J. O. Holloszy. 1991. Effects of gender, age, and fitness level on response of Vo2max to training in 60–71 yr olds. *J. Appl. Physiol.* 71:2004–2011.
51. LaCroix, A. Z., S. G. Leveille, J. A. Hecht, L. C. Grothaus, and E. H. Wagner. 1996. Does walking decrease the risk of cardiovascular disease hospitalizations and death in older adults? *J. Am. Geriatr. Soc.* 44:113–120.
52. Blair, S. N., H. W. Kohl III, C. E. Barlow, R. S. Paffenbarger Jr., L. W. Gibbons, and C. A. Macera. 1995. Changes in physical fitness and all-cause mortality: a prospective study of healthy and unhealthy men. *JAMA* 273:1093–1098.
53. Paffenbarger, R. S., Jr., R. T. Hyde, A. L. Wing, and C.-C. Hsieh. 1986. Physical activity, all-cause mortality, and longevity of college alumni. *N. Engl. J. Med.* 314:605–613.
54. Leon, A. S., J. Connett, D. R. Jacobs Jr., and R. Rauramaa. 1987. Leisure-time physical activity levels and risk of coronary heart disease and death: the Multiple Risk Factor Intervention Trial. *JAMA* 258:2388–2395.
55. Slattery, M. L., D. R. Jacobs Jr., and M. Z. Nichaman. 1989. Leisure-time physical activity and coronary heart disease death: the U.S. Railroad Study. *Circulation* 79:304–311.
56. Helmrich, S. P., D. R. Ragland, R. W. Leung, and R. S. Paffenbarger Jr. 1991. Physical activity and reduced occurrence of non-insulin-dependent diabetes mellitus. *N. Engl. J. Med.* 325:147–152.

In Depth: Disordered Eating

1. American Psychiatric Association. 1994. Diagnostic and Statistical Manual of Mental Disorders (DSM-IV). 4th ed. Washington, DC: American Psychiatric Association.
2. Treasure J., Claudino A. M., Zucker N. Eating Disorders. 2010. *Lancet* 375:583–593.
3. Vandereycken, W. 2002. Families of patients with eating disorders. In: Fairburn, D. G., and K. D. Brownell, eds. Eating Disorders and Obesity: A Comprehensive Handbook. 2nd ed. New York Guilford Press, pp. 215–220.
4. Patrick, L. 2002. Eating disorders: A review of the literature with emphasis on medical complication and clinical nutrition. *Altern. Med. Rev.* 7(3):184–202.
5. Striegel-Moore, R. H., and L. Smolak. 2002. Gender, ethnicity, and eating disorders. In: Fairburn, D. G., and K. D. Brownell, eds. Eating Disorders and Obesity: A Comprehensive Handbook. 2nd ed. New York: Guilford Press, pp. 251–255.
6. Steinberg, L. 2002. Adolescence. 6th ed. New York: McGraw-Hill.
7. Stice E. 2002. Sociocultural influences on body image and eating disturbances. In: Fairburn, D. G., and K. D. Brownell, eds. Eating Disorders and Obesity: A Comprehensive Handbook. 2nd ed. New York: Guilford Press, pp. 103–107.
8. Wonderlich, S. A. 2002. Personality and eating disorders. In: Fairburn, D. G., and K. D. Brownell, eds. Eating Disorders and Obesity: A Comprehensive Handbook. 2nd ed. New York: Guilford Press, pp. 204–209.
9. Robb, A. S., and M. J. Dadson. 2002. Eating disorders in males. Child Adolesc. *Psychiatric. Clin. N. Am.* 11:399–418.
10. American Psychiatric Association, 2000. Diagnostic and Statistical Manual of Mental Disorders, Text Revision.
11. Beals, K. A. 2004. Disordered Eating in Athletes: A Comprehensive Guide for Health Professionals. Champaign, IL: Human Kinetics Publishers.
12. Andersen, A. E. 2001. Eating disorders in males: Gender divergence management. Currents 2(2). University of Iowa Health Care. Available at http://www.uihealthcare.com/news/currents/vol2issue2/eatingdisordersinmen.html.
13. Pope H. G., K. A. Phillips, and R. Olivardia. 2000. The Adonis Complex: The Secret Crisis of Male Body Obsession. New York: The Free Press.
14. Garfinkel, P. E. 2002. Classification and diagnosis of eating disorders. In: Fairburn D. G., and K. D. Brownell, eds. Eating Disorders and Obesity: A Comprehensive Handbook. 2nd ed. New York: Guilford Press, pp. 155–161.
15. Grilo, C. M. 2002. Binge eating disorder. In: D. G. Fairburn and K. D. Brownell, eds. Eating Disorders and Obesity: A Comprehensive Handbook. 2nd ed. New York: Guilford Press, pp. 178–182.
16. Stunkard, A. J. 2002. Night eating syndrome. In: DG Fairburn and KD Brownell, eds. Eating Disorders and Obesity: A Comprehensive Handbook. 2nd ed. New York: Guilford Press, pp. 183–187.
17. Nattiv A., A. B. Loucks, M. M. Manore, C. F. Sanborn, J. Sundgot-Borgen, and M. P. Warren. 2007. The female athlete triad. *Medicine and Science in Sport and Exercise.* 39(10):1867–1882.
18. National Eating Disorders Association. 2005. What should I say? Tips for talking to a friend who may be struggling with an eating disorder. Available at http://www.nationaleatingdisorders.org/p.asp?WebPage_ID5322&Profile_ID541174.

Chapter 13

1. Centers for Disease Control and Prevention (CDC). March 17, 2009. Investigation Update: Outbreak of Salmonella typhimurium Infections, 2008–2009. Available at www.cdc.gov/salmonella/

typhimurium/update.html; U.S. Food and Drug Administration (FDA). FDA Urges Consumers Not to Eat Hundreds of Products Recalled Because of Contaminated Peanuts and Peanut Ingredients. FDA Hot Topics. Available at www.fda.gov/oc/opacom/hottopics/salmonellatyph/article.html.

2. Centers for Disease Control and Prevention (CDC). Salmonella Outbreak Investigations. March 3, 2010. Available at www.cdc.gov/salmonella/outbreaks.html.
3. Centers for Disease Control and Prevention (CDC), Division of Bacterial and Mycotic Diseases (DFBMD). Salmonellosis. May 21, 2008. Available at www.cdc.gov/nczved/dfbmd/disease_listing/salmonellosis_gi.html#8.
4. Doering, C. Foodborne illness costs $152 billion annually. Reuters. March 4, 2010. Available at www.reuters.com/article/idUSTRE6220NO20100304.
5. Centers for Disease Control and Prevention (CDC), Division of Bacterial and Mycotic Diseases (DFBMD). 2005. Disease Listing. Foodborne Illness. Available at http://www.cdc.gov/ncidod/dbmd/diseaseinfo/foodborneinfections_g.htm.
6. Centers for Disease Control and Prevention (CDC). CDC Report Points to Need for New Foodborne Illness Strategies. April 10, 2008. Available at www.cdc.gov/media/pressrel/2008/r080410.htm.
7. Centers for Disease Control and Prevention (CDC). April 9, 2009. Annual Report Indicates Salmonella Continues to Show Least Improvement. Available at www.cdc.gov/media/pressrel/2009/r090409.htm.
8. Harris, G. President Promises to Bolster Food Safety. March 15, 2009. The New York Times. Available at www.nytimes.com/2009/03/15/us/politics/15address.html.
9. Doering, C. Foodborne illness costs $152 billion annually. Reuters. March 4, 2010. Available at www.reuters.com/article/idUSTRE6220NO20100304.
10. Centers for Disease Control and Prevention (CDC). Foodborne Illness. January 10, 2005. Available at www.cdc.gov/ncidod/dbmd/diseaseinfo/foodborneinfections_g.htm.
11. Ibid.
12. Centers for Disease Control and Prevention (CDC), Division of Viral Diseases Norovirus: Q&A. February 23, 2010. Avilable at www.cdc.gov/ncidod/dvrd/revb/gastro/norovirus-qa.htm.
13. Norovirus Blog. January 14, 2009. Michigan Continues to Be a Hotspot for Norovirus. Available at www.noroblog.com/2009/01/articles/norovirus-outbreaks/michigan-continues-to-be-a-hotspot-for-norovirus/.
14. United States Department of Agriculture (USDA) Food Safety and Inspection Service. Parasites and Foodborne Illness. May, 2001. Available at http://origin-www.fsis.usda.gov/Fact_Sheets/Parasites_and_Foodborne_Illness/index.asp.
15. Bauman, R.W. 2009. Microbiology. San Francisco: Pearson Benjamin Cummings.
16. International Society for Infectious Diseases. Prion Disease Update 2010. March 4, 2010. Available at http://promedmail.oracle.com/pls/otn/pm?an=20100304.0709.
17. Bauman, R.W. 2009. Ibid.
18. Preidt, R. Predicted "Red Tide" Could Make Shellfish a Dangerous Dish. National Library of Medicine's Medline Plus: Health Day. February 26, 2010. Available at www.nlm.nih.gov/medlineplus/print/news/fullstory_95794.html.
19. Centers for Disease Control and Prevention (CDC), Division of Bacterial and Mycotic Diseases (DFBMD). Marine Toxins. October 12, 2005. Available at www.cdc.gov/ncidod/dbmd/diseaseinfo/marinetoxins_g.htm.
20. Ibid.
21. Pavlista, A. D. 2001. Green potatoes: The problem and solution. NebGuide. The University of Nebraska-Lincoln Cooperative Extension. Available at http://ianrpubs.unl.edu/horticulture/g1437.htm.
22. Food and Drug Administration (FDA). FDA Finalizes Report on 2006 Spinach Outbreak. March 23, 2007. FDA News. Available at www.fda.gov/bbs/topics/NEWS/2007/NEW01593.html
23. U.S. Department of Agriculture (USDA). Partnership for Food Safety Education (PFSE). Fight Bac! Safe Food Handling. 2006. www.fightbac.org/content/view/6/11/.
24. National Digestive Diseases Information Clearinghouse (NDDIC). May, 2007. Bacteria and foodborne illness. NIH Publication No. 07-4730. Available at http://digestive.niddk.nih.gov/ddiseases/pubs/bacteria/index.htm.
25. Ibid.
26. Food and Drug Administration (FDA) 2005c. Eating defensively: Food safety advice for persons with AIDS. Available at http://www.cfsan.fda.gov/∼dms/aidseat.html.
27. U.S. Department of Agriculture (USDA). Food Product Dating. February 8, 2007. Fact Sheets: Food Labeling. Available at www.fsis.usda/gov/Factsheets/Food_Product_Dating/index.asp
28. U.S. Department of Agriculture (USDA). Partnership for Food Safety Education (PFSE). Fight Bac! Safe Food Handling. 2006. Op cit.
29. Ibid.
30. Ibid.
31. Food Marketing Institute. 2003. A Consumer Guide to Food Quality and Safe Handling: Meat, Poultry, Seafood, Eggs [pamphlet]. Washington, DC: Food Marketing Institute, pp. 1–5.
32. Ibid.
33. Food and Drug Administration (FDA) 2003. Anisakis simplex and related worms. Foodborne Pathogenic Microorganisms and Natural Toxins Handbook. Available at www.cfsan.fda.gov/~mow/chap25.html.
34. Center for Science in the Public Interest (CSPI). 2006b. Tips to prevent food poisoning: CSPI's "eggspert" egg advice. Available at http://www.cspinet.org/foodsafety/eggspert_advice.html.
35. U.S. Department of Agriculture (USDA). 2003. Safe Food Handling. Barbecue Food Safety. Available at http://www.fsis.usda.gov/Fact_Sheets/Barbecue_Food_Safety/index.asp.
36. Shephard, S. 2000. Pickled, Potted and Canned: The Story of Food Preserving. London: Headline Publishing.
37. Aseptic Packaging Council. 2005. The award-winning, Earth smart packaging for a healthy lifestyle. Available at http://www.aseptic.org/main.shtml.
38. United States Food and Drug Administration (FDA). News & Events. Bisphenol A (BPA). January 2010. Available at www.fda.gov/NewsEvents/PublicHealthFocus/ucm064437.htm; Centers for Disease Control and Prevention (CDC) Fact Sheet: Bisphenol A (BPA). February 11, 2010. Available at www.cdc.gov/exposurereport/BisphenolA_FactSheet.html; Kristof, N. Chemicals in Our Food, and Bodies. November 8, 2009. *New York Times*. Available at www.nytimes.com/2009/11/08/opinion/08Kristof.html.
39. United States Department of Health and Human Services (USDHHS). Bisphenol A (BPA) Information for Parents. February 12, 2010. Available at www.hhs.gov/safety/bpa/.
40. Loaharanu, P. 2003. Irradiated Foods. New York: American Council on Science & Health Booklets.
41. Center for Science in the Public Interest (CSPI). 2006a. Food safety. Chemical cuisine. CSPI's guide to food additives. Available at http://www.cspinet.org/reports/chemcuisine.htm.
42. Geha, R. S., A. Beiser, C. Ren, R. Patterson, P. A. Greenberger, L. C. Grammer, A. M. Ditto, K. E. Harris, M. A. Shaughnessy, P. R. Yarnold, et al. 2000. Review of alleged reaction to monosodium glutamate and outcome of a multicenter double-blind placebo-controlled study. *J. Nutr.* 130(4S Suppl):1058S–1062S.
43. World Health organization (WHO). 2010. Twenty Questions on Genetically Modified (GM) Foods. Available at www.who.int/foodsafety/publications/biotech/20questions/en/.

44. U.S. Department of Agriculture (USDA), Economic Research Service. 2005. Data. Adoption of Genetically Engineered Crops in the U.S. Available at http://www.ers.usda.gov/Data/BiotechCrops/.

45. McHughen, A. 2000. Pandora's Picnic Basket: The potential and hazards of genetically modified foods. Oxford: Oxford University Press, pp. 17–45.

46. President's Cancer Panel. 2010. Reducing environmental cancer risk: What we can do now: 2008-2009 annual report. Available online at: http://deainfo.nci.nih.gov/advisory/pcp/pcp.htm.

47. Schafer, K. S., and S. E. Kegley. 2002. Persistent toxic chemicals in the U.S. food supply. J. Epidemiol. *Community Health* 56:813–817.

48. Food and Drug Administration (FDA). March 2004. Update 11/23/2009. What You Need to Know About Mercury in Fish and Shellfish. Available at www.fda.gov/Food/ResourcesForYou/Consumers/ucm110591.htm.

49. Ibid.

50. U.S. Food and Drug Administration (FDA). Questions and Answers About Dioxins. 09/21/2009. www.fda.gov/Food/FoodSafety/FoodContaminantsAdulteration/ChemicalContaminants/DioxinsPCBs/ucm077524.htm.

51. Ibid.

52. Environmental Protection Agency (EPA). 2005c. Pesticides: Health and Safety: Human Health Issues. Available at www.epa.gov/pesticides/health/human.htm.

53. Environmental Protection Agency (EPA). 2005d. Pesticides: Health and Safety: Pesticides and Food: Health Problems Pesticides May Pose. Available at http://www.epa.gov/pesticides/food/risks.htm.

54. Environmental Protection Agency (EPA). 2005e. Pesticides: Health and Safety: Pesticides and Food: Why Children May Be Especially Sensitive to Pesticides. Available at http://www.epa.gov/pesticides/food/pest.htm.

55. Environmental Protection Agency (EPA). 2005a. About Pesticides. Available at http://www.epa.gov/pesticides/about/index.htm.

56. Environmental Protection Agency (EPA). 2005b. Pesticides and Food: Healthy, Sensible Food Practices. Available at http://www.epa.gov/pesticides/food/tips.htm.

57. LeSage, L. 1999. News Release. Health Canada rejects bovine growth hormone in Canada. Health Canada Online. Available at http://www.hc-sc.gc.ca/ahc-asc/media/nr-cp/1999/1999_03_e.html.

58. Hankinson, S. E., W. C. Willett, G. A. Colditz, D. J. Hunter, D. S. Michaud, B. Deroo, B. Rosner, F. E. Speizer, and M. Pollak. 1998. Circulating concentrations of insulin-like growth factor-I and risk of breast cancer. *Lancet* 351(9113):1393–1396.

59. Chan, J. M., M. J. Stampfer, E. Giovannucci, P. H. Gann, J. Ma, P. Wilkinson, C. H. Hennekens, and M. Pollak. 1998. Plasma insulin-like growth factor-I and prostate cancer risk: A prospective study. *Science* 279(5350):563–566.

60. Smith T. C., M. J. Male, A. L. Harper, J. S. Kroeger, G. P. Tinkler, et al. (2009). Methicillin-Resistant Staphylococcus aureus (MRSA) Strain ST398 Is Present in Midwestern U.S. Swine and Swine Workers. PLoS ONE 4(1): e4258. Doi: 10.1371/journal.pone.0004258.

61. Centers for Disease Control and Prevention (CDC). October 17, 2007. Invasive MRSA. Available at www.cdc.gov/ncidod/dhqp/ar_mrsa_Invasive_FS.html.

62. Smith T. C., et al. (2009). Op. cit.

63. Organic Trade Association. 2009. OTA's 2009 Organic Industry Survey. May, 2009. Available at www.ota.com/pics/documents/01a_OTAExecutiveSummary.pdf.

64. Ibid.

65. United States Department of Agriculture (USDA). Agricultural Marketing Service. National Organic Program. 02/05/2010. Understanding Organic. Available at www.ams.usda.gov/AMSv1.0/ams.fetchTemplateData.do?template=TemplateA&leftNav=NationalOrganicProgram&page=NOPUnderstandingOrganic&description=Understanding%20Organic&acct=nopgeninfo.

66. Heaton, S. 2003. Organic Farming, Food Quality and Human Health: A Review of the Evidence. Soil Association. Bristol: Briston House.

67. Asami, D. K., Y. J. Hong, D. M. Barrett, and A. E. Mitchell. 2003. Comparison of the total phenolic and ascorbic acid content of freeze-dried and air-dried marionberry, strawberry, and corn grown using conventional, organic, and sustainable agricultural practices. *J. Agric. Food Chem.* 51(5):1237–1241.

68. Carbonaro, M., M. Mattera, S. Nicoli, P. Bergamo, and M. Cappelloni. 2002. Modulation of antioxidant compounds in organic vs conventional fruit (peach, Prunus persica L., and pear, Pyrus communis L.). *J. Agric. Food Chem.* 50(19):5458–5462.

69. Grinder-Pedersen, L., S. E. Rasmussen, S. Bügel, L. O. Jørgensen, D. Vagn Gundersen, and B. Sandström. 2003. Effect of diets based on foods from conventional versus organic production on intake and excretion of flavonoids and markers of antioxidative defense in humans. *Agric. Food Chem.* 51(19):5671–5676.

70. Dangour, A. D., S. K. Dodhia, A. Hayter, E. Allen, K. Lock, and R. Uauy. 2009. Nutritional quality of organic foods: a systematic review. *American Journal of Clinical Nutrition*. July 29, 2009. Doi:10.3945/ajcn.2009.28041.

71. Severson, K. and A. Martin. 2009. It's organic, but does that mean it's safer? *New York Times*. March 4. Available at www.nytimes.com/2009/03/04/dining/04cert.html.

72. World Health organization (WHO). 2010. Twenty Questions on Genetically Modified (GM) Foods. Available at www.who.int/foodsafety/publications/biotech/20questions/en/.

73. Neuman, W. 2010. Justice Dept. Tells Farmers It Will Press Agriculture Industry on Antitrust. *New York Times*. March 12. Available at www.nytimes.com/2010/03/13/business/13seed.html.

74. James, C. 2004. Preview: Global Status of Commercialized Biotech/GM Crops: 2004. ISAAA Briefs No. 32. Ithaca, NY: ISAAA.

In Depth: Global Nutrition

1. Associated Press. 2005. Malawi drought highlights food shortage. *New York Times*, October 17.

2. Food and Agriculture Organization (FAO). 2009. The State of Food Insecurity in the World 2009. FAO Media Centre, October 14, 2009. Available at www.fao.org/news/story/en/item/36207/icode/.

3. World Health Organization (WHO). 2010. What are the key health dangers for children? July 24, 2008. Geneva: World Health Organization. Available at www.who.int/features/qa/13/en/.

4. National Aeronautics and Space Administration (NASA). 2005. Earth observatory: Famine in Niger and Mali. http://earthobservatory.nasa.gov/NaturalHazards/natural_hazards_v2.php3?img_id=13028. (Accessed August 2007.)

5. Central Intelligence Agency. 2010. The World Factbook: Sudan. February 15, 2010. Available at www.cia.gov/library/publications/the-world-factbook/geos/su.html; and Stroehlein, A. 2004. Darfur starvation will be televised . . . eventually. *Christian Science Monitor*, June 8. www.csmonitor.com/2004/0608/p09s02-coop.htm.

6. Friends of the World Food Program. 2010. Number of Hungry Quadruples in Southern Sudan Amidst Conflict and Drought. February 2. Available at www.friendsofwfp.org/site/apps/nlnet/content2.aspx?c=hrKJI.

7. UNICEF. 2008. Basic education and gender equity. February, 2008. Available at www.unicef.org/girlseducation/index_bigpicture.html.

8. UNAIDS/WHO. 2009. AIDS Epidemic Update: Global Facts & Figures: December. http://data.unaids.org/pub/FactSheet/2009/20091124_FS_global_en.pdf.

9. Squires, N. 2009. At UN food summit, Ban Ki-Moon warns of rise in child hunger deaths. *The Christian Science Monitor*. October 16, 2009. Available at www.csmonitor.com/World/Europe/2009/1116/p06s04-woeu.html.

10. Ezra, M., and G. E. Kiros. 2000. Household vulnerability to food crisis and mortality in the drought-prone areas of northern Ethiopia. *J. Biosoc. Sci.* 32:395–409.

11. Black, R. E., S. S. Morris, and J. Bryce. 2003. Where and why are 10 million children dying every year? *Lancet* 361:2226–2234.

12. UNICEF. 2009. The State of the World's Children 2009. UNICEF. Available at http://www.unicef.org/sowc09/press/fastfacts.php.

13. Kristof, N. D. World's Healthiest Food. 2010. *New York Times*, January 3. Available at www.nytimes.com/2010/01/03/opinion/03kristof.html.

14. Drewnowski, A. 2004. Poverty and obesity. www.niehs.nih.gov/drcpt/beoconf/postconf/overview/drewnowski2.pdf.

15. Adair, L. S., and A. M. Prentice. 2004. A critical evaluation of the fetal origins hypothesis and its implications for developing countries. *J. Nutr.* 134:191–193.

16. Yajnik, C. S. 2004. Early life origins of insulin resistance and type 2 diabetes in India and other Asian countries. *J. Nutr.* 134:205–210.

17. World Health Organization. Obesity and Overweight. September 2006. Available at http://www.who.int/dietphysicalactivity/publications/facts/obesity/en/.

18. Food Research and Action Center (FRAC). July, 2006. Hunger in the U.S.: The Paradox of Obesity and Hunger. Available at www.frac.org.html/hunger_in_the_us/hunger&obesity.htm.

19. U.S. Department of Agriculture (USDA). 2009. Economic Research Service. Food Security in the United States: Key Statistics and Graphics. November 16, 2009. www.ers.usda.gov/Briefing/FoodSecurity/Stats_Graphs.htm.

20. Zinn, H. 2006. Original Zinn, p. 167. New York: Harper Perennial.

21. United States Department of Agriculture (USDA) Food and Nutrition Service. 2010. Supplemental Nutrition Assistance Program. January 26, 2010. Available at www.fns.usda.gov/FSP/faqs.htm.

Chapter 14

1. Centers for Disease Control and Prevention (CDC). December 22, 2009. Births and Natality. Available at www.cdc.gov/nchs/fastats/births.htm.

2. Davidson, M. R., M. L. London, and P. W. Ladewig. 2008. Olds' Maternal-Newborn Nursing and Women's Health Across the Life-span, 8th ed. Upper Saddle River, NJ: Prentice Hall Health.

3. Viswanathan, M., A. M. Siega-Riz, M-K. Moos, A. Deierlein, S. Mumford, J. Knaack, P. Thieda, L. J. Lux, and K. N. Lohr. 2008. Outcomes of Maternal Weight Gain, Evidence Report/Technology Assessment No. 168. AHRQ Publication No. 08-E009. Rockville, MD: Agency for Healthcare Research and Quality.

4. Rasmussen, K. M., and A. L. Yaktine, eds. 2009. Weight Gain During Pregnancy: Reexamining the Guidelines. Institute of Medicine; National Research Council. Washington, DC: National Academy Press.

5. Wrotniak, B. H., J. Shults, S. Butts, and N. Stettler. 2008. Gestational weight gain and risk of overweight in the offspring at age 7 in a multicenter, multiethnic cohort study. *Am J. Clin. Nutr.* 87:1818–1824.

6. Institute of Medicine, Food and Nutrition Board, Board on Children, Youth, and Families. 2006. Influence of Pregnancy Weight on Maternal and Child Health: Workshop Report Influence of Pregnancy Weight on Maternal and Child Health. Washington, DC: National Academies Press.

7. U.S. Department of Health & Human Services. 2007. Breastfeeding, Maternal & Infant Health Outcomes in Developed Countries. www.ahrq.gov/clinic/tp/brfouttp.htm. (Accessed March 2010.)

8. Centers for Disease Control and Prevention (CDC). 2009. Facts about folic acid: Folic acid home page. Available at http://www.cdc.gov/ncbddd/folicacid/about.html. (Accessed March 2010.)

9. Institute of Medicine, Food and Nutrition Board. 1998. Dietary Reference Intakes for Thiamin, Riboflavin, Niacin, Vitamin B6, Folate, Vitamin B12, Pantothenic Acid, Biotin, and Choline. Washington, DC: National Academies Press.

10. Institute of Medicine, Food and Nutrition Board. 1997. Dietary Reference Intakes for Calcium, Phosphorus, Magnesium, Vitamin D, and Fluoride. Washington, DC: National Academies Press.

11. Office of Dietary Supplements. 2007. Dietary supplement fact sheet: Iron. National Institutes of Health. Available at http://dietary-supplements.info.nih.gov/factsheets/Iron_pf.asp. (Accessed March 2010).

12. Institute of Medicine, Food and Nutrition Board. 2004. Dietary Reference for Water, Potassium, Sodium, Chloride, and Sulfate. Washington, DC: National Academies Press.

13. Lacasse, A., E. Rey, E. Ferreira, C. Morin, and A. Bérard. 2009. Epidemiology of nausea and vomiting of pregnancy: prevalence, severity, determinants, and the importance of race/ethnicity. *BMC Pregnancy and Childbirth* 9:26.

14. Francis, J. J. Pregnancy: Preparation for the Next Generation. In: Wilson, T, G. A. Bray, N. J. Temple, and M. B. Struble. Nutrition Guide for Physicians. 2010. Humana Press.

15. Clausen, T. D., E. R. Mathiesen, T. Hansen, O. Pedersen, D. M. Jensen, J. Lauenborg, L. Schmidt, and P. Bamm. 2009. Overweight and the metabolic syndrome in adult offspring of women with diet-treated gestational diabetes mellitus or type 1 diabetes. *J. Clin. Endocrinology Metab.* 94:2464–2470.

16. Reece, E. A. 2010. The fetal and maternal consequences of gestational diabetes. *J. Maternal–Fetal Neonatal Med.* 23:199-203.

17. Leeman, L., and P. Fontaine. 2008. Hypertenisve disorders of pregnancy. *Am. Fam. Physician.* 78:93–100.

18. Stewart, A., J. Walsh, and N. Van Eyk. 2008. Adverse outcomes associated with adolescent pregnancy. *J. Ped. Adolesc. Gynecol.* 21:59–60.

19. Craig, W. J., A. R. Mangels, and the American Dietetic Association. 2009. Position of the American Dietetic Association: vegetarian diets. *J. Am. Diet. Assoc.* 109:1266–1282.

20. American Dietetic Association. 2008. Position of the American Dietetic Association: nutrition and lifestyle for a healthy pregnancy outcome. 108:553–561.

21. National Organization on Fetal Alcohol Syndrome (NOFAS). 2001–2004. FAQs. What are fetal alcohol spectrum disorders? Available at http://www.nofas.org/faqs.aspx?id=15. Accessed March 2010.

22. National Center for Health Statistics. 2009. Health, United States, 2008 with Chartbooks. Hyattsvilee, MD: U.S. Government Printing Office.

23. Substance Abuse and Mental Health Services Administration. 2008. Results from the 2007 National Survey on Drug Use and Health: National Findings. NSDUH Series H-34, DHHS Publication No. SMA 08-4343. Rockville, MD.

24. U.S. Department of Health and Human Services and U.S. Department of Agriculture. 2010. Dietary Guidelines for Americans 2010, 7th edn. Washington, DC: U.S. Government Printing Office. www.healthierus.gov/dietaryguidelines.

25. World Health Organization (WHO). November, 2007. Dioxins and their effects on human health. Available at www.who.int/mediacentre/factsheets/fs225/en/index.html.

26. Gavard, J. A. and R. Artal. 2008. Effect of exercise on pregnancy outcome. *Clin. Obstet. Gynec.* 51:467–480.

27. Centers for Disease Control and Prevention. 2009. Breastfeeding among U.S. Children born 1999–2005, CDC National Immunization Survey. Available at www.cdc.gov/breastfeeding/data/NIS_data/.

28. Jana, A. K. Interventions for promoting the initiation of breastfeeding: RHL commentary. 2009. The WHO Reproductive Health Library; Geneva: World Health Organization. Available at http://apps.who.int/rhl/pregnancy_childbirth/care_after_childbirth/cd001688_JanaAK_com/en/.

29. Mayo Clinic. Induced lactation: Can I breast-feed my adopted baby? October 29, 2008. Available at www.mayoclinic.com/health/induced-lactation/AN01882.

30. ESPGHAN Committee on Nutrition: Agostoni, C., C. Braegger, T. Decsi, S. Kolacek, B. Koletzko, K.F. Michaelsen, W. Mihatsch, L.A. Moreno, J. Puntis, R. Shamir, H. Szajewska, D. Turck, and J. van Goudoever. 2009. Breast-feeding: a commentary by the ESPGHAN Committee on Nutrition. *J. Ped. Gastroentrerol Nutr.* 49:112–125.

31. American Academy of Pediatrics (AAP), Section on Breastfeeding. 2005. Breastfeeding and the use of human milk policy statement. *Pediatrics* 115:496–506.

32. Collaborative Group on Hormonal Factors in Breast Cancer. 2003. Breast cancer and breastfeeding: collaborative reanalysis of individual data from 47 epidemiological studies in 30 countries, including 50,302 women with breast cancer and 96,973 women without the disease. *Lancet* 360:187–195.

33. Agency for Healthcare Research and Quality. 2007. Breastfeeding and Maternal and Infant Health Outcomes in Developed Countries. U.S. Department of Health and Human Services. Rockville, MD. AHRQ Publication No. 07-E007.

34. Nickerson, K. 2006. Environmental contaminants in breast milk. *J. Midwifery Women's Health* 51:26–34.

35. Kline, M.W. 2009. Early exclusive breastfeeding: still the cornerstone of child survival. *Am. J. Clin. Nutr.* 89:1281–1282.

36. Adams, C., R. Berger, P. Conning, L. Cruikshank, and K. Dore. 2001. Breastfeeding trends at a community breastfeeding center: an evaluative survey. *J. Obstet. Gynecol. Neonatal Nurs.* 30(4):392–400.

37. American Academy of Pediatrics, Section on Breastfeeding. 2005. Breastfeeding and the use of human milk policy statement. *Pediatrics* 115:496–506.

38. ESPGHAN Committee on Nutrition: C. Agostoni, I. Axelsson, O. Goulet, B. Koletzko, K.F. Michaelsen, J. Puntis, D. Rieu, J. RIgo, R. Shamir, H. Szajewska, and D. Turck. 2006. Soy protein infant formulae and follow-on formulae: a commentary by the ESPGHAN committee on nutrition. *J. Ped. Gastroenterol Nutr.* 42:352–361.

39. Grummer-Strawn, L. M., and M. Zuguo. 2004. Does breastfeeding protect against pediatric overweight? Analysis of longitudinal data from the Centers for Disease Control and Prevention Pediatric Nutrition Surveillance System. *Pediatrics* 113e:e81–e86.

40. Weyerman, M., D. Rothenbacher, and H. Brenner. 2006. Duration of breastfeeding and risk of overweight in childhood: A prospective birth cohort study from Germany. *Int. J. Obesity.* (London) 30:1281–1287.

41. Koletzko, B., Scaglioni, R. von Kries, R. Closa Monasterolo, J. Excribano Subias, S. Scaglioni, M. Giovannini, J. Beyer, et al., for the European Childhood Obesity Trial Study Group, 2009. Can infant feeding choices modulate later obesity rates? *Am. J. Clin. Nutr.* 89 (suppl):1502S–1580S.

42. Gillman, M. W., S. L. Rifas-Shiman, C. A. Camargo Jr., C. S. Berkey, A. L. Frazier, H. R. Rockett, A. E. Field, and G. A. Colditz. 2001. Risk of overweight among adolescents who were breastfed as infants. *JAMA* 285:2461–1467.

43. Owen, C. G., R. M. Martin, P. H. Whincup, D. Smith, and D. G. Cppk. 2005. Effect of infant feeding on the risk of obesity across the life course: A quantitative review of published evidence. *Pediatrics* 115:1367–1377.

44. O'Tierney, P. F., D. J. P. Barker, C. Osmond, E. Kajantie, and J. G. Eriksson. 2009. Duration of breastfeeding and adiposity in adult life. *J. Nutr.* 139:422S–425S.

45. Ludwig, D. S., and H. A. Pollack. 2009. Obesity and the economy: From crisis to opportunity. *JAMA* 301:533–535.

In Depth: The Fetal Environment: A Lasting Impression

1. Lussana, F., R. C. Painter, M. C. Ocke, H. R. Buller, P. M. Bossuyt, and T. J. Roseboom. 2008. Prenatal exposure to the Dutch famine is associated with a preference for fatty foods and a more atherogenic lipid profile. *Am. J. Clin. Nutr.* 88:1648–1652.

2. Lumey, L. H., A. D. Stein, H. S. Kahn, and J. A. Romijn. 2009. Lipid profiles in middle-aged men and women after famine exposure during gestation: the Dutch Hunger Winter Families Study. *Am. J. Clin. Nutr.* 90:1737–1743.

3. Kaijser, M., A. K. E. Bonamy, O. Akre, S. Cnattingius, F. Granath, M. Norman, and A. Ekbom. 2009. Perinatal risk factors for diabetes in later life. *Diabetes* 58:523–526.

4. Jaddoe, V. W. V. 2008. Fetal nutritional origins of adult diseases: challenges for epidemiological research. *Eur. J. Epidemiol.* 23:767–771.

5. Stanner, S. A., K. Bulmer, C. Andres, O. E. Lantseva, V. Borodina, V. V. Poteen, and J. S. Yudkin. 1997. Does malnutrition in utero determine diabetes and coronary heart disease in adulthood? Results from the Leningrad siege study, a cross sectional study. *Brit. Med. J.* 315:1342–1348.

6. Stanner, S. A., and J. S. Yudkin. 2001. Fetal programming and the Leningrad siege study. *Twin Research* 4:287–292.

7. Barker, D. J., C. Osmond, T. J. Forsen, E. Kajantie, and J. G. Eriksson. 2005. Trajectories of growth among children who have coronary events as adults. *N. Engl. J. Med.* 353:1802–1809.

8. Miranda, J. J., S. Kinra, J. P. Casas, G. Davey Smith, and S. Ebrahim. 2008. Non-communicable diseases in low- and middle-income countries: context, determinants and health policy. *Trop. Med. Int. Health.* 13: 1225–1234.

9. Oken, E., J. S. Radesky, R. O. Wright, D. C. Bellinger, C. J. Amarasiriwardena, K. P. Kleinman, H. Hu, and M. W. Gillman. 2008. Associations of maternal fish intake during pregnancy and breastfeeding duration with attainment of developmental milestones in early childhood. *Am. J. Clin. Nutr.* 88:789–796.

10. Maret, W., and H. H. Sandstead. 2008. Possible roles of zinc nutriture in the fetal origins of disease. *Experimental Gerontology* 43:378–381.

11. Catalano, P. M., K. Farrell, A. Thomas, L. Huston-Presley, P. Mencin, S. Hauguel de Mouson, and S. B. Amini. 2009. Perinatal risk factors for childhood obesity and metabolic dysregulation. *Am. J. Clin. Nutr.* 90:1303–1313.

12. Stuebe, A. M., M. R. Forman, and K. B. Michels. 2009. Maternal-recalled gestational weight gain, pre-pregnancy body mass index, and obesity in the daughter. *Int.l J. Obesity.* 33:743–752.

13. Bouret, S. G. 2010. Role of early hormonal and nutritional experiences in shaping feeding behavior and hypothalamic development. *J. Nutr.* 140:653–657.

14. Stothard, K. J., P. W. G. Tennant, R. Bell, and J. Rankin. 2009. Maternal overweight and obesity and the risk of congenital anomalies: a systematic review and meta-analysis. *JAMA* 301:636–650.

15. Clausen, T. D., E. R. Mathiesen, T. Hansen, O. Pedersen, D. M. Jensen, J. Lauenborg, and P. Damm. 2008. High prevalence of type 2 diabetes and pre-diabetes in adult offspring of women with gestational diabetes mellitus or type 1 diabetes. *Diab. Care* 31:340–346.

16. Clausen, T. D., E. R. Mathiesen, T. Hansen, O. Pedersen, D. M. Jensen, J. Lauenborg, L. Schmidt, and P. Damm. 2009. Overweight and the metabolic syndrome in adult offspring of women with diet-treated gestational diabetes mellitus or type 1 diabetes. *J. Clin. Endocrinology. Metab.* 94:2464–2470.

17. Jenkins, K. J., A. Correa, J. A. Feinstein, L. Botto, A. E. Britt, S. R. Daniels, M. Elixson, C. A. Warnes, and C. L. Webb. 2007.

Noninherited risk factors and congenital cardiovascular defects: current knowledge. *Circulation* 115:2995–3014.
18. Cetin, I., C. Berti, and S. Calabrese. 2009. Role of micronutrients in the periconceptual period. *Hum. Reproduction Update* 16:80–95.
19. Lie, R. T., A. J. Wilxoc, J. Taylor, H. K. Gjessing, L. D. Saugstad, F. Aabyholm, and H. Vindenes. 2008. Maternal smoking and oral clefts: the role of detoxification pathway genes. *Epidemiology* 55:382–288.
20. Zucker, M. 2002. Smoking during pregnancy: even worse than you think. Pulmonary Reviews.com 7(3). Available at http://www.pulmonaryreviews.com/march02/smoking.html. Accessed March 2010.
21. March of Dimes. 2007. Quick Reference Fact Sheets: Environmental Risks and Pregnancy. http://www.marchofdimes.com/professionals/14332_9146.asp. Accessed March 2010.
22. Centers for Disease Control and Prevention. Chronic Disease and Health Promotion. 2009. Chronic Disease Overview. December 17. Available at www.cdc.gov/chronicdisease/overview/index.htm#2. Accessed March 2010.

Chapter 15

1. Ogden, C. L., M. D. Carroll, L. R. Curtin, M. M. Lamb, and K. M. Flegal. 2010. Prevalence of high body mass index in U.S. children and adolescents, 2007–2008. *JAMA* 303:242–249.
2. Institute of Medicine, Food and Nutrition Board. 2002. Dietary Reference Intakes for Energy, Carbohydrates, Fiber, Fat, Protein and Amino Acids (Macronutrients). Washington, DC: National Academies Press.
3. Kleinman, R. E. (ed.) 2009. Pediatric Nutrition Handbook, 6th edn. Elk Grove Village, IL: American Academy of Pediatrics.
4. Institute of Medicine, Food and Nutrition Board. 1997. Dietary Reference Intakes for Calcium, Phosphorus, Magnesium, Vitamin D, and Fluoride. Washington, DC: National Academies Press.
5. Institute of Medicine, Food and Nutrition Board. 2001. Dietary Reference Intakes for Vitamin A, Vitamin K, Arsenic, Boron, Chromium, Copper, Iodine, Iron, Manganese, Molybdenum, Nickel, Silicon, Vanadium, and Zinc. Washington, DC: National Academies Press.
6. Institute of Medicine, Food and Nutrition Board. 2004. Dietary Reference Intakes for Water, Potassium, Sodium, Chloride, and Sulfate. Washington, DC: National Academies Press.
7. King, L. 2010. Vegan Children Malnutrition Myths. Available at http://www.associatedcontent.com/article/2917766/vegan_children_malnutrition_myths.html.
8. Stern, R. 2007. Diet from hell. *Phoenix New Times*, May 10, 2007. www.phoenixnewtimes.com/2007-05-10/news/diet-from-hell/.
9. Anon. 2009. Vegetarian Diets — Is it safe for children to be vegetarians? Available at http://www.webmd.com/food-recipes/tc/vegetarian-diets-is-it-safe-for-children-to-be-vegetarians. (Accessed June 2010.)
10. Craig, W. C., and A. R. Mangels. 2009. Position of the American Dietetic Association: Vegetarian Diets. *J. Am. Diet. Assoc* 109:1266–1282.
11. Sanders, T. A. B., and J. Manning. 2008. The growth and development of vegan children. *J. Hum. Nutr. Diet.* 5:11–21.
12. Food and Nutrition Board. Institute of Medicine. 1989. Recommended Dietary Allowances, 10th edn. Washington, DC: National Academies Press.
13. Story, M. 2009. The Third School Nutrition Dietary Assessment Study: Findings and policy implications for improving the health of U.S. children. *J. Am. Diet. Assoc.* 109:S7–S13.
14. Hoyland, A., L. Dye, and C. L. Lawton. 2009. A systematic review of the effect of breakfast on the cognitive performance of children and adolescents. *Nutr. Res. Rev.* 22:220–243.
15. Ingwersen, J., M. A. Defeyter, D. O. Kennedy, K. A.Wesnes, and A. B. Scholey. 2007. A low glycaemic index breakfast cereal preferentially prevents children's cognitive performance from declining throughout the morning. *Appetite* 49:240–244.
16. Stallings, V. A., and A. L. Yaktine (eds.) 2007. Nutrition Standards for Foods in Schools: Leading the Way Toward Healthier Youth. Washington, DC: National Academies Press.
17. Miller, C. H. 2009. A practice perspective on the third School Nutrition Dietary Assessment Study. *J. Am. Diet. Assoc.* 109:S14–S17.
18. Murphy, M. M., J. S. Douglass, R. K. Johnson, and L. A. Spence. 2008. Drinking flavored or plain milk is positively associated with nutrient intake and is not associated with adverse effects on weight status in U.S. children and adolescents. *J. Am. Diet. Assoc.* 108:631–639.
19. C. M. Weaver. 2010. Consequences of excluding dairy, milk avoiders, calcium requirements in children. Lactose Intolerance and Health: NIH Consensus Development Conference Program and Abstracts. National Institutes of Health. Bethesda, MD.
20. Nord, M., M. Andrews, and S. Carlson. 2009. Household Food Security in the United States, 2008. U.S.D.A. Economic Research Service Report No. (ERR-66). Available at http://www.ers.usda.gov/publications/err83/.
21. Strang, J., and M. Story. 2005. Adolescent growth and development. In: Stang, J. and M. Story (eds). Guidelines for Adolescent Nutrition Services. Minneapolis, MN. University of Minnesota.
22. Striegel-Moore, R. H., D. Thompson, S. G. Affenito, D. L. Franko, E. Obarzanek, B. A. Barton, G. B. Schreiber, S. R. Daniels, M. Schmidt, and P. B. Crawford. 2006. Correlates of beverage intake in adolescent girls: The National Heart, Lung, and Blood Institute growth and health study. *J. Pediatr.* 148:183–187.
23. World Health organization (WHO). 2010. Health effects of smoking among young people. Retrieved from www.who.int/tobacco/research/youth/health_effects/en/index.html.
24. Centers for Disease Control and Prevention. 2009. Childhood overweight and obesity: Use of BMI to screen for overweight and obesity in children. Available at http://www.cdc.gov/obesity/childhood/defining.html.
25. Ludwig, D. S. 2007. Childhood obesity — the shape of things to come. *New Engl. J. Med.* 357:2325–2327.
26. Ogden, C. L., M. D. Carroll, and K. M. Flegal. 2008. High body mass index for age among U.S. children and adolescents, 2003-2006. *JAMA* 299:2401–2405.
27. Agras, W. S., L. D. Hammer, F. McNicholas, and H. C. Kraemer. 2004. Risk factors for childhood overweight: A prospective study from birth to 9.5 years. *J. Pediatr.* 145:19–24.
28. Zeller, M., and S. Daniels. 2004. The obesity epidemic: Family matters. *J. Pediatr.* 145:3–4.
29. Ritchie, L. D., G. Welk, D. Styne, D. E. Gerstein, and P. B. Crawford. 2005. Family environment and pediatric overweight: What is a parent to do? *J. Am. Diet. Assoc.* 105:S70–S79.
30. U.S. Department of Health and Human Services. 2008. 2008 Physical Activity Guidelines for Americans. Washington, DC. Available at http://www.health.gov/paguidelines/pdf/paguide.pdf.
31. National Center for Health Statistics. 2010. Health, United States 2009: With Special Feature on Medical Technology. Hyattsville, MD.
32. Robinson, K. 2007. Trends in health status and health care use among older women. Aging Trends, No 7. Hyattsville, MD: National Center for Health Statistics.
33. The American Dietetic Association National Center for Nutrition and Dietetics, Kids Activity Pyramid. www.fitness.gov/10tips.htm.
34. Jarosz, P. A., and A. Bellar. 2008. Sarcopenic obesity: An emerging cause of frailty in older adults. *Ger. Nursing.* 30:64–70.
35. Campbell, W. W., C. A. Johnson, G. P. McCabe, and N. S. Carnell. 2008. Dietary protein requirements of younger and older adults. *Am. J. Clin. Nutr.* 88:1322–1329.
36. Houston, D. K., B. J. Nicklas, J. Ding, T. B. Harris, F. A. Tylavsky, A. B. Newman, J. Sun Lee, N. R. Sahyoun, M. Visser, and S. B. Kritchevsky for the Health ABC Study. 2008. Dietary protein intake is associated with lean mass change in older, community-dwelling

adults: The Health, Aging, and Body Composition (Health ABC) Study. *Am. J. Clin. Nutr.* 87:150–155.

37. Institute of Medicine, Food and Nutrition Board. 1998. Dietary Reference Intakes for Thiamin, Riboflavin, Niacin, Vitamin B6, Folate, Vitamin B12, Pantothenic Acid, Biotin, and Choline. Washington, DC: National Academies Press.

38. Hackam, D. G., and S. S. Anand. 2003. Emerging risk factors for atherosclerotic vascular disease: a critical review of the evidence. *J. Am. Med. Assoc.* 290:932–940.

39. Zoico, E., V. DiFrancesco, J. M. Guralmik, G. Mazzali, A. Bortolani, S. Guariento, G. Sergi, O. Bosello, and M. Zamboni. 2004. Physical disability and muscular strength in relation to obesity and different body composition indexes in a sample of healthy elderly women. *International J. Obesity* 28:234–241.

40. Dolan, C. M., H. Kraemer, W. Browner, K. Ensrud, and J. L. Kelsy. 2007. Associations between body composition, anthropometry, and mortality in women aged 65 years and older. *Am. J. Public Health* 97:913–918.

41. Qato, D. M., G. C. Alexander, R. M. Conti, M. Johnson, P. Schumm, and S. T. Lindau. 2008. Use of prescription and over-the-counter medications and dietary supplements among older adults in the United States. *JAMA* 300:2867–2878.

42. National Eye Institute, National Institutes of Health. November 2003. Photos, Images, and Videos. Ref. no. EDS05. www.nei.nih.gov/photo/search/keyword.asp?keyword5macular; and National Eye Institute, National Institutes of Health. November 2003. Photos, Images, and Videos. Ref. no. EDS03. www.nei.nih.gov/photo/search/keyword.asp?keyword cataract.

43. Nord, M., M. Andrews, and S. Carlson. 2009. Household Food Security in the United States, 2008. U.S.D.A. Economic Research Service Report No. (EER-83). Available at http://www.ers.usda .gov/publications/err83/

44. Schoenborn, C.A. and P.F. Adams. 2010. Health behaviors of adults: United States, 2005-2007. National Center for Health Statistics. Vital Health State 10(245). Available at http://www.cdc .gov/nchs/data/series/sr_10/sr10_245.pdf.

45. Centers for Disease Control and Prevention. 2010. How much physical activity do older adults need? Available at http://www .cdc.gov/physicalactivity/everyone/guidelines/olderadults.html.

46. Thompson, P. D., B. A. Franklin, G. J. Balady, S. N. Blair, D. Corrado, N.A. M. Estes III, J. E. Fulton, N. F. Gordon, W. L. Haskell, M. S. Link, B. J. Maron, M. A. Mittleman, A. Pelliccia, N. K. Wenger, S. N. Willich, and F. Costa. 2007. Exercise and acute cardiovascular events: placing the risks into perspective. A scientific statement from the American Heart Association Council on Nutrition, Physical Activity, and Metaoblism and the Council on Clinical Cardiology. *Circulation* 115:2358–2368.

In Depth: Searching for the Fountain of Youth

1. Mayo Clinic. 2009. Calorie-restriction diet for anti-aging. www.mayoclinic.com/health/calorie-restriction-diet/MY00578.

2. Fontana, L., L. Partridge, and V. D. Longo. 2010. Extending healthy life span — from yeast to humans. *Science* 328:321–226.

3. Speakman, J. 2010. Can calorie restriction increase the human lifespan? Experimental Biology 2010. April 24.

4. Fontana, L.. and S. Klein. 2007. Aging, adiposity, and calorie restriction. *J. Am. Med. Assoc.* 297:986–994.

5. Masoro, E. J. 2005. Overview of caloric restriction and ageing. *Mech. Ageing Dev.* 126:913–922.

6. Helibron, L. K., and E. Ravussin. 2003. Calorie restriction and aging: review of the literature and implications for studies in humans. *Am. J. Clin. Nutr.* 78(3):361–369.

7. Kostoff, R. N. 2001. Energy restriction. *Am. J. Clin. Nutr.* 74(4):556–557.

8. Heilbronn, L. K., S. R. Smith, C. K. Martin, S. D. Anton, and E. Ravussin. 2005. Alternate-day fasting in nonobese subjects: effects on body weight, body composition, and energy metabolism. *Am. J. Clin. Nutr.* 81:69–73.

9. Ames, B. 2005. Increasing longevity by tuning up metabolism. *EMBO Reports* 6:S20–S23.

10. Thomas, D. R. 2006. Vitamins in aging, health, and longevity. *Clinical Interventions in Aging* 1:81–91.

11. Bjelakovic, G., D. Nikolova, L. Lotte Gluud, R. G. Simonetti, and C. Gluud. 2007. Mortality in randomized trials of antioxidant supplements for primary and secondary prevention: Systemic review and analysis. *JAMA* 297:842–857.

12. National Center for Complementary and Alternative Medicine. 2008. Herbs at a Glance: Ginkgo. Available at http://nccam.nih .gov/health/ginkgo.

13. Mayo Clinic 2009. Human growth hormone (HGH): Does it slow aging? Available at: www.mayoclinic.com/health/ growth-hormone/HA00030. (Accessed June 2010)

14. Mayo Clinic 2009. DHEA: Evidence for anti-aging claims is weak. Available at: www.mayoclinic.com/health/dhea/HA00084.

15. Centers for Disease Control and Prevention (CDC). 2009. Chronic disease overview. Available at: www.cdc.gov/chronicdisease/ overview/.

16. Centers for Disease Control and Prevention (CDC). 2010. Smoking and Tobacco Use: Fast Facts, April 30, 2010. Available at www.cdc.gov/tobacco/data_statistics/fact_sheets/fast_facts/ index.htm#toll.

ANSWERS TO REVIEW QUESTIONS

Answers to Review Questions 11-15 (essay questions) for each chapter are located on the Companion Website at **www.pearsonhighered.com/thompsonmanore**

Chapter 1

1. **d.** micronutrients.
2. **b.** National Institutes of Health.
3. **c.** contain 90 kcal of energy.
4. **d.** "A high-protein diet increases the risk for porous bones" is an example of a hypothesis.
5. **d.** all of the above
6. False. Vitamins do not provide any energy, although many vitamins are critical to the metabolic processes that assist us in generating energy from carbohydrates, fats, and proteins.
7. True.
8. True.
9. True.
10. True.

Chapter 2

1. **d.** The % Daily Values of select nutrients in a serving of the packaged food.
2. **b.** provides enough of the energy, nutrients, and fiber to maintain a person's health.
3. **a.** at least half your grains as whole grains each day.
4. **c.** Being physically active each day.
5. **b.** Foods with a lot of nutrients per Calorie, such as fish, are more nutritious choices than foods with fewer nutrients per Calorie, such as candy.
6. False. There is no standardized definition for a serving size for foods.
7. False. Structure-function claims can be made wihout FDA approval.
8. True.
9. True.
10. False. A Pew Research Center report states that about one-third of Americans eat out about once a week, and another one-third eat out two or more times per week.

Chapter 3

1. **c.** atoms, molecules, cells, tissues, organs, systems
2. **d.** emulsifies fats.
3. **c.** hypothalamus.
4. **a.** seepage of gastric acid into the esophagus.
5. **c.** small intestine.
6. True.
7. True.
8. False. Vitamins and minerals are not really "digested" the same way that macronutrients are. These compounds do not have to be broken down because they are small enough to be readily absorbed by the small intestine. For example, fat-soluble vitamins, such as vitamins A, D, E, and K, are soluble in lipids and are absorbed into the intestinal cells along with the fats in our foods. Water-soluble vitamins, such as the B vitamins and vitamin C, typically undergo some type of active transport process that helps assure the vitamin is absorbed by the small intestine. Minerals are absorbed all along the small intestine, and in some cases in the large intestine as well, by a wide variety of mechanisms.
9. False. If you have diarrhea, bowel rest is recommended. In contrast, increasing your fiber might be advised if you're prone to constipation.
10. False. Cells are the smallest units of life. Atoms are the smallest units of matter in nature.

Chapter 4

1. **b.** the potential of foods to raise blood glucose and insulin levels.
2. **d.** carbon, hydrogen, and oxygen.
3. **d.** sweetened soft drinks.
4. **a.** monosaccharides.
5. **a.** phenylketonuria.
6. False. Sugar alcohols are considered nutritive sweeteners because they contain 2 to 4 kcal of energy per gram.
7. True.
8. False. Adults need at least 25 grams of fiber daily.
9. False. Plants store glucose as starch.
10. False. Salivary amylase breaks starches into maltose and shorter polysaccharides.

Chapter 5

1. **d.** found in leafy green vegetables, flax seeds, soy milk, and fish.
2. **b.** exercise regularly.
3. **a.** lipoprotein lipase.
4. **d.** all of the above.
5. **a.** monounsaturated fats.
6. True.
7. False. Fat is an important source of energy during rest and during exercise, and adipose tissue is our primary storage site for fat. We rely significantly on the fat stored in our adipose tissue to provide energy during rest and exercise.
8. False. A triglyceride is a lipid comprised of a glycerol molecule and three fatty acids. Thus, fatty acids are a component of triglycerides.
9. False. While most trans fatty acids result from the hydrogenation of vegetable oils by food manufacturers, a small amount of trans fatty acids are found in cow's milk.
10. False. A serving of food labeled reduced fat has at least 25% less fat than a standard serving, but may not have fewer Calories than a full-fat version of the same food.

Chapter 6

1. **d.** mutual supplementation.
2. **a.** Rice, pinto beans, acorn squash, soy butter, and almond milk.
3. **c.** protease.
4. **b.** amine group.
5. **c.** carbon, oxygen, hydrogen, and nitrogen.
6. True.
7. False. Both shape and function are lost when a protein is denatured.
8. False. Some hormones are made from lipids.
9. False. Buffers help the body maintain acid-base balance.
10. False. Depending upon the type of sport, athletes may require the same or up to two times as much protein as nonactive people.

Chapter 7

1. **b.** It can be found in fresh fruits and vegetables.
2. **d.** A healthy infant of average weight.
3. **a.** extracellular fluid.
4. **d.** It is freely permeable to water but impermeable to solutes.
5. **d.** all of the above.
6. False. In addition to water, the body needs electrolytes, such as sodium and potassium, to prevent fluid imbalances during long-distance events such as a marathon. As purified water contains no electrolytes, this would not be the ideal beverage to prevent fluid imbalances during a marathon.

7. False. Our thirst mechanism is triggered by an increase in the concentration of electrolytes in our blood.
8. False. Hypernatremia is commonly caused by a rapid intake of high amounts of sodium.
9. False. Quenching our thirst does not guarantee adequate hydration. Urine that is clear or light yellow in color is one indicator of adequate hydration.
10. False. These conditions are associated with decreased fluid loss or an increase in body fluid. Diarrhea, blood loss, and low humidity are conditions that increase fluid loss.

Chapter 8

1. **d.** It is destroyed by exposure to high heat.
2. **b.** an atom loses an electron.
3. **a.** cardiovascular disease.
4. **d.** all of the above.
5. **a.** vitamin A.
6. True.
7. True.
8. False. Vitamin C helps regenerate vitamin E.
9. True.
10. False. Pregnant women should not consume beef liver very often, as it can lead to vitamin A toxicity and potentially serious birth defects.

Chapter 9

1. **a.** calcium and phosphorus.
2. **c.** has normal bone density as compared to an average, healthy 30-year-old.
3. **d.** It provides the scaffolding for cortical bone.
4. **c.** a fair-skinned retired teacher living in a nursing home in Ohio
5. **d.** structure of bone, nerve transmission, and muscle contraction.
6. True.
7. True.
8. False. Our body makes vitamin D by converting a cholesterol compound in our skin to the active form of vitamin D that we need to function. We do not absorb vitamin D from sunlight, but when the ultraviolet rays of the sun hit our skin, they react to eventually form calcitriol, which is considered the primary active form of vitamin D in our bodies.
9. False. Magnesium is a major mineral.
10. True.

Chapter 10

1. **d.** thiamin, pantothenic acid, and biotin.
2. **b.** vitamin K.
3. **b.** Iron is a component of hemoglobin, myoglobin, and certain enzymes.
4. **c.** an amino acid.
5. **d.** Choline is necessary for the synthesis of phospholipids and other components of cell membranes.
6. True.
7. True.
8. False. Non-heme iron is found in both plant-based and animal-based foods.
9. False. Neural tube defects occur during the first four weeks of pregnancy; this is often before a woman even knows she is pregnant. Thus, the best way for a woman to protect her fetus against neural tube defects is to make sure she is consuming adequate folate before she is pregnant.
10. False. Wilson's disease is a rare disorder that causes copper toxicity.

Chapter 11

1. **d.** body mass index.
2. **a.** basal metabolic rate, thermal effect of food, and effect of physical activity.
3. **b.** take in more energy than they expend.
4. **c.** all people have a genetic set-point for their body weight.
5. **a.** hunger.
6. False. It is the apple-shaped fat patterning, or excess fat in the trunk region, that is known to increase a person's risk for many chronic diseases.
7. True.
8. True.
9. False. Healthful weight gain includes eating more energy than you expend and also exercising both to maintain aerobic fitness and to build muscle mass.
10. True.

Chapter 12

1. **c.** 50 to 70% of your estimated maximal heart rate.
2. **a.** 1 to 3 seconds.
3. **b.** fat
4. **c.** seems to increase strength gained in resistance exercise.
5. **d.** drink a beverage containing carbohydrate and electrolytes both before and during the event in amounts that balance hydration with energy, carbohydrate, and electrolyte needs.
6. True.
7. False. A dietary fat intake of 15 to 25% of total energy intake is generally recommended for athletes.
8. False. Carbohydrate loading involves altering duration and intensity of exercise and intake of carbohydrate such that the storage of carbohydrate is maximized.
9. False. Sports anemia is not true anemia, but a transient decrease in iron stores that occurs at the start of an exercise program. This is a result of an initial increase in plasma volume (or water in our blood) that is not matched by an increase in hemoglobin.
10. True.

Chapter 13

1. **c.** within 2 hours of serving.
2. **c.** a type of fungus used to ferment foods.
3. **b.** a flavor enhancer used in a variety of foods.
4. **a.** contain only organically produced ingredients, excluding water and salt.
5. **d.** all of the above.
6. False. The appropriate temperature for cooking foods varies according to the food.
7. False. The ARMS was established by the FDA, not the CDC.
8. True.
9. True.
10. True.

Chapter 14

1. **b.** neural tube defects
2. **c.** oxytocin
3. **a.** fiber
4. **b.** women who begin their pregnancy underweight.
5. **d.** iron-fortified rice cereal.
6. False. These issues are most likely to occur in the first trimester of pregnancy.
7. True.
8. True.
9. False. Caffeine does enter breast milk.
10. False. If uncontrolled, gestational diabetes can result in a baby that is too large as a result of receiving too much glucose across the placenta during fetal life. It can also result in preeclampsia.

Chapter 15

1. **b.** vitamin D
2. **c.** 45 to 65%
3. **d.** allergies
4. **a.** 1/2 cup of iron-fortified cooked oat cereal, two tablespoons of mashed pineapple, and one cup of whole milk

5. **a.** Cigarette smoking can interfere with the metabolism of nutrients.
6. False. Preschool children are able to understand the basic information about which foods are more nutritious and those that should be eaten in moderation. Also, parents are important role models for preschool children.
7. True.
8. False. There are several prescription acne medications that contain vitamin A derivatives, but vitamin A taken in supplement form is not effective in acne treatment and, due to its risk for toxicity, vitamin A should not be used in amounts that exceed 100 percent of the Daily Value.
9. True.
10. True.

GLOSSARY

24-hour recall A data collection tool that assesses everything a person has consumed over the past 24 hours.

A

absorption The physiologic process by which molecules of food are taken from the gastrointestinal tract into the circulation.
Acceptable Daily Intake (ADI) An FDA estimate of the amount of a non-nutritive sweetener that someone can consume each day over a lifetime without adverse effects.
Acceptable Macronutrient Distribution Range (AMDR) The range of macronutrient intakes that provides adequate levels of essential nutrients and is associated with a reduced risk for chronic disease.
acetylcholine A neurotransmitter that is involved in many functions, including muscle movement and memory storage.
acidosis A disorder in which the blood becomes acidic; that is, the level of hydrogen in the blood is excessive. It can be caused by respiratory or metabolic problems.
added sugars Sugars and syrups that are added to food during processing or preparation.
adenosine triphosphate (ATP) The common currency of energy for virtually all cells of the body.
adequate diet A diet that provides enough of the energy, nutrients, and fiber needed to maintain a person's health.
Adequate Intake (AI) A recommended average daily nutrient intake level based on observed or experimentally determined estimates of nutrient intake by a group of healthy people.
alcohol Chemically, a compound characterized by the presence of a hydroxyl group; in common usage, a beverage made from fermented fruits, vegetables, or grains and containing ethanol.
alcohol abuse The excessive consumption of alcohol, whether chronically or occasionally.
alcohol hangover A consequence of drinking too much alcohol; symptoms include headache, fatigue, dizziness, muscle aches, nausea and vomiting, sensitivity to light and sound, extreme thirst, and mood disturbances.
alcohol poisoning A potentially fatal condition in which an overdose of alcohol results in cardiac and/or respiratory failure.
alcoholic hepatitis Inflammation of the liver caused by alcohol; other forms of hepatitis can be caused by a virus or toxin.
alcoholism A disease state characterized by chronic dependence on alcohol.
alkalosis A disorder in which the blood becomes basic; that is, the level of hydrogen in the blood is deficient. It can be caused by respiratory or metabolic problems.
alpha-linolenic acid An essential fatty acid found in leafy green vegetables, flaxseed oil, soy oil, fish oil, and fish products; an omega-3 fatty acid.
amenorrhea The absence of menstruation. In females who had previously been menstruating, it is defined as the absence of menstrual periods for 3 or more months.
amino acids Nitrogen-containing molecules that combine to form proteins.
amniotic fluid The watery fluid contained within the innermost membrane of the sac containing the fetus. It cushions and protects the growing fetus.
anabolic The term applied to a substance that builds muscle and increases strength.
anaerobic Means "without oxygen," the term used to refer to metabolic reactions that occur in the absence of oxygen.
anencephaly A fatal neural tube defect in which there is partial absence of brain tissue, most likely caused by failure of the neural tube to close.
anorexia nervosa A serious, potentially life-threatening eating disorder characterized by self-starvation, which eventually leads to a deficiency in energy and the essential nutrients the body requires to function normally.
anorexia An absence of appetite.
antibodies Defensive proteins of the immune system. Their production is prompted by the presence of bacteria, viruses, toxins, allergens, and so on.
antioxidant A compound that has the ability to prevent or repair the damage caused by oxidation.
appetite A psychological desire to consume specific foods.
ariboflavinosis A condition caused by riboflavin deficiency.
atherosclerosis A condition characterized by accumulation of deposits of lipids and scar tissue on artery walls. These deposits build up to such a degree that they impair blood flow.
atrophic gastritis A condition that results in low stomach acid secretion; is estimated to occur in about 10–30% of adults older than 50 years.

B

bacteria Microorganisms that lack a true nucleus and have a chemical called peptidoglycan in their cell walls.
balanced diet A diet that contains the combinations of foods that provide the proper proportions of nutrients.
basal metabolic rate (BMR) The energy the body expends to maintain its fundamental physiologic functions.
beriberi A disease of muscle wasting and nerve damage caused by thiamin deficiency.
bile Fluid produced by the liver and stored in the gallbladder; it emulsifies fats in the small intestine.
binge drinking The consumption of five or more alcoholic drinks on one occasion for men, or four or more for women.
binge eating Consumption of a large amount of food in a short period of time, usually accompanied by a feeling of loss of self-control.
binge-eating disorder A disorder characterized by binge eating an average of twice a week or more, typically without compensatory purging.
bioavailability The degree to which our body can absorb and utilize any given nutrient.
biopesticides Chemicals—primarily insecticides—that are derived naturally in order to reduce crop damage.
blood volume The amount of fluid in blood.
body composition The ratio of a person's body fat to lean body mass.
body image A person's perception of his or her body's appearance and functioning.
body mass index (BMI) A measurement representing the ratio of a person's body weight to his or her height.

bolus A mass of food that has been chewed and moistened in the mouth.
bone density The degree of compactness of bone tissue, reflecting the strength of the bones. *Peak bone density* is the point at which a bone is strongest.
brown adipose tissue A type of adipose tissue that has more mitochondria than white adipose tissue, and which can increase energy expenditure by uncoupling oxidation from ATP production. It is found in significant amounts in animals and newborn humans.
brush border The microvilli-covered lining cells of the small intestine's villi. These microvilli tremendously increase the small intestine's absorptive capacity.
buffers Proteins that help maintain proper acid–base balance by attaching to, or releasing, hydrogen ions as conditions change in the body.
bulimia nervosa A serious eating disorder characterized by recurrent episodes of binge eating and recurrent inappropriate compensatory behaviors in order to prevent weight gain, such as self-induced vomiting, fasting, excessive exercise, or misuse of laxatives, diuretics, enemas, or other medications.

C

calcitonin A hormone secreted by the thyroid gland when blood calcium levels are too high. Calcitonin inhibits the actions of vitamin D, preventing reabsorption of calcium in the kidneys, limiting calcium absorption in the small intestine, and inhibiting the osteoclasts from breaking down bone.
calcitriol The primary active form of vitamin D in the body.
calcium rigor A failure of muscles to relax, which leads to a hardening or stiffening of the muscles; caused by high levels of blood calcium.
calcium tetany A condition in which muscles experience twitching and spasms as a result of inadequate blood calcium levels.
cancer A group of diseases characterized by cells that reproduce spontaneously and independently and may invade other tissues and organs.
carbohydrate One of the three macronutrients, a compound made up of carbon, hydrogen, and oxygen that is derived from plants and provides energy.
carbohydrate loading Also known as glycogen loading. A process that involves altering training and carbohydrate intake, so that muscle glycogen storage is maximized.
carcinogen Any substance capable of causing the cellular mutations that lead to cancer, such as certain pesticides, industrial chemicals, and pollutants.
cardiovascular disease A general term that refers to abnormal conditions involving dysfunction of the heart and blood vessels; cardiovascular disease can result in heart attack or stroke.
carotenoid A fat-soluble plant pigment that the body stores in the liver and adipose tissues. The body is able to convert certain carotenoids to vitamin A.
cash crops Crops grown to be sold rather than eaten, such as cotton, tobacco, jute, and sugarcane.
celiac disease An autoimmune disorder characterized by an inability to absorb a component of gluten called gliadin. This causes an inflammatory immune response that damages the lining of the small intestine.
cell The smallest unit of matter that exhibits the properties of living things, such as growth, reproduction, and metabolism.
cell differentiation The process by which immature, undifferentiated stem cells develop into highly specialized functional cells of discrete organs and tissues.
cell membrane The boundary of an animal cell that separates its internal cytoplasm and organelles from the external environment.
Centers for Disease Control and Prevention (CDC) The leading federal agency in the United States that protects the health and safety of people. Its mission is to promote health and quality of life by preventing and controlling disease, injury, and disability.
cephalic phase The earliest phase of digestion, in which the brain thinks about and prepares the digestive organs for the consumption of food.
chronic diseases Diseases that come on slowly and can persist for years, often despite treatment.
chylomicron A lipoprotein produced in the mucosal cell of the intestine; transports dietary fat out of the intestinal tract.
chyme A semifluid mass consisting of partially digested food, water, and gastric juices.
cirrhosis of the liver Endstage liver disease characterized by significant abnormalities in liver structure and function; may lead to complete liver failure.
coenzyme A molecule that combines with an enzyme to activate it and help it do its job.
cofactor A mineral or other substance that is needed to allow enzymes to function properly.
colic A condition of inconsolable infant crying that lasts for hours at a time.
collagen A protein found in all the connective tissues in our body.
colostrum The first fluid made and secreted by the breasts from late in pregnancy to about a week after birth. It is rich in immune factors and protein.
complementary proteins Two or more foods that together contain all nine essential amino acids necessary for a complete protein. It is not necessary to eat complementary proteins at the same meal.
complete proteins Foods that contain all nine essential amino acids.
complex carbohydrate A nutrient compound consisting of long chains of glucose molecules, such as starch, glycogen, and fiber.
conception (also called *fertilization*) The uniting of an ovum (egg) and sperm to create a fertilized egg, or zygote.
constipation A condition characterized by the absence of bowel movements for a period of time that is significantly longer than normal for the individual. When a bowel movement does occur, stools are usually small, hard, and difficult to pass.
cool-down Activities done after an exercise session is completed; should be gradual and allow your body to slowly recover from exercise.
cortical bone (compact bone) A dense bone tissue that makes up the outer surface of all bones as well as the entirety of most small bones of the body.
creatine phosphate (CP) A high-energy compound that can be broken down for energy and used to regenerate ATP.
cretinism A form of mental retardation that occurs in children whose mothers experienced iodine deficiency during pregnancy.
cross-contamination Contamination of one food by another via the unintended transfer of microbes through physical contact.
cytoplasm The interior of an animal cell, not including its nucleus.

D

danger zone The range of temperature at which many microorganisms capable of causing human illness thrive; about 40°F to 140°F (4°C to 60°C).
DASH diet The diet developed in response to research into hypertension funded by the National Institutes of Health: DASH stands for "Dietary Approaches to Stop Hypertension."
deamination The process by which an amine group is removed from an amino acid. The nitrogen is then transported to the kidneys for excretion in the urine, while the carbon and other components are metabolized for energy or used to make other compounds.
dehydration The depletion of body fluid that results when fluid excretion exceeds fluid intake.
denaturation The process by which proteins uncoil and lose their shape and function when they are exposed to heat, acids, bases, heavy metals, alcohol, and other damaging substances.
denature The action of the unfolding of proteins in the stomach. Proteins must be denatured before they can be digested.
dental caries Dental erosion and decay caused by acid-secreting bacteria in the mouth and on the teeth. The acid produced is a by-product of bacterial metabolism of carbohydrates deposited on the teeth.
diabetes A chronic disease in which the body can no longer regulate glucose normally.
diarrhea A condition characterized by the frequent passage of loose, watery stools.
dietary fiber The nondigestible carbohydrate parts of plants that form the support structures of leaves, stems, and seeds.
Dietary Guidelines for Americans A set of principles developed by the U.S. Department of Agriculture and the U.S. Department of Health and Human Services to assist Americans in designing a healthful diet and lifestyle. These Guidelines are updated every 5 years.
Dietary Reference Intakes (DRIs) A set of nutritional reference values for the United States and Canada that applies to healthy people.
dietary supplement A product taken by mouth that contains a "dietary ingredient" intended to supplement the diet.
digestion The process by which foods are broken down into their component molecules, either mechanically or chemically.
disaccharide A carbohydrate compound consisting of two sugar molecules joined together.
diseases of aging Conditions that typically occur later in life as a result of lifelong accumulated risk, such as exposure to high-fat diets, a lack of physical activity, and excess sun exposure.
disordered eating A variety of abnormal or atypical eating behaviors that are used to keep or maintain a lower body weight.
diuretic A substance that increases fluid loss via the urine. Common diuretics include alcohol, some prescription medications, and many over-the-counter weight-loss pills.
docosahexaenoic acid (DHA) Another metabolic derivative of alpha-linolenic acid; together with EPA, it appears to reduce our risk for a heart attack.
drink The amount of an alcoholic beverage that provides approximately 0.5 fl. oz of pure ethanol.
dual energy x-ray absorptiometry (DXA or DEXA) Currently, the most accurate tool for measuring bone density.

E

eating disorder A clinically diagnosed psychiatric disorder characterized by severe disturbances in body image and eating behaviors.
edema A disorder in which fluids build up in the tissue spaces of the body, causing fluid imbalances and a swollen appearance.
eicosapentaenoic acid (EPA) A metabolic derivative of alpha-linolenic acid.
electrolyte A substance that disassociates in solution into positively and negatively charged ions and is thus capable of carrying an electrical current.
electron A negatively charged particle orbiting the nucleus of an atom.
elimination The process by which undigested portions of food and waste products are removed from the body.
embryo The human growth and developmental stage lasting from the third week to the end of the eighth week after fertilization.
empty calories A term used by the USDA to indicate Calories from solid fats and/or added sugars.
energy cost of physical activity The energy that is expended on body movement and muscular work above basal levels.
energy expenditure The energy the body expends to maintain its basic functions and to perform all levels of movement and activity.
energy intake The amount of food a person eats; in other words, it is the number of kilocalories consumed.
enriched foods Foods in which nutrients that were lost during processing have been added back, so that the food meets a specified standard.
enteric nervous system The nerves of the GI tract.
enzymes Small chemicals, usually proteins, that act on other chemicals to speed up body processes but are not apparently changed during those processes.
epiphyseal plates Plates of cartilage located toward the end of long bones that provide for growth in the length of long bones.
ergogenic aids Substances used to improve exercise and athletic performance.
erythrocytes The red blood cells, which are the cells that transport oxygen in our blood.
esophagus A muscular tube of the GI tract connecting the back of the mouth to the stomach.
essential amino acids Amino acids not produced by the body that must be obtained from food.
essential fatty acids (EFAs) Fatty acids that must be consumed in the diet because they cannot be made by our bodies. The two essential fatty acids are linoleic acid and alpha-linolenic acid.
Estimated Average Requirement (EAR) The average daily nutrient intake level estimated to meet the requirement of half the healthy individuals in a particular life stage or gender group.
Estimated Energy Requirement (EER) The average dietary energy intake that is predicted to maintain energy balance in a healthy adult.
ethanol A specific alcohol compound (C_2H_5OH) formed from the fermentation of dietary carbohydrates and used in a variety of alcoholic beverages.

evaporative cooling Another term for sweating, which is the primary way in which we dissipate heat.
exercise A subcategory of leisure-time physical activity; any activity that is purposeful, planned, and structured.
extracellular fluid The fluid outside the body's cells, either in the body's tissues or as the liquid portion of blood, called *plasma*.

F

famine A widespread severe food shortage that causes starvation and death in a large portion of a population in a region.
fat-soluble vitamins Vitamins that are not soluble in water but are soluble in fat, including vitamins A, D, E, and K.
fats An important energy source for our body at rest and during low-intensity exercise.
fatty acids Long chains of carbon atoms bound to each other as well as to hydrogen atoms.
fatty liver An early and reversible stage of liver disease often found in people who abuse alcohol and characterized by the abnormal accumulation of fat within liver cells; also called alcoholic steatosis.
female athlete triad A serious syndrome that consists of three clinical conditions in some physically active females: low energy availability (with or without eating disorders), amenorrhea, and osteoporosis.
fermentation A process in which an agent causes an organic substance to break down into simpler substances and results in the production of ATP.
ferritin A storage form of iron in our body, found primarily in the intestinal mucosa, spleen, bone marrow, and liver.
fetal adaptation The process by which a fetus's metabolism, hormone production, and other physiologic processes shift in response to factors, such as inadequate energy intake, in the maternal environment.
fetal alcohol effects (FAE) A set of subtle consequences of maternal intake of alcohol, such as impaired learning and behavioral problems.
fetal alcohol spectrum disorders (FASD) A range of conditions that result from maternal intake of alcohol.
fetal alcohol syndrome (FAS) A set of serious, irreversible alcohol-related birth defects characterized by certain physical and mental abnormalities.
fetus The human growth and developmental stage lasting from the beginning of the ninth week after conception to birth.
FIT principle The principle used to achieve an appropriate overload for physical training; FIT stands for frequency, intensity, and time of activity.
fluid A substance composed of molecules that move past one another freely. Fluids are characterized by their ability to conform to the shape of whatever container holds them.
fluorosis A condition marked by staining and pitting of the teeth; caused by an abnormally high intake of fluoride.
food additives Substances intentionally put into food to enhance appearance, palatability, and quality.
food allergy An inflammatory reaction to food caused by an immune system hypersensitivity.
food insecurity Circumstances in which households are uncertain of having, or unable to acquire, enough food to meet the needs of all their members because they have insufficient money or other resources for food.
food intolerance Gastrointestinal discomfort caused by certain foods that is not a result of an immune system reaction.
food preservatives Chemicals that help prevent microbial spoilage and enzymatic deterioration.
food-borne illness An illness transmitted through food or water, either by an infectious agent, a poisonous substance, or a protein that causes an immune reaction.
fortified foods Foods in which nutrients are added that did not originally exist in the food, or which existed in insignificant amounts.
free radical A highly unstable atom with an unpaired electron in its outermost shell.
frequency The number of activity sessions per week you perform.
fructose The sweetest natural sugar; a monosaccharide that occurs in fruits and vegetables; also called levulose, or fruit sugar.
functional fiber The nondigestible forms of carbohydrates that are extracted from plants or manufactured in a laboratory and have known health benefits.
functional food A food or food component that provides a health benefit beyond basic nutrition.
fungi Plantlike, spore-forming organisms that can grow either as single cells or multicellular colonies.

G

galactose A monosaccharide that joins with glucose to create lactose, one of the three most common disaccharides.
gallbladder A tissue sac beneath the liver that stores bile and secretes it into the small intestine.
gastric juice Acidic liquid secreted within the stomach; it contains hydrochloric acid, pepsin, and other compounds.
gastroesophageal reflux disease (GERD) A more painful type of GER that occurs more than twice per week.
gastrointestinal (GI) tract A long, muscular tube consisting of several organs: the mouth, esophagus, stomach, small intestine, and large intestine.
gene expression The process of using a gene to make a protein.
Generally Recognized as Safe (GRAS) A designated list established by Congress that identifies several hundred substances that either have been tested and found to be safe and approved by the FDA for use in the food industry or are deemed safe as a result of consensus among experts qualified by scientific training and experience.
genetic modification The process of changing an organism by manipulating its genetic material.
gestation The period of intrauterine development from conception to birth.
gestational diabetes Insufficient insulin production or insulin resistance that results in consistently high blood glucose levels, specifically during pregnancy; the condition typically resolves after birth occurs.
ghrelin A protein, synthesized in the stomach, that acts as a hormone and plays an important role in appetite regulation by stimulating appetite.
glucagon The hormone secreted by the alpha cells of the pancreas in response to decreased blood levels of glucose; it causes the breakdown of liver stores of glycogen into glucose.
gluconeogenesis The generation of glucose from the breakdown of proteins into amino acids.

glucose The most abundant sugar molecule, a monosaccharide generally found in combination with other sugars; it is the preferred source of energy for the brain and an important source of energy for all cells.
glycemic index The system that assigns ratings (or values) for the potential of foods to raise blood glucose and insulin levels.
glycemic load The amount of carbohydrate in a food multiplied by the glycemic index of the carbohydrate.
glycerol An alcohol composed of three carbon atoms; it is the backbone of a triglyceride molecule.
glycogen A polysaccharide; the storage form of glucose in animals.
glycolysis The breakdown of glucose; yields two ATP molecules and two pyruvic acid molecules for each molecule of glucose.
goiter Enlargement of the thyroid gland; can be caused by either iodine toxicity or deficiency.
grazing Consistently eating small meals throughout the day; done by many athletes to meet their high energy demands.

H

healthful diet A diet that provides the proper combination of energy and nutrients and is adequate, moderate, balanced, and varied.
heartburn (gastroesophageal reflux [GER]) A painful sensation that occurs over the sternum when hydrochloric acid backs up into the lower esophagus.
heat cramps Involuntary, spasmodic, and painful muscle contractions that are caused by electrolyte imbalances occurring as a result of strenuous physical activity in high environmental heat.
heat exhaustion A serious condition, characterized by heavy sweating, pallor, nausea and vomiting, dizziness, and moderately elevated body temperature, that develops from dehydration in high heat.
heat stroke A potentially fatal response to high temperature characterized by failure of the body's heat-regulating mechanisms, also commonly called *sunstroke*.
helminth A multicellular microscopic worm.
heme The iron-containing molecule found in hemoglobin.
heme iron Iron that is a part of hemoglobin and myoglobin; found only in animal-based foods, such as meat, fish, and poultry.
hemoglobin The oxygen-carrying protein found in our red blood cells; almost two-thirds of all the iron in our body is found in hemoglobin.
hemosiderin A storage form of iron in our body, found primarily in the intestinal mucosa, spleen, bone marrow, and liver.
herb A plant or plant part used for its scent, flavor, and/or therapeutic properties (also called a *botanical*).
hidden fats Fats that are hidden in foods, such as the fats found in baked goods, regular-fat dairy products, marbling in meat, and fried foods.
high-density lipoprotein (HDL) A lipoprotein made in the liver and released into the blood. HDLs function to transport cholesterol from the tissues back to the liver. Often called the "good cholesterol."
homocysteine An amino acid that requires adequate levels of folate, vitamin B_6, and vitamin B_{12} for its metabolism. High levels of homocysteine in the blood are associated with an increased risk for vascular diseases, such as cardiovascular disease.
hormone A chemical messenger secreted into the bloodstream by one of the many glands of the body, which acts as a regulator of physiologic processes at a site remote from the gland that secreted it.
hunger A physiologic sensation that prompts us to eat.
hydrogenation The process of adding hydrogen to unsaturated fatty acids, making them more saturated and thereby more solid at room temperature.
hypercalcemia A condition marked by an abnormally high concentration of calcium in the blood.
hyperkalemia A condition in which blood potassium levels are dangerously high.
hypermagnesemia A condition marked by an abnormally high concentration of magnesium in the blood.
hypernatremia A condition in which blood sodium levels are dangerously high.
hypertension A chronic condition characterized by above-average blood pressure readings—specifically, systolic blood pressure over 140 mm Hg or diastolic blood pressure over 90 mm Hg.
hypocalcemia A condition characterized by an abnormally low concentration of calcium in the blood.
hypoglycemia A condition marked by blood glucose levels that are below normal fasting levels.
hypokalemia A condition in which blood potassium levels are dangerously low.
hypomagnesemia A condition characterized by an abnormally low concentration of magnesium in the blood.
hyponatremia A condition in which blood sodium levels are dangerously low.
hypothalamus A region of forebrain above the pituitary gland, where visceral sensations, such as hunger and thirst, are regulated.
hypothesis An educated guess as to why a phenomenon occurs.

I

impaired fasting glucose Fasting blood glucose levels that are higher than normal but not high enough to lead to a diagnosis of type 2 diabetes; also called *pre-diabetes*.
incomplete proteins Foods that do not contain all of the essential amino acids in sufficient amounts to support growth and health.
insensible water loss The loss of water not noticeable by a person, such as through evaporation from the skin and exhalation from the lungs during breathing.
insoluble fibers Fibers that do not dissolve in water.
insulin The hormone secreted by the beta cells of the pancreas in response to increased blood levels of glucose; it facilitates the uptake of glucose by body cells.
intensity The amount of effort expended during the activity, or how difficult the activity is to perform.
intracellular fluid The fluid held at any given time within the walls of the body's cells.
intrinsic factor A protein secreted by cells of the stomach that binds to vitamin B_{12} and aids its absorption in the small intestine.
ion An electrically charged particle, either positively or negatively charged.

iron-deficiency anemia A form of anemia that results from severe iron deficiency.
irradiation A sterilization process using gamma rays or other forms of radiation, but which does not impart radiation to the food being treated.
irritable bowel syndrome (IBS) A bowel disorder that interferes with normal functions of the colon.

K

Keshan disease A heart disorder caused by selenium deficiency. It was first identified in children in the Keshan province of China.
ketoacidosis A condition in which excessive ketones are present in the blood, causing the blood to become very acidic, which alters basic body functions and damages tissues. Untreated ketoacidosis can be fatal. This condition is found in individuals with untreated diabetes mellitus.
ketones Substances produced during the breakdown of fat when carbohydrate intake is insufficient to meet energy needs. Ketones provide an alternative energy source for the brain when glucose levels are low.
ketosis The process by which the breakdown of fat during fasting states results in the production of ketones.
kwashiorkor A form of protein–energy malnutrition that is typically seen in developing countries in infants and toddlers who are weaned early because of the birth of a subsequent child. Denied breast milk, they are fed a cereal diet that provides adequate energy but inadequate protein.

L

lactase A digestive enzyme that breaks lactose into glucose and galactose.
lactation The production of breast milk.
lacteal A small lymph vessel located inside the villi of the small intestine.
lactic acid A compound that results when pyruvic acid is metabolized in the presence of insufficient oxygen.
lactose A disaccharide consisting of one glucose molecule and one galactose molecule. It is found in milk, including human breast milk; also called *milk sugar*.
lactose intolerance A disorder in which the body does not produce enough lactase enzyme to break down the sugar lactose, which is found in milk and milk products.
large intestine The final organ of the GI tract, consisting of the cecum, colon, rectum, and anal canal and in which most water is absorbed and feces are formed.
leisure-time physical activity Any activity not related to a person's occupation; includes competitive sports, recreational activities, and planned exercise training.
leptin A hormone, produced by body fat, that acts to reduce food intake and to decrease body weight and body fat.
leukocytes The white blood cells, which protect us from infection and illness.
limiting amino acid The essential amino acid that is missing or in the smallest supply in the amino acid pool and is thus responsible for slowing or halting protein synthesis.
linoleic acid An essential fatty acid found in vegetable and nut oils; also known as omega-6 fatty acid.
lipids A diverse group of organic substances that are insoluble in water; lipids include triglycerides, phospholipids, and sterols.
lipoprotein A spherical compound in which fat clusters in the center and phospholipids and proteins form the outside of the sphere.
lipoprotein lipase An enzyme that sits on the outside of cells and breaks apart triglycerides, so that their fatty acids can be removed and taken up by the cell.
liver The largest auxiliary organ of the GI tract and one of the most important organs of the body. Its functions include the production of bile and processing of nutrient-rich blood from the small intestine.
low birth weight Having a weight of less than 5.5 pounds at birth.
low-density lipoprotein (LDL) A lipoprotein formed in the blood from VLDLs that transports cholesterol to the cells of the body. Often called the "bad cholesterol."
low-intensity activities Activities that cause very mild increases in breathing, sweating, and heart rate.

M

macrocytic anemia A form of anemia manifested as the production of larger than normal red blood cells containing insufficient hemoglobin, which inhibits adequate transport of oxygen; also called megaloblastic anemia. Macrocytic anemia can be caused by a severe folate deficiency.
macronutrients Nutrients that our body needs in relatively large amounts to support normal function and health. Carbohydrates, fats, and proteins are macronutrients.
major minerals Minerals that must be consumed in amounts of 100 mg/day or more and that are present in the body at the level of 5 g or more.
malnutrition A state of poor nutritional health that can be improved by adjustments in nutrient intake.
maltase A digestive enzyme that breaks maltose into glucose.
maltose A disaccharide consisting of two molecules of glucose. It does not generally occur independently in foods but results as a by-product of digestion; maltose is also called *malt sugar.*
marasmus A form of protein–energy malnutrition that results from grossly inadequate intakes of protein, energy, and other nutrients.
maximal heart rate The rate at which your heart beats during maximal-intensity exercise.
meat factor A special factor found in meat, fish, and poultry that enhances the absorption of non-heme iron.
megadose A dose of a nutrient that is 10 or more times greater than the recommended amount.
megadosing Consuming nutrients in amounts that are ten or more times higher than recommended levels.
metabolic syndrome A cluster of risks factors that increase one's risk for heart disease, type 2 diabetes, and stroke, including abdominal obesity, higher than normal triglyceride levels, lower than normal HDL-cholesterol levels, higher than normal blood pressure (greater than or equal to 130/85 mm Hg), and elevated fasting blood glucose levels.
metabolic water The water formed as a by-product of our body's metabolic reactions.
metabolism The process by which large molecules, such as carbohydrates, fats, and proteins, are broken down via chemical reactions into smaller molecules that can be used as fuel, stored, or assembled into new compounds the body needs.
metabolites The form that nutrients take when they have been used by the body. For example, lactate is a metabolite of

carbohydrate that is produced when we use carbohydrate for energy.
micronutrients Nutrients needed in relatively small amounts to support normal health and body functions. Vitamins and minerals are micronutrients.
minerals Inorganic substances that are not broken down during digestion and absorption and are not destroyed by heat or light. Minerals assist in the regulation of many body processes and are classified as major minerals or trace minerals.
moderate-intensity activities Activities that cause moderate increases in breathing, sweating, and heart rate.
moderation Eating any foods in moderate amounts—not too much and not too little.
monosaccharide The simplest of carbohydrates, consisting of one sugar molecule, the most common form of which is glucose.
monounsaturated fatty acids (MUFAs) Fatty acids that have two carbons in the chain bound to each other with one double bond; these types of fatty acids are generally liquid at room temperature.
morbid obesity A condition in which a person's body weight exceeds 100% of normal, putting him or her at very high risk for serious health consequences.
morning sickness Varying degrees of nausea and vomiting associated with pregnancy, most commonly in the first trimester.
multifactorial disease Any disease that may be attributable to one or more of a variety of causes.
mutual supplementation The process of combining two or more incomplete protein sources to make a complete protein.
myoglobin An iron-containing protein similar to hemoglobin except that it is found in muscle cells.
MyPlate The USDA interactive food guidance system based on the 2010 Dietary Guidelines for Americans and the Dietary Reference Intakes. MyPlate (chooseMyPlate.gov) was introduced in 2011 and is the visual representation of the USDA Food Patterns.
MyPyramid The previous (2005) graphic representation of the USDA Food Guide. MyPyramid was replaced with MyPlate in 2011.

N

National Institutes of Health (NIH) The world's leading medical research center and the focal point for medical research in the United States.
neural tube Embryonic tissue that forms a tube, which eventually becomes the brain and spinal cord.
neural tube defects The most common malformations of the central nervous system that occur during fetal development. A folate deficiency can cause neural tube defects.
night blindness A vitamin A deficiency disorder that results in loss of the ability to see in dim light.
night-eating syndrome A disorder characterized by intake of the majority of the day's energy between 8:00 PM and 6:00 AM. Individuals with this disorder also experience mood and sleep disorders.
non-heme iron Iron that is not part of hemoglobin or myoglobin; found in both animal-based and plant-based foods.
non-nutritive sweeteners Manufactured sweeteners that provide little or no energy; also called *alternative sweeteners.*
nonessential amino acids Amino acids that can be manufactured by the body in sufficient quantities and therefore do not need to be consumed regularly in our diet.
nucleus The positively charged, central core of an atom. It is made up of two types of particles—protons and neutrons—bound tightly together. The nucleus of an atom contains essentially all of its atomic mass.
nutrient density The relative amount of nutrients per amount of energy (or number of Calories).
nutrient-dense foods Foods that provide the most nutrients for the least amount of energy (Calories).
nutrients Chemicals found in foods that are critical to human growth and function.
nutrition The science that studies food and how food nourishes our body and influences our health.
Nutrition Facts Panel The label on a food package that contains the nutrition information required by the FDA.
nutrition transition A shift in dietary pattern toward greater food security, greater variety of foods, and more foods with high energy density; associated with increased incidence of obesity and chronic disease.
nutritive sweeteners Sweeteners, such as sucrose, fructose, honey, and brown sugar, that contribute Calories (energy).

O

obesity Having an excess of body fat that adversely affects health, resulting in a person weighing substantially more than an accepted standard for a given height.
organ A body structure composed of two or more tissues and performing a specific function; for example, the esophagus.
organelle A tiny "organ" within a cell that performs a discrete function necessary to the cell.
organic A substance or nutrient that contains the elements carbon and hydrogen.
osmosis The movement of water (or any solvent) through a semipermeable membrane from an area where solutes are less concentrated to areas where solutes are highly concentrated.
osteoblasts Cells that prompt the formation of new bone matrix by laying down the collagen-containing component of bone, which is then mineralized.
osteoclasts Cells that erode the surface of bones by secreting enzymes and acids that dig grooves into the bone matrix.
osteomalacia A vitamin D–deficiency disease in adults, in which bones become weak and prone to fractures.
osteoporosis A disease characterized by low bone mass and deterioration of bone tissue, leading to increased bone fragility and fracture risk.
ounce-equivalent (oz-equivalent) A serving size that is 1 ounce, or equivalent to an ounce, for the grains section and the meats and beans section of the USDA Food Guide.
overload principle Placing an extra physical demand on your body in order to improve your fitness level.
overnutrition Malnutrition defined by an absolute excess of calories leading to overweight. Diet may be high quality or poor quality.
overpopulated A term used to describe a region that has insufficient resources to support the number of people living there.
overweight Having a moderate amount of excess body fat, resulting in a person weighing more than an accepted standard for a given height, but not considered obese.
ovulation The release of an ovum (egg) from a woman's ovary.
oxidation A chemical reaction in which molecules of a substance are broken down into their component atoms. During oxidation, the atoms involved lose electrons.

P

pancreas A gland located behind the stomach that secretes digestive enzymes.

pancreatic amylase An enzyme secreted by the pancreas into the small intestine that digests any remaining starch into maltose.
parasite A microorganism that simultaneously derives benefit from and harms its host.
parathyroid hormone (PTH) A hormone secreted by the parathyroid gland when blood calcium levels fall. Also known as parathormone, it increases blood calcium levels by stimulating the activation of vitamin D, increasing reabsorption of calcium from the kidneys, and stimulating osteoclasts to break down bone, which releases more calcium into the bloodstream.
pasteurization A form of sterilization using high temperatures for short periods of time.
pellagra A disease that results from severe niacin deficiency.
pepsin An enzyme in the stomach that begins the breakdown of proteins into shorter polypeptide chains and single amino acids.
peptic ulcer An area of the GI tract that has been eroded away by the acidic gastric juice of the stomach.
peptide bonds Unique types of chemical bonds in which the amine group of one amino acid binds to the acid group of another in order to manufacture dipeptides and all larger peptide molecules.
peptide YY (PYY) A protein, produced in the gastrointestinal tract, that is released after a meal in amounts proportional to the energy content of the meal; it decreases appetite and inhibits food intake.
percent Daily Values (%DV) Information on a Nutrition Facts Panel that identifies how much a serving of food contributes to your overall intake of the nutrients listed on the label; based on an energy intake of 2,000 Calories per day.
peristalsis Waves of squeezing and pushing contractions that move food in one direction through the length of the GI tract.
pernicious anemia A form of anemia that is the primary cause of a vitamin B_{12} deficiency; occurs at the end stage of a disorder that causes the loss of certain cells in the stomach.
persistent organic pollutants (POPs) Chemicals released into the environment as a result of industry, agriculture, or improper waste disposal; automobile emissions also are considered POPs.
pesticides Chemicals used either in the field or in storage to destroy plant, fungal, and animal pests.
pH Stands for percentage of hydrogen. It is a measure of the acidity—or level of hydrogen—of any solution, including human blood.
phospholipids A type of lipid in which a fatty acid is combined with another compound that contains phosphate; unlike other lipids, phospholipids are soluble in water.
photosynthesis The process by which plants use sunlight to fuel a chemical reaction that combines carbon and water into glucose, which is then stored in their cells.
physical activity Any movement produced by muscles that increases energy expenditure; includes occupational, household, leisure-time, and transportation activities.
Physical Activity Pyramid A pyramid-shaped graphic that suggests types and amounts of activity that should be done weekly to increase physical activity levels.
physical fitness The ability to carry out daily tasks with vigor and alertness, without undue fatigue, and with ample energy to enjoy leisure-time pursuits and meet unforeseen emergencies.
phytic acid The form of phosphorus stored in plants.
phytochemicals Compounds found in plants that are believed to have health-promoting effects in humans.
pica An abnormal craving to eat non-food substances such as clay, paint, or chalk.
placenta A pregnancy-specific organ formed from both maternal and embryonic tissues. It is responsible for oxygen, nutrient, and waste exchange between mother and fetus.
plasma The fluid portion of the blood; needed to maintain adequate blood volume, so that the blood can flow easily throughout our body.
platelets Cell fragments that assist in the formation of blood clots and help stop bleeding.
polysaccharide A complex carbohydrate consisting of long chains of glucose.
polyunsaturated fatty acids (PUFAs) Fatty acids that have more than one double bond in the chain; these types of fatty acids are generally liquid at room temperature.
preeclampsia High blood pressure that is pregnancy-specific and accompanied by protein in the urine, edema, and unexpected weight gain.
preterm The birth of a baby prior to 38 weeks' gestation.
prion An infectious, self-replicating protein.
processed foods Foods that are manipulated mechanically or chemically during their production or packaging. Processed foods may or may not resemble the original ingredients in their final form.
proof A measure of the alcohol content of a liquid; 100 proof liquor is 50% alcohol by volume, 80 proof liquor is 40% alcohol by volume, and so on.
prooxidant A nutrient that promotes oxidation and oxidative cell and tissue damage.
proteases Enzymes that continue the breakdown of polypeptides in the small intestine.
protein–energy malnutrition A disorder caused by inadequate consumption of protein. It is characterized by severe wasting.
proteins Large, complex molecules made up of amino acids and found as essential components of all living cells.
protozoa Single-celled, mobile microorganisms.
provitamin An inactive form of a vitamin that the body can convert to an active form. An example is beta-carotene.
puberty The period of life in which secondary sexual characteristics develop and people become biologically capable of reproducing.
purging An attempt to rid the body of unwanted food by vomiting or other compensatory means, such as excessive exercise, fasting, or laxative abuse.
pyruvic acid The primary end product of glycolysis.

R

recombinant bovine growth hormone (rBGH) A genetically engineered hormone injected into dairy cows to enhance their milk output.
recombinant DNA technology A type of genetic modification in which scientists combine DNA from different sources to produce a transgenic organism that expresses a desired trait.
Recommended Dietary Allowance (RDA) The average daily nutrient intake level that meets the nutrient requirements of 97–98% of healthy individuals in a particular life stage and gender group.
remodeling The two-step process by which bone tissue is recycled; includes the breakdown of existing bone and the formation of new bone.

residues Chemicals that remain in foods despite cleaning and processing.
resistance training Exercises in which our muscles act against resistance.
resorption The process by which the surface of bone is broken down by cells called osteoclasts.
resveratrol A potent phenolic antioxidant found in red wine as well as grapes and nuts.
retina The delicate, light-sensitive membrane lining the inner eyeball and connected to the optic nerve. It contains retinal.
retinal An active, aldehyde form of vitamin A that plays an important role in healthy vision and immune function.
retinoic acid An active, acid form of vitamin A that plays an important role in cell growth and immune function.
retinol An active, alcohol form of vitamin A that plays an important role in healthy vision and immune function.
rhodopsin A light-sensitive pigment found in the rod cells that is formed by retinal and opsin.
ribose A five-carbon monosaccharide that is located in the genetic material of cells.
rickets A vitamin D–deficiency disease in children. Signs include deformities of the skeleton, such as bowed legs and knocked knees. Severe rickets can be fatal.

S

saliva A mixture of water, mucus, enzymes, and other chemicals that moistens the mouth and food, binds food particles together, and begins the digestion of carbohydrates.
salivary amylase An enzyme in saliva that breaks starch into smaller particles and eventually into the disaccharide maltose.
salivary glands A group of glands found under and behind the tongue and beneath the jaw that release saliva continually as well as in response to the thought, sight, smell, or presence of food.
saturated fatty acids (SFAs) Fatty acids that have no carbons joined together with a double bond; these types of fatty acids are generally solid at room temperature.
sensible water loss Water loss that is noticed by a person, such as through urine output and visible sweating.
set-point theory The theory that the body raises or lowers energy expenditure in response to increased or decreased food intake and physical activity. This action maintains an individual's body weight within a narrow range.
simple carbohydrate Commonly called *sugar;* can be either a monosaccharide (such as glucose) or a disaccharide.
small intestine The longest portion of the GI tract, where most digestion and absorption takes place.
soluble fibers Fibers that dissolve in water.
solvent A substance that is capable of mixing with and breaking apart a variety of compounds. Water is an excellent solvent.
sphincter A tight ring of muscle separating some of the organs of the GI tract and opening in response to nerve signals indicating that food is ready to pass into the next section.
spina bifida The embryotic neural tube defect that occurs when the spinal vertebrae fail to completely enclose the spinal cord, allowing it to protrude.
spontaneous abortion (also called *miscarriage*) The natural termination of a pregnancy and expulsion of pregnancy tissues because of a genetic, developmental, or physiologic abnormality that is so severe that the pregnancy cannot be maintained.
starch A polysaccharide stored in plants; the storage form of glucose in plants.
sterols A type of lipid found in foods and the body that has a ring structure; cholesterol is the most common sterol that occurs in our diets.
stomach A J-shaped organ where food is partially digested, churned, and stored until it is released into the small intestine.
stunting Low height for age.
sucrase A digestive enzyme that breaks sucrose into glucose and fructose.
sucrose A disaccharide composed of one glucose molecule and one fructose molecule; sucrose is sweeter than lactose or maltose.
sudden infant death syndrome (SIDS) The sudden death of a previously healthy infant; the most common cause of death in infants over 1 month of age.
sustainable agriculture Techniques of food production that preserve the environment indefinitely.
system A group of organs that work together to perform a unique function; for example, the gastrointestinal system.

T

T-score A comparison of an individual's bone density to the average peak bone density of a 30-year-old healthy adult.
teratogen A compound known to cause fetal harm or danger.
theory A conclusion drawn from repeated experiments.
thermic effect of food (TEF) The energy expended as a result of processing food consumed.
thirst mechanism A cluster of nerve cells in the hypothalamus that stimulate our conscious desire to drink fluids in response to an increase in the concentration of salt in our blood or a decrease in blood pressure and blood volume.
thrifty gene theory The theory that some people possess a gene (or genes) that causes them to be energetically thrifty, resulting in their expending less energy at rest and during physical activity.
time of activity How long each exercise session lasts.
tissue A grouping of like cells that performs a function; for example, muscle tissue.
tocopherol The active form of vitamin E in our body.
Tolerable Upper Intake Level (UL) The highest average daily nutrient intake level likely to pose no risk of adverse health effects to almost all individuals in a particular life stage and gender group.
total fiber The sum of dietary fiber and functional fiber.
toxin A harmful substance; specifically, a chemical produced by a microorganism that harms tissues or causes adverse immune responses.
trabecular bone (spongy bone) A porous bone tissue that makes up only 20% of our skeleton and is found within the ends of the long bones, inside the spinal vertebrae, inside the flat bones (sternum, ribs, and most bones of the skull), and inside the bones of the pelvis.
trace minerals Minerals that must be consumed in amounts of less than 100 mg/day and that are present in the body at the level of less than 5 g.
transamination The process of transferring the amine group from one amino acid to another in order to manufacture a new amino acid.
transcription The process through which messenger RNA copies genetic information from DNA in the nucleus.

transferrin The transport protein for iron.
transgenic crops Plant varieties that have had one or more genes altered through the use of genetic technologies; also called genetically modified organisms, or GMOs.
translation The process that occurs when the genetic information carried by messenger RNA is translated into a chain of amino acids at the ribosome.
transport proteins Protein molecules that help transport substances throughout the body and across cell membranes.
triglyceride A molecule consisting of three fatty acids attached to a three-carbon glycerol backbone.
trimester Any one of three stages of pregnancy, each lasting 13 to 14 weeks.
tumor Any newly formed mass of undifferentiated cells.
type 1 diabetes A disorder in which the body cannot produce enough insulin.
type 2 diabetes A progressive disorder in which body cells become less responsive to insulin.

U

umbilical cord The cord containing the arteries and veins that connect the baby (from the navel) to the mother via the placenta.
undernutrition Malnutrition defined by an absolute lack of adequate energy leading to underweight.
underweight Having too little body fat to maintain health, causing a person to weigh less than an acceptably defined standard for a given height.
urinary tract infection A bacterial infection of the urethra, the tube leading from the bladder to the body exterior.
USDA Food Patterns A template for healthy eating built around the USDA 2010 Dietary Guidelines for Americans. Previously was called the USDA Food Guide.

V

variety Eating a lot of different foods each day.
vegetarianism The practice of restricting the diet to food substances of plant origin, including vegetables, fruits, grains, and nuts.
very-low-density lipoprotein (VLDL) A lipoprotein made in the liver and intestine that functions to transport endogenous lipids, especially triglycerides, to the tissues of the body.
vigorous-intensity activities Activities that produce significant increases in breathing, sweating, and heart rate; talking is difficult when exercising at a vigorous intensity.
viruses A group of infectious agents that are much smaller than bacteria, lack independent metabolism, and are incapable of growth or reproduction apart from living cells.
viscous Having a gel-like consistency; viscous fibers form a gel when dissolved in water.
visible fats Fat we can see in our foods or see added to foods, such as butter, margarine, cream, shortening, salad dressings, chicken skin, and untrimmed fat on meat.
vitamins Organic compounds that assist in regulating body processes.

W

warm-up Activities that prepare you for an exercise bout, including stretching, calisthenics, and movements specific to the exercise bout; also called preliminary exercise.
wasting Very low weight for height.
water-soluble vitamins Vitamins that are soluble in water, including vitamin C and the B-complex vitamins.
wellness A multidimensional, lifelong process that includes physical, emotional, social, occupational, and spiritual health.

Z

zygote A fertilized egg (ovum) consisting of a single cell.

INDEX

A

abortion, spontaneous, 504
absorption, nutrients, 81, 85, 92–96, 103–105, 298
Academy of Pediatrics, 548
Acceptable Daily Intake (ADI), 130–132. *See also* dietary reference intake (DRI); specific nutrient names
Acceptable Macronutrient Distribution Range (AMDR), 13, 15, 122–123, 157–158
accessory factors, 217, 328
Accutane, 272, 558
acesulfame-K, 130–132
acetylcholine, 343
acid-base balance, 194–195, 346
acidity, food safety, 464
acidosis, 195
acne, 272, 558
activity
  adolescents, 555
  benefits of, 412–413
  cancer risk, 283–284, 288
  carbohydrate intake, 114, 426–429
  cardiovascular disease, 176
  childhood obesity, prevention of, 561
  dehydration, preventing, 251–252
  Dietary Guidelines for Americans, 48
  energy needs, 378–379, 380, 419–423
  ergogenic aids, 434–438
  fats, energy from, 152–153, 429
  female athlete triad, 451–452
  fitness program, components of, 413–418
  FIT principle, 415–417
  fluid intake, 243
  fluid loss, 235
  heat illnesses, 252–253
  levels of, debate about, 439
  muscle dysmorphia, 447
  nutrition needs, overview, 424–425
  older adults, 571
  osteoporosis, risk of, 322
  pregnancy and, 516–517
  protein requirements, 199, 200, 202, 429–430
  serving size and, 59
  social influences, 385–386
  sports beverages, 247
  vitamin and mineral needs, 432–434
  water, intake recommendations, 237
  web resources, 441
  for weight loss, 394–396
  wellness and, 5–6
added sugars, 123–125
addiction, 36. *See also* alcohol use and abuse; drug use and abuse
Addison, Thomas, 339
additives, food safety, 476–478
adenosine triphosphate (ATP)
  creatine supplements, 436
  energy from, 419–423
  fermentation, 110
  mitochondria, 81
  phosphorus intake, 245
  ribose supplements, 437–438
adequate intake (AI)
  calcium, 297–298
  chloride, 245
  fiber, 126–127
  magnesium, 311
  overview, 13, 14–15
  potassium, 242
  sodium, 240
  vitamin K, 308–309
adipose tissue
  body composition measurement, 372–374
  brown adipose, 383–384
  energy from, 10–11
  function of, 154
  overview, 156–157
adolescents
  food choices, 556–557
  growth and activity patterns, 554–555
  nutrition needs, 555–556
  nutrition-related concerns, 558–559
  pregnancy, 514–515
adrenaline, 152–153
adult day-care, 569–570
adult-onset diabetes, 140
Adverse Reaction Monitoring System (ARMS), 478
advertising, 20–21, 444, 446
aerobic metabolism, 420–421, 422. *See also* metabolism
aflatoxin, 461
African Americans, 50, 56, 372
age-related macular degeneration, 569
aging
  body fluid, 228
  dehydration, risk of, 251
  nutrition needs, 564–567
  nutrition-related concerns, 567–570
  osteoporosis, 320–321
  physical activity level, 571
  physiologic changes, 562–563
  phytochemicals and, 68–71
  slowing the process of, 574–579
  statistics on, 561–562
agouti gene, 25
agriculture
  food-borne illness, 456–457, 458
  food insecurity, 492–493
  genetically modified organisms, 479–480, 487
  growth hormones, use of, 484–485
  pesticides and herbicides, 482–483
  sustainability, 496
AIDS/HIV, 524
alanine, 187
Al-Anon, 36, 37
Alateen, 36
albumin, 153
alcohol, fermentation, 110
alcohol, in breast milk, 523
alcoholic hepatitis, 34
Alcoholics Anonymous, Inc., 37
alcohol related birth defects (ARBD), 35, 515
alcohol-related neurodevelopmental disorder (ARND), 35, 515
alcohol use and abuse
  adolescents, 558–559
  brain function, 33
  cancer risk, 283–284, 287–288
  Dietary Guidelines for Americans, 50
  effect on liver, 89–90
  energy from, 10
  fluid loss, 235
  hangovers, 32
  health effects, 31–36
  hypokalemia, 245
  liver and, 33–34
  metabolism of alcohol, 30–31
  moderate intake, 29–30
  myths about, 31
  niacin deficiency, 333
  osteoporosis, risk of, 320–321
  overview, 9
  poisoning, 33
  pregnancy, 515, 538–539
  self-assessment, 35–36
  thiamin intake, 332
  ulcers, causes of, 94
alendronate, 323
alkalosis, 195
allergies
  Adverse Reaction Monitoring System (ARMS), 478
  breastfeeding, 522
  food coloring, 478
  to foods, 101–103
  infants and, 531
  milk, 101
  sulfites, 475
  toddlers and, 546
  web resources, 99, 105
alpha-linolenic acid, 150–151, 159
alpha-tocopherol, 260–262, 477
Alpha-Tocopherol Beta-Carotene Cancer Prevention Study, 277
alternative medicine, 363–364
altitude, fluid loss, 235
Alzheimer's disease, 7
Amanita phalloides, 462
amaranth, 205
amenorrhea, 322, 446, 451
American College of Sports Medicine (ACSM), 24, 27
American Dental Association, 135
American Dietetic Association (ADA), 22, 24, 65, 366, 548
American Heart Association, 149, 399
American Journal of Clinical Nutrition, 24
American Society for Nutrition (ASN), 24, 27
amino acids
  energy from, 114, 423
  folate and, 337

amino acids, *(cont.)*
  limiting amino acid, 192
  proteins and, 11, 186–192
  selenium and, 274
  sulfur intake, 345–346
  supplements, 202
  transport of, 197–198
  vitamin B_6, 334–336
amniotic fluid, 231, 512
amylase, 82, 116–117
anabolic steroids, 435
anaerobic metabolism, 422
anaerobic reactions, 419–420
anal canal, 90–91
analysis, research, 18
anaphylactic shock, 103
androstenedione, 435–436
anemia
  folate intake, 338–339
  infants, 531–532
  iron-deficiency, 6, 352–354, 543
  macrolytic anemia, 510
  microcytic anemia, 353
  sports anemia, 433
  vitamin C deficiency, 266
  vitamin E, 262
anencephaly, 510
angina pectoris, 174
animal products, fat content, 162, 163
animal research studies, 19
anorexia, defined, 74
anorexia nervosa, 443, 446–448, 452
antacids, 324
antacids, food interactions, 570
antibiotics, 484–485, 570
antibodies, 103, 195–196
anticoagulants, 262, 570
anticonvulsants, food interactions, 570
antidepressants, food interactions, 570
antioxidants
  beta-carotene, 259, 267–269
  cancer prevention, 288–289
  copper, iron, zinc and manganese, 276
  food or supplements, debate about, 277
  food preservation, 474
  function of, 258–259
  older adults, nutrition needs, 565
  oxidation process and free radicals, 256–258
  phytochemicals, 68–71
  selenium, 259, 274–276
  vegetarian diet, 207
  vision and, 569
  vitamin A, 259, 269–274
  vitamin C, 259, 262–267
  vitamin E, 259, 260–262
antiretroviral agents, 570
appetite, 74–77, 82, 114
appetite-supressing drugs, 407
apple-shaped fat distribution, 374
aquifers, 237
arginine, 187
ariboflavinosis, 332
ARMS (Adverse Reaction Monitoring System), 478
Aronson, Emme, 369, 370
artificial sweeteners, 128–132
ascending colon, 90–91
ascorbic acid. *See* vitamin C (ascorbic acid)
aseptic packaging, 474
Asian Diet Pyramid, 56, 57
Asians, body mass index, 372
asparagine, 187
aspartame, 130–132
aspartic acid, 131–132, 186, 187
Aspergillus flavus, 461
aspirin, 94, 570
atherosclerosis, 174, 412
athletes. *See also* exercise
  body mass index, 372
  carbohydrate intake, 426–429
  energy needs, 424–425
  ergogenic aids, 434–438
  fats, energy from, 429
  female athlete triad, 322
  fluid intake, 243
  heat illnesses, 252–253
  protein requirements, 200, 202, 429–430
  sports beverages, 247
  vitamin and mineral needs, 432–434
  water, intake recommendations, 237
  web resources, 441
Atkins' diet, 389, 399
atoms, oxidation, 256–257
ATP (adenosine triphosphate)
  creatine supplements, 436
  energy from, 419–423
  fermentation, 110
  mitochondria, 81
  phosphorus intake, 245
  ribose supplements, 437–438
atrophic gastritis, 340
autoimmune diseases
  celiac disease, 103–105
  diabetes, 139
aversions, pregnancy, 513
avidin, 341

B

Bacillus thuringiensis (Bt), 482–483
bacteria, 90–91, 457, 459, 460
balanced diet, 41. *See also* diet
barley, 103
basal metabolic rate (BMR), 377–378, 380, 381–382
beans, 53, 182–183, 192
beet extract, 477
Behavioral Risk Factor Surveillance System (BRFSS), 23
beriberi, 217, 331–332
Bernstein, Leslie, 327
best if used by date, 466
beta-carotene
  food additive, 477
  food or supplements, debate about, 277
  functions and sources, 259, 267–269
  older adults, 566–567
Beta-Carotene and Retinol Efficacy Trial, 277
beta-endorphins, 384
BHA (butylated hydroxyanisole), 474, 477
BHT (butylated hydroxytoluene), 474, 477
bicarbonate, 87
bile, 87, 156
binge drinking, 31–32
binge eating, 448–450, 450
bioaccumulation, 481–482
bioavailability, 298
bioelectrical impedance analysis (BIA), 373
biopesticides, 482–483
biotin (vitamin B_7)
  energy metabolism, 328–329
  functions and sources, 341–342
  intake recommendations, 330
  overview, 12, 218–220
biphosphates, 323
birth defects, alcohol and, 35, 515
birth weight, 505
bisphenol A (BPA), 475
black tea, antioxidants in, 277
blastocyst, 503
blindness, 272–274
blood
  coagulation, 347
  copper intake, 355–356
  donation of, 235
  iron, 348–354
  nutrient needs, summary chart, 347
  nutrient transport, 88–89
  overview of, 346–347
  vitamin K, 347–348
  volume, fluid balance, 230, 234
  zinc intake, 354–355
blood alcohol concentration (BAC), 30–31, 33
blood glucose
  alcohol and, 30
  breakfast, importance of, 552
  glycemic index, 121–122
  high-protein diets, 399
  regulation of, 119–120
  Zone Diet, 430
blood lipids, 125, 176–177. *See also* cholesterol
blood pressure
  alcohol use and, 30
  blood volume and, 230
  body weight and, 371
  diet and, 6
  fat distribution patterns, 374–375
  fluid balance, 234
  health claims, food labels, 46
  hypertension, overview, 174–175
  physical activity and, 412
  potassium intake, 244
  pregnancy and, 514
  reducing, 182–183
  sodium consumption, 241
  vegetarian diet, 207
BMI (body mass index), 370–372
Bod Pod, 373
body composition, 412, 555, 563
body fat, 153, 372–375, 421–422, 563
body image, 443, 553–554, 558
body mass index (BMI), 370–372, 374, 507, 560
body temperature
  dehydration, 251
  fluid balance and, 230, 430–432
  heat illnesses, 252–253
body weight
  adolescents, 555
  body composition, 372–374
  body mass index (BMI), 370–372, 374
  breastfeeding, 519, 533

carbohydrates and, 114–115
children and adolescents, 560–561
cultural and economic factors, 384–385
diabetes and, 139–140
diet plans, creating, 393–397
diets for weight loss, 388–389, 392–393
early childhood, nutrition needs, 553–554
energy balance, 375–380, 380
fat blockers, 169
fat distribution patterns, 374–375
fat intake and, 158
fetal environment, 538
fiber and, 115
food choices, fat storage and, 382
genetic factors, 381–382
healthy body weight, 370
high-fructose corn syrup, 133
obesity, In Depth, 402–409
older adults, 567–568
physical activity and, 412
physiology, influence of, 382–384
pregnancy, 505, 507
psychological and social factors, 385–387
sugar intake, 125
toddlers, 546
underweight, 397–398
web resources, 401, 409
weight loss, readiness for, 390–392
bolus, 83–84
bonding, mother-infant, 523
bones
adolescents, 554–555
bone density, 293–294, 558, 563
calcium, function of, 296–301
composition of, 292–293
early childhood, nutrition needs, 553
female athlete triad, 433
fluoride, 312–313
functions of, 292
growth and modeling, 293–294
health of, 295–296
magnesium, functions and sources, 310–312
manganese intake, 344
osteoporosis, In Depth, 318–325
phosphorus, 245, 309–310
protein consumption, 210
vitamin A, 271
vitamin D, 301–308
vitamin K, 308–309
bottled water, 238
botulism, 461
bovine spongiform encephalopathy (BSE), 461, 462
BPA (bisphenol A), 475
branched-chain amino acids, 331
breads, fiber, 125–128
breakfast, importance of, 551, 552
breast cancer, 167, 283, 284
breastfeeding
advantages and challenges, 521–525
calcium intake, 298
fluid loss, 235
herbal supplement use, 364
iron status and, 351
nutrition needs, 517–524
vitamin D content, 307
brown adipose tissue, 383–384
brown bread, 126
brown sugar, 124
brush border, 87
buffers, acid-base balance, 195
bulimia nervosa, 443, 448–450, 452
burns, dehydration, 251
butter, 149

C

caffeine
breast milk, 523
exercise and, 436–437
fluid loss, 235
osteoporosis, risk of, 320–321
pregnancy, consumption during, 515
calcitonin, 296, 323
calcitriol, 302, 303
calcium
adolescents, nutrition needs, 555–556, 558
bones, composition of, 292–293
breastfeeding, intake for, 520
early childhood, nutrition needs, 553
exercise, intake for, 433
fiber and, 127
food additives, 478
functions and sources, 296–301
health claims, 225
iron absorption and, 350
lactose intolerance, 101
muscle fatigue and, 422
older adults, nutrition needs, 564–566, 565, 568
osteoporosis, risk of, 321–322
overview, 12, 221
physical activity, intake for, 424
pregnancy, intake requirements, 509, 511
protein consumption, 210
supplements, 324
toddlers, nutrition needs, 542, 546–547
vegan diet, 208
calcium carbonate, 324
calcium chloride, 477, 478
calcium citrate, 324
calcium citrate malate, 324
calcium lactate, 324
calcium phosphate, 324
calcium propionate, 475, 477
calcium rigor, 297
calcium tetany, 297
Calories. *See also* energy
adolescents, nutrition needs, 555–556
alcohol and, 30
balancing, 48
carbohydrates, 113–115
defined, 9
Dietary Guidelines for Americans, 48
early childhood, nutrition needs, 549–550
empty, 52
energy balance, 375–380
fast-food meals, 58, 60, 61
fats, 160, 161
fats, energy from, 152–153
low and reduced fat foods, 162
Nutrition Facts Panel, 43
older adults, nutrition needs, 564
pregnancy, need for, 508
restriction of, 575–577
serving size and, 59
thermic effect of food (TEF), 378
toddlers, nutrition needs, 542–544
USDA Food Patterns, 52
Campylobacter jejuni, 459, 460
cancer
alcohol use and, 34
breast cancer, 283
colorectal, 115, 310
definition and classification, 282–283
diet and, 6
fat intake and, 167
food residues, 480–486
health claims, food labels, 46
lung cancer, 283
mortality rates, 7
physical activity and, 413
phytochemicals, 71
prevention, 287–289
risk factors, 283–286
signs and symptoms, 286–287
treatment, 287
vegetarian diet, 208
vitamin A, 270
vitamin D, 302
canning, food preservation, 473–474
capillaries, 87
carageenan, 113, 477
caramel, 477
Carbohydrate Addict's Diet, 389
carbohydrate loading, 118
carbohydrates
adolescents, nutrition needs, 555
alternative sweeteners, 128–132
blood glucose levels, 119–120
breastfeeding, intake for, 520
in breast milk, 521
carbohydrate loading, 428–429
complex, 110–113
Dietary Guidelines for Americans, 50
dietary recommendations, 122–128
Dietary Reference Intake (DRI), 15
diets for weight loss, 389
digestion of, 87, 116–118
early childhood, nutrition needs, 550
energy from, 113–115, 377, 420–421
fat storage and, 382
fiber, 115
fiber-rich carbohydrates, 125–128
glycemic index, 121–122
infant formula, 528
metabolism of, 335, 341
older adults, nutrition needs, 564–565
overview, 8, 9–10, 108–110
physical activity, intake for, 424
pregnancy, intake requirements, 508–509
simple, 109–110
sources of, 427–428
toddlers, nutrition needs, 542–544
carbonated beverages, 238
carcinogens, 208, 283, 284. *See also* cancer
cardiorespiratory fitness, 412, 416–417
cardiovascular disease
body weight and, 371
diet and, 6
fat distribution patterns, 374–375
fat intake and, 167
fiber and, 115

cardiovascular disease, *(cont.)*
  folate intake, 338
  health claims, food labels, 46
  high-protein diets, 399
  mortality rate, 7
  overview, 173–183
  physical activity and, 412
  potassium, role of, 243
  prevention of, 179–183
  protein consumption, 210
  risks factors, 175–179
  trans fats, 164
  vegetarian diet, 207
  vitamin intake and, 335
cardiovascular system, nutrient transport, 88–89
carnitine, 263, 335, 437
carotenoderma, 268
carotenoids, 68–71, 267–269
carotenosis, 268
carpal tunnel syndrome, 336
cartilage, 344
case control studies, 19–20
casein, 102, 528
cash crops, 493
cashews, 147
catalase, 276
cataracts, 332, 569
cavities, teeth, 123–124, 553
cecum, 90–91
celiac disease, 103–105, 274, 307, 308, 348
cell differentiation, 271
cell membrane, 80, 154, 258, 260–262
cells
  fats, function of, 154
  free radicals, damage from, 258
  growth, repair and maintenance, 193–194
  intracellular fluid, 228
  structures and functions, 79–81
  vitamin E, 260–262
cellulose, 113, 477
Centers for Disease Control and Prevention (CDC)
  food-borne illness, 455, 456, 463
  information from, 23
  website, 27, 457
central nervous system, 91–92
cephalic phase, digestion, 82
cereals, fiber, 125–128
cerebral arteries, 174
cerebrospinal fluid, 231
ceruloplasmin, 355
cervical cancer, 284–285
chaparral, 367
charbroiled meats, 284
cheese, 468
chewing, 82, 83, 84
childhood obesity, 404–405
child mortality, 493–494
children. *See also* adolescents; infants
  early childhood, food choices, 551–553
  early childhood, nutrition needs, 547–550
  nutrition-related concerns, 546–547
  toddlers, food choice, 545–546
  toddlers, nutrition needs, 542–545
  web resources, 573
Chinese ephedra, 367, 437
chitosan, 169
chloride, 12, 221, 229, 236, 245. *See also* electrolytes
chlorine, water and, 237
chlorophyll, 108, 463
choking, infants and toddlers, 530
cholecalciferol, 218, 302, 303, 304
cholecystokinin (CCK), 86–87, 384
cholesterol
  cardiovascular disease and, 176–177
  cell membranes, 80
  Dietary Guidelines for Americans, 50
  fat digestion, 156
  fiber and, 115
  food labeling, 45
  high-protein diets, 399
  overview, 10–11
  physical activity and, 412
  protein consumption, 210
  saturated and trans fats, 163–164
  structure of, 151–152
  sugar intake and, 125
  vitamin D and, 302, 303
choline, 330, 343
chromium
  functions and sources, 222, 344
  health claims, 225
  intake recommendations, 330
  overview, 12
  supplements, 345, 437
chronic disease, 4, 34
chylomicron, 156
chyme, 85, 87, 90
cigarette smoking
  adolescents, 558–559
  cancer risk, 283, 284
  cardiovascular disease, 176
  osteoporosis, risk of, 320–321
  pregnancy and, 516, 538–539
ciguatoxins, 462–463
circulatory system, nutrient transport, 88–89
cirrhosis of the liver, 34
cis fatty acid, 147–148
claims, food labels, 44
clinical trials, 20
Clostridium botulinum, 459, 461, 464, 473–474, 530
clotting, blood, 347
coagulation, blood, 347
cobalamin. *See* vitamin B_{12} (cobalamin)
coenzymes, 328–329, 332, 347–348
cofactors, 259, 310–312, 355–356
cold, common, 264, 357
colic, 531
collagen, 263
colon, 90–91, 96, 97
colon cleansing, 91, 97
colonic irrigation, 91, 97
colorectal cancer
  exercise, 284
  fat intake and, 167
  fiber and, 115
  magnesium intake, 310
  mortality, 283
  physical activity and, 413
coloring agents, 477–478
colostrum, 518
comfrey, 367
Commodity Supplemental Food Program, 570
common bile duct, 87
common cold, 264, 357
compact bone, 292
complementary proteins, 192
complete proteins, 192. *See also* protein
complex carbohydrates, 108. *See also* carbohydrates
conception, 502
conditionally essential amino acid, 187
confectioner's sugar, 124
congestive heart failure, 241
constants, research, 18
constipation, 95–96, 115, 350, 513–514
control group, research, 18
cooking, foods safety, 469–470
cool-down, physical activity, 418
cooling, food preservation, 473
copper
  antioxidant function, 259
  functions and sources, 222, 355–356
  overview, 12
  recommended intake, 347
  superoxide dismutase antioxidant enzyme system, 276
  zinc and, 356
corn sweetener, 124
corn syrup, 124, 530
coronary heart disease, 46, 174
cortical bone, 292
cortisol, 119–120
cost, food choice and, 386, 554, 569–570
cravings, pregnancy, 513
creatine, metabolism of, 339
creatine phosphate (CP), 419–420, 422, 436
creatine supplements, 436
cretinism, 276, 344
Creutzfeldt-Jakob disease, 462
Crohn's disease, 274, 307, 308, 348
cross-contamination, 465, 466
culture
  body weight and, 384–385
  eating disorders and, 444–445
  food choices and, 76–77
cured meats, 284
cylomicrons, 177
cysteine, 187, 192, 193, 210, 345–346
cystic fibrosis, 274, 307, 308, 348
cytochromes, 348
cytoplasm, cell, 80

D

dairy
  food labels, 102
  toddlers, nutrition needs, 543
dairy foods
  adolescents, nutrition needs, 556, 558
  calcium sources, 298–300, 306
  DASH diet, 182–183
  early childhood, nutrition needs, 553
  growth hormones, 484–485
  lactose intolerance, 101
  MyPlate, 52, 53
  riboflavin, 332
  serving size, 54
  vitamin D, 305

danger zone, food safety, 463
DASH diet, 182–183, 389
data collection, research, 18
dates, food labels, 466
deamination, 196
Dean Ornish's Program for Reversing Heart Disease, 392–393
death, causes of, 7
deathcap mushroom, 462
dehydration
  alcohol consumption, 32
  colon cleansing, 97
  diarrhea, 95
  infants, 531
  older adults, 567
  overview of, 238, 251–252
  physical activity and, 430–432
dehydroascorbic acid, 262–267
dehydroepiandrosteron (DHEA), 435–436
Delaney Clause, 478
denaturation, proteins, 190–192
denature, defined, 85
dental caries
  added sugars, 123–124
  early childhood, nutrition needs, 553
  health claims, food labels, 46
  infants, 532
dental health. *See* teeth
deoxyribonucleic acid (DNA)
  cell nucleus, 80
  metabolism of, 344
  phosphorus intake, 245
  synthesis of, 339
  vitamin C, 263
depolarization, 232
dermatitis herpetiformis, 104
descending colon, 90–91
desiccants, food additives, 478
detox liquid diet, 97
dexfenfluramine, 407
dextrose, 124
DHEA (dehydroepiandrosterone), 435–436
diabetes
  alcohol and, 30
  blood glucose, regulation of, 119–120
  body weight and, 371
  cardiovascular disease and, 176
  childhood obesity and, 404
  dehydration, 251
  diet and, 6
  fat distribution patterns, 374–375
  fiber and, 115
  gestational diabetes, 514
  glycemic index, 121–122
  mortality rates, 7
  overview of, 137–141
  physical activity and, 412
  protein consumption, 210–211
  sugar intake and, 125
diabetic acidosis, 244
diarrhea, 95, 235, 245, 251
diastolic blood pressure, 175
diatoms, 483
diet
  Dietary Guidelines for Americans, 48–51
  fat storage, food choices and, 382
  food labels and, 41–47
  healthful, defined, 40–41
  for weight gain, 397–398
  for weight loss, creating, 393–397
dietary fiber, 112–113
Dietary Guidelines for Americans, 29, 48–51, 65, 122–123, 389
dietary reference intake (DRI). *See also* specific nutrient names
  early childhood, nutrition needs, 547–550
  essential fatty acids, 159
  older adults, 564–566
  overview, 13–16
  toddlers, 542
Dietary Supplement Health and Education Act (DSHEA), 361
dietary supplements. *See* supplements
diets, for weight loss, 388–389, 392–393
digestion. *See also* gastrointestinal system
  carbohydrates, 116–118
  disorders of, 92–96
  fats, 154–157
  large intestine, 90–91
  neuromuscular system and, 91–92
  overview, 81–83
  proteins, 197–199
  small intestine, 86–90
  vegetarian diet, 207–208
Dilantin, 308
dining out, 58, 60–62, 165–166, 168, 470–471, 560
dinoflagellates, 462–463
dioxins, food safety, 482
dipeptide, 188
disaccharidase, 109–110
disease, food insecurity and, 493
disordered eating
  adolescents, 558
  binge-eating, 450
  bulimia nervosa, 448–450
  continuum of, 443
  contributing factors, 443–446
  female athlete triad, 451–452
  night-eating syndrome, 450–451
  treatment for, 452
  vegetarian diet and, 208
  web resources, 453
distilled water, 238
diuretics
  alcohol, 32
  dehydration, 251
  fluid loss, 235
  food interactions, 570
  potassium intake, 244
diverticulosis, 115
DNA (deoxyribonucleic acid)
  cell nucleus, 80
  metabolism of, 344
  phosphorus intake, 245
  synthesis of, 339
  vitamin C, 263
docosahexaenoic acid (DHA), 151, 509
dowager's hump, 319, 320
drug-alcohol interactions, 30
drug use and abuse, 516, 538–539, 558–559
drying, food preservation, 473
dual energy x-ray absorptiometry (DEXA), 295–296, 373
duodenal ulcers, 94
duodenum, 86
Dutch Famine Study, 537

E

early childhood, nutrition needs
  food choices, 551–553
  nutrient needs, 549–550
  nutrition-related concerns, 553–554
eating disorders
  adolescents, 558
  anorexia nervosa, 443, 446–448
  binge-eating, 450
  bulimia nervosa, 448–450
  continuum of, 443
  contributing factors, 443–446
  female athlete triad, 322, 433, 451–452
  night-eating syndrome, 450–451
  treatment for, 452
  vegetarian diet, 208
  web resources, 453
eating patterns, Dietary Guidelines for Americans, 51
eclampsia, 514
economic factors, 384–385, 386, 569–570. *See also* food insecurity
edema, protein intake, 194, 195
EDTA (ethylenediaminetetraacedtic acid), 474, 477
eggs, 102, 469–470
eicosanoids, 148, 150, 159
eicosapentaenoic acid (EPA), 151
Eijkman, Christiaan, 331
elderly. *See* aging
electrolytes
  bulimia nervosa, 449
  chloride, function and sources, 245
  function of, 231–233
  heat illnesses, 252–253
  overview, 228–231
  phosphorus, function and sources, 245–246
  potassium, functions and sources, 242–245
  protein and, 194, 196
  sodium, functions and sources, 240–242
  sports beverages, 247
electrons, oxidation, 256–257
elimination
  defined, 81
  digestive disorders, 92–96
embryo, 503
emotional health, defined, 6
emotions, food choices and, 76–77
empty Calories, 52
emulsifiers, food additives, 478
endoplasmic reticulum (ER), 80
endurance, muscular, 412
enemas, 97
energy
  adolescents, nutrition needs, 555–556
  biotin, 341–342
  calculating, 10
  Calorie restriction, 575–577
  carbohydrates, 113–115, 426–429
  choline, 343
  chromium, 344, 345
  Dietary Guidelines for Americans, 48, 49
  diets for weight loss, 389, 392–393
  early childhood, nutrition needs, 549–550

energy, *(cont.)*
Estimated Average Requirement (EAR), 13, 14
fats, 152–153, 161, 429
folate, 336–339
food labeling, 45
intake/expenditure balance, 375–380
iodine, 343–344
iron, 348
low and reduced fat foods, 162
macronutrients, 9–11
manganese, 344–345
marasmus, 493–494
metabolism, regulation of, 328–329
mitochondria, 81
niacin, 333–334
nutrients for, chart of, 330
older adults, nutrition needs, 564
pantothenic acid, 341
physical activity, energy cost of, 378–379
physical activity, energy sources, 419–423
physical activity, nutrition for, 424–425
physical activity, weight loss, 394–396
pregnancy, need for, 508
protein-energy malnutrition, 211–212
protein intake, 429–430
proteins as source, 196–197
sources of, 50
sulfur, 345–346
thermic effect of food (TEF), 378
toddlers, energy needs, 542–543
vitamins and, 11–12, 331–332, 334–336, 339–341
energy density, 394, 395
energy drinks, 436–437
enriched foods, 126
enteric nervous system, 91–92
enterotoxins, 461
environment
appetite cues, 76–77
fetal development, 536–539
fluid loss, 235
Environmental Protection Agency (EPA), 237–238, 456, 457, 483
enzymes
antioxidants, 259
coenzymes, 328–329
copper intake, 355–356
digestion, 82–83, 87, 116–117
glutathione peroxidase, 274
iron and, 348
lactose intolerance, 101
lipoprotein lipase, 157
pancreatic amylase, 117
protein digestion, 197
proteins as, 194
salivary amylase, 116–117
superoxide dismutase antioxidant enzyme system, 276
zinc intake, 354
Ephedra, 437
ephedra, 367
ephedrine, 437
epidemiological studies, 19
epiglottis, 83
epinephrine, 103, 119–120, 263
epiphyseal plates, 555
epitonin, 367
ergocalciferol, 304
ergogenic aids, 434–438
erythrocyte hemolysis, 262
erythrocytes. *See also* blood
iron-deficiency anemia, 6, 352–353, 543
overview, 346–347
protein structure, 190–191
synthesis of, 337
vitamin E, 260–262
Escherichia coli, 459, 460
esophageal sphincter, 83
esophagus, 83–84
essential amino acids, 187
essential fatty acids, 148, 150
essential hypertension, 175
Estimated Average Requirement (EAR), 13, 14
Estimated Energy Requirement (EER), 13, 15, 542, 549–550
estrogen, 320, 554–555, 563
estrogen receptor modulators, 323
ethics, vegetarian diet and, 206–207
Ethiopians, 372
ethnicity
body mass index calculation, 372
diabetes and, 138
Food Guide Pyramid variations, 56, 57, 58
vegetarian diet, 206–207
evaporation, fluid balance, 234–235
evaporative cooling, 230, 431
exercise
adolescents, 555
benefits of, 412–413
cancer risk, 283–284, 288
carbohydrates and, 114, 426–429
cardiovascular disease, 176
childhood obesity, prevention of, 561
dehydration, preventing, 251–252
energy needs, 378–379, 380, 419–423
ergogenic aids, 434–438
fats, energy from, 152–153, 429
female athlete triad, 322, 433, 451–452
fitness program, components of, 413–418
FIT principle, 415–417
fluid intake, 243
fluid loss, 235
heat illnesses, 252–253
levels of, debate about, 439
muscle dysmorphia, 447
nutrition needs, overview, 424–425
older adults, 571
osteoporosis, risk of, 322
pregnancy and, 516–517
protein requirements, 199, 200, 202, 429–430
serving size and, 59
social influences, 385–386
sports beverages, 247
vitamin and mineral needs, 432–434
water, intake recommendations, 237
web resources, 441
for weight loss, 394–396
wellness and, 5–6
exhalation, fluid balance, 234–235
experimental design, 17–18
extracellular fluid, 228, 229
extrusion reflex, 530
eyes
aging and, 563
beta-carotene, 267
older adults, 569
vitamin A, benefits of, 270–271, 272–274

F

fad diets, 388–389
family, influences of, 444–445
family history, cancer risk, 283
famine, 491–492, 537–538
farming practices
food-borne illness, 456–457, 458
food insecurity, 492–493
genetically modified organisms, 479–480, 487
growth hormones, use of, 484–485
pesticides and herbicides, 482–483
sustainability, 496
fast-food restaurants, 58, 60–62
fat, body, 153, 372–375, 421–422, 563
fat, dietary
adolescents, nutrition needs, 555
beneficial fats, 164–165
in breast milk, 521
cancer risk, 283–284
chronic disease and, 167
DASH diet, 182–183
defined, 144
dietary recommendations, 15, 50, 157–166
digestion of, 87
dining out, 165–166, 168
early childhood, nutrition needs, 549–550
energy from, 377
fast-food meals, 60, 61
fat blockers, 169
fat replacers, 166
food labeling, 45
importance of, 152–154
low-fat diets, 392–393
metabolism of, 154–157, 341
Nutrition Facts Panel, 43
older adults, nutrition needs, 564
overview, 8, 10–11
phospholipids, 151
physical activity, intake for, 424
pregnancy, intake requirements, 509
saturated and trans, 163–164
sources of, 160, 163
sterols, 151–152
storage of, 156–157, 382
toddlers, nutrition needs, 542–544
triglycerides, 144–150
fat distribution patterns, 374–375
fat-free, defined, 160
fatigue, 287
fat-modified foods, 160, 162
fat-soluble vitamins, 12, 153–154, 217–218
fat substitutes, 274
fatty acids, 144–150, 520
fatty liver, 34
feces, 91, 234–235
female athlete triad, 322, 433, 451–452
fenfluramine, 407
fermentation, 110
ferritin, 349, 352–354
fetal adaptation, 537
fetal alcohol effects (FAE), 35, 515
fetal alcohol spectrum disorders (FASD), 35, 515
fetal alcohol syndrome (FAS), 35, 515
fetal development
alcohol, effects on, 35
fetal environment, In Depth, 536–539

first trimester, 503–504
folate intake, 338
second trimester, 504–505
third trimester, 505
timeline, 506
fever, 235, 251. *See also* temperature, body
fiber
adolescents, nutrition needs, 555
constipation, 96
dietary guidelines for, 125–128
digestion of, 118
food labeling, 45
importance of, 115
older adults, nutrition needs, 564
overview, 112–113
sources of, 127–128
toddlers, nutrition needs, 543, 547
zinc absorption and, 354
fibrous proteins, 190–192
FightBAC!, 465
fight-or-flight reaction, 119
filtered water, 239
fish
food labels, 102
omega fatty acids, 164–165
pregnancy, consumption during, 509
raw, consumption of, 469
toxins, 462, 463, 481–482
vitamin D, 304
fitness, 412, 413–418, 441. *See also* exercise
FIT principle (frequency, intensity, time), 415–417
flavin adenine dinucleotide (FAD), 329, 332
flavin mononucleotide (FMN), 329, 332
flavonoids, 69, 71
flavor, fats and, 154
flavoring agents, food additives, 476–477
FlavrSavr tomato, 479–480
flexibility, 412, 415
flexitarian diet, 206
flour, terminology, 126
fluid balance
bulimia nervosa, 449
chloride, function and sources, 245
dehydration, 250–252
electrolytes, function of, 231–233
heat illnesses, 252–253
maintaining, 233–235
overview, 228–231
phosphorus, function and sources, 245–246, 309–310
potassium, functions and sources, 242–245
protein and, 194, 211
sodium, functions and sources, 240–242
water intake, 236–240
fluid intake
adolescents, nutrition needs, 556
breastfeeding, 520–521
early childhood, nutrition needs, 550
infant needs, 528
older adults, nutrition needs, 567
physical activity and, 430–432
pregnancy, 512
toddlers, nutrition needs, 542, 543
flukes, 460
fluoride
bone health and, 298
early childhood, 553
functions and sources, 222, 312–313
overview, 12
toddlers, 543
fluorohydroxyapatite, 312
fluorosis, 313
flushing, 333
folate/folic acid
energy metabolism, 328–329
food additives, 478
functions and sources, 336–339
homocysteine levels and, 277
intake recommendations, 330
overview, 12, 218–220
pregnancy, intake requirements, 509–510
recommended intake, 347
riboflavin and, 332
vitamin B_6 and, 335
food allergies. *See* allergies
Food and Agriculture Organization of the United Nations (FAO), 476
Food and Drug Administration (FDA). *See* U.S. Food and Drug Administration
food banks, 569–570
food-borne illness
causes of, 457–464
overview of, 456–457
prevention, 464–472
spoilage, preventing, 472–476
tracking of, 455
food chain, bioaccumulation, 481–482
food choice
adolescents, 556–557
cost and, 386
cultural and economic factors, 384–385
early childhood, 551–553
toddlers, 545–546
food coloring, 477–478
food distribution, 493
food infections. *See* food-borne illness
food insecurity, 491–496, 554, 569–570
food intolerance, 101
food intoxications, 457. *See also* food-borne illness
food labels
carbohydrates, recognizing, 129
dates on, 466
fats, 160, 161
food allergens, 102
grain and cereal terms, 126
Nutrition Facts Panel, 43–44
overview, 41–47
supplements, 362
Food Patterns, USDA, 51–52
empty Calories, 52
ethnic variations, 56–58
food groups, 52, 53
serving sizes, 54–56
food poisoning. *See* food-borne illness
food production, 456–457, 458
food safety. *See also* food-borne illness
diarrhea, 95, 96
Dietary Guidelines for Americans, 51
dining out, 470–471
food additives, 476–478
food storage, 466–468, 472–476
genetically modified foods, 479–480
government agencies, 456
growth hormones, 484–485
organic foods, 485–486
pregnancy and, 516
residues, 480–486
toxins, 470
travel and, 471–472
vegetarian diet, 206–207
web resources, 489
formula, infant, 526–529
fortified foods, 126
fractures. *See* osteoporosis
free radicals
copper intake, 355
iron and, 348
manganese, 344
phytochemicals, 68–71
sources of, 257–258
zinc intake, 354
freeze-drying, food preservation, 473
freezing, food safety, 467–468
frequency, physical activity, 415–416
fructose, 109, 124, 125, 129
fruitarian diet, 207, 208
fruit juice sweetener, 124
fruits
beta-carotene, 268
DASH diet, 182–183
Dietary Guidelines for Americans, 51
MyPlate, 52, 53
pesticides in, 484
serving size, 54
vitamin C, 262–267
fruit sugar, 109
functional fiber, 112–113
functional foods, debate about, 63
functional tolerance, alcohol, 31
function claims, food labels, 44–45
fungi, food-borne illness, 461, 468
fungicides, 482–483
Funk, Casimir, 331

G

galactose, 109
gallbladder, 86–87, 155, 156
gamma-butyrolactone (GBL), 436
gamma-hydroxybutyric acid (GHB), 436
gamma rays, 475–476
gastric banding, 408
gastric bypass surgery, 408
gastric juice, 85–86
gastric lipase, 85
gastric phase, digestion, 85
gastric ulcers, 94
gastrin, 85, 197
gastroenteritis, 460
gastroesophageal reflux disease (GERD), 92–94, 513
gastroesophageal reflux (GER), 92–94
gastroesophageal sphincter, 84
gastrointestinal system. *See also* digestion
aging and, 563
celiac disease, 103–105
colon cleansing, 97
constipation, 95–96
defined, 81
diarrhea, 95, 96
disorders of, 92–96
fiber, importance of, 115
food intolerance, 101
irritable bowel syndrome, 96

gastrointestinal system, *(cont.)*
neuromuscular system, 91–92
probiotics, 63
gastroplasty, 408
GBL (gamma-butyrolactone), 436
gelatin, 477
gender differences, 228, 374–375
gene library, 479
Generally Recognized as Safe (GRAS), 478
genetically modified organisms, 479–480, 487
genetic factors
body weight, 381–382, 383, 404
cancer, 283
celiac disease, 103
eating disorders, 444
nutrigenomics, debate about, 25
osteoporosis, 320
protein synthesis, 188–189
germander, 367
germanium, 367
gestation, 505. *See also* fetal development; pregnancy
gestational diabetes, 514
gestational hypertension, 514
GHB (gamma-hydroxybutyric acid), 436
ghrelin, 383, 404
Giardia duodenalis, 460
Giardia lamblia, 460
gliadin, 103
global nutrition, 490–499
globular proteins, 190–192
glucagon, 74–75, 87, 119–120
glucocorticoid medications, 308
glucogenesis, 341
glucometers, 139
gluconeogenesis, 114, 119, 196
glucose
added sugars, 124
carbohydrate digestion, 117–118
defined, 108
glycemic index, 121–122
overview, 109
glucose, blood levels. *See also* diabetes
alcohol and, 30
breakfast, importance of, 552
high-protein diets, 399
Zone Diet, 430
glutamic acid, 187
glutamine, 187
glutathione peroxidase, 332
glutathione peroxidase antioxidant enzyme system, 274
gluten, 103
glycemic index, 121–122
glycemic load, 121–122
glycerin, 477
glycerol, 144–150, 151
glycine, 186, 187, 337
glycogen, 112, 118, 420–421, 422, 426
glycolysis, 420–421, 422
goals, weight loss, 393
goat's milk, 530
goiter, 344
Goldberger, Joseph, 5
government, information sources, 23. *See also* Centers for Disease Control and Prevention (CDC); U.S. Department of Agriculture; U.S. Department of Health and Human Services; U.S. Food and Drug Administration
grains
amino acid content, 193
celiac disease, 103–105
DASH diet, 182–183
fat content, 162, 163
fiber-rich carbohydrates, 125–128
MyPlate, 52, 53
protein from, 205
serving size, 54
granulated sugar, 124
GRAS (generally recognized as safe), 478
gravity, food transport and, 84
grazing, 425
Grijns, Gerrit, 331
grilling, food safety, 469–470
groundwater, 237
growth chart, infants and toddlers, 526
growth hormone, 119–120, 484–485
guar gum, 477
gum arabic, 477
gum disease, 123–124, 568
gums, soluble fiber, 112–113

H

hand washing, 465–466
hangovers, alcohol, 32
health claims, 44, 225
Health Claims Report Card, 44, 46
healthful diet. *See* diet
health inspections, food safety, 470–471
hearing, sense of, 76
heartburn, 92–94
heart disease
body weight and, 371
diet and, 6
fat distribution patterns, 374–375
fat intake and, 167
fiber and, 115
folate intake, 338
health claims, food labels, 46
high-protein diets, 399
mortality rate, 7
overview, 173–183
physical activity and, 412
potassium, role of, 243
prevention of, 179–183
protein consumption, 210
risk factors, 175–179
trans fats, 164
vegetarian diet, 207
vitamin intake and, 335
heart rate, maximal and training, 416–417
heat cramps, 252
heat exhaustion, 252–253
heat-related illness, 431
heat stroke, 253
Helicobacter pylori, 94, 285
helminths, 460
heme, 335, 348
heme iron, 223, 350
hemicellulose, 113
hemochromatosis, 266
hemoglobin, 348–354, 354–355
hemorrhagic stroke, 30, 262
hemorrhoids, 115
hemosiderin, 349
hepatitis, 34, 460
herbal supplements, 363–364
herbicides, 482–483
heredity. *See* genetic factors
hidden fats, 160
high-density lipoproteins (HDLs), 125, 178, 412. *See also* cholesterol
high-fructose corn syrup, 109, 124, 133, 238
high-pressure processing, 474
hindmilk, 522
Hispanics, body mass index, 372
histidine, 187, 337
HIV/AIDS, 524
Hodgkin, Dorothy Crowfoot, 339
homocysteine, 277, 335, 338, 339, 343
honey, 111, 124, 129, 530
Hopkins, F. G., 328
hormone replacement therapy, 323
hormones
adolescents, 554–555
aging and, 563
blood glucose regulation, 119–120
fat metabolism, 152–153
gastrin, 85
hunger and, 74–75
micronutrients and, 329
parathyroid hormone (PTH), 296
proteins as, 194
selenium and, 274
thirst mechanism, 234
vitamin C, 263
vitamin D, 301–302
Hot Topic
acne and vitamin A, 272
amino acid supplements, 202
appetite suppressants, 77
breastfeeding adopted children, 520
diet supplements, 398
ergogenic aids, 435
high-Calorie beverages, 238
hypoglycemia, 119
insulin pumps, 139
Mediterranean diet, 56, 58
muscle dysmorphia, 447
nuts, 147
packaging, toxins in, 475
premenstrual syndrome, 336
resveratrol, 71
spam, 22
supplements, older adults, 567
tobacco use, 284
24-hour recall interview, 23
Human papillomavirus, 284–285
human research studies, 19–20
humectant, food additives, 478
humidity, food safety, 464
hunger, 74–77, 82, 119, 382–383
hydration. *See* fluid balance; fluid intake
hydrochloric acid (HCl), 85, 92–94, 197
hydrogenation, 147–148
hydrogen breath test, 101
hydroxyapatite, 292
hyperactivity, sugar and, 124
hypercalcemia, 300–301, 307
hyperkalemia, 243
hypermagnesemia, 311

hypernatremia, 241
hypertension
  alcohol use and, 30
  blood volume and, 230
  body weight and, 371
  diet and, 6
  fat distribution patterns, 374–375
  fluid balance, 234
  health claims, food labels, 46
  overview, 174–175
  physical activity and, 412
  potassium intake, 244
  pregnancy and, 514
  reducing blood pressure, 182–183
  sodium consumption, 241
hypocalcemia, 301
hypoglycemia, 119, 141
hypokalemia, 244–245
hypomagnesemia, 312
hyponatremia, 227, 238, 242, 243
hypotension, 230, 234
hypothalamus, 74, 233–234
hypothesis, research, 17, 18
hypothyroidism, 344

I

ibuprofen, ulcers and, 94
ileocecal valve, 86, 90–91
ileum, 86
illness, fluid balance, 235
immune system
  beta-carotene, 267
  chromium intake, 344
  food allergies, 101–103
  free radical production, 257–258
  iron intake, 348
  irritable bowel syndrome, 96
  physical activity and, 413
  protein, function of, 195–196
  vitamin A, 271
  vitamin B_6, 335
  zinc and, 354, 357
impaired fasting glucose, 139–140
incomplete proteins, 192
In Depth
  alcohol use and abuse, 28–37
  cancer, 281–289
  cardiovascular disease, 173–183
  diabetes, 137–141
  dietary supplements, 360–365
  disordered eating, 442–453
  fetal environment, 536–539
  fluid imbalance, 250–253
  food related disorders, 100–105
  fountain of youth, search for, 574–579
  global nutrition, 490–499
  obesity, 402–409
  osteoporosis, 318–325
  phytochemicals, 67–71
  vitamins and minerals, 216–225
industrial canning, food preservation, 473–474
infant mortality, 493–494, 501
infants
  dehydration, 251
  fetal alcohol spectrum disorder, 35
  nutrition needs, 525–533
  nutrition-related concerns, 531–532
  solid foods, introducing, 528, 530
  vitamin K, 348
  web resources, 535
infectious agents, cancer and, 284–285
inflammation, 176, 257–258
influenza, mortality rates, 7
information sources, reliability of, 16–24
insecticides, 482–483
insensible water loss, 234–235
insoluble fiber, 113
insulin. *See also* diabetes
  adrenaline, effect on, 153
  alcohol and, 30
  blood glucose regulation, 119–120
  chromium and, 344
  diabetes, In Depth, 137–141
  hunger and, 74–75
  pancreas and, 87
  Zone Diet, 430
insulin insensitivity, 139
insulin-like growth factor (IGF-1), 484–485
intensity, physical activity, 416–417
International Atomic Energy Agency (IAEA), 476
International Food Information Council Foundation (IFIC), 105, 135
interstitial fluid, 228
intestinal flora, 91
intestines
  celiac disease, 103–105
  colon cleansing, debate about, 97
  constipation, 95–96
  diarrhea, 95
  digestive process, large intestine, 85, 90–91
  digestive process, small intestine, 85, 86–90
  fat digestion, 155
  fiber, 115, 118
  irritable bowel syndrome, 96
  probiotics, 63
  protein digestion, 197–198
intolerance, food, 101
intracellular fluid, 228, 229
intravascular fluid, 228
intrinsic factor, 341
invert sugar, 124
iodine
  deficiency, 494
  food additives, 478
  functions and sources, 222, 343–344
  intake recommendations, 330
  overview, 12
  pregnancy, intake requirements, 509, 512
ions, electrolyte balance, 229
iron
  adolescents, nutrition needs, 555–556
  antioxidant function, 259
  breastfeeding, intake for, 520
  exercise, intake for, 433
  fiber and, 127
  functions and sources, 222, 348–354
  infant needs, 527
  older adults, nutrition needs, 565
  overview, 12
  physical activity, intake for, 424
  pregnancy, intake requirements, 509, 511
  recommended intake, 347
  superoxide dismutase antioxidant enzyme system, 276
  toddlers, nutrition needs, 542, 546–547
  vegan diet, 208
  vitamin C intake, 266
iron-deficiency anemia, 6, 352–354, 543
irradiation, food preservation, 475–476
irritable bowel syndrome (IBS), 96
isoleucine, 187, 192, 193, 331
isomalt, 129
isotretinoin, 272

J

jejunum, 86
Jenny Craig, 389
joints, 6, 344
Journal of Nutrition Education and Behavior, 24
Journal of the American Dietetic Association, 24

K

Kashin-Beck disease, 275–276
kava kava, 367
Keshan disease, 274
ketoacidosis, 114, 399
ketones, 114, 399
ketosis, 114
kidney disease
  mortality rates, 7
  potassium intake, 244
  protein consumption, 210–211
  sodium consumption, 241
  vegetarian diet, 208
  vitamin C intake, 266
  vitamin D intake, 307
kidneys. *See also* kidney disease
  failure, potassium consumption, 243
  fluid balance, 234–235
  kidney stones, 266, 300–301
  thirst mechanism, 234
kilocalories. *See also* energy
  carbohydrates, 113–115
  defined, 9
  fats, 152–153, 160, 161
  low and reduced fat foods, 162
kwashiorkor, 211–212, 494
kyphosis, 319, 320

L

labels, food
  carbohydrates, recognizing, 129
  dates on, 466
  fats, 160, 161
  food allergens, 102
  Nutrition Facts Panel, 43–44
  overview, 41–47
labels, supplements, 362
lactalbumin, 521
lactase, 101, 117
lactation, 298, 517–525
lacteal, 87
lactic acid, 420–421, 422
lacto-ovo-vegetarian diet, 207, 546–547

lactose, 109–110, 124, 521, 528
lactose intolerance, 101
large intestine, 63, 90–91, 96, 118
Latin American Diet Pyramid, 56, 57
laxatives, 97, 245, 251, 570
lead, 324, 482, 532, 539
learned response, food choice and, 77
lecithin, 151, 477
legumes, 193, 203
leisure-time physical activity, 412. *See also* physical activity
Leningrad famine, 537
leptin, 383, 404
less fat, defined, 160
leucine, 186, 187, 331
leukocytes, overview, 263, 346–347. *See also* blood
levulose, 109, 124
licensed nutritionist (LN), 22
lifestyle choices
  body weight and, 384–385
  cancer risk, 284
  cardiovascular disease, 179–183
  diabetes and, 140–141
  obesity, prevention of, 561
Life Without Bread, 389
light, defined, 160
lignins, 113
limiting amino acid, 192
linoleic acid, 150, 159
lipase, 157
lipids, 10–11. *See also* fat, dietary
lipoprotein lipase (LPL), 157
lipoproteins, 156
liposuction, 408–409
Listeria monocytogenes, 459, 473
Live Active Culture seal, 63
liver
  alcohol, effects of, 33–34
  alcohol metabolism, 30
  blood glucose regulation, 119–120
  digestion, carbohydrates, 117–118
  fat digestion, 156
  nutrient regulation, 89–90
  protein digestion, 197–198
  sulfur intake, 345–346
liver disease, 307
livestock production, 213
lobelia, 367
locust gum, 477
low birth weight, 505
low-density lipoproteins (LDLs). *See also* cholesterol
  free radicals, damage from, 258
  high-protein diets, 399
  overview of, 177–178
  sugar intake and, 125
  vitamin A, 270
  vitamin C, 263
  vitamin E, 260–262
low-fat, defined, 160, 162
low-intensity activities, 416–417
L-tryptophan, 367
lung cancer, 283
lymph, 87, 88–89
lymphatic system, 88–89
lymph nodes, 88–89
lysine, 187, 192, 193

M

macrobiotic diet, 207, 208
macrocytic anemia, 338–339
macrolytic anemia, 510
macular degeneration, 569
mad cow disease, 461, 462
magnesium, 12, 221, 225, 298, 310–312
magnolia-stephania, 367
ma huang, 367, 437
major minerals, defined, 12, 220–221. *See also* minerals
malabsorption, celiac disease, 103–105
malnutrition
  alcohol use and, 34
  celiac disease, 104
  global issues, 491–496
  health effects, 493–494
  protein-energy malnutrition, 211–212
  solutions for, 496–497
  in United States, 495–496
maltase, 117
maltol, 477
maltose, 109–110, 124
malt sugar, 110
manganese
  antioxidant function, 259
  functions and sources, 222, 344–345
  intake recommendations, 330
  overview, 12
  superoxide dismutase antioxidant enzyme system, 276
mannitol, 124, 129
maple sugar, 124
marasmus, 211–212, 493–494
March of Dimes, 37, 539
margarine, 149
maternal iron deficiency, 511
maximal heart rate, 416–417
McGwire, Mark, 435
meat, 54, 182–183, 461, 462. *See also* protein
meat factor, 350
meconium, 518
media
  eating disorders and, 444, 446
  research reporting, 20–21
medications
  acne treatment, 558
  alcohol interactions, 30
  appetite suppressants, 77
  blood lipids, lowering, 183
  breast milk, 523
  fluid loss, 235
  nutrition, interactions with, 569
  osteoporosis, 323
  ulcers and, 94
  vitamin D, interactions, 308
  weight loss, 406–408
Medicine and Science in Sports and Exercise, 24
Mediterranean diet, 51, 56, 58
megadosing, vitamins, 217–218, 266
megaloblastic anemia, 339
megaloblasts, 339
men. *See also* eating disorders
  alcohol use and, 31–32
  body fluid, 228
  calcium intake, 298
  fat distribution patterns, 374–375
  fertility, 502
  fluoride intake, 298
  magnesium intake, 298, 311
  muscle dysmorphia, 447
  osteoporosis, 320
  phosphorus intake, 246, 298
  potassium requirements, 244
  selenium intake, 275
  vitamin A intake, 271–272
  vitamin C intake, 265
  vitamin D intake, 298, 305
  vitamin E intake, 261
  vitamin K intake, 298, 308–309
  water, recommended intake, 236
menadione, 218
menaquinone, 218, 308–309
menopause, 296, 320
menstruation, 322, 446, 451
mercury, 481–482, 539
Meridia, 407
messenger RNA (mRNA), 188–189
metabolic syndrome, 140, 403–404
metabolic tolerance, alcohol, 31
metabolic water, 234
metabolism
  basal metabolic rate (BMR), 377–378
  biotin, 341–342
  choline, 343
  chromium, 344, 345
  energy for muscles, 419–423
  fat distribution patterns, 374–375
  folate and, 336–339
  iodine, 343–344
  manganese, 344–345
  niacin, 333–334
  pantothenic acid, 341
  regulation of, 328–329
  sulfur, 345–346
  thermic effect of food (TEF), 378
  vitamin B_{12} (cobalamin), 339–341
  vitamin B_6 (pyridoxine), 334–336
  vitamin B_2 (riboflavin), 332
  vitamin B_1 (thiamin), 331–332
  vitamins and, 11–12
metabolites, phytochemicals, 68–71
methicillin-resistant *Staphylococcus aureus* (MRSA), 484–485
methionine
  bone loss and, 210
  metabolism of, 335, 337, 339
  overview, 187
  sources, 192, 193
  sulfur and, 345–346
  vitamin B_6 and, 336
micelle, 156
microbial biopesticides, 482–483
microcytic anemia, 338–339, 353
micron filtration, 239
micronutrients. *See also* specific vitamin and mineral names
  absorption of, 223
  adolescents, nutrition needs, 555–556
  controversies about, 223–225
  early childhood, nutrition needs, 550
  minerals, 220–221
  older adults, nutrition needs, 565
  overview, 11–12
  toddlers, nutrition needs, 543

use of, 221–223
vitamins, overview, 217–220
microwave cooking, food safety, 469–470, 475
milk. *See also* dairy foods
adolescents, nutrition needs, 556, 558
calcium sources, 298–300, 306
DASH diet, 182–183
early childhood, nutrition needs, 553
food labels, 102
growth hormones, 484–485
infant needs, 530
lactose intolerance, 101
riboflavin, 332
toddlers, nutrition needs, 543
vitamin D, 305
Milk Matters, 558
milk sugar, 109–110
millet, 205
minerals. *See also* specific mineral names
absorption of, 87
antioxidants, 259
calcium overconsumption, 300–301
energy metabolism, 328–329
fiber and, 127
infant needs, 527
overview, 8, 220–223
mineral water, 238
miscarriage, 504. *See also* pregnancy
mitochondria, 81, 348
model systems, research, 19
moderate-intensity activities, 416–417
moderation, defined, 40
modified atmosphere packaging, 474
molasses, 111, 124
mold, 461, 468
mold, inhibitors of, 474–475
molybdenum, 12
monosaccharides, 109, 116–117
monosodium glutamate (MSG), 477
monounsaturated fatty acids (MUFAs), 145. *See also* fat, dietary
morbid obesity, 370–372
morning sickness, 512–513
mortality
infant mortality rates, 501
leading causes of death, 7
undernutrition, 493–494
Mothers Against Drunk Driving, 37
mouth, 81–83, 155, 198
mouthwash, 313
MSG (monosodium glutamate), 477
mucilage, 113
mucus, 85, 87, 231
muscle dysmorphia, 447
muscles
amino acid supplements, 202
anabolic steroids, 435
androsterone, 435–436
body mass index and, 372
calcium, function of, 297
chromium intake, 344, 345
contraction, 232–233
dehydroeplandrosterone, 435–436
endurance, 412
energy sources in, 419–420
gastrointestinal tract, 91–92
GHB (gamma-hydroxybutyric acid), 436
heat cramps, 252
lactic acid buildup, 422
musculoskeletal fitness, 412
protein structure, 190
strength training, 415
mushrooms, 461–462
mutual supplementation, 192
mycotoxins, 461
myelin, 349
myoglobin, 348
MyPlate, 51–52
empty Calories, 52
ethnic variations, 56–58
ethnic versions, 56, 57, 58
food groups, 52, 53
for children, 549
older adults, 565, 566
serving sizes, 54–56
vegetarian diet, 209–210
website, 58, 65

N

naproxen sodium, 94
National Cancer Institute (NCI), 23
National Center for Complementary and Alternative Medicine (NCCAM), 23, 65, 363–364
National Center for Health Statistics, 27
National Council on Alcoholism and Drug Dependence, Inc., 37
National Digestive Diseases Clearinghouse, 104
National Health and Nutrition Examination Survey (NHANES), 23
National Heart, Lung, and Blood Institute (NHLBI), 23
National Institute of Child Health and Human Development, 558
National Institute of Dental and Craniofacial Research, 135
National Institute of Diabetes and Digestive and Kidney Diseases (NIDDK), 23
National Institute on Alcohol Abuse and Alcoholism, 37
National Institute on Alcoholism and Alcohol Abuse, 36
National Institutes of Health, 23, 27
National Organic Program (NOP), 485
National School Breakfast Program, 496
National School Lunch Program (NSLP), 496, 551
National Student Campaign Against Hunger and Homelessness, 497
National Weight Control Registry, 395
National Yogurt Association, 63
Native Americans, MyPyramid, 56
natural disasters, food insecurity, 491–496
natural sweetener, 124
nausea and vomiting of pregnancy (NVP), 512–513
nervous system
calcium, function of, 297
electrolytes, function of, 232, 233
gastrointestinal system, 91–92
hunger and, 74
mercury, 481–482
nutrients for function, 236
vitamin B_{12} and, 339
neural tube defects, 46, 338, 359, 510
neuromuscular system, 91–92, 236, 349
neuropeptide Y, 384
neurotoxins, 461
neurotransmitters, 263, 331, 334–335, 339
New Pritikin Program, 392–393
niacin
energy metabolism, 328–329
functions and sources, 333–334
intake recommendations, 330
overview, 12, 218–220
pellagra, 5
riboflavin and, 332
toxicity, 367
vitamin B_6 and, 335
nicotinamide, 219, 330, 333
nicotine, in breast milk, 523
nicotinic acid, 219, 330, 333
night blindness, 272, 273
night-eating syndrome, 450–451
nitrates, food preservation, 475
nitrites, 475
nitrogen, 11, 196
nitrogen balance, 199–201
nitrosamines, 263
nonessential amino acids, 187
non-heme iron, 223, 350
non-nutritive sweeteners, 130–132
nonsteroidal anti-inflammatory drugs (NSAIDs), 94
norepinephrine, 119–120, 263
norovirus, 460
nucleotide synthesis, 336–337
nucleus, atoms, 256–257
nucleus, cells, 80
nursing bottle syndrome, 532
nutraceuticals, debate about, 63
nutrient-dense foods, defined, 48
nutrient density, 48, 49
nutrients. *See also* specific nutrient names
Dietary Guidelines for Americans, 48–51
intake recommendations, 13–16
macronutrients, 9–11
micronutrients, 11–12
Nutrition Facts Panel, 43
overview, 8–13
nutrient transport, 329
nutrigenomics, 25, 225
nutrition. *See also* diet; nutrients
advice about, 21–24
contributions to health, overview, 4–7
defined, 4
dining out, 58, 60–62
disease prevention and, 6–7
early childhood, nutrition needs, 547–550
MyPlate, 51–58
nutrigenomics, debate about, 25
professional organizations, 24
research, evaluating, 16–21
USDA Food Patterns, 51–58
Nutrition Debate
antioxidants, food or supplements, 277
breastfeeding, 533
colon cleansing, 97
fat blockers, 169
functional foods, 63
genetically modified organisms, 487
high-fructose corn syrup, 133
high-protein diets, 399
meat consumption and global warming, 213

Nutrition Debate, *(cont.)*
nutrigenomics, 25
older adults, physical activity level, 571
physical activity, levels of, 439
sports beverages, 247
vitamin D deficiency, 315
zinc and the common cold, 357
Nutrition Facts Panel, 43–44, 123
nutritionists, 22
Nutrition Label Activity
calcium intake, 306
carbohydrates, recognizing, 129
fat content, 161
food allergens, 102
health claims, 47
infant formula, 529
serving sizes, 55
Nutrition Labeling and Education Act, 41
Nutrition Myth or Fact
athletes, proteins needs of, 199
breakfast, importance of, 552
chromium supplements, 345
fluid intake during exercise, 243
healthy eating, cost of, 386
honey, nutritional value, 111
lactic acid and muscle fatigue, 422
mad cow disease, beef consumption, 462
margarine *vs.* butter, 149
pellagra, 5
ulcers, causes of, 94
vegan diets, children and, 548
vitamin C and the common cold, 264
Nutrition Services Incentive Program, 570
nutrition transition, 495
nutritive sweeteners, 129
nuts
amino acid content, 193
DASH diet, 182–183
food labels, 102
overview, 147
protein content, 203–204

O

obesity
body composition, 372–374
body mass index (BMI), 370–372, 374
breastfeeding and, 533
cardiovascular disease, 176
causes of, 404–405
children and adolescents, 560–561
cultural and economic factors, 384–385
developing nations, 495
diabetes and, 139–140
diet and, 6
diet plans, creating, 393–397
diets for weight loss, 388–389, 392–393
dining out and, 58, 60–62
early childhood, nutrition needs, 553–554
energy balance, 375–380, 380
fat distribution patterns, 374–375
fetal environment, 538
genetic factors, 381–382
health effects, 403–404
high-fructose corn syrup, 133
older adults, 567–568
physical activity and, 412
physiology, influence of, 382–384
psychological and social factors, 385–387
rates of, 7
sugar intake and, 125
toddlers, 546
treatment for, 405–409
vegetarian diet, 207
vitamin D, 304, 315
web resources, 401, 409
weight loss, readiness for, 390–392
observation, research, 17, 19
obsessive-compulsive behaviors, 444
occupational health, defined, 6
oils. *See also* fat, dietary
DASH diet, 182–183
defined, 144
Dietary Guidelines for Americans, 50
Dietary Reference Intake (DRI), 15
overview, 8, 10–11
Old Ways Preservation and Exchange Trust, 65
older adults
nutrition needs, 564–567
nutrition-related concerns, 567–570
physical activity level, 571
physiologic changes, 562–563
slowing the aging process, 574–579
statistics on, 561–562
olestra, 166, 274
oligopeptide, 188
omega fatty acids, 148, 150–151, 159, 164–165
oral contraceptives, iron absorption and, 351
organelles, cells, 80
organic, defined, 8
organic food, 386, 485–486
organic pollutants, food safety, 481–482
organosulfur compounds, 69
orlistat, 407
Ornish diet, 392–393
osmosis, 231–232
osteoarthritis, diet and, 6
osteoblasts, 294
osteocalcin, 308
osteoclasts, 294
osteomalacia, 307
osteoporosis
adolescents, nutrition needs, 558
aging and, 563
assessment of, 295–296
calcium intake and, 301
defined, 319
diet and, 6
early childhood, nutrition needs, 553
fluoride intake, 312
health claims, food labels, 46
physical activity and, 413
prevention of, 324–325
risk for, 294, 320–322
treatment of, 322–324
vitamin K intake, 308
ounce-equivalent, 55
Overeaters Anonymous, 409
overload principle, 415
overnutrition, 495
overpopulation, food insecurity, 492
overweight
body composition, 372–374
body mass index (BMI), 370–372, 374
breastfeeding and, 533
cardiovascular disease, 176
causes of, 404–405
children and adolescents, 560–561
cultural and economic factors, 384–385
developing nations, 495
diet plans, creating, 393–397
diets for weight loss, 388–389, 392–393
early childhood, nutrition needs, 553–554
energy balance, 375–380, 380
fat distribution patterns, 374–375
fetal environment, 538
genetic factors, 381–382
health effects, 403–404
older adults, 567–568
physical activity and, 412
physiology, influence of, 382–384
pregnancy weight gain, 505, 507
psychological and social factors, 385–387
toddlers, 546
treatment for, 405–409
web resources, 401, 409
weight loss, readiness for, 390–392
ovovegetarian diet, 207
ovulation, 503
oxidation, 256–258
oxygen, food safety and, 464
oxygen transport, iron and, 348
oxytocin, 518

P

packaging, food safety, 474
pain relievers, 94
palmitic acid, 421
pancreas
adrenaline, effect on, 153
alcohol use, 34
digestive process, 86–87
fat digestion, 156
insulin production, 119–120
pancreatic amylase, 87, 117
pancreatic lipase, 87
pantothenic acid
energy metabolism, 328–329
functions and sources, 219, 341
intake recommendations, 330
overview, 12, 218–220
parasites, 460, 469
parathyroid hormone (PTH), 296, 301
Pasteur, Louis, 474
pasteurization, 474
Peanut Corporation of America (PCA), 455
peanuts, 13, 102–103
pear-shaped fat distribution, 374
pectin, 112–113, 477
peer pressure, food choice and, 551
pellagra, 5, 6, 333–334
pepsin, 197
pepsinogen, 85, 197
peptic ulcers, 94
peptide bonds, 188
peptide YY (PYY), 383
peptidoglycan, 457, 460
percent daily values, 44
perfectionism, 444
performance enhancers, 434–438
peripheral nervous system, 91–92. *See also* nervous system

peristalsis, 84
pernicious anemia, 339
persistent organic pollutants, 481–482
pescovegetarian diet, 207
pesticides, 482–483, 484, 485, 489
pH, body, 194–195
phen-fen, 407
phenobarbital, 308
phenolic acids, 69
phenomenon, research, 17
phentermine, 407
phenylalanine, 131–132, 187
phenylketonuria (PKU), 131–132, 187
phosphate, 422
phosphofructokinase (PFK), 194
phospholipids, 80, 151, 339
phosphorus
  bone health and, 298, 309–310
  bones, composition of, 292–293
  electrolyte balance, 229
  function and sources, 245–246
  neuromuscular function, 236
  overview, 12, 221
photosynthesis, 108
phylloquinone, 218, 308–309
physical activity
  adolescents, 555
  benefits of, 412–413
  cancer risk, 283–284, 288
  carbohydrates, 114, 426–429
  cardiovascular disease, 176
  childhood obesity, prevention of, 561
  dehydration, preventing, 251–252
  Dietary Guidelines for Americans, 48
  energy needs, 378–379, 380, 419–423
  ergogenic aids, 434–438
  fats, energy from, 152–153, 429
  female athlete triad, 322, 433, 451–452
  fitness program, components of, 413–418
  FIT principle, 415–417
  fluid intake, 243
  fluid loss, 235
  heat illnesses, 252–253
  levels of, debate about, 439
  muscle dysmorphia, 447
  nutrition needs, overview, 424–425
  older adults, 571
  osteoporosis, risk of, 322
  pregnancy and, 516–517
  protein requirements, 199, 200, 202, 429–430
  serving size and, 59
  social influences, 385–386
  sports beverages, 247
  vitamin and mineral needs, 432–434
  water, intake recommendations, 237
  web resources, 441
  for weight loss, 394–396
  wellness and, 5–6
Physical Activity Pyramid, 414–415
physical fitness, 412. *See also* physical activity
phytates, 350, 354
phytic acid, 246
phytochemicals, 51, 67–71, 259
phytoestrogens, 69
pica, 513
placebo-controlled research studies, 20
placebo effect, 20
placenta, 504
plants, carbohydrates from, 110–113
plaque, atherosclerosis, 174
plasma, 228, 346–347
platelets, 174, 346–347
pleural fluid, 231
poison, 33, 461–462
pollutants, food safety, 481–482
Polynesians, body mass index, 372
polypeptide, 188, 197
polyphenols, 350
polysaccharides, 110–113
polyunsaturated fatty acids (PUFAs), 145
Pondimin, 407
portal vein, 89–90
portion size, 393–394, 545
potassium. *See also* electrolytes
  Dietary Guidelines for Americans, 51
  electrolyte balance, 194, 195, 229
  functions and sources, 242–245
  muscle contraction, 232–233
  nerve impulses, 232, 233
  neuromuscular function, 236
  overview, 12, 221
potassium sorbate, 477
potatoes, 463
poverty, food insecurity, 386, 554, 569–570
pre-diabetes, 140
preeclampsia, 514
pregnancy
  acne treatments, 558
  adolescent pregnancy, 514–515
  alcohol use and abuse, 35, 515
  breastfeeding, advantages and challenges, 521–525
  caffeine, 515
  calcium intake, 298
  constipation, 513–514
  cravings and aversions, 513
  drug use and abuse, 516
  exercise, 516–517
  fetal development timeline, 506
  fetal environment, In Depth, 536–539
  fluid loss, 235
  folate intake, 338
  food safety, 516
  gastroesophageal reflux (GERD), 513
  gestational diabetes, 514
  herbal supplements, 364
  hypertension, 514
  iodine intake, 344
  lactation, 517–524
  macronutrient needs, 508–509
  micronutrient needs, 509–512
  morning sickness, 512–513
  nutritional needs, 502–505
  physical activity and, 413
  selenium intake, 276
  smoking and, 284, 516
  vegetarian diet and, 515
  vitamin A, 272
  web resources, 535
  weight gain, 505, 507
prehypertension, 175
premenstrual syndrome, 336
preschoolers
  food choices, 551–553
  nutrition needs, 549–550
  nutrition-related concerns, 553–554
prescription medications
  acne treatment, 558
  alcohol interactions, 30
  appetite suppressants, 77
  blood lipids, lowering, 183
  breast milk, 523
  fluid loss, 235
  nutrition, interactions with, 569
  osteoporosis, 323
  ulcers and, 94
  vitamin D, interactions, 308
  weight loss, 406–408
preservation, food, 473–476
preterm birth, 505
primary hypertension, 175
primary structure, proteins, 190–192
prion, 461, 462
Pritikin diet, 392–393
probiotics, 63
processed foods, food safety, 472–476, 473–476
processes foods, added sugar, 123
procoagulants, 347
professional organizations, overview of, 24
prolactin, 518
proline, 187
proof, alcohol, 29
prooxidant, 266
Propionic acid, 475
propylene glycol, 477
propyl gallate, 474, 477
prostate cancer, 167
proteases, 87, 197–198
protein
  adolescents, nutrition needs, 555
  amino acids, 186–187
  breastfeeding, intake for, 520
  in breast milk, 521
  complete and incomplete, 192
  DASH diet, 182–183
  defined, 186
  dietary recommendations, 199–205
  Dietary Reference Intake (DRI), 15
  diets for weight loss, 389
  digestion of, 197–199
  early childhood, nutrition needs, 550
  energy from, 10, 114, 377
  as energy source, 423
  fat storage and, 382
  functions of, 193–197
  high-protein diets, 389, 399
  kwashiorkor, 494
  metabolism of, 341
  MyPlate, 52, 53
  older adults, nutrition needs, 565
  osteoporosis, risk of, 321
  over consumption of, 210–211
  overview, 8, 11
  physical activity, intake for, 424, 429–430
  pregnancy, intake requirements, 508–509
  protein-energy malnutrition, 211–212
  protein turnover, 189–190
  satiation and, 75
  sources of, 202–205
  structure of, 190–192
  sulfur intake, 345–346
  synthesis of, 188–192
  toddlers, nutrition needs, 542–544, 546–547
  vegetarian diets, 205–210
  zinc and, 354

Protein Power diet, 389
prothrombin, 308–309, 347
protozoa, 460
provitamins, 267, 302, 303
psychological influences, body weight, 385–387
psychosomatic effect, 20
psyllium, 113
puberty, growth and activity patterns, 554–555. *See also* adolescents
publications, nutrition profession, 24
purging, 448–450
pyloric sphincter, 86
pyridoxal, 219, 334–336
pyridoxamine, 219, 334–336
pyridoxine, 219
  functions and sources, 334–336
  intake recommendations, 330
pyruvic acid, 420–421

Q

quackery
  Find the Quack, 26
  health claims, 64
  media reports, 20–21
quaternary structure, proteins, 190–192
Quetelet's index, 370–372
Quick Tips
  alcohol intake, 31
  beta-carotene intake, 269
  calcium, sources of, 300
  cancer risk, reducing, 288
  dining out, 61
  eating out, limiting fat, 168
  fiber, sources for, 127
  food behaviors, modifying, 397
  food safety, barbecues, 470
  iron intake, increasing, 352
  legumes, adding to diet, 205
  media hype, 21
  pesticide exposure, 483
  physical activity, barriers, 395
  physical activity, increasing, 418
  portion size, 394
  saturated and trans fats, reducing, 166
  sodium, reducing intake, 242
  stocking your first kitchen, 557
  supplements, safety of, 363
  traveler's diarrhea, 96
  vitamin C, sources of, 265
  vitamin E, 261
  vitamins, food preparation, 343
quinoa, 205
quinones, 308–309
quorn, 205

R

race
  diabetes and, 138
raw fish, 469
raw sugar, 124
recombinant bovine growth hormone (rBGH), 484–485
recombinant bovine somatotropin (rBST), 484–485
recombinant DNA technology, 479–480
recommended daily allowance (RDA)
  early childhood, nutrition needs, 550
  older adults, 564–566
  toddlers, nutrition needs, 542–543
Recommended Dietary Allowance (RDA)
  beta-carotene, 267–268
  carbohydrates, 122–128
  magnesium, 311
  overview, 13, 14
  phosphorus, 309–310
  protein, 199, 201–202
  selenium, 275
  vitamin A, 271–272
  vitamin C, 265
  vitamin D, 302–303
  vitamin E, 261
  vitamin K, 308–309
red blood cells (RBCs). *See also* blood
  iron-deficiency anemia, 6, 352–353, 543
  overview, 346–347
  protein structure, 190–191
  synthesis of, 337
  vitamin E, 260–262
red tide, 462
reduced fat, defined, 160, 162
Redux, 407
refined flour, 126
refrigeration, food safety, 467
registered dietitian, 22
religion, diet and, 56, 206–207
remodeling, bone, 293–294
reproduction, human. *See* pregnancy
research studies
  evaluating, 16–21
  media and, 20–21
  types of, 19–21
residues, food safety, 480–486
resistance training, 415
resorption, bone, 294
respiratory disease
  mortality rates, 7
restaurant dining, 58, 60–62, 165–166, 168, 470–471, 560
resveratrol, 29–30, 71
retina, 270–271
Retin-A, 272
retinal, 269
retinoic acid, 218, 269
retinoids, 269
retinol, 218, 267, 269–274, 277
Retinol Activity Equivalents (RAE), 269–270
retinol-binding protein, 269
reverse osmosis, 239
rhodopsin, 270–271
riboflavin
  energy metabolism, 328–329
  exercise, intake for, 433
  functions and sources, 332
  intake recommendations, 330
  overview, 12, 218–220
  vegan diet, 208
ribonucleic acid (RNA), 245, 339, 344
ribose, 109, 437–438
ribosomes, 80
rice, 192
rickets, 307
RNA (ribonucleic acid), 245, 339, 344
roundworms, 460
running, energy use, 421
rye, 103

S

saccharin, 130–132
safety, food. *See* food safety
saliva, 82, 231, 563
salivary amylase, 116–117
salivary glands, 82, 83
Salmonella, 455, 459, 460, 470
salt, intake, 48, 50
salting, food preservation, 473
sample size, research, 17–18
satiety, 75, 154, 382–383
saturated fats. *See also* fat, dietary
  Dietary Guidelines for Americans, 50
  dietary recommendations, 163–164
  overview, 145
  reducing in diet, 165, 166
saturated fatty acids, 145
school lunches, 549–550
scientific method, 16–20
scratch test, food allergies, 103
scurvy, 4, 6, 262, 266
seafood, 462, 463
Sears, Barry, 430
secondary structure, proteins, 190–192
sedentary lifestyle, 384–385
selective breeding, 479–480
selenium
  antioxidant function, 259
  functions and sources, 222, 274–276
  health claims, 225
  overview, 12
sell by date, 466
semivegetarian diet, 207
Senior Farmers' Market Nutrition Program, 570
senses, 76, 562–563
sensible water loss, 234–235
sensory neuropathy, 336
serine, 187, 337
serotonin, 384
serving size
  MyPlate, 54–56
  NIH quiz about, 65
  Nutrition Facts Panel, 43
  Nutrition Label Activity, 55
  toddlers, 545
  weight management and, 393–394
  You Do The Math, 59
set-point theory, 381–382
shelf-life, food safety, 466
shellfish, food labels, 102
sibutramine, 407
sickle cell anemia, 338–339
sigmoid colon, 90–91
simple carbohydrates, 108–109. *See also* carbohydrates
skin, 267, 302, 303, 558
skin cancer, 285–286, 287
skinfold measurement, 373
Slow Food USA, 489
small intestine
  celiac disease, 103–105
  digestive process, 85, 86–90
  fat digestion, 155
  probiotics, 63
  protein digestion, 197–198
smell, sense of, 76, 562–563
smoking, food preservation, 473

smoking tobacco
- adolescents, 558–559
- cancer risk, 283, 284
- cardiovascular disease, 176
- osteoporosis, risk of, 320–321
- pregnancy and, 516, 538–539

social health, defined, 6
social influences, body weight and, 385–387, 405
social influences, food choices, 76–77
Society for Nutrition Education (SNE), 24, 27, 401
socioeconomic status
- body weight and, 384–385
- food insecurity, 554
- healthy eating, cost of, 386
- older adults, 569–570

sodium. *See also* electrolytes
- Dietary Guidelines for Americans, 48, 50
- electrolyte balance, 194, 195, 229
- fast-food meals, 60, 61
- food labeling, 45
- functions and sources, 240–242
- hypertension and, 182–183
- muscle contraction, 232–233
- nerve impulses, 232, 233
- neuromuscular function, 236
- osteoporosis, risk of, 322
- overview, 12, 221
- pregnancy, intake requirements, 509, 512

sodium ascorbate, 478
sodium benzoate, 477
sodium bisulfite, 475, 477
sodium chloride (salt), food preservation, 477
sodium nitrate, 477
sodium nitrite, 477
sodium propionate, 475, 477
soft drinks, 123, 125, 133, 238, 310
solanine, 463
soluble fiber, 112–113
solutes, 231–232
solvents, 230, 231–232
sorbic acid, 477
sorbitol, 124, 129
sorghum, 205
soy-based infant formula, 528
soybeans, 102, 192, 203, 350
soy milk, 547
Special Supplemental Nutrition Program for Women, Infants and Children (WIC), 496
sphincters, 81, 83
spina bifida, 510
spiritual health, defined, 6
spongy bone, 293
spontaneous abortion, 504
sports anemia, 433
sports beverages, 237, 247
stabilizers, food additives, 478
Staphylococcus, 459, 484–485
starch, 110–112
steroid hormones, 263
steroids, anabolic, 435
sterols, overview, 151–152. *See also* cholesterol
stomach
- alcohol metabolism, 30
- digestive disorders, 92–94
- digestive process, 85–86
- fat digestion, 155
- protein digestion, 197
- ulcers, 92–94

stone ground, defined, 126
storage, food safety, 466–468, 472–476
strength, amino acid supplements, 202
stress, 94, 96, 413
Stringer, Korey, 250–251, 253
stroke, 6, 7, 174
structure-function claims, food labels, 44–46
sucralose, 130, 132
sucrase, 117
sucrose, 109–110, 129
sudden infant death syndrome (SIDS), 522
sugar, 45, 50, 109, 111, 122–125. *See also* carbohydrates; glucose
sugar alcohols, 129
Sugar Busters, 389
sugaring, food preservation, 473
sulfites, 475, 477
sulfur, 12, 221, 345–346
sulfur amino acids, 210
sulfur dioxide, 475, 477
Summer Food Service Program, 496
sunburn, dehydration, 251
sunlight, 301–304, 314, 315, 565
superoxide dismutase, 354, 355
Supplementary Nutrition Assistance Program (SNAP), 496, 554, 569
supplements
- amino acids, 202
- anti-aging, 577–578
- antioxidants, 277
- beta-carotene, 267–268
- breastfeeding, 520
- chromium, 345
- debate about, 63
- fat blockers, 169
- herbal, 363–364
- illness and injury from, 367
- infant needs, 527–528
- micronutrients, value of, 224–225
- need for, 364–366
- older adults, 566–567
- osteoporosis prevention, 324–325
- performance enhancers (ergogenic aids), 434–438
- phytochemicals, 71
- pregnancy and, 512
- safety of, 362–363
- silver supplements, 567
- types and regulation of, 361–362
- web resources, 225, 367
- weight loss, 388–389
- zinc, 357

surface water, 237
surgery
- fluid loss, 235
- weight loss, 408–409

sushi, 469
swallowing, 84
sweat, fluid balance, 234–235
sweeteners, alternative, 128–132
synovial fluid, 231
synthetic pesticides, 483
synthetic pheromones, 482–483
systems, organs, 81
systolic blood pressure, 175
systolic hypertension, 174

T

Takaki, Kanehiro, 331
tapeworms, 460, 461
tartrazine, 477, 478
taste, sense of, 76, 563
T cells, 271
tea, 277, 367
tears, 231
teens. *See* adolescents
teeth
- digestion, process of, 83
- early childhood, nutrition needs, 553
- fluoride, 312–313
- gum disease, 123–124, 568
- infants, 532
- older adults, 568
- sugar and, 123–124

teff, 205
temperature, body
- dehydration, 251
- fluid balance and, 230, 430–432
- heat illnesses, 252–253

temperature, food safety
- cooking, 469–470
- danger zone, 463
- storage, 467–468

teratogen, defined, 34, 35, 502
tertiary structure, proteins, 190–192
testosterone, 320, 554–555, 563
texture, 76, 154, 478
thalassemia, 338–339
thawing, food safety, 467–468
theory, research, 18–19
thermic effect of food (TEF), 378
thiamin pyrophosphate (TPP), 329, 331
thiamin (vitamin B_1)
- energy metabolism, 328–329
- exercise, intake for, 433
- functions and sources, 331–332
- intake recommendations, 330
- overview, 12, 218–220

thickening agents, 478
thirst, 233–234
threonine, 187
thrifty gene theory, 381
thyroid gland, 296
thyroid hormone, 274, 343–344
thyroxine, 263, 274
time of activity, FIT principle, 417
tissue fluid, 228
tissues, 81
tobacco use
- adolescents, 558–559
- cancer risk, 283, 284
- cardiovascular disease, 176
- osteoporosis, risk of, 320–321
- pregnancy and, 516, 538–539

tocopherols, 218, 260–262
tocotrienols, 260–262
toddlers
- food choices, 545–546
- nutrition needs, 542–545
- nutrition-related concerns, 546–547

tofu, 213
Tolerable Upper Intake Level (UL), 13, 15
tongue, 83
toothpaste, 313

total fiber, 112–113
total serum cholesterol, 178–179. *See also* cholesterol
toxins, 97, 457, 461, 470
trabecular bone, 292
trace minerals, defined, 12, 220–221. *See also* minerals
trachea, 83
transamination, 187
transcription, protein synthesis, 188–189
trans fats. *See also* fat, dietary
  dietary recommendations, 163–164
  overview, 147–148
  reducing in diet, 165, 166
transferrin, 352, 353
transgenic crops, 496
translation, protein synthesis, 188–189
transportation, food safety, 458
transport proteins, 194, 196
transverse colon, 90–91
traumatic injury, 34, 235
travel, food safety and, 471–472
traveler's diarrhea, 95, 96
tretinoin, 272
triglycerides, 144–150, 412. *See also* fat, dietary
trimester, defined, 502. *See also* pregnancy
tripeptide, 188
triticale, 103
tryptophan, 187, 333, 384
T-score, 295–296
Tufts Modified MyPyramid for Older Adults, 565, 566
tumors, 282
turbinado sugar, 124
type 1 diabetes. *See* diabetes
type 2 diabetes. *See* diabetes
tyrosine, 187

U

ulcers, 94
ultrafiltration, 239
ultraviolet radiation, 285–286, 314
umbilical cord, 504
unbleached flour, 126
uncoupling proteins, 383–384
undernutrition
  fetal development, 537–538
  global issues, 491–496
  health effects, 493–494
  in United States, 495–496
underwater weighing, 373
underweight
  body mass index (BMI), 370–372
  healthy weight gain, 397–398
  older adults, 567–568
  pregnancy weight gain, 505, 507
  social factors, 386–387
unsaturated fatty acids, 145. *See also* fat, dietary
upper esophageal sphincter, 83
urea, 196, 211, 344
urinary tract infections, 512
urine, 234–235, 252
U.S. Department of Agriculture
  Food Patterns, 51–58
  Dietary Guidelines for Americans, 48–51, 389
  food safety, 456, 465
  MyPlate, 51–58
  organic farming, 485
  website, 457
U.S. Department of Health and Human Services, 23, 558
U.S. Environmental Protection Agency, 456
U.S. Food and Drug Administration
  food allergens, labels and, 102
  food labels, 41
  food safety, 455
  prescription appetite suppressants, 77
  supplements, 361
  water, regulation of, 238
  website, 65, 457
U.S. Pharmacopoeia (USP), 363
use by date, 466

V

valine, 187, 331
vanillin, 476
variables, research, 18
variant Creutzfeldt-Jakob disease, 462
variety, defined, 41
vegan diet. *See also* vegetarian diet
  challenges of, 208
  children, debate about, 548
  exercise and, 430, 433
  health benefits, 207
  supplements for, 365
  toddlers, needs of, 546–547
  web resources, 573
vegetable-based oils, 149, 162, 164
vegetables
  amino acid content, 193
  beta-carotene, 268
  calcium source, 298–299, 306
  DASH diet, 182–183
  Dietary Guidelines for Americans, 51
  MyPlate, 52, 53
  pesticides in, 484
  serving size, 54
  vitamin C, 264–265
vegetarian diet
  exercise and, 430, 433
  Food Guide Pyramid, 209–210
  mutual supplementation, protein, 192, 193
  pregnancy, 515
  protein and, 185, 205–210
  supplements for, 365
  toddlers, needs of, 546–547
  vitamin E, 260–261
  web resources, 573
Vegetarian Food Guide Pyramid, 209–210
vertical banded gastroplasty, 408
very-low-density lipoproteins, 177. *See also* cholesterol
vigorous-intensity activities, 416–417
villi, 87
viruses, food-borne illness, 460
visible fat, 160
vision
  aging and, 563
  appetite stimulation, 76
  beta-carotene, 267
  older adults, 569
  vitamin A, benefits of, 270–271, 272–274
vitamin A
  acne treatments, 558
  adolescents, nutrition needs, 555–556
  antioxidant function, 259
  beta-carotene, 267–269
  deficiency, 217, 494
  early childhood, nutrition needs, 550
  food or supplements, debate about, 277
  function and sources, 269–274
  health claims, 225
  older adults, nutrition needs, 566–567
  overview, 12, 217–218
  pregnancy, intake requirements, 509, 511
  sources, 272
  toddlers, nutrition needs, 542
  toxicity, 367
  transport of, 153–154
  zinc and, 354
vitamin B_7 (biotin)
  energy metabolism, 328–329
  functions and sources, 341–342
  intake recommendations, 330
  overview, 12, 218–220
vitamin B_{12} (cobalamin)
  energy metabolism, 328–329
  exercise, intake for, 433
  functions and sources, 339–341
  intake recommendations, 330
  older adults, nutrition needs, 564–566
  overview, 12, 218–220
  pregnancy, intake requirements, 509, 510
  recommended intake, 347
  toddlers, nutrition needs, 547
  vegan diet, 208
vitamin B_9 (folate/folic acid)
  energy metabolism, 328–329
  food additives, 478
  functions and sources, 336–339
  homocysteine levels and, 277
  intake recommendations, 330
  overview, 12, 218–220
  pregnancy, intake requirements, 509–510
  recommended intake, 347
  vitamin B_6 and, 335
vitamin B_6 (pyridoxine)
  energy metabolism, 328–329
  exercise, intake for, 433
  functions and sources, 334–336
  intake recommendations, 330
  older adults, nutrition needs, 564–566
  overview, 12, 218–220
  riboflavin and, 332
  toxicity, 367
vitamin B_2 (riboflavin)
  energy metabolism, 328–329
  exercise, intake for, 433
  functions and sources, 332–333
  intake recommendations, 330
  overview, 12, 218–220
  vegan diet, 208

vitamin B_1 (thiamin)
energy metabolism, 328–329
exercise, intake for, 433
functions and sources, 331–332
intake recommendations, 330
overview, 12, 218–220
vitamin C (ascorbic acid)
antioxidant function, 259
common cold and, 264
early childhood, nutrition needs, 550
food preservatives, 474, 477, 478
function and sources, 262–267
older adults, nutrition needs, 565, 568
overview, 12, 218–220
pregnancy, intake requirements, 509, 510
toddlers, nutrition needs, 542
vision and, 569
vitamin D
bone health and, 296, 298
deficiency, debate about, 315
food additives, 478
functions and sources, 301–308
health claims, 225
infant needs, 527
older adults, nutrition needs, 564, 565, 566, 568
osteoporosis, risk of, 321–322
overview, 12, 217–218
pregnancy, intake requirements, 509, 511
supplements, 324–325
toddlers, nutrition needs, 547
transport of, 153–154
vegan diet, 208
vitamin E
antioxidant function, 259, 260–262
early childhood, nutrition needs, 550
food additives, 478
food or supplements, debate about, 277
health claims, 225
older adults, nutrition needs, 565
overview, 12, 217–218
sources of, 261
toddlers, nutrition needs, 542
transport of, 153–154
vision and, 569
vitamin K
bone health and, 298, 308–309
functions and sources, 347–348
health claims, 225
overview, 12, 217–218
recommended intake, 347
riboflavin and, 332
transport of, 153–154
vitamins. *See also* supplements; specific vitamin name
absorption of, 87
antioxidants, 258–259
celiac disease, 104
classification of, 217–220
energy metabolism, 328–329
fat-soluble, 153–154
fiber and, 127
infant needs, 527
overview, 8, 11–12
pellagra, 5
physical activity, intake for, 424
provitamins, 267
special needs populations, 365
vomiting, 235, 245, 251

W

waist-to-hip ratio, 374–375
walking, energy use, 421
walnuts, 147
warm-up, physical activity, 418
washing, food safety, 465–466
water. *See also* fluid balance
absorption, intestines, 87
alcohol consumption, 32
dietary recommendations, 236–240
fluoride, 312–313
overhydration/dehydration, 238
overview, 8, 13
physical activity, intake for, 424, 430–432
safety of, 472
water-soluble vitamins, 12, 218–220
web resources
aging, 579
alcohol use and abuse, 37
anemia, 359
calcium, 317
cancer risk and prevention, 289
cardiovascular disease, 183
Centers for Disease Control and Prevention (CDC), 27, 457
children's nutrition, 573
diabetes, 141
dietary fats, 169
dietary supplements, 225, 279, 367
diet guidelines, 65
digestive disorders, 99, 105
eating disorders, 453
electrolyte balance, 249
Environmental Protection Agency, 457
exercise, 441
fetal development, 539
fluoride, 317
food insecurity, 499
food safety, 489
general nutrition information, 27
heat illnesses, 252–253
infant nutrition, 535
longevity, 579
MyPlate, 58, 65
National Center for Health Statistics, 27
National Institutes of Health (NIH), 27
neural tube defects, 359
obesity, 409
oral health, 135
osteoporosis, 325
pregnancy, 535
protein consumption, 215
supplements, 441
U.S. Department of Agriculture, 457
U.S. Food and Drug Administration, 457
vegetarian diet, 215, 573
vitamin D, 317
water, 249
weight management, 401
weight-for-age growth chart, 526
weight loss
body fluid loss, 252
breastfeeding, 519
diets for, 388–389, 392–393
supplements, 169
unexplained, 286
weight management
adolescents, 555
alcohol, Calories in, 30
body composition, 372–374
body mass index (BMI), 370–372, 374
breastfeeding, 519, 533
carbohydrates, 114–115
children and adolescents, 560–561
cultural and economic factors, 384–385
diabetes and, 139–140
Dietary Guidelines for Americans, 48
diet plans, creating, 393–397
early childhood, nutrition needs, 553–554
energy balance, 375–380, 380
fat blockers, 169
fat distribution patterns, 374–375
fat intake, 158
fiber and, 115
food choices, fat storage and, 382
genetic factors, 381–382
healthy body weight, 370
high-fructose corn syrup, 133
obesity, In Depth, 402–409
older adults, 567–568
physical activity and, 412
physiology, influence of, 382–384
pregnancy, 505, 507
psychological and social factors, 385–387
sports beverages, 247
sugar intake, 125
underweight, 397–398
web resources, 401, 409
weight loss, readiness for, 390–392
Weight Watchers, 389
wellness, 5–6, 15
well water, 237–238
Wernicke-Korsakoff syndrome, 332
What About You
alcohol abuse, 35
blood lipid levels, 179
bottled water, 239
cancer risks, lifestyle and, 285
cues for eating, 78
diabetes, risk for, 140
disordered eating, risk of, 444
global food insecurity, 498
osteoporosis, risk of, 323
protein consumption, 204
vitamin D intake, 305
weight loss, readiness, 390–392
wheat, 102, 103, 126
Whipple's disease, 307
white blood cells (WBCs), 263, 346–347. *See also* blood
white flour, 126
white sugar, 124
whole-grain flour, 126
whole-wheat flour, 126
WIC (Special Supplemental Nutrition Program for Women, Infants, and Children), 496

willow bark, 367
Wilson's disease, 356
women. *See also* eating disorders; pregnancy
  alcohol use and, 30, 31–32
  body fluid, 228
  breastfeeding, 517–524
  calcium intake, 298, 300
  fat distribution patterns, 374–375
  female athlete triad, 433, 451–452
  fluoride intake, 298
  iron intake, 433
  magnesium intake, 298, 311
  phosphorus intake, 246, 298
  potassium requirements, 244
  selenium intake, 275
  vitamin A intake, 271–272
  vitamin C intake, 265
  vitamin D intake, 298, 305
  vitamin E intake, 261
  vitamin K intake, 298, 308–309
  water, recommended intake, 236
World Health Organization, 272, 476
wormwood, 367
wound healing, 263

X

xanthan gum, 477
Xenical, 407
xylitol, 124, 129

Y

yeast, 461
yogurt, probiotics, 63
You Do The Math
  basal metabolic rate and daily energy needs, 380
  body mass index calculation, 374
  energy from carbohydrates, fats, proteins, 10
  heart rate, maximal and training, 417
  protein needs, 201
  serving size, 59
  toddlers, menu planning, 544

Z

zinc
  antioxidant function, 259
  common cold, debate about, 357
  copper and, 356
  deficiency, 494
  fiber and, 127
  functions and sources, 222, 354–355
  older adults, nutrition needs, 565
  overview, 12
  pregnancy, intake requirements, 509, 511
  recommended intake, 347
  superoxide dismutase antioxidant enzyme system, 276
  toddlers, nutrition needs, 542, 546–547
  vegan diet, 208
  vision and, 569
Zone Diet, 430
zygote, 503

CREDITS

Chapter 1

Opener Agencja FREE/Alamy; **p 4:** Brian Chase/Bvdc/Dreamstime; **p 5:** Lester V. Bergman/Corbis; 1.1 Wrangel/Dreamstime; **p 9:** Tom Stewart/Corbis; **p 10:** Ana Strack/Corbis; **p 12:** Bluehill/Dreamstime; **p 13:** Scott Rothstein/Webking/Dreamstime; **p 14:** Comstock Images/Thinkstock; **p 19:** Stockbyte/Getty Images; **p 21:** Kristin Piljay; **p 22:** Liquidlibrary/Thinkstock; **p 23:** Michael Donne/Photo Researchers; **p 24:** Rubberball/Getty Images; **p 25:** Randy Jirtle

In-Depth: Alcohol

Opener Ljupco/iStockphoto; Fig 1 Kristin Piljay; **p 30:** Michael Newman/PhotoEdit; **p 32:** top Jemma Jones/Alamy; **p 32:** bottom Edie Layland/Laylandmasuda/Dreamstime; **p 33:** Stockbyte/Getty Images; Fig 2a Science Photo Library/Photo Researchers; Fig 2b Martin Rotker/Photo Researchers; **p 34:** Enigma/Alamy; **p 35:** George Steinmetz Photography

Chapter 2

Opener Dan Kenyon/Taxi/Getty Images; **p 40:** top Adams Picture Library t/a apl/Alamy; **p 40:** bottom left Photosani/Shutterstock; **p 40:** bottom right Forest Badger/Shutterstock; **p 41:** iStockphoto; **p 42:** AP Photo; **p 44:** Sky Bonillo/Photo Edit; **p 47:** Ned Frisk Photography/Corbis; 2.4 Creative Digital Visions; **p 48:** Kzenon/Shutterstock; **p 50:** top Alexander Walter/Taxi/Getty Images; **p 50:** bottom Andrew Whittuck/Dorling Kindersley; 2.6 top to bottom ALEAIMAGE/iStockphoto; Kelly Cline/iStockphoto; Lew Robertson/iStockphoto; Morgan Lane Photography/Shutterstock; Natalia Mylova/Fotolia; **p 55:** iStockphoto/Thinkstock; 2.8 Kristin Piljay; **p 56:** Dorling Kindersley; 2.11a left Image Source Pink/Alamy; 2.11a right Envision/Corbis; 2.11b right F. Schussler/PhotoLink/Getty Images; 2.11b right Ragnar Schmuck/Getty Images; **p 60:** top Joe Raedle/Getty Images; **p 60:** bottom Sigrid Estrada/Getty Images; 2.12 Creative Digital Visions; **p 62:** Koichi Kamoshida/Getty Images; **p 63:** Kristin Piljay

In Depth: Phytochemicals

Opener Tooga/Getty Images; **p 68:** Ian O'Leary/Dorling Kindersley; Fig 1 top to bottom Southern Illinois University/Photo Researchers; Lew Robertson/Foodpix/Jupiter Images; Image **p 70:** top Photodisc/Getty Images; Source Pink/Getty Images; Pixtal/AGE Fotostock; Joy Brown/Shutterstock; **p 70:** bottom Rob Bartee/Alamy; **p 71:** Kurt Wilson/Foodpix/Jupiter Images

Chapter 3

Opener JGI/Jamie Grill/Getty Images; **p 74:** top Jean Luc Morales/Getty Images; **p 74:** bottom Howard Kingsnorth/Getty Images; 3.2 Jon Riley/Stone/Getty Images; **p 77:** Paul Poplis/Foodpix/Jupiter Images; **p 78:** George Doyle & Ciaran Griffin/Stockbyte/Getty Images; **p 82:** Jonelle Weaver/Taxi/Getty Images; **p 87:** Bon Appetit/Alamy; 3.11 left Steve Gschmeissner/Photo Researchers; 3.11 right Dr. David M. Phillips/Getty Images; **p 88:** Bruce Shippee/Shutterstock; **p 91:** SPL/Photo Researchers; **p 92:** David Sacks/Stone/Getty Images; **p 93:** Getty Images; **p 94:** MedicalRF.com/Alamy; 3.15 Dr. E. Walker/Science Photo Library/Photo Researchers; **p 95:** Susan Van Etten/Photo Edit; **p 96:** Nataliya Peregudova/Fotolia; **p 97:** Annabella Bluesky/Margie Finchell/Photo Researchers

In Depth: Disorders Related to Specific Foods

Opener Roberto A Sanchez/iStockphoto; **p 101:** Dorling Kindersley; **p 102:** David Murray and Jules Selmes/Dorling Kindersley; **p 103:** top Rubberball/Getty Images; **p 103:** bottom Cordelia Molloy/Photo Researchers; **p 104:** top Scott Indermaur/Jupiter Images; **p 104:** bottom iStockphoto

Chapter 4

Opener Suzannah Skelton/iStockphoto; **p 109:** Brocreativ/Shutterstock; **p 111:** left Foodcollection/Getty Images; **p 111:** right Rimglow/Dreamstime; **p 112:** Monkey Business Images/Shutterstock; **p 113:** top Kristin Piljay; **p 113:** bottom Rob Lewine/Bettmann/Corbis; 4.5 top to bottom Richard Smith/Masterfile; Doug Menuez/Getty Images; Technotr/iStockphoto; **p 115:** top Peter Weber/Shutterstock; **p 115:** bottom Dorling Kindersley; **p 121:** left Steve Shott/Dorling Kindersley; **p 121:** right Ryan McVay/Getty Images; **p 122:** Ian O'Leary/Dorling Kindersley; **p 123:** Joe Raedle/Getty Images; **p 125:** Dorling Kindersley; **p 126:** top left John Shepherd/iStockphoto; **p 126:** top right Dusan Zidar/Shutterstock; **p 126:** bottom left Dorling Kindersley; **p 126:** bottom right Bgphoto/Dreamstime; 4.13 Alexandr Vlassyuk/Dreamstime; **p 128:** Kristin Piljay; 4.14a-b iStockphoto; **p 132:** PhotoDisc/Getty Images; **p 133:** Brian Buckley/Alamy Images

In Depth: Diabetes

Opener Volkan Taner/iStockphoto; **p 138:** Scott Camazine/Alamy; **p 139:** Scott Camazine/Photo Researchers; Fig 2 Roche Diagnostics Corporation; **p 141:** top George Doyle & Ciaran Griffin/Stockbyte/Getty Images; **p 141:** bottom Getty Images

Chapter 5

Opener sasimoto/iStockphoto; **p 144:** top Frances Roberts/Alamy; **p 144:** bottom Dorling Kindersley; **p 147:** top Sailorr/Dreamstime; **p 147:** bottom Fotolia; **p 148:** AP Photos; **p 149:** Comstock/Thinkstock; **p 150:** Lyudmila Suvorova/iStockphoto; **p 152:** Andersen Floss/Photodisc/Getty Images; **p 153:** top Doug Pensinger/Getty Images; **p 153:** bottom Odd Anderdsen/Getty Images; **p 154:** top Danny E. Hooks/Shutterstock; **p 154:** bottom Kip Peticolas/Fundamental Photographs, NYC; **p 158:** top PhotoDisc/Getty Images; **p 158:** bottom Jeff Greenberg/AGE Fotostock; **p 159:** Wilmy van Ulft/Shutterstock; 5.13 Foodfolio/Alamy; **p 163:** Joe Gough/iStockphoto; **p 167:** top left Shutterstock; **p 167:** top right iStockphoto/Thinkstock; **p 167:** bottom left Jacek Chabraszewski/Shutterstock; **p 167:** bottom right Scott Karcich/Dreamstime; **p 168:** James Leynse/Bettmann/Corbis; **p 169:** Alex Potemkin/iStockphoto

In Depth: Cardiovascular Disease

Opener Science Photo Library/Getty Images; **p 174:** Creatas Images/Jupiter Images; Fig 1a Science Photo Library/Photo Researchers; Fig 1b Wikipedia; **p 175:** Ned Frisk Photography/Corbis; **p 176:** Gabe Palmer/Alamy; **p 177:** AP Photos; **p 181:** top Shutterstock; **p 181:** bottom Clive Streeter/Dorling Kindersley

Chapter 6

Opener Melissa Mai Yee Lo/iStockphoto; **p 186:** Shutterstock; **p 190:** Nicholas Rjabow/iStockphoto; 6.7b Andrew Syred/Photo Researchers; 6.8 Creative Digital Visions; 6.10a Medical-on-Line/Alamy; 6.10b Geri Engberg; **p 198:** Ian O'Leary/Dorling Kindersley; **p 199:** AP Photos; 6.13a Jupiter Images; 6.13b Andrew Holdbrooke/Corbis; 6.13c Alan K. Bailey/Getty Images; **p 203:** Ranald MacKechnie/Dorling Kindersley; **p 206:** top left Barbara Petrick/Dreamstime; **p 206:** top right Stockstudios/Shutterstock; **p 206:** middle left Lauri Patterson/iStockphoto; **p 206:** middle right Elena Elisseeva/Dreamstime; **p 207:** Banana Stock/Alamy; **p 208:** Shutterstock; **p 209:** Stockbyte/Getty

Images; **p 210:** Dorling Kindersley; 6.15a Paul Almasy/Corbis; 6.15b AP Photos; p 213a Glowimages/Getty Images; p 213b Kevin Schafer/Danita Delimont Photography

In Depth: Vitamins and Minerals: Micronutrients with Macro Powers

Opener Tatar/iStockphoto; **p 217:** top Simon Smith/Dorling Kindersley; **p 217:** bottom Alexandr Makarov/Shutterstock; **p 218:** Paul Prescott/ Shuttesrtock; **p 220:** Barbara Helgason/Dreamstime; **p 223:** left Safia Fatimi/Getty Images; **p 223:** right Matt Jeacock/iStockphoto; **p 224:** top Rubberball/Getty Images; **p 224:** bottom Nancy R. Cohen/Getty Images

Chapter 7

Opener Iaroslav Danylchenko/iStockphoto; **p 228:** Arthur Tilley/Getty Images; **p 230:** Jupiterimages/Thinkstock; **p 234:** Jill Chen/iStockphoto; **p 235:** top photo25th/Shutterstock; **p 235:** bottom Stockbyte/Getty Images; **p 236:** Corbis; 7.7 Photodisc/Getty Images; **p 238:** Network Productions/The Image Works; **p 239:** top Kristin Piljay; **p 239:** bottom George Doyle & Ciaran Griffin/Stockbyte/Getty Images; **p 240:** Andrea Skjold/Shutterstock; **p 241:** top left iStockphoto; **p 241:** top right Lorraine Kourafas/Shutterstock; **p 241:** middle left barbaradudzinska/ shutterstock; **p 241:** middle right FotografiaBasica/iStockphoto; **p 241:** bottom Rachel Weill/Foodpix/Jupiter Images; **p 243:** top Al Bello/ Getty Images; **p 243:** bottom Michael Pohuski/Jupiter Images; 7.8 Kenishirotie/iStockphoto; **p 245:** top Foodcollection/Getty Images; **p 245:** bottom Fotogiunta/Shutterstock; 7.9 Peter Zijlstra/Shutterstock; **p 247:** Tobias Titz/Getty Images

In Depth: Fluid Imbalance

Opener Dave & Les Jacobs/Getty Images; **p 251:** left Rick Stewart/Getty Images; **p 251:** right Eyewire Collection/Photodisc/Getty images; **p 253:** top Ned Frisk Photography/Corbis

Chapter 8

Opener Kelly Cline/iStockphoto; **p 258:** Walter Bibikow/Alamy; **p 260:** Valentyn Volkov/Shutterstock; 8.6 Eyewave/iStockphoto; **p 262:** Dorling Kindersley; **p 263:** top left Paul Blundell/Alamy; **p 263:** top right Foodfolio/Alamy; **p 263:** bottom left Le Do/iStockphoto; **p 263:** bottom right Stock Foundry/Alamy; **p 264:** Steve Gorton/Dorling Kindersley; 8.7 Uyen Le/iStockphoto; **p 265:** Philip Wilkins/Dorling Kindersley; 8.8 Medical-on-Line/Alamy; **p 266:** PhotoDisc/Getty Images; **p 268:** Corbis; 8.9 Norman Chan/iStockphoto; **p 270:** JLP/Sylvia Torres/Corbis; **p 271:** Dorling Kindersley; 8.12 Leonid Nyshko/iStockphoto; 8.13 Kristin Piljay; 8.14 Denis Pepin/iStockphoto; **p 275:** Dorling Kindersley; 8.15 Miranda Mimi Kuo; **p 277:** Ukrphoto/Dreamstime

In Depth: Cancer

Opener Jack Kunnen/iStockphoto; Fig 2 St. Bartholomew's Hospital/ Photo Researchers; **p 283:** Dave King/Dorling Kindersley; Fig 3a Edward H. Gill/Custom Medical Stock Photo; Fig 3b Lauren Shear/ Photo Researchers; **p 284:** Wolfgang Amri/iStockphoto; Fig 4 Custom Medical Stock Photo/Newscom; **p 286:** Paul Souders/Corbis; Fig 5 Dr. P. Marazzi/Photo Researchers; **p 288:** Suzannah Skelton/ iStockphoto; **p 289:** Ned Frisk Photography/Corbis

Chapter 9

Opener Diane Diederich/iStockphoto; 9.4 left Science Photo Library/ Photo Researchers; 9.4 right Pascal Alix/Photo Researchers; **p 294:** Richard Ross/Getty Images; **p 296:** Dave King/Dorling Kindersley; 9.6 Clint Scholz/iStockphoto; **p 297:** left Peter Anderson/Dorling Kindersley; **p 297:** right Polka Dot Images/Jupiter Images; **p 298:** top to bottom Brand Z Food/Alamy; Comstock Images/Jupiter Images; Bill Varie/ Workbook Stock/Jupiter Images; Dorling Kindersley; Paul Poplis/ Foodpix/Jupiter Images; **p 299:** top left Heike Brauer/Dreamstime; **p 299:** top right SoFood/Alamy; **p 299:** bottom left Igor Dutina/ Shutterstock; **p 299:** bottom right Alejandro Rivera/iStockphoto; **p 302:** Peter Turnley/Corbis; 9.10 Jiri Hera/Shutterstock; **p 304:** top Dorling Kindersley; 9.11 Biophoto Associates/Photo Researchers; **p 305:** Stockbyte/Getty Images; **p 306:** top Philip Dowell/Dorling Kindersley; **p 306:** bottom Dorling Kindersley; 9.12 vm/iStockphoto; **p 308:** Catherine Ledner/Getty Images; **p 308:** Spencer Jones/Photodisc/Getty Images; 9.13 CanuckStock/Shutterstock; **p 310:** Larry Williams/ Bettmann/Corbis; 9.14 National Institute of Dental Research; **p 313:** Johner Images/Getty Images

In Depth: Osteoporosis

Opener Lilli Day/Getty Images; Fig 1 Michael Klein/Peter Arnold, Inc./ PhotoLibrary; Fig 2a Robert Destefano/Alamy; Fig 2b Living Art Enterprises/Photo Researchers; Fig 2c Custom Medical Stock Photo/ Newscom; Fig 3 ZUMA Press/Newscom; **p 319:** Larry Mulvehill/Science Source/Photo Researchers; **p 319:** Spencer Platt/Getty Images; **p 320:** Duomo/Corbis; **p 321:** Frances Roberts/Alamy; **p 322:** Kristin Piljay; **p 323:** top Ned Frisk Photography/Corbis; **p 323:** bottom Marc Romanelli/Getty Images

Chapter 10

Opener Donald Erickson/iStockphoto; **p 326:** PhotoDisc/Getty Images; **p 329:** Nayashkova Olga/Shutterstock; 10.2 Fuat Kose/iStockphoto; **p 330:** Barry Gregg/Corbis; 10.4 Burwell and Burwell Photography/ iStockphoto; **p 331:** Paul Johnson/iStockphoto; 10.5 Alex Staroseltsev/ Shutterstock; **p 333:** Shutterstock; 10.6 Alasdair Thomson/iStockphoto; **p 334:** Creatas Images/Jupiter Unlimited; 10.7 Serhiy Shullye/ iStockphoto; **p 338:** Food Features/Alamy; 10.9 Kari Høglund/ iStockphoto; **p 339:** David Murray/Dorling Kindersley; **p 340:** Shutterstock; **p 341:** top Corbis; **p 341:** bottom Andy Crawford/Dorling Kindersley; **p 342:** top Alison Wright/Corbis; **p 342:** bottom Monique le Luhandre/Dorling Kindersley; 343 top Kristin Piljay; 343 bottom Kati Molin/Shutterstock; 10.11bViktar Malyshchyts/Shutterstock; **p 346:** top Sebastian Kaulitzki/Shutterstock; **p 346:** bottom Dorling Kindersley; **p 347:** Burke/Triolo Productions/Foodpix/Jupiter Images; 10.14 Shutterstock; **p 351:** top left Joshua Morris/iStockphoto; **p 351:** top right Shutterstock; **p 351:** middle left Robyn Mackenzie/iStockphoto; **p 351:** middle right Andy Dean Photography/Shutterstock; **p 351:** bottom Rubberball/Getty Images; **p 352:** Isabelle Rozenbaum & Frederic Cirou/ Getty Images; 10.16 Shutterstock; 10.17 Stefanie Timmermann/ iStockphoto; **p 354:** Ian O'Leary/Dorling Kindersley; **p 355:** Kristin Piljay

In Depth: Dietary Supplements: Necessity or Waste?

Opener Don Wilkie/iStockphoto; **p 359:** Cordelia Molloy/Photo Researchers; **p 361:** Kristin Piljay; **p 362:** kanusommer/Shutterstock; **p 364:** top Digital Vision/Getty Images; **p 364:** bottom Stockbyte/Getty Images

Chapter 11

Opener Alena Dvorakova/iStockphoto; **p 368:** Eugene Gologursky/ WireImage/Getty Images; **p 369:** Photodisc/Getty Images; **p 370:** R H Production/Robert Harding World Imagery; 11.3 top to bottom PhotoEdit; Custom Medical Stock Photo, Inc; SPL/Photo Researchers; Phanie/Photo Researchers;; Life Measurement, Inc.; 11.5 Kristin Piljay; 11.6a Stockbyte/Getty Images; 11.6b ML Harris/Getty Images; 11.6c LWA/Sharie Kennedy/Getty Images; **p 375:** Dorling Kindersley; **p 377:** Stockbyte/Thinkstock; **p 380:** Alvis Upitis/Getty Images; **p 381:** iStockphoto; **p 383:** Bruce Dale/Getty Images; **p 384:** Norma Joseph/ Alamy; **p 385:** top PhotoDisc/Getty Images; **p 385:** bottom Mark Douet/Getty Images; **p 387:** Jacek Chabraszewski/Shutterstock; **p 391:** BananaStock/Jupiter Images; 11.10 Creative Digital Visions; **p 395:** Fotolia; **p 397:** Chris Hondros/Getty Images

In Depth: Obesity

Opener hartphotography1/iStockphoto; **p 401:** Andrew Hancock/The New York Times/Redux; **p 402:** doc-stock/Alamy; **p 404:** top Digital Vision/Thinkstock; **p 404:** bottom Obesity/Alamy; **p 405:** top William Thomas Cain/Getty Images; **p 405:** bottom Ryan McVay/Getty Images; **p 407:** top George Doyle & Ciaran Griffin/Stockbyte/Getty Images; **p 407:** bottom LIU Jin/APF/Corbis

Chapter 12

Opener Redlink/Corbis; **p 410:** Robert W. Ginn/AGE Fotostock; **p 411:** top Caleb Kennal/PNI/Aurora Photos; **p 411:** bottom Photodisc/Getty Images; **p 412:** AP Photos; **p 413:** Will & Deni McIntyre/Photo Researchers; 12.2 top to bottom BananaStock/Jupiter Images; Alan Jakubek/Corbis; Comstock Images/Jupiter Images; **p 416:** Moodboard/Alamy; **p 417:** Image Source/Jupiter Images; 12.5 top to bottom Stock Foundry/Alamy; Shutterstock; iStockphoto; mylife photos/Alamy; Shutterstock;; Image Source/Corbis; **p 420:** Corbis Super RF/Alamy; **p 422:** Stephen Oliver/Dorling Kindersley; 12.8 Laura Murray; **p 424:** Jens Schlueter/Getty Images; **p 426:** Photodisc/Getty Images; **p 427:** Scott T. Smith/Corbis; **p 428:** Dave King/Dorling Kindersley; **p 429:** David Young-Wolff/Getty Images; 12.10 left Lily Valde/Pixland/Jupiter Images; 12.10 right Dominic Burke/Alamy; **p 432:** Stockbyte/Getty Images; **p 433:** Altrendo/Getty Images; **p 435:** Derek Hall/Dorling Kindersley; **p 437:** Stockbyte/Getty Images

In Depth: Disordered Eating

Opener Image Source/Corbis; **p 441:** Eugenio Savio/AP Photo; **p 442:** Digital Vision/Getty Images; Fig 2 Laura Murray; Fig 3 Karl Prouse/Catwalking/Getty Images; Fig 4 Kendall Samantha Alon/SIPA; **p 445:** Blake Little/Getty Images; **p 447:** top Roel Loopers/Photolibrary; Fig 6 Baumgartner Olivia/Corbis; **p 448:** D. Hurst/Alamy; **p 449:** Photodisc/Thinkstock; **p 450:** AP Photos; **p 451:** Rubberball/Getty Images

Chapter 13

Opener Russ Schleipman/Corbis; **p 04:** matka_Wariatka/Shutterstock; 13.1 top to bottom Exactostock/SuperStock; Fotolia; David Wei/Alamy; Frank Rumpenhorst/Newscom; Huntstock, Inc/Alamy; 13.2a Barry Dowsett/Photo Researchers; 13.2b Dr. Tony Brain/Photo Researchers; 13.2c Martin Oeggerli/Photo Researchers; 13.3 Andrew Syred/Photo Researchers; 13.4 Matt Meadows/Peter Arnold, Inc./PhotoLibrary; **p 10:** StockFood/Getty Images; 13.5 Neil Fletcher/Dorling Kindersley Media Library; **p 11:** Jean-Louis Vosgien/Shutterstock; **p 12:** top Vanessa Davies/Dorling Kindersley; **p 12:** bottom Justin Sullivan/Getty Images; **p 13:** Digital Vision/Getty Images; **p 14:** Kristin Piljay; **p 18:** Alan Richardson/Foodpix/Jupiter Images; **p 20:** Stockbyte/Getty Images; **p 21:** top Owen Franken/Corbis; **p 21:** bottom Hulton Archive Photos/Getty Images; **p 22:** top Digital Vision/Getty Images; **p 22:** bottom AKG/Photo Researchers; **p 23:** Lon C. Diehl/PhotoEdit; **p 25:** AbleStock .com/Thinkstock; **p 28:** Image100/Corbis; 13.12 left Brian Hagiwara/Foodpix/Jupiter Images; 13.12 right Carl Walsh/Aurora Photos; **p 30:** top Corbis; **p 30:** bottom Red Cover/Alamy; **p 33:** Abbott Laboratories; **p 35:** Oby Talbot/AP Photo

In Depth: Global Nutrition

Opener Cover/Getty Images; **p 39:** left Brennan Linsley/AP Photo; **p 39:** right Reuters/Corbis; **p 40:** Peter Turnley/Corbis; **p 41:** Nik Wheeler/Corbis; **p 42:** Neil Cooper/Alamy; **p 43:** David Turnley/Corbis; **p 45:** top Getty Images; **p 45:** bottom George Doyle & Ciaran Griffin/Stockbyte/Getty Images

Chapter 14

Opener Adam Borkowski/iStockphoto; **p 04:** David Phillips/The Population Council/Photo Researchers; 14.4a-b Lennart Nilsson/Scanpix; 14.4c Neil Bromhall/Photo Researchers; 14.4d Tom Galliher/Corbis; 14.5 Ron Sutherland/Photo Researchers; **p 09:** Ian O'Leary/Getty Images; 14.6 Ingret/Shutterstock; 14.7a Biophoto Associates/Science Source/Photo Researchers; **p 12:** Dave King/Dorling Kindersley; **p 13:** Juanmonino/iStockphoto; **p 14:** Allana Wesley White/Corbis; **p 15:** Brand X Pictures/Photodisc/Getty Images; **p 16:** top Dorling Kindersley; **p 16:** bottom Jim Craigmyle/Corbis; **p 18:** Phanie/Photo Researchers; **p 19:** George Doyle & Ciaran Griffin/Stockbyte/Getty Images; 14.9 Brigitte Sporrer/Getty Images; **p 23:** Rick Gomez/AGE Fotostock; **p 24:** Darama/Corbis; **p 26:** top Chris Craymer/Getty Images; **p 26:** bottom Philip Gould/Corbis; **p 27:** top Jose Luis Pelaez, Inc./Corbis; **p 27:** bottom Mel Yates/Getty Images; **p 30:** Pixland/Getty Images; **p 32:** Corbis; **p 33:** top Tom Stewart/Corbis; **p 33:** bottom Anne Flinn Powell/Photolibrary; 14.12 Dr. Pamela R. Erickson; **p 35:** Richard Levine/Alamy

In Depth: The Fetal Environment: A Lasting Impression

Opener Nugene Chiang/AsiaPix/Corbis; Fig 1 Kent PAGE/Newscom; **p 41:** PhotoDisc/Getty Images

Chapter 15

Opener Monkey Business Images/Shutterstock; **p 04:** top Blend Images/Superstock; **p 04:** bottom Michael Newman/PhotoEdit; 15.1 Dave King/Dorling Kindersley; **p 07:** Shutterstock; **p 08:** top Roger Phillips/Dorling Kindersley; **p 08:** bottom Foodfolio/Alamy; **p 09:** top Jaume Gual/AGE Fotostock; **p 10:** debr22pics/Shutterstock; **p 12:** top Laura Murray; **p 12:** bottom Creatas Images/Thinkstock; **p 13:** Bob Daemmrich/The Image Works; **p 14:** Shutterstock; **p 15:** Paul Barton/Corbis; **p 18:** top George Doyle/Thinkstock; **p 18:** bottom Adam Gault/Getty Images; **p 21:** top Tome & Dee Ann McCarthy/Corbis; **p 21:** bottom Rubberball/Getty Images; **p 22:** iStockphoto; **p 23:** top ImageState/Alamy; **p 23:** bottom Gabe Palmer/Alamy; **p 24:** Claro Cortes IV/Reuters/Corbis; **p 25:** top Raymond Gehman/Corbis; **p 25:** bottom Ariel Skelley/Corbis; **p 26:** Don Smetzer/Getty Images; **p 27:** Richard Koek/Getty Images; **p 29:** top Jed Share/Getty Images; **p 29:** bottom Deborah Jaffe/Foodpix/Jupiter Images; 15.9 National Institute of Health; **p 31:** Mark Richards/PhotoEdit; **p 32:** Karen Pruess/The Image Works; **p 33:** Donna Day/Getty Images

In Depth: Searching for the Fountain of Youth

Opener Thomas Schweizer/Corbis; **p 37:** The Art Archive/Alamy; **p 38:** IPS/Jupiter Images; **p 39:** Andreas Pollok/Getty Images; **p 40:** top Ned Frisk Photography/Corbis; **p 40:** bottom Dorling Kindersley